FIFTH EDITION

PRESCRIPTION
for
Nutritional Healing

PHYLLIS A. BALCH, CNC

AVERY
a member of Penguin Group (USA) Inc. · New York

AVERY

Published by the Penguin Group
Penguin Group (USA) Inc., 375 Hudson Street, New York, New York 10014, USA • Penguin Group (Canada),
90 Eglinton Avenue East, Suite 700, Toronto, Ontario M4P 2Y3, Canada (a division of Pearson Penguin Canada Inc.)
• Penguin Books Ltd, 80 Strand, London WC2R 0RL, England • Penguin Ireland, 25 St Stephen's Green, Dublin 2,
Ireland (a division of Penguin Books Ltd) • Penguin Group (Australia), 250 Camberwell Road, Camberwell, Victoria
3124, Australia • (a division of Pearson Australia Group Pty Ltd) • Penguin Books India Pvt Ltd, 11 Community
Centre, Panchsheel Park, New Delhi–110 017, India • Penguin Group (NZ), 67 Apollo Drive, Rosedale, North Shore
0632, New Zealand (a division of Pearson New Zealand Ltd) • Penguin Books (South Africa) (Pty) Ltd,
24 Sturdee Avenue, Rosebank, Johannesburg 2196, South Africa

Penguin Books Ltd, Registered Offices: 80 Strand, London WC2R 0RL, England

Most Avery books are available at special quantity discounts for bulk purchase for sales promotions, premiums,
fund-raising, and educational needs. Special books or book excerpts also can be created to fit specific needs.
For details, write Penguin Group (USA) Inc. Special Markets, 375 Hudson Street, New York, NY 10014.

Library of Congress Cataloging-in-Publication Data

Balch, Phyllis A., 1930–2004.
Prescription for nutritional healing : a practical A-to-Z reference to drug-free remedies using vitamins,
minerals, herbs & food supplements / Phyllis A. Balch.—5th ed.
p.   cm.
Includes bibliographical references and index.
ISBN 978-1-58333-400-3 (alk. paper)
1. Nutrition—Popular works.   2. Dietary supplements—Popular works.   3. Herbs—Therapeutic use—
Popular works.   I. Title.
RA784.B2483   2010   2010021746
615.8'54—dc22

Printed in the United States of America
7   9   10   8   6

Neither the publisher nor the author is engaged in rendering professional advice or services to the individual reader. The ideas, procedures, and suggestions contained in this book are not intended as a substitute for consulting with your physician. All matters regarding your health require medical supervision. Neither the author nor the publisher shall be liable or responsible for any loss or damage allegedly arising from any information or suggestion in this book.

The recipes contained in this book are to be followed exactly as written. The publisher is not responsible for your specific health or allergy needs that may require medical supervision. The publisher is not responsible for any adverse reactions to the recipes contained in this book.

While the author has made every effort to provide accurate telephone numbers and Internet addresses at the time of publication, neither the publisher nor the author assumes any responsibility for errors, or for changes that occur after publication. Further, the publisher does not have any control over and does not assume any responsibility for author or third-party websites or their content.

CONTENTS

Part Three   Remedies and Therapies

Appendix

AUTHOR'S ACKNOWLEDGMENTS
from the Fourth Edition

There are many people who have come and gone in my life and have contributed to my books in many different ways, but I want to dedicate this to three loyal and true friends who are no longer with me: Judge Wendell W. Mayer, Charles R. Cripe, and Skeeners Balch. I also wish to acknowledge the following people, who both advised and supported me as I prepared and wrote the fourth edition of this book: my daughters, Ruby Hines and Cheryl Keene; my grandchildren, Lisa, Ryan, and Rachel; my brother, Al Henning; and my research and editing staff, Jeffrey W. Hallinger and Gary L. Loderhose and editor Amy Tecklenburg.

My gratitude also extends to Laurence Royse, D.Sc.; Aftab J. Ahmad, Ph.D., consulting molecular biologist; Philip Domenico, Ph.D., microbiologist and nutrition editor; Deborah A. Edson, R.Ph.; James J. Gormley, editor-in-chief, *Remedies Magazine*; and also to members of the faculty of Southwest College of Naturopathic Medicine, Paul Mittman, N.D., president, and Mona Morstein, N.D., associate professor, all of whom graciously assisted in preparing and reviewing this book.

Finally, I would like to thank all the readers who have remained loyal throughout the years.

Phyllis A. Balch

PREFACE

Socrates once said, "There is only one good, knowledge, and one evil, ignorance." This statement should guide us in all of our actions, especially where our health is concerned. Too many of us do not have the slightest idea of how to maintain good health. When illness strikes, we rely on our doctors to cure us. What we fail to realize is that "the cure" comes from within. Nature has provided us with a wondrous immune system, and all we have to do is take proper care of this inner healing force.

Does this sound too simple? Basically, it is simple; our modern lifestyles have gotten us off the right track, with fast foods, alcohol abuse, drug dependencies, a polluted environment, and high-tech stress. Nature intended to fuel our inner healing force with the right natural substances to enable the body to function up to its fullest potential. Nature's resources—whole foods, vitamins, minerals, enzymes, amino acids, phytochemicals, and other natural bounties—are designed for use in our immune systems. However, because most of us have a profound lack of knowledge as to what our bodies need to function properly, we find ourselves out of balance and susceptible to all sorts of illnesses.

All individuals should take an active role in the maintenance of their health, the prevention of disease, and the treatment of their disorders with the guidance of a health care professional. The more we take it upon ourselves to learn about nutrition, the better prepared we will be to take that active role. A good diet coupled with medical advice offers the best chance of living a healthy life. Attitude is also an important factor in the processes of health maintenance and healing. We must have a positive state of mind in order to bring harmony to the body. The realization that body (lifestyle), spirit (desire), and mind (belief) must come together is the first step to better health.

This book is the culmination of half a lifetime of study, work, and research. It is intended to provide you and your health care professional with a more natural approach to healing, which may be used in conjunction with your current medical treatment. A number of the suggestions offered, such as intravenous therapy, can be administered only by or under the supervision of a licensed physician. Also, because our body chemistries differ, some of us may have allergic reactions to certain supplements.

Before taking any nutritional supplement, check with your health care professional regarding its appropriateness. For your children, always check with their pediatrician first.

Should you experience an allergic reaction, especially abnormal bowel function (such as diarrhea), to any supplement, immediately discontinue use of the supplement. You should never attempt to treat yourself without professional advice.

No statement in this publication should be construed as a claim for cure, treatment, or prevention of any disease. It is also important to point out that you should not reject mainstream medical methods. Learn about your condition, and don't be afraid to ask questions. Feel free to get second and even third opinions from qualified health professionals. It is a sign of wisdom, not cowardice, to seek more knowledge through your active participation as a patient.

Every effort has been made to include the latest research available on nutritional healing. We also have added new disorders at the suggestions of our readers. All the information in this book has been carefully researched, and the data have been reviewed and updated throughout the production process. Because this body of knowledge promises to continue growing and changing, we suggest that when questions arise, you refer to one of the health or medical organizations in the Appendix for up-to-date information on treatment and prevention of disorders, or ask your health care provider. We will strive to keep abreast of new scientific information, treatments, and supplements.

Nearly nine hundred years ago, Moses Maimonides said, "The physician should not treat the ailment, but the patient who is suffering from it." This book was designed to meet the differing needs of individuals and to help each person create his or her own nutritional program.

HOW TO USE THIS BOOK

This is a comprehensive in-home guide that will help you achieve and maintain the highest level of health and fitness through careful dietary planning and nutritional supplementation.

Even if you are healthy, you will benefit from this book because it gives advice on how to achieve and maintain optimum health, build up your immune system, and increase your energy level. Written by a certified nutritionist, this book blends the latest scientific research with traditional treatments. It provides all the information you need to design your own personal nutritional program. In addition, the author offers traditional and up-to-date home remedies, and suggests healthful modifications in diet and lifestyle.

It is important to stress that the suggestions offered in this book are not intended to replace appropriate medical investigation and treatment. The supplements and medications recommended for a particular disorder should be approved and monitored by your medical doctor or trained health care professional. If surgery or other conventional medical interventions are crucial and cannot be avoided, the nutritional supplements can shorten healing time.

The book is divided into three parts. Part One discusses the basic principles of nutrition and health, and lists and explains the various types of nutrients, food supplements, enzymes, antioxidants, and herbs found in health food shops and drugstores. Part Two is divided into sections on common disorders, from acne to cancer to yeast infection, arranged in alphabetical order. Each section discusses how to identify the symptoms and suggests ways to correct or treat the disorder through dietary guidelines and a supplementation program. Some contain helpful diagnostic self-tests to help you determine whether or not you have the condition in question. Part Three offers descriptions and explanations of traditional therapies and conventional treatments that can be used in conjunction with a nutritional program. Also discussed in Part Three are a number of alternative therapy approaches, such as acupressure and acupuncture, aromatherapy, Ayurvedic medicine, Chinese medicine, chiropractic, color therapy, fasting, glandular therapy, homeopathy, hydrotherapy, hyperbaric oxygen therapy, light therapy, magnet therapy, massage therapy, and music/sound therapy. In addition, there are insets throughout the book providing in-depth coverage of important topics. The ramifications of different drug therapies are discussed and the latest medical updates are provided.

Also included, in an appendix, is information on how to find some of the products recommended in this book, along with a recommended reading list and a list of health organizations and the addresses and/or phone numbers at which they can be reached for information. In a nod to current technology, website addresses are given as well. A glossary is provided for easy reference.

Although a healthy diet is the backbone of any nutritional program, we believe that most if not all people should supplement their diets with the proper nutrients to achieve wellness. Nutritional deficiency diseases such as scurvy are rare, but these are only the tip of the iceberg when it comes to the problems a lack of adequate nutrition can cause. Nutritional deficiencies can cause a variety of symptoms, in addition to weakening the body's defenses against serious illness. Moreover, nutritional requirements can be influenced by many factors. People who are heavy alcohol drinkers, cigarette smokers, prescription or recreational drug users, and/or dieters are at a greater than normal risk for deficiencies, as are adolescents, elderly people, pregnant and nursing women, women who take oral contraceptives, people with certain genetic disorders, people who eat poor diets, and people with diabetes or other chronic illnesses. Unfortunately, a large percentage of the population fits into one or more of these categories.

The supplementation programs recommended in this book should be followed for three to twelve months, depending upon your individual needs and the recommendations of your health care provider. Start by taking nutrients classified "essential" and "very important" for the relevant disorder. Many times, the nutrients recommended for a particular disorder can be found in a single product. Before you start taking them on a regular basis, test the supplements one at a time to find out if you have a reaction to any of them. If you do not find relief within thirty days, add the supplements from the "helpful" list to your program. Each of us is unique; you may need all the nutrients listed, or you may be deficient in only a few. If you still do not notice an improvement after a month, consult your health care provider. You may suffer from malabsorption.

Always take supplements with a full glass of water. Nutritional supplements are concentrated and can overburden the liver if not enough liquid is consumed with the supplements. Water enhances absorption and is needed to aid in carrying the nutrients to the cells.

If you follow a nutritional supplementation program for longer than a year, change brands periodically so that you do not develop an intolerance or build up a resistance to one or more of the ingredients in one supplement. You can become intolerant to the ingredients in vitamins and other supplements just as you can to foods. Learn to listen to your body. Given time, you will notice changes in your body and be able to identify their cause. After the supplementation period for a certain disorder is completed, decrease supplement dosages gradually so that your body has a chance to adjust. Keep in mind, though, that virtually all of us need to supplement our diets with the basic nutrients for optimum wellness and illness prevention.

PART ONE

Understanding *the* Elements of Health

Introduction

The body is a complex organism that has the ability to heal itself—if only you listen to it and respond with proper nourishment and care. In spite of all the abuse our bodies endure—whether through exposure to environmental toxins, poor nutrition, cigarette smoking, alcohol consumption, or inactivity—they still usually serve us well for many years before signs of illness may start to appear. Even then, with a little help, they respond and continue to function.

The human body is the greatest machine on earth. Nerve signals travel through muscles at speeds as fast as 200 miles per hour. The brain puts out enough electric power to light a 20-watt lightbulb. If your leg muscles moved as fast as your eye muscles, you could walk over fifty miles in one day. According to scientists, bone is among the strongest building materials known to humankind.

Think of your body as being composed of millions of tiny little engines. Some of these engines work in unison; some work independently. All are on call twenty-four hours a day. In order for the engines to work properly, they require specific fuels. If the type of fuel given is the wrong blend, the engine will not perform to its maximum capacity. If the fuel is of a poor grade, the engine may sputter, hesitate, and lose power. If the engine is given no fuel at all, it will stop.

The fuel we give our bodies' engines comes directly from the things we consume. The foods we eat contain nutrients. These nutrients come in the form of vitamins, minerals, enzymes, water, amino acids, carbohydrates, and lipids. It is these nutrients that sustain life by providing us with the basic materials our bodies need to carry on their daily functions.

Individual nutrients differ in form and function, and in the amount needed by the body; however, they are all vital to our health. The actions that involve nutrients take place on microscopic levels, and the specific processes differ greatly. Nutrients are involved in all body processes, from combating infection to repairing tissue to thinking. Although nutrients have different specific functions, their common function is to keep us going.

Research has shown that each part of the body contains high concentrations of certain nutrients. A deficiency of those nutrients will cause the body part to malfunction and eventually break down—and, like dominos, other body parts will follow. To keep this from happening, we need a proper diet and appropriate nutritional supplements. Brain function, memory, skin elasticity, eyesight, energy, the ratio of lean-to-fat tissue in the body, and overall health are all indications of how well the body is functioning. With the help of the proper nutrients, exercise, and a balanced diet, we can slow the aging process and greatly improve our chances for a healthier, pain-free—and possibly longer—life.

If we do not give ourselves the proper nutrients, we can impair the body's normal functions and cause ourselves great harm. Even if we show no signs of illness, we may not necessarily be healthy. It simply may be that we are not yet exhibiting any overt symptoms of illness. One problem most of us have is that we do not get the nutrients we need from our diets because most of the foods we consume are cooked and/or processed. Cooking food at high temperatures and conventional food processing destroy vital nutrients the body needs to function properly. The organic raw foods that supply these elements are largely missing from today's diet.

The past decade has brought to light much new knowledge about nutrition and its effects on the body, and the role it plays in disease. Phytochemicals, also known as phytonutrients, are one example of the results of this research.

Phytochemicals are compounds present in plants that make the plants biologically active. All fruits and vegetables contain phytochemicals. However, since few people eat enough fruits and vegetables to get the optimum amount of phytochemicals from diet alone, supplementation is recommended. Phytochemicals are not nutrients in the classic sense, but they determine a plant's color, flavor, and ability to resist disease. Researchers have identified literally thousands of phytochemicals and also have developed the technology to extract these chemical compounds and concentrate them into pills, powders, and capsules. These products are included under the term "nutraceuticals." The FDA uses the term "dietary supplement" to define natural compounds like phytochemicals.

Your body's nutritional needs are as unique to you as your appearance is. The first essential step toward wellness is to be sure you are getting the correct amounts of the proper nutrients. By understanding the principles of holistic nutrition and knowing what nutrients you need, you can improve the state of your health, ward off disease, and maintain a harmonious balance in the way nature intended. Part One of this book should provide you with a clear understanding of the vitamins, minerals, amino acids, enzymes, phytochemicals, and other nutrients you need, as well as important information on natural food supplements, herbs, and products that enhance nutrient activity. Eating a healthful diet and supplementing your diet with appropriate nutrients will help to assure that your organs, cells, and tissues get the fuel they need to operate properly.

The nutrients suggested in this book promote healing and wellness by allowing the body to heal and reinvigorate itself.

Nutrition, Diet, and Wellness

UNDERSTANDING THE BASICS OF NUTRITION

Good nutrition is the foundation of good health. Everyone needs the four basic nutrients—water, carbohydrates, proteins, and fats—as well as vitamins, minerals, and other micronutrients.

To be able to choose the proper foods, and to better understand why those foods should be supported with supplements, you need to have a clear idea of the components of a healthy diet.

It is now a requirement in the United States that all packaged foods have a nutrition label that tells the consumer what is actually inside the package. This system may not be perfect, but it is a big improvement over no labeling at all, the situation that existed only a generation ago. Keep in mind that all fresh, minimally processed foods, such as grains purchased in bulk, meats, fruits, and vegetables, do not carry labels. However, they are inherently healthier than packaged foods because they have more beneficial nutrients and fewer harmful ones. For example, unlike processed items, these foods are naturally high in potassium and low in sodium.

Let's look at one of these labels and see what it tells us. Look at Figure 1.1 below, which happens to be a label for a package of macaroni and cheese:

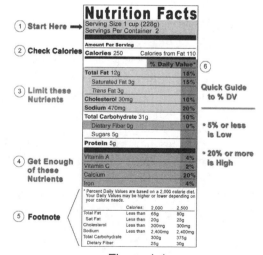

Figure 1.1

- The serving size is listed at the top of the label. All of the daily value percentages are based on this amount. It's good to keep in mind that the serving size listed on the label may not correspond with what many people consider a serving or portion of the product.

- There are 250 calories in this product, and 110 calories (almost half the calories in the product) come from fat (panel 2). This is not a good sign. A rule of thumb is that fat should contribute no more than 30 percent of the total calories per serving.

- Note the total fat, cholesterol, and sodium information (panel 3). The amount of total fat (bad) is shown, as are the amounts of saturated fat (bad). It's also important to pay attention to how much sodium the product contains and to maintain total intake below the suggested daily value.

- Panel 3 also gives the amount of dietary fiber (good), sugars (bad), and protein (you need some at each meal), and panel 4, selected vitamins and minerals (good).

- The footnote panel (5) gives target information for various nutrients based on a diet containing a total of 2,000 or 2,500 calories per day. This may or may not be useful to you, depending on your particular situation and calorie goal. It is important to be aware also that the percentages given in the preceding are percentages of a 2,000-calorie diet and are *not* a percentage of the amount we actually recommend for good health or to maintain a healthy weight.

There is still some question as to the benefits of the current food labeling system. Some are calling for a thorough assessment of whether the new labeling has actually enabled consumers to make healthier food choices. Some of the major food companies such as Kraft Foods and major grocery store chains such as Stop & Shop are already creating new labeling systems to help consumers make better choices. This section of the book will discuss the items shown on the nutrition label—and more—and also how they affect your health.

The Four Basic Nutrients

Water, carbohydrates, proteins, and fats are the basic building blocks of a good diet. By choosing the healthiest forms of each of these nutrients and eating them in the proper balance, you enable your body to function at its optimal level.

Water

The human body is two-thirds water. Water is an essential nutrient that is involved in every function of the body. It helps transport nutrients and waste products in and out of cells. It is necessary for all digestive, absorptive, circulatory, and excretory functions, as well as for the utilization of the water-soluble vitamins. It is also needed for the maintenance of proper body temperature. Each day the body loses up to 1 quart of water each from the kidneys and skin, about 1 cup from the lungs, and ½ cup from feces—a total of about 6 to 10 cups. To replace the water lost, males need to consume about 15 cups of fluid and females about 11 cups.

Ingesting an adequate amount of water each day—whether by food or water—is essential to maintain good health. Usually urine will be pale yellow in color if the body is sufficiently hydrated. It is possible to get a good portion of your daily intake of water—at least ten 8-ounce glasses—not from the tap, but from fruits and vegetables, which are loaded with water, some up to 90 percent water. Although recent studies have shown that beverages such as juices and sodas can be counted toward the daily fluid requirement, obtaining proper levels of fluids from fruits and vegetables and noncaloric beverages such as water and herbal tea is preferable, especially for weight control. For details on choosing the best water, *see* WATER in Part One.

Carbohydrates

Carbohydrates supply the body with the energy it needs to function. They are found almost exclusively in plant foods, such as fruits, vegetables, peas, grains, and beans. Milk and milk products are the only foods derived from animals that contain carbohydrates.

Carbohydrates are divided into two groups—simple carbohydrates and complex carbohydrates. *Simple carbohydrates,* sometimes called simple sugars, include fructose (fruit sugar), sucrose (table sugar), and lactose (milk sugar), as well as several other sugars. Fruits are one of the richest natural sources of simple carbohydrates. *Complex carbohydrates* are also made up of sugars, but the sugar molecules are strung together to form longer, more complex chains. Complex carbohydrates include fiber and starches. Foods rich in complex carbohydrates include vegetables, whole grains, peas, and beans.

Newer classifications for carbohydrates are based on their glycemic indexes (GI). The index is a scoring system to show how much glucose appears in the blood after eating a carbohydrate-containing food—the higher the number, the greater the blood sugar response. So a low GI food will cause a small rise, while a high GI food will trigger a dramatic spike. A GI of 70 or more is high, a GI of 56 to 69 is medium, and a GI of 55 or less is low. Most simple carbohydrates raise blood sugar levels more than complex ones, but not always. For example, white bread raises blood sugar more than table sugar because sugar has a lower GI. Eating foods with high glycemic indexes can lead to obesity, heart disease, and diabetes. (The glycemic index of foods can be found on www.mendosa.com/gilists.htm and glycemicindex.ca.) Simply put, adopting a low–glycemic index diet is healthier. Low–glycemic index foods include fruits, vegetables, meat, oils, and dairy products. Most grain-based foods, especially those that are highly processed, have high glycemic indexes.

Carbohydrates are the main source of blood glucose, which is a major fuel for all of the body's cells and the only source of energy for the brain and red blood cells. Both simple and complex carbohydrates are converted into glucose. The glucose is then either used directly to provide energy for the body or stored in the liver for future use. If a person consumes more calories than his or her body is using, a portion of the carbohydrates consumed may be stored in the body as fat.

Due to complex chemical reactions in the brain, eating carbohydrates has a mild tranquilizing effect, and can be beneficial for people who suffer from seasonal affective disorder and/or depression.

When choosing carbohydrate-rich foods for your diet, choose unrefined foods such as fruits, vegetables, peas, beans, and whole-grain products, instead of refined, processed foods such as soft drinks, desserts, candy, and sugar. Refined foods offer few, if any, of the vitamins and minerals that are important to your health. Foods that are rich in nutrients are called nutrient-dense foods. A healthy diet should consist mainly of these foods and avoid those that are nutrient-poor. In addition, eating large amounts of simple carbohydrates found in refined foods, especially over a period of many years, can lead to a number of disorders, including diabetes and hypoglycemia (low blood sugar). Yet another problem is that foods high in refined simple sugars are often also high in fats, which should be limited in a healthy diet. This is why such foods—which include most cookies and cakes, as well as many snack foods—are usually loaded with calories.

A word is in order here regarding fiber, a very important form of carbohydrate. Referred to in the past as "roughage," dietary fiber is the part of a plant that is resistant to the body's digestive enzymes. As a result, only a relatively small amount of fiber is digested or metabolized in the intestines. Instead, most of it moves through the gastrointestinal tract and ends up in the stool.

Although most fiber is not digested, it delivers several important health benefits. First, fiber retains water, resulting in softer and bulkier stools that prevent constipation and hemorrhoids. A high-fiber diet also reduces the risk of colon cancer, perhaps by speeding the rate at which stool passes through the intestine and by keeping the digestive tract clean. In addition, fiber binds with certain substances that would normally result in the production of cholesterol, and eliminates these substances from the body. In this way, a high-fiber diet helps lower blood cholesterol levels, reducing the risk of heart disease.

It is recommended that about 50 to 60 percent of your total daily calories come from carbohydrates. If much of your diet consists of healthy complex carbohydrates, you should easily fulfill the recommended daily minimum of 25 grams of fiber. Fiber should come primarily from a wide variety of fruits and vegetables. Whole grains are better than highly processed ones because they contain more fiber. Fiber is either soluble or insoluble. The soluble type is broken down in the large intestine (colon). Insoluble fiber is not digested and is simply excreted in the stool.

Protein

Protein is essential for growth and development. It provides the body with energy, and is needed for the manufacture of hormones, antibodies, enzymes, and tissues. It also helps maintain the proper acid-alkali balance in the body.

When protein is consumed, the body breaks it down into amino acids, the building blocks of all proteins. Since protein is essential for life, other foods such as fruits and vegetables, which are alkaline-producing, need to be consumed to balance the body. Some of the amino acids from proteins are designated *nonessential*. This does not mean that they are unnecessary, but rather that they do not have to come from the diet because they can be synthesized by the body from other amino acids. Other amino acids are considered *essential*, meaning that the body cannot synthesize them, and therefore must obtain them from the diet.

Whenever the body *makes* a protein—when it builds muscle, for instance—it needs a variety of amino acids for the protein-making process. These amino acids may come from dietary protein or from the body's own pool of amino acids. If a shortage of amino acids becomes chronic, which can occur if the diet is deficient in essential amino acids, the building of protein in the body stops, and the body suffers. The brain will trigger the muscle cells to release vital proteins to support the body. However, in extreme cases, some patients develop cachexia, which presents as weight loss, muscle atrophy, and severe fatigue and can result from a poor dietary protein intake. (For more information about amino acids, *see* AMINO ACIDS in Part One.)

Because of the importance of consuming proteins that provide all of the necessary amino acids, dietary proteins are considered to belong to two different groups, depending on the amino acids they provide. *Complete proteins,* which constitute the first group, contain ample amounts of all the essential amino acids. These proteins are found in meat, fish, poultry, cheese, eggs, and milk. *Incomplete proteins,* which constitute the second group, contain only some of the essential amino acids. These proteins are found in a variety of foods, including grains, legumes, and leafy green vegetables.

Although it is important to consume the full range of amino acids, both essential and nonessential, it is not necessary to get them from meat, fish, poultry, and other complete-protein foods. In fact, because of their high fat content—as well as the use of antibiotics and other chemicals in the raising of poultry and cattle—most of those foods should be eaten only in moderation. Many animal proteins are now available without hormones, or the animals are organically fed and hormone-free, so this risk can be mitigated by choosing these meats. It is best to trim all visible fat—including skin—from animal proteins and use low-fat or nonfat dairy products. Doing this will help reduce the risk of heart disease while still allowing for adequate intake of protein.

Fortunately, the dietary strategy called *mutual supplementation* enables you to combine partial-protein foods to make *complementary protein*—proteins that supply adequate amounts of all the essential amino acids. For instance, although beans and brown rice are both quite rich in protein, each lacks one or more of the necessary amino acids. However, when you combine beans and brown rice with each other, or when you combine either one with any of a number of protein-rich foods, you form a complete protein that is a high-quality substitute for meat. To make a complete protein, combine *beans* with any one of the following:

- Brown rice
- Corn
- Nuts
- Seeds
- Wheat

Or combine *brown rice* with any one of the following:

- Beans
- Nuts
- Seeds

Recent research indicates that it is possible to adequately meet your essential amino acid needs by eating an assortment of protein-containing foods over the course of the day and that there may be no need to combine proteins in one meal.

The problem is that many Americans eat too much protein, especially at one sitting, largely as the result of a diet high in meat and dairy products. Protein synthesis (manufacturing of new proteins for the body) works best when the protein is consumed on a regular basis throughout the day. However, if you have reduced the amount of meat and dairy foods in your diet, you should make sure to get 50 to 60 grams of protein a day. To make sure that you are getting enough variety of amino acids in your diet, add protein-rich foods to meals and snacks as often as possible. Eat bread with nut butters, for instance, or add nuts and seeds to salads and vegetable casseroles. Be aware that a combination of any grains, any nuts and seeds, any legumes (such as beans, peanuts, and peas), and a variety of mixed vegetables will make a complete protein. In addition, cornmeal fortified with the amino acid L-lysine makes a complete protein.

All soybean products, such as tofu and soymilk, are complete proteins. These foods have high levels of fiber, and soy has been found to be the healthiest source of protein, more so than any other food. Soybean protein makes up 35 to 38 percent of its total calories, offers all eight essential amino acids, and is high in vitamin B_6. The average American consumes only about 10 milligrams of soy protein per day, although the American Heart Association suggests that consuming at least 25 grams per day may reduce the risk of heart disease. Available in health food stores, tofu, soy oil, soy flour, soy-based meat substitutes, soy cheese, and many other soy products are healthful ways to complement the meatless diet. Fermented soy products, such as miso, tempeh, fermented tofu, and soymilk, are now widely available and are loaded with isoflavones, which are immediately bioavailable, and they have more genistein (soy isoflavones) and nutrients than regular soy. They also fit in with Asian dietary practices. Fermentation yields more nutrients such as beta-glucan, glutathione, and the B-vitamins than standard products.

Low-fat yogurt is the only animal-derived complete-protein source recommended for frequent use in the diet. Full-fat yogurt is loaded with saturated fats and should be avoided or used as a treat. Yogurt is made from milk that is curdled by bacteria; it contains *Lactobacillus acidophilus* and other "friendly" bacteria needed for the digestion of foods and the prevention of many disorders, including candidiasis. Yogurt is also a good source of calcium and other essential nutrients. Some yogurts have other healthy bacterial strains added to them.

Do not buy the sweetened, flavored yogurts that are sold in supermarkets. These products contain added sugar and, often, preservatives. Instead, either purchase fresh unsweetened yogurt from a health food store or make the yogurt yourself and sweeten it with fruit juices and other wholesome ingredients. Yogurt makers are relatively inexpensive and easy to use, and are available at most health food stores.

Fats

Although much attention has been focused on the need to reduce dietary fat, the body does need fat. During infancy and childhood, fat is necessary for normal brain development. Throughout life, it is essential to provide energy and support growth. Fat is, in fact, the most concentrated source of energy available to the body. However, after about two years of age, the body requires only small amounts of fat—much less than is provided by the average American diet. If you are an adult, about one-third of your calories should come from fat. Of that total, one-third should be saturated, one-third polyunsaturated (corn oil and fish oil), and one-third monounsaturated (olive oil).

Excessive fat intake is a major causative factor in obesity, high blood pressure, coronary heart disease, and colon cancer, and has been linked to a number of other disorders as well. To understand how fat intake is related to these health problems, it is necessary to understand the different types of fats available and the ways in which these fats act within the body.

Fats are composed of building blocks called *fatty acids*. There are three major categories of fatty acids—saturated, polyunsaturated, and monounsaturated. These classifications are based on the number of hydrogen atoms in the chemical structure of a given molecule of fatty acid.

Saturated fatty acids are found primarily in animal products, including dairy items such as whole milk, cream, butter, and cheese, and fatty meats like beef, veal, lamb, pork, and ham. The fat marbling you can see in beef and pork is composed of saturated fat. Some vegetable products—including coconut oil and palm kernel oil—are also high in saturates. The liver uses saturated fats to manufacture cholesterol. The excessive dietary intake of saturated fats can significantly raise the blood cholesterol level, especially the level of low-density lipoproteins (LDLs), or "bad cholesterol." (For more information about cholesterol, *see* HIGH CHOLESTEROL in Part Two.) Guidelines issued by the National Cholesterol Education Program (NCEP), and widely supported by most experts, recommend that the daily intake of saturated fats be kept below 10 percent of total caloric intake. However, for people who have severe problems with high blood cholesterol, even that level may be too high.

Polyunsaturated fatty acids are found in greatest abundance in corn, soybean, safflower, and sunflower oils. Certain fish oils are also high in polyunsaturates. Unlike the saturated fats, polyunsaturates may actually lower the total blood cholesterol level. In doing so, however, large amounts of polyunsaturates also have a tendency to reduce levels of high-density lipoproteins (HDLs), or "good cholesterol." For this reason—and because polyunsaturates, like all fats, are high in calories for their weight and volume—the NCEP guidelines state that an individual's intake of polyunsaturated fats should not exceed 10 percent of total caloric intake.

Recently the concept of "good" and "bad" fats has surfaced. Good fats are polyunsaturated and include those listed above. Newly added to this list are the omega-3 fats, which don't affect cholesterol levels, but may reduce the risk of heart disease by keeping blood flowing freely. Omega-3 fats are essential for life, but since the 1900s people have been eating fewer of the foods that contain them. The polyunsaturated fats commonly consumed in the United States come from vegetable-based oils like corn, sunflower, and cottonseed oil and contain omega-6s. Although they are also essential, you only need to consume a teaspoon a day of these oils to meet your total omega-6 needs.

Over time, the intake of omega-6s has dwarfed that of omega-3s; our ancestors used to eat these fats in a one-to-one ratio. Many scientists believe that this shift in dietary intake of fats has led to many of the chronic diseases of aging seen today like heart disease, diabetes, and arthritis, and depression. The best way to balance your omega-3 to omega-6 ratio is to eat fish at least twice a week, and use canola oil rather than omega-6–rich vegetable oils. Most people have a ten-year store of omega-6 fats in their bodies. Therefore, it doesn't make sense to worry about getting enough every day. Olive oil contains hardly any essential fatty acids. Flax oil is rich in omega-3 fats, but only about 5 to 10 percent of the omega-3s in flax is usable by the body. Nevertheless, it is low in omega-6s, so it can be used, but only in uncooked items, as heat destroys the omega-3s.

Another caveat concerning polyunsaturated fats: vegetable shortening and stick margarine are made of liquid polyunsaturated fats, which means they should be healthful, but they are so highly processed that they are not. It is preferable to substitute soft-tub margarine, which is less processed than stick margarine, on your toast. It does not perform well when heated, however, so use stick margarine and vegetable shortenings when cooking—they are still preferable to butter.

Monounsaturated fatty acids are found mostly in vegetable and nut oils such as olive, peanut, and canola. These fats appear to reduce blood levels of LDLs without affecting HDLs in any way. However, this positive impact upon LDL cholesterol is relatively modest. The NCEP guidelines recommend that intake of monounsaturated fats be kept between 10 and 15 percent of total caloric intake.

Although most foods—including some plant-derived foods—contain a combination of all three types of fatty acids, one of the types usually predominates. Thus, a fat or oil is considered "saturated" or "high in saturates" when it is composed primarily of saturated fatty acids. Such saturated fats are usually solid at room temperature. Similarly, a fat or oil composed mostly of polyunsaturated fatty acids is called "polyunsaturated," while a fat or oil composed mostly of monounsaturated fatty acids is called "monounsaturated."

One other element, *trans-fatty acids,* which used to be in many food products, is thought to play a role in blood cholesterol levels and other factors that increase the risk of heart disease. Also called *trans fats,* these substances occur when polyunsaturated oils are altered through hydrogenation, a process used to harden liquid vegetable oils into solid foods like margarine and shortening. As of January 2006, the FDA has required all food manufacturers to list the trans-fat content on the nutrition label. Almost immediately products free of trans fats emerged on the market. Today you won't find many products that contain trans fats. If you do see trans fats on the label, you should avoid products where there is more than 0.5 gram per serving. Your total intake should be less than 1 percent of total caloric intake or about 2 grams per 1,800-calorie diet.

It is clear that if your goal is to lower blood cholesterol, polyunsaturated and monounsaturated fats are more desirable than saturated fats or products with trans-fatty acids. Just as important, your total calories from fat should range between 20 to 35 percent of daily calories.

The Micronutrients: Vitamins and Minerals

Like water, carbohydrates, protein, and fats, and the enzymes required to digest them, vitamins and minerals are essential to life. They are therefore considered nutrients, and are often referred to as *micronutrients* simply because they are needed in relatively small amounts compared with the four basic nutrients.

Recommended Dietary Allowances (RDAs) were instituted in 1941 by the National Academy of Sciences' U.S. Food and Nutrition Board as a standard for the daily amounts of vitamins and minerals needed by a healthy person. These RDAs were the basis for the U.S. Recommended Daily Allowances (U.S. RDAs) adopted by the Food and Drug Administration (FDA). The U.S. RDA used to be the term that was used on food labels. However, the provisions of the Nutrition Labeling and Education Act and the Dietary Supplement Act of 1992 required a change in food product labeling to use a new reference term, Daily Value (DV), which began to appear on FDA-regulated product labels in 1994. Today you can look at any food or dietary supplement label and see the percent DV of all essential nutrients contained in the product. DVs are made up of two sets of references: Daily Reference Values (DRVs) and Reference Daily Intakes (RDIs).

DRVs are a set of dietary references that apply to fat, saturated fat, cholesterol, carbohydrate, protein, fiber, sodium, and potassium. RDIs are a set of dietary references based on the Recommended Dietary Allowances for essential vitamins and minerals and, in selected groups, protein. The term *RDI* replaces *U.S. RDA.*

In 1998 the Food and Nutrition Board published new guidelines for healthy eating and called them Dietary Reference Intakes (DRIs). These can be used for planning and assessing diets for healthy people.

The goal is to have these guidelines, which make up the DRI, replace the previous RDA standard.

The amounts of these nutrients defined by the DRI give us about twice the amount needed to ward off vitamin deficiency diseases such as beriberi, rickets, scurvy, and night blindness. What they do not account for are the amounts needed to maintain maximum health, rather than borderline health. Moreover, they are not good at providing an individual's need but rather population norms.

Scientific studies have shown that taking dosages of vitamins above the DRIs helps our body work better. The DRIs therefore are not very useful for determining what our intake of different vitamins should be. We prefer to speak in terms of *optimum daily intakes* (ODIs)—the amounts of nutrients needed for vibrant good health. This entails consuming larger amounts of vitamins than the DRIs. The nutrient doses recommended on page 11 are ODIs. By providing our bodies with an optimum daily amount of necessary vitamins, we can enhance our health. The dosages outlined in this book will enable you to design a vitamin program that is custom-tailored for the individual. Many nutrients with a DRI also have a corresponding Tolerable Upper Level of Intake (UL), which is higher than the DRI but that has been found to be safe (to learn the ULs for all vitamins and minerals, go to http://fnic.nal.usda.gov). Do not take more than the UL for any nutrient (unless your health care provider recommends that you do) because it is not safe to do so based on what we know today. The ULs are constantly under scrutiny. For example, scientists have called for the FDA to increase the UL for vitamin D.

FDA'S NEW GOOD MANUFACTURING PRACTICES

Ideally, all of us would get all the nutrients we need for optimal health from fresh, healthful foods. In reality, however, this is often difficult, if not impossible. In our chemically polluted and stress-filled world, our nutritional requirements have been increasing, but the number of calories we require has been *decreasing,* as our general level of physical activity has declined. This means we are faced with needing somehow to get more nutrients from less food. At the same time, many of our foods are depleted of certain nutrients. Modern farming practices have resulted in soils that are lacking in selenium and other nutrients.

Harvesting and shipping practices are dictated not by nutritional considerations but by marketing demands. Add to this extensive processing, improper storage, and other factors, and it is little wonder that many of the foods that reach our tables cannot meet our nutritional needs. Getting even the DRI of vitamins from today's diet has become quite hard to do. This means that for optimum health, it is necessary to take nutrients in supplement form. Dr. Bruce Ames, a well-known nutritional scientist, argues that low dietary intakes of vitamins and minerals is widespread in the United States and that this may accelerate chronic diseases of aging like cancer.

Everyone would benefit from taking dietary supplements given the nature of the food supply. And supplements have become much safer. As of July 2008, all companies that manufacture dietary supplements must follow Good Manufacturing Practices (GMPs). The FDA has established guidelines for manufacturing procedures so that you actually get the nutrients that are advertised on the label. Also, the new requirements dictate that the products are clean and free of harmful bacteria and other toxins. The FDA now requires manufacturers to store all the ingredients used in a product after the product has been sold. Each product must have a name and phone number to call if a user becomes ill. The batch number of the product then can be matched to the stored product to help figure out why someone has had an adverse reaction.

Nutrients and Dosages for Maintaining Good Health

The table on the following page—which includes not just vitamin and mineral supplements, but other supplements as well—should be used as a guideline. Although the amounts listed as ODIs are safe (they will not cause toxicity), they should be varied according to a person's size and body weight. People who are active and exercise; those who are under great stress, on restricted diets, or mentally or physically ill; women who take oral contraceptives; those on medication; those who are recovering from surgery; and smokers and those who consume alcoholic beverages—all may need larger-than-normal amounts of certain nutrients.

In addition to a proper diet, exercise and a positive attitude are two important elements that are needed to prevent sickness and disease. If your lifestyle includes each of these, you will feel good and have more energy—something we all deserve. Nature has the answers we need to maintain our health, but you need to know what nutrients you are taking to make sure all the pieces of the puzzle fit together.

If you are not used to taking supplements, especially in larger-than-normal doses, your body may need time to adjust. Always take a multivitamin/multimineral supplement with food—if possible, with the biggest meal of the day—to avoid stomach upset and foster better absorption of the nutrients. Otherwise, if the tablet can be split in two, take half in the morning and half at the evening meal.

Daily dosages are suggested; however, before using any supplements, you should consult with your health care provider. The dosages given here are for adults and children weighing 100 pounds and over. Appropriate dosages for children vary according to age and weight. A child weighing between 70 and 100 pounds should be given three-quarters the adult dose; a child weighing less than 70 pounds (and *over* the age of six years) should be given one-half the adult dose. A child under the age of six years should be given nutritional formulas designed specifically for young children. Follow the dosage directions on the product label. Many products have not been directly tested for use by children, so be sure to check with the child's health care provider before giving any supplement to a child. Besides vitamins and minerals, other nutrients that have been tested in children include *Andrographis Paniculata,* cranberry, echinacea, evening primrose oil, garlic, ivy leaf, and valerian.

I recommend using only quality supplements from a reputable source. Lower-priced supplements can mean lower quality, with higher levels of fillers and other undesirable ingredients. Give your body the best—it deserves it. Of course it is better to take the supplements than not, so if you can't afford the higher-quality vitamins, then use the lower-cost ones. If you cannot locate one or more of the supplements recommended in this book, you can call, write, or e-mail one of the sources listed in the Appendix.

For your reference, both milligrams (mg) and micrograms (mcg) refer to specific weights. An international unit (IU), by contrast, is the amount of a vitamin, mineral, or other substance agreed upon by the International Conference for Unification of Formulae to elicit a certain biological activity. Thus, an international unit of one vitamin will be of a different weight than an international unit of a different vitamin. It is a useful gauge for how much of a particular vitamin or mineral you are taking, but in terms of weight it is meaningful only for that particular substance and no other. Studies have found that people who regularly take supplements typically have a better quality of life, a lower risk of heart attack and diabetes, and lower blood pressure compared to those who do not take supplements.

Vitamins	Optimum Daily Intakes*
Vitamin A (retinol)	5,000–10,000 IU
Carotenoid complex containing beta-carotene	5,000–25,000 IU
Vitamin B_1 (thiamine)	50–100 mg
Vitamin B_2 (riboflavin)	15–50 mg
Vitamin B_3 (niacin)	15–50 mg
(niacinamide)	50–100 mg
Vitamin B_5 (pantothenic acid)	50–100 mg
Vitamin B_6 (pyridoxine)	50–100 mg
Vitamin B_{12}	200–400 mcg
Biotin	400–800 mcg
Choline	50–200 mg
Folic acid	400–800 mcg
Inositol	50–200 mg
Para-aminobenzoic acid (PABA)	10–50 mg
Vitamin C with mineral ascorbates (Ester-C)	1,000–3,000 mg
Bioflavonoids (mixed)	200–500 mg
Hesperidin	50–100 mg
Rutin	25 mg
Vitamin D_3 (cholecalciferol)	400 IU
Vitamin E (d-alpha-tocopherol)	200 IU
Vitamin K (use natural sources such as alfalfa, green leafy vegetables)	100–500 mcg
Essential fatty acids (EFAs) (primrose oil, flaxseed oil, salmon oil, and fish oil are good sources)	As directed on label.

Minerals	Optimum Daily Intakes
Boron (picolinate or citrate)	3–6 mg
Calcium (citrate, ascorbate, or malate)	1,500–2,000 mg
Chromium (GTF, picolinate, or polynicotinate)	150–400 mcg
Copper	2–3 mg
Iodine (kelp is a good source)	100–225 mcg
Iron** (ferrous gluconate, fumarate, citrate, or amino acid chelate; avoid inorganic forms such as ferrous sulfate, which can oxidize vitamin E)	18–30 mg
Magnesium	750–1,000 mg
Manganese	3–10 mg
Molybdenum (ascorbate, aspartate, or picolinate)	30–100 mcg
Potassium (citrate)	99–500 mg
Selenium	100–200 mcg
Vanadium (vanadyl sulfate)	200 mcg–1 mg
Zinc	30–50 mg

Amino Acids***	Optimum Daily Intakes
Acetyl-L-carnitine	100–500 mg
Acetyl-L-cysteine	100–500 mg
L-carnitine	500 mg
L-cysteine	50–100 mg
L-lysine	50–100 mg
L-methionine	50–100 mg
L-tyrosine	500 mg
Taurine	100–500 mg

Optional Supplements****	Optimum Daily Intakes
Chondroitin sulfate	As directed on label.
Coenzyme Q_{10}	30–100 mg
Cryptoxanthin	110 mcg
Flavonoids (citrus fruits and berries)	As directed on label.
Garlic	As directed on label.
Ginkgo biloba (herb)	As directed on label.
Glucosamine sulfate	As directed on label.
Lecithin	200–500 mg
Lutein/lycopene	As directed on label.
Pectin	50–100 mg
Phosphatidyl choline	As directed on label.
Phosphatidyl serine	As directed on label.
Pycnogenol or grape seed extract (OPCs)	As directed on label.
Quercetin	70–140 mg
RNA-DNA	100 mg
Silicon	As directed on label.
Soy isoflavones (genistein)	As directed on label.
Superoxide dismutase (SOD)	As directed on label.
Zeaxanthin	90 mcg

*Be careful not to confuse milligrams (mg) with micrograms (mcg). A microgram is 1/1,000 of a milligram, or 1/1,000,000 of a gram.

**You should take iron supplements only if you have been diagnosed with a deficiency of this mineral. Always take iron supplements separately, rather than in a multivitamin and mineral formula.

***See AMINO ACIDS for more information. You should not take individual amino acids on a regular basis unless you are using them for the treatment of a specific disorder.

****See NATURAL FOOD SUPPLEMENTS for more information.

Other supplements that you may wish to take for increased energy include the following:

- Bee pollen.

- Coenzyme A.

- Coenzyme 1 (nicotinamide adenine dinucleotide with high-energy hydrogen, or NADH; sold under the brand name Enada).

- Free form amino acid.

- Kyo-Green from Wakunaga of America.

- N, N-Dimethylglycine (DMG).

- Octacosanol.

- Siberian ginseng.

- Spirulina.

- Wheat germ.

In addition, there are many good formulas on the market specifically formulated to help meet the nutritional needs of infants and children, among them Mycel Baby Vites from Ethical Nutrients, a highly absorbable liquid multivitamin formula.

Synergy and Deficiency

Data compiled by the U.S. Department of Agriculture indicate that at least 40 percent of the people in this country routinely consume a diet containing only 60 percent of the Recommended Daily Allowance (RDA) of each of ten selected nutrients. This means that close to half of the population (and very likely more) suffer from a deficiency of at least one important nutrient. A poll of 37,000 Americans conducted by Food Technology found that half of them were deficient in vitamin B_6 (pyridoxine), 42 percent did not consume sufficient amounts of calcium, 39 percent had an insufficient iron intake, and 25 to 39 percent did not obtain enough vitamin C. Additional research has shown that a vitamin deficiency may not affect the whole body, but only specific cells. For example, those who smoke may suffer from a vitamin C deficiency, but only in the lung area.

Whenever you seek to correct a vitamin or mineral deficiency, you must recognize that nutrients work synergistically. This means that there is a cooperative action between certain vitamins and minerals, which work as catalysts, promoting the absorption and assimilation of other vitamins and minerals. Correcting a deficiency in one vitamin or mineral requires the addition of others, not simply replacement of the one in which you are deficient. This is why taking a single vitamin or mineral may be ineffective, or even dangerous, and why a balanced vitamin and mineral preparation should always be taken in addition to any single supplements. The following table indicates which vitamins and minerals are necessary to correct certain deficiencies. The best way to avoid interfering with the natural synergies among nutrients is to take supplements with meals, unless otherwise instructed. Food stimulates the natural digestive processes and contains natural nutrients to foster the digestion and absorption of nutrients from food and supplements.

Vitamins	Supplements Needed for Assimilation
Vitamin A	Choline, essential fatty acids, zinc, vitamins C, D, and E.
Vitamin B complex	Calcium, vitamins C and E.
Vitamin B_1 (thiamine)	Manganese, vitamin B complex, vitamins C and E.
Vitamin B_2 (riboflavin)	Vitamin B complex, vitamin C.
Vitamin B_3 (niacin)	Vitamin B complex, vitamin C.
Vitamin B_5 (pantothenic acid)	Vitamin B complex, vitamins A, C, and E.
Vitamin B_6 (pyridoxine)	Potassium, vitamin B complex, vitamin C.
Biotin	Folic acid, vitamin B complex, pantothenic acid (vitamin B_5), vitamin B_{12}, vitamin C.
Choline	Vitamin B complex, vitamin B_{12}, folic acid, inositol.
Inositol	Vitamin B complex, vitamin C.
Para-aminobenzoic acid (PABA)	Vitamin B complex, folic acid, vitamin C.
Vitamin C	Bioflavonoids, calcium, magnesium.
Vitamin D	Calcium, choline, essential fatty acids, phosphorus, vitamins A and C.
Vitamin E	Essential fatty acids, manganese, selenium, vitamin A, vitamin B_1 (thiamine), inositol, vitamin C.
Essential fatty acids	Vitamins A, C, D, and E.

Minerals	Supplements Needed for Assimilation
Calcium	Boron, essential fatty acids, lysine, magnesium, manganese, phosphorus, vitamins A, C, D, and E.
Copper	Cobalt, folic acid, iron, zinc.
Iodine	Iron, manganese, phosphorus.
Magnesium	Calcium, phosphorus, potassium, vitamin B_6 (pyridoxine), vitamins C and D.
Manganese	Calcium, iron, vitamin B complex, vitamin E.
Phosphorus	Calcium, iron, manganese, sodium, vitamin B_6 (pyridoxine).
Silicon	Iron, phosphorus.
Sodium	Calcium, potassium, sulfur, vitamin D.
Sulfur	Potassium, vitamin B_1 (thiamine), pantothenic acid (vitamin B_5), biotin.
Zinc	Calcium, copper, phosphorus, vitamin B_6 (pyridoxine).

There are certain cautions that you should take into account when taking supplements. Antibiotics interfere with the natural balance of normal intestinal flora needed to produce vitamin K, which is necessary for normal blood clotting and maintaining the integrity of the bones. Too much coffee and/or caffeine-containing soft drinks can interfere with calcium metabolism. Aspirin can irritate the gastrointestinal tract, and may cause gastrointestinal bleeding.

Aspirin can also interfere with the absorption of B vitamins and vitamin C. If you are taking aspirin daily for cardiovascular health, it is better to take baby aspirin—studies have shown that it is less irritating to the gastrointestinal tract, and it works just as well as ordinary aspirin. Baby aspirin usually has 80 milligrams of aspirin, but check with your health care provider before using aspirin in this way.

BASIC GUIDELINES FOR SELECTING AND PREPARING FOODS

Clearly, a healthy diet must provide a proper balance of the four essential nutrients, as well as a rich supply of vitamins, minerals, and other micronutrients. However, it is not enough simply to purchase foods that are high in complex carbohydrates with low-glycemic indexes, fiber, and complementary proteins, and low in saturated fats. Food also must be free of harmful additives, and it must be prepared in a way that preserves its nutrients and avoids the production of harmful substances.

When nutritionists talk about diet, they are referring to live whole foods—unprocessed food with nothing added or taken away. Whole foods are more healthful because they contain no potentially harmful ingredients. In addition, plant foods are full of hundreds of phytochemicals that can help prevent disease and keep the body healthy. These are our front-line defenders against cancer and free radicals (see Phytochemicals on page 14). Foods known to supply important phytochemicals include soybeans and soy products, broccoli, citrus peels, flax, garlic, green tea, grapes, and tomatoes. In order to optimize your phytochemical intake, it's important to consume a biodiverse diet. To achieve biodiversity in your diet, simply eating a lot of fruits and vegetables is not enough. A biodiverse diet not only includes consuming at least 8 to 10 servings (½ cup per serving) per day, but also making sure there is as much diversity within food groups as possible.

Avoid Foods That Contain Additives and Artificial Ingredients

Additives are placed in foods for a number of reasons: to lengthen shelf life; to make a food more appealing by enhancing color, texture, or taste; to facilitate food preparation; or to otherwise make the product more marketable.

Certain additives, like sugar, are derived from natural sources. Other additives, like aspartame (in NutraSweet and Equal), are made synthetically. Sweeteners derived from natural sources include sucralose, the compound used in Splenda. Sucralose is synthesized from sucrose (sugar) and appears to be inert metabolically, which would make it ideal for people with diabetes. However, sucralose might be stored in the body simply because this synthetic molecule is never found in nature and the body is not equipped to metabolize it. We would advise limiting the use of this additive/artificial sweetener. Although many additives are used in very small amounts, it has been estimated that the average American consumes about 5 pounds of additives per year. If you include sugar—the food-processing industry's most used additive—the number jumps to 135 pounds a year. Anyone whose diet is high in processed products clearly consumes a significant amount of additives and artificial ingredients.

At their best, additives and artificial ingredients simply add little or no nutritional value to a food product. At their worst, some additives could pose a threat to your health. The history of additive use includes a number of products that were once deemed safe but later were banned or allowed only if accompanied by warnings. The artificial sweeteners cyclamate and saccharin are just two examples of such products. Other additives, like monosodium glutamate (MSG) and aspartame, are used without warnings per se, but packages of food that contain them are now marked in the United States with sometimes cryptic statements, such as "PHENYLKETONURICS: CONTAINS PHENYLALANINE," which appears on packets of Equal, NutraSweet, and other products containing aspartame. These products may cause problems for some sensitive people. The warning is there to protect children born with PKU (phenylketonuria). This condition is identified at birth so those who have it know they have it. The long-term effects of most sugar-substitute additives, including sucralose, are unknown. A safer sugar substitute is an extract made from the herb *Stevia rebaudiana*, which is available in health food stores. Stevia is derived from the leaf of a plant and has recently become commercially available. It is a natural sweetener that does not affect blood sugar levels and yields a pleasant sweet taste. In 2009, the FDA granted stevia GRAS (Generally Recognized as Safe) status.

Increase Your Consumption of Raw Produce

The most healthful fruits and vegetables are those that have been grown organically—without the use of insecticides, herbicides, artificial fertilizers, or growth-stimulating chemicals. Organic produce can be found in select health food stores, as well as in some supermarkets and greenmarkets and through food co-ops.

When choosing your produce, look for fruits and vegetables that are at the peak of ripeness. These contain more vitamins and enzymes than do foods that are underripe or overripe, or that have been stored for any length of time. The longer a food is kept in storage, the more nutrients it loses.

Once you get your organic produce home, running water and a vegetable brush are probably all that will be needed to get it ready for the table. If the produce is not organic, however, you will want to wash it more thoroughly to rid it of any chemical residues. Use a soft vegetable brush to scrub the foods, and then let them soak in water for ten minutes.

You can also clean produce with nontoxic rinsing preparations, which are available in reputable health food stores. If the products are waxed, peel them, because wax cannot be washed away. Remove as thin a layer of peel as possible.

Most fruits and vegetables should be eaten in their entirety, as all of the parts, including the skin, contain valuable nutrients. When eating citrus fruits, remove the rinds, but eat the white part inside the skin for its vitamin C and bioflavonoid content.

Although most people usually cook their vegetables before eating, both fruits and vegetables should be eaten raw if possible. All enzymes and most vitamins are extremely sensitive to heat, and are usually destroyed in the cooking process.

If fresh produce is unavailable, use frozen fruits and vegetables instead. Avoid highly processed food items be-

Phytochemicals

For many years, researchers have recognized that diets high in fruits, vegetables, grains, and legumes appear to reduce the risk of a number of diseases, including cancer, heart disease, diabetes, and high blood pressure when compared with diets high in meat. More recently, it was discovered that the disease-preventing effects of these foods are partly due to antioxidants—specific vitamins, minerals, and enzymes that help prevent cancer and other disorders by protecting cells against damage from oxidation. Now, researchers have discovered that fruits, vegetables, grains, and legumes contain yet another group of health-promoting nutrients. Called *phytochemicals,* these substances appear to be powerful ammunition in the war against cancer and other disorders.

Phytochemicals are the biologically active substances in plants that are responsible for giving them color, flavor, and natural disease resistance. To understand how phytochemicals protect the body against cancer, it is necessary to understand that cancer formation is a multistep process. Phytochemicals seem to fight cancer by blocking one or more of the steps that lead to cancer.

For instance, cancer can begin when a carcinogenic molecule—from the food you eat or the air you breathe—invades a cell. But if sulforaphane, a phytochemical found in broccoli, also reaches the cell, it activates a group of enzymes that whisk the carcinogen out of the cell before it can cause any harm.

Other phytochemicals are known to prevent cancer in other ways. Flavonoids, found in citrus fruits and berries, keep cancer-causing hormones from latching on to cells in the first place. Genistein, found in soybeans, kills tumors by preventing the formation of the capillaries needed to nourish them. Indoles, found in cruciferous vegetables such as Brussels sprouts, cauliflower, and cabbage, increase immune activity and make it easier for the body to excrete toxins. Saponins, found in kidney beans, chickpeas, soybeans, and lentils, may prevent cancer cells from multiplying. P-coumaric acid and chlorogenic acid, found in tomatoes, interfere with certain chemical unions that can create carcinogens. The list of these protective substances goes on and on. Tomatoes alone are believed to contain an estimated 10,000 different phytochemicals.

Although no long-term human studies have shown that specific phytochemicals stop cancer, research on phytochemicals supports the more than two hundred studies that link lowered cancer risk with a diet rich in grains, legumes, fruits, and vegetables. Moreover, animal and in vitro studies have demonstrated how some phytochemicals prevent carcinogens from promoting the growth of specific cancers. For instance, the phytochemical phenethyl isothiocyanate (PEITC), found in cabbage and turnips, has been shown to inhibit the growth of lung cancer in rats and mice. Among other things, PEITC protects the cells' DNA from a potent carcinogen found in tobacco smoke.

Researchers have been able to isolate some phytochemicals, and a number of companies are now selling concentrates that contain phytochemicals obtained from vegetables such as broccoli. These may be used as supplemental sources of some of these nutrients.

However, such pills should *not* be seen as replacements for fresh whole foods. Because several *thousand* phytochemicals are currently known to exist, and because new ones are being discovered all the time, no supplement can possibly contain all of the cancer-fighters found in a shopping basket full of fruits and vegetables.

Fortunately, it is easy to get a healthy dose of phytochemicals at every meal. Almost every grain, legume, fruit, and vegetable tested has been found to contain these substances. Moreover, unlike many vitamins, these substances do not appear to be destroyed by cooking or other processing. Genistein, the substance found in soybeans, for instance, is also found in soybean products such as tofu and miso soup. Similarly, the phytochemical PEITC, found in cabbage, remains intact even when the cabbage is made into coleslaw or sauerkraut. Of course, by eating much of your produce raw or only lightly cooked, you will be able to enjoy the benefits not just of phytochemicals, but of all the vitamins, minerals, and other nutrients that fresh whole foods have to offer.

cause they usually contain significant amounts of salt and sugar and other unhealthy additives. If raw produce does not agree with you, steam your vegetables lightly in a steamer, cooking pan, or wok just until slightly tender.

If fresh fruits and vegetables are not an option, it is still better to eat them than not—regardless of the form they come in. Many of the published studies on the health benefits of fruits and vegetables were based on consumption of any type (organic and nonorganic) and any state (fresh, frozen, canned, and juice).

Avoid Overcooking Your Foods

As just discussed, cooking foods for all but brief periods of time can destroy many valuable nutrients. More alarming is that when foods are cooked to the point of browning or charring, the organic compounds they contain undergo changes in structure, producing carcinogens.

Barbecued meats seem to pose the worst health threat in this regard. When burning fat drips onto an open flame, polycyclic aromatic hydrocarbons (PAHs)—dangerous carcinogens—are formed. When amino acids and other chemicals found in muscle are exposed to high temperatures, other carcinogens, called heterocyclic aromatic amines (HAAs), are cre-

Is Aspartame a Safe Sugar Substitute?

Due to America's obsession with dieting, the popularity of aspartame (found in Equal and NutraSweet, as well as many processed food products) has soared. Because it is about two hundred times sweeter than sugar, much smaller amounts of aspartame are needed to sweeten the taste of foods. This artificial sweetener pervades supermarket shelves. It is especially prevalent in diet foods, and can be found in a number of products, including instant breakfasts, breath mints, cereals, sugar-free chewing gum, cocoa mixes, coffee beverages, frozen desserts, gelatin desserts, juice beverages, laxatives, milk drinks, multivitamins, nonprescription pharmaceuticals, shake mixes, soft drinks, tabletop sweeteners, tea beverages, instant teas and coffees, topping mixes, wine coolers, and yogurt.

Upon digestion, aspartame breaks down into three components. The first two are the amino acids phenylalanine and aspartic acid and the third is methanol, or methyl alcohol.

Ever since it was introduced, aspartame has been the center of controversy. Supposedly, a significant number of people have reported suffering ill effects as a result of aspartame consumption. According to the 1990 book *Aspartame (NutraSweet): Is It Safe?* by H. J. Roberts, reactions included headaches, mood swings, changes in vision, nausea and diarrhea, sleep disorders, memory loss and confusion, and even convulsions. People with phenylketonuria (PKU) lack an enzyme needed to convert phenylalanine into tyrosine. Because of this, they accumulate phenylalanine, and at high levels it can be toxic to them. Consequently, these people almost certainly should not use aspartame. But how about the rest of us?

By now, the subject has become so emotional that it is difficult to separate fact from fancy. An entire cottage industry exists to educate people on the safety (or non-safety) of this one sweetener. Proponents claim that neither aspartame nor its components accumulate in the body and that the chemical components are used in the body in exactly the same way as those derived from "natural" foods. The amounts of the chemicals are also quite small compared to those gained from other food sources. For instance, a serving of low-fat milk contains about six times more phenylalanine and thirteen times more aspartic acid than does the same quantity of diet soda sweetened with 100 percent aspartame. In the same vein, a serving of tomato juice has six times more methanol than an equivalent diet soda.

Other voices claim that the sale of aspartame must be stopped and the conspiracy between the manufacturer, the FDA, and an entire cast of players, some quite unlikely, needs to be exposed.

Actually, aspartame has been tested for more than thirty years in over two hundred studies, and so far all have concluded that it is a safe product, and can be used by almost everyone, including children and pregnant women. This is true not only in the United States, but also in France, Great Britain, and Europe as a whole.

In summary, earlier fears about safety centered on the components of aspartame being ingested in very high doses by laboratory animals. Some flaws in original studies were taken to be conspiratorial rather than simple mistakes. Subsequent research has shown that it just isn't possible for a normal human being to ingest enough aspartame to raise plasma concentrations of its metabolic constituents to toxic or dangerous levels.

Needless to say, however, there are sensitive people who have allergic reactions to many products. If you have experienced any type of reaction to aspartame, you should refrain from using foods that contain this additive. Better yet, avoid the controversy by avoiding all additives, and enjoy a diet rich in fruits and fresh juices. These foods are naturally sweet, free of artificial coloring and preservatives, and full of the nutrients needed for good health. An herbal sweetener called stevia is also available.

---

ated. In fact, many of the chemicals used to produce cancer in laboratory animals have been isolated from cooked proteins.

It is important to note, though, that cooked meats do not pose the only threat. Even browned or burned bread crusts contain a variety of carcinogenic substances.

The dangers posed by the practice of cooking foods at high temperatures or until browned or burned should not be dismissed. Although eating habits vary widely from person to person, it seems safe to assume that many people consume many grams of overcooked foods a day. By comparison, only half a gram of this same dangerous burned material is inhaled by someone who smokes two packs of cigarettes a day. Clearly, by eating produce raw or only lightly cooked, and by greatly limiting your consumption of meat, you will be doing much to decrease your risk of cancer and, possibly, other disorders.

Use the Proper Cooking Utensils

Although raw foods have many advantages over cooked ones, nourishing soups and a variety of other dishes can be made healthfully. One of the ways to ensure wholesome cooked food is the careful selection of cookware.

When preparing foods, use only glass, stainless steel, or iron pots and pans. Do not use aluminum cookware or utensils. Foods cooked or stored in aluminum produce a substance that neutralizes the digestive juices, leading to acidosis and ulcers. Worse, the aluminum in the cookware can leach from the pot into the food. When the food is consumed, the aluminum is absorbed by the body, where it accumulates in the brain and nervous system tissues. Excessive amounts of these aluminum deposits have been implicated in Alzheimer's disease.

Basic Nutritional Guide

A diet high in nutrients is the key to good health. Use the following table as a guide when deciding which types of food to include in your diet and which ones to avoid in order to maintain good health.

Type of Food	Foods to Avoid	Acceptable Foods
Beans	Canned pork and beans, canned beans with salt or preservatives, frozen beans.	All beans (especially soy) cooked without animal fat or salt.
Beverages	Alcoholic drinks, coffee, cocoa, pasteurized and/or sweetened juices and fruit drinks, sodas, tea (except herbal and green tea).	Herbal teas, fresh vegetable and fruit juices, grain beverages (often sold as coffee substitutes), mineral or distilled water.
Dairy products	All soft cheeses, all pasteurized or artificially colored cheese products, ice cream.	Raw goat cheese, nonfat cottage cheese, kefir, unsweetened yogurt, goat's milk, raw or skim milk, buttermilk.
Eggs	Fried or pickled.	Boiled or poached (limit of four weekly).
Fish	All fried fish, all shellfish, salted fish, anchovies, herring, fish canned in oil.	All freshwater whitefish, salmon, broiled or baked fish, water-packed tuna. (Limit tuna to two servings a week to avoid excessive mercury intake.)
Fruits	Canned, bottled, or frozen fruits with sweeteners added; oranges.	All fresh, frozen, stewed, or dried fruits without sweeteners (except oranges, which are acidic and highly allergenic), unsulfured fruits, home-canned fruits.
Grains	All white flour products, white rice, pasta, crackers, cold cereals, instant types of oatmeal and other hot cereals.	All whole grains and products containing whole grains: cereals, breads, muffins, whole-grain crackers, cream of wheat or rye cereal, buckwheat, millet, oats, brown rice, wild rice. (Limit yeast breads to 3 servings per week.)
Meats	Beef; all forms of pork; hot dogs; luncheon meats; smoked, pickled, and processed meats; corned beef; duck; goose; spare ribs; gravies; organ meats.	Skinless turkey and chicken, lamb. (Limit meat to three 3-oz. servings per week.)
Nuts	All salted or roasted nuts; peanuts (if suffering from a related disorder).	All fresh raw nuts (peanuts in moderation only).
Oils (fats)	All saturated fats, hydrogenated margarine, refined processed oils, shortenings, hardened oils.	All cold-pressed oils: corn, safflower, sesame, olive, flaxseed, soybean, sunflower, and canola oils; margarine made from these oils; eggless mayonnaise.
Seasonings	Black or white pepper, salt, hot red peppers, all types of vinegar except pure natural apple cider vinegar.	Garlic, onions, cayenne, Spike, all herbs, dried vegetables, apple cider vinegar, tamari, miso, seaweed, dulse.
Soups	Canned soups made with salt, preservatives, MSG, or fat stock; all creamed soups.	Homemade bean (salt- and fat-free), lentil, pea, vegetable, barley, brown rice, onion.
Sprouts and seeds	All seeds cooked in oil or salt.	All slightly cooked sprouts (except alfalfa, which should be raw and washed thoroughly), wheatgrass, all raw seeds.
Sweets	White, brown, or raw cane sugar, corn syrups, chocolate, sugar candy, fructose (except that in fresh whole fruit), all syrups (except pure maple syrup), all sugar substitutes, jams and jellies made with sugar.	Barley malt or rice syrup, small amounts of raw honey, pure maple syrup, stevia, unsulfured blackstrap molasses.
Vegetables	All canned or frozen with salt or additives.	All raw, fresh, frozen (no additives), or home-canned without salt (undercook vegetables slightly).

Other cookware to be avoided includes all pots and pans with nonstick coatings. Too often, the metals and other substances in the pots' finish flakes or leaches into the food. Ultimately, these chemicals end up in your body.

Limit Your Use of Salt

Although some sodium is essential for survival, inadequate sodium intake is a rare problem. (Symptoms of salt deficiency include lightheadedness and muscles fatigue.) We need at least 1,000 to 1,500 milligrams of sodium a day to stay healthy. This is enough to accomplish all the vital functions that sodium performs in the body—helping maintain normal fluid levels, healthy muscle function, and proper acidity (pH) of the blood. Excessive sodium intake can cause fluid to be retained in the tissues, which can lead to hypertension (high blood pressure) and can aggravate many medical disorders, including congestive heart failure, certain forms of kidney disease, and premenstrual syndrome (PMS).

One of the best ways to limit the sodium in your diet is to limit your consumption of processed and fast foods, which often contain excessively high amounts of sodium. Cooking at home is a perfect opportunity to control your salt intake. Last, if you can see it, avoid it—for example, in salty snacks such as pretzels and potato chips.

Vitamins

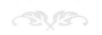

INTRODUCTION

Vitamins are essential to life. They contribute to good health by regulating the metabolism and assisting the biochemical processes that release energy from digested food. They are considered micronutrients because the body needs them in relatively small amounts compared with nutrients such as carbohydrates, proteins, fats, and water.

Enzymes are essential chemicals that are the foundation of human bodily functions. (*See* ENZYMES in Part One.) They are catalysts (activators) in the chemical reactions that are continually taking place within the body. As coenzymes, vitamins work with enzymes, thereby allowing all the activities that occur within the body to be carried out as they should be. Whole, fresh raw foods are a good source of enzymes.

Of the major vitamins, some are soluble in water and others in oil. Water-soluble vitamins must be taken into the body daily, as they cannot be stored and are excreted within four hours to one day. These include vitamin C and the B-complex vitamins. Oil-soluble vitamins can be stored for longer periods of time in the body's fatty tissue and the liver. These include vitamins A, D, E, and K. Both types of vitamin are needed by the body for proper functioning.

SYNTHETIC VERSUS NATURAL

Make sure you are getting at least 100 percent of all essential vitamins from the foods you eat with a diet rich in fruits and vegetables. Once this has been accomplished, most people will need more from supplements to achieve optimal health. Vitamin supplements can be divided into two groups—synthetic and natural. Synthetic vitamins are produced in laboratories from isolated chemicals that mirror their counterparts found in nature. Natural vitamins are derived from food sources. Although there are no major chemical differences between a vitamin found in food and one created in a laboratory, synthetic supplements contain the isolated vitamins only, while natural supplements may contain other nutrients not yet discovered. This is because these vitamins are in their natural state. If you are deficient in a particular nutrient, the chemical source will work, but you will not get the benefits of the vitamin as found in whole foods. Supplements that are not labeled natural also may include coal tars, artificial coloring, preservatives, sugars, and starch, as well as other additives. You should beware of such harmful elements.

However, you should also note that a bottle of "natural" vitamins might contain vitamins that have not been extracted from a natural food source. It is necessary to read labels carefully to make sure the products you buy contain nutrients from food sources, with none of the artificial additives mentioned above.

Studies have shown that protein-bonded vitamins, as found in natural whole food supplements, are absorbed, utilized, and retained in the tissues better than supplements that are not protein-bonded. Chemical-derived vitamins are not protein-bonded. Vitamins and minerals in food are bonded to proteins, lipids, carbohydrates, and bioflavonoids.

Dr. Abram Hoffer, one of the "founding fathers" of orthomolecular medicine (a school of medicine that emphasizes the role of nutrition in health), explains:

> Components [of food] do not exist free in nature; nature does not lay down pure protein, pure fat, or pure carbohydrates. Their molecules are interlaced in very complex three-dimensional structures, which even now have not been fully described. Intermingled are the essential nutrients such as vitamins and minerals, again not free, but combined in complex molecules.
>
> Using a natural form of vitamins and minerals in nutritional supplements is the objective of the protein-bonding process. Taking supplements with meals helps to assure a supply of other nutrients needed for better assimilation as well.

WHAT'S ON THE SHELVES?

Over-the-counter vitamin supplements come in various forms, combinations, and amounts. They are available in tablet, capsule, gel-capsule, powder, sublingual (under the tongue), lozenge, and liquid forms. They can also be administered by injection.

In most cases, it is a matter of personal preference as to how you take them; however, due to slight variations in how rapidly the supplements are absorbed and assimilated into the body, we will sometimes recommend one form over another. These recommendations are given throughout the book.

Vitamin supplements are usually available as isolated vitamins or in combination with other nutrients. It is important to select your vitamins based upon what you really need. A program designed for health maintenance would be different from one designed to overcome a specific disorder. Some 59 percent of Americans are now taking supplements on a regular basis.

If you find one supplement that meets your needs, remember to take it daily. If it does not contain a large enough quantity of what you want, you may consider taking more than one. Just make sure that you are aware of the increased dosage of the other nutrients it may contain. If there is no single supplement that provides you with what you are looking for, consider taking a combination of different supplements. This book lists each supplement separately, so you will know what each does and the amount needed. But you may find a supplement that contains several needed nutrients in one tablet or capsule. In fact, a good multivitamin (and multimineral) should be a part of everyone's diet after he or she reaches a certain age, with additional supplements as necessary.

Because the potency of most vitamins may be decreased by sunlight, make sure that the container holding your vitamins is dark enough to shield its contents properly. Some people may be sensitive to plastic, and may need to purchase vitamins in glass containers. Vitamin supplements should be kept in a cool, dark place.

All vitamin supplements work best when taken in combination with food. Unless specified otherwise, oil-soluble vitamins should be taken before meals, and water-soluble ones should be taken after meals. (This applies when you are taking individual supplements only. Multivitamins have both water-soluble and oil-soluble elements.) If you are concerned about getting the full potency from your supplements, you may want to try using raw food–created vitamins made from a single-cell yeast, *Saccharomyces cerevisiae*. This yeast creates vitamins and minerals that are not isolated or synthesized, but that come from nutrient-dense whole foods. One of the best sources of raw food–created vitamins is Garden of Life.

VITAMINS FROM A TO Z

Vitamin A and the Carotenoids

Vitamin A prevents night blindness and other eye problems, as well as some skin disorders, such as acne. It enhances immunity, may help to heal gastrointestinal ulcers, and is needed for the maintenance and repair of epithelial tissue, of which the skin and mucous membranes are composed.

It is important in the formation of bones and teeth, aids in fat storage, and protects against colds, flu, and infections of the kidneys, bladder, lungs, and mucous membranes. Vitamin A acts as an antioxidant, helping to protect the cells against cancer and other diseases (*see* ANTIOXIDANTS in Part One) and is necessary for new cell growth. It guards against heart disease and stroke, and lowers cholesterol levels. People receiving radiation treatment for cervical cancer, prostate cancer, or colorectal cancer have benefited from taking oral vitamin A. Radiation-induced anal ulcers can be a problem with such treatment programs, and a

vitamin A megadose (100,000 international units daily) significantly reduced symptoms in 88 percent of people undergoing such regimens. This important vitamin also slows the aging process. The body cannot utilize protein without vitamin A. Vitamin A is a well-known wrinkle eliminator. Applied topically in the form of tretinoin (the active ingredient in Retin-A and Renova), vitamin A reduces fine lines in the skin and helps to fade age spots.

A deficiency of vitamin A can cause dry hair and/or skin, dryness of the conjunctiva and cornea, poor growth, and/or night blindness. Other possible results of vitamin A deficiency include abscesses in the ears; insomnia; fatigue; reproductive difficulties; sinusitis, pneumonia, and frequent colds and other respiratory infections; skin disorders, including acne; and weight loss.

The *carotenoids* are a class of compounds related to vitamin A. In some cases, they can act as precursors of vitamin A; some act as antioxidants or have other important functions.

The best-known subclass of the carotenoids is the carotenes, of which beta-carotene is the most widely known. Also included in this group are alpha-carotene, gamma-carotene, and lycopene. When food or supplements containing beta-carotene are consumed, the beta-carotene is converted into vitamin A in the liver. According to recent reports, beta-carotene appears to aid in cancer prevention by scavenging, or neutralizing, free radicals. One study reported in the *Journal of the National Cancer Institute*, published in May 2003, found that people who took beta-carotene supplements and who smoked and drank alcohol doubled their risk of precancerous colorectal tumors, while for those who also took the supplements but who didn't smoke or drink there was a 44 percent *decrease* in their risk. Other types of carotenoids that have been identified are the xanthophylls (including beta-cryptoxanthin, canthaxanthin, lutein, and zeaxanthin); the limonoids (including limonene); and the phytosterols (including perillyl alcohol). Evidence suggests that greater consumption of lutein reduces the risk of cataracts and age-related macular degeneration (AMD), and that taking lutein supplements can slow the progress of these disorders, although it does not appear to reverse them if they are already established. High lutein consumption has also been reported to decrease the incidence of prostate cancer.

Science has not yet discovered all of the carotenoids, although one source documents six hundred different carotenoids identified so far. Combinations of carotenoids have been shown to be more beneficial than individual carotenoids taken alone.

Taking large amounts of vitamin A, more than 100,000 international units daily, over long periods can be toxic to the body, mainly to the liver. Toxic levels of vitamin A are associated with abdominal pain, amenorrhea (cessation of menstruation), enlargement of the liver and/or spleen, gastrointestinal disturbances, hair loss, itching, joint pain, nausea and vomiting, water on the brain, elevated liver enzymes, and small cracks and scales on the lips and at the corners of the mouth. Excessive intake of vitamin A during pregnancy has been linked to birth defects, including cleft palate and heart defects. It is better to take beta-carotene during pregnancy. If you have a particular disorder that calls for taking high doses of vitamin A, use an emulsified form, which puts less stress on the liver.

No overdose can occur with beta-carotene, although if you take too much, your skin may turn slightly yellow-orange in color. Beta-carotene does not have the same effect as vitamin A in the body and is not harmful in larger amounts unless your liver cannot convert beta-carotene into vitamin A. There is mixed evidence (mostly from studies done in Europe) as to whether too much vitamin A may increase the risk of osteoporosis. In the United States women usually don't have a problem with getting too much vitamin A because manufacturers mix beta-carotene with vitamin A. However, women who are worried about osteoporosis should consult a health care provider before taking vitamin A. It is important to take only *natural* beta-carotene or a natural carotenoid complex. Betatene is the trade name for a type of carotenoid complex extracted from sea algae. Different manufacturers use it as an ingredient in various products.

Sources

Vitamin A can be obtained from animal livers, fish liver oils, and green and yellow fruits and vegetables. Foods that contain significant amounts include apricots, asparagus, beet greens, broccoli, cantaloupe, carrots, collards, dandelion greens, dulse (a red seaweed), fish liver and fish liver oil, garlic, kale, mustard greens, papayas, peaches, pumpkin, red peppers, spinach, spirulina, sweet potatoes, Swiss chard, turnip greens, watercress, and yellow squash. It is also present in the following herbs: alfalfa, borage leaves, burdock root, cayenne (capsicum), chickweed, eyebright, fennel seed, hops, kelp, lemongrass, mullein, nettle, oat straw, paprika, parsley, peppermint, plantain, raspberry leaf, red clover, rose hips, sage, uva ursi, violet leaves, watercress, and yellow dock. Animal sources of vitamin A are up to six times as strong as vegetable sources, but you should exercise caution if you choose to eat organ meats. A plant-based diet better promotes overall health.

Comments

Antibiotics, laxatives, and some cholesterol-lowering drugs interfere with the absorption of vitamin A.

Cautions

If you have liver disease, do not take a daily dose of over 10,000 international units of vitamin A in pill form, or any amount of cod liver oil. If you are pregnant, do not take more than 10,000 international units of vitamin A daily because of reported problems in fetal development. Children should not take more than 18,000 international units of vi-

tamin A on a daily basis for over one month. For most people, beta-carotene is the best source of vitamin A because it is converted by the liver into only the amount of vitamin A that the body actually needs. However, if you have diabetes or hypothyroidism, there is a good possibility your body cannot convert beta-carotene into vitamin A. Consuming large amounts of beta-carotene may therefore place unnecessary stress on your liver.

Vitamin B Complex

The B vitamins help to maintain the health of the nerves, skin, eyes, hair, liver, and mouth, as well as healthy muscle tone in the gastrointestinal tract and proper brain function.

B-complex vitamins act as coenzymes, helping enzymes to react chemically with other substances, and are involved in energy production. They may be useful for alleviating depression or anxiety as well. Adequate intake of the B vitamins is very important for elderly people because these nutrients are not as well absorbed as we age. There have even been cases of people diagnosed with Alzheimer's disease whose problems were later found to be due to a deficiency of vitamin B_{12} plus the B complex vitamins. The B vitamins should always be taken together, but up to two to three times more of one B vitamin than another can be taken for a period of time if needed for a particular disorder. There are spray and sublingual forms that are absorbed more easily, which are good choices for older adults and those with absorption problems.

Because the B vitamins work together, a deficiency in one often indicates a deficiency in another. Although the B vitamins are a team, they will be discussed individually.

Vitamin B_1 (Thiamine)

Thiamine (thiamine hydrochloride) enhances circulation and assists in blood formation, carbohydrate metabolism, and in the production of hydrochloric acid, which is important for proper digestion. Thiamine also optimizes cognitive activity and brain function. It has a positive effect on energy, growth, normal appetite, and learning capacity, and is needed for proper muscle tone of the intestines, stomach, and heart. Thiamine also acts as an antioxidant, protecting the body from the degenerative effects of aging, alcohol consumption, and smoking.

Beriberi, a nervous system disease that is rare in developed nations, is caused by a deficiency of thiamine. Other symptoms that can result from thiamine deficiency include constipation, edema, enlarged liver, fatigue, forgetfulness, gastrointestinal disturbances, heart changes, irritability, labored breathing, loss of appetite, muscle atrophy, nervousness, numbness of the hands and feet, pain and sensitivity, poor coordination, tingling sensations, weak and sore muscles, general weakness, and severe weight loss.

Benfotiamine is a fat-soluble form of the water-soluble vitamin B_1. Its use is reserved for cases such as alcoholic peripheral neuropathy, a disorder involving decreased nerve functioning caused by damage from excessive drinking of alcohol. It is found naturally in small quantities in roasted, crushed garlic, as well as in onions, shallots, and leeks. This variant of the vitamin lasts longer in the body, yielding potentially therapeutic benefits that regular vitamin B_1 cannot achieve. Benfotiamine may be more effective than thiamine in controlling damage from diabetes because it is a better activator of the enzyme transketolase. This enzyme assists in keeping glucose-derived compounds out of healthy vascular (blood vessel) and nerve cells. The normal supplemental dose is 150 to 600 milligrams per day, taken under the guidance of a doctor or other qualified health care practitioner.

Sources

The richest food sources of thiamine include brown rice, egg yolks, fish, legumes, liver, peanuts, peas, pork, poultry, rice bran, wheat germ, and whole grains. Other sources include asparagus, brewer's yeast, broccoli, Brussels sprouts, dulse, kelp, most nuts, oatmeal, plums, dried prunes, raisins, spirulina, and watercress. Herbs that contain thiamine include alfalfa, bladderwrack, burdock root, catnip, cayenne, chamomile, chickweed, eyebright, fennel seed, fenugreek, hops, nettle, oat straw, parsley, peppermint, raspberry leaf, red clover, rose hips, sage, yarrow, and yellow dock.

Comments

Antibiotics, phenytoin (Dilantin, a drug used to prevent seizures), sulfa drugs, and oral contraceptives, as well as heavy alcohol or caffeine consumption, may decrease thiamine levels in the body. A high-carbohydrate diet increases the need for thiamine. Alcoholics are among those most often deficient in thiamine because the alcohol inhibits its storage. This is sometimes manifested as a disorder known as Wernicke-Korsakoff syndrome, which is characterized by memory problems, abnormal movements, confusion, drowsiness, and other symptoms.

Vitamin B_2 (Riboflavin)

Riboflavin is necessary for red blood cell formation, antibody production, cell respiration, and growth. It alleviates eye fatigue and is important in the prevention and treatment of cataracts. It aids in the metabolism of carbohydrates, fats, and proteins. Together with vitamin A, it maintains and improves the mucous membranes in the digestive tract. Riboflavin also facilitates the use of oxygen by the tissues of the skin, nails, and hair; eliminates dandruff; and helps the absorption of iron and vitamin B_6 (pyridoxine).

Consumption of adequate amounts of riboflavin is important during pregnancy, because a lack of this vitamin can damage a developing fetus even if a woman shows no signs of deficiency. Riboflavin is needed for the metabolism of the amino acid tryptophan, which is converted into niacin

in the body. Carpal tunnel syndrome may benefit from a treatment program that includes riboflavin and vitamin B_6.

Deficiency symptoms include cracks and sores at the corners of the mouth, eye disorders, inflammation of the mouth and tongue, and skin lesions, a group of symptoms collectively referred to as *ariboflavinosis*. Other possible deficiency symptoms include dermatitis, dizziness, hair loss, insomnia, light sensitivity, poor digestion, retarded growth, and slowed mental response.

Sources

High levels of vitamin B_2 are found in the following foods: cheese, egg yolks, fish, legumes, meat, milk, poultry, spinach, whole grains, and yogurt. Other sources include asparagus, avocados, broccoli, Brussels sprouts, currants, dandelion greens, dulse, kelp, leafy green vegetables, mushrooms, molasses, nuts, and watercress. Herbs that contain vitamin B_2 include alfalfa, bladderwrack, burdock root, catnip, cayenne, chamomile, chickweed, eyebright, fennel seed, fenugreek, ginseng, hops, mullein, nettle, oat straw, parsley, peppermint, raspberry leaves, red clover, rose hips, sage, and yellow dock.

Comments

Factors that increase the need for riboflavin include the use of oral contraceptives and strenuous exercise. This B vitamin is easily destroyed by light, antibiotics, and the consumption of alcohol. Taking too much riboflavin (over 50 milligrams daily) over a long period of time may lead to cataracts and retinal diseases. Taking high doses also may turn urine a deep yellow.

Vitamin B_3 (Niacin, Nicotinic Acid, Niacinamide)

Vitamin B_3 is needed for proper circulation and healthy skin. It aids in the functioning of the nervous system; in the metabolism of carbohydrates, fats, and proteins; and in the production of hydrochloric acid for the digestive system. It is involved in the normal secretion of bile and stomach fluids, and in the synthesis of sex hormones. Niacin (nicotinic acid) lowers cholesterol and improves circulation. It is helpful for schizophrenia and other mental illnesses, and is also a memory-enhancer.

Pellagra is a disease caused by niacin deficiency. Other symptoms of niacin deficiency include canker sores, dementia, depression, diarrhea, dizziness, fatigue, halitosis, headaches, indigestion, insomnia, limb pains, loss of appetite, low blood sugar, muscular weakness, skin eruptions, and inflammation.

Sources

Niacin and niacinamide are found in beef liver, brewer's yeast, broccoli, carrots, cheese, corn flour, dandelion greens, dates, eggs, fish, milk, nuts, peanuts, pork, potatoes, rabbit, tomatoes, wheat germ, and whole wheat products. Herbs that contain niacin include alfalfa, burdock root, catnip, cayenne, chamomile, chickweed, eyebright, fennel seed, hops, licorice, mullein, nettle, oat straw, parsley, peppermint, raspberry leaf, red clover, rose hips, slippery elm, and yellow dock. A cup of coffee provides about 3 milligrams of niacin.

Comments

A flush, usually harmless, may occur after you take a niacin supplement; you might develop a red rash on your skin and a tingling sensation may be experienced as well. Usually, these symptoms last only a few minutes.

There are two forms of this vitamin: niacin (or nicotinic acid) and niacinamide. In the form of niacinamide, it does not cause flushing. However, niacinamide does not have all the same properties of niacin. Specifically, it is not effective for lowering blood cholesterol.

Taking high doses of special, extended-release niacin for cholesterol control is a relatively recent phenomenon. The intent is to lower levels of low-density lipoproteins (LDL, or "bad," cholesterol), raise levels of high-density lipoproteins (HDL, or "good," cholesterol), and to reduce triglyceride levels. This type of niacin is *not* dietary niacin. A product called Niaspan, produced by Abbott Laboratories, is an extended-release type of niacin approved for cholesterol control.

Cautions

Dietary niacin should *not* be substituted for Niaspan. Taking high doses of dietary niacin (more than 500 milligrams daily) can damage the liver. People who are pregnant or who suffer from diabetes, glaucoma, gout, liver disease, or peptic ulcers should use niacin supplements with caution. Niacin can elevate blood sugar levels.

Vitamin B$_5$ (Pantothenic Acid)

Known as the antistress vitamin, pantothenic acid plays a role in the production of the adrenal hormones and the formation of antibodies, aids in vitamin utilization, and helps to convert fats, carbohydrates, and proteins into energy.

Pantothenic acid is required by all cells in the body and is concentrated in the organs. It is also involved in the production of neurotransmitters. This vitamin is an essential element of coenzyme A, a vital body chemical involved in many necessary metabolic functions. Pantothenic acid is also a stamina enhancer and prevents certain forms of anemia. It is needed for normal functioning of the gastrointestinal tract and may be helpful in treating depression and anxiety. A deficiency of pantothenic acid may cause fatigue, headache, nausea, and tingling in the hands. Pantothenic acid is also needed for proper functioning of the adrenal glands.

Sources

The following foods contain pantothenic acid: avocados, beef, brewer's yeast, eggs, fresh vegetables, kidney, legumes, liver, lobster, mushrooms, nuts, pork, royal jelly, saltwater fish, torula yeast, whole rye flour, and whole wheat.

Vitamin B$_6$ (Pyridoxine)

Pyridoxine is involved in more bodily functions than almost any other single nutrient. It affects both physical and mental health. It is beneficial if you suffer from water retention, and is necessary for the production of hydrochloric acid and the absorption of fats and protein. It also aids in maintaining sodium and potassium balance, and promotes red blood cell formation.

Pyridoxine is required by the nervous system and is needed for normal brain function and for the synthesis of the nucleic acids RNA and DNA, which contain the genetic instructions for the reproduction of all cells and for normal cellular growth. It activates many enzymes and aids in the absorption of vitamin B$_{12}$, in immune system function, and in antibody production.

Vitamin B$_6$ plays a role in cancer immunity and aids in the prevention of arteriosclerosis. It inhibits the formation of a toxic chemical called homocysteine, which attacks the heart muscle and allows the deposition of cholesterol around the heart muscle. Pyridoxine acts as a mild diuretic, reducing the symptoms of premenstrual syndrome, and it may be useful in preventing calcium oxalate kidney stones as well. It is helpful in the treatment of allergies, arthritis, and asthma.

A deficiency of vitamin B$_6$ can result in anemia, convulsions, headaches, nausea, flaky skin, a sore tongue, and vomiting. Other possible signs of deficiency include acne, anorexia, arthritis, conjunctivitis, cracks or sores on the mouth and lips, depression, dizziness, fatigue, hyperirritability, impaired wound healing, inflammation of the mouth and gums, learning difficulties, impaired memory or memory loss, hair loss, hearing problems, numbness, oily facial skin, stunted growth, and tingling sensations. Carpal tunnel syndrome has been linked to a deficiency of vitamin B$_6$ as well.

Sources

All foods contain some vitamin B$_6$; however, the following foods have the highest amounts: brewer's yeast, carrots, chicken, eggs, fish, meat, peas, spinach, sunflower seeds, walnuts, and wheat germ. Other sources include avocado, bananas, beans, blackstrap molasses, broccoli, brown rice and other whole grains, cabbage, cantaloupe, corn, dulse (a red seaweed), plantains, potatoes, rice bran, soybeans, and tempeh. Herbs that contain vitamin B$_6$ include alfalfa, catnip, and oat straw.

Comments

Antidepressants, estrogen therapy, and oral contraceptives may increase the need for vitamin B_6. Diuretics and cortisone drugs block the absorption of this vitamin by the body.

Prolonged use of high doses of vitamin B_6 (over 1,000 milligrams per day) can be toxic, and may result in nerve damage and loss of coordination.

Vitamin B_{12} (Methylcobalamin)

Vitamin B_{12} is the most chemically complex of all the vitamins and is the general name for a group of essential biological compounds known as cobalamins. The cobalamins are similar to hemoglobin in the blood except that instead of iron they contain cobalt. Vitamin B_{12} comes in several forms. Not all forms are equally effective. The most effective form is *methyl*cobalamin. However, the most common form is *cyano*cobalamin, because it is easier to manufacture and is therefore less expensive.

Unfortunately, the very commmon and inexpensive cyanocobalamin form is difficult for the body to absorb, and the small amount that is absorbed usually fails to find its way into the cells, where it can perform its intended tasks. The liver does, however, convert a small amount of cyanocobalamin into methylcobalamin, but much larger amounts than can be converted are needed to carry out the normal functions of vitamin B_{12}. As a result, many people who take large doses of cyanocobalamin continue to be deficient in the vitamin. They often find themselves resorting to vitamin B_{12} injections, which are available from a doctor by prescription only. Vitamin B_{12} deficiency caused by malabsorption is most common in elderly people. A simple alternative is to take the methylcobalamin form in the first place, either swallowed in tablet form or sublingually. Those with severe digestive disorders may have no choice but to resort to vitamin B_{12} injections. Injections usually are administered every two to three months.

Methylcobalamin is active in the growth and protection of the nervous system. Larger quantities are especially necessary to protect against neurological deterioration as we age. One Danish study found that daily supplementation with 6 micrograms per day (the DRI is 2.4 micrograms) appeared to be sufficient to correct deficiencies in women aged forty-one to seventy-five years.

Vitamin B_{12}, in the methylcobalamin form, may help prevent Parkinson's disease and slow the progression in those who already have the disease by protecting against neural toxicity caused by excess L-dopa, a probable cause of the disease. The vitamin has been shown to reverse the symptoms of such rare neurological diseases as Bell's palsy (see page 682), and shows promise in the treatment of multiple sclerosis and other neurological diseases. Very few substances are known to have any impact on regenerating damaged nerves in humans. However, a 1994 study in the *Journal of Neurological Science* suggested that the methylcobalamin form of vitamin B_{12} could increase the synthesis of certain proteins that help regenerate nerves. The study showed that very high doses of methylcobalamin produced nerve regeneration in rats. No substantive human studies on nerve regeneration are known to date, but as new research is reported it will be included in future editions of this book.

Methylcobalamin is essential in converting homocysteine into methionine, which is used to build protein. As such, it plays an important role in protein synthesis necessary for cardiovascular function. It has been found that high levels of homocysteine that have gone unconverted may be toxic to the lining of the blood vessels and may increase clotting factors, which can result in the buildup of plaque and eventually lead to heart disease and stroke. As such, vitamin B_{12} plays an important role in protein synthesis necessary for cardiovascular function.

Vitamin B_{12} is needed to prevent anemia; it aids folic acid in regulating the formation of red blood cells, and helps in the utilization of iron. This vitamin is also required for proper digestion, absorption of foods, and the metabolism of carbohydrates and fats. It aids in cell formation and cellular longevity. In addition, vitamin B_{12} prevents nerve damage, maintains fertility, and promotes normal growth and development by maintaining the fatty sheaths that cover and protect nerve endings. A study reported in the *American Journal of Obstetrics and Gynecology* in 2004 found that women who gave birth to children with spina bifida had vitamin B_{12} levels that were 21 percent lower than those of mothers who had had healthy children. Vitamin B_{12} is also linked to the production of acetylcholine, a neurotransmitter that assists memory and learning. Vitamin B_{12} supplementation has been shown to enhance sleep patterns, allowing for more restful and refreshing sleep.

A vitamin B_{12} deficiency can be caused by malabsorption, which is most common in older adults and in people with digestive disorders. Deficiency can cause abnormal gait, bone loss, chronic fatigue, constipation, depression, digestive disorders, dizziness, drowsiness, enlargement of the liver, eye disorders, hallucinations, headaches (including migraines), inflammation of the tongue, irritability, labored breathing, memory loss, moodiness, nervousness, neurological damage, palpitations, pernicious anemia, ringing in the ears, and spinal-cord degeneration.

Researchers caution that all patients with unexplained anemia and/or neurological symptoms, as well as patients at risk of developing low B_{12} levels like the elderly and those with intestinal disorders, should have blood levels measured. In addition, those with cognitive impairment may want to be tested for low B_{12} levels.

Strict vegetarians must remember that they require vitamin B_{12} supplementation, as this vitamin is found almost exclusively in animal tissues. Although people who follow a strictly vegetarian diet may not see any signs of the deficiency for some time—the body can store up to five years' worth of vitamin B_{12}—signs eventually will develop. Those who have followed a vegetarian diet for a long time (more than five years) should have B_{12} blood levels measured yearly.

Sources

The largest amounts of vitamin B_{12} are found in meats, brewer's yeast, clams, eggs, herring, kidney, liver, mackerel, milk and dairy products, and seafood. Vitamin B_{12} is not found in many vegetables; it is available only from sea vegetables, such as dulse, kelp, kombu, bladderwrack, and nori, and soybeans and soy products. It is believed that bacteria present in the large intestine synthesize most B_{12}. It is also present in the herbs alfalfa and hops.

Comments

Antigout medications, anticoagulant drugs, and potassium supplements may block the absorption of vitamin B_{12} from the digestive tract. Taking vitamin B_{12} in sublingual tablets, which are dissolved under the tongue rather than swallowed, can be a good option for those who have difficulty absorbing this vitamin. *Intrinsic factor* is a protein produced in the gastrointestinal tract that is necessary for absorption of vitamin B_{12}. People who lack intrinsic factor must use a sublingual form (or injections) for absorption. A blood test called the Schilling test can be used to determine the body's ability to absorb vitamin B_{12}.

At this time there are still some health food stores that do not stock the methylcobalamin form of vitamin B_{12}. It is expected that as research results become more widely known, the methylcobalamin form will become easier to find in your local health food store under various brand names.

Biotin

Biotin aids in cell growth; in fatty acid production; in the metabolism of carbohydrates, fats, and proteins; and in the utilization of the other B-complex vitamins. Sufficient quantities are needed for healthy hair and skin. One hundred milligrams of biotin daily may prevent hair loss in some men. Biotin also promotes healthy sweat glands, nerve tissue, and bone marrow. In addition, it helps to relieve muscle pain.

In infants, a condition called *seborrheic dermatitis*, or cradle cap, which is characterized by a dry, scaly scalp, may occur as a result of biotin deficiency. In adults, deficiency of this B vitamin is rare because it can be produced in the intestines from foods such as those mentioned below. However, if a deficiency does occur, it can cause anemia, depression, hair loss, high blood sugar, inflammation or pallor of the skin and mucous membranes, insomnia, loss of appetite, muscular pain, nausea, and soreness of the tongue.

Sources

Biotin is found in brewer's yeast, cooked egg yolks, meat, milk, poultry, saltwater fish, soybeans, and whole grains.

Comments

Raw egg whites contain a protein called avidin, which combines with biotin in the intestinal tract and depletes the body of this needed nutrient. Fats and oils that have been subjected to heat or exposed to the air for any length of time inhibit biotin absorption. Antibiotics, sulfa drugs, and saccharin also threaten the availability of biotin.

Choline

Choline is needed for the proper transmission of nerve impulses from the brain through the central nervous system, as well as for gallbladder regulation, liver function, and lecithin formation. It aids in hormone production and minimizes excess fat in the liver because it aids in fat and cholesterol metabolism. Without choline, brain function and memory are impaired. Choline is beneficial for disorders of the nervous system such as Parkinson's disease and tardive dyskinesia. A deficiency may result in fatty buildup in the liver, as well as in cardiac symptoms, gastric ulcers, high blood pressure, an inability to digest fats, kidney and liver impairment, and stunted growth.

Research in the last decade indicates that choline plays an important role in cardiovascular health, as well as in reproduction and fetal development. One study showed a need for choline for both prevention and treatment of arteriosclerosis and the metabolism of homocysteine. This is such an important nutrient that it recently was added to the list of essential compounds. People who have a high choline intake have the lowest levels of inflammation in the body, which reduces their risk of heart disease.

Sources

The following foods contain significant amounts of choline: broccoli, oat bran, egg yolks, lecithin (about 13 percent choline by weight), legumes, liver, meat, milk, shrimp, soybeans, and whole-grain cereals. If you are managing your cholesterol levels, using one egg yolk for every two egg whites will help you get enough choline.

Folate

Also known as folacin, folic acid, or pteroylglutamic acid (PGA), folate is considered a brain food, and is needed for energy production and the formation of red blood cells. It also strengthens immunity by aiding in the proper formation and functioning of white blood cells. Because it functions as a coenzyme in DNA and RNA synthesis, it is important for healthy cell division and replication. It is involved in protein metabolism and has been used in the prevention and treatment of folic acid anemia. This nutrient may also help depression and anxiety, and may be effective in the treatment of uterine cervical dysplasia.

Folate may be the most important nutrient in regulating homocysteine levels. Homocysteine is an amino acid that is naturally formed in the body as the result of the breakdown of another amino acid, methionine. In recent years, high levels of homocysteine have been found to be associated with an increased risk of atherosclerosis (hardening of the arteries due to the accumulation of fatty plaques). Normally, homocysteine is converted to other, non-harmful amino acids in the body. In order for this conversion to take place as it should, the body needs an adequate supply of folate, as well as of vitamins B_6 and B_{12}. Homocysteine levels in red blood cells have been shown to have an inverse relationship to levels of these three important B vitamins—that is, the lower the levels of these vitamins, the higher the level of homocysteine.

Folate is very important in pregnancy. It helps to regulate embryonic and fetal nerve cell formation, which is vital for normal development. Studies have shown that a daily intake of 400 micrograms of folate in early pregnancy may prevent the vast majority of neural tube defects, such as spina bifida and anencephaly. It may also help to prevent premature birth. To be effective, this regimen must begin *before* conception and continue for at least the first three months of pregnancy; if a woman waits until she knows she is pregnant, it may be too late, because critical events in fetal development occur during the first six weeks of pregnancy—before many women know that they have conceived. In the mid-1990s, the government required that enriched grain products be fortified with folic acid. This was an attempt to achieve an across-the-board reduction in neural-tube birth defects such as spina bifida. Since the program started, there has also been a decline in stroke-related deaths that appears to be related. Researchers attribute this decline to the reduction of serum homocysteine levels in the population as a whole. However, some researchers worry that the higher folic acid intake may mask B_{12} deficiencies. If you are worried about low B_{12} (see B_{12}, above), consult your health care practitioner before taking folic acid supplements.

Many experts still recommend that every woman of childbearing age take a folate supplement daily as a matter of course. Folate works best when combined with vitamin B_{12} and vitamin C. Another option is to simply take a good-quality multivitamin; most have at least 400 micrograms of folic acid and these other nutrients.

A sore, red tongue is one sign of folate deficiency. Other possible signs include anemia, apathy, digestive disturbances, fatigue, graying hair, growth impairment, insomnia, labored breathing, memory problems, paranoia, weakness, and birth defects in one's offspring. Folate deficiency may be caused by inadequate consumption of fresh fruits and vegetables; consumption of only cooked or microwaved vegetables (cooking destroys folate); and malabsorption problems.

Sources

The following foods contain significant quantities of folate: asparagus, barley, beef, bran, brewer's yeast, brown rice, cheese, chicken, dates, green leafy vegetables, lamb, legumes, lentils, liver, milk, mushrooms, oranges, split peas, pork, root vegetables, salmon, tuna, wheat germ, whole grains, and whole wheat. Unlike most other nutrients, synthetic folic acid from a supplement is more bioavailable than folic acid from food. It is best to eat folate-rich foods and take a supplement, especially if you are a woman of childbearing age.

Comments

Oral contraceptives may increase the need for folate. Alcohol also can act as an enemy to folate absorption.

Cautions

Do not take high doses of folate for extended periods if you have a hormone-related cancer or seizure disorder.

Inositol

Inositol is vital for hair growth. This vitamin has a calming effect and helps to reduce cholesterol levels. It helps prevent hardening of the arteries and is important in the formation of lecithin and the metabolism of fat and cholesterol. It also helps remove fats from the liver. Deficiency can lead to arteriosclerosis, constipation, hair loss, high blood cholesterol, irritability, mood swings, and skin eruptions. Research has also shown that high doses of inositol may help in the treatment of depression, obsessive-compulsive disorder, and anxiety disorders, without the side effects of prescription medications.

Sources

Inositol is found in brewer's yeast, fruits, lecithin, legumes, meats, milk, unrefined molasses, raisins, vegetables, and whole grains.

Comments

Consuming large amounts of caffeine may cause a shortage of inositol in the body.

Para-Aminobenzoic Acid (PABA)

PABA is one of the basic constituents of folate and also helps in the assimilation of pantothenic acid. PABA can be converted into folate by intestinal bacteria. This antioxidant helps protect against sunburn by reducing the absorption of ultraviolet-B (UV-B) radiation. Consequently, it helps to prevent skin cancer. It also acts as a coenzyme in the breakdown and utilization of protein; and assists in the formation of red blood cells.

PABA also aids in the maintenance of healthy intestinal flora. Supplementing the diet with PABA may restore gray hair to its original color if the graying was caused by stress or a nutritional deficiency. Other benefits of PABA include protection against secondhand smoke, ozone, and other air pollutants; reduced inflammation in arthritis; and enhanced flexibility.

A deficiency of PABA may lead to depression, fatigue, gastrointestinal disorders, graying of the hair, irritability, nervousness, and patchy areas of white skin.

Sources

Foods that contain PABA include kidney, liver, molasses, mushrooms, spinach, and whole grains.

Comments

Sulfa drugs may cause a deficiency of PABA.

Vitamin C (Ascorbic Acid)

Vitamin C is an antioxidant that is required for at least three hundred metabolic functions in the body, including tissue growth and repair, adrenal gland function, and healthy gums. It also aids in the production of antistress hormones and interferon, an important immune system protein, and is needed for the metabolism of folic acid, tyrosine, and phenylalanine. Studies have shown that taking vitamin C can reduce symptoms of asthma. It protects against the harmful effects of pollution, helps to prevent cancer, protects against infection, and enhances immunity. Vitamin C increases the absorption of iron. It can combine with toxic substances, such as certain heavy metals, and render them harmless so that they can be eliminated from the body.

Most people know of vitamin C and its perceived ability to prevent the common cold. But over the years there has been conflicting data on vitamin C and its effect on colds. And the data remains conflicting. Recently, a group of researchers with the Cochrane Collaboration Reviews, the largest medical literature database, looked at the effect of vitamin C and its use in the treatment of the common cold in over 11,000 people. They found that for intakes of vitamin C greater than 200 milligrams, vitamin C reduced the duration and severity of common cold symptoms but not the number of colds someone gets in a year. However, in extreme physical stress as experienced by marathon runners and skiers, vitamin C reduced the common cold risk by half. Another group of scientists found that vitamin C (when individuals used 500 milligrams per day) reduced the frequency of the common cold but did not affect the duration or severity.

This vitamin also may reduce levels of low-density lipo-

proteins (LDL, the so-called "bad cholesterol"), while increasing levels of high-density lipoproteins (HDL, or "good cholesterol"), as well as lowering high blood pressure and helping to prevent atherosclerosis. Essential in the formation of collagen, vitamin C protects against abnormal blood clotting and bruising, may reduce the risk of cataracts, and promotes the healing of wounds and burns. It may even boost your love life by causing more of the hormone oxytocin to be released.

Vitamin C has been useful in managing *Helicobacter pylori* (commonly known as *H. pylori*). *H. pylori* is a bacteria that grows in the stomach and may result in pain, gas, and bloating. Using 1,000 milligrams of vitamin C, in combination with drugs to treat the condition, allowed for less of the drugs to be used, which resulted in a cost savings to the patients.

Vitamin C works synergistically with both vitamin E and beta-carotene—that is, when these vitamins work together, they have an effect even greater than the sum of their individual effects, and taking them together may counter potential adverse effects of taking these vitamins alone. Long-term users of vitamins E and C in combination seem to have higher cognitive abilities as they age, as reported by a 2003 study.

Vitamin E scavenges for dangerous free radicals in cell membranes, while vitamin C attacks free radicals in biologic fluids. These vitamins reinforce and extend each other's antioxidant activity.

Because the body cannot manufacture vitamin C, it must be obtained through the diet or in the form of supplements.

It was once thought that most of the vitamin C consumed in the diet was lost in the urine, although this idea is being challenged because initial studies apparently failed to account for the half-life, or consistent decreasing rate of elimination from the blood, of the vitamin in the original calculations.

If you require larger-than-normal amounts of vitamin C due to serious illness, such as cancer, it is more effective to take it intravenously, under the supervision of a physician, than it is to take high doses orally.

Scurvy is a disease caused by vitamin C deficiency. It is characterized by poor wound healing, soft and spongy bleeding gums, edema, extreme weakness, and "pinpoint" hemorrhages under the skin. Fortunately, this condition is rare in Western societies. More common are signs of lesser degrees of deficiency, including gums that bleed when brushed; increased susceptibility to infection, especially colds and bronchial infections; joint pains; lack of energy; poor digestion; prolonged wound healing time; a tendency to bruise easily; and tooth loss.

Sources

Vitamin C is found in berries, citrus fruits, and green vegetables. Good sources include asparagus, avocados, beet greens, black currants, broccoli, Brussels sprouts, cantaloupe, collards, dandelion greens, dulse, grapefruit, kale, lemons, mangos, mustard greens, onions, oranges, papayas, green peas, sweet peppers, persimmons, pineapple, radishes, rose hips, spinach, strawberries, Swiss chard, tomatoes, turnip greens, and watercress. Orange juice is an excellent source of vitamin C, but *only* if it is freshly squeezed or has been processed by methods that don't involve heating or pasteurization. While freshly squeezed juice is best, frozen juices are often processed by nonthermal methods and can be good sources of vitamin C. Some so-called fruit drinks have added vitamin C, and although they are not as good a choice as real fruit juices, they are preferable to carbonated beverages that are devoid of any nutrients.

Herbs that contain vitamin C include alfalfa, burdock root, cayenne, chickweed, eyebright, fennel seed, fenugreek, hops, kelp, peppermint, mullein, nettle, oat straw, paprika, parsley, pine needle, plantain, raspberry leaf, red clover, rose hips, skullcap, violet leaves, yarrow, and yellow dock.

Comments

Alcohol, analgesics, antidepressants, anticoagulants, oral contraceptives, and steroids may reduce levels of vitamin C in the body. Smoking causes a serious depletion of vitamin C.

Diabetes medications such as chlorpropamide (Diabinese) and sulfa drugs may not be as effective if taken with vitamin C. Taking high doses of vitamin C may cause a false-negative reading in tests for blood in the stool. It is thought that for some people taking too much vitamin C may cause it to act as a pro-oxidant (creating damaging oxygen particles) rather than an antioxidant (negating the harmful effect of oxygen free radicals). For example, patients with kidney failure had increased oxidation of tissues by taking only 214 milligrams per day.

For maximum effectiveness, supplemental vitamin C should be taken in divided doses, twice daily. Esterified vitamin C (Ester-C) is an effective form of vitamin C. Recently, however, some investigators have found that Ester-C may be no more bioavailable than regular vitamin C (ascorbic acid). We will have to wait to see what is discovered in future studies. Ester-C is created by having the vitamin C react with a necessary mineral, such as calcium, magnesium, potassium, sodium, or zinc. This results in a form of the vitamin that is nonacidic and that contains vitamin C metabolites identical to those produced by the body. Esterified vitamin C enters the bloodstream and tissues four times faster than standard forms of vitamin C because it moves into the blood cells more efficiently and also stays in the body tissues longer. The levels of vitamin C in white blood cells achieved by taking esterified vitamin C are four times higher than those achieved with standard vitamin C. Further, only one-third as much is lost through excretion in the urine. A variety of manufacturers produce supplements containing Ester-C, either by itself or in combination with other valuable nutrients, including the antioxidants Pycnogenol and proanthocyanidins, and the herbs echinacea and garlic.

Cautions

If aspirin and standard vitamin C (ascorbic acid) are taken together in large doses, stomach irritation can occur, possibly leading to ulcers. If you take aspirin regularly, use an esterified form of vitamin C, and take it separately from the aspirin.

If you are pregnant, do not take more than 5,000 milligrams of vitamin C daily. A developing infant may become dependent on this supplement and develop scurvy when deprived of the accustomed megadoses after birth. If you have a bruise or sprained muscle, temporarily cut back on vitamin C to less than 90 milligrams daily. Larger amounts may combine with iron produced by the injuries to cause more damage.

Avoid using chewable vitamin C supplements, because these can damage tooth enamel.

Vitamin D

Vitamin D, a fat-soluble vitamin that has properties of both a vitamin and a hormone, is required for the absorption and utilization of calcium and phosphorus. It is necessary for growth, and is especially important for the normal growth and development of bones and teeth in children. It protects against muscle weakness and is involved in regulation of the heartbeat. It is also important in the prevention and treatment of breast and colon cancer, osteoarthritis, osteoporosis, and hypocalcemia; enhances immunity; and is necessary for thyroid function and normal blood clotting.

There are several forms of vitamin D, including vitamin D_2 (ergocalciferol), which comes from food sources; vitamin D_3 (cholecalciferol), which is synthesized in the skin in response to exposure to the sun's ultraviolet rays; and a synthetic form identified as vitamin D_5. Of the three, vitamin D_3 is considered the natural form of vitamin D and was thought to be the most active. Newer data shows that D_2 is as effective as D_3 in maintaining vitamin D levels in the blood.

The form of vitamin D that we get from food or supplements is not fully active. It requires conversion by the liver, and then by the kidneys, before it becomes fully active. This is why people with liver or kidney disorders are at a higher risk for osteoporosis. When the skin is exposed to the sun's ultraviolet rays, a cholesterol compound in the skin is transformed into a precursor of vitamin D. Exposing the face and arms to the sun for fifteen minutes three times a week is an effective way to ensure adequate amounts of vitamin D in the body.

Vitamin D has been the ignored vitamin until recently. Studies have shown that at least 40 percent of people have less-than-optimal levels of the vitamin in their blood. As much as 70 to 80 percent of Hispanic-Americans and African-Americans may be deficient in vitamin D. Those with more coloring in the skin have a harder time absorbing vitamin D from sunlight. In addition, those who live above the 37th latitude obtain virtually no vitamin D from sunlight between November and March.

Not getting enough vitamin D in the diet or from direct sunlight has been linked to the development of several diseases including heart disease, osteoporosis, diabetes, and cancers such as breast and colon. As baby boomers age, the risk of osteoporosis increases. Taking more than 400 IU of vitamin D has been shown to reduce the risk of fractures by 20 percent in those over sixty-five years of age. But how much is needed to optimize health is still open for debate. Some have argued that it is necessary to consume very high amounts of vitamin D—in excess of the UL for safety—in order to maintain blood levels associated with reducing the risk of disease. Before the FDA considers increasing the UL for vitamin D, more research is needed to assure that there is no risk of toxicity at the upper levels. We do not recommend exceeding the UL for vitamin D until further research has been conducted.

Sources

Fish liver oils, fatty saltwater fish (especially mackerel), dairy products, and eggs all contain vitamin D. It is also found in butter, cod liver oil, dandelion greens, egg yolks, halibut, liver, milk, shiitake and chanterelle mushrooms, oatmeal, oysters, salmon, sardines, sweet potatoes, tuna, and vegetable oils. Herbs that contain vitamin D include alfalfa, nettle, and parsley.

Vitamin D is also formed by the body in response to the action of sunlight on the skin. Of all the nutrients, this is one of a few that is difficult to reach the DRI from food alone and supplementation may be needed. It may make sense to take serial blood tests each year with a physical examination to see if you are getting enough vitamin D to maintain healthy levels.

Comments

Intestinal disorders and liver and gallbladder malfunctions interfere with the absorption of vitamin D. Some cholesterol-lowering drugs, antacids, mineral oil, and steroid hormones such as cortisone also interfere with absorption.

Thiazide diuretics such as chlorothiazide (Diuril) and hydrochlorothiazide (Esidrix, HydroDIURIL, Oretic) disturb the body's calcium/vitamin D ratio. Taking excessive amounts of vitamin D (over 1,000 international units) daily may cause a decrease in bone mass.

Cautions

Toxicity may result from taking excessive amounts of supplemental vitamin D.

Vitamin E

Vitamin E is actually a family of eight antioxidant compounds. These consist of four tocopherols (alpha, beta, gamma, and delta) and four tocotrienols (also alpha through delta). The alpha-tocopherol form is the one found in the largest quantities in human blood and tissue. Small amounts of the gamma form are also found.

Alpha-tocopherol acts as an antioxidant in the human body. As an antioxidant, vitamin E prevents cell damage by inhibiting the oxidation of lipids (fats) and the formation of free radicals. It protects other fat-soluble vitamins from destruction by oxygen and aids in the utilization of vitamin A. It protects the low-density lipoproteins (LDL cholesterol) from oxidation as well. Oxidized LDL has been implicated in the development of cardiovascular disease. It is also known to inhibit blood platelet aggregation (clotting) and has other functions related to the activity of the immune system.

Vitamin E is essential for life, and Americans typically don't get enough of it from their diet. Only 8 percent of men and 2.4 percent of women consume the amount the government recommends. You at least need the DRI for vitamin E, and perhaps more. It is hard to get this nutrient from foods alone, so supplementation is recommended. We don't recommend taking unsafe doses; that is, doses in excess of the UL of safety. None of the dosages given in previous editions of this book seriously exceed the maximums (upper levels or ULs) published by the Office of Dietary Supplements of the National Institutes of Health. These upper limits were established based on the possibility of hemorrhage rather than any perceived problem with the vitamin itself.

The most common dietary form of vitamin E is the gamma-tocopherol form. However, this form is not taken up by the body in any quantity because the liver selectively incorporates alpha-tocopherol into blood lipoproteins for delivery to the tissues. About ten times more alpha-tocopherol than gamma-tocopherol is found in the blood. However, the gamma form may have some unique benefits in suppressing colon cancer, according to recent animal studies, making a sufficient amount of *dietary* vitamin E even more important to good health.

Vitamin E deficiency may result in damage to red blood cells and destruction of nerves. Signs of deficiency can include infertility (in both men and women), menstrual problems, neuromuscular impairment, shortened red blood cell life span, spontaneous abortion (miscarriage), and uterine degeneration. People with impaired balance and coordination and/or damage to the retina (pigmented retinopathy) may also be deficient. Individuals with severe malnutrition, genetic defects affecting a liver protein known as alpha-tocopherol transfer protein (alpha-TTP), or fat malabsorption problems such as those caused by cystic fibrosis, cholestatic liver disease, or Crohn's disease may have a vitamin E deficiency. True vitamin E deficiency is rare, but

The Vitamin E Controversy

A common complaint among consumers of nutritional information is that researchers are always changing their minds about what is good for you. The problem is that two different studies using the same nutrient have the potential to produce contradictory data. This is because nutrients are consumed in varying amounts, making it almost impossible to determine the exact intake of a single compound. Moreover, the only way to completely isolate a nutrient for study would be to remove it entirely, and this would risk making the person ill. Vitamin E serves as a perfect example of these challenges and why there is often conflicting data among nutritional research studies. In 2004 a group of researchers reported that consuming vitamin E in supplement form in excess of 200 IUs per day actually increased the chances of dying. Previous studies, and these were numerous, had been fairly unanimous in their findings that 400 IUs of vitamin E actually reduced the risk of heart disease and prostate cancer. How is it possible that researchers came up with such different conclusions about the same vitamin? First, in the 2004 study, participants were rarely given vitamin E on its own. Usually it was given with beta-carotene and vitamin C. Other studies have shown that beta-carotene increases the risk of death in smokers. So some of the increased risk of death attributed to vitamin E was likely related to smokers who took both nutrients. Second, the study included all forms of vitamin E. Sometimes vitamin E was given as alpha-tocopherol and sometimes as mixed tocopherols. and since each has distinct biological effects, they cannot be lumped together. Third, because most participants were over 60, and a majority had preexisting conditions, such as heart disease, the study's application to younger, healthy adults may be limited.

low intake (lower than required) is relatively common. One study showed that 27 to 41 percent of people studied had blood levels of alpha-tocopherol less than 20 micromoles per liter (μmoles/L), the level below which there appears to be an increased risk for cardiovascular disease. Low levels of vitamin E in the body have been linked to both bowel cancer and breast cancer.

The d-alpha-tocopherol form of vitamin E is the most potent, and is the one we recommend. Also, natural sources of vitamin E are better than synthetic vitamin E because natural vitamin E is more available for use by the body than the synthetic form. Synthetic vitamin E is only 67 percent as active as the natural form. Read labels closely. The natural form of vitamin E is listed as *d-alpha-tocopherol, rrr-alpha-tocopherol, d-alpha-tocopherol acetate or d-alpha-tocopherol succinate.* The synthetic form is listed as *dl-alpha-tocopherol* or *all-rac alpha-tocopherol* (watch out for the *l* after the *d*). The synthetic form costs only about half as much as the natural form, but it has significantly less activity, or potency. Some vitamin manufacturers have been known to mix 10 percent natural and 90 percent synthetic vitamin E, then label the product *natural.* Your responsibility is to check the label and make sure it says *100 percent potency* or *100 percent natural vitamin E.*

If you cannot absorb fat, there is a special water-soluble form of vitamin E available from various suppliers.

Sources

Vitamin E is found in the following food sources: avocados, cold-pressed vegetable oils (olive, soybean, corn, canola, safflower, and sunflower), dark green leafy vegetables, legumes, nuts (almonds, hazelnuts, peanuts), seeds, and whole grains. Significant quantities of this vitamin are also found in brown rice, cornmeal, dulse, eggs, kelp, desiccated liver, milk, oatmeal, organ meats, soybeans, sweet potatoes, watercress, wheat, and wheat germ. Herbs that contain vitamin E include alfalfa, bladderwrack, dandelion, dong quai, flaxseed, nettle, oat straw, raspberry leaf, and rose hips.

Comments

The body needs zinc in order to maintain the proper level of vitamin E in the blood. Vitamin E that has oxidized a free radical can be revitalized by vitamin C and enabled to battle additional free radicals, according to Lester Packer, Ph.D., noted researcher and professor of molecular and cell biology at the University of California–Berkeley. Adding vitamin E to fats and oils prevents them from becoming rancid. The oxidation of fats is a key factor in the formation of plaque adhering to blood vessel walls.

If you take both vitamin E and iron supplements, take them at different times of the day. Inorganic forms of iron (such as ferrous sulfate) destroy vitamin E. Organic iron (ferrous gluconate or ferrous fumarate) leaves vitamin E intact.

Cautions

If you are taking an anticoagulant medication (blood-thinner), do not take more than 200 international units of vitamin E daily. If you suffer from diabetes, rheumatic heart disease, or an overactive thyroid, do not take more than the recommended dose. If you have high blood pressure, start with a small amount, such as 100 international units daily, and increase slowly to the desired amount. If you have retinitis pigmentosa that is *not* associated with vitamin E deficiency, do not take any supplemental vitamin E.

Vitamin K

Vitamin K is needed for the production of prothrombin, which is necessary for blood clotting. It is also essential for bone formation and repair; it is necessary for the synthesis of osteocalcin, the protein in bone tissue on which calcium crystallizes. Consequently, it may help prevent osteoporosis. In addition, it may protect the vascular system by preventing calcification in the arteries. The liver is a very efficient extractor of vitamin K, which it uses to make clotting factors for the blood. Some investigators have argued that the current DRIs may be insufficient to meet the needs of other tissues in the body.

Vitamin K plays an important role in the intestines and aids in converting glucose into glycogen for storage in the liver, promoting healthy liver function. It may increase resistance to infection in children and help prevent cancers that target the inner linings of the organs. It aids in promoting longevity. A deficiency of this vitamin can cause abnormal and/or internal bleeding.

There are three forms of vitamin K. The first is vitamin K_1 (phylloquinone or phytonadione), which comes from plants and makes up your dietary vitamin K. The second is vitamin K_2, a family of substances called menaquinones, which are made by intestinal bacteria and also found in butter, cow liver, chicken, egg yolks, fermented soybean products, and some cheeses. Third, there is vitamin K_3 (menadione), which is a synthetic, man-made substance.

Sources

Vitamin K_1 is found in some foods, including asparagus, blackstrap molasses, broccoli, Brussels sprouts, cabbage, cauliflower, chicken, dark green leafy vegetables, egg yolks, leaf lettuce, liver, oatmeal, oats, rye, safflower oil, soybeans, wheat, and yogurt. Herbs that can supply vitamin K_1 include alfalfa, green tea, kelp, nettle, oat straw, and shepherd's purse. However, the majority of the body's supply of this vitamin is synthesized by the "friendly" bacteria normally present in the intestines, which comes as a result of consuming soluble fiber.

Comments

Antibiotics increase the need for dietary or supplemental vitamin K. Because bacteria in the intestines synthesize vitamin K, taking antibiotics—which kill the bacteria—interferes with this process. Antibiotics also interfere with the absorption of vitamin K. Vitamin K deficiency can be caused by any of the following:

- A poor or restricted diet lacking in fiber.
- Crohn's disease, ulcerative colitis.
- Liver disease that interferes with vitamin K storage.
- The use of antibiotics, cholesterol-lowering drugs, mineral oil, aspirin, and/or blood-thinners.

Low levels of vitamin K are associated with insulin release and glucose regulation problems, and may lead to low bone density in women. Supplementing the diet with this vitamin enhances the bone-building process by attracting calcium to the bone. Supplemental vitamin K also reduces the amount of calcium in the urine and frees up more calcium to be used by the bone-building process.

Cautions

Do not take large doses of synthetic vitamin K during the last few weeks of pregnancy. It can result in a toxic reaction in the newborn. If you are taking anticoagulant (blood-thinning) drugs, consult with your health care provider before taking any supplemental vitamin K, as it can interfere with the action of these medications. Megadoses of this vitamin can accumulate in the body and cause flushing and sweating.

Bioflavonoids

Although bioflavonoids are not true vitamins in the strictest sense, they are sometimes referred to as vitamin P. Bioflavonoids are essential for the absorption of vitamin C, and the two should be taken together. There are many different bioflavonoids, including citrin, eriodictyol, flavones, hesperetin, hesperidin, quercetin, quercetrin, and rutin. The human body cannot produce bioflavonoids, so they must be supplied in the diet.

Bioflavonoids are used extensively in the treatment of athletic injuries because they relieve pain, bumps, and bruises. They also reduce pain located in the legs or across the back, and lessen symptoms associated with prolonged bleeding and low serum calcium. Bioflavonoids act synergistically with vitamin C to protect and preserve the structure of capillaries. In addition, bioflavonoids have an antibacterial effect and promote circulation, stimulate bile production, lower cholesterol levels, and treat and prevent cataracts. When taken with vitamin C, bioflavonoids also reduce the symptoms of oral herpes.

Quercetin, a bioflavonoid available in supplement form, may effectively treat and prevent asthma symptoms. Activated Quercetin from Source Naturals is a good source of quercetin. It also contains two other ingredients that increase its efficacy: bromelain, an enzyme from pineapple, and vitamin C, in the nonacidic form of magnesium ascorbate. Bromelain and quercetin are synergists, and should be taken in conjunction to enhance absorption.

Sources

Peppers, buckwheat, black currants, and the white material just beneath the peel of citrus fruits contain bioflavonoids. Sources of bioflavonoids include apricots, blackberries, cherries, grapefruit, grapes, lemons, oranges, plums, and prunes. Herbs that contain bioflavonoids include chervil, elderberries, hawthorn berry, rose hips, and shepherd's purse.

Comments

Extremely high doses of bioflavonoids may cause diarrhea.

Coenzyme Q_{10}

Coenzyme Q_{10} is a vitamin-like substance found in all parts of the body, the action of which resembles that of vitamin E. It may be an even more powerful antioxidant. It is also called ubiquinone. There are ten common substances designated coenzyme Qs, but coenzyme Q_{10} is the only one found in human tissue. This substance plays a critical role in the production of energy in every cell of the body. It aids circulation, stimulates the immune system, increases tissue oxygenation, and has vital anti-aging effects. Deficiencies of coenzyme Q_{10} have been linked to periodontal disease, diabetes, and muscular dystrophy.

Research has revealed that supplemental coenzyme Q_{10} has the ability to counter histamine, and therefore is beneficial for people with allergies, asthma, or respiratory disease. Many people also use it when taking cholesterol-lowering drugs in the statin family to reduce leg cramps. Medical literature does not support this practice, but coenzyme Q_{10} is not harmful and there is enough anecdotal information that it may relieve cramping, so it can't hurt to try it.

Coenzyme Q_{10} is used by many health care professionals to treat anomalies of mental function, such as those associated with schizophrenia and Alzheimer's disease. It is also beneficial in fighting obesity, candidiasis, multiple sclerosis, and diabetes. Other conditions—such as heart disease, migraines, and Parkinson's disease—are related to a defect in the body's ability to turn food into energy, and coenzyme Q_{10} may help.

Coenzyme Q_{10} appears to be a giant step forward in the treatment and prevention of cardiovascular disease. A six-year study conducted by scientists at the University of Texas found that people being treated for congestive heart failure who took coenzyme Q_{10} in addition to conventional therapy had a 75 percent chance of survival after three years, compared with a 25 percent survival rate for those using conventional therapy alone. In a similar study by the University of Texas and the Center for Adult Diseases in Japan, coenzyme Q_{10} was shown to be able to lower high blood pressure without medication or dietary changes.

In addition to its use in fighting cardiovascular disease, coenzyme Q_{10} has been shown to be effective in reducing mortality in experimental animals afflicted with tumors and leukemia. Some doctors give their patients coenzyme Q_{10} to reduce the side effects of cancer chemotherapy.

Coenzyme Q_{10} is widely used in Japan. More than 12 million people in that country are reportedly taking it at the direction of their physicians for treatment of heart disease (it strengthens the heart muscle) and high blood pressure, and also to enhance the immune system. Research in Japan has shown that coenzyme Q_{10} also protects the stomach lining and duodenum, and may help heal duodenal ulcers.

The amount of coenzyme Q_{10} present in the body declines with age, so it should be supplemented in the diet, especially by people who are over the age of fifty. A chewable form containing 50 milligrams or more of this vital nutrient, available from FoodScience of Vermont, is an especially easy to assimilate supplement. Nature's Plus and Carlson Labs both make soft gel-capsules of coenzyme Q_{10} in dosage levels up to 300 milligrams. Oil-based forms are best.

Sources

Mackerel, salmon, and sardines contain the largest amounts of coenzyme Q_{10}. It is also found in beef, peanuts, and spinach. People consume about 10 to 15 milligrams a day, mainly from meat and fish. Vegetarians should be aware that their intake may be less than optimal and should consider supplementation.

Comments

Coenzyme Q_{10} is oil soluble and is best absorbed when taken with oily or fatty foods, such as fish. Be cautious when purchasing coenzyme Q_{10}. Not all products offer it in its purest form. Its natural color is dark bright yellow to orange, and it has very little taste in the powdered form. It should be kept away from heat and light. Pure coenzyme Q_{10} is perishable and deteriorates in temperatures above 115°F. A liquid or oil form is preferable.

Minerals

INTRODUCTION

Every living cell on this planet depends on minerals for proper function and structure. Minerals are needed for the proper composition of body fluids, the formation of blood and bone, the maintenance of healthy nerve function, and the regulation of muscle tone, including that of the muscles of the cardiovascular system. Like vitamins, minerals function as coenzymes, enabling the body to perform its functions, including energy production, growth, and healing. Because all enzyme activities involve minerals, minerals are essential for the proper utilization of vitamins and other nutrients.

The human body, as with all of nature, must maintain its proper chemical balance. This balance depends on the levels of different minerals in the body and especially the ratios of certain mineral levels to one another. The level of each mineral in the body has an effect on every other one, so if one is out of balance, all mineral levels are affected. If not corrected, this can start a chain reaction of imbalances that leads to illness.

Minerals are naturally occurring elements found in the earth. Rock formations are made up of mineral salts. Rock and stone are gradually broken down into tiny fragments by erosion, a process that can take literally millions of years.

The resulting dust and sand accumulate, forming the basis of soil. The soil is teeming with microbes that utilize these tiny crystals of mineral salts, which are then passed from the soil to plants. Herbivorous animals eat the plants. We obtain these minerals by consuming plants or herbivorous animals.

Nutritionally, minerals belong to two groups: bulk minerals (also called macrominerals) and trace minerals (microminerals).

Bulk minerals include calcium, magnesium, sodium, potassium, and phosphorus. These are needed in larger amounts than trace minerals. Although only minute quantities of trace minerals are needed, they are nevertheless important for good health. Trace minerals include boron, chromium, copper, germanium, iodine, iron, manganese, molybdenum, selenium, silicon, sulfur, vanadium, and zinc.

Because minerals are stored primarily in the body's bone and muscle tissue, it is possible to develop mineral toxicity if extremely large quantities are consumed. Such situations are rare, however, because toxic levels of minerals generally accumulate only if massive amounts are ingested for a prolonged period of time.

WHAT'S ON THE SHELVES

As with vitamins, it can be difficult, if not impossible, to obtain the amounts of minerals needed for optimum health through diet alone. Mineral supplements can help you to make sure you are getting all the minerals your body requires.

Minerals are often found in multivitamin formulas. Minerals also are sold as single supplements. These are available in tablet, capsule, powder, and liquid forms. Some are available in chelated form, which means that the minerals are bonded to protein molecules that transport them to the bloodstream and enhance their absorption. When mineral supplements are taken with a meal, they are usually automatically chelated in the stomach during digestion. There is some controversy over which mineral supplements are best, but we prefer the chelated preparations. Our experience with the various chelated formulas available has shown that, in general, arginate forms of minerals make the most effective supplements.

Once a mineral is absorbed, it must be carried by the blood to the cells and then transported across the cell membranes in a form that can be utilized by the cells. After minerals enter the body, they compete with one another for absorption. For example, too much zinc can deplete the body of copper; excessive calcium intake can affect magnesium absorption (and vice versa). Consequently, supplemental minerals should always be taken in balanced amounts. Otherwise, they will not be effective and may even be harmful. The absorption of minerals can also be affected by the use of fiber supplements. Fiber decreases the body's absorption of minerals. Therefore, supplemental fiber and minerals should be taken at different times.

THE ABCs OF MINERALS

Boron

Boron is needed in trace amounts for healthy bones and muscle growth because it assists in the production of natural steroid compounds within the body. It is also necessary for the metabolism of calcium, phosphorus, and magnesium.

Boron enhances brain function, promotes alertness, and plays a role in how the body utilizes energy from fats and sugars. Most people are not deficient in boron. However, elderly people usually benefit from taking a supplement of 2 to 3 milligrams daily because they have greater problems with calcium absorption. Boron deficiency accentuates vitamin D deficiency.

Boron helps to prevent postmenopausal osteoporosis and build muscle. New research indicates that taking supplemental boron can shrink prostate tumor size, lower blood levels of prostate-specific antigen (PSA, a marker for prostate cancer), and may help prevent prostate cancer. Boron alleviates joint discomfort by reducing levels of both COX-2 and LOX enzymes (see ARTHRITIS in Part Two) and helps to preserve cognitive function. Studies have shown that in areas of the world where the level of boron in the soil is low there are a greater number of people suffering from arthritis. A study conducted by the U.S. Department of Agriculture indicated that within eight days of supplementing their daily diet with 3 milligrams of boron, a test group of postmenopausal women lost 40 percent less calcium, one-third less magnesium, and slightly less phosphorus through their urine than they had before beginning boron supplementation.

Sources

Boron is found naturally in apples, carrots, grapes, dark green leafy vegetables, raw nuts, pears, and whole grains.

Cautions

Do not take more than 3 to 6 milligrams of supplemental boron daily unless it is prescribed by a health care professional. Boron is toxic in high doses (15 milligrams or more daily for adults, less for children) but is not carcinogenic or mutagenic. Many supplements for bone health contain 3 milligrams of boron. If you are also using a multivitamin/multimineral supplement, be sure that your total intake through diet and supplements does not exceed 20 milligrams.

Calcium

Calcium is vital for the formation of strong bones and teeth and for the maintenance of healthy gums. It is also important in the maintenance of a regular heartbeat and in the transmission of nerve impulses. Calcium lowers cholesterol levels and helps prevent cardiovascular disease. It is needed for muscular growth and contraction, and for the prevention of muscle cramps. It may increase the rate of bone growth and bone mineral density in children. Recently, calcium from dairy products or supplements has been shown to promote weight loss, especially in terms of fat loss. However, these findings are not universally accepted.

This important mineral is also essential in blood clotting and helps prevent cancer. It may lower blood pressure and prevent bone loss associated with osteoporosis as well. Calcium provides energy and participates in the protein structuring of RNA and DNA. It is also involved in the ac-

tivation of several enzymes, including lipase, which breaks down fats for utilization by the body. In addition, calcium maintains proper cell membrane permeability, aids in neuromuscular activity, helps to keep the skin healthy, and protects against the development of preeclampsia during pregnancy, the number-one cause of maternal death. If high blood pressure develops due to pregnancy, it can be reduced by calcium intake.

Calcium protects the bones and teeth from lead by inhibiting absorption of this toxic metal. If there is a calcium deficiency, lead can be absorbed by the body and deposited in the teeth and bones.

Calcium deficiency can lead to the following problems: aching joints, brittle nails, eczema, elevated blood cholesterol, heart palpitations, hypertension (high blood pressure), insomnia, muscle cramps, nervousness, numbness in the arms and/or legs, a pasty complexion, rheumatoid arthritis, rickets, and tooth decay. Deficiencies of calcium are also associated with cognitive impairment, convulsions, depression, delusions, and hyperactivity.

Sources

Calcium is found in dairy foods, salmon (with bones), sardines, seafood, and dark green leafy vegetables. Other food sources include almonds, asparagus, blackstrap molasses, brewer's yeast, broccoli, buttermilk, cabbage, carob, cheese, collards, dandelion greens, dulse, figs, filberts, goat's milk, kale, kelp, milk, mustard greens, oats, prunes, sesame seeds, soybeans, tofu, turnip greens, watercress, whey, and yogurt.

Herbs that contain calcium include alfalfa, burdock root, cayenne, chamomile, chickweed, chicory, dandelion, eyebright, fennel seed, fenugreek, flaxseed, hops, kelp, lemongrass, mullein, nettle, oat straw, paprika, parsley, peppermint, plantain, raspberry leaves, red clover, rose hips, shepherd's purse, violet leaves, yarrow, and yellow dock. The amount of calcium in these herbs is so small, however, that they should not be considered as contributing to dietary intake.

Comments

The amino acid lysine is needed for calcium absorption. Food sources of lysine include cheese, eggs, fish, lima beans, milk, potatoes, red meat, soy products, and brewer's yeast. Lysine is also available in supplement form.

Female athletes and menopausal women need greater amounts of calcium than other women because their estrogen levels are lower. Estrogen protects the skeletal system by promoting the deposition of calcium in bone.

Heavy exercising hinders calcium uptake, but moderate exercise promotes it. Insufficient vitamin D intake, or the ingestion of excessive amounts of phosphorus and magnesium, also hinders the uptake of calcium.

If you are taking medication for osteoporosis, a supplement containing vitamin D and calcium is required to help the medicine work properly. Other types of prescription medicines, such as steroids and anticonvulsants (antiseizure drugs), interfere with bone metabolism, and taking supplemental calcium will help with that.

If calcium is taken with iron, they bind together, preventing the optimal absorption of both minerals. It is therefore best to take calcium and iron at different times. Too much calcium can interfere with the absorption of zinc, and excess zinc can interfere with calcium absorption (especially if calcium intake is low). For most people, the best ratio between supplemental calcium and zinc is up to 2,500 milligrams of calcium with 50 milligrams of zinc daily. A hair analysis can determine the levels of these and other minerals in the body.

A diet that is high in protein, fat, and/or sugar affects calcium uptake. The average American diet of meats, refined grains, and soft drinks (which are high in phosphorus) leads to increased excretion of calcium. Consuming alcoholic beverages, coffee, junk foods, excess salt, and/or white flour also leads to the loss of calcium by the body. A diet based on foods such as vegetables, fruits, and whole grains, which contain significant amounts of calcium but lower amounts of phosphorus, is preferable.

Oxalic acid (found in almonds, beet greens, cashews, chard, cocoa, rhubarb, soybeans, and spinach) interferes with calcium absorption by binding with it in the intestines and producing insoluble salts that cannot be absorbed. The normal consumption of foods containing oxalic acid should not pose a problem, but overindulgence in these foods inhibits the absorption of calcium. Oxalic acid can also combine with calcium to form calcium-oxalate kidney stones. Studies have shown, however, that taking magnesium and potassium supplements can prevent the formation of this type of stone.

Calcium supplements are more effective when taken in smaller doses spread throughout the day and before bedtime. This mineral works *less* effectively when taken in a single megadose. Most experts agree that no more than 500 milligrams should be taken at one time, as this is the maximum amount the body can absorb in one dose. However, because calcium also promotes a sound sleep when taken at night, and because a high-fiber diet can interfere with calcium absorption, some recommend taking a single dose at bedtime. The National Academy of Sciences recommends an intake of at least 1,000 to 1,300 milligrams of calcium per day, particularly for those who have or are at risk of developing osteoporosis. Because the body is more likely to absorb a higher percentage of the calcium when taken in smaller doses, we recommend taking 1,500 to 2,000 milligrams in divided doses with food throughout the day.

Some vitamin companies use a compound called D_1-calcium phosphate in their products. This form of calcium is insoluble and interferes with the absorption of the nutrients in a multinutrient supplement. Antacids such as Tums are *not* recommended as a source of calcium. While they do contain calcium, if taken in quantities sufficient to serve as a source of this mineral, they could neutralize the stomach acid needed for calcium absorption. Additionally, a significant percentage (estimates range from 20 to 40 percent) of people over the age of sixty may have a condition called *atrophic gastritis*. This is a chronic inflammation of the stomach, and it reduces the ability to break down the calcium carbonate contained in Tums. People under sixty are more likely to have an overproduction of acid; in that case, calcium carbonate could neutralize some of the excess and reduce the associated symptoms of belching, gas, and bloating.

Since the amount of calcium required per day is large, some people find it difficult to swallow the pills. Chewable versions are available; these are ideal for children who do not meet calcium needs from dairy products. It is best to match the percentage Daily Value for calcium and vitamin D. For example, a good product would have 50 percent DV for calcium and vitamin D in a single unit. Then you can take two or more depending upon your need.

Cautions

Calcium may interfere with the effects of verapamil (Calan, Isoptin, Verelan), a calcium channel blocker sometimes prescribed for heart problems and high blood pressure.

Calcium can also interfere with the effectiveness of tetracycline, thyroid hormone, certain anticonvulsants, and steroids. Consult your health care provider before taking supplemental calcium if you must take any of these drugs.

Phenobarbital and diuretics may cause a deficiency of calcium. Although several major studies have shown that added calcium in the diet does not appear to increase the risk for either a first or repeat attack of kidney stones, persons with a history of kidney stones or kidney disease should not take calcium supplements except on the advice of a physician. The maximum safe dosage of supplemental calcium is now placed at 2,500 milligrams per day.

Newer data has shown that calcium from dairy and supplements increases the risk of prostate cancer. Men in the United States who consumed more than 2½ servings a day of dairy products (about 600 milligrams) had a 32 percent increase in prostate cancer. Studies done in Europe found a relationship between dairy product consumption and the nonaggressive form of prostate cancer but not the aggressive form. The low-fat dairy products were more harmful than those with more fat or than calcium-containing foods that are not dairy products. Dairy products may also lead to an increased risk when used in conjunction with a high-protein diet.

Chromium

Because it is involved in the metabolism of glucose, chromium (sometimes also called glucose tolerance factor or GTF) is needed for energy. It is also vital in the synthesis of

Is Chromium Picolinate Safe?

An Australian study published in *Angewandte Chemie International Edition* in 2004 warned that trivalent chromium compounds like those used as supplements (chromium picolinate) can be converted into a carcinogenic form by means of oxidation in the body. This flies in the face of a wealth of data in more than sixty other published studies that found such chromium compounds to be safe and nontoxic. At this point, there appears to be no cause for alarm.

cholesterol, fats, and proteins. This essential mineral maintains stable blood sugar levels through proper insulin utilization, and can be helpful both for people with diabetes and those with hypoglycemia. Studies have shown that low plasma chromium levels can be an indication of coronary artery disease. Additional chromium is needed during pregnancy because the developing fetus increases demand for this mineral. Chromium supplements can help an expectant mother maintain healthy blood sugar levels during pregnancy.

The average American diet is chromium deficient. Only one in ten Americans has an adequate amount of chromium in his or her diet. There are five main reasons for this: The form of chromium in many foods is not easily absorbed (only 0.4 to 2.5 percent of dietary chromium is absorbed); not enough foods containing chromium are consumed; much of the chromium content is lost during processing; many people do not like the foods that are the best sources of chromium; and high quantities of sugar in the diet cause a loss of chromium from the body. Researchers estimate that two out of every three Americans have glucose regulation issues including hypoglycemia, pre-hypoglycemia, or diabetes. The ability to maintain normal blood sugar levels is jeopardized by the lack of chromium in our soil and water supply and by a diet high in refined white sugar, flour, and junk foods. A number of human and animal studies have found that chromium supplements can improve insulin sensitivity and blood sugar control in the face of insulin resistance, elevated blood glucose levels, impaired glucose tolerance, and diabetes.

A deficiency of chromium can lead to anxiety, fatigue, glucose intolerance (particularly in people with diabetes), inadequate metabolism of amino acids, and an increased risk of arteriosclerosis. Excessive intake (the level depends upon individual tolerance) can lead to chromium toxicity, which has been associated with dermatitis, gastrointestinal ulcers, and kidney and liver impairment. No toxicities have been reported, and thus chromium does not have an Upper Limit of Safety (UL). (See the chart on page 11 for this book's recommended chromium intake.) As depicted in the movie *Erin Brockovich*, people can become ill from chromium, but it is important to note that this was a different form of the mineral. The form that is obtained through diet is called divalent and the one that is toxic is hexavalent.

Supplemental chromium is best absorbed by the body when it is taken in a form called *chromium picolinate* (chromium chelated with picolinate, a naturally occurring amino acid metabolite). Picolinate enables chromium to readily enter into the body's cells, where the mineral can then help insulin do its job much more effectively.

Chromium picolinate has been used successfully to control blood cholesterol and blood glucose levels. The NIH funded a study to look at the benefits of chromium picolinate for patients with diabetes and heart disease. Preliminary data shows it lowers blood sugar and cholesterol. It also promotes the loss of fat and an increase in lean muscle tissue. Studies show it may increase longevity and help to fight osteoporosis. In addition, when combined with biotin, chromium picolinate reduces insulin resistance and reduces "bad" (LDL) cholesterol in patients with type 2 diabetes.

Chromium polynicotinate (chromium bonded to niacin) is an effective form of this mineral as well.

Sources

Chromium is found in the following food sources: beef, beer, brewer's yeast, brown rice, cheese, turkey, fish, and whole grains. It may also be found in dried beans, blackstrap molasses, broccoli, calf liver, chicken, corn and corn oil, dairy products, dried liver, dulse, eggs, green beans, mushrooms, and potatoes. Herbs that contain chromium include catnip, licorice, nettle, oat straw, red clover, sarsaparilla, wild yam, and yarrow.

Comments

Active, athletic individuals—people who engage in vigorous aerobic activities and consume higher amounts of carbohydrates than the general population—have higher chromium requirements than nonathletes. Chromium levels start to decrease as we age, starting in our early forties.

Some smaller studies have confirmed that added chromium in the diet can reduce total body fat and increase the percentage of muscle.

Cautions

If you have insulin-dependent diabetes, you should not use chromium unless your health care practitioner prescribes it. Chromium supplements can make insulin function more effectively and, in effect, reduce insulin requirements. People with diabetes therefore have to monitor their blood sugar levels very carefully when using chromium. Chromium requirements differ from person to person; consult your health care provider to determine the correct amount of this mineral for you.

Some people experience light-headedness or a slight skin rash when taking chromium. If you feel light-headed, stop taking the supplement and consult your health care provider. If you develop a rash, either try switching brands or discontinue use.

Copper

Among its many functions, copper aids in the formation of bone, hemoglobin, and red blood cells, and works in balance with zinc and vitamin C to form elastin, an important skin protein. It is involved in the healing process, energy production, hair and skin coloring, and taste sensitivity.

This mineral is also needed for healthy nerves and joints. One of the early signs of copper deficiency is osteoporosis.

Copper is essential for the formation of collagen, one of the fundamental proteins making up bones, skin, and connective tissue. Other possible signs of copper deficiency include anemia, baldness, diarrhea, general weakness, impaired respiratory function, and skin sores. A lack of copper can also lead to increased blood fat levels. (*See* COPPER DEFICIENCY in Part Two.)

Excessive intake of copper can lead to toxicity, which has been associated with depression, irritability, nausea and vomiting, nervousness, and joint and muscle pain. Ingesting a quantity as small as 10 milligrams usually causes nausea. Sixty milligrams generally results in vomiting, and just 3.5 grams (3,500 milligrams) can be fatal. Children can be affected at much smaller dosage levels. (*See* COPPER TOXICITY in Part Two.)

Sources

Besides its use in cookware and plumbing, copper is also widely distributed in foods. Food sources include almonds, avocados, barley, beans, beets, blackstrap molasses, broccoli, garlic, lentils, liver, mushrooms, nuts, oats, oranges, pecans, radishes, raisins, salmon, seafood, soybeans, and green leafy vegetables.

Comments

The level of copper in the body is related to the levels of zinc and vitamin C. Copper levels are reduced if large amounts of zinc or vitamin C are consumed. If copper intake is too high, levels of vitamin C and zinc drop.

The consumption of high amounts of fructose (fruit sugar) can make a copper deficiency significantly worse. In a study conducted by the U.S. Department of Agriculture, people who obtained 20 percent of their daily calories from fructose showed decreased levels of red blood cell super-oxide dismutase (SOD), a copper-dependent enzyme critical to antioxidant protection within the red blood cells.

Cautions

Excessive copper in the body can promote destruction of eye tissue through oxidation. Persons with eye problems should be especially careful to balance their intake of copper with that of iron, zinc, and calcium. In one study, elderly individuals who consumed a high-fat diet, rich in saturated fat and trans fat, and had high copper intakes (greater than 1.6 milligrams per day), seemed to experience greater cognitive impairment compared to those who ate a diet low in these fats or a diet lower in copper (0.88 mg per day) with high amounts of these dietary fats. In this study, it was best to get copper from foods rather than supplements.

Germanium

Germanium improves cellular oxygenation, but is not an essential nutrient. It helps to fight pain, keep the immune system functioning properly, and rid the body of toxins and poisons. Researchers have shown that consuming foods containing organic germanium is an effective way to increase tissue oxygenation, because, like hemoglobin, germanium acts as a carrier of oxygen to the cells. A Japanese scientist, Kazuhiko Asai, found that an intake of 100 to 300 milligrams of germanium per day improved many illnesses, including rheumatoid arthritis, food allergies, elevated cholesterol, candidiasis, chronic viral infections, cancer, and AIDS.

Sources

Germanium is found in all organic material, of both plant and animal origin. The following foods contain the greatest concentrations of germanium: broccoli, celery, garlic, shiitake mushrooms, milk, onions, rhubarb, sauerkraut, tomato juice, and the herbs aloe vera, comfrey, ginseng, and suma.

Comments

Germanium is best obtained through the diet.

Cautions

Although it is rare, some individuals may have a toxic reaction to this mineral if they take it in excessive amounts. People have been known to develop kidney problems, and there have been some deaths associated with germanium. Speak to a health care professional before using it, particularly if you have kidney problems.

Iodine

Needed only in trace amounts, iodine helps to metabolize excess fat and is important for physical and mental development. It is also needed for a healthy thyroid gland and for the prevention of goiter, a grossly swollen gland rarely seen these days. Certain parts of the country have little or no iodine in the soil, and isolated agrarian cultural groups that refrained from using iodized salt and cattle feed were subject to this disorder. Iodine deficiency in children may result in mental retardation. In addition, iodine deficiency has been linked to breast cancer and is associated with fatigue, neonatal hypothyroidism, and weight gain.

Excessive iodine intake (sometimes as little as 750 micrograms daily) may inhibit the secretion of thyroid hormone and can produce a metallic taste and sores in the mouth, swollen salivary glands, diarrhea, and vomiting. If you have any problem with your thyroid, speak with your physician about iodine. In most cases, however, the small risk of chronic iodine excess is far outweighed by the hazards of a low-iodine diet. It is especially important for women of childbearing age and children to get adequate amounts of iodine.

Sources

Foods that are high in iodine include dairy products (from cattle fed iodine-supplemented feed and salt licks), iodized salt, seafood, saltwater fish, and kelp. It may also be found in asparagus, dulse, garlic, lima beans, mushrooms, sea salt (which provides nature's own balance of minerals), sesame seeds, soybeans, spinach (*see* Comments, below), summer squash, Swiss chard, and turnip greens. Most fruits and vegetables grown near the coasts contain more iodine than those grown inland.

Comments

Some foods block the uptake of iodine into the thyroid gland when eaten raw in large amounts. These include Brussels sprouts, cabbage, cauliflower, kale, peaches, pears, spinach, and turnips. If you have an underactive thyroid, you should limit your consumption of these foods.

Iron

Perhaps the most important of iron's functions in the body is the production of hemoglobin and myoglobin (the form of hemoglobin found in muscle tissue), and the oxygenation of red blood cells. Iron is the mineral found in the largest amounts in the blood. It is essential for many enzymes, including catalase, and is important for growth. Iron is also required for a healthy immune system and for energy production.

Iron deficiency is most often caused by insufficient intake. However, it may result from intestinal bleeding, a diet high in phosphorus, poor digestion, long-term illness, ulcers, prolonged use of antacids, excessive coffee or tea consumption, and other causes. Menstruating women may become iron deficient, especially if they have heavy or pro-

longed periods and/or short menstrual cycles. In some cases, a deficiency of vitamin B_6 (pyridoxine) or vitamin B_{12} can be the underlying cause of anemia. Strenuous exercise and heavy perspiration also deplete iron from the body. Strict vegetarians are susceptible to iron deficiency and should have regular blood tests to check iron levels.

Iron deficiency symptoms include anemia, brittle hair, difficulty swallowing, digestive disturbances, dizziness, fatigue, fragile bones, hair loss, inflammation of the tissues of the mouth, nails that are spoon-shaped or that have ridges running lengthwise, nervousness, obesity, pallor, and slowed mental reactions.

Because iron is stored in the body, excessive iron intake can also cause problems. Too much iron in the tissues and organs leads to the production of free radicals and increases the need for vitamin E. High levels of iron were once thought to be associated with heart disease and cancer. Newer data indicates that having high iron stores does not seem to predict who will get cancer but may predict who will get heart disease. However, ferritin, a protein in the body that binds to iron, was associated with an increased risk of cancer in women when the level was greater than 160 micrograms per liter.

The buildup of iron in the tissues has been associated with a rare disease known as hemochromatosis, a hereditary disorder of iron metabolism that is found mostly in men and postmenopausal women and that causes excessive absorption of iron from both foods and supplements, leading to bronze skin pigmentation, arthritis, cirrhosis of the liver, diabetes, and heart disorders.

Sources

Iron is found in eggs, fish, liver, meat, poultry, green leafy vegetables, whole grains, and enriched breads and cereals. Other food sources with lesser amounts include almonds, avocados, beets, blackstrap molasses, brewer's yeast, dates, dulse, kelp, kidney and lima beans, lentils, millet, peaches, pears, dried prunes, pumpkins, raisins, rice and wheat bran, sesame seeds, soybeans, and watercress. Herbs that contain very small amounts of iron include alfalfa, burdock root, catnip, cayenne, chamomile, chickweed, chicory, dandelion, dong quai, eyebright, fennel seed, fenugreek, kelp, lemongrass, licorice, milk thistle seed, mullein, nettle, oat straw, paprika, parsley, peppermint, plantain, raspberry leaf, rose hips, sarsaparilla, shepherd's purse, uva ursi, and yellow dock. Foods are distinguished between heme iron (only from animal sources) and non-heme sources. The heme iron foods present iron in a form that is more readily absorbed into the body.

Comments

Unless you are diagnosed as anemic, are menstruating, or are of childbearing age, you should not take iron supplements. If you take a multivitamin and mineral supplement, choose a product that does not contain iron. Be sure to read labels. Some products contain iron below the DRI and should be avoided by everyone; the amount in these products is too low if you are anemic or require iron and too high if you don't need more. If you do need to take iron supplements, do not take them at the same time as vitamin E, and choose an organic form of iron such as ferrous gluconate or ferrous fumarate. Inorganic forms of iron, such as ferrous sulfate, can oxidize vitamin E. The RDA for iron is 8 milligrams per day for adult men, 12 milligrams a day for male children above age ten, and 18 milligrams per day for adult women and girls over eleven years of age (27 milligrams for pregnant women).

There must be sufficient hydrochloric acid (HCl) present in the stomach in order for iron to be absorbed. Copper, manganese, molybdenum, vitamin A, and the B-complex vitamins are also needed for complete iron absorption. Taking vitamin C can increase iron absorption by as much as 30 percent.

Taking calcium with meals can inhibit the absorption of iron from dietary sources. If you are iron deficient, take calcium supplements at bedtime or at other times when you are not consuming foods containing iron. Excessive amounts of zinc and vitamin E can also interfere with iron absorption. The utilization of iron may be impaired by rheumatoid arthritis and cancer. These diseases can result in anemia despite adequate amounts of iron stored in the liver, spleen, and bone marrow. Iron deficiency is more prevalent in people with candidiasis or chronic herpes infections.

Cautions

Do not take iron supplements if you have an infection. Because bacteria require iron for growth, the body "hides" iron in the liver and other storage sites when an infection is present. Taking extra iron at such times encourages the proliferation of bacteria in the body. Iron may cause constipation.

Magnesium

Magnesium is a vital catalyst in enzyme activity, especially the activity of those enzymes involved in energy production. It also assists in calcium and potassium uptake. A deficiency of magnesium interferes with the transmission of nerve and muscle impulses, causing irritability and nervousness. Supplementing the diet with magnesium can help prevent depression, dizziness, muscle weakness and twitching, and premenstrual syndrome (PMS), and also aids in maintaining the body's proper pH balance and normal body temperature.

Magnesium is necessary to prevent the calcification of soft tissue. This essential mineral protects the arterial linings from stress caused by sudden blood pressure changes, and plays a role in the formation of bone and in carbohydrate and mineral metabolism. With vitamin B_6 (pyridoxine), magnesium helps to reduce and dissolve calcium-phosphate kidney stones, and may prevent calcium-oxalate kidney stones. Research has shown that magnesium may help prevent cardiovascular disease, osteoporosis, and certain forms of cancer, and it may reduce cholesterol levels. It is effective in preventing premature labor and convulsions in pregnant women.

Studies have shown that taking magnesium supplements during pregnancy has a dramatic effect in reducing birth defects. A study reported by the *Journal of the American Medical Association* reported a 70 percent lower incidence of mental retardation in the children of mothers who had taken magnesium supplements during pregnancy. The incidence of cerebral palsy was 90 percent lower.

Possible manifestations of magnesium deficiency include confusion, insomnia, irritability, poor digestion, rapid heartbeat, seizures, and tantrums; often, a magnesium deficiency can be synonymous with diabetes. Magnesium deficiencies are at the root of many cardiovascular problems.

Magnesium deficiency may be a major cause of fatal cardiac arrhythmia, hypertension, and sudden cardiac arrest, as well as asthma, chronic fatigue and chronic pain syndromes, depression, insomnia, irritable bowel syndrome, and pulmonary disorders. Research has also shown that magnesium deficiency may contribute to the formation of kidney stones. To test for magnesium deficiency, a procedure called an intracellular (mononuclear cell) magnesium screen should be performed. This is a more sensitive test than the typical serum magnesium screen, and can detect a deficiency with more accuracy. Magnesium screening should be a routine test, as a low magnesium level makes nearly every disease worse. It is particularly important for individuals who have, or who are considered at risk for developing, cardiovascular disease. Muscle biopsies give a better picture of your magnesium status than blood tests do.

Sources

Magnesium is found in most foods, especially dairy products, fish, meat, and seafood. Other rich food sources include apples, apricots, avocados, bananas, black-eyed peas, blackstrap molasses, brewer's yeast, brown rice, cantaloupe, dulse, figs, garlic, grapefruit, green leafy vegetables, kelp, lemons, lima beans, millet, nuts, peaches, salmon, sesame seeds, soybeans, tofu, torula yeast, watercress, wheat, and whole grains. Herbs that contain magnesium include alfalfa, bladderwrack, catnip, cayenne, chamomile, chickweed, dandelion, eyebright, fennel seed, fenugreek, hops, lemongrass, licorice, mullein, nettle, oat straw, paprika, parsley, peppermint, raspberry leaf, red clover, sage, shepherd's purse, yarrow, and yellow dock.

Comments

The consumption of alcohol, the use of diuretics, diarrhea, the presence of fluoride, and high levels of zinc and vitamin D all increase the body's need for magnesium. The consumption of large amounts of fats, cod liver oil, calcium, vitamin D, and protein decrease magnesium absorption. Fat-soluble vitamins also hinder the absorption of magnesium, as do foods high in oxalic acid, such as almonds, chard, cocoa, rhubarb, spinach, and tea.

Manganese

Minute quantities of manganese are needed for protein and fat metabolism, healthy nerves, a healthy immune system, and blood sugar regulation. Manganese is used in energy production and is required for normal bone growth and for reproduction. In addition, it is used in the formation of cartilage and synovial (lubricating) fluid of the joints. It is also necessary for the synthesis of bone.

Manganese is essential for people with iron-deficiency anemia and is needed for the utilization of vitamin B_1 (thiamine) and vitamin E. Manganese works well with the B-complex vitamins to give an overall feeling of well-being. It aids in the formation of mother's milk and is a key element in the production of enzymes needed to oxidize fats and to metabolize purines, including the antioxidant enzyme superoxide dismutase (SOD).

A deficiency of manganese (which is extremely rare) may lead to atherosclerosis, confusion, convulsions, eye problems, hearing problems, heart disorders, high cholesterol levels, hypertension, irritability, memory loss, muscle contractions, pancreatic damage, profuse perspiration, rapid pulse, teeth grinding, tremors, and a tendency toward breast ailments.

Sources

The largest quantities of manganese are found in avocados, nuts and seeds, seaweed, and whole grains. This mineral may also be found in blueberries, egg yolks, legumes, dried peas, pineapples, and green leafy vegetables. Herbs that contain manganese include alfalfa, burdock root, catnip, chamomile, chickweed, dandelion, eyebright, fennel seed, fenugreek, ginseng, hops, lemongrass, mullein, parsley, peppermint, raspberry, red clover, rose hips, wild yam, yarrow, and yellow dock.

Molybdenum

This essential mineral is required in extremely small amounts for nitrogen metabolism. It aids in the final stages of the conversion of purines to uric acid. It promotes normal cell function, aids in the activation of certain enzymes, and is a component of the metabolic enzyme xanthine oxidase.

Molybdenum is found in the liver, bones, and kidneys. It supports bone growth and strengthening of the teeth. A low intake is associated with mouth and gum disorders and cancer. A molybdenum deficiency may cause impotence in older men. People whose diets are high in refined and processed foods are at risk for deficiency.

Sources

This trace mineral is found in beans, beef liver, cereal grains, dark green leafy vegetables, legumes, and peas.

Comments

Heat and moisture can change the action of supplemental molybdenum. A high intake of sulfur may decrease molybdenum levels. Excess amounts of molybdenum (more than 15 milligrams daily) may interfere with copper metabolism.

Cautions

Do not take more than 15 milligrams of molybdenum daily. Higher doses may lead to the development of gout.

Phosphorus

Phosphorus is needed for blood clotting, bone and tooth formation, cell growth, contraction of the heart muscle, normal heart rhythm, and kidney function. It also assists the body in the utilization of vitamins and the conversion of food to energy. A proper balance of magnesium, calcium, and phosphorus should be maintained at all times. If one of these minerals is present in either excessive or insufficient amounts, this will have adverse effects on the body.

Deficiencies of phosphorus are rare, but can lead to such symptoms as anxiety, bone pain, fatigue, irregular breathing, irritability, numbness, skin sensitivity, trembling, weakness, and weight changes.

Sources

Phosphorus deficiency is rare because this mineral is found in most foods, especially processed cooked foods and carbonated soft drinks. Significant amounts of phosphorus are contained in asparagus; bran; brewer's yeast; corn; dairy products; eggs; fish; dried fruit; garlic; legumes; nuts; sesame, sunflower, and pumpkin seeds; meats; poultry; salmon; and whole grains.

Comments

Excessive amounts of phosphorus interfere with calcium uptake. A diet high in processed cooked foods and junk food such as carbonated beverages is a common culprit. Vitamin D increases the effectiveness of phosphorus.

Potassium

This mineral is important for a healthy nervous system and a regular heart rhythm. It helps prevent stroke, aids in proper muscle contraction, and works with sodium to control the body's water balance. Potassium is important for chemical reactions within the cells and aids in maintaining stable blood pressure and in transmitting electrochemical impulses. A 1997 review of earlier studies showed that low potassium intake might be a significant factor in the development of high blood pressure. A high intake of potassium protects several body systems, including cardiovascular, kidney, and bone. The potassium in fruits and vegetables contains organic salts such as malate and citrate, which neutralize the acid urine that can cause kidney stones. Potassium also regulates the transfer of nutrients through cell membranes. This function of potassium has been shown to decrease with age, which may account for some of the circulatory damage, lethargy, and weakness experienced by older people. Together with magnesium, potassium can help prevent calcium-oxalate kidney stones.

In one study, healthy individuals with normal blood pressure experienced lower blood pressure from both potassium chloride and potassium citrate. The levels were still normal, but on the lower side of normal, which is desirable. The amount of potassium given in this study was the equivalent of what is found in five half-cup servings of fruits and vegetables. Anyone with high blood pressure would benefit from lowered blood pressure to reduce heart disease risk.

Signs of potassium deficiency include abnormally dry skin, acne, chills, cognitive impairment, constipation, depression, diarrhea, diminished reflex function, edema, nervousness, insatiable thirst, fluctuations in heartbeat, glucose intolerance, growth impairment, high cholesterol levels, insomnia, low blood pressure, muscular fatigue and weakness, nausea and vomiting, periodic headaches, proteinuria (protein in the urine), respiratory distress, and salt retention.

Sources

Food sources of potassium include dairy foods, fish, fruit, legumes, meat, poultry, vegetables, and whole grains. High amounts are found in apricots, avocados, bananas, lima beans, blackstrap molasses, brewer's yeast, brown rice, dates, dulse, figs, dried fruit, garlic, nuts, potatoes, raisins, spinach, torula yeast, wheat bran, winter squash, yams, and yogurt. Herbs that contain potassium include catnip, hops, nettle, plantain, red clover, sage, and skullcap. In general, if it is grown in the ground—for example, fruits and vegetables—it is rich in potassium. In addition, these foods are very low in sodium. It is desirable to consume 2.5 to 3.5 grams of potassium per day from your diet.

Comments

Kidney disorders, diarrhea, and the use of diuretics or laxatives all disrupt potassium levels. Tobacco and caffeine reduce potassium absorption. Using large amounts of licorice over long periods can deplete the body's potassium supply.

Potassium is needed for hormone secretion. The secretion of stress hormones causes a decrease in the potassium-to-sodium ratio both inside and outside the cells. As a result, stress increases the body's potassium requirements.

Too much potassium from supplements could be harmful. Check with your health care professional before using potassium supplements.

Selenium

Selenium's principal function is to inhibit the oxidation of lipids (fats) as a component of the enzyme glutathione peroxidase. It is a vital antioxidant, especially when combined with vitamin E. It protects the immune system by preventing the formation of free radicals that can damage the body. (*See* ANTIOXIDANTS in Part One.) It plays a vital role in regulating the effects of thyroid hormone on fat metabolism.

Selenium has also been found to function as a preventive against the formation of certain types of tumors. One study found that men who took 200 micrograms of selenium daily over a ten-year period had roughly half the risk of developing lung, prostate, and colorectal cancer as compared with men who did not.

Selenium and vitamin E act synergistically to aid in the production of antibodies and to help maintain a healthy heart and liver. This trace element is needed for pancreatic function and tissue elasticity. When combined with vitamin E and zinc, it may also provide relief from an enlarged prostate. Selenium supplementation has been found to protect the liver in people with alcoholic cirrhosis. Studies conducted at the University of Miami indicate that taking supplemental selenium may enhance the survival of people with AIDS by increasing both red and white blood cell counts. It has shown promise in the treatment of arthritis, cardiovascular disease, male infertility, cataracts, AIDS, and high blood pressure. For very sick patients in the intensive care unit, selenium appears to reduce mortality rates. In one study, the death rate was 14 percent lower in those getting a high dose of selenium (1,000 micrograms a day). Selenium is incorporated into over twenty-five proteins, called selenoproteins, that play pivotal roles in a number of bodily activities, from activating thyroid hormones to regenerating vitamin C.

Selenium deficiency has been linked to cancer and heart disease. It has also been associated with exhaustion, growth impairment, high cholesterol levels, infections, liver impairment, pancreatic insufficiency, and sterility. There is some thought that selenium deficiency might be linked to a host of viral outbreaks, from new strains of influenza to Ebola, wrought by the rapidly mutating virus's interaction with selenium-deficient hosts in places like Africa and China where there is little or no selenium in the soil.

Some have found selenium to be related to cognitive function. One study found that lower selenium content in fingernails was related to poorer cognitive function in a group of elderly Chinese. This finding supports the hypothesis that a lifelong low selenium level is associated with lower cognition.

Sources

Selenium can be found in meat and grains, depending on the selenium content of the soil where the food is raised. Because New Zealand soils are low in selenium, cattle and sheep raised there have suffered a breakdown of muscle tissue, including the heart muscle. However, human intake of selenium there is adequate because of imported Australian wheat. The soil of much American farmland is low in selenium, resulting in selenium-deficient produce.

Selenium can be found in Brazil nuts (the only truly concentrated natural source), brewer's yeast, broccoli, brown rice, chicken, dairy products, dulse, garlic, kelp, liver, molasses, onions, salmon, seafood, torula yeast, tuna, vegetables, wheat germ, and whole grains. Herbs that contain selenium include alfalfa, burdock root, catnip, cayenne, chamomile, chickweed, fennel seed, fenugreek, garlic, ginseng, hawthorn berry, hops, lemongrass, milk thistle, nettle, oat straw, parsley, peppermint, raspberry leaf, rose hips, sarsaparilla, uva ursi, yarrow, and yellow dock.

Comments

The typical dietary intake of selenium is 80 to 150 micrograms. Taking up to 200 micrograms per day is considered safe for most people. This is half the maximum allowable dose.

Cautions

Symptoms of selenosis (excessively high selenium levels) can include arthritis, brittle nails, garlicky breath, gastrointestinal disorders, hair loss, irritability, liver and kidney impairment, a metallic taste in the mouth, pallor, skin eruptions, tooth loss, and yellowish skin. Unless your health care provider prescribes it, do *not* take more than 400 micrograms daily. One ounce of Brazil nuts can contain as much as 544 micrograms of selenium. If you take supplemental selenium, do not consume Brazil nuts. If you are pregnant, you should *not* take more than 40 micrograms of supplemental selenium daily, nor should you consume Brazil nuts.

Silicon

Silicon is the second most abundant element on the planet (oxygen is the first). It is necessary for the formation of collagen for bones and connective tissue; for healthy nails, skin, and hair; and for calcium absorption in the early stages of bone formation. It is needed to maintain flexible arteries, and plays a major role in preventing cardiovascular disease. Silicon counteracts the effects of aluminum on the body and is important in the prevention of Alzheimer's disease and osteoporosis. It stimulates the immune system and inhibits the aging process in tissues. Silicon levels decrease with aging, so elderly people need larger amounts.

A seven-year study in French women showed that higher silicon intakes, primarily from drinking water, appeared to be protective against developing Alzheimer's disease.

Sources

Foods that contain silicon include alfalfa, beets, brown rice, rice bran, rice hulls, whole and rolled oats, bell peppers, soybeans, leafy green vegetables, and whole grains.

Comments

Silicon is most commonly found in the form of silica, a compound of silicon and oxygen also known as silicon dioxide (SiO_2). One form of silicon, called silicic acid (actually, orthosilicic acid or OSA), appears to be extremely absorbable and useful as a silicon transport agent in the body. Two good sources of silicon are Body Essential Silica Gel from NatureWorks and Jarrosil from Jarrow Formulas. The minerals boron, calcium, magnesium, manganese, and potassium are needed for the efficient utilization of silicon.

Sodium

Sodium is necessary for maintaining proper water balance and blood pH. It is also needed for stomach, nerve, and muscle function. Although sodium deficiency is rare—most people have adequate (if not excessive) levels of sodium in their bodies—it can occur. This condition is most likely to affect people who take diuretics for high blood pressure, especially if they simultaneously adhere to low-sodium diets.

Some experts estimate that as many as 20 percent of elderly people who take diuretics may be deficient in sodium. In some cases of disorders such as fibromyalgia, studies have shown that moderate amounts of sodium may be needed as well (natural sea salt is recommended). Symptoms of sodium deficiency can include abdominal cramps, anorexia, confusion, dehydration, depression, dizziness, fatigue, flatulence, hallucinations, headache, heart palpitations, an impaired sense of taste, lethargy, low blood pressure, memory impairment, muscular weakness, nausea and vomiting, poor coordination, recurrent infections, seizures, and weight loss. Excessive sodium intake can result in edema, high blood pressure, potassium deficiency, and liver and kidney disease.

Sources

Virtually all foods contain some sodium.

Comments

A proper balance of potassium and sodium is necessary for good health. Because most people consume too much sodium, they typically need more potassium as well. An imbalance between sodium and potassium can lead to heart disease. If you sweat excessively from exercise or heat, you will need to make sure to replace salt lost in perspiration through foods or beverages with added salt.

Sulfur

An acid-forming mineral that is part of the chemical structure of the amino acids methionine, cysteine, taurine, and glutathione, sulfur disinfects the blood, helps the body to resist bacteria, and protects the protoplasm of cells. It aids in necessary oxidation reactions in the body, stimulates bile secretion, and protects against toxic substances. Because of its ability to protect against the harmful effects of radiation and pollution, sulfur slows the aging process. It is found in all body tissues, and is needed for the synthesis of collagen, a principal protein that gives the skin its structural integrity.

Sources

Brussels sprouts, dried beans, cabbage, eggs, fish, garlic, kale, meats, onions, soybeans, turnips, and wheat germ contain sulfur, as do the amino acids cysteine, cystine, and methionine. Sulfur is also available in tablet and powder forms. Methylsufonylmethane (MSM) is a good form of sulfur.

Comments

Moisture and heat may destroy or change the action of sulfur in the body. Sulfur is one of the key substances that makes garlic the "king of herbs."

Vanadium

Vanadium is needed for cellular metabolism and for the formation of bones and teeth. It plays a role in growth and reproduction, and inhibits cholesterol synthesis. Vanadium has been shown to have the ability to improve insulin utilization, resulting in improved glucose tolerance. A vanadium deficiency may be linked to cardiovascular and kidney disease, impaired reproductive ability, and increased infant mortality. Vanadium is not easily absorbed. Athletes may require more of this trace mineral than nonathletes.

Sources

Vanadium is found in dill, fish, olives, meat, radishes, snap beans, vegetable oils, and whole grains.

Comments

There may be an interaction between vanadium and chromium. If you take supplemental chromium and vanadium, take them at different times. Tobacco use decreases the uptake of vanadium.

Zinc

This essential mineral is important in prostate gland function and the growth of the reproductive organs. Zinc may help prevent acne and regulate the activity of oil glands. It is required for protein synthesis and collagen formation, and promotes a healthy immune system and the healing of wounds. Zinc also enhances acuity of taste and smell. It protects the liver from chemical damage and is vital for bone formation. It is a constituent of insulin and many vital enzymes, including the antioxidant enzyme superoxide dismutase (SOD). It also helps to fight and prevent the formation of free radicals in other ways. A form of zinc called zinc monomethionine (zinc bound with the amino acid methionine), sold under the trademark OptiZinc, has been found to have antioxidant activity comparable to that of vitamin C, vitamin E, and beta-carotene. Zinc lozenges have been reported to be effective in relieving symptoms of the common cold and reducing the duration of colds.

Sufficient intake and absorption of zinc are needed to maintain the proper concentration of vitamin E in the blood. In addition, zinc increases the absorption of vitamin A. For optimum health, a proper 1-to-10 balance between copper and zinc levels should be maintained.

A deficiency of zinc may result in the loss of the senses of taste and smell. It can also cause fingernails to become thin, peel, and develop white spots. Other possible signs of zinc deficiency include acne, delayed sexual maturation, fatigue, growth impairment, hair loss, high cholesterol levels, impaired night vision, impotence, increased susceptibility to infection, infertility, memory impairment, a propensity to diabetes, prostate trouble, recurrent colds and flu, skin lesions, and slow wound healing.

Sources

Zinc is found in the following food sources: brewer's yeast, dulse, egg yolks, fish, kelp, lamb, legumes, lima beans, liver, meats, mushrooms, oysters, pecans, poultry, pumpkin seeds, sardines, seafood, soy lecithin, soybeans, sunflower seeds, torula yeast, and whole grains. Herbs that contain zinc include alfalfa, burdock root, cayenne, chamomile, chickweed, dandelion, eyebright, fennel seed, hops, milk thistle, mullein, nettle, parsley, rose hips, sage, sarsaparilla, skullcap, and wild yam.

Comments

Zinc levels may be lowered by diarrhea, kidney disease, cirrhosis of the liver, diabetes, or the consumption of fiber, which causes zinc to be excreted through the intestinal tract. A significant amount of zinc is lost through perspiration.

The consumption of hard water also can upset zinc levels. Compounds called phytates that are found in grains and legumes bind with zinc so that it cannot be absorbed.

If you take both zinc and iron supplements, take them at different times. If these two minerals are taken together, they interfere with each other's activity.

Cautions

Do not take a total of more than 100 milligrams of zinc daily. While daily doses less than 100 milligrams enhance the immune response, doses of more than 100 milligrams can depress the immune system.

Air

INTRODUCTION

Air is what we breathe. It is made up almost entirely of nitrogen, oxygen, argon, carbon dioxide, some water vapor, and tiny amounts of inert gases such as krypton, neon, and helium. The part essential for life is oxygen, which makes up about 21 percent of the air. The nitrogen component is basically 78 percent and argon is less than 1 percent. The remaining gases are found in very small quantities, measured as parts per million.

Water vapor can exist in varying amounts (0 to 5 percent) in any given location, depending on the air temperature and other factors. Without getting too technical, it is enough to say that as the air temperature rises, its ability to hold water vapor increases.

Nonstandard components can include particulates, chemical vapors, methane, sulfur dioxide, oxides of nitrogen, ammonia, and carbon monoxide, among others. Levels of these compounds can vary from place to place, and are collectively called *air pollution.*

AIR POLLUTION—WHAT IS IT?

Air pollution is basically contamination of the air caused by the discharge of harmful substances. It can cause immediate health problems, such as burning eyes and nose, an itchy irritated throat, and/or breathing difficulties. Over long periods, exposure to some of the chemicals and particulates found in polluted air can cause cancer, birth defects, brain and nerve damage, and injury to the lungs and breathing passages. Dust and particulates from smokestacks, and especially from diesel exhaust, are suspected of increasing the number of deaths from heart attacks by affecting the heart's ability to maintain its rhythm. The very young and the very old suffer the most from the effects of air pollution, but the duration of the exposure and the concentration of the chemical pollutants are important. Certain contaminants can, at high levels, cause severe injury or even death in short order.

Air pollution also causes damage to the environment and to the infrastructure. Trees, lakes, crops, and animals (both wild and domestic) are affected, as are buildings, bridges, monuments, and other man-made structures. Air pollution almost certainly has thinned the protective ozone layer above the earth, allowing dangerous radiation from the sun's rays to cause cancers, birth defects, and other injuries to humans throughout the world.

Smog is a type of large-scale air pollution caused by chemical reactions in the air between different pollutants from vehicle exhaust and industrial sources. Smog can have a different specific cause depending on location, wind, and weather, but the effect is essentially the same. Smog becomes a real problem when a phenomenon known as *temperature inversion* occurs. That is, the air near the ground is cooler than the air above, which holds down the pollution so it can't disperse. Cities surrounded by mountains, such as Los Angeles, are particularly prone to this phenomenon. If the inversion happens in the winter, it traps mostly particulates and carbon monoxide. If it happens in the summer, expect smog.

Indoor air pollution, including secondhand smoke, is almost as big a problem as outdoor air pollution. In the United States, most people now spend between 80 and 90 percent of their time indoors. It sounds unbelievable until you actually do the math. We live in sealed buildings, our kids go to school in sealed buildings, and we commute in air-conditioned cars to work in sealed offices. It's no wonder that indoor pollution has such an effect on our health. And the effect may be even more serious in northern climates, where the weather keeps people indoors in the winter. Defective air-handling equipment, faulty air-conditioning and building design, poor maintenance of air-conditioning and heating systems, plus gas emissions from carpeting, paints, paneling, computers, copying machines, plastic furniture—all contribute to an ever-growing problem.

THE MAJOR POLLUTANTS

There are thousands of potential air pollutants. Some of the major ones are as follows.

Carbon Monoxide

Carbon monoxide (CO) is colorless, odorless, and poisonous. After it is inhaled, the carbon monoxide molecules enter the bloodstream via the lungs. They bind with the red blood cells, preventing them from picking up oxygen. Because the cells throughout the body are then starved of oxygen, serious problems result. Low concentrations cause dizziness, headaches, and fatigue. Exposure to high concentrations is usually fatal.

Carbon monoxide is created for the most part by automobile engines as a product of incomplete combustion, although even a wood-burning stove emits plenty of the gas. Home-testing kits are available to test the levels at home.

44

Carbon Dioxide

Carbon dioxide (CO_2) is a greenhouse gas that is normally found in the atmosphere. As we use oxygen, we generate carbon dioxide, which is exhaled with each breath. Luckily for us, plants that use photosynthesis need this carbon dioxide to live. They take it in, use it, and excrete oxygen. This has been a good relationship. At present, the concentration in the air is around 360 parts per million (ppm). This varies with location and season (it's a bit higher in the summer). This so-called "natural" concentration has been trending upward for the last 11,000 years, since the end of the last ice age. About the time the ice sheets began to retreat, the concentration of CO_2 in the air was around 200 ppm.

The oceans hold most of the CO_2 on the planet—at least fifty times more than is in the air and ten times more than in all the plant and soil sources. Circulation patterns, or megacurrents, transport the CO_2 up and down in the oceans—most of the CO_2 is held in deep, cold waters—and there is a constant interchange of CO_2 between the oceans and the atmosphere. As the oceans have warmed up, they are giving up their CO_2 to the air. By the late 1700s, the atmospheric CO_2 level was up to 280 ppm, by 1960 it was up to 315 ppm, and today it is approximately 390 ppm. Over the past fifty years, atmospheric CO_2 has been increasing by about 1 ppm per year, which is an indicator not only of the natural processes taking place but also the rapidly increasing burning of fossil fuels.

Why is this important? Because CO_2 is a greenhouse gas, the more of it there is in the atmosphere, the warmer the climate will become.

Chlorofluorocarbons (CFCs)

These CFCs, used widely in industry and especially as a refrigerant in air-conditioning systems, are commonly known as *freon*. There are several commercial forms of freon; all are greenhouse gases. The latest form of freon being used extensively is designated R134. An older form, R12, was used as a solvent and in air conditioners through the 1990s (and is still used in some countries). When released into the atmosphere, all forms of freon eventually rise into the stratosphere. Through reaction with other atmospheric chemicals, freon has reduced the amount of ozone (O_3). This ozone layer is a protective shield against harmful solar ultraviolet (UV) radiation. Increased skin cancers and other related problems caused by an increased level of UV radiation at the earth's surface have been the result.

In addition, the reduction in the ozone layer has lowered the temperature of the stratosphere, and the temperature differential between it and the troposphere (the layer closest to the ground) has caused an increase in both stratospheric and surface wind speeds, and has the potential for altering the climate.

In a vicious cycle, the lowered stratospheric temperature can further reduce the ozone layer because as the temperature drops, the amount of ozone naturally decreases.

Hazardous Air Pollutants (HAPs)

This is a general class of chemicals that can cause serious health and environmental effects. Health effects can include cancer, birth defects, nervous system disorders, respiratory problems, and even death at high concentrations. There are literally thousands of these chemicals, and almost 200 of them have been positively identified as potential hazards. Most are produced in chemical plants for industrial use or as intermediate products used to manufacture other chemicals.

Examples of these chemicals are acrolein, formaldehyde, acetaldehyde, beryllium, and arsenic, among others. The greatest hazard still comes from diesel emissions.

Lead

Lead is a highly toxic metal that produces a number of problems, especially neurological disorders in young children. Lead has been phased out of gasoline and consumer products, but there are still quantities of lead in the environment as lead paint and lead piping, and lead-contaminated dust and soil from years of lead emission is still a problem. Luckily, the number of children with elevated blood levels of lead has dropped significantly. More information on lead can be obtained from the National Lead Information Center (NLIC) at www.epa.gov/lead/nlic.htm.

Ozone (O_3)

Ozone is beneficial only if it remains in the stratosphere, where a layer of it shields us from ultraviolet radiation. This form of oxygen, having three atoms rather than two, is toxic and can damage our health, the environment, trees, and crops. It is also corrosive to many materials. Normally, the health problems most experienced by ozone exposure include respiratory tract irritation, chest pain, coughing, increased susceptibility to lung infections, and an inability to catch one's breath. Ozone at ground level comes from the oxidation of organic compounds given up naturally by vegetation, auto emissions, electrical discharges (brush-type motors, generators, and lightning), and the burning of coal.

Oxides of Nitrogen (NO_x)

There are several significant oxides of nitrogen (the subscript x denotes any number of oxygen atoms) that affect air pollution. These nitrogen compounds react with many volatile organic compounds, both man-made and natural, to form what we call smog. Smog causes breathing difficulties, coughing, and general respiratory system distress.

One by-product is acid rain, which kills vegetation and sterilizes lakes. The burning of fossil fuels, either gasoline in automobiles or coal and oil in power plants, predominantly produces these oxides of nitrogen. As energy demands increase we can expect NO_x emissions to increase, and consequently more ozone and smog will be created.

Particulate Matter

The term *particulate matter* refers to any type of solid material in the air in the form of dust, smoke, or vapor, which can remain suspended for a long time. Breathing in these microscopic particles is one of the major causes of lung damage and respiratory disease. Particles from diesel engines have been rated as the most hazardous pollutant in an entire arsenal of pollutants, simply on the basis of tonnage emitted. Nobody is exempt. People in urban areas are subjected to heavy traffic and industrial pollution. Farmers who don't have to contend with heavy traffic nevertheless work amid clouds of soil dust, chemical vapors, fertilizer, and flour and grain dust. Industrial processes, mining, road construction, and any number of other modern activities contribute to the problem. New evidence suggests that as many as 50,000 Americans may die each year from inhaling these microscopic specks. The World Health Organization has estimated that deaths worldwide could be as high as 2.8 million annually. People with existing respiratory problems are naturally more prone to feel the effects when air quality is bad.

Many others have been dying from sudden heart failure, which may be caused by abnormalities in the heart rhythm in response to changing demands. When the air is thick with dust and soot, the heart is less able to adjust its rhythm. These pollutants also reduce lung capacity, depending on the particulate level: the greater the particle density, the less the lung capacity. Smaller particles appear to be more hazardous than larger ones.

Particulates also pick up hitchhikers, such as toxic metals, acidic aerosols, and other particles of different chemical composition than themselves. Particles of dust from the sub-Saharan region of Africa have reached all the way into Arizona and Texas, causing asthma problems for people there and all throughout the Caribbean basin.

Sulfur Dioxide (SO₂)

Sulfur dioxide is a pungent, toxic gas produced by the burning of coal, usually in power plants. More than 65 percent, or 13 million tons a year, comes from our electric utilities. This takes into account the large number of domestic power plants that have installed scrubbers. Worldwide, the problem is almost out of control. Coal-fired power plants in China and other areas of Asia are not even equipped with rudimentary stack scrubbers. A few other industrial processes, including some paper mills and smelters, also produce SO_2 (from the odor, people generally know where they are). Like the oxides of nitrogen, sulfur dioxide is a major contributor to acid rain and smog. Corrosive acids (such as sulfurous acid and sulfuric acid) formed in the air can rain down to cause massive damage to wildlife, vegetation, streams, rivers, and lakes. Lung problems are caused by breathing sulfur dioxide, including permanent lung damage from long-term exposure (or exposure for shorter times at higher doses).

Volatile Organic Compounds (VOCs)

There are many volatile organic compounds. Volatile chemicals form vapors easily at normal room temperature. Many of the VOCs we find in the air are natural, and are excreted as part of natural processes by vegetation. Others are not found in nature, and are escapees from a petrochemical plant (a source site) or somewhere downstream where the chemical is being utilized. An example is gasoline. Vapor can escape right at the refinery, during transfer to storage, during delivery to the distributor and gas station, or right at the pump when it is being pumped into the gas tank.

Other VOCs include benzene, one of the most prevalent chemicals known. Solvents such as toluene, xylene, and perchlorethylene are VOCs, as are a host of other products. VOCs are also released as combustion products, such as during the burning of coal, natural gas, oil, and even wood. Vehicle emissions are a major source of VOCs, as are vapors from industrial glues, solvents, paints, and many other consumer products.

Water

INTRODUCTION

Human beings can survive without food for thirty to forty days—about five weeks—but without water, life would end in three to five days. The average person's body is composed of approximately 70 percent water, although the water content varies considerably from person to person and even from one body part to another. The body's water supply is responsible for and involved in nearly every bodily process, including digestion, absorption, circulation, and excretion. Water is also the primary transporter of nutrients throughout the body and so is necessary for all building functions in the body. Water helps maintain normal body temperature and is essential for carrying waste material out of the body. Therefore, replacing the water that is continually being lost through sweating and elimination is very important.

A drop in the body's water content causes a decline in blood volume. The lowering of blood volume in turn triggers the hypothalamus, which is the brain's thirst center, to send out the demand for a drink. This causes a slight rise in the concentration of sodium in the blood. These changes quickly trigger a sensation of thirst. Unfortunately, people often consume only enough liquid to quench a dry or parched throat—not enough to cover all of their water loss.

As a result, they can become dehydrated. As we age, the sense of thirst becomes dulled. At the same time, we have a lower percentage of reserve body water than we had when we were younger. This is why it is important to drink water even when you do not feel thirsty. Drinking water can also help control overeating, as thirst is sometimes mistaken for hunger.

Quality water is beneficial for virtually all disorders known to humankind. Bowel and bladder problems, as well as headaches, can be reduced by drinking water. If not enough water is consumed, toxins can build up in the system, causing headaches. Water flushes out these toxins.

Anxiety attacks, food intolerances, "acid stomach" and heartburn, muscle pains, colitis pain, hot flashes, and many other discomforts and disorders can be eased quickly by drinking a full glass of water. Chronic fatigue syndrome (CFS) is another disorder that necessitates consuming plenty of quality water daily to flush out toxins and other substances that contribute to muscle aches and extreme fatigue.

Without adequate water, we would poison ourselves with our own metabolic wastes. The kidneys remove waste products, such as uric acid, urea, and lactic acid, all of which must be dissolved in water. If there is not enough water available to remove these substances effectively, they may cause damage to the kidneys. Digestion and metabolism also rely on water for certain enzymatic and chemical reactions in the body. Water carries nutrients and oxygen to cells through the blood and is involved in the regulation of body temperature through perspiration. Water is especially important for people who have musculoskeletal problems such as arthritis, or who are athletic, as it lubricates the joints. Because lung tissue must be moist to facilitate oxygen intake and carbon dioxide excretion, water is essential for breathing. Approximately one pint of liquid is lost each day through exhaling. If you do not take in enough water to maintain fluid balance, every bodily function can be impaired. And the more active you are, the more water you must consume in order to keep your body's water level in balance.

Inadequate water consumption may contribute to excess body fat; poor muscle tone; digestive problems; poor functioning of many organs, including the brain; joint and muscle soreness; and, paradoxically, water retention. Consuming plenty of quality water can slow the aging process, and can prevent or improve arthritis, kidney stones, constipation, arteriosclerosis, obesity, glaucoma, cataracts, diabetes, hypoglycemia, and many other diseases. It is not expensive, and you should feel a difference quickly, but you must drink about ten full glasses of quality water (80 ounces) daily.

Obtaining quality water would seem to be an easy matter. However, due to the numerous types of classifications water is given, the average consumer can easily be confused about what is available. This section offers a guide to understanding what the most commonly used classifications of water mean and how these different kinds of water may help or harm the body.

TAP WATER

Water that comes out of household taps or faucets is generally obtained either from surface water or from ground water. Surface water is water that has run off from ponds, creeks, streams, rivers, and lakes, and is collected in reservoirs. Ground water is water that has filtered through the ground to the water table and is extracted by means of a well. Approximately half of the tap water in the United States comes from lakes, rivers, or other surface sources. Underground aquifers and municipal wells provide 35 percent of tap water, and the remaining 15 percent comes from private wells.

The Safety of Tap Water

Most people assume that when they turn on the kitchen tap, they are getting clean, safe, healthy drinking water. Unfortunately, this often is not the case. Regardless of the original source of tap water, it is vulnerable to a number of different types of impurities, and may be full of harmful chemicals and inorganic minerals that the body cannot use.

Some undesirable substances found in water—including radon, fluoride, and arsenic, as well as iron, lead, copper, and other heavy metals—can occur naturally. Other contaminants, such as fertilizers, asbestos, cyanides, herbicides, pesticides, and industrial chemicals, may leach into ground water through the soil, or into any tap water from plumbing pipes. Many of these chemicals have been linked to cancer and other disorders. Water can also contain biological contaminants, including viruses, bacteria, and parasites.

Still other substances—including chlorine, fluorides, carbon, lime, phosphates, soda ash, and aluminum sulfate—are intentionally added to public water supplies to kill bacteria, adjust pH, and eliminate cloudiness, among other things. Even if the levels of individual substances in water are well within "allowable" limits, the total of all contaminants present may still be harmful to your health. And private wells may not be regulated at all, except at the local level.

The greatest concerns about water quality today focus on chlorine, arsenic, atrazine and other compounds known as triazenes, perchlorate, organophosphate pesticides, trihalomethanes, lead, herbicides such as acetochlor, and parasites. Chlorine has long been added to public water supplies to kill disease-causing bacteria. However, the levels of chlorine in drinking water today can be quite high, and some by-products of chlorine are known carcinogens. As a result, the U.S. Environmental Protection Agency (EPA) is considering steps to reduce the level of chlorine in drinking water, but is facing opposition from industry groups.

Pesticides pose a risk in any area where the tap water is extracted from an underground source. These chemicals are suspected of causing, or at least contributing to, an increased incidence of cancer, especially breast cancer. The pesticide problem is a particular concern in areas where agriculture is (or was) a major part of the economy. These chemicals are persistent. Residues from pesticides used decades ago may still be present in water coming out of the tap today, and may pose a risk to health.

Long considered a problem limited to poor, developing countries, the presence of bacteria and parasites in drinking water—especially a parasite called *cryptosporidium*—is becoming a serious problem in the United States. In April 1993, as many as 370,000 people in and around Milwaukee, Wisconsin, were stricken by the parasite *Cryptosporidium parvum* from the city's water supply. Thousands suffered from severe diarrhea, and up to 100 deaths were attributed to the outbreak. These "unacceptable" levels of cryptosporidia, most likely from agricultural runoff, forced users of the public water system to boil their tap water before using it. The same organism has created controversy over the safety of the water in New York City; many people with weakened immune systems have charged that cryptosporidia in the city water have made them sick, even though local officials insist that the water is safe to drink. For people with HIV or AIDS, cryptosporidia can be lethal.

The chlorine added to water to kill bacteria is not effective at killing these parasites. Like cryptosporidiosis, giardiasis is caused by an intestinal parasite and can be contracted through drinking water. And like cryptosporidia, giardia resists the effects of chlorine (outbreaks have occurred in areas where the water is routinely chlorine-treated) and poses a more serious problem for people with diminished immune response. Indeed, because of increasing concern over the danger contaminated drinking water poses for people with compromised immune systems, the U.S. Centers for Disease Control and Prevention (CDC) and the EPA have issued suggestions that immune-compromised individuals boil tap water for at least one minute before use, use an appropriate filtration system, or buy quality bottled drinking water.

The biggest problem is that even when municipalities comply with EPA regulations, the regulations themselves are weak and have been written in such a way that it is relatively easy to comply. For instance, there is no safe level for arsenic in drinking water, per se, according to recent studies. The EPA sets its limits based on the risk of developing cancer as 1 in every 10,000 people. This still may represent too great a risk for some people. Average levels of arsenic in drinking water are around 5 parts per billion (ppb). In 2002, the EPA upgraded the standard for arsenic from 50 to 10 ppb (the lower the amount the better the standard). The National Academy of Sciences has found that even at 10 ppb, the lifetime risk of developing life-threatening cancer is 1 in 333. This is thirty times higher than the EPA's own standard for what it says is acceptable risk. The good news about drinking city water is that the contaminants are published on the EPA website. With bottled water, you need to contact the manufacturer to get such information. The risk of getting sick may be lower with public water because more people become exposed and word gets out faster.

Whatever the source of your water, it is important to know some warning signs of bad water. Watch for cloudiness or murkiness in water. Chlorination can cause some cloudiness, but it usually clears if the water is left to stand, whereas bacterial or sedimentary cloudiness will remain. Foaming may be caused by bacterial contamination, by floating particles of sediment, or by soaps or detergents.

Bacteria can be destroyed by boiling water for at least five minutes, while sediment should settle out if you let the water stand for several hours. Strange smells or tastes in water that was previously fine could mean chemical contamination. However, many toxic hazards that work their way into water do not change its taste, smell, or appearance.

Hard versus Soft Water

Hard water, found in various parts of the country, contains relatively high concentrations of the minerals calcium and magnesium. The presence of these minerals prevents soap from lathering and results in filmy sediment being deposited on hair, clothing, pipes, dishes, washtubs, and anything else that comes into regular contact with the water. It also affects the taste. Hard water can be annoying, and though some studies have shown that deaths from heart disease may be lower in areas where the drinking water is hard, we believe that the calcium found in hard water is not good for the heart, arteries, or bones. Hard water deposits its calcium and other minerals on the *outside* of these structures, while it is the calcium and magnesium found *within* these structures that are beneficial to the body.

Soft water can be naturally soft or it may be hard water that has been treated to remove the calcium and magnesium. Standard water-softening systems work by using pressure to pass the water through exchange media to exchange "hard" calcium and magnesium ions for "soft" sodium or potassium ions. Most use either sodium chloride or potassium chloride for this purpose. The primary benefit of softening is in improved cleaning properties for the water and less mineral buildup inside household pipes and equipment. One potentially serious problem with artificially softened water is that it is more likely than hard water to dissolve the lining of pipes. This poses an especially significant threat if pipes are made of lead. Another threat comes from certain plastic and galvanized pipes, which contain cadmium, a toxic heavy metal. These types of pipes are rarely used in construction today, but they may be present in older buildings that have not undergone extensive renovation. But leaching from pipes can be a problem with today's copper pipes as well. Dangerous levels of copper, iron, zinc, and arsenic can leach into softened water from copper pipes. Another potential problem with artificially softened water is of concern to people with kidney failure. People with kidney failure must restrict their intake of potassium. Potassium-based water-softening systems can therefore pose a danger to such individuals.

Fluoridation

For many years now, controversy has raged over whether fluoride should be added to drinking water. As early as 1961, as recorded in the Congressional Record, fluoride was exposed as a lethal poison in our nation's water supply.

Proponents say that fluoride occurs naturally and helps develop and maintain strong bones and teeth. Opponents to fluoridation contend that when fluoridated water is consumed regularly, toxic levels of fluorine, the poisonous substance from which fluoride is derived, build up in the body, causing irreparable harm to the immune system. The Delaney Congressional Investigation Committee, the government body charged with monitoring additives and other substances in the food supply, has stated "fluoridation is mass medication without parallel in the history of medicine." Meanwhile, no convincing scientific proof has ever been generated that fluoridated water makes for stronger bones and teeth. It is known, however, that chronic fluoride use can result in health problems, including osteoporosis and osteomalacia, and also damages teeth and leaves them mottled. But this only occurs with very high doses. Fluorine is never found in elemental form in nature because it is so reactive. Numerous compounds of fluorine can, however, exist. These are notoriously toxic compounds, so much so that they are used in rat poison and insecticides. The naturally occurring form of fluoride, calcium fluoride, is not toxic—but this form of fluoride is not used to fluoridate water. Sodium fluoride (NaF) is added to city water supplies in the proportion of about one part per million to help prevent tooth decay. Sodium fluoride (NaF), stannous fluoride (SnF_2), and sodium monofluorophosphate (Na_2PO_3F) are also added to toothpaste, also to help prevent tooth decay.

Today, more than half the cities in the United States fluoridate their water supplies. In fact, in many states it is required. Although many ailments and disorders—including Down syndrome, mottled teeth, and cancer—have been linked to fluoridated water, fluoridation has become the standard rather than the exception.

Individuals have different levels of tolerance for toxins such as fluoride. In addition, many water sources have levels of fluoride higher than one part per million, the level generally recognized as safe and originally set as the acceptable limit by the EPA. After the EPA learned that water in many towns had natural fluoride levels much higher than this, the permissible fluoride limit was raised—quadrupled, in fact—to four parts per million. And this is in addition to fluoride encountered from other sources. Since so many local water supplies are fluoridated, there is a good chance that virtually any packaged food product made with water, such as soft drinks and reconstituted juices, contains fluoride. It is easy to see how many Americans may be ingesting excessive amounts of this potentially toxic substance.

If your tap water contains fluoride, and you wish to remove it, you can use a reverse osmosis, distillation, or activated alumina filtration system to eliminate almost all of the fluoride from your water.

MTBE and Drinking Water

Since 1979, methyl tertiary-butyl ether (MTBE) has been added to gasoline to increase its oxygen content. It took the place of lead as an octane enhancer, and was supposed to reduce the problems of both smog and carbon monoxide in the atmosphere. The Clean Air Act of 1990 required the use of reformulated gasoline, or RFG, in certain parts of the country, with the goal of reducing air pollution in those areas. RFG accounts for some 30 percent of gasoline sold in the United States, and MTBE is now added to over 80 percent of RFG fuel.

According to a disturbing report aired on the CBS television program *60 Minutes* on January 16, 2000, this measure to improve air quality has, ironically, given Americans yet another reason to be concerned about the safety of their drinking water supply. MTBE has been seeping into all our water supplies, both surface and underground, at an alarming rate. It has been found in storm water in 592 samples collected in sixteen cities between 1991 and 1995. The primary sources of the MTBE that ends up in water systems are leaking gasoline tanks, and reservoirs, drinking water lakes, and rivers where gasoline-powered recreational watercraft are permitted. Less than one-tenth of a gallon (roughly 12 ounces) of MTBE is capable of contaminating 13 million gallons of drinking water. It is estimated that more than 1 million gallons of fuel are deposited, un-burned, into the water supply each year as a result of recreational boating.

Few long-term studies have been done on this chemical, but what little research there is indicates that MTBE is a likely human carcinogen and immune-system depressant. Certainly, tests on rats have provided evidence that MTBE is a cancer-causing agent. To date, drinking water supplies in the states of California, New York, Maine, Pennsylvania, Connecticut, and Rhode Island have been closed down due to contamination by MTBE (boiling drinking water does not help purge it of this agent). MTBE-contaminated tap water can cause problems even if you do not drink it. This chemical can also be absorbed through the skin when showering and can be inhaled as a vapor in the air. Possible effects of inhaling MTBE include headaches, burning of the nose and throat, dizziness, nausea, asthma, and respiratory problems. The possible effects on wildlife have not yet been documented.

If you have a private well, your local health department may be able to tell you if MTBE has been found in your area. To get your water tested, call the EPA's Safe Drinking Water Hotline at 800-426-4791. The EPA still has not made a determination on the continued use of MTBE.

Water Analysis

Not all drinking water contains significant amounts of toxic substances. Some places rate higher in water safety than others. In addition, not all cities and towns process their water supplies the same way. Some do nothing at all to their water. Others add chemicals to the water to kill bacteria. Still others filter their water. It is up to the individual to find out how local drinking water is treated and to determine how safe the water coming out of the tap is.

The EPA has defined pure water as "bacteriologically safe" water, and it recommends—but does not require—that tap water have a pH between 6.5 and 8.5. This allows for a great deal of leeway in what passes as acceptable water. If you are concerned about the safety of the water coming out of your tap, you can contact your local water officials or local health department, which may test your tap water free of charge. In some cases, you may have to contact your state's water supply or health department. Typically, however, these agencies test the water only for bacteria levels, not for toxic substances. Therefore, you might want to contact a commercial laboratory or local state university laboratory to test your water for its chemical content. If you find that your tap water is unacceptable either because of its taste or because of its toxic chemical content, you may choose to use one of the alternative water supplies described in this section.

The Water Quality Association (*see* Health and Medical Organizations in the Appendix) is prepared to answer questions about the various types of water and methods of water treatment. In addition, the EPA operates the toll-free Safe Drinking Water Hotline, which can help you to locate an office or laboratory in your area that does certified water testing. There are also a number of laboratories that will send a self-addressed container for you to fill and return by mail for testing. Results are usually available in two to three weeks.

To help you understand the results of water testing, you should obtain information on the EPA's Recommended Maximum Contaminant Levels. This and other water quality information is available from NSF International at www.nsf.org or 800-673-6275.

Improving Tap Water

Tap water can be improved in several ways. Heating tap water to a rolling boil and keeping it there for three to five minutes will kill bacteria and parasites. However, most people find boiling their drinking water too impractical and time-consuming. In addition, this procedure has the effect of concentrating whatever lead is present in the water, and the water must then be refrigerated if it is to be used for drinking. The taste of chlorinated tap water can be improved by keeping the water in an uncovered pitcher for several hours to allow the chlorine taste and odor to dissipate.

Water can also be aerated in a blender to remove chlorine and other chemicals. Nevertheless, neither of these last two methods will improve the quality of the water—only the taste.

Filtration is a means by which contaminants in water are removed, rendering the water cleaner and better tasting. There are many different ways in which water can be filtered.

Nature filters water as the water runs through streams and as it seeps down through the soil and rocks to the water table. As water passes through the earth or over the rocks in a stream, the bacteria in the water leach into the rocks and are replaced with minerals such as calcium and magnesium.

There are also man-made ways of filtering water. There are three basic types of filter available:

- Absorbent types, which use materials such as carbon to pick up impurities.

- Microfiltration systems, which run water through filters with tiny pores to catch and eliminate contaminants (the filter may be made of any of a number of different materials).

- Special media such as ion-exchange resins that are designed to remove heavy metals.

Filters are often arranged in series, so that the filtering media that are most effective for specific types of contaminants can be used. The primary advantages of filters are relatively low cost and ease of use.

Water filtration systems vary in effectiveness. Two types that are considered good are reverse osmosis and ceramic filtration systems. In reverse osmosis filtering, the water is forced through a semipermeable membrane, while charged particles and larger molecules are repelled. It is the best system for treating water that is brackish (high in salt), high in nitrates, and loaded with inorganic heavy metals such as iron and lead. However, no filter can remove absolutely all contaminants. Each pore of even the finest filter is large enough for some viruses to permeate. To remove parasites such as cryptosporidia, the EPA and CDC recommend purchasing a filter that has an NSF rating for parasite reduction *and* that has an absolute pore size of one micron or smaller (a micron is 1310^{26} meter).

Other water treatment systems that remove various contaminants include distillers and ultraviolet treatment units. The latter are used to kill bacteria and viruses in water. Each treatment method has its advantages and disadvantages (*see* Home Water Treatment Methods, page 52). Costs can vary from under fifty dollars for faucet-mounted units to many thousands of dollars for whole-house reverse osmosis systems. Using a combination of methods can result in the best overall quality drinking water. Even

the quality and taste of distilled water can be improved by passing the water through a charcoal/carbon filter as a final step.

Before you purchase a water treatment unit, contact NSF International or the Water Quality Association. These nonprofit testing and certification organizations verify manufacturers' claims and certify that the materials used are nontoxic and structurally sound. They conduct periodic unannounced audits of the products they certify to ensure that the products still comply with standards.

BOTTLED WATER

Because of concerns over the safety and health effects of tap water, many people today are turning to bottled water. Bottled water is usually classified by its source (spring, spa, geyser, public water supply, etc.), by its mineral content (containing at least 250 parts per million of dissolved solids), and/or by the type of treatment it has undergone (deionized, steam-distilled, etc.). Because there is a lot of overlap, some water falls into more than one classification. In addition, most states have no rules governing appropriate labeling, so some bottled water claims may be misleading or incorrect. The biggest problem with bottled water is its threat to the environment from the improper disposal of the bottles. Only 20 percent of Americans recycle bottles. Americans drink 18 gallons of bottled water per capita. This equals 144 16-ounce bottles per person per year, which mostly goes to the garbage or incinerator. Incineration causes toxic by-products such as chloride gas and ash, containing heavy metals. Energy is needed to transport these empty bottles as well. If you use bottled water, buy it in bulk and transfer water to reusable containers.

While the EPA is charged with the regulation of public water supplies, it is the FDA that has responsibility for overseeing the quality and safety of bottled drinking water. Recently, there has been concern over the possible leaching of plastic particles into the water that comes in plastic bottles. Researchers from the Harvard School of Public Health found that people who drank from clear plastic polycarbonate bottles had an increase in bisphenol A (BPA) of 69 percent. BPA is used to make reusable hard plastic—such as those used in water cooler bottles—more durable. The harder the bottle, the more BPA in it. BPA is used in hundreds of everyday products. The health effects on adults are not well understood, though a recent large human study linked BPA concentrations in people's urine to an increased prevalence of diabetes, heart disease, and liver toxicity. For adults, most BPA is flushed from the body in a matter of hours. The real risk in terms of developing these diseases actually comes from what we eat and drink, not the BPA in the containers.

The FDA defined the terms used to describe bottled drinking waters in specific requirements in April 1997, making the choices for the consumer somewhat clearer than in the past. The FDA regulations for bottled water al-

Home Water Treatment Methods

Treatment Type	Configurations	How It Works	What It Does
Activated Carbon	Faucet-Mounted Pour-Through Countertop Under Sink Whole House	Water is filtered through a carbon trap that absorbs the contaminants.	Reduces levels of chlorine, herbicides, lead, hydrogen sulfide, and VOCs (volatile organic compounds). Also improves color and reduces turbidity.
Carbon Filtration	Faucet-Mounted Under Sink or Counter	Water is passed through charcoal granules or a solid block of charcoal that captures contaminants. When carbon is used up or plugged, cartridge is replaced.	Reduces levels of chlorine, organic chemicals, and pesticides. Improves taste and odor.
Distillation	Countertop Freestanding Whole House	Raises water temperature to boiling, leaving contaminants behind. Pure condensate is collected.	Reduces levels of arsenic, cadmium, chromium, iron, lead, giardia cysts, nitrates, and sulfates. Reduces turbidity.
Reverse Osmosis	Countertop Under Sink Whole House	Forces pressurized water through a semipermeable membrane and sends improved water to a holding tank.	Reduces levels of arsenic, cadmium, iron, chlorine, lead, giardia cysts, nitrates, sulfates, and radium. Reduces color and turbidity.
Water Softener	Whole House	Replaces calcium and magnesium with sodium to "soften" the water.	Reduces levels of calcium, magnesium, iron, and radium.

low for the various terms that have been defined to be used with one another if bottled water meets more than one definition, so it is possible for some water labels to include a number of different terms.

All the terms that are legally necessary to describe bottled drinking water are discussed in the paragraphs that follow. Any term you find on a label that is *not* defined or included here is a marketing slogan added to entice the consumer to buy the product. It can mean anything that the manufacturer of the product says it means.

Artesian Water

Artesian water, or artesian well water, is water drawn from a well where the water is brought to the surface by natural pressure or flow.

Bottled Water

Bottled water, or bottled drinking water, is water that is intended for human consumption and that is sealed in bottles or other containers with no added ingredients except for optional antimicrobial agents. These must be identified on the label. If bottled water comes from a community water system or from a municipal source, this information must appear on the label. About 25 percent of bottled waters now sold come from the same water supplies that flow into some areas' household taps.

Deionized or Demineralized Water

When the electric charge of a molecule of water has been neutralized by the addition or removal of electrons, the resulting water is called *deionized* or *demineralized*. The deionization process removes nitrates and the minerals calcium and magnesium, in addition to the heavy metals cadmium, barium, lead, mercury, and some forms of radium.

Ground Water

This is water that comes from underground, in the water table, that is under pressure equal to or greater than atmospheric pressure, and that does not come into contact with surface water. Ground water must be pumped mechanically for bottling.

Mineral Water

Mineral water is water containing not less than 250 parts per million total dissolved solids (TDS), originating from a geologically and physically protected underground water source or spring that has been tapped at the spring opening or through a borehole. Mineral water is distinguished from other types of water by constant levels and relative proportions of minerals and trace elements at its source, allowing for seasonal variations. No minerals may be added to this water. If the TDS content of mineral water is below 500 parts per million, the water may be labeled *low mineral content*. If it is greater than 1,500 parts per million, the label *high mineral content* may be used.

Depending on where the source is, the minerals the water contains will vary. If you are suffering from a deficiency of certain minerals and are drinking mineral water for therapeutic reasons, you must be aware of which minerals are in the particular brand of water you drink. If you are drinking mineral water containing minerals that you do not lack, you could be doing yourself more harm than good.

Most mineral waters are carbonated. However, some sparkling waters, such as club soda, are called mineral waters because the manufacturer added bicarbonates, citrates, and sodium phosphates to filtered or distilled tap water.

Natural Spring Water

The term *natural spring water* on a bottled water label doesn't tell you where the water came from, only that the mineral content of the water has not been altered. It may or may not have been filtered or otherwise treated. While the number of gallons of "natural spring water" flowing through watercoolers and from bottles has more than doubled in recent years, the meaning of these words on a label has been firmly defined only since the final changes in the FDA bottled drinking water regulations have been in place.

Spring water is water that comes from an underground formation from which water flows naturally to the surface of the earth. It must be collected at the spring or through a borehole tapping the underground formation that feeds the spring. To meet the definition of *spring*, there must be natural force bringing the water to the surface opening. The location of the spring must be identified on the label of any water labeled as spring water.

If you use a watercooler for bottled spring water, you should be sure to clean the cooler once a month to destroy bacteria. Run a 50-50 mixture of hydrogen peroxide and baking soda through the reservoir and spigots, then remove the residue by rinsing the cooler with four or more gallons of tap water.

Sparkling Water

This is bottled water that contains the same amount of carbon dioxide that it had at emergence from the water source. It can be a healthful alternative to soda and alcoholic beverages, but if it is loaded with fructose and other sweeteners, it may be no better than soda pop. Read labels before you buy. Soda water, seltzer water, and tonic water are *not* considered bottled waters. They are regulated separately, may contain sugar and calories, and are considered soft drinks.

Understanding where the carbonation in sparkling water comes from isn't always easy. So-called naturally sparkling water must get its carbonation from the same source as the water. If water is labeled *carbonated natural water*, that means the carbonation came from a source other than the one that supplied the water. That doesn't mean the water is of poor quality. It can still be called natural because its mineral content is the same as when it came from the ground, even though it has been carbonated from a separate source. People suffering from intestinal disorders or ulcers should avoid drinking carbonated water because it may be irritating to the gastrointestinal tract.

Steam-Distilled Water

Distillation involves vaporizing water by boiling it. The steam rises, leaving behind most of the bacteria, viruses, chemicals, minerals, and pollutants from the water. The steam is then moved into a condensing chamber, where it is cooled and condensed to become distilled water.

Once consumed, steam-distilled water leaches inorganic minerals rejected by the cells and tissues out of the body.

We believe that only steam-distilled or reverse-osmosis-filtered water should be consumed. This water should be used not only for drinking, but also for cooking, because foods such as pasta, rice, and beans can absorb chemicals found in unpurified water.

Flavor can be added to distilled water by adding 1 to 2 tablespoons of raw apple cider vinegar (obtained from a health food store) per gallon of distilled water. Vinegar is an excellent solvent and aids in digestion. Lemon juice is another good flavoring agent, and has cleansing properties as well. For added minerals, you can add mineral drops to steam-distilled water. Concentrace from Trace Minerals Research is a good product for this purpose. Add 1¼ teaspoons of mineral drops to every 5 gallons of water.

Amino Acids

INTRODUCTION

Amino acids are the chemical units, or "building blocks," as they are popularly called, that make up proteins. They also are the end products of protein digestion, or *hydrolysis*.

Amino acids contain about 16 percent nitrogen. Chemically, this is what distinguishes them from the other two basic nutrients, sugars and fatty acids, which do not contain nitrogen.

To understand how vital amino acids are, you must understand how essential proteins are to life. It is protein that provides the structure for all living things. Every living organism, from the largest animal to the tiniest microbe, is composed of protein. In its various forms, protein participates in the vital chemical processes that sustain life.

Proteins are a necessary part of every living cell in the body. Next to water, protein makes up the greatest portion of our body weight. In the human body, protein substances make up the muscles, ligaments, tendons, organs, glands, nails, hair, and many vital body fluids, and are essential for the growth of bones. The enzymes and hormones that catalyze and regulate all bodily processes are proteins. Proteins help to regulate the body's water balance and maintain the proper internal pH. They assist in the exchange of nutrients between the intercellular fluids and the tissues, blood, and lymph. A deficiency of protein can upset the body's fluid balance, causing edema. Proteins form the structural basis of chromosomes, through which genetic information is passed from parents to offspring. The genetic "code" contained in each cell's DNA is actually information for how to make that cell's proteins.

Proteins are chains of amino acids linked together by what are called *peptide bonds*. Each individual type of protein is composed of a specific group of amino acids in a specific chemical arrangement. It is the particular amino acids present and the way in which they are linked together in sequence that gives the proteins that make up the various tissues their unique functions and characters. Each protein in the body is tailored for a specific need; proteins are not interchangeable.

The proteins that make up the human body are not obtained directly from the diet. Rather, dietary protein is broken down into its constituent amino acids, which the body then uses to build the specific proteins it needs. Thus, it is the amino acids rather than protein that are the essential nutrients.

In addition to those that combine to form the body's proteins, there are other amino acids that are important in metabolic functions. Some, such as citrulline, glutathione, ornithine, and taurine, can be similar to (or by-products of) the protein-building amino acids. Some act as neurotransmitters or as precursors of neurotransmitters, the chemicals that carry information from one nerve cell to another. Certain amino acids are thus necessary for the brain to receive and send messages. Unlike many other substances, neurotransmitters are able to pass through the *blood-brain barrier*. This is a kind of defensive shield designed to protect the brain from toxins and foreign invaders that may be circulating in the bloodstream. The endothelial cells that make up the walls of the capillaries in the brain are much more tightly meshed together than are those of capillaries elsewhere in the body. This prevents many substances, especially water-based substances, from diffusing through the capillary walls into brain tissue. Because certain amino acids can pass through this barrier, they can be used by the brain to communicate with nerve cells elsewhere in the body.

Amino acids also enable vitamins and minerals to perform their jobs properly. Even if vitamins and minerals are absorbed and assimilated by the body, they cannot be effective unless the necessary amino acids are present. For example, low levels of the amino acid tyrosine may lead to iron deficiency. Deficiency and/or impaired metabolism of the amino acids methionine and taurine has been linked to allergies and autoimmune disorders. Many elderly people suffer from depression or neurological problems that may be associated with deficiencies of the amino acids tyrosine, tryptophan, phenylalanine, and histidine, and also of the *branched-chain amino acids*—valine, isoleucine, and leucine.

These are amino acids that can be used to provide energy directly to muscle tissue. High doses of branched-chain amino acids have been used in hospitals to treat people suffering from trauma and infection. Some people are born with an inability to metabolize the branched-chain amino acids. This potentially life-threatening condition, branched-chain ketoaciduria (often referred to as *maple syrup urine disease* because keto acids released into the urine cause it to smell like maple syrup), can result in neurological damage and necessitates a special diet, including a synthetic infant formula that does not contain leucine, isoleucine, or valine.

There are approximately twenty-eight commonly known amino acids that are combined in various ways to create the hundreds of different types of proteins present in all living things. In the human body, the liver produces about 80 percent of the amino acids needed. The remaining 20 percent must be obtained from the diet. These are called the *essential amino acids.* The essential amino acids that must enter the body through diet are histidine, isoleucine, leucine, lysine, methionine, phenylalanine, threonine, tryptophan, and valine. Although infants need to obtain histidine from their diet, most adult bodies can make enough. The *nonessential amino acids,* which can be manufactured in the body from other amino acids obtained from dietary sources, include alanine, arginine, asparagine, aspartic acid, citrulline, cysteine, cystine, gamma-aminobutyric acid, glutamic acid, glutamine, glycine, ornithine, proline, serine, taurine, and tyrosine.

The fact that they are termed *nonessential* does not mean that they are not necessary, only that they need not be obtained through the diet because the body can manufacture them as needed. Nonessential amino acids can indeed become essential under certain conditions. For instance, the nonessential amino acids cysteine and tyrosine are made from the essential amino acids methionine and phenylalanine. If methionine and phenylalanine are not available in sufficient quantities, cysteine and tyrosine then become essential in the diet. Also, in times of stress such as an illness, both arginine and glutamine are considered to be "conditionally essential." Hospitalized patients have benefitted from amino acid supplements of each to enhance the functioning of their immune systems. Arginine is popular with body builders, who claim they feel a rush of blood flow, which helps them lift heavier weights.

The processes of assembling amino acids to make proteins, and of breaking down proteins into individual amino acids for the body's use, are continuous ones. When we need more enzyme proteins, the body produces more enzyme proteins; when we need more cells, the body produces more proteins for cells. These different types of proteins are produced as the need arises. Should the body become depleted of its reserves of any of the essential amino acids, it would not be able to produce the proteins that require those amino acids. An inadequate supply of even one essential amino acid can hinder the synthesis, and reduce body levels, of necessary proteins. This can result in negative nitrogen balance, an unhealthy condition in which the body excretes more nitrogen than it assimilates. Further, *all* of the essential amino acids must be present simultaneously in the diet in order for the other amino acids to be utilized—otherwise, the body remains in negative nitrogen balance. A lack of vital proteins in the body can cause problems ranging from indigestion to depression to stunted growth.

How could such a situation occur? More easily than you might think. Many factors can contribute to deficiencies of essential amino acids, even if you eat a well-balanced diet that contains enough protein. Impaired absorption, infection, trauma, stress, drug use, age, and imbalances of other nutrients can all affect the availability of essential amino acids in the body. Insufficient intake of vitamins and minerals, especially vitamin C, can interfere with the absorption of amino acids in the lower part of the small intestines. Vitamin B_6 is needed also, for the transport of amino acids in the body.

If your diet is not properly balanced—that is, if it fails to supply adequate amounts of the essential amino acids—sooner or later, this will become apparent as some type of physical disorder. When the brain senses the lack of any of the essential amino acids, it immediately sends a signal to the muscles to release some of their tissue. Human muscle is rich in essential amino acids, so it can support the vital organs like the liver and heart during times of poor intake. Sometimes in the case of cancer patients who are unable to eat, a massive muscle wasting called cachexia will occur. This condition can be reversed with food, but it takes a long time.

This does not mean, however, that eating a diet containing enormous amounts of protein is the answer. In fact, it is unhealthy to consume a diet that is deficient in protein or one that contains too much. Excess protein puts undue stress on the kidneys and the liver, which are faced with processing the waste products of protein metabolism. Nearly half of the amino acids in dietary protein are transformed into glucose by the liver and utilized to provide needed energy to the cells. This process results in a waste product, ammonia. Ammonia is toxic to the body, so the body protects itself by having the liver turn the ammonia into a much less toxic compound, urea, which is then carried through the bloodstream, filtered out by the kidneys, and excreted.

As long as protein intake is not too great and the liver is working properly, ammonia is neutralized almost as soon as it is produced, so it does no harm. However, if there is too much ammonia for the liver to cope with—as a result of too much protein consumption, poor digestion, and/or a defect in liver function—toxic levels may accumulate.

Strenuous exercise also tends to promote the accumulation of excess ammonia. This may put a person at risk for serious health problems, including encephalopathy (brain disease) or hepatic coma. Abnormally high levels of urea can also cause problems, including inflamed kidneys and back pain. (*See* NUTRITION, DIET, AND WELLNESS in Part One.)

It is possible to take supplements containing amino acids, both essential and nonessential. For certain disorders, taking supplements of specific amino acids can be very beneficial. When you take a specific amino acid or amino acid combination, it supports the metabolic pathway involved in your particular illness. Vegetarians, especially vegans, would be wise to take a formula containing all of the essential amino acids to ensure that their protein requirements are met.

WHAT'S ON THE SHELVES

Supplemental amino acids are available in combination with various multivitamin formulas, as protein mixtures, in a wide variety of food supplements, and in a number of amino acid formulas. They can be purchased as capsules, tablets, liquids, and powders. Most amino acid supplements are derived from animal protein, yeast protein, or vegetable protein. Crystalline free form amino acids are generally extracted from a variety of grain products. Brown rice bran is a prime source, although cold-pressed yeast and milk proteins are also used.

Free form means the amino acid is in its purest form. Free form amino acids need no digestion and are absorbed directly into the bloodstream. These white crystalline amino acids are stable at room temperature and decompose when heated to temperatures of 350°F to 660°F (180°C to 350°C). They are rapidly absorbed and do not come from potentially allergenic food sources. For best results, choose encapsulated powders or powder.

When choosing amino acid supplements, look for products that contain USP (U.S. Pharmacopeia) pharmaceutical-grade L-crystalline amino acids. A good company is Ajinomoto. It manufactures amino acids for intravenous use as well as orally for the public. Most of the amino acids (except for glycine) can appear in two forms, the chemical structure of one being the mirror image of the other. These are called the D- and L- forms—for example, D-cystine and L-cystine. The "D" stands for *dextro* (Latin for "right") and the "L" for *levo* (Latin for "left"); these terms denote the direction of the rotation of the spiral that is the chemical structure of the molecule. Proteins in animal and plant tissue are made from the L- forms of amino acids (with the exception of phenylalanine, which is also used in the form of DL-phenylalanine, a mixture of the D- and L- forms). Thus, with respect to supplements of amino acids, products containing the L- forms of amino acids are considered to be more compatible with human biochemistry.

Each amino acid has specific functions in the body. The many functions and possible symptoms of deficiency of twenty-eight amino acids and related compounds are described below. When taking amino acids individually for healing purposes, take them on an empty stomach to avoid making them compete for absorption with the amino acids present in foods. When taking individual amino acids, it is best to take them in the morning or between meals, with small amounts of vitamin B_6 and vitamin C to enhance absorption.

When taking an amino acid complex that includes all of the essential amino acids, it is best to take it a half hour away from a meal, either before or after. If you are taking individual amino acids, it is wise also to take a full amino acid complex, including both essential and nonessential amino acids, at a different time. This is the best way to assure you have adequate amounts of all the necessary amino acids.

Be aware that individual amino acids should not be taken for long periods of time. A good rule to follow is to alternate the individual amino acids that fit your needs and back them up with an amino acid complex, taking the supplements for two months and then discontinuing them for two months. Moderation is the key. Some amino acids have potentially toxic effects when taken in high doses (over 6,000 milligrams per day) and may cause neurological damage. These include aspartic acid, glutamic acid, homocysteine, serine, and tryptophan. Cysteine can be toxic if taken in amounts over 1,000 milligrams per day. Do not give supplemental amino acids to a child, or take doses of any amino acid in excess of the amount recommended unless specifically directed to do so by your health care provider.

Some recommended amino acid products include the following:

- A/G-Pro from Miller Pharmacal Group, a complete amino acid and mineral supplement.

- Anabolic Amino Balance and Muscle Octane from Anabol Naturals. Anabolic Amino Balance is a complex of twenty-three free form amino acids. Muscle Octane is a blend of free form branched-chain amino acids (L-leucine, L-valine, and L-isoleucine). Anabol Naturals also produces free form single amino acids.

- Super Daily Amino Blend from Carlson Laboratories, a complex containing twenty amino acids, both essential and nonessential.

THE ABCs OF AMINO ACIDS

Alanine

Alanine plays a major role in the transfer of nitrogen from peripheral tissue to the liver. It aids in the metabolism of glucose, a simple carbohydrate that the body uses for energy.

Alanine also guards against the buildup of toxic substances that are released in the muscle cells when muscle protein is broken down to meet energy needs quickly, such as happens with aerobic exercise. Epstein-Barr virus and chronic fatigue syndrome have been associated with excessive alanine levels and low levels of tyrosine and phenylalanine. One form of alanine, beta-alanine, is a constituent of pantothenic acid (vitamin B_5) and coenzyme A, a vital catalyst in the body.

Research has found that for people with insulin-dependent diabetes, taking an oral dose of L-alanine can be more effective than a conventional bedtime snack in preventing nighttime hypoglycemia.

Arginine

Arginine retards the growth of tumors and cancer by enhancing immune function. It increases the size and activity of the thymus gland, which manufactures T lymphocytes (T cells), crucial components of the immune system. Arginine may therefore benefit those suffering from AIDS and malignant diseases that suppress the immune system. It is also good for liver disorders such as cirrhosis of the liver and fatty liver; it aids in liver detoxification by neutralizing ammonia. It may also reduce the effects of chronic alcohol toxicity.

Seminal fluid contains arginine. Studies suggest that sexual maturity may be delayed by arginine deficiency; conversely, arginine is useful in treating sterility in men. It is found in high concentrations in the skin and connective tissues, making it helpful for healing and repair of damaged tissue.

Arginine is important for muscle metabolism. It helps to maintain a proper nitrogen balance by acting as a vehicle for transportation and storage, and aiding in the excretion, of excess nitrogen. Studies have shown that it also reduces nitrogen losses in people who have undergone surgery, and improves the function of cells in lymphatic tissue. This amino acid aids in weight loss because it facilitates an increase in muscle mass and a reduction of body fat. It is also involved in a variety of enzymes and hormones. It aids in stimulating the pancreas to release insulin, is a component of the pituitary hormone vasopressin, and assists in the release of growth hormones. Because arginine is a component of collagen and aids in building new bone and tendon cells, it can be good for arthritis and connective tissue disorders.

Scar tissue that forms during wound healing is made up of collagen, which is rich in arginine. A variety of functions, including insulin production, glucose tolerance, and liver lipid metabolism, are impaired if the body is deficient in arginine.

This amino acid can be produced in the body; however, in newborn infants, production may not occur quickly enough to keep up with requirements. It is therefore deemed essential early in life. Foods high in arginine include carob, chocolate, coconut, dairy products, gelatin, meat, oats, peanuts, soybeans, walnuts, white flour, wheat, and wheat germ. Eating watermelon can increase plasma arginine levels because watermelon is rich in citrulline, which is a precursor to arginine. Some people who engage in strength-training activities might want to increase nitric oxide levels to increase blood flow and enhance performance. One study showed that taking 3 grams of arginine a day with a protein supplement slightly increased nitric oxide production and did not cause harm.

People with viral infections such as herpes should *not* take supplemental arginine, and should avoid foods rich in arginine and low in the amino acid lysine (see page 62), as this appears to promote the growth of certain viruses. Pregnant and lactating women should avoid L-arginine supplements. Persons with schizophrenia should avoid amounts over 30 milligrams daily. Long-term use, especially of high doses, is not recommended. One study found that several weeks of large doses might result in thickening and coarsening of the skin.

Asparagine

Asparagine, created from another amino acid, aspartic acid, is needed to maintain balance in the central nervous system; it prevents you from being either overly nervous or overly calm. As it is converted back into aspartic acid, asparagine releases energy that brain and nervous system cells use for metabolism. It promotes the process by which one amino acid is transformed into another in the liver.

Aspartic Acid

Because aspartic acid increases stamina, it is good for fatigue and depression, and plays a vital role in metabolism. Chronic fatigue syndrome may result from low levels of aspartic acid, because this leads to lowered cellular energy. In proper balance, aspartic acid is beneficial for neural and brain disorders; it has been found in increased levels in persons with epilepsy and in decreased levels in people with some types of depression. It is good for athletes and helps to protect the liver by aiding in the removal of excess ammonia.

Aspartic acid combines with other amino acids to form molecules that absorb toxins and remove them from the bloodstream. It also helps to move certain minerals across the intestinal lining and into the blood and cells, aids cell function, and aids the function of RNA and DNA, which are the carriers of genetic information. It enhances the production of immunoglobulins and antibodies (immune system proteins). Plant protein, especially that found in sprouting seeds, contains an abundance of aspartic acid. The artificial sweetener aspartame is made from aspartic acid and phenylalanine, another amino acid.

Carnitine

Carnitine is not an amino acid in the strictest sense (it is actually a substance related to the B vitamins). However, because it has a chemical structure similar to that of amino acids, it is usually considered together with them.

Unlike true amino acids, carnitine is not used for protein synthesis or as a neurotransmitter. Its main function in the body is to help transport long-chain fatty acids, which are burned within the cells, mainly in the mitochondria, to provide energy. This is a major source of energy for the muscles. Carnitine thus increases the use of fat as an energy source. This prevents fatty buildup, especially in the heart, liver, and skeletal muscles. Carnitine may be useful in treating chronic fatigue syndrome (CFS), because a disturbance in the function of the mitochondria (the site of energy production within the cells) may be a factor in fatigue. Studies have shown decreased carnitine levels in many people with CFS.

Carnitine reduces the health risks posed by poor fat metabolism associated with diabetes; inhibits alcohol-induced fatty liver; and lessens the risk of heart disorders.

Studies have shown that damage to the heart from cardiac surgery can be reduced by treatment with carnitine. According to *The American Journal of Cardiology*, one study showed that proprionyl-L-carnitine, a carnitine derivative, helps to ease the severe pain of intermittent claudication, a condition in which a blocked artery in the thigh decreases the supply of blood and oxygen to leg muscles, causing pain, especially with physical activity. Carnitine has the ability to lower blood triglyceride levels, aid in weight loss, improve the motility of sperm, and improve muscle strength in people with neuromuscular disorders. It may be useful in treating Alzheimer's disease. Conversely, carnitine deficiency may be a contributor to certain types of muscular dystrophy, and it has been shown that these disorders lead to losses of carnitine in the urine. People with such conditions need greater-than-normal amounts of carnitine. Carnitine has also been shown to reduce fatigue, which is common in many diseases. In studies, people with celiac disease (an autoimmune disorder of the small intestine) and people with cancer had more energy with carnitine supplementation.

Carnitine also enhances the effectiveness of the antioxidant vitamins E and C. It works with antioxidants to help slow the aging process by promoting the synthesis of carnitine acetyl-transferase, an enzyme in the mitochondria of brain cells that is vital for the production of cellular energy there. Supplemental carnitine has been shown to reduce damage to the bad cholesterol, LDL, in patients with type 2 diabetes. This shows that carnitine is effective at limiting the oxidative stress that is common in diabetes and many other conditions.

The body can manufacture carnitine if sufficient amounts of iron, vitamin B_1 (thiamine), vitamin B_6 (pyridoxine), and the amino acids lysine and methionine are available. The synthesis of carnitine also depends on the presence of adequate levels of vitamin C. Inadequate intake of any of these nutrients can result in a carnitine deficiency. Carnitine can also be obtained from food, primarily meats and other foods of animal origin.

Many cases of carnitine deficiency have been identified as partly genetic in origin, resulting from an inherited defect in carnitine synthesis. Possible symptoms of deficiency include confusion, heart pain, muscle weakness, and obesity.

Because of their generally greater muscle mass, men need more carnitine than do women. Vegetarians are more likely than nonvegetarians to be deficient in carnitine because it is not found in vegetable protein. Moreover, neither methionine nor lysine, two of the key constituents from which the body makes carnitine, are obtainable from vegetable sources in sufficient amounts. To ensure adequate production of carnitine, vegetarians should take supplements or should eat grains, such as cornmeal, that have been fortified with lysine.

Supplemental carnitine is available in different forms, including D-carnitine, L-carnitine, and DL-carnitine. DL-carnitine is not recommended, as it may cause toxicity.

Acetyl-L-carnitine (ALC), a carnitine derivative produced naturally in the body, is involved in carbohydrate and protein metabolism and in the transport of fats into the mitochondria. It increases levels of carnitine in tissues and even surpasses the metabolic potency of carnitine. ALC has become one of the most studied compounds for its antiaging effects, particularly with regard to degeneration of the brain and nervous system. Several major studies have shown that daily supplementation with ALC significantly slows the progression of Alzheimer's disease, resulting in less deterioration in memory, attention and language, and spatial abilities.

It also can be used to treat other cognitive disorders, as well as depression. ALC provides numerous other benefits to many of the body's systems. It helps to limit damage caused by oxygen starvation, enhance the immune system, protect against oxidative stress, stimulate the antioxidant activity of certain enzymes, protect membranes, slow cerebral aging, prevent nerve disease associated with diabetes and sciatica, modulate hormonal changes caused by physical stress, and increase the performance-enhancing benefits of branched-chain amino acids.

Total brain levels of ALC (and carnitine) decline with age. In most of the studies of ALC done with humans, subjects took 500 to 2,500 milligrams daily, in divided doses. No toxic or serious side effects have been reported.

Carnosine

L-carnosine is a dipeptide composed of two bonded amino acids—alanine and histidine. It is found naturally in the body, particularly in brain tissue, the heart, skin, muscles, kidneys, and stomach. Carnosine levels in the body decline with age. This compound has the ability to help prevent glycosylation, the cross linking of proteins with sugars to form advanced glycosylation end products, or AGEs. This effect may be beneficial for combating diabetes, kidney failure, neuropathy, and aging in general.

To date, no serious side effects have been noted in trials. The normal oral dose is 100 to 500 milligrams daily (with occasional breaks). Avoid megadosing. This is the oral form, not the eyedrop form used in Russia for cataract treatment (that is N-alpha-acetylcarnosine).

Citrulline

The body makes citrulline from another amino acid, ornithine. Citrulline promotes energy, stimulates the immune system, is metabolized to form L-arginine, and detoxifies ammonia, which damages living cells. Citrulline is found primarily in the liver. It is helpful in treating fatigue.

Cysteine and Cystine

These two amino acids are closely related; each molecule of cystine consists of two molecules of cysteine joined together.

Cysteine is very unstable and is easily converted to L-cystine; however, each form is capable of converting into the other as needed. Both are sulfur-containing amino acids that aid in the formation of skin and are important in detoxification.

Cysteine is present in alpha-keratin, the chief protein constituent of the fingernails, toenails, skin, and hair. Cysteine aids in the production of collagen and promotes the proper elasticity and texture of the skin. It is also found in a variety of other proteins in the body, including several of the digestive enzymes.

Cysteine helps to detoxify harmful toxins and protect the body from radiation damage. It is one of the best free radical destroyers, and works best when taken with selenium and vitamin E. Cysteine is also a precursor to glutathione, a substance that detoxifies the liver by binding with potentially harmful substances there. It helps to protect the liver and brain from damage due to alcohol, drugs, and toxic compounds in cigarette smoke.

Since cysteine is more soluble than cystine, it is used more readily in the body and is usually best for treating most illnesses. This amino acid is formed from L-methionine in the body. Vitamin B_6, vitamin B_{12}, and folate are necessary for cysteine synthesis, which may not take place as it should in the presence of chronic disease. Therefore, people with chronic illnesses may need higher-than-normal doses of cysteine, as much as 1,000 milligrams three times daily for a month at a time.

Supplementation with L-cysteine is recommended in the treatment of rheumatoid arthritis, hardening of the arteries, and mutogenic disorders such as cancer. It promotes healing after surgery and severe burns, chelates heavy metals, and binds with soluble iron, aiding in iron absorption. This amino acid also promotes the burning of fat and the building of muscle. Because of its ability to break down mucus in the respiratory tract, L-cysteine is often beneficial in the treatment of bronchitis, emphysema, and tuberculosis. It promotes healing from respiratory disorders and plays an important role in the activity of white blood cells, which fight disease.

Cystine or the N-acetyl form of cysteine (N-acetylcysteine, or NAC) may be used in place of L-cysteine. NAC aids in preventing side effects from chemotherapy and radiation therapy. Because it increases glutathione levels in the lungs, kidneys, liver, and bone marrow, it has an antiaging effect on the body—reducing the accumulation of age spots, for example. NAC has been shown to be more effective at boosting glutathione levels than supplements of cystine or even of glutathione itself.

People who have diabetes should be cautious about taking supplemental cysteine because it is capable of inactivating insulin. Persons with cystinuria, a rare genetic condition that leads to the formation of cystine kidney stones, also should not take cysteine.

Gamma-Aminobutyric Acid

Gamma-aminobutyric acid (GABA) is an amino acid that acts as a neurotransmitter in the central nervous system. It is essential for brain metabolism, aiding in proper brain function. GABA is formed in the body from another amino acid, glutamic acid. Its function is to decrease neuron activity and inhibit nerve cells from overfiring. Together with niacinamide and inositol, it prevents anxiety- and stress-related messages from reaching the motor centers of the brain by occupying their receptor sites.

GABA can be taken to calm the body in much the same way as diazepam (Valium), chlordiazepoxide (Librium), and other tranquilizers, but without the fear of addiction. It has been used in the treatment of epilepsy and hypertension.

GABA is good for depressed sex drive because of its ability as a relaxant. It is also useful for enlarged prostate glands, probably because it plays a role in the mechanism regulating the release of sex hormones. GABA is effective in treating attention deficit disorder and may reduce cravings for alcohol. It is also thought to promote growth hormone secretion.

Too much GABA, however, can cause increased anxiety, shortness of breath, numbness around the mouth, and tingling in the extremities. Further, abnormal levels of GABA unbalance the brain's message-delivery system and may cause seizures.

Glutamic Acid

Glutamic acid is an excitatory neurotransmitter that increases the firing of neurons in the central nervous system. It is a major excitatory neurotransmitter in the brain and spinal cord. It is converted into either glutamine or GABA.

This amino acid is important in the metabolism of sugars and fats, and aids in the transportation of potassium into the spinal fluid and across the blood-brain barrier. Although it does not pass the blood-brain barrier as readily as glutamine does, it is found at high levels in the blood and may infiltrate the brain in small amounts. The brain can use glutamic acid as fuel. Glutamic acid can detoxify ammonia by picking up nitrogen atoms, in the process creating another amino acid, glutamine. The conversion of glutamic acid into glutamine is the only means by which ammonia in the brain can be detoxified.

Glutamic acid helps to correct personality disorders and is useful in treating childhood behavioral disorders. It is used in the treatment of epilepsy, mental retardation, muscular dystrophy, ulcers, and hypoglycemic coma, a complication of insulin treatment for diabetes. It is a component of folate (folic acid), a B vitamin that helps the body break down amino acids. Because one of its salts is monosodium glutamate (MSG), glutamic acid should be avoided by anyone who is allergic to MSG.

Glutamine

Glutamine is the most abundant free amino acid found in the muscles of the body. Because it can readily pass the blood-brain barrier, it is known as brain fuel. In the brain, glutamine is converted into glutamic acid—which is essential for cerebral function—and vice versa. It also increases the amount of GABA, which is needed to sustain proper brain function and mental activity. It assists in maintaining the proper acid/alkaline balance in the body, and is the basis of the building blocks for the synthesis of RNA and DNA. It promotes mental ability and the maintenance of a healthy digestive tract.

When an amino acid is broken down, nitrogen is released. The body needs nitrogen, but free nitrogen can form ammonia, which is especially toxic to brain tissues. The liver can convert nitrogen into urea, which is excreted in the urine, or nitrogen may attach itself to glutamic acid. This process forms glutamine. Glutamine is unique among the amino acids in that each molecule contains not one nitrogen atom but two. Thus, its creation helps to clear ammonia from the tissues, especially brain tissue, and it can transfer nitrogen from one place to another.

Glutamine is found in large amounts in the muscles and is readily available when needed for the synthesis of skeletal muscle proteins. Because this amino acid helps to build and maintain muscle, supplemental glutamine is useful for dieters and bodybuilders. More important, it helps to prevent the kind of muscle wasting that can accompany prolonged bed rest or diseases such as cancer and AIDS. This is because stress and injury (including surgical trauma) cause the muscles to release glutamine into the bloodstream. In addition, glutamine helps strengthen the lining of the intestinal tract, so that nutrients are more efficiently absorbed. This is important for wasting diseases such as cancer.

In fact, during times of stress, as much as one third of the glutamine present in the muscles may be released. As a result, stress and/or illness can lead to the loss of skeletal muscle. If enough glutamine is available, however, this can be prevented.

Supplemental L-glutamine can be helpful in the treatment of arthritis, autoimmune diseases, fibrosis, intestinal disorders, peptic ulcers, connective tissue diseases such as polymyositis and scleroderma, and tissue damage due to radiation treatment for cancer. L-glutamine can enhance mental functioning and has been used to treat a range of problems, including developmental disabilities, epilepsy, fatigue, impotence, depression, schizophrenia, and senility.

It preserves glutathione in the liver and protects that organ from the effects of acetaminophen overdose. It enhances antioxidant protection. L-glutamine decreases sugar cravings and the desire for alcohol, and is useful for recovering alcoholics.

Many plant and animal substances contain glutamine, but cooking easily destroys it. If eaten raw, spinach and parsley are good sources. Supplemental glutamine must be kept absolutely dry or the powder will degrade into ammonia and pyroglutamic acid. Glutamine should *not* be taken by persons with cirrhosis of the liver, kidney problems, Reye's syndrome, or any type of disorder that can result in an accumulation of ammonia in the blood. For such individuals, taking supplemental glutamine may only

cause further damage to the body. Be aware that although the names sound similar, glutamine, glutamic acid (also sometimes called glutamate), glutathione, gluten, and monosodium glutamate are all different substances.

Glutathione

Like carnitine, glutathione is not technically one of the amino acids. It is a compound classified as a tripeptide, and the body produces it from the amino acids cysteine, glutamic acid, and glycine. Because of its close relationship to these amino acids, however, it is usually considered together with them.

Glutathione is a powerful antioxidant that is produced in the liver. The largest stores of glutathione are found in the liver, where it detoxifies harmful compounds so that they can be excreted through the bile. Some glutathione is released from the liver directly into the bloodstream, where it helps to maintain the integrity of red blood cells and protect white blood cells. Glutathione is also found in the lungs and the intestinal tract. It is needed for carbohydrate metabolism and appears to exert antiaging effects, aiding in the breakdown of oxidized fats that may contribute to atherosclerosis.

It can mitigate some of the damage caused by tobacco smoke because it modifies the harmful effects of aldehydes, chemicals present in cigarette smoke that damage cells and molecules, and it may protect the liver from alcohol-induced damage.

A deficiency of glutathione first affects the nervous system, causing such symptoms as lack of coordination, mental disorders, tremors, and difficulty maintaining balance. These problems are believed to be due to the development of lesions in the brain. A study sponsored in part by the National Cancer Institute found that people with HIV disease who had low glutathione levels had a lower survival rate over a three-year period than those whose glutathione levels were normal. As we age, glutathione levels decline, although it is not known whether this is because we use it more rapidly or produce less of it to begin with. Unfortunately, if not corrected, the lack of glutathione in turn accelerates the aging process.

Supplemental glutathione is expensive, and the effectiveness of oral formulas is questionable. To raise glutathione levels, it is better to supply the body with the raw materials it uses to make this compound: cysteine, glutamic acid, and glycine. The N-acetyl form of cysteine, N-acetylcysteine (NAC), is considered particularly effective for this purpose.

Glycine

Glycine retards muscle degeneration by supplying additional creatine, a compound that is present in muscle tissue and is utilized in the construction of DNA and RNA. It improves glycogen storage, thus freeing up glucose for energy needs. It is essential for the synthesis of nucleic acids, bile acids, and other nonessential amino acids in the body.

Glycine is used in many gastric antacid agents. Because high concentrations of glycine are found in the skin and connective tissues, it is useful for repairing damaged tissues and promoting healing.

Glycine is necessary for central nervous system function and a healthy prostate. It functions as an inhibitory neurotransmitter and as such can help prevent epileptic seizures. It has been used in the treatment of manic (bipolar) depression, and can also be effective for hyperactivity.

Having too much of this amino acid in the body can cause fatigue, but having the proper amount produces more energy. If necessary, glycine can be converted into the amino acid serine in the body.

Histidine

Histidine is an essential amino acid that is significant in the growth and repair of tissues. It is important for the maintenance of the myelin sheaths, which protect nerve cells, and is needed for the production of both red and white blood cells. Histidine also protects the body from radiation damage, helps lower blood pressure, aids in removing heavy metals from the system, and may help in the prevention of AIDS.

Histidine levels that are too high may lead to stress and even psychological disorders such as anxiety and schizophrenia; people with schizophrenia have been found to have high levels of histidine in their bodies. Inadequate levels of histidine may contribute to rheumatoid arthritis and may be associated with nerve deafness. Methionine has the ability to lower histidine levels.

Histamine, an important immune system chemical, is derived from histidine. Histamine aids in sexual arousal.

Because the availability of histidine influences histamine production, taking supplemental histidine—together with vitamins B_3 (niacin) and B_6 (pyridoxine), which are required for the transformation from histidine to histamine—may help improve sexual functioning and pleasure.

Because histamine also stimulates the secretion of gastric juices, histidine may be helpful for people with indigestion resulting from a lack of stomach acid.

Persons with manic (bipolar) depression should not take supplemental histidine unless a deficiency has been identified. Natural sources of histidine include rice, wheat, and rye.

Homocysteine

Homocysteine is an amino acid that is produced in the body in the course of methionine metabolism. This amino acid has been the focus of increasing attention in recent years, because high levels of homocysteine in the blood are associated with an increased risk of cardiovascular disease.

Further, it is known that homocysteine has a toxic effect on cells lining the arteries, makes the blood more prone to clotting, and promotes the oxidation of low-density lipoproteins (LDL, the so-called "bad cholesterol"), which makes it more likely that cholesterol will be deposited as plaque in the blood vessels.

Like other amino acids, homocysteine does perform a necessary function in the body. It is then usually broken down quickly into the amino acid cysteine and other important compounds, including adenosine triphosphate (ATP, an important source of cellular energy) and S-adenosylmethionine (SAMe). However, a genetic defect or, more commonly, deficiencies of vitamins B_6 and B_{12} and folate (folic acid) can prevent homocysteine from converting rapidly enough. As a result, high levels of the amino acid accumulate in the body, damaging cell membranes and blood vessels, and increasing the risk of cardiovascular disease, particularly atherosclerosis. Vitamins B_6 and B_{12} and folate work together to facilitate the breakdown of homocysteine, and thus help protect against heart disease.

Isoleucine

Isoleucine, one of the essential amino acids, is needed for hemoglobin formation and also stabilizes and regulates blood sugar and energy levels. It is metabolized in muscle tissue. It is one of the three branched-chain amino acids. These amino acids are valuable for athletes because they enhance energy, increase endurance, and aid in the healing and repair of muscle tissue.

Isoleucine has been found to be deficient in people suffering from many different mental and physical disorders. A deficiency of isoleucine can lead to symptoms similar to those of hypoglycemia.

Food sources of isoleucine include almonds, cashews, chicken, chickpeas, eggs, fish, lentils, liver, meat, rye, most seeds, and soy protein. It is also available in supplemental form. Supplemental L-isoleucine should always be taken with a correct balance of the other two branched-chain amino acids, L-leucine and L-valine—approximately 2 milligrams of leucine for each milligram of valine and isoleucine. Combination supplements that provide all three of the branched-chain amino acids are available and may be more convenient to use.

Leucine

Leucine is an essential amino acid and one of the branched-chain amino acids (the others are isoleucine and valine). These work together to protect muscle and act as fuel. Leucine plus other dietary proteins fosters muscle growth even without the other two branched-chain amino acids. They promote the healing of bones, skin, and muscle tissue, and are recommended for those recovering from surgery. Leucine also lowers elevated blood sugar levels and aids in increasing growth hormone production.

Natural sources of leucine include brown rice, beans, meat, nuts, soy flour, and whole wheat. Supplemental L-leucine must be taken in balance with L-isoleucine and L-valine (*see* Isoleucine in this section), and it should be taken in moderation, or symptoms of hypoglycemia may result. An excessively high intake of leucine may also contribute to pellagra, and may increase the amount of ammonia present in the body.

Lysine

Lysine is an essential amino acid that is a necessary building block for all protein. It is needed for proper growth and bone development in children; it helps calcium absorption and maintains a proper nitrogen balance in adults. This amino acid aids in the production of antibodies, hormones, and enzymes, and helps in collagen formation and tissue repair. Because it helps to build muscle protein, it is good for those recovering from surgery and sports injuries. It also lowers high serum triglyceride levels.

Another very useful ability of this amino acid is its capacity for fighting cold sores and herpesviruses. Taking supplemental L-lysine, together with vitamin C with bioflavonoids, can effectively fight and/or prevent herpes outbreaks, especially if foods containing the amino acid arginine are avoided (*see* HERPESVIRUS INFECTION in Part Two). Supplemental L-lysine also may decrease acute alcohol intoxication.

Lysine is an essential amino acid, and so cannot be manufactured in the body. It is therefore vital that adequate amounts be included in the diet. Deficiencies can result in anemia, bloodshot eyes, enzyme disorders, hair loss, an inability to concentrate, irritability, lack of energy, poor appetite, reproductive disorders, retarded growth, and weight loss. Food sources of lysine include cheese, eggs, fish, lima beans, milk, potatoes, red meat, soy products, and yeast.

Methionine

Methionine is an essential amino acid that assists in the breakdown of fats, thus helping to prevent a buildup of fat in the liver and arteries that might obstruct blood flow to the brain, heart, and kidneys. The synthesis of the amino acids cysteine and taurine may depend on the availability of methionine. This amino acid helps the digestive system; helps to detoxify harmful agents such as lead and other heavy metals; helps diminish muscle weakness, prevent brittle hair, and protect against radiation; and is beneficial for people with osteoporosis or chemical allergies. It is useful also in the treatment of rheumatic fever and toxemia of pregnancy.

Methionine is a powerful antioxidant. It is a good source of sulfur, which inactivates free radicals and helps to prevent skin and nail problems. It is also good for people with Gilbert's syndrome, an anomaly of liver function, and is required for the synthesis of nucleic acids, collagen, and proteins found in every cell of the body. It is beneficial for women who take oral contraceptives because it promotes the excretion of estrogen. It reduces the level of histamine in the body, which can be useful for people with schizophrenia, whose histamine levels are typically higher than normal.

As levels of toxic substances in the body increase, the need for methionine increases. The body can convert methionine into the amino acid cysteine, a precursor of glutathione. Methionine thus protects glutathione; it helps to prevent glutathione depletion if the body is overloaded with toxins. Since glutathione is a key neutralizer of toxins in the liver, this protects the liver from the damaging effects of toxic compounds.

An essential amino acid, methionine is not synthesized in the body and so must be obtained from food sources or from dietary supplements. Good food sources of methionine include beans, eggs, fish, garlic, lentils, meat, onions, soybeans, seeds, and yogurt. Because the body uses methionine to derive a brain food called choline, it is wise to supplement the diet with choline or lecithin (which is high in choline) to ensure that the supply of methionine is not depleted.

Ornithine

Ornithine helps to prompt the release of growth hormone, which promotes the metabolism of excess body fat. This effect is enhanced if ornithine is combined with arginine and carnitine. Ornithine is necessary for proper immune-system and liver function. This amino acid also detoxifies ammonia and aids in liver regeneration. High concentrations of ornithine are found in the skin and connective tissue, making it useful for promoting healing and repairing damaged tissues.

Ornithine is synthesized in the body from arginine, and in turn serves as the precursor of citrulline, proline, and glutamic acid. Children, pregnant women, nursing mothers, or anyone with a history of schizophrenia should not take supplemental L-ornithine, unless they are specifically directed to do so by a physician.

Phenylalanine

Phenylalanine is an essential amino acid. Because it can cross the blood-brain barrier, it can have a direct effect on brain chemistry. Once in the body, phenylalanine can be converted into another amino acid, tyrosine, which in turn is used to synthesize two key neurotransmitters that promote alertness: dopamine and norepinephrine. Because of its relationship to the action of the central nervous system, this amino acid can elevate mood, decrease pain, aid in memory and learning, and suppress the appetite. It can be used to treat arthritis, depression, menstrual cramps, migraines, obesity, Parkinson's disease, and schizophrenia.

Phenylalanine is available in three different forms, designated L-, D-, and DL-. The L- form is the most common type and is the form in which phenylalanine is incorporated into the body's proteins. The D- form acts as a painkiller. The DL- form is a combination of the D- and the L-. Like the D- form, it is effective for controlling pain, especially the pain of arthritis; like the L- form, it functions as a building block for proteins, increases mental alertness, suppresses the appetite, and helps people with Parkinson's disease. It has been used to alleviate the symptoms of premenstrual syndrome (PMS) and various types of chronic pain.

Supplemental phenylalanine, as well as products containing aspartame (an artificial sweetener made from phenylalanine and another amino acid, aspartic acid), should *not* be taken by pregnant women or by people who suffer from anxiety attacks, diabetes, high blood pressure, phenylketonuria (PKU), or preexisting pigmented melanoma, a type of skin cancer.

Proline

Proline improves skin texture by aiding in the production of collagen and reducing the loss of collagen through the aging process. It is needed to repair tissue after a major sunburn or severe burn. It also helps in the healing of cartilage and the strengthening of joints, tendons, and heart muscle. It works with vitamin C to promote healthy connective tissue.

Proline is obtained primarily from meat sources, dairy products, and eggs.

Serine

Serine is needed for the proper metabolism of fats and fatty acids, the growth of muscle, and the maintenance of a healthy immune system. It is a component of brain proteins and the protective myelin sheaths that cover nerve fibers. It is important in RNA and DNA function, cell membrane formation, and creatine synthesis. It also aids in the production of immunoglobulins and antibodies. However, too-high serine levels in the body may have adverse effects on the immune system.

Serine can be made from glycine in the body, but this process requires the presence of sufficient amounts of vitamins B_3 and B_6 and folic acid. Food sources of serine include meat and soy foods, as well as many foods that often cause allergic reactions, such as dairy products, wheat gluten, and peanuts. It is included as a natural moisturizing agent in many cosmetics and skin-care preparations.

Taurine

High concentrations of taurine are found in the heart muscle, white blood cells, skeletal muscle, and central nervous system. It is a building block of all the other amino acids as well as a key component of bile, which is needed for the digestion of fats, the absorption of fat-soluble vitamins,

and the control of serum cholesterol levels. Taurine can be useful for people with atherosclerosis, edema, heart disorders, hypertension, or hypoglycemia. It is vital for the proper utilization of sodium, potassium, calcium, and magnesium, and it has been shown to play a particular role in sparing the loss of potassium from the heart muscle. This helps to prevent the development of potentially dangerous cardiac arrhythmias.

Taurine has a protective effect on the brain, particularly if the brain is dehydrated. It is used to treat anxiety, epilepsy, hyperactivity, poor brain function, and seizures.

Taurine is found in concentrations up to four times greater in the brains of children than in those of adults. It may be that a deficiency of taurine in the developing brain is involved in seizures. Zinc deficiency also is commonly found in people with epilepsy, and this may play a part in the deficiency of taurine. Taurine is also associated with zinc in maintaining eye function; a deficiency of both may impair vision. Taurine supplementation may benefit children with Down syndrome and muscular dystrophy. This amino acid is also used in some clinics for breast cancer treatment.

Excessive losses of taurine through the urine can be caused by many metabolic disorders. Cardiac arrhythmias, disorders of platelet formation, intestinal problems, an overgrowth of candida, physical or emotional stress, a zinc deficiency, and excessive consumption of alcohol are all associated with high urinary losses of taurine. Excessive alcohol consumption also causes the body to lose its ability to utilize taurine properly. Taurine supplementation may reduce symptoms of alcohol withdrawal. Diabetes increases the body's requirements for taurine; conversely, supplementation with taurine and cystine may decrease the need for insulin.

Taurine is found in eggs, fish, meat, and milk, but not in vegetable proteins. It can be synthesized from cysteine in the liver and from methionine elsewhere in the body, as long as sufficient quantities of vitamin B_6 are present. For vegetarians, synthesis by the body is crucial. For individuals with genetic or metabolic disorders that prevent the synthesis of taurine, taurine supplementation is required.

Threonine

Threonine is an essential amino acid that helps to maintain the proper protein balance in the body. It is important for the formation of collagen, elastin, and tooth enamel, and aids liver and lipotropic function when combined with aspartic acid and methionine. A precursor of the amino acids glycine and serine, threonine is present in the heart, central nervous system, and skeletal muscle, and helps to prevent fatty buildup in the liver. It enhances the immune system by aiding in the production of antibodies, and may be helpful in treating some types of depression.

Because the threonine content of grains is low, vegetarians are more likely than others to have deficiencies.

Tryptophan

Tryptophan is an essential amino acid that is necessary for the production of vitamin B_3 (niacin). It is used by the brain to produce serotonin, a necessary neurotransmitter that transfers nerve impulses from one cell to another and is responsible for normal sleep. Consequently, tryptophan helps to combat depression and insomnia and to stabilize moods. But it is most commonly used to treat sleep problems.

Tryptophan helps to control hyperactivity in children, alleviates stress, is good for the heart, aids in weight control by reducing appetite, and enhances the release of growth hormone. It is good for migraine headaches and may reduce some of the effects of nicotine. Sufficient amounts of vitamins B_6 (pyridoxine) and C, folate, and magnesium are necessary for the formation of tryptophan, which, in turn, is required for the formation of serotonin. A study reported in the *Archives of General Psychiatry* found that women with a history of bulimia nervosa, an eating disorder, experienced relapses after they took an amino acid mixture lacking tryptophan. Researchers believe that insufficient tryptophan altered brain serotonin levels and, consequently, the transmission of nerve impulses. A lack of tryptophan and magnesium may contribute to coronary artery spasms.

The best dietary sources of tryptophan include brown rice, cottage cheese, meat, peanuts, and soy protein. In November 1989, the U.S. Centers for Disease Control (CDC) reported evidence linking L-tryptophan supplements to a blood disorder called eosinophilia-myalgia syndrome (EMS). Several hundred cases of this illness—which is characterized by an elevated white blood cell count and can also cause such symptoms as fatigue, muscular pain, respiratory ailments, edema, and rash—were reported. After the CDC established an association between the blood disorder and products containing L-tryptophan in New Mexico, the U.S. Food and Drug Administration (FDA) first warned consumers to stop taking L-tryptophan supplements, then recalled all products in which L-tryptophan was the sole or a major component. According to the FDA, at least thirty-eight deaths could be attributed to the tryptophan supplements.

Subsequent research showed that it was contaminants in the supplements, *not* the tryptophan, that was probably responsible for the problem. In 2005, tryptophan supplements were sold again in the United States after the FDA carefully reviewed the new source of tryptophan and deemed it acceptable.

Tyrosine

Tyrosine is important to overall metabolism. It is a precursor of adrenaline and the neurotransmitters norepinephrine and dopamine, which regulate mood and stimulate metabolism and the nervous system. Tyrosine acts as a mood elevator; a lack of adequate amounts of tyrosine leads to a deficiency of norepinephrine in the brain, which in turn can result in depression. It also acts as a mild anti-oxidant, suppresses the appetite, and helps to reduce body fat. It aids in the production of melanin (the pigment responsible for skin and hair color) and in the functions of the adrenal, thyroid, and pituitary glands. It is also involved in the metabolism of the amino acid phenylalanine.

Tyrosine attaches to iodine atoms to form active thyroid hormones. Not surprisingly, low plasma levels of tyrosine have been associated with hypothyroidism. Symptoms of tyrosine deficiency can also include low blood pressure, low body temperature (such as cold hands and feet), and restless leg syndrome.

Supplemental L-tyrosine has been used for stress reduction, and research suggests it may be helpful against chronic fatigue and narcolepsy. It has been used to help individuals suffering from anxiety, depression, low sex drive, allergies, and headaches, as well as persons undergoing withdrawal from drugs. It may also help people with Parkinson's disease.

Natural sources of tyrosine include almonds, avocados, bananas, dairy products, lima beans, pumpkin seeds, and sesame seeds. Tyrosine can also be produced from phenylalanine in the body. Supplements of L-tyrosine should be taken at bedtime or with a high-carbohydrate meal so that it does not have to compete for absorption with other amino acids.

Persons taking monoamine oxidase (MAO) inhibitors, commonly prescribed for depression, must strictly limit their intake of foods containing tyrosine and should *not* take any supplements containing L-tyrosine, as it may lead to a sudden and dangerous rise in blood pressure. Anyone who takes prescription medication for depression should discuss necessary dietary restrictions with his or her physician.

Valine

Valine, an essential amino acid, has a stimulant effect. It is needed for muscle metabolism, tissue repair, and the maintenance of a proper nitrogen balance in the body. Valine is found in high concentrations in muscle tissue. It is one of the branched-chain amino acids, which means that it can be used as an energy source by muscle tissue. It may be helpful in treating liver and gallbladder disease, and it is good for correcting the type of severe amino acid deficiencies that can be caused by drug addiction. An excessively high level of valine may lead to such symptoms as a crawling sensation in the skin and even hallucinations.

Dietary sources of valine include dairy products, grains, meat, mushrooms, peanuts, and soy protein. Supplemental L-valine should always be taken in balance with the other branched-chain amino acids, L-isoleucine and L-leucine (*see* Isoleucine in this section).

Antioxidants

INTRODUCTION

Antioxidants are natural compounds that help protect the body from harmful free radicals. These are atoms or groups of atoms that can cause damage to cells, impairing the immune system and leading to infections and various degenerative diseases such as heart disease and cancer. Antioxidants therefore play a beneficial role in the prevention of disease. Free radical damage is thought by scientists to be the basis for the aging process as well. (*See* Free Radicals on page 67.)

There are a number of known free radicals that occur in the body, the most common of which are oxygen-derived free radicals, such as superoxide radicals and hydroxyl radicals, hypochlorite radicals, hydrogen peroxide, various lipid peroxides, and nitric oxide. They may be formed by exposure to radiation, including exposure to the sun's rays; exposure to toxic chemicals such as those found in cigarette smoke, polluted air, and industrial and household chemicals; and various metabolic processes, such as the process of breaking down stored fat molecules for use as an energy source.

Free radicals are normally kept in check by the action of *free radical scavengers* that occur naturally in the body. These scavengers neutralize the free radicals. Certain enzymes serve this vital function. Four important enzymes that neutralize free radicals are superoxide dismutase (SOD), methionine reductase, catalase, and glutathione peroxidase.

The body makes these as a matter of course. There are also a number of phytochemicals and nutrients that act as antioxidants, including vitamin A, beta-carotene and other carotenoids, flavonoids, vitamins C and E, and the mineral selenium. Researchers have recently found that eggplant contains high levels of chlorogenic acid, which has proven to be a highly effective antioxidant. Another antioxidant is the hormone melatonin, which is a powerful free radical neutralizer. Certain herbs have antioxidant properties as well.

Although many antioxidants can be obtained from food sources such as sprouted grains and fresh fruits and vegetables, it is difficult to get enough of them from these sources to hold back the free radicals constantly being generated in our polluted environment. We can minimize free radical damage by taking supplements of key nutrients. A high intake of antioxidant nutrients appears to be especially protective against cancer.

Antioxidants work synergistically in giving protection against free radical damage, so it is better to take smaller doses of several different antioxidants than a large amount of only one. For example, while beta-carotene by itself is an excellent antioxidant, a mix of natural carotenoids provides more health benefits than beta-carotene alone. There are many good combination formulas available that make it easy to take multiple antioxidants every day. Similarly, taking antioxidants together, for example beta-carotene with vitamin E and vitamin C, appears to be more effective than taking any one alone.

Some of the major antioxidants are described in the sections that follow.

THE ANTIOXIDANTS

Alpha-Lipoic Acid

Alpha-lipoic acid (ALA) is a powerful antioxidant—both on its own and as a "recycler" of vitamin E and vitamin C. It can restore the antioxidant properties of these vitamins after they have neutralized free radicals. ALA also stimulates the body's production of glutathione and aids in the absorption of coenzyme Q_{10}, both important antioxidants. Because ALA is soluble in both water and fat, it can move into all parts of cells to deactivate free radicals.

Supplemental ALA has been used for almost three decades in Europe to treat peripheral nerve degeneration and to help control blood sugar levels in people with diabetes. It also helps to detoxify the liver of metal pollutants, block cataract formation, protect nerve tissues against oxidative stress, and reduce blood cholesterol levels. It can be used with carnitine to provide an antiaging effect. ALA is known also as a metabolic antioxidant, because without it, cells cannot use sugar to produce energy. The body does not produce large amounts of ALA, but because it is found naturally in only a few foods, including spinach, broccoli, potatoes, brewer's yeast, and organ meats, supplementation may be necessary.

Bilberry

The herb bilberry (*Vaccinium myrtillus*), a European relative of the American blueberry, contains natural antioxidants that keep capillary walls strong and flexible. They also help to maintain the flexibility of the walls of red blood cells and allow them to pass through the capillaries more freely. Everyone knows that vitamins C and E are good sources of antioxidants, but bilberry, which contains anthocyanidins phytochemicals, also acts as an antioxidant. It also helps to lower blood pressure, inhibit clot formation, and enhance blood supply to the nervous system. Studies indicate that anthocyanidins can provide up to fifty times the antioxidant protection of vitamin E and ten times the protection of vitamin C. In addition, this herb protects the eyes and may enhance vision; supports and strengthens collagen structures; inhibits the growth of bacteria; acts as an anti-inflammatory; and has antiaging and anticarcinogenic effects. One study that looked at the effects of bilberry on night vision found that vision was not improved with the amounts that are typically sold. Tests have shown that the compound glucoquinine, found in bilberry leaves, helps to lower blood sugar levels.

Burdock

The herb burdock (*Arctium lappa*) was tested by researchers at the Chia Nan College of Pharmacy and Science in Taiwan for its antioxidant properties. They found that burdock is a powerful antioxidant, capable of scavenging hydrogen peroxide and superoxide radicals. It also showed a marked scavenging effect against hydroxyl radicals. The study showed also that burdock and vitamin E quench more free radicals when used in combination. Burdock also might protect against cancer by helping to control cell mutation.

Carotenoids

See under Vitamin A and the Carotenoids.

Coenzyme Q$_{10}$

Coenzyme Q$_{10}$ is an antioxidant that is structurally similar to vitamin E. It plays a crucial role in the generation of cellular energy, is a significant immunologic stimulant, increases circulation, has antiaging effects, and is beneficial for the cardiovascular system. Also known as *ubiquinone* (from *quinone*, a type of coenzyme, and *ubiquitous*, because it exists everywhere in the body), coenzyme Q$_{10}$ is found in highest concentrations in the heart, followed by the liver, kidney, spleen, and pancreas. Within the mitochondria, the cells' energy-production centers, coenzyme Q$_{10}$ helps to metabolize fats and carbohydrates. It also helps to maintain the flexibility of cell membranes.

Various research reports suggest that coenzyme Q$_{10}$ also may be beneficial in treating cancer, AIDS, muscular dystrophy, allergies, gastric ulcers, myopathy, Parkinson's disease, and deafness.

Natural sources of coenzyme Q$_{10}$ include meats, peanuts, sardines, and spinach. (*See* Natural Food Supplements later in Part One for more on coenzyme Q$_{10}$.)

Curcumin (Turmeric)

Found in the spice turmeric, the phytochemical curcumin has antioxidant properties that prevent the formation of

and neutralize existing free radicals. It stops precancerous changes within DNA and interferes with enzymes necessary for cancer progression. Curcumin stops the oxidation of cholesterol, thus protecting against the formation of plaque in the arteries. In a study of chronic smokers, those who took curcumin excreted a substantially lower level of mutagens (substances that induce cells to mutate) in their urine, a reflection of how well the body is dealing with these cancer-causing substances. Curcumin has been shown to be of benefit to some patients with advanced pancreatic cancer. It may also calm an overactive immune system in patients with ulcerative colitis, reducing inflammation, redness, and soreness. In one study, curcumin helped keep patients with ulcerative colitis from experiencing intestinal flare-ups. But it does not seem to be effective for other inflammatory conditions such as psoriasis. Curcumin also blocks toxic compounds from reaching or reacting with body tissues, and may prevent cataracts.

Curcumin should not be taken by anyone who has biliary tract obstruction or is taking anticoagulants, as curcumin stimulates bile secretion and acts as a blood-thinner.

Flavonoids

Flavonoids are especially potent antioxidants and metal chelators. They are the largest category of plant compounds called polyphenols. They are chemical compounds that plants produce to protect themselves from parasites, bacteria, and cell injury. More than 4,000 chemically unique flavonoids are known; they occur in fruits, vegetables, spices, seeds, nuts, flowers, and bark. Wine (particularly red wine), apples, blueberries, bilberries, onions, soy products, and tea are some of the best food sources of flavonoids. Certain flavonoids in fruits and vegetables have much greater antioxidant activity than vitamins C and E or beta-carotene. In fact, flavonoids protect the antioxidant vitamins from oxidative damage.

Numerous medicinal herbs contain therapeutic amounts of flavonoids; they often are a major component of an herb's medicinal activity, which include helping prevent heart disease and cancer, and reducing the incidence of neurodegenerative diseases.

Natural sources of the flavonoids include almonds, apples, broccoli, citrus fruits, tea, tomatoes, onions, soybeans, and red wine. In the United States, the greatest intake of flavonoids comes from citrus fruits, tea, and wine.

Garlic

This versatile healing herb also has antioxidant properties. The sulfhydryl (sulfur and hydrogen) compounds in garlic are potent chelators of toxic heavy metals, binding with them so that they can be excreted. These same compounds are effective protectants against oxidation and free radicals.

Garlic aids in the detoxification of peroxides such as hydrogen peroxide and helps to prevent fats from being oxi-

Free Radicals

A free radical is an atom or group of atoms that contains at least one unpaired electron. Electrons are negatively charged particles that usually occur in pairs, forming a chemically stable arrangement. If an electron is unpaired, another atom or molecule can easily bond with it, causing a chemical reaction. Because they join so readily with other compounds, free radicals can effect dramatic changes in the body, and they can cause a lot of oxidative damage. Each free radical may exist for only a tiny fraction of a second, but the damage it leaves behind can be irreversible, particularly damage to heart muscle cells, nerve cells, and certain immune system sensor cells.

Free radicals are normally present in the body in small numbers. Oxygen-charged particles are created in the body as we breathe. Diets rich in antioxidants can more than neutralize these particles. Dietary supplements rich in antioxidants act in the same way. Biochemical processes naturally lead to the formation of free radicals, and under normal circumstances the body can keep them in check. Indeed, not all free radicals are bad. Free radicals produced by the immune system destroy viruses and bacteria. Other free radicals are involved in producing vital hormones and activating enzymes that are needed for life. We need free radicals to produce energy and various substances that the body requires. If there is excessive free radical formation, however, damage to cells and tissues can occur. The formation of a large number of free radicals stimulates the formation of more free radicals, leading to even more damage.

Many different factors can lead to an excess of free radicals. Exposure to radiation, whether from the sun or small amounts from medical x-rays, activates the formation of free radicals, as does exposure to environmental pollutants such as tobacco smoke and automobile exhaust. Diet also can contribute to the formation of free radicals. When the body obtains nutrients through the diet, it utilizes oxygen and these nutrients to create energy. In this oxidation process, oxygen molecules containing unpaired electrons are released. These oxygen free radicals can cause damage to the body if produced in extremely large amounts. Being overweight or consuming a diet that is high in fat can increase free radical activity because oxidation occurs more readily in fat molecules than it does in carbohydrate or protein molecules. Cooking fats at high temperatures, particularly frying foods in oil, can produce large numbers of free radicals.

The presence of a dangerous number of free radicals can alter the way in which the cells code genetic material.

Changes in protein structure can occur as a result of errors in protein synthesis. The body's immune system may then see this altered protein as a foreign substance and try to destroy it. The formation of mutated proteins can eventually damage the immune system and lead to leukemia and other types of cancer, as well as to many other diseases.

In addition to damaging genetic material, free radicals can destroy the protective cell membranes. Calcium levels in the body may be upset as well. Over time, the body produces more free radicals than it does scavengers. The resulting imbalance contributes to the aging process.

Substances known as antioxidants neutralize free radicals by binding to their free electrons. Antioxidants available in supplement form include the enzymes superoxide dismutase and glutathione peroxidase; vitamin A, beta-carotene, and vitamins C and E; the minerals selenium and zinc; and the hormone melatonin. By destroying free radicals, antioxidants help to detoxify and protect the body.

---

dized and deposited in tissues and arteries. Garlic also contains antioxidant nutrients such as vitamins A and C and selenium.

Studies on aged garlic extract (AGE) have shown that the aging process substantially boosts garlic's antioxidant potential. AGE protects against DNA damage, keeps blood vessels healthy, and guards against radiation and sunlight damage. According to researcher and nutritionist Robert I-San Lin, Ph.D., aged garlic extract can prevent liver damage caused by carbon tetrachloride, a common indoor pollutant and free radical generator. Overall, aged garlic supplements provide a greater concentration of garlic's beneficial compounds. It is particularly helpful to reduce oxidation associated with aging. If you're worried about "garlic breath" putting a strain on your social life, choose an odorless and tasteless form such as Kyolic aged garlic extract from Wakunaga of America. Aged garlic extract reduces blood cholesterol levels, thus lowering the risk of heart attack; provides protection from heart disease by pre-venting clots that can lead to heart attacks and strokes; and helps lower high blood pressure. Timed-released garlic has been shown to reduce blood cholesterol levels, and to lower fasting blood sugar levels in patients with type 2 diabetes.

Ginkgo Biloba

Ginkgo biloba is an herb with powerful antioxidant effects in the brain, retina, and cardiovascular system. It is well known for its ability to enhance circulation, and a study reported in the *Journal of the American Medical Association* showed that it has a measurable effect on dementia in people with Alzheimer's disease and people recovering from strokes. Other studies indicate that it can improve both long- and short-term memory and enhance concentration.

Ginkgo biloba has also been used to treat hearing problems, impotence, and macular degeneration.

Anyone who takes prescription anticoagulant (blood-thinning) medication or who uses over-the-counter painkillers regularly should consult a health care provider before using ginkgo biloba, as the combination may result in internal bleeding.

Glutathione

Glutathione is a protein that is produced in the liver from the amino acids cysteine, glutamic acid, and glycine. It is a powerful antioxidant that inhibits the formation of, and protects against cellular damage from, free radicals. It helps to defend the body against damage from cigarette smoking, exposure to radiation, cancer chemotherapy, and toxins such as alcohol. As a detoxifier of heavy metals and drugs, it aids in the treatment of blood and liver disorders.

Glutathione protects cells in several ways. It neutralizes oxygen molecules before they can harm cells. Together with selenium, it forms the enzyme glutathione peroxidase, which neutralizes hydrogen peroxide. It is also a component of another antioxidant enzyme, glutathione-S-transferase, which is a broad-spectrum liver-detoxifying enzyme.

Glutathione protects not only individual cells but also the tissues of the arteries, brain, heart, immune cells, kidneys, lenses of the eyes, liver, lungs, and skin against oxidant damage. It plays a role in preventing cancer, especially liver cancer, and may actually target carcinogens, make them water-soluble, and then help escort them from the body. It may also have an antiaging effect. The rate at which we age is directly correlated with reduced concentrations of glutathione in cellular fluids; as we grow older, glutathione levels drop, resulting in a decreased ability to deactivate free radicals.

Glutathione can be taken in supplement form. The production of glutathione by the body can be boosted by taking supplemental dehydroepiandrosterone (DHEA), a hormone; N-acetylcysteine or L-cysteine; and L-methionine. Studies suggest that this may be a better way of raising glutathione levels than taking glutathione itself, but check with your health care professional if you have any hormonal problems.

Grape Seed Extract

See under Oligomeric Proanthocyanidins *in this section.*

Green Tea

Tea is the most commonly consumed beverage around the world after water. Green tea contains compounds known as polyphenols, including phytochemicals that have antioxidant, antibacterial, antiviral, and health-enhancing properties. Tests on epigallocatechin gallate (EGCG), a particular type of polyphenol in green tea, have shown that it is able to penetrate the body's cells and shield DNA from hydrogen peroxide, a potent free radical. Epidemiological studies have shown that green tea protects against cancer, lowers cholesterol levels, and reduces the clotting tendency of the blood. Because green tea boosts immune function and acts as an antiviral and anti-inflammatory agent, it may help prevent cancer. In one study, it was shown to prevent symptoms associated with colds and flu, and even reduced the number of these illnesses. It also shows promise as a weight-loss aid that can promote the burning of fat and help to regulate blood sugar and insulin levels. Instead of drinking green tea, a supplement containing known quantities of it can produce weight loss—especially as fat—and lower blood pressure and "bad" (LDL) cholesterol.

Green tea is simply the dried leaves of the tea plant. All green teas are from the species *Camellia sinensis*, but depending on the locale where they are grown and on the processing they can be quite different. Chinese teas are predominant, and comprise about 90 percent of what is sold. There are numerous regional Chinese teas, the best known being *lung ching* (dragon well).

Other teas from Japan are equally good. Japanese green teas are of two basic types, *sencha* or *gyokuro*. Sencha is grown in the full sun, while gyokuro is shaded a few weeks before it is harvested. While there are many brands, the basic difference is that gyokuro makes a sweeter, darker green tea than sencha, which is somewhat grassy in flavor. It also costs over twice as much. Gyokuro is the source of the special handmade powdered tea used in the traditional tea ceremony.

Green tea is not fermented and has more polyphenols than black tea. Black tea undergoes natural fermentation, which converts tannins, astringent phytochemicals, into more complex compounds. This fermentation process destroys some of black tea's polyphenols, and it was once thought that it was thus rendered less effective as an antioxidant. Tests have shown, however, that both green and black teas contain about the same amount of antioxidant polyphenols, but that there are different combinations of antioxidants between black and green teas depending on the method of processing. Black tea lowers blood sugar and raises insulin levels after a meal. The polyphenolic content of black tea is thought to stimulate the pancreas to release insulin.

Green tea does contain caffeine (15 to 25 milligrams per 3/4 cup), but it is less than in similar amounts of coffee (80 to 115 milligrams per 3/4 cup) or caffeinated carbonated beverages (38 to 46 milligrams per can). Those who have heart problems or sensitivity to caffeine, or are pregnant may want to limit their intake of caffeine. Green tea contains vitamin K, which can make anticoagulant medication less effective. Consult your health provider if you are using them.

Methionine

A unique amino acid, methionine neutralizes hydroxyl radicals, one of the most dangerous types of free radicals. Most often a by-product of reactions between heavy metals and less toxic free radicals, hydroxyl radicals can be formed also during strenuous exercise or exposure to high levels of radiation, and can damage any type of body tissue.

N-Acetylcysteine (NAC)

The sulfur-containing amino acid cysteine is needed to produce the free radical fighter glutathione and to help maintain it at adequate levels in the cells. N-acetylcysteine (NAC) is a more stable form of cysteine that can be taken in supplement form.

NAC is used by the liver and the lymphocytes to detoxify chemicals and other poisons. It is a powerful detoxifier of alcohol, tobacco smoke, and environmental pollutants, all of which are immune suppressors. Taking supplemental NAC can boost the levels of protective enzymes in the body, thus slowing some of the cellular damage that is characteristic of aging. NAC supplementation may also decrease both the frequency and duration of infectious diseases. It has been used in the management of AIDS and chronic bronchitis.

People with diabetes should not take supplemental NAC without first consulting a health care provider, as it can interfere with the effectiveness of insulin.

Nicotinamide Adenine Dinucleotide (NADH)

Also known as coenzyme 1, nicotinamide adenine dinucleotide with high-energy hydrogen, or NADH, is the "spark" that ignites energy production in the body's cells.

NADH's high antioxidant capacity derives from its ability to reduce levels of substances. NADH plays a central role in DNA repair and maintenance, and in the cellular immune defense system. Studies report that NADH also can inhibit the auto-oxidation of the neurotransmitter dopamine, which causes the release of toxic chemicals that may damage sensitive parts of the brain.

Oligomeric Proanthocyanidins

Oligomeric proanthocyanidins (OPCs) are naturally occurring substances present in a variety of food and botanical sources. They are unique phytochemicals known as flavonoids that have powerful antioxidant capabilities. OPCs are highly water soluble, so the body is able to absorb them rapidly. Clinical tests suggest that OPCs may be as much as fifty times more potent than vitamin E and twenty times more potent than vitamin C in terms of bioavailable antioxidant activity. What's more, OPCs work with the antioxidant glutathione to recycle and restore oxidized vitamin C, thus increasing the vitamin's effectiveness. Because they are able to cross the blood-brain barrier, OPCs can protect the brain and spinal nerves against free radical damage. In addition to their antioxidant activity, OPCs protect the liver from damage caused by toxic doses of acetaminophen, a nonprescription pain reliever; they strengthen and repair connective tissue, including that of the cardiovascular system; and they support the immune system and slow aging. They also moderate allergic and inflammatory responses by reducing histamine production.

OPCs are found throughout plant life; however, the two main sources are pine bark extract (Pycnogenol), produced from a French coastal pine tree, and grape seed extract, made from the seeds of the wine grape (*Vitis vinifera*). Pycnogenol was the first source of OPCs discovered, and the process for extracting it was patented in the 1950s. Pycnogenol is a trademarked name for pine bark extract, not a generic term for OPCs from other sources.

Pycnogenol

See under Oligomeric Proanthocyanidins above.

Selenium

Selenium is an essential trace mineral that functions as an antioxidant in partnership with vitamin E to protect tissues and cell membranes. Among other things, it increases antioxidant enzyme levels in cells. Selenium is also an integral component of the antioxidant enzyme glutathione peroxidase (each molecule of this enzyme contains four atoms of selenium). Glutathione peroxidase targets harmful hydrogen peroxide in the body and converts it into water. It is a particularly important guardian of blood cells and of the heart, liver, and lungs.

Numerous plants contain selenium, including garlic, asparagus, and grains, but the levels depend on soil content, which varies from one geographic region to another.

Use caution when taking supplemental selenium. A maximum safe dose is 400 micrograms (mcg) daily. Amounts higher than 1,000 micrograms (1 milligram) daily may be toxic.

The best natural sources of selenium include Brazil nuts (over 500 micrograms per ounce!), brown rice, seafood, eggs, tuna, and buckwheat.

Silymarin

Extracted from the seeds of the herb milk thistle, silymarin has been used for centuries to treat liver disease. The active ingredients in milk thistle are several types of flavonoids (powerful antioxidants), known collectively as silymarin.

Silymarin guards the liver from oxidative damage. It also protects the liver from toxins, drugs, and the effects of alcohol, and promotes the growth of new liver cells. In addition, silymarin increases levels of glutathione, superoxide dismutase, and catalase, potent antioxidant enzymes that protect the liver. It also has been shown to reduce insulin resistance, which may help patients with diabetes. In one study, patients with diabetes who received silymarin experienced blood glucose control and better blood tests related to liver function.

Superoxide Dismutase

Superoxide dismutase (SOD) is an enzyme. SOD revitalizes cells and reduces the rate of cell destruction. It neutralizes the most common, and possibly the most dangerous, free radicals—superoxide radicals. Superoxide radicals instigate the breakdown of synovial fluid, the lubricant for the body's joints. This leads to friction and, ultimately, inflammation.

SOD works synergistically with the enzyme catalase, which is abundant throughout the body. Catalase removes hydrogen peroxide by-products created by SOD reactions.

SOD also aids in the body's utilization of zinc, copper, and manganese. Its levels tend to decline with age, while free radical production increases. Its potential as an anti-aging treatment is currently being explored.

Chemically speaking, there are two forms of this enzyme. The copper/zinc form (known as Cu/Zn SOD) exerts its antioxidant properties in the cytoplasm of cells. This is the watery fluid that surrounds all the other cellular components. Metabolic activity that takes place in the cytoplasm results in the production of free radicals, and Cu/Zn neutralizes them. The manganese form (Mn SOD) is active in the mitochondria, structures within cells where energy is produced. The production of cellular energy also leads to the creation of free radicals.

SOD occurs naturally in barley grass, broccoli, Brussels sprouts, cabbage, wheatgrass, and most green plants. It is also available in supplement form. SOD supplements in pill form must be enteric coated—that is, coated with a protective substance that allows the pill to pass intact through the stomach acid into the small intestines to be absorbed. Cell Guard from Biotec Food Corporation and KAL SOD-3 from Nutraceutical International Corporation are good sources of SOD.

Vitamin A and the Carotenoids

A class of phytochemicals, carotenoids are fat-soluble pigments found in yellow, red, green, and orange vegetables and fruits. They are a potent family of antioxidants that include alpha-carotene, beta-carotene, lycopene, lutein, and zeaxanthin. Of the more than five hundred carotenoids found in nature, about fifty can be converted into vitamin A in the body.

Carotenoids quench singlet oxygen, which is not, chemically speaking, a free radical, but is nevertheless highly reactive and can damage body molecules. Carotenoids also act as anticancer agents, decrease the risk of cataracts and age-related macular degeneration, and inhibit heart disease.

Studies have shown that carotenoids found in tomato juice (lycopene), carrots (alpha- and beta-carotene), and spinach (lutein) may help to protect against cancer by reducing oxidative and other damage to DNA. Together, the antioxidants alpha-lipoic acid, coenzyme Q_{10}, vitamin C, and vitamin E help conserve carotenoids in tissues. Another carotenoid, astaxanthin, when taken as a supplement, was shown to be well-absorbed and tended to reduce damage to fat particles floating in the blood. This means that astaxanthin may be a beneficial supplement to reduce the risk of heart disease.

The body converts beta-carotene into vitamin A as needed. Any leftover beta-carotene then acts as an antioxidant, breaking free radical chain reactions and preventing the oxidation of cholesterol. It reduces the oxidation of DNA and disables reactive oxygen species molecules generated by exposure to sunlight and air pollution, preventing damage to eyes, lungs, and skin.

A recent laboratory study found that taking very high doses of supplemental beta-carotene alone (50,000 international units or more daily) may interfere with the normal control of cell division. It is best to take a carotenoid complex containing a variety of carotenoids.

Natural sources of vitamin A include liver, whole milk, whole eggs, cheddar cheese, and beta-carotene foods. Natural sources of the carotenoids in general include sweet potatoes, carrots, spinach, corn, sweet peppers, spirulina, and kale.

Vitamin C

Vitamin C is a very powerful antioxidant that also recharges other antioxidants, such as vitamin E, to keep them potent. Its water solubility makes it an efficient free radical scavenger in body fluids. Some studies have shown that vitamin C is the first line of antioxidant defense in plasma against many different kinds of free radicals. The cells of the brain and spinal cord, which frequently incur free radical damage, can be protected by significant amounts of vitamin C. This vitamin also guards against atherosclerosis by preventing damage to artery walls. Vitamin C acts as a more potent free radical scavenger in the presence of the phytochemical hesperidin.

Natural sources of vitamin C include citrus fruits, papaya, Brussels sprouts, broccoli, and strawberries.

Vitamin E

Vitamin E is a powerful antioxidant that prevents the oxidation of lipids (fats). Fat oxidation has been implicated in the process that leads to atherosclerosis. Vitamin E is fat soluble and, since cell membranes are composed of lipids, it effectively prevents the cells' protective coatings from becoming rancid as a result of the assault of free radicals.

Vitamin E also improves oxygen utilization, enhances immune response, plays a role in the prevention of cataracts caused by free radical damage, and may reduce the risk of coronary artery disease.

The natural form of vitamin E (d-alpha-tocopherol) is superior to the synthetic version (dl-alpha-tocopherol).

New evidence suggests that zinc is needed to maintain normal blood concentrations of vitamin E. Selenium enhances vitamin E uptake.

For information regarding dosage and safety of vitamin E supplements, consult the Vitamins section in Part One of this book. Natural sources of vitamin E include nuts, soybeans, spinach, sunflower seeds, asparagus, and sweet potatoes.

Zinc

Zinc's main antioxidant function is in the prevention of fat oxidation. In addition, it is a constituent of the antioxidant enzyme superoxide dismutase (SOD). Zinc is also needed for proper maintenance of vitamin E levels in the blood and aids in the absorption of vitamin A.

Enzymes

INTRODUCTION

The late Dr. Edward Howell, a physician and pioneer in enzyme research, called enzymes the "sparks of life." These energized protein molecules play a necessary role in virtually all of the biochemical activities that go on in the body.

They are essential for digesting food, for stimulating the brain, for providing cellular energy, and for repairing all tissues, organs, and cells. Life as we know it could not exist without the action of enzymes, even in the presence of sufficient amounts of vitamins, minerals, water, and other nutrients.

In their primary role, enzymes are catalysts—substances that accelerate and precipitate the hundreds of thousands of biochemical reactions in the body that control life's processes. If it were not for the catalytic action of enzymes, most of these reactions would take place far too slowly to sustain life. Enzymes are not consumed in the reactions they facilitate.

Each enzyme has a specific function in the body that no other enzyme can fulfill. The chemical shape of each enzyme is specialized so that it can initiate a reaction only in a certain substance, or in a group of closely related substances, and not in others. The substance on which an enzyme acts is called the *substrate*. Because there must be a different enzyme for every substrate, the body must produce a great number of different enzymes.

THE FUNCTIONS OF ENZYMES

Enzymes assist in practically all bodily functions. Digestive enzymes break down food particles for energy. This chemical reaction is called *hydrolysis*, and it involves using water to break the chemical bonds to turn food into energy. The stored energy is later converted by other enzymes for use by the body as required. Iron is concentrated in the blood by the action of enzymes; other enzymes in the blood help the blood to coagulate in order to stop bleeding. Uricolytic enzymes catalyze the conversion of uric acid into urea. Respiratory enzymes aid in eliminating carbon dioxide from the lungs. Enzymes assist the kidneys, liver, lungs, colon, and skin in removing wastes and toxins from the body. Enzymes also utilize the nutrients ingested by the body to construct new muscle tissue, nerve cells, bone, skin, and glandular tissue. One enzyme can take dietary phosphorus and convert it into bone. Enzymes prompt the oxidation of glucose, which creates energy for the cells. Enzymes also protect the blood from dangerous waste mate-

rials by converting these substances to forms that are easily eliminated by the body. Indeed, the functions of enzymes are so many and so diverse that it would be impossible to name them all.

Enzymes are often divided into two groups: digestive enzymes and metabolic enzymes. Digestive enzymes are secreted along the gastrointestinal tract and break down foods, enabling the nutrients to be absorbed into the bloodstream for use in various bodily functions. If you don't make enough digestive enzymes, you will experience any or all of the following symptoms: bloating, gas, indigestion, diarrhea, and pain. Of the macronutrients—carbohydrate, protein, and fat—people have the most trouble digesting fat, followed by protein and carbohydrate. Those who are lactose intolerant lack the enzymes needed to break down milk sugar. When choosing an enzyme supplement, make sure that it addresses your specific digestion needs. There are three main categories of digestive enzymes: amylase, protease, and lipase.

- *Amylase*, found in saliva and in the pancreatic and intestinal juices, breaks down carbohydrates. It begins to act as soon as you start chewing (this is why it is important to chew your food well). Different types of amylase break down specific types of sugars. For example, lactase breaks down lactose (milk sugar), maltase breaks down maltose (malt sugar), and sucrase breaks down sucrose (cane and beet sugar).

- *Protease*, found in the stomach juices and also in the pancreatic and intestinal juices, helps to digest protein.

- *Lipase*, found in the stomach and pancreatic juices, and also present in fats in foods, aids in fat digestion.

Another component of the digestive process is hydrochloric acid. While not technically an enzyme itself, it interacts with digestive enzymes as they perform their functions.

Metabolic enzymes are enzymes that catalyze the various chemical reactions within the cells, such as energy production and detoxification. Metabolic enzymes govern the activities of all the body's organs, tissues, and cells. They are the workers that build the body from proteins, carbohydrates, and fats. Metabolic enzymes are found doing their specific work in the blood, organs, and tissues. Each body tissue has its own specific set of metabolic enzymes.

Two particularly important metabolic enzymes are superoxide dismutase (SOD) and its partner, catalase. SOD is an antioxidant that protects the cells by attacking a common free radical, superoxide. (*See* Superoxide Dismutase *under* ANTIOXIDANTS in Part One.) Catalase breaks down hydrogen peroxide, a metabolic waste product, and liberates oxygen for the body to use.

The body uses most of its enzyme-producing potential to produce about two dozen enzymes. These control the breakdown and utilization of proteins, fats, and carbohydrates to create the hundreds of metabolic enzymes necessary to maintain the rest of the tissues and organs in their functions.

FOOD ENZYMES

While the body manufactures a supply of enzymes, it also can, and should, obtain enzymes from food. In fact, the body's ability to manufacture enzymes is being seriously taxed by our diet of processed and highly cooked food. Unfortunately, enzymes are extremely sensitive to heat. Low to moderate heat (118°F or above) destroys most enzymes in food. To obtain enzymes from the diet, some people find benefit from eating raw foods. Eating raw foods or, alternatively, taking enzyme supplements, helps prevent depletion of the body's own enzymes and thus reduces the stress on the body. Since enzymes are made from protein, it is essential to consume adequate amounts of protein in the diet.

Who should take enzyme supplements? Anyone who has a malabsorption problem, a yeast infection (candidiasis), or is over age sixty and whose digestive process seems to be stalling out, resulting in unpleasant symptoms. Ingredients should include pancreatin, lipase, amylase, and protease. This combination ensures digestion and absorption of amino acids, fat-soluble nutrients, and carbohydrates. Bromelain, derived from pineapple stems, along with papain, derived from the papaya fruit, also are welcome. Specific problems can be addressed by the addition of specific enzymes. For instance, people who have trouble with dairy sugars should consider lactase; people who can't digest legumes might try legumase. Hydrochloric acid supplements also might be necessary in the form of betaine hydrochloride taken as capsules at the start of each meal.

Enzymes can be found naturally in many different foods, from both plant and animal sources. Avocados, papayas, pineapples, bananas, and mangos are all high in enzymes. Sprouts are the richest source. Unripe papaya and pineapple are excellent sources of enzymes. The enzymes extracted from papaya and pineapple—papain and bromelain, respectively—are proteolytic enzymes, which break down proteins. Many fat-containing foods also supply lipase, which breaks down fats. In fact, fat in food exposed only to pancreatic lipase (the lipase produced by the body) in the intestines is not as well digested as fat that is first worked on in the stomach by food lipase. Pancreatic lipase digests fat in a highly alkaline environment (the intestines), whereas lipase found in food fats works in a more acidic environment (the stomach). The optimal extraction of nutrients from fats depends on the work of different fat-digesting enzymes in successive stages.

Hydrochloric acid (HCl) comes in several different forms, including lysine HCl and betaine HCl. Betaine HCl is derived from sugar beets. When new, HCl capsules and tablets are almost white in color, but sometimes they can turn a deep purple color when they age. Supplemental HCl is not sold in powder or liquid form because contact with the teeth can damage tooth enamel. HCl has a sulfurlike odor.

Superoxide dismutase occurs naturally in a variety of food sources, including alfalfa, barley grass, broccoli, Brussels sprouts, cabbage, wheatgrass, and most dark green plants.

As powerful as they are, enzymes cannot act alone. They require adequate amounts of other substances, known as coenzymes, to be fully active. Among the most important coenzymes are the B-complex vitamins, vitamin C, vitamin E, and zinc.

COMMERCIALLY AVAILABLE ENZYMES

The majority of commercially available enzymes are digestive enzymes extracted from various sources. Enzymes are not manufactured synthetically. Most commercial enzyme products are made from animal enzymes, such as pancreatin and pepsin, which help in the digestion of food once it has reached the lower stomach and the intestinal tract. Some companies make their supplements from enzymes extracted from aspergillus, a type of fungus. Be sure to read labels. Those from animals are usually more concentrated than those grown from this fungus.

These enzymes begin their predigestive work in the upper stomach. All of these products are used primarily to aid the digestion of foods and absorption of nutrients, especially protein. If proteins are not completely digested, undigested protein particles may make their way into the bloodstream through the intestinal wall with other nutrients. This phenomenon is known as *leaky gut syndrome*, and it can result in allergic reactions that may be more or less severe, depending upon the strength of the immune system. This is one reason why the proper digestion of proteins is so important.

Any enzyme that acts on protein and prepares it for absorption is called a proteolytic enzyme. Proteolytic enzymes available in supplement form include pepsin, trypsin, rennin, pancreatin, chymotrypsin, bromelain, and papain. In addition to aiding digestion, proteolytic enzymes have been shown to be beneficial as anti-inflammatory agents. Pancreatin, derived from secretions of animal pancreas, is a focus of cancer research, because people with cancer are often deficient in this enzyme. Pancreatin is used in the treatment of digestive problems, viral infections, and sports injuries, as well as pancreatic insufficiency, food allergies, cystic fibrosis, autoimmune disorders, and other chronic illnesses.

Also available in supplement form are the antioxidant enzymes superoxide dismutase (SOD) and catalase.

The following table lists some common enzymes and their substrates (the substance acted upon).

Enzyme	Substrate
Amylase	Carbohydrates
Bromelain	Proteins
Cellulase	Fiber
Chymopapain	Proteins
Diastase	Carbohydrates
Glucoamylase	Carbohydrates
Hemicellulase	Carbohydrates
Hyaluronidase	Proteins, adhesions, fibrin
Invertase	Carbohydrates
Lactase	Lactose (milk sugar)
Lipase	Fats
Maltase	Carbohydrates
Pancreatin	Proteins, fats, carbohydrates
Papain	Proteins, fats, carbohydrates
Pectinase	Carbohydrates
Pepsin	Proteins
Phytase	Carbohydrates
Plasmin	Proteins
Protease	Proteins
Rennin	Proteins
Trypsin	Proteins

If you decide to supplement, keep in mind that the way you respond to an enzyme may vary depending on the manufacturer. The good thing about digestive enzymes is that they work right away, so if you find you are not digesting a certain food—even after you have taken the enzyme—try another brand. Enzyme supplements may not be for everyone. During pregnancy, it is a rule to be careful with supplements in general. Nursing mothers also should be careful about supplements, to avoid affecting their milk. People who have hemophilia or who take anticoagulants (blood-thinners) should consult their health care providers before taking large amounts of enzymes. Anyone contemplating surgery where there is a high risk of bleeding should ask his or her physician for advice before taking any supplement.

WHAT'S ON THE SHELVES

Enzymes are available over the counter in tablet, capsule, powder, and liquid forms. They may be sold in combination with each other or as separate items. Some enzyme products also contain garlic to aid digestion.

For maximum benefit, any digestive enzyme supplement you choose should contain all of the major enzyme groups—amylase, protease, and lipase. Digestive enzymes should be taken with meals. You can make your own di-

gestive enzymes by drying papaya seeds, placing them in a pepper grinder, and sprinkling them on your foods. These have a peppery taste.

If you take supplemental superoxide dismutase (SOD), make sure to choose a product that is enteric coated—that is, coated with a protective substance that allows the SOD to pass intact through the stomach acid to be absorbed in the small intestine. Do not crush or chew these pills. All forms of enzymes should be kept in a reasonably cool place to ensure potency because they are susceptible to moisture.

Research has shown that as we grow older, the body's ability to produce enzymes decreases. At the same time, malabsorption of nutrients, tissue breakdown, and chronic health conditions increase. Taking supplemental enzymes can help to ensure that you continue to get the full nutritional value from your foods. We believe that enzyme supplementation is vital for elderly persons. In addition, most patients with cystic fibrosis require enzyme supplements. This disease affects the pancreas and renders it unable to make adequate amounts of all digestive enzymes. Be sure to check with your health care provider to determine what product is right for you.

The following are a few recommended enzyme complex products:

- AbsorbAid from Nature's Sources is made from plant enzymes and includes lipase, amylase, and protease from bromelain, as well as cellulase and lactase. It has been shown to significantly improve the absorption of nutrients, especially essential fatty acids and zinc.

- Acid-Ease from Enzymatic Therapy is a digestive aid from natural plant sources that includes amylase, lipase, and cellulase, as well as the soothing herbs marshmallow root and slippery elm.

- All Complete Enzymes from TriMedica, Inc., is a blend of plant enzymes that provide a full range of essential enzymes, plus coenzymes for added effectiveness. It is designed to adapt to various body temperatures and pH levels without losing potency. Ingredients include amylase, lipase, bromelain, papain, protease, cellulase, acidophilus, bifidus, and trace minerals.

- Bio-Gestin from Biotec Foods (a division of AgriGenic Food Corporation) is freeze-dried mature green papaya containing papain and chymopapain. The naturally sweet taste of the papaya makes these especially good capsules to open and sprinkle over food before eating.

- Digestive Aid #34 Food Enzymes from Carlson Laboratories contains pancreatin and ox bile, with enough capability in each tablet to digest 34 grams of protein, 120 grams of carbohydrate, and 21 grams of fat. Ox bile is a beneficial supplement for people with gallbladder disorders.

- Essential Enzymes from Source Naturals is a full-spectrum digestive enzyme supplement containing protease (acid stable), lipase, amylase, cellulase, and lactase. The powder in the capsules has very little taste of its own, and the contents may be added to food that is not hot (over 110°F) by sprinkling over food (this is a good option for vegetarians who want to avoid gelatin capsules). This supplement is designed to work in both the acidic environment of the stomach and the more alkaline environment of the intestines.

- Digest Support from Natrol is a multienzyme formula containing all three classes of digestive enzymes (proteolytic, amyolytic, and lipolytic), including protease 1 and 2, amylase, cellulase, lipase, maltase, and sucrase. It also contains A-galactosidase, an enzyme that acts on galactose, a breakdown product of lactose (milk sugar), and fights gas.

- Inf-Zyme Forte from American Biologics is a combination of enzymes and antioxidants for people requiring supplemental digestive enzymes to aid in the breakdown of proteins, fats, and carbohydrates. It may also be helpful for chronic or acute inflammation. Its ingredients include amylase, bromelain, catalase, chymotrypsin, L-cysteine, lipase, pancreatin, papain, rutin, superoxide dismutase, trypsin, and zinc. If taken as a digestive aid, the recommended dosage is 1 to 3 tablets following each meal; if you use it for other purposes, such as illness, inflammation, and/or injury, take 3 to 6 tablets one hour before each meal or between meals. Inf-Zyme Forte may be taken by persons on sodium-restricted diets.

- Mega-Zyme from Enzymatic Therapy is an extra-strength pancreatic and digestive enzyme tablet. Each tablet contains protease, amylase, lipase, trypsin, papain, bromelain, and lysozyme.

- MegaZymes from MegaFood is a vegetarian enzyme and herbal formula made from plant-based enzymes, including amylase, cellulase, glucoamylase, invertase, lactase, lipase, and protease, blended with the tonic herbs caraway, gentian, and ginger, plus acidophilus to support healthy intestinal flora.

- Metazyme from Metagenics is a plant-derived enzyme supplement that contains protease, amylase, lipase, and cellulase.

- Multi-Zyme from FoodScience of Vermont is an enteric-coated tablet containing pepsin, bromelain, ox bile, pancreas extract, papain, proteases, amylase, lipases, cellulase, and hydrochloric acid (HCl). HCl is another component of the digestive process that works with enzymes to break down foods.

- Vegetarian Enzyme Complex from Futurebiotics contains protease, amylase, cellulase, lipase, papain, and bromelain.

Other sources for quality enzyme supplements include the National Enzyme Company and Miller Pharmacal Group. Miller Pharmacal products, available through health care professionals only, include:

- Milco-zyme, a two-part enzyme supplement with glutamic acid HCl, betaine HCl, papain, pepsin, and an enteric-coated side of the same tablet with pancreatin, lipase, amylase, and bromelain.

- Carozyme, which contains betaine HCl, trypsin, chymotrypsin, bromelain, pancreatin, mannitol, thymus extract, lipase, amylase, and papain.

- Proteolytic Enzymes, made with enteric-coated trypsin and chymotrypsin.

- Karbozyme (not to be confused with the sound-alike product above), which contains pancreatin, sodium bicarbonate, and potassium bicarbonate.

- MM-Zyme, which contains pancreatic lipase, bromelain, amylase, raw pancreas extract, papain, trypsin, chymotrypsin, and selenium.

Finally, while not technically an enzyme product, Bioperine 10 from Nature's Plus also enhances the digestion and absorption of nutrients. It contains an extract of black pepper (*Piper nigrum*), and when taken with food or with vitamin, mineral, or herbal supplements, it may help food to digest and accelerates the distribution of nutrients throughout the body. However, not all vitamin, mineral, and herbal supplements have been tested in clinical studies.

Natural Food Supplements

INTRODUCTION

Natural food supplements include a wide variety of products. Almost all health food stores carry them, and a number of drugstores, supermarkets, and mass market/club stores stock them on their shelves as well. In general, natural food supplements are composed of, derived from, or by-products of foods that provide health benefits. In some cases, health benefit claims made by manufacturers are based upon a supplement's use in traditional healing; in other cases, they are based on modern scientific research. Today, label claims are regulated by the FDA and FTC to be true, not misleading, and based on science.

Food supplements can be high in certain nutrients, contain active ingredients that aid digestive or metabolic processes, or provide a combination of nutrients and active ingredients. It is important to point out that some unscrupulous manufacturers make false promises. It is therefore vital to be an informed consumer.

Many natural food supplements have been known to work for years; these products are medically endorsed only when they are "discovered" by researchers deemed acceptable by these groups. Such recent discoveries include garlic, aloe vera, fiber, and fish oils—substances that have been used for centuries in many parts of the world. In a review by the head of the American Botanical Council, Mark Blumenthal, several herbs have not only been used a long time but have also stood up to rigorous scientific testing. He makes an argument for the strong science behind St. John's wort to help with depression, garlic to help people with heart disease, ginseng to improve sexual function in males, and echinacea to boost immunity.

WHAT'S ON THE SHELVES

Food supplements come in many shapes and forms—tablets, capsules, powders, liquids, jellies, creams, biscuits, wafers, granules, and more. Product packaging depends entirely on the nature of the food supplement's composition.

The potency of these products varies. Because they are made up of perishable foods, food derivatives, or food by-products, their potency may be affected by the length of time they sit on a shelf or by the temperature at which they are kept. If you don't understand how a product is to be used, ask questions or read the available literature on the particular supplement. All products sold today need to have a "sell-by" date on the label. If there isn't one, contact the manufacturer and tell them the code on your box.

If you have never used a natural food supplement, you may be uncomfortable about buying and using one for the first time. This is normal. Keep in mind that once you become familiar with its use and benefits, you won't give the idea of using it a second thought.

In this section, we describe some of the types of food supplements that are recommended for use in dealing with the various disorders discussed in Part Two of this book.

Acidophilus

See Lactobacillus Acidophilus in this section.

Adenosine Triphosphate (ATP)

Adenosine triphosphate (ATP) is a compound that serves as the immediate source of energy for the body's cells, notably muscle cells. It increases energy and stamina, builds muscular density, increases muscular strength, buffers lactic-acid buildup (the reason for sore, achy muscles after physical activity), delays fatigue, and preserves muscle fibers. ATP is produced naturally in the body from adenine, a nitrogen-containing compound; ribose, a type of sugar; and phosphate units, each containing one phosphorus atom and four oxygen atoms.

Alfalfa

One of the most mineral-rich foods known, alfalfa has roots that grow as much as 130 feet into the earth. Alfalfa is available in liquid extract form and is good to use while fasting because of its chlorophyll and nutrient content. It contains digestive-aiding enzymes, amino acids, and carbohydrates. It also contains calcium, magnesium, phosphorus, potassium, plus virtually all known vitamins. The minerals are in a balanced form, which promotes absorption. These minerals are alkaline, but have a neutralizing effect on the intestinal tract.

If you need a mineral supplement, alfalfa is a good choice. It has helped many arthritis sufferers. Alfalfa, wheatgrass, barley, and spirulina, all of which contain chlorophyll, have been found to aid in the healing of intestinal ulcers, gastritis, liver disorders, eczema, hemorrhoids, asthma, high blood pressure, anemia, constipation, body and breath odor, bleeding gums, infections, burns, athlete's foot, and cancer.

Aloe Vera

This plant is known for its healing effect and is used in many cosmetic and hair care products. There are over two hundred different species of aloe that grow in dry regions around the world.

Aloe vera is commonly known as a skin healer, moisturizer, and softener. It is dramatically effective on burns of all types, and is also good for cuts, insect stings, bruises, acne and blemishes, poison ivy, welts, skin ulcers, and eczema.

Taken internally, 98 or 99 percent pure aloe vera juice is known to aid in the healing of stomach disorders, ulcers, constipation, hemorrhoids, rectal itching, colitis, and all colon problems.

Aloe vera can also be helpful against infections, varicose veins, skin cancer, and arthritis, and is used in the management of AIDS.

We have had excellent results using colon cleansers containing psyllium husks in combination with aloe vera juice. We have found this combination to be good for food allergy and colon disorder sufferers. Psyllium keeps the folds and pockets in the colon free of toxic material that gathers there. The aloe vera not only has a healing effect, but if constipation or diarrhea is present, it will return the stools to normal.

It takes a few weeks to cleanse the colon, but regular, periodic use will keep the colon clean. As with any substance, it is possible to develop intolerance to aloe vera juice and/or psyllium husks, so this treatment should not be used on an ongoing basis.

Barley Grass

Barley grass contains small amounts of calcium, iron, all the essential amino acids, chlorophyll, flavonoids, vitamin B_{12}, vitamin C, and many minerals, plus enzymes. This food heals stomach, duodenal, and colon disorders as well as pancreatitis, and is an effective anti-inflammatory.

Bee By-products

See Bee Pollen, Bee Propolis, Honey, and Royal Jelly, all in this section.

Bee Pollen

Bee pollen is a powderlike material that is produced by the anthers of flowering plants and gathered by bees. It is composed of 10 to 15 percent protein and also contains B-complex vitamins, vitamin C, essential fatty acids, enzymes, carotene, calcium, copper, iron, magnesium, potassium, manganese, sodium, plant sterols, and simple sugars.

Like other bee products, bee pollen has an antimicrobial effect. In addition, it is useful for combating fatigue, depression, cancer, and colon disorders. It is also helpful for people with allergies because it strengthens the immune system.

It is best to obtain bee pollen from a local source, as this increases its antiallergenic properties. Fresh bee pollen should not cling together or form clumps, and it should be sold in a tightly sealed container. Some people (an estimated 0.05 percent of the population) may be allergic to bee pollen. It is best to try taking a small amount at first and watch for a developing rash, wheezing, discomfort, or any other signs of a reaction. If such symptoms occur, discontinue taking bee pollen.

Bee Propolis

Bee propolis is a resinous substance collected from various plants by bees. Bees use propolis, together with beeswax, in the construction of hives. As a supplement, it is an excellent aid against bacterial infections. Bee propolis is believed to stimulate phagocytosis, the process by which some white blood cells destroy bacteria.

Propolis is beneficial as a salve for abrasions and bruises because of its antibacterial effect. Good results have been reported on the use of propolis against inflammation of the mucous membranes of the mouth and throat, dry cough and throat, halitosis, tonsillitis, ulcers, and acne, and for the stimulation of the immune system.

Be sure that any bee products you use smell and taste fresh. All bee products should be in tightly sealed containers. It is best to purchase these products from a manufacturer who specializes in bee products. If you are using bee products for allergies, it is best to obtain products that are produced within a ten-mile radius of your home. This way, you get a minute dose of pollen to desensitize you to the local pollen in the area.

Beta-1,3-Glucan

Beta-1,3-glucan is a polysaccharide (a complex type of carbohydrate molecule) with immune-stimulating properties. Specifically, it stimulates the activity of macrophages (immune cells that destroy cellular debris), microorganisms, and abnormal cells by surrounding and digesting them.

Beta-1,3-D-glucan is a supplemental form of beta-1,3-glucan made from the cell walls of baker's yeast. Despite its origin, it does not contain any yeast proteins. It is useful for treating many bacterial, viral, and fungal diseases. It can also kill tumor cells and increase bone marrow production.

Because of its ability to protect the immune system, beta-1,3-D-glucan may protect against the effects of aging. Studies done as early as the 1970s have found that it can reduce the size of cancerous tumors in rats. Further investigation has shown beta-1,3-D-glucan to be a potent agent for healing sores and ulcers in women who have undergone mastectomies.

Bifidobacterium Bifidum

Bifidobacterium bifidum aids in the synthesis of the B vitamins by creating healthy intestinal flora. *B. bifidum* is the predominant healthy organism in the intestinal flora and establishes a healthy environment for the manufacture of the B-complex vitamins and vitamin K.

When you take antibiotics, the "friendly" bacteria in your digestive tract are destroyed along with the harmful bacteria. Supplementing your diet with *B. bifidum* helps you maintain healthy intestinal flora and helps strengthen the intestinal wall. Unhealthy flora can result in the liberation of abnormally high levels of ammonia as protein-containing foods are digested. This irritates the intestinal membranes. In addition, the ammonia is absorbed into the bloodstream and must be detoxified by the liver, or it will cause nausea, a decrease in appetite, vomiting, and other toxic reactions. By promoting the proper digestion of foods, the friendly bacteria also aid in preventing digestive disorders such as constipation and gas, as well as food allergies. If digestion is poor, the activity of intestinal bacteria on undigested food may lead to excessive production of the body chemical histamine, which triggers allergic symptoms.

Yeast infections of the vaginal tract respond very favorably to douching with *B. bifidum* preparations. These microorganisms destroy the pathogenic organisms. When used as an enema, *B. bifidum* also helps establish a healthy intestinal environment. It improves bowel function by aiding peristalsis, and results in the production of a softer, smoother stool. Harmful bacteria are kept in check, and toxic wastes that have accumulated in the intestines are destroyed and/or eliminated from the body.

B. bifidum may be useful in the treatment of cirrhosis of the liver and chronic hepatitis; by improving digestion, it reduces the strain on the liver. Many people who do not respond to *L. acidophilus* react positively to *B. bifidum*. Many experts consider *B. bifidum* to be preferable to *L. acidophilus* for children and for adults with liver disorders. This product needs to be taken every day or the body will go back to its usual state of bacteria growth.

Bifidus

See Bifidobacterium Bifidum above.

Bovine Cartilage

Cleaned, dried, and powdered bovine cartilage is a supplement that helps to accelerate wound healing and reduce inflammation. Like shark cartilage, it has been shown to be helpful for psoriasis, all types of arthritis, and ulcerative colitis. Bovine Cartilage from FoodScience of Vermont is a good source made from hormone-free, organically raised cattle.

Brewer's Yeast

See Yeast in this section.

Cellulose

See under Fiber in this section.

Cerasomal-cis-9-cetylmyristoleate

This is a modified version of a medium-chain fatty acid, cetylmyristoleate, which is found in nuts, vegetables, and animal tissue. It appears to be a very promising development in arthritis research. Studies in laboratory rats have shown it to have anti-inflammatory effects, and early clinical studies in people suggest it may be beneficial for many with osteoarthritis, rheumatoid arthritis, and psoriatic arthritis, as well as psoriasis. It is believed to work by normalizing the functioning of the immune system and reducing the production of pro-inflammatory prostaglandins.

Chlorella

Chlorella is a tiny, single-celled water-grown alga containing a nucleus and an enormous amount of readily available chlorophyll. It also contains protein (approximately 58 percent), carbohydrates, all of the B vitamins, vitamins C and E, amino acids, and rare trace minerals. In fact, it is virtually a complete food. It contains more vitamin B_{12} than liver, plus a considerable amount of beta-carotene. It has a strong cell wall, however, which makes it difficult to gain access to its nutrients. Consequently, it requires factory processing to be effective.

Chlorella is one of the few edible species of water-grown algae. The chlorophyll in chlorella can help speed the cleansing of the bloodstream. Chlorella is very high in RNA and DNA, and has been found to protect against the effects of ultraviolet radiation. Studies show that chlorella is an excellent source of protein, especially for people who cannot or who choose not to eat meat. It is available from Sun Chlorella USA. (*See* Manufacturer and Distribution Information in the Appendix for further information.)

Chlorophyll

See under Chlorella and "Green Drinks" in this section.

Chondroitin Sulfate

Chondroitin sulfate is an important element in the creation of cartilage. Cartilage is the tough yet flexible connective tissue found in the joints, where it acts as a cushion, and in other parts of the body, such as the tip of the nose and the outer ear.

Chemically, chondroitins belong to a group of substances classified as *glycosaminoglycans* (also referred to as *mucopolysaccharides*), which are complex types of carbohydrate molecules. Glycosaminoglycans in turn attach to proteins such as collagen and elastin, forming even more complex substances designated *proteoglycans*, which are a vital component of cartilage tissue. Chondroitin sulfate attracts water to the proteoglycans and holds it there, which is important for maintaining healthy joint cartilage. It can also protect existing cartilage from premature degeneration by blocking certain enzymes that destroy cartilage and prevent nutrients from being transported to the cartilage for repair. In one study of patients with osteoarthritis of the knee who used chondroitin, the diseased progressed more slowly and they had less pain compared to a group that was not treated. It was more effective in patients with mild knee pain than in those with severe pain.

Taking supplemental chondroitin sulfate, usually derived from powdered shark cartilage or cow trachea cartilage, has been shown to be helpful in the treatment of osteoarthritis. Many times it is used in conjunction with glucosamine for even more effective therapy. The supplements are usually taken together in pill form. Neither chondroitin sulfate nor glucosamine has shown any toxic effects, but there are potential side effects for certain people. The Arthritis Foundation recommends exercising caution in taking these supplements for treatment of osteoarthritis. Let your physician know you are taking these supplements, and discuss any allergies or potential reactions. Use caution in taking chondroitin sulfate if you are taking anticoagulants (blood-thinners) or daily aspirin, as it is chemically similar to the blood-thinner heparin. Pregnant women should not take these supplements, as there has not been sufficient study regarding their safety and potential side effects during pregnancy.

Twinlab manufactures a few good products containing chondroitin sulfate. Glucosamine Chondroitin Sulfate from Only Natural, Inc. is a good combination source of glucosamine and chondroitin sulfate.

Citrin

Citrin is a trademarked name for a standardized herbal extract from the fruit of the *Garcinia cambogia* plant (Indian berry). It inhibits the synthesis of fatty acids in the liver, promotes the burning of body fat as fuel, and suppresses the appetite. Its main usefulness is in treating obesity; it may also aid in preventing or slowing atherosclerosis and heart disease. It does not affect the nervous system or have any known side effects. Citrin is found in a number of products sold by various manufacturers. Recent studies suggest that Garcitrin, a similar extract made from *Garcinia cambogia*, may be more effective for weight loss than Citrin.

Coenzyme A

Coenzyme A, a substance manufactured by body cells from pantothenic acid (vitamin B$_5$), is at the center of the whole metabolic process. It performs a vital role in the process by which the cells generate energy from glucose. Indeed, it helps produce around 90 percent of the energy the body needs to function. Coenzyme A also begins the metabolism

of fatty acids. A lack of sufficient coenzyme A can result in stiff, sore muscles and a decrease in energy. Taken as a supplement, coenzyme A increases energy, supports the manufacture of substances critical for the brain and adrenal glands, helps with the manufacture of connective tissue, and supports the immune system. Studies suggest that coenzyme A may be as, if not more, beneficial than coenzyme Q$_{10}$.

Coenzyme Q$_{10}$

Coenzyme Q$_{10}$ is present in the mitochondria of all the cells in the body. It is vital because it carries into the cells the energy-laden protons and electrons that are used to produce adenosine triphosphate (ATP), the immediate source of cellular energy. (*See* Adenosine Triphosphate [ATP] earlier in this section.) This is a constant process because the body can store only a small quantity of ATP at any one time. It is believed that as many as 75 percent of people over fifty may be deficient in coenzyme Q$_{10}$. A lack of sufficient coenzyme Q$_{10}$ can lead to cardiovascular disease. Without enough of it, the heart cannot circulate the blood effectively. Coenzyme Q$_{10}$ has varied applications, including migraine prevention, improving energy levels, lowering blood pressure, and the management of chronic cardiac failure. It has *not* been shown to help with glucose management, prevent oxidation of bad cholesterol, enhance blood flow from the heart, or inhibit periodontal disease. In Japan, coenzyme Q$_{10}$ has been approved for use in treating congestive heart failure. (*See* ANTIOXIDANTS earlier in this chapter for a discussion of coenzyme Q$_{10}$ as an antioxidant.)

Colostrum

Colostrum is a thin, yellowish fluid secreted by the mammary glands of mammalian mothers in the first days after giving birth, before the production of true milk begins. It contains high levels of protein and growth factors, as well as immune factors that help to protect the newborn against infection. Taken as a supplement, colostrum can boost the immune system by enhancing the ability of the thymus gland to create T cells and also can help the body to burn fat and build lean muscle. It may also accelerate the healing of injuries, increase vitality and stamina, and have an anti-aging effect.

Supplemental colostrum usually contains bovine (cow) colostrum. Good sources include Colostrum Plus from Symbiotics and Colostrum Prime Life from Jarrow Formulas.

Corn Germ

Using a process that isolates the embryo of the corn plant, which contains the most usable nutrients, corn germ is made. Corn germ has a longer shelf life than wheat germ and is higher in some nutrients, especially zinc. Corn germ contains ten times the amount of zinc found in wheat germ.

You can use corn germ to bread chicken or fish. It is also good when added to cereals and used as a topping.

Creatine

Creatine (creatine monohydrate) is a compound produced by metabolic processes in the body. When muscles are in use, the compound adenosine triphosphate (ATP) is broken down into two other compounds—adenosine diphosphate (ADP) and inorganic phosphate. This process produces the body's cellular energy, which, among other things, powers the muscles. Each such burst of energy is very fleeting.

However, with the addition of creatine, ADP can be transformed back to ATP, the source of cellular energy. Taken as a supplement, creatine can increase both endurance and strength, making possible extended workout time. Longer workouts in turn can result in a real increase in lean muscle mass, and do not simply puff up the muscle with water.

Creatine is particularly popular with athletes. The use of creatine for muscle-depleting illnesses and the natural wasting of muscles that comes with age is also being studied. In one study, elderly men and women had improved upper body grip strength and lower body muscle endurance after using creatine. They were less fatigued in general and experienced no side effects from the supplement.

Creatine should be used in combination with a balanced, nutritionally complete diet. Vegetarians do not get enough dietary creatine—since it comes exclusively from animal-based foods—and may need supplementation, especially if they exercise. Those who eat animal-based foods consume about 2 grams a day. You should not take it with fruit juices, as this combination results in the production of creatinine, which is difficult for the kidneys to process. Never exceed the recommended dose. Smaller doses (about 2.5 grams) rather than 5 or more grams seemed to be just as effective in growing new muscles during a workout.

Dehydroepiandrosterone (DHEA)

Dehydroepiandrosterone (DHEA) is a hormone that is produced primarily by the adrenal glands and is found naturally in the human body. It is an important base from which other key substances, including the hormones testosterone, progesterone, and corticosterone, can be derived, either directly or indirectly. The amount of DHEA produced by the body declines with age, particularly after age forty. Research indicates that taking DHEA supplements may help to prevent cancer, arterial disease, multiple sclerosis, and Alzheimer's disease; may be beneficial in the treatment of lupus and osteoporosis; may enhance the activity of the immune system; and may help to improve memory.

Caution should be exercised when taking this supplement. Some physicians believe that taking high doses of DHEA suppresses the body's natural ability to synthesize this hormone. Further, laboratory studies have shown that high doses can lead to liver damage. If you take supplemental DHEA, it is important also to take supplements of the antioxidant vitamins C and E and the antioxidant mineral selenium to prevent oxidative damage to the liver. Possible side effects of taking DHEA include excess growth of facial hair in women. This can often be avoided by starting with a dose of 10 milligrams daily. 7-Keto DHEA is a derivative of DHEA that is not converted into estrogen or testosterone, which is good for women concerned about breast cancer and for men concerned about prostate cancer. 7-Keto DHEA is a good and safer alternative to DHEA and has the same benefits.

Desiccated Liver

Desiccated liver is concentrated dried liver that is put into powdered or tablet form. This form of liver contains vitamins A, D, and C; the B-complex vitamins; and the minerals calcium, copper, phosphorus, and iron. Desiccated liver is good for people with anemia, and aids in building healthy red blood cells. It is known to increase energy, aid in liver disorders, and help relieve stress in the body. Use only a product made from liver derived from beef that is raised organically.

Dimethylglycine (DMG)

Dimethylglycine (DMG) is a derivative of glycine, the simplest of the amino acids. It acts as a building block for many important substances, including the amino acid methionine, choline, a number of important hormones and neurotransmitters, and DNA.

Low levels of DMG are present in meats, seeds, and grains. It is a safe, nontoxic food substance that does not build up in the body. No deficiency symptoms are associated with a lack of DMG in the diet, but taking supplemental DMG can have a wide range of beneficial effects, including helping the body maintain high energy levels and boosting mental acuity. DMG has been found to enhance the immune system and to reduce elevated blood cholesterol and triglyceride levels. It improves oxygen utilization by the body, helps to normalize blood pressure and blood glucose levels, and improves the functioning of many important organs. It may also be useful for controlling epileptic seizures. Some people have used DMG as a substitute for pangamic acid, a supplement that is no longer available in the United States but that is widely used in Russia to treat heart disease, liver disease, alcohol and drug addiction, and other problems. DMG is thought to increase pangamic acid levels in the body. Aangamik DMG from FoodScience of Vermont is a good source of supplemental DMG.

Dimethylsulfoxide (DMSO)

Dimethylsulfoxide (DMSO) is a by-product of wood processing for papermaking. It is a somewhat oily liquid that looks like mineral oil and has a slightly garlicky odor. Because it is an excellent solvent, it is widely used as a degreaser, paint thinner, and antifreeze. However, it also has remarkable therapeutic properties, especially for the healing of injuries. Applying DMSO on sprained ankles, pulled muscles, dislocated joints, and even at the site of simple fractures can virtually eliminate the pain. It also promotes immune system activity.

DMSO is absorbed through the skin and enters the bloodstream by osmosis through capillary walls. It is then distributed through the circulatory system and ultimately is excreted through the urine. Because of the properties of DMSO, it will take any contaminants on the skin or in the product directly into the bloodstream. For this reason, only pure DMSO from a health food source can be used. The use of hardware store DMSO could cause serious health problems. DMSO has been used successfully in the treatment of brain and spinal cord damage, arthritis, Down syndrome, sciatica and other back problems, keloids, acne, burns, musculoskeletal problems, sports injuries, cancer, sinusitis, headaches, skin ulcers, herpes, and cataracts. The use of DMSO may result in a garlicky body odor. This is temporary and is not a cause for concern.

Essential Fatty Acids (EFAs)

Fatty acids are the basic building blocks of which fats and oils are composed. Contrary to popular myth, the body does need some of the right kind of fat. The fatty acids that are necessary for health and that cannot be made by the body are called *essential fatty acids* (EFAs). EFAs must be supplied through the diet.

EFAs have desirable effects on many disorders. They improve the skin and hair, reduce blood pressure, aid in the prevention of arthritis, lower cholesterol and triglyceride levels, and reduce the risk of blood clot formation. They are beneficial for candidiasis, cardiovascular disease, eczema, and psoriasis. Found in high concentrations in the brain, EFAs aid in the transmission of nerve impulses, and are needed for the normal development and functioning of the brain. A deficiency of EFAs can lead to an impaired ability to learn and recall information. Infant formulas now contain ARA and DHA, essential fats for infants, which may promote better learning.

Every living cell in the body needs EFAs. They are essential for rebuilding and producing new cells. They are also used by the body for the production of prostaglandins, hormonelike substances that act as chemical messengers and regulators of various body processes.

There are two basic categories of EFAs, designated *omega-3* and *omega-6,* based on their chemical structures. Omega-3 EFAs, including alpha-linolenic and eicosapen-

taenoic acid (EPA), are found in fresh deepwater fish, fish oil, and certain vegetable oils, among them canola oil, flaxseed oil, and walnut oil. Omega-6 EFAs, which include linoleic and gamma-linolenic acids, are found primarily in raw nuts, seeds, and legumes, and in unsaturated vegetable oils, such as borage oil, grape seed oil, primrose oil, sesame oil, and soybean oil. A recent study reported in the British medical journal *Lancet* has shown that omega-3 fatty acids, which create a more stable arterial plaque, are better for your heart than the omega-6 variety. We recommend that you try to increase your consumption of omega-3s at the expense of the omega-6s. In order to supply EFAs, these oils must be consumed in pure liquid or supplement form and must not be subjected to heat, either in processing or cooking. Heat destroys EFAs. Worse, it results in the creation of dangerous free radicals. (*See* ANTIOXIDANTS in Part One.) If oils are hydrogenated (processed to make the oil more solid, as is commonly done in the production of margarine), the linoleic acid is converted into trans-fatty acids, which are not beneficial to the body.

The daily requirement for EFAs is satisfied by an amount equivalent to 10 to 20 percent of total fat intake. The most essential of the EFAs is linoleic acid.

A number of sources of EFAs are recommended in this book, among them fish oils, flaxseeds and flaxseed oil, and primrose oil. If you are taking any of these oils, you need to cut back on linoleic-rich oils such as corn, sunflower, and cottonseed oil to avoid getting too much of the omega-6 fats.

Emu Oil

Emu oil is an excellent source of linoleic acid, linolenic acid, and oleic acid. Linolenic acid has anti-inflammatory properties. It can be used topically for the relief of rashes, hemorrhoids, poison ivy, insect bites, arthritis, joint aches, and muscle strains, and it has been known to stop the pain of burns. It can also be used as a facial moisturizer to reduce wrinkles and lines. Thunder Ridge Emu is a good source for emu oil.

Fish Oil

Fish oil is a good source of omega-3 EFAs. Salmon, herring, tuna (limit to 1 serving per week), and sardines are good sources of fish oil because they have a higher fat content and provide more omega-3 factors than other fishes.

For instance, 4 ounces of salmon contains 1,000 to 4,600 milligrams of omega-3 fatty acids, while 4 ounces of cod (a low-fat fish) contains only about 300 milligrams. Menhaden, another type of fish, supplies most of the oil used in dietary supplements because it is rich in omega-3s.

Carlson Laboratories markets a good Norwegian salmon oil that we recommend. Cod liver oil from Norway is the most commonly used fish oil and is milder tasting than other varieties. Author Dale Alexander claims it is excellent for arthritis. He has marketed an oil containing 13,800 international units of vitamin A and 1,380 international units of vitamin D per tablespoon. However, we do not recommend that you rely on cod liver oil as a source of the EFAs. You would have to overdose on vitamins A and D to obtain the amount of fatty acids you need.

People with diabetes have been cautioned not to take fish oil supplements because fish oil may slightly raise blood cholesterol levels. However, the benefit of such oils in reducing triglyceride levels outweighs this risk. People with diabetes should check with their health care provider, but they should consume fish anyway for its EFAs.

Flaxseeds and Flaxseed Oil

Flaxseeds are rich in omega-3 EFAs, magnesium, potassium, and fiber. The omega-3s in plant-based foods are not in a bioactive form, which means the body has to process them before it can use them. In contrast, omega-3s from fish are ready for the body to use. Most experts agree that the body uses only 10 percent or less of omega-3s from plant-based foods. Both seeds and oils are also a good source of the B vitamins, protein, and zinc. They are low in saturated fats and calories, and contain no cholesterol. The nutty taste of ground flaxseeds is pleasant, and they can be mixed with water or any fruit or vegetable juice. They can also be added to salads, soups, yogurt, cereals, baked goods, or fresh juices. You can grind these tiny seeds in a coffee grinder.

If you prefer not to eat the seeds, you can use flaxseed oil as an alternative. Like the seeds from which it is extracted, organic cold-pressed flaxseed oil is rich in EFAs. Several studies have shown that it can reduce the pain, inflammation, and swelling of arthritis. It has been found to lower blood cholesterol and triglyceride levels, and to help reduce the hardening effects of cholesterol on cell membranes.

Grape Seed Oil

Of the many natural sources of EFAs, grape seed oil is among the highest in linoleic acid and among the lowest in saturated fats. Grape seed oil is rich in omega-6 oils, which are essential, but usually we get more than enough omega-6s in our diet, so use it sparingly. It contains no cholesterol and no sodium. It has a light, nutty taste that brings out the flavor in many foods. Unlike most other oils, it can be heated to temperatures as high as 485°F without producing dangerous and possibly carcinogenic free radicals. These features make it good for use in cooking. Buy only grape seed oil that is cold-pressed and contains no preservatives.

Primrose Oil

Primrose oil (also known as evening primrose oil) contains 9 to 10 percent gamma-linolenic acid (GLA). It is an anti-inflammatory fatty acid and may help reduce the likelihood of developing cancer, diabetes, heart disease, and Alzheimer's disease. It relieves pain and inflammation; enhances the release of sex hormones, including estrogen and testosterone; aids in lowering cholesterol levels; and is beneficial for cirrhosis of the liver.

Many women have found that primrose oil supplements relieve unpleasant menopausal symptoms such as hot flashes. Because it promotes the production of estrogen, women suffering from breast cancer that is diagnosed as estrogen-receptor positive (estrogen-related) should avoid or limit their intake of primrose oil. Black currant seed oil is a good substitute.

Evening Primrose Oil

See Primrose Oil above.

Fiber

Found in many foods, fiber helps to lower blood cholesterol levels and stabilize blood sugar levels. It helps prevent colon cancer, constipation, hemorrhoids, obesity, and many other disorders. Fiber is also good for removing certain toxic metals from the body. Because the refining process has removed much of the natural fiber from our foods, the typical American diet is lacking in fiber.

There are seven basic classifications of fiber: bran, cellulose, gum, hemicellulose, lignin, mucilages, and pectin. Each form has its own function. It is best to rotate among several different supplemental fiber sources. Start with small amounts and gradually increase your intake until your stools are the proper consistency. Also, be aware that while today's average diet is lacking in fiber, consuming excessive amounts may decrease the absorption of zinc, iron, and calcium. Always take supplemental fiber separately from other medications or supplements. Otherwise, it can lessen their strength and effectiveness.

In addition to using a fiber supplement, you should make sure to get fiber through your diet. Make sure your diet contains these high-fiber foods:

- Whole-grain cereals and flours.
- Brown rice.
- Agar agar (made from the algae species *gelidium*; also called dai choy goh).
- All kinds of bran.
- Fresh fruit.
- Dried prunes.
- Nuts.

- Seeds (especially flaxseeds)
- Beans.
- Lentils.
- Peas.
- Fresh, raw vegetables.

Eat several of these foods daily. When eating organic produce, leave the skin on apples and potatoes. Coat chicken in corn bran or oats for baking. Add extra bran to cereals and breads. Unsalted, unbuttered popcorn is also excellent for added fiber.

Bran, Gums, and Mucilages

Both gums and mucilages help to regulate blood glucose levels, aid in lowering cholesterol, and help in the removal of toxins. They are found in oatmeal, oat bran, sesame seeds, and dried beans. Gums and mucilages are soluble fibers that foster the growth of healthy bacteria, which in turn discourage the growth of harmful ones. If you are taking any probiotics, for example, bifidobacteria, it is best to take it with one of these fibers.

One of the following should be part of your daily dietary plan:

- *Fennel seed.* Fennel is an herb that is helpful for digestive purposes. The seeds of this plant help to rid the intestinal tract of mucus and aid in relieving flatulence.
- *Glucomannan.* Derived from the tuber of the amorphophallis plant, it picks up and removes fat from the colon wall. This substance is good for diabetes, as it has been recognized for normalizing blood sugar and is good for people with hypoglycemia. Glucomannan expands to sixty times its own weight, thereby helping to curb the appetite. Taking 2 to 3 capsules with a large glass of water thirty minutes before meals is helpful for reducing allergic reactions and some symptoms associated with high and low blood sugar disorders. Always be sure to drink a large glass of water when taking glucomannan in capsule or pill form, as capsules can lodge in the throat and expand there, causing breathing problems. Glucomannan is tasteless and odorless, and can be added to foods to help normalize blood sugar.
- *Guar gum.* Extracted from the seeds of the guar plant, guar gum is good for the treatment of diabetes and for curbing the appetite. It also has the ability to reduce the levels of cholesterol, triglycerides, and low-density lipoproteins in the blood, and binds with toxic substances and carries them out of the body. Guar gum tablets must be chewed thoroughly or sucked gradually, not swallowed whole, and should be taken with lots of water, because guar gum has a tendency to ball up in the throat when mixed with saliva. It should not be used by individuals who have difficulty swallowing or who have

had gastrointestinal surgery. Some persons with colon disorders may have trouble using guar gum.

- *Oat bran and rice bran.* Bran is the broken coat of the seed of cereal grain that has been separated from the flour or meal by sifting or bolting. It helps to lower cholesterol.
- *Psyllium seed.* Psyllium is a grain grown in India that is utilized for its fiber content. A good intestinal cleanser and stool softener, it is one of the most popular fibers used. It thickens very quickly when mixed with liquid, and must be consumed immediately. Some doctors recommend Metamucil, which contains psyllium hydrophilic mucilloid, as a laxative and fiber supplement. However, we prefer less processing and all-natural products.

Cellulose

Cellulose is an indigestible carbohydrate (or insoluble fiber) found in the outer layer of vegetables and fruits. It is good for hemorrhoids, varicose veins, colitis, and constipation, and for the removal of cancer-causing substances from the colon wall.

It is found in apples, beets, Brazil nuts, broccoli, carrots, celery, green beans, lima beans, pears, peas, and whole grains.

Hemicellulose

Hemicellulose is an indigestible complex carbohydrate that absorbs water. It is good for promoting weight loss, relieving constipation, preventing colon cancer, and controlling carcinogens in the intestinal tract. Hemicellulose is found in apples, bananas, beans, beets, cabbage, corn, green leafy vegetables, pears, peppers, and whole-grain cereals.

Lignin

This form of fiber is good for lowering cholesterol levels. It helps to prevent the formation of gallstones by binding with bile acids and removing cholesterol before stones can form. It is beneficial for persons with diabetes or colon cancer. Those who eat a lot of dietary lignins have been shown to have better cognitive function compared to those who eat a low-lignin diet.

Lignins are found in all plants but especially in alfalfa, berries, Brazil nuts, broccoli, carrots, green beans, peaches, peas, potatoes, seed oils, strawberries, tomatoes, and whole grains.

Pectin

Because it slows the absorption of food after meals, pectin is good for people with diabetes. It also removes unwanted metals and toxins, reduces the side effects of radiation therapy, helps lower cholesterol, and reduces the risk of heart disease and gallstones. Pectin is found in apples, bananas, beets, cabbage, carrots, citrus fruits, dried peas, and okra.

Combination Fiber Supplements

There are many products available that combine two or more different types of fiber, or that combine fiber with other ingredients. Be sure you buy one that has both soluble and insoluble fiber. Two products of this kind that we recommend are:

- Colon Care Plus from Aerobic Life Industries. This formula contains psyllium and oat bran, and provides approximately 3 grams of soluble fiber and 4 grams of insoluble fiber per serving.

- Ultimate Cleanse from Nature's Secret. This formula combines gums with cellulose, hemicellulose, pectin, and lignin, plus herbs that support and cleanse the blood and internal organs.

Fish Oil

See under Essential Fatty Acids in this section.

5-Hydroxy L-Tryptophan (5-HTP)

5-HTP is a substance that is created naturally in the body from the amino acid tryptophan, and that in turn is used by the body to produce serotonin, an important neurotransmitter. Supplemental 5-HTP is derived from the seeds of the griffonia plant (*Griffonia simplicifolia*), which is native to western Africa. It can be used to aid in weight loss, insomnia, and depression.

5-HTP should be used together with a high-carbohydrate food or liquid such as orange juice, and as part of a comprehensive nutritional program. It may not benefit everyone who takes it. If you regularly take large doses of 5-HTP (more than 300 milligrams daily), you should undergo blood testing for eosinophil (a type of white blood cell) levels every three months. HTP.Calm from Natural Balance is a good source of 5-HTP. You should avoid this supplement if you are taking antidepressants.

Flaxseeds and Flaxseed Oil

See under Essential Fatty Acids in this section.

Garlic

Garlic is one of the most valuable foods on this planet. It has been used since biblical times and is mentioned in the literature of the ancient Hebrews, Greeks, Babylonians, Romans, and Egyptians. The builders of the pyramids supposedly ate garlic daily for endurance and strength.

Garlic lowers blood pressure through the actions of one of its components, methyl-allyl-trisulfide, which dilates blood vessels. It thins the blood by inhibiting platelet aggregation, which reduces the risk of blood clots and aids in preventing heart attacks. It also lowers serum cholesterol levels and aids in digestion. Garlic is useful for many diseases and illnesses, including cancer. It is a potent immune system stimulant and a natural antibiotic. It should be consumed daily. It can be eaten fresh, taken in supplement form, or used to prepare garlic oil.

Garlic contains an amino acid derivative, alliin. When garlic is consumed, the enzyme alliinase, which converts alliin to allicin, is released. Allicin has an antibiotic effect; it exerts an antibacterial effect estimated to be equivalent to 1 percent of that of penicillin. Because of its antibiotic properties, garlic was used to treat wounds and infections and to prevent gangrene during World War I.

Garlic is also effective against fungal infections, including athlete's foot, systemic candidiasis, and yeast vaginitis. There is some evidence that it may also destroy certain viruses, such as those associated with fever blisters, genital herpes, a form of the common cold, smallpox, and a type of influenza.

Garlic oil is good for the heart and colon, and is effective in the treatment of arthritis, candidiasis, and circulation problems. To make garlic oil, add peeled whole garlic cloves to a quart of olive or canola oil. Experiment to find the number of cloves that gives the degree of flavor you like. Be sure to wash your hands thoroughly and rinse the garlic after peeling and before placing it in the oil. The peel may contain mold and bacteria that can contaminate the oil.

Keep garlic oil refrigerated. This mixture will keep for up to a month before you need to replace it with fresh oil. Garlic oil can be used for sautéing, in salad dressings, and in a variety of other ways. If you find the odor too strong after you eat garlic, chew some sprigs of parsley or mint, or caraway or fennel seeds.

An alternative to fresh garlic is Kyolic from Wakunaga of America. Kyolic is an odorless, "sociable" garlic product, and is available in tablet, capsule, and oil extract forms.

Ginkgo Biloba

The ornamental tree *Ginkgo biloba* originated in China thousands of years ago, and now grows in temperate climates throughout the world. The extract of its fan-shaped leaves is one of the world's most popular herbal products. It has been reported in scientific journals to enhance blood circulation and to increase the supply of oxygen to the heart, brain, and all bodily parts. This makes it useful for improving memory and relieving muscle pains. It also acts as an antioxidant, has antiaging effects, reduces blood pressure, inhibits blood clotting, and is helpful for tinnitus, vertigo, hearing loss, impotence, and Raynaud's disease.

Ginkgo biloba is widely known as the "smart herb" of our time. It has even been said to slow the early progression of Alzheimer's disease in some individuals. In one study of the very old (over eighty-five years of age), ginkgo biloba was shown to slow the progression of dementia and memory decline. There also was no increased risk of bleeding, as had been reported in earlier studies.

Ginseng

Ginseng is used throughout the Far East as a general tonic to combat weakness and give extra energy. There are a number of different varieties of ginseng:

- Eleutherococcus senticosus (Siberian ginseng),

- Panax quinquefolium (American ginseng),

- Panax ginseng (Chinese or Korean ginseng), and

- Panax japonicum (Japanese ginseng).

Panax ginseng is the most widely used species. Early Native Americans were familiar with ginseng. They called it *gisens* and used it for stomach and bronchial disorders, asthma, and neck pain. Russian scientists claim that the ginseng root stimulates both physical and mental activity, improves endocrine gland function, and has a positive effect on the sex glands. It has been shown to help men regain sexual function. Ginseng is beneficial for fatigue because it spares glycogen (the form of glucose stored in the liver and muscle cells) by increasing the use of fatty acids as an energy source. It is used to enhance athletic performance, to rejuvenate, to increase longevity, and to detoxify and normalize the entire system. Many studies have shown ginseng to be effective at improving energy levels, endurance, and alertness. Cancer patients who used ginseng reported a better quality of life, especially related to mood and socialization.

In lower doses, ginseng seems to raise blood pressure, while higher amounts appear to reduce blood pressure. Research suggests that high doses of ginseng may be helpful for inflammatory diseases such as rheumatoid arthritis, without the side effects of steroids, and may also protect against the harmful effects of radiation. Ginseng is beneficial for people with diabetes because it decreases the level of the hormone cortisol in the blood (cortisol interferes with the function of insulin). Normal individuals who were tested with one of several specially prepared ginseng formulas experienced less blood sugar response after a meal, but the level was not low enough to be harmful. Other parts of the ginseng plant used in this study had no effect on blood sugar levels. A portion of the ginseng rootlet referred to as Rg1 seemed to be the most important regulator of blood sugar response to foods. Nevertheless, people with hypoglycemia should avoid using large amounts of ginseng.

The root is sold in many forms: as a whole root or root pieces, which are either untreated or blanched; as a powder or powdered extract; as a liquid extract or concentrate; in granules for instant tea; as a tincture; in an oil base; and in tablets and capsules. These products should not contain sugar or added color, and should be pure ginseng. Many supplement manufacturers add ginseng to combination products, but these often contain such low amounts that they may not be effective.

We advise following the Russian approach to using ginseng: Take it for fifteen to twenty days, followed by a rest period of two weeks. Avoid long-term usage of high doses. Ginseng should not be used by people with high blood pressure, or during pregnancy or lactation.

Glucomannan

See under Fiber in this section.

Glucosamine

This is one of a number of substances classified as an *amino sugar*. Unlike other forms of sugar in the body, amino sugars are components of carbohydrates that are incorporated into the structure of body tissues, rather than being used as a source of energy. Glucosamine is thus involved in the formation of the nails, tendons, skin, eyes, bones, ligaments, and heart valves. It also plays a role in the mucous secretions of the digestive, respiratory, and urinary tracts.

Glucosamine is made in the body from the simple carbohydrate glucose and the amino acid glutamine. It is found in high concentrations in joint structures. It is also available as a supplement, in the form of glucosamine sulfate, which helps to combat both the causes and symptoms of osteoarthritis. Glucosamine has been studied in nearly 200 clinical trials. Although not all the participants in these studies responded to the supplements, most did. For patients with osteoarthritis of the knee, glucosamine was more effective than taking nothing, and reduced the likelihood of needing a knee replacement. Glucosamine was also shown to help with acute injuries such as one would get from exercise. Athletes with recent knee injuries healed faster in terms of knee flexion and extension when using glucosamine compared to a group who took nothing.

It can also slightly reduce the destruction of cartilage and depression caused by taking nonsteroidal anti-inflammatory drugs (NSAIDs), which are commonly prescribed for people with arthritis. Glucosamine may be taken in conjunction with chondroitin sulfate for an even greater effect on osteoarthritis (*see* Chondroitin Sulfate in this section).

In addition to having benefits for people with osteoarthritis, supplemental glucosamine can be helpful for asthma, bursitis, candidiasis, food allergies, osteoporosis, respiratory allergies, tendinitis, vaginitis, and various skin problems. The product GS-500 from Enzymatic Therapy is a good source of glucosamine. GlucosaMend from Source Naturals and Glucosamine Plus from FoodScience of Vermont are other recommended products. A related compound is N-acetylglucosamine (NAG), available as N-A-G from Source Naturals.

Grape Seed Oil

See under Essential Fatty Acids in this section.

"Green Drinks"

"Green drinks" are natural food formulas made from plants that are good detoxifiers and blood cleansers, as well as sources of chlorophyll, minerals, enzymes, and other important nutrients. Greens help neutralize acid buildup in the blood. Eating a Western diet, which is high in meat, dairy, and grains, produces an excess of hydrogen ions in the blood, making it acidic. An adequate intake of fruits and vegetables can counteract this effect, but few of us consume enough of these foods. The green drinks leave an alkaline residue upon digestion, just like fruits and vegetables. This neutralizes the acid from the other foods. Generally, green drinks are sold in powdered form to be mixed just before use. Many different companies market green drink formulas. We recommend buying organic green drinks. In addition, those that provide the greatest number of different plants offer a broader range of antioxidant protection. The following are some recommended products:

- BarleyLife from AIM International. This product contains a combination of barley juice and kelp.

- Earthsource Greens & More from Solgar. This formula combines four organically grown grasses (alfalfa, barley, kamut, and wheat), Hawaiian blue-green spirulina, and Chinese chlorella with three potent immune-stimulating mushrooms (maitake, reishi, and shiitake), plus powdered broccoli, carrots, and red beets, which supply phytonutrients. Its fruit flavor comes from fresh fruit powders.

- Green Magma from Green Foods Corporation. Green Magma is a pure, natural juice of young barley leaves that are organically grown in Japan and are pesticide-free. Brown rice is added to supply vitamins B_1 (thiamine) and B_3 (niacin) and linoleic acid. Green Magma contains thousands of enzymes, which play an important role in the metabolism of the body (*see* ENZYMES in Part One), plus a high concentration of superoxide dismutase (SOD). The powdered product may be added to juice or quality water.

- Kyo-Green from Wakunaga of America. This is a combination of barley, wheatgrass, kelp, and the green algae chlorella. The barley and wheatgrass are organically grown. It is a highly concentrated natural source of chlorophyll, amino acids, vitamins and minerals, carotene, and enzymes. Chlorella is a rich natural source of vitamin A, and kelp supplies iodine and other valuable minerals. (*See* Chlorella and Kelp in this section.)

- ProGreens from NutriCology (Allergy Research Group). ProGreens includes organic alfalfa, barley, oat, and wheat-grass juice powders; natural fiber; wheat sprouts; blue-green algae; sea algae; fructooligosaccharides (FOS); lecithin; standardized bioflavonoid extracts; along with royal jelly and bee pollen; beet and spinach extracts; acerola juice powder; natural vitamin E; and the herbs astragalus, echinacea, licorice, Siberian ginseng, and suma.

Green Papaya

Green (unripe) papaya is an excellent source of vitamins, minerals, and enzymes. Ounce for ounce, it contains more vitamin A than carrots and more vitamin C than oranges, as well as abundant B vitamins and vitamin E. The complex of enzymes it contains helps to digest proteins, carbohydrates, and fats.

Green papaya can be eaten fresh or taken in supplement form. Papain is the most abundant, most active enzyme in both the fresh fruit and the powdered supplement form. Papain possesses very powerful digestive action.

Guar Gum

See under Fiber in this section.

Hemicellulose

See under Fiber in this section.

Honey

Bees produce honey by mixing nectar, which is a sweet substance secreted by flowers, with bee enzymes. Honey is a highly concentrated source of many essential nutrients, including large amounts of carbohydrates (sugars), some minerals, B-complex vitamins, and vitamins C, D, and E.

Honey is used to promote energy and healing. It has been shown to be an effective treatment for relieving symptoms of coughing from an upper respiratory tract infection in people two to eighteen years of age. The FDA and leading medical groups have called the effectiveness of most cold and flu preparations into question. Honey offers a natural and effective alternative. It is a natural antiseptic and makes a good salve for burns and wounds. Honey is also used for sweetening foods and beverages. It varies somewhat in color and taste depending on the origin of the flower and nectar, but in general it is approximately twice as sweet as sugar, so not as much is needed for sweetening purposes.

People who have diabetes or hypoglycemia should be careful when consuming honey and its by-products. These substances affect blood sugar levels in the same way that refined sugars do. Tupelo honey contains more fructose than other types of honey and it is absorbed at a slower rate, so some people with hypoglycemia can use this type sparingly without ill effects.

Buy only unfiltered, unheated, unprocessed honey, and

never give honey to an infant under one year of age. In its natural form, honey can contain spores of the bacteria that cause botulism. This poses no problem for adults and older children, but in infants and those with compromised immune systems, the spores can colonize the digestive tract and produce the deadly botulin toxin there. Honey is safe for babies after age one.

Inosine

Inosine occurs naturally in the human body. It is involved in the rebuilding of adenosine triphosphate (ATP; see page 76, and stimulates the production of a compound designated 2,3-disphosphoglycerate (2,3-DPG), which is needed in the transportation of oxygen to muscle cells for the production of energy. Weight and endurance trainers have found supplemental inosine to be beneficial; it is believed to increase muscle development and blood circulation. It also enhances immune function.

If you have kidney problems or gout, you should not take inosine because it can increase the production of uric acid. For best results, use the dosage recommended by the manufacturer for your body size, and take it forty-five to sixty minutes prior to exercising.

Inositol Hexaphosphate (IP_6)

Inositol hexaphosphate (IP_6, also known as phytic acid) is a compound consisting of the B vitamin inositol plus six phosphate groups. Found naturally in many foods, including wheat, rice, and legumes, it is a powerful antioxidant that has many positive effects on the body. Laboratory studies suggest it may fight cancer, prevent and treat heart disease, prevent kidney stones and liver disease, and also reduce cholesterol levels and prevent the inappropriate formation of blood clots, a major cause of heart attacks. IP_6 inhibits the activity of free radicals in the body, which slows the type of abnormal cell division associated with cancer and tumor growth. It works best very early in the development of malignant tumors, before the malignancy can even be recognized by the immune system. The cells are then normalized and begin to grow in the usual manner again.

IP_6 contains a substance designated beta-1,3-D-glucan, which helps to maintain a strong immune system in people undergoing chemotherapy and radiation. IP_6 protects the heart by preventing the formation of blood clots in blood vessels and reducing the levels of cholesterol and triglycerides (fats) in the bloodstream. It protects the liver by preventing fatty deposits from accumulating there. Studies have shown that a diet high in IP_6 is associated with a lower incidence of cancer of the breast, colon, and prostate.

Significant amounts of IP_6 are found in foods such as beans, brown rice, whole-kernel corn, sesame seeds, wheat bran, cornbread, grape juice, raisins, and mulberries. It can also be taken in supplement form. Some studies have shown that IP_6 may interfere with the body's absorption of minerals, so supplements should not be taken within one hour of meals. IP_6 from Jarrow Formulas and Cell Forté with IP-6 and Inositol from Enzymatic Therapy are recommended sources of IP_6.

Kelp

Kelp is a type of seaweed that can be eaten raw, but it is usually dried, granulated, or ground into powder. It is also available in a liquid form that can be added to drinking water. Granulated or powdered kelp can be used as a condiment and for flavoring, as a salt substitute. If you find the taste unappealing, you can purchase it in tablet form.

Kelp is a rich source of vitamins, especially the B vitamins, as well as of many valuable minerals and trace elements. It is reported to be very beneficial to brain tissue, the membranes surrounding the brain, the sensory nerves, and the spinal cord, as well as the nails and blood vessels. It has been used in the treatment of thyroid problems because of its iodine content, and is useful for other conditions as varied as hair loss, obesity, and ulcers. It protects against the effects of radiation and softens stools. Kelp is recommended as a daily dietary supplement, especially for people with mineral deficiencies.

Kombucha Tea

The kombucha, or Manchurian, "mushroom" has reputedly been used in Asian countries and in Russia for centuries. The kombucha itself is not eaten. Rather, a tea is made by fermenting it for about a week in a mixture of water, sugar, and green or black tea, with apple cider vinegar or a bit of previously made tea added. Kept in this mixture, the kombucha reproduces, and the daughter mushrooms can then be used to produce more tea.

Although commonly referred to as a mushroom, the kombucha is actually a combination of a number of different elements, including lichen, bacteria, and yeast. Kombucha tea contains a variety of different nutrients and other health-promoting substances. It is a natural energy booster and detoxifier that may also help slow or reverse the aging process.

Because of the way in which it has traditionally been propagated (one at a time, by individual users), kombucha may be difficult to find. Many people who have them received a daughter mushroom as a gift from a friend, although there are some herbal companies that sell both the mushrooms and the bottled tea commercially.

Lactobacillus Acidophilus

Lactobacillus acidophilus is a type of "friendly" bacteria that assists in the digestion of proteins, a process in which lactic acid, hydrogen peroxide, enzymes, B vitamins, and antibiotic substances that inhibit pathogenic organisms are produced. Acidophilus has antifungal properties, helps to reduce blood cholesterol levels, aids digestion, and enhances the absorption of nutrients.

The flora in the healthy colon should consist of at least 85 percent lactobacilli and 15 percent coliform bacteria. However, the typical colon bacteria count today is the reverse. This can result in gas, bloating, intestinal and systemic toxicity, constipation, and malabsorption of nutrients, and is conducive to an overgrowth of candida. Taking an acidophilus supplement helps to combat all of these problems by returning the intestinal flora to a healthier balance. In addition, acidophilus may help to detoxify harmful substances. Between 5 and 30 percent of those who take antibiotics develop antibiotic-associated diarrhea, and *Lactobacillus acidophilus* may prevent it.

There are many good acidophilus supplements available. Acidophilus products come in tablet, capsule, and powdered forms. We recommend using the powdered form. Natren, Inc., markets quality products that contain very high numbers of organisms. Other good nondairy acidophilus supplements include Primadophilus from Nature's Way, Probiotic All-Flora from New Chapter, and Flora from DaVinci Labs.

Acidophilus can die at high temperatures. Whatever product you choose, keep it in a cool, dry place—refrigerate but do not freeze it. Take acidophilus on an empty stomach in the morning and one hour before each meal. If you are taking antibiotics, do not take the antibiotics and acidophilus simultaneously.

Lactoferrin

Lactoferrin is a protein that occurs naturally in human bile, tears, mucus, saliva, and milk. Because it binds with free iron in the body, it plays an important role in regulating iron levels (and, in turn, growth) and aids in preventing and fighting infection by depriving disease-causing organisms of the iron they need to grow and multiply. It also plays a role in the functioning of lymphocytes, a type of white blood cell important for immunity. Taken in supplement form, it may boost immune function and help in combating both infectious and inflammatory conditions. It may also benefit intestinal health.

Lecithin

Lecithin is a type of lipid that is needed by every living cell in the human body. Cell membranes, which regulate the passage of nutrients into and out of the cells, are largely composed of lecithin. The protective sheaths surrounding the brain are composed of lecithin, and the muscles and nerve cells also contain this essential fatty substance.

Lecithin consists mostly of the B vitamin choline, and also contains linoleic acid and inositol. Although lecithin is a lipid, it is partly soluble in water and thus acts as an emulsifying agent. This is why many processed foods contain lecithin.

This nutrient helps to prevent arteriosclerosis, protects against cardiovascular disease, improves brain function, and aids in the absorption of thiamine by the liver and vitamin A by the intestine. It is also known to promote energy and is needed to help repair damage to the liver caused by alcoholism. Lecithin enables fats, such as cholesterol and other lipids, to be dispersed in water and removed from the body. The vital organs and arteries are thus protected from fatty buildup.

Lecithin would be a wise addition to anyone's diet. It is especially valuable for older adults. Anyone who is taking niacin for high serum cholesterol and triglycerides should also include lecithin in his or her program. Two tablespoons of lecithin granules can be sprinkled on cereals and soups or added to juices or breads. Lecithin also comes in capsule form. Taking one 1,200-milligram capsule before each meal helps in the digestion of fats and the absorption of fat-soluble vitamins. More recently, a mixture of lecithin and soy stanols has been shown to be an effective cholesterol-lowering supplement. It can reduce the amount of cholesterol absorbed from the diet, thereby reducing both total cholesterol and LDL (bad cholesterol).

Most lecithin is derived from soybeans, but recently egg lecithin has become popular. This type of lecithin is extracted from the yolks of fresh eggs. Egg lecithin may hold promise for those suffering from AIDS, herpes, chronic fatigue syndrome, and immune disorders associated with aging. Studies have shown that it works better for people with these disorders than soy lecithin does. Other sources of lecithin include brewer's yeast, grains, legumes, fish, and wheat germ.

Lignin

See under Fiber in this section.

Maitake

Maitake (*Grifola frondosa*) is a mushroom that has a long history of use in traditional Chinese and Japanese herbology and cooking. It grows wild in Japan, as well as in some wooded areas in eastern North America. Because maitake is difficult to cultivate, however, only relatively recently have the mushrooms become widely available.

Maitake is considered an adaptogen, which means that it helps the body adapt to stress and normalizes bodily functions. Its healing properties are thought to be related to its high content of a polysaccharide called beta-1,6-glucan, which is considered very powerful. In laboratory studies, this substance has been shown to prevent carcinogenesis, inhibit the growth of cancerous tumors, kill HIV, and enhance the activity of key immune cells known as T-helper cells or CD4 cells. Maitake may also be useful for diabetes, chronic fatigue syndrome, chronic hepatitis, obesity, and high blood pressure.

Maitake can be eaten in food or taken as a supplement.

Buy organically grown dried mushrooms (when using them in cooking, soak them in water or broth for half an hour first), or purchase maitake in capsule, extract, or tea form. Some of the capsule supplements contain a small amount of vitamin C, which enhances the effectiveness of the active ingredient in maitake by aiding in its absorption.

Melatonin

The hormone melatonin is naturally produced by the pineal gland, a cone-shaped structure in the brain. The body's pattern of melatonin production is similar to that of the other "antiaging" hormones, human growth hormone (HGH) and dehydroepiandrosterone (DHEA). Throughout early life, melatonin is produced in abundance. It was thought for some time that the production of melatonin begins to drop at puberty, and then continues to decline steadily as we age. This may not be true, according to research done at the Harvard Medical School. Researchers say that older people who were on aspirin therapy might have skewed the results because taking aspirin reduces melatonin levels in the body.

Research has demonstrated that melatonin may have several profound long-term effects on the body. As one of the most powerful antioxidants ever discovered—with a greater range of effectiveness than vitamin C, vitamin E, or beta-carotene—melatonin helps prevent harmful oxidation reactions from occurring. In this way, melatonin may prevent the changes that lead to hypertension and heart attack, and may reduce the risk of certain kinds of cancer. Melatonin also has been found to stimulate the immune system; have a major role in the production of estrogen, testosterone, and possibly other hormones, helping to prevent cancers involving the reproductive system; and slow the growth of existing malignancies. Recent studies suggest that if melatonin is taken in the mornings, tumor growth may be stimulated, but if it is taken in the evenings, tumor growth tends to be slowed. In addition, as melatonin is secreted cyclically, in response to the fall of darkness at the end of each day, the hormone helps our bodies keep in sync with the rhythms of day and night. Thus, melatonin helps regulate sleep.

Research on melatonin continues, and with it, knowledge is increasing about the functions of melatonin in the body and the effects of melatonin supplementation. Melatonin is the internal sleep facilitator in humans. Both human research studies and anecdotal evidence indicate that melatonin supplements can be an effective and side effect–free sleep aid both for adults suffering from insomnia and for children with autism, epilepsy, Down syndrome, cerebral palsy, and other problems that can cause sleep disorders. There is evidence that supplemental melatonin can induce sleep by reducing restlessness before sleep, and correct sleep patterns during sleep so you feel rested upon awakening. Sleeping disorders increase with age, and melatonin has been shown to help. Subjects over fifty-five years of age who used 2 milligrams of time-released melatonin had better quality of sleep and felt more alert in the morning. It has been shown to be effective in those who suffer from minor sleep disorders when used on a regular basis, and episodically for jet lag or shift workers. In addition, in a rare condition resulting in nocturnal hypertension, patients using melatonin experienced a reduction in blood pressure while they slept. For patients with mild cognitive impairment, melatonin allowed for better performance on several tests that assess cognitive function. Mental acuity was thought to improve because the patients slept better and felt refreshed in the morning.

Animal and other laboratory research indicates that melatonin supplementation may help prevent age-related disorders, and perhaps extend life. Melatonin can be taken to ease PMS symptoms; stimulate the immune system; prevent memory loss, arteriosclerosis, and stroke; and treat cancer and Alzheimer's disease.

Although no toxic levels of melatonin have been found, it is a powerful hormone, and some researchers feel that certain people probably should not use this supplement until further information is available. Included in this category are pregnant and nursing women; people with severe allergies or autoimmune diseases; people with immune system cancers, such as lymphoma and leukemia; and healthy children, who already produce sufficient amounts of the hormone. Because high doses of melatonin have been found to act as a contraceptive, women who wish to become pregnant also might want to avoid taking this supplement.

Melatonin should be taken two hours or less before bedtime. This schedule is designed to release the added hormone at the same time that natural production peaks. A sustained-release form is best if you frequently awaken after several hours' sleep; a sublingual form is best if you are very ill or suffer from malabsorption. When you awaken after melatonin-assisted sleep, you should feel refreshed—not tired or groggy. If you do experience grogginess, you should reduce the dosage. (To learn how you can maintain or increase your melatonin levels through daily routines, *see* Maintaining Your Melatonin Level Naturally on page 90.) For information on other antiaging hormones, *see* DHEA THERAPY and GROWTH HORMONE THERAPY in Part Three.

Methylsulfonylmethane (MSM)

Methylsulfonylmethane (MSM, also known as dimethylsulfone) is a naturally occurring organic sulfur compound found in plant and animal tissues that is essential for optimum health. It is a derivative of dimethylsulfoxide (DMSO), which has remarkable therapeutic properties, especially for the healing of injuries. It can also help to detoxify the body on a cellular level. MSM helps to nourish the hair, skin, and nails; relieve pain and inflammation; reduce allergy problems; and promote gastrointestinal health. It has also been found to aid immune function, and there have

---

Maintaining Your Melatonin Level Naturally

As darkness falls at the end of each day, melatonin production rises. In the morning, when daylight hits the retina, neural impulses cause production of the hormone to slow. Clearly, light and darkness are the primary factors that set the rhythms of melatonin production. However, they are not the only factors involved. In fact, it has been found that a variety of regular daily routines can strengthen the rhythm of melatonin production. Here are a few simple ways in which you can help your body maintain high levels of this important hormone:

- Eat regular meals. The rhythm of melatonin production is strengthened by regular daily routines. Keep your mealtimes as regular as possible to keep your body in sync with the rhythms of the day.
- Keep your diet light at night. When melatonin production begins after nightfall, the digestive process is slowed.

Thus, any heavy foods eaten close to bedtime may lead to digestive problems, which can make it difficult to sleep. To get the sleep you need, eat small, light meals in the late evening.

- Avoid stimulants. Stimulants such as coffee, tea, and caffeine-containing medications and soft drinks can interfere with melatonin production by interfering with your sleep. As much as possible, eliminate these stimulants from your diet and lifestyle. Or, at the very least, allow at least four to five hours between the time you consume them and bedtime.
- Avoid exercising late at night. Vigorous activity delays melatonin secretion. If you exercise in the morning, you will reinforce healthful sleeping habits that lead to regular melatonin production. For best results, do your morning exercise outdoors, in the morning light.

---

been reports of benefits to patients with heartburn, arthritis, lung problems, migraines, and muscle pain. MSM is present naturally in foods such as fresh fish, meat, plants, fruit, and milk. However, it can be eliminated by even moderate processing, including drying or heating.

Most North Americans today eat considerable amounts of processed food, and MSM is normally either not present at all or present only in very small amounts in the typical diet. Most people therefore would probably benefit from supplementation.

Research suggests that we require a constant supply of MSM for optimum good health, as sulfur is one of the essential minerals. Commonly recommended dosage levels are about 2,000 milligrams (2 grams) per day taken in divided doses, with the morning and evening meals, but it is best to start out at 1,000 milligrams (1 gram) per day to avoid a too-rapid rate of detoxification. Higher doses (3,000 milligrams twice a day) were shown to be safe and effective at helping patients with osteoarthritis perform daily activities and feel better in general. The positive effects in this study occurred in eighty-four days. However, benefits could become evident in as few as two to twenty-one days, and can be enhanced by vitamin C supplementation. In addition, when MSM was combined with sternum collagen II, pain and soreness decreased in a group of patients with osteoarthritis. MSM is found in a variety of products from the following companies: Aerobic Life Industries, Allergy Research Group, Bluebonnet, Country Life, Jarrow, and Natrol.

Mucilage

See under Fiber in this section.

Nicotinamide Adenine Dinucleotide (NADH)

NADH is a form of vitamin B_3 (niacin) that is essential for the production of various neurotransmitters and cellular energy. NADH, which is also known as coenzyme 1, also acts as an antioxidant (*see under* ANTIOXIDANTS in Part One).

As we age, natural levels of NADH decline, which can lead to reduced levels of both energy and significant brain chemicals. Taking supplemental NADH can result in improvements in the biochemistry of energy production, especially in the brain and nervous systems. NADH shows promise as a therapy for Parkinson's disease because it results in an increase in brain levels of the neurotransmitter dopamine, which is deficient in people with this disorder.

People with Alzheimer's disease may be helped by this supplement as well. Some people suffering from chronic fatigue syndrome (CFS) have shown significant improvement with NADH therapy.

Oat Bran

See under Fiber in this section.

Octacosanol

Octacosanol is a naturally derived wheat germ oil concentrate. Although it would be possible to extract octacosanol from whole wheat, 10 pounds of wheat would be needed to obtain just 1,000 micrograms of octacosanol. Wheat germ has long been known for its many benefits. Today, extracts of wheat germ weighing only 2 milligrams offer remarkable benefits as well.

Octacosanol has been clinically proven to increase oxygen utilization during exercise and improve glycogen stores in muscle tissue. As a result, it increases physical endurance, improves reaction time, reduces high-altitude stress, and aids in tissue oxygenation. This substance can greatly benefit those who experience muscle pain after exercise or have a lowered endurance level. It is good for muscular dystrophies and other neuromuscular disorders as well. It also reduces blood cholesterol levels.

Olive Leaf Extract

Olive leaf extract is an herbal supplement that has been shown to be effective against virtually all the viruses and bacteria on which it has been tested. Laboratory studies suggest that olive leaf extract interferes with viral infection becoming established and/or spreading, either by rendering viruses incapable of infecting cells or by preventing them from reproducing. It has been shown to help protect against infection by such viruses as human immunodeficiency virus (HIV), herpesviruses, and influenza viruses. It is useful for such disorders as pneumonia, sore throat, sinusitis, and skin diseases such as chronic infections and rashes, as well as for fungal and bacterial infections. Olivir from DaVinci Laboratories is a good source of olive leaf extract that has been tested in clinical trials.

Pectin

See under Fiber in this section.

Perilla

Perilla (*Perilla frutescens*) is an Asian plant that is a member of the mint family. It has been prescribed by Asian herbalists for the relief of cough and lung ailments, and for certain types of food poisoning, as well as to prevent the flu and restore energy balance. It may aid in increasing learning ability and is also used as a culinary herb.

Perilla comes in several forms, including seed oil. This is an unsaturated oil that contains linolenic, linoleic, and oleic acids. Perilla oil is available in capsule form. Studies suggest that it may be an effective and safe source of essential omega-3 fatty acids.

Phosphatidyl Choline

Phosphatidyl choline (PC) is a component of lecithin. (*See* Lecithin in this section.) Taken as a supplement, it helps to break down fats and can be helpful in preventing atherosclerosis (hardening of the arteries due to fatty plaques in the blood vessels), heart disease, gallstones, and liver problems. It has also shown substantial benefits for people with neurological disorders, memory loss, and depression.

PC is known to be safe and effective; however, people with bipolar mood disorder should not take large amounts.

Phosphatidyl Serine

Phosphatidyl serine (PS) is a substance classified as a phospholipid (a phosphorus-containing lipid) that is needed by every cell in the body, and is especially abundant in nerve cells. PS is the most important of the phospholipids and is crucial for the maintenance of healthy cell membranes. Although the brain normally produces enough PS, production dwindles as we age, which can result in deficiency.

Supplemental PS, which is compounded from soybean oil in products sold in the United States, has been said to reduce symptoms of depression and Alzheimer's disease, and to enhance memory and learning abilities. Some of the earlier studies on this product focused on PS from cow brains, which is no longer sold in the United States. That was a different product chemically from the soy-based product sold today and results may not be the same. Some people have experienced nausea as a result of taking PS; however, taking it with food can help to avoid this. No danger has been reported with long-term use of the soy-based supplement. Its safety for pregnant women has not been determined.

Primrose Oil

See under Essential Fatty Acids in this section.

Probiotics

Probiotics are beneficial bacteria normally present in the digestive tract. They are vital for proper digestion and also perform a number of other useful functions, such as preventing the overgrowth of yeast and other pathogens, and synthesizing vitamin K. The probiotics most often used as supplements are acidophilus and bifidobacteria. (*See Lactobacillus acidophilus* and/or *Bifidobacterium bifidum* in this section.)

Cultured, or fermented, foods also contain various types and amounts of beneficial bacteria. These foods include buttermilk, cheese, kefir, miso, sauerkraut, tempeh, umeboshi, and yogurt.

Progesterone Cream

Progesterone is a hormone that is produced primarily by the ovaries and also by the adrenal glands. It works in partnership with estrogen to regulate menstrual cycles and is important for the maintenance of pregnancy. In addition to its role in the female reproductive system, it has a number of other important effects: it stimulates the activity of bone-building cells called osteoblasts; exerts an antidepressant and calming effect in the brain; helps to regulate blood sugar levels; and plays a role in maintaining the myelin sheaths that protect nerve cells. It can be used by the body to produce other hormones, including DHEA, estrogen, testosterone, and cortisol, as needed. A deficiency of pro-gesterone, on the other hand, can exacerbate symptoms of premenstrual syndrome (PMS) and menopausal discomfort, and may increase the risk of osteoporosis. Progesterone deficiency becomes increasingly common in women as they approach menopause, and can start as early as age thirty-five. Symptoms can include night sweats, hot flashes, depression, and premenstrual discomfort.

Supplemental progesterone is available in cream form. The hormone is absorbed through the skin after the cream is applied, and it passes directly into the bloodstream for transport to sites where progesterone is needed. As these are biologically active substances, consult your health care professional before using them.

Propolis

See Bee Propolis in this section.

Psyllium Seed

See under Fiber in this section.

Red Yeast Rice

Red yeast rice is a food product created by fermenting rice with a strain of red yeast (*Monascus purpureus* Went yeast). It is also sometimes referred to as Monascus rice or, in Chinese, *Hung-chu* or *Hong-Qu*. It has long been used in China and Japan as a food and as a remedy for digestive ailments and poor circulation. More recently, red yeast rice extract, taken in supplement form, has been found both to reduce overall blood cholesterol levels and to improve the ratio of HDL ("good cholesterol") to LDL ("bad cholesterol"). A study conducted by the University of California–Los Angeles, School of Medicine found that people who took red yeast rice and maintained a low-fat diet reduced their overall cholesterol levels by an average of 40 points over a period of twelve weeks. The extract contains a number of cholesterol-lowering compounds known as *statins.* One of these is lovastatin, a substance also sold as a prescription drug under the brand name Mevacor. Lovastatin acts to lower cholesterol by inhibiting the action of an enzyme designated HMG-CoA reductase, which in turn limits the rate at which the body produces cholesterol. Studies have shown statins to lower cholesterol levels and reduce the risk of heart attack. Unlike prescription products, red yeast rice extract has shown no serious adverse side effects in clinical trials. Smaller amounts of lovastatin from a plant as opposed to drugs are required to be effective. This is because it is thought that the natural compounds in the plant work synergistically with the active ingredient. Merck, which sells Mevacor, asked the FDA to ban red yeast rice extract. The FDA considered Merck's request, but decided to allow companies to continue to sell it. However, the FDA did mandate that there cannot be any mention of lowering cholesterol levels or reducing heart disease risk. Check with your health care professional before using red yeast rice.

Reishi

See Shiitake and Reishi in this section.

Rice Bran

See under Fiber in this section.

Royal Jelly

Royal jelly is a thick, milky substance that is secreted from the pharyngeal glands of a special group of young nurse bees between their sixth and twelfth days of life. When honey and pollen are combined and refined within the young nurse bee, royal jelly is naturally created. This substance contains all of the B-complex vitamins, including a high concentration of pantothenic acid (vitamin B_5) and vitamin B_6 (pyridoxine), and is the only natural source of pure acetylcholine. Royal jelly also contains minerals, enzymes, hormones, eighteen amino acids, antibacterial and antibiotic components, and vitamins A, C, D, and E. It is useful for bronchial asthma, liver disease, pancreatitis, insomnia, stomach ulcers, kidney disease, bone fractures, and skin disorders, and it strengthens the immune system. This product must be combined with honey to preserve its potency. Royal jelly spoils easily. Keep it refrigerated and make sure it is tightly sealed when purchased.

S-Adenosylmethionine (SAMe)

S-adenosylmethionine (SAMe) is a derivative of the amino acid methionine that is formed in the body when methionine combines with adenosine triphosphate (ATP), the major source of cellular energy. Taken as a supplement, SAMe has a variety of positive effects:

- It is an effective antidepressant.
- It is beneficial for disorders of the joints and connective tissue, including arthritis and fibromyalgia.
- It promotes the health of the liver.
- It may lower levels of homocysteine, an amino acid that is associated with cardiovascular disease.
- It may help to slow the aging process.

SAMe works closely with folic acid, choline, and vitamins B_6 and B_{12}. It is one of a class of substances called *methyl donors.* As the name implies, methyl donors are compounds that "donate" units called methyl groups, which contain hydrogen and carbon atoms, to other substances. This process is called *methylation,* and it is one way in which the body protects itself from damage on the cellular level.

Among other things, methyl donors help to protect against such serious disorders as cancer, heart disease, neurological disorders, and many age-related problems, and facilitate the manufacture of DNA and brain neurotransmitters. SAMe increases catechol-O-methyltransferase (COMT) enzyme activity, which has been shown to somewhat lessen aggressive symptoms in schizophrenia. In addition, brain waves of elderly patients with depression responded favorably with SAMe at different doses. The effect was observed at one hour and lasted up to six. In patients with AIDS, depressive symptoms were improved with SAMe, and the change was noted after one week of treatment. SAMe has also been shown to be effective when coupled with drugs classified as selective serotonin reuptake inhibitors (SSRIs). If you are taking medications for depression, check with your health care provider before using SAMe.

Taking supplemental SAMe may also increase natural levels of glutathione, an antioxidant; phosphatidyl choline, which aids in the metabolism of fats; and the hormone melatonin. A small number of people have experienced minor nausea, gastrointestinal disturbances, and headaches as a result of taking high doses, but otherwise no notable side effects have been reported. Although SAMe is considered very safe, anyone with bipolar mood disorder should consult a physician before taking this supplement. Do not give to a child under twelve. SAMe should always be taken on an empty stomach. Be sure what you purchase is SAMe because there have been some knockoffs. It is rather costly.

Sea Cucumber

Sea cucumbers, also known as *bêche de mer* and *trepang*, are not actually cucumbers, but are marine animals related to starfishes and sea urchins. They have been used in China for thousands of years as a treatment for arthritis. Modern research has confirmed they are beneficial for musculoskeletal inflammatory diseases, especially rheumatoid arthritis, osteoarthritis, and ankylosing spondylitis, a rheumatic disease that affects the spine.

Researchers believe that sea cucumbers improve the balance of prostaglandins, which regulate the inflammatory process. They also contain substances known as chondroitins, which are often lacking in people with arthritis and connective tissue disorders (*see* Chondroitin Sulfate in this section). In addition, sea cucumbers provide vitamins A, B_1 (thiamine), B_2 (riboflavin), B_3 (niacin), and C, as well as the minerals calcium, iron, magnesium, and zinc.

Sea Mussel

The green-lipped mussel (*Perna canaliculus*) is a species of edible shellfish. These mussels contain numerous amino acids, the building blocks of body proteins, in addition to enzymes and essential trace elements. The minerals they contain are present in a balance similar to that in blood plasma, and these minerals are naturally chelated by the amino acids, making for better assimilation into the body.

Sea mussel aids in the functioning of the cardiovascular system, the lymphatic system, the endocrine system, the eyes, connective tissues, and mucous membranes. They help to reduce inflammation and relieve the pain and stiffness of arthritis. They also promote the healing of wounds and burns.

Shark Cartilage

The tough, elastic material that makes up the skeleton of the shark is dried and pulverized (finely powdered) to make this food supplement. Shark cartilage contains a number of active components, the most important of which is a type of protein that acts as an angiogenesis inhibitor—that is, it supposedly acts to suppress the development of new blood vessels. This would make it valuable in fighting a number of disorders. Many cancerous tumors, for instance, are able to grow only because they induce the body to develop new networks of blood vessels to supply them with nutrients.

Shark cartilage is said to suppress this process, so that tumors are deprived of their source of nourishment and, often, begin to shrink. Many patients with advanced stages of cancer of the breast, colon, prostate, and others have sought shark cartilage as a means to avoid disease progression. To date, however, studies show that shark cartilage has no impact on disease progression, and many patients had adverse side effects from using the product.

There are certain eye disorders, such as diabetic retinopathy and macular degeneration, that are characterized by the growth of new blood vessels within the eye; because they grow in inappropriate places, the presence of these blood vessels can lead to blindness. Such diseases also may respond well to shark cartilage. Other conditions for which shark cartilage is useful include arthritis, psoriasis, and regional enteritis (inflammation of the lining of the bowels). In addition to angiogenesis-inhibiting protein, shark cartilage contains calcium (approximately 16 percent) and phosphorus (approximately 8 percent), which are absorbed as nutrients, and mucopolysaccharides that act to stimulate the immune system.

Shark cartilage is available in powder and capsule forms. Exercise caution when buying shark cartilage, as the purity and correct processing of the product are vital to its effectiveness. Not all shark cartilage products contain only 100 percent pure shark cartilage, so read labels carefully.

Pure shark cartilage is white in color. If you are taking large quantities of shark cartilage, it may be wise to increase your supplementation of certain minerals, especially magnesium and potassium, to maintain a proper mineral balance in the body. Shark cartilage should *not* be taken by pregnant women or children, or by persons who have recently undergone surgery or suffered a heart attack.

Shiitake and Reishi

Shiitake and reishi are Japanese mushrooms with a delicate texture, strong stems, and well-defined undersides. They are attractive and have impressive health-promoting properties.

Shiitake (*Lentinus edodes*) contain a polysaccharide, lentinan, that strengthens the immune system by increasing T cell function. Shiitake mushrooms contain eighteen amino acids, seven of which are essential amino acids. They are rich in B vitamins, especially vitamins B_1 (thiamine), B_2 (riboflavin), and B_3 (niacin). When sun-dried, they contain high amounts of vitamin D. Their effectiveness in treating cancer has been reported in a joint study by the Medical Department of Koibe University and Nippon Kinoko Institute in Japan. These mushrooms are considered delicacies and are entirely edible.

Reishi (*Ganoderma lucidum*) have been popular for at least two thousand years in the Far East. They were rated number one on ancient Chinese lists of superior medicines, and were believed to give eternal youth and longevity.

Today, both shiitake and reishi mushrooms are used to treat a variety of disorders and to promote vitality. They are used to prevent high blood pressure and heart disease, to control and lower cholesterol, to build resistance to disease, and to treat fatigue and viral infections. They are also known to have anti-tumor properties valuable in treating cancer.

The mushrooms are available fresh or dried for use in foods (soak dried mushrooms in warm water or broth for thirty minutes before using), as well as in supplements in capsule, pill, and extract form.

Spirulina

Spirulina is a microalgae that thrives in hot, sunny climates and in alkaline waters around the world, and produces twenty times as much protein as soybeans growing on an equal-sized area of land. It contains concentrations of nutrients unlike any other single grain, herb, or plant. Among its valuable components are gamma-linolenic acid (GLA), linoleic and arachidonic acids, vitamin B_{12} (needed, especially by vegetarians, for healthy red blood cells), iron, a high level of protein (60 to 70 percent), essential amino acids, and the nucleic acids RNA and DNA, along with chlorophyll, and phycocyanin, a blue pigment that is found only in blue-green algae and that has increased the survival rate of mice with liver cancer in laboratory experiments. Spirulina has been clinically tested and has shown a variety of effects. Those with the common cold experienced less sneezing and congestion. Others showed lowered cholesterol levels and blood pressure. Finally, those who used spirulina as part of their regular diet had reduced post-exercise muscle soreness that may have allowed them to have longer workout sessions.

Spirulina is a naturally digestible food that aids in pro-

tecting the immune system, in cholesterol reduction, and in mineral absorption. Because it supplies nutrients needed to help cleanse and heal, while also curbing the appetite, it is beneficial for people who are fasting. A person with hypoglycemia may benefit from using this food supplement between meals because its high protein content helps stabilize blood sugar levels.

Torula Yeast

See Yeast in this section.

Wheat Germ

Wheat germ is the embryo of the wheat berry. It is a good source of vitamin E; most of the B vitamins; the minerals calcium, magnesium, and phosphorus; and several trace elements.

One problem with wheat germ is that it spoils easily. If you purchase wheat germ separately from the flour, make sure the product is fresh. It should be either vacuum packed or refrigerated, with a packing date or a label stating the date by which the product should be used. Toasted wheat germ has a longer shelf life, but the raw product is better because it is unprocessed. Wheat germ oil capsules are also available.

Wheatgrass

Wheatgrass is a rich nutritional food that was popularized by the late Dr. Ann Wigmore, an educator and founder of the Hippocrates Health Institute in Boston. Wheatgrass contains a great variety of vitamins, minerals, and trace elements. According to Dr. Wigmore, 1 pound of fresh wheatgrass is equal in nutritional value to nearly 25 pounds of the choicest vegetables.

Dr. Wigmore reported that wheatgrass therapy, along with "living foods," helped to eliminate cancerous growths and helped many other disorders, including mental health problems. The molecular structure of chlorophyll resembles that of hemoglobin, the oxygen-carrying protein of red blood cells, and this may be the reason for the effectiveness of wheatgrass. The key difference between the two is that the metallic atom in the middle of each molecule of human hemoglobin is iron, while the metallic atom at the center of a molecule of chlorophyll is magnesium. In experiments on anemic animals, blood counts returned to normal after four to five days of receiving chlorophyll.

Whey Protein

Whey is a normal by-product of cheesemaking; it is the liquid that is left when the solids in milk come together and are pressed into solid form. Filtering and purifying produces whey protein, then the water is removed to produce a powder that, while high in quality protein, is free of fat and lactose (milk sugar).

This supplement helps to build lean body mass by increasing the body's production of muscle protein. A 30-gram serving of whey protein contains nearly all of the essential amino acids necessary each day. For this reason, it is popular among athletes and bodybuilders, and may also help to protect against muscle wasting in people with such diseases as AIDS and cancer. In addition to its effect on muscles, it appears to inhibit the proliferation of cancer cells, protect against free radical damage, and enhance immune function. Compared to soy protein, whey seems more effective at promoting weight loss. Some recommended whey protein supplements include Biochem Whey Pro from Country Life, Enhanced Life Extension Whey Protein from Life Extension, Molkosan from A. Vogel/Bioforce, and Whey to Go from Solgar.

Yeast

Yeast are single-celled organisms that can multiply at extremely rapid rates, doubling in number in two hours. Yeast is rich in many basic nutrients, such as the B vitamins (except for vitamin B_{12}), sixteen amino acids, and at least fourteen different minerals. The protein content of yeast is responsible for 52 percent of its weight. Yeast is also high in phosphorus.

There are various media on which yeast may be grown. Brewer's yeast, also known as nutritional yeast, is grown on hops, a bitter herb that is also used as an ingredient in beer. Torula yeast is grown on blackstrap molasses or wood pulp. A liquid yeast product from Switzerland called Bio-Strath, distributed by A. Vogel/Bioforce USA, is derived from herbs, honey, and malt. It is a natural product that we highly recommend.

Live baker's yeast should be avoided. Live yeast cells actually deplete the body of B vitamins and other nutrients. In nutritional yeast, these live cells are destroyed, leaving the beneficial nutrients behind.

Yeast may be consumed in juice or water, and is a good energy booster between meals. It can also be added to the diet to aid in treating certain disorders. It helps in sugar metabolism and is good for eczema, heart disorders, gout, nervousness, and fatigue. By enhancing the immune system, yeast is useful for people undergoing radiation therapy or chemotherapy for cancer. Yeast also seems to increase mental and physical efficiency.

Specialty Supplements

In addition to the substances discussed above, there are many natural food supplements designed for specific circumstances.

There are too many of these products for us to discuss all of them here, but some that we feel are to be highly recommended are the following:

- Allergy Relief formulas from bioAllers. These are eight homeopathic formulas designed to relieve allergies by combining homeopathic remedies with specific allergens to help strengthen resistance to those allergens. Formulas include Animal Hair/Dander; Grain/Dairy; Grass Pollen; Mold/Yeast/Dust; Pollen/Hayfever; Sinus & Allergy Nasal Spray; and Tree Pollen.

- Herbal Actives Artichoke from Nature's Plus. This supplement contains artichoke extract standardized to a minimum of 2.5 to 5 percent caffeoylquinic acids, and also contains sesquiterpene lactones and the highly active flavonoids scolymoside, inulin, and taraxasterol. It is designed to support the liver and circulatory system and assists in cholesterol output reduction and conversion of cholesterol into bile acids.

- Betatene. This is a dietary supplement of mixed carotenoids, including alpha- and beta-carotene, lutein, lycopene, zeaxanthin, and cryptoxanthin. It is intended to help maintain a healthy and strong immune system.

- Bone Maximizer from Metabolic Response Modifiers. This is a combination supplement that contains microcrystalline hydroxyapatite concentrate (MCHC). MCHC is a source of bone proteins and highly absorbable calcium. Other ingredients include glucosamine, pregnenolone, vitamin D, magnesium, methylsulfonylmethane (MSM, a source of bioavailable sulfur), and other nutrients vital for bone health.

- Bone Support with Ostivone from Twinlab. This is a combination supplement designed to help maintain healthy bones. Ingredients include ipriflavone, calcium, vitamin D, magnesium, boron, and purified soy phytoestrogen extracts.

- Cardiaforce from A. Vogel/Bioforce USA. This hawthorn berry extract promotes healthy cardiovascular function, circulation, and heart muscle strength. It is a liquid supplement that is meant to be added to water and taken three times a day, before meals. It has no known interactions with other medications, and should be taken over a period of several months, with periodic short interruptions.

- Cold, flu, and allergy season formulas from ZAND. This is a line of products designed to support health through the various allergy seasons of the year. Individual formulas include Insure Herbal, an echinacea and goldenseal formula; Decongest Herbal, a natural decongestant formula; Herbal-Mist throat spray; and Allergy Season Formula, which contains bromelain, nettle extract, quercetin, and vitamin B_5 (pantothenic acid). These formulas can be used individually or on a rotating basis.

- Diamond Mind from Diamond-Herpanacine Associates. This product combines a number of herbal extracts and nutrients, including ginkgo biloba, gotu kola, ginseng, garlic, phosphatidyl serine, and phosphatidyl choline, in a supplement intended to support and improve memory, concentration, and mental energy and alertness.

- Diamond Trim from Diamond-Herpanacine Associates. This is a supplement program intended to promote weight loss by helping control appetite, reduce food cravings, increase the burning of calories, and reduce the absorption of fats. It also contains minerals to replenish those often lost through dieting. Ingredients include fiber, digestive enzymes, the herbs St. John's wort and griffonia, the minerals calcium and potassium, and a trace mineral complex.

- Noni from Earth's Bounty. Noni (*Morinda citrifolia*) is a small tree that grows in Hawaii and other tropical regions. The fruit of this plant has a long history of use for a wide variety of problems, including joint problems, pain, inflammation, digestive problems, and cardiovascular disorders. Its active compounds include phytochemicals, designated anthraquinones, enzymes, and alkaloids.

- Echinaforce from Bioforce, USA. This is a liquid echinacea supplement that promotes natural disease resistance during the winter season and helps to maintain a healthy immune system.

- Fibroplex from Metagenics. This supplement contains vitamins B_1 (thiamine) and B_6 (pyridoxine), magnesium, manganese, and malic acid. It is designed to provide nutritional support for the nerves and muscles.

- GastroSoothe from Enzymatic Therapy. GastroSoothe is a natural antacid that contains calcium carbonate, deglycyrrhizinated licorice extract (DGL), and the amino acid glycine for the relief of indigestion and heartburn.

- Herbal Mood Boost from Country Life. This supplement contains a complex of herbs and nutrients known for their positive effects on mood and anxiety, including St. John's wort, 5-hydroxytryptophan (5-HTP), Siberian ginseng, kava kava, and passionflower.

- Hyper-C Serum from Jason Natural Cosmetics. This is an oil-based moisturizing formula that contains vitamin C, an antioxidant, to protect the skin from free radical damage. It also reduces the appearance of existing fine lines and wrinkles, evens out skin tones, and makes the skin softer and smoother in texture.

- HyperiCalm from Enzymatic Therapy. This supplement contains St. John's wort extract standardized to provide 0.3 percent hypericin. It is designed to support mental and nervous system function (*see* St. John's Wort under Herbs and Their Uses in HERBS in Part One).

- Instant Enerjetz from Superior Source (Continental Vitamin Company). This is a convenient, easy-to-take form of vitamin B_{12} that is placed on or under the tongue (not swallowed). Vitamin B_{12} is needed to prevent anemia and maintain a healthy nervous system, and it boosts energy and combats fatigue (*see* VITAMINS in Part One).

- Jerusalem artichoke tablets. Jerusalem artichoke whole tuber flour (JAF) tablets are a good source of fructo-oligosaccharides (FOS), which support the growth of healthy intestinal flora.

- Kyolic Neuro Logic from Wakunaga of America. This supplement contains aged garlic extract, ginkgo biloba extract, lecithin, acetyl-L-carnitine, and phosphatidyl serine in a formula designed to improve memory and mental activity.

- Miracle 2000 from Century Systems, Inc., is a combination supplement that contains twenty-seven vitamins and minerals, eighteen herbs, eight amino acids, and numerous ionic trace minerals.

- Nature's Answer line of herbal extracts designed for children. They are made using alcohol, like standard extracts, but the alcohol is then removed and replaced with glycerin, which is a preservative and a natural sweetener. Formulas include Bubble B-Gone, a combination colic remedy containing catnip, chamomile, fennel, and lemon balm; KidCatnip; KidChamomile; E-KID-nacea, an echinacea extract; E-KID-nacea Plus, which contains echinacea and goldenseal; and KID-B-Well, an immune-system tonic containing astragalus, burdock, and dandelion.

- Quick Cleanse Program from ZAND (Nutraceuticals International Corp.). This is a program utilizing three separate supplements: Cleansing Fiber formula, a fiber supplement containing psyllium seed and husk, plus bentonite and kaolin; Cleansing Laxative formula, with cascara sagrada (an herbal stimulant laxative) and kaolin; and Thistle Cleanse formula, a milk thistle supplement. This combination of formulas is designed to cleanse the intestinal tract, eliminate toxins, and support liver function.

- Remifemin from Enzymatic Therapy. Remifemin is a standardized extract of black cohosh that has been used in Europe for over forty years for the treatment of menopausal symptoms. (*see* Black Cohosh under Herbs and Their Uses in HERBS in Part One). This supplement does not affect hormone levels.

- Soy-Licious from Country Life. This dietary supplement is a high-protein soy-based drink mix with added genistein and daidzein (soy isoflavones), essential vitamins and minerals, antioxidants, and adaptogenic herbs (adaptogens are herbs that help the body adapt to and cope with the effects of stress).

- Sub-Adrene from American Biologics. This is a highly concentrated whole adrenal-cortical extract of bovine origin. Designed for sublingual administration, it has a peppermint taste and supplies a balance of natural steroids.

- Ultra Juice Green from Nature's Plus (Natural Organics). This is a supplement based on marine algae and containing a total of twenty different green foods in tablet form. It contains a wide range of vitamins, minerals, and phytonutrients.

- VitaSerum from ABRA, Inc. This is a skin care product designed to protect against free radicals, stimulate cell renewal, and reduce the visible signs of aging. It contains vitamin C from acerola berries; herbal extracts of elder flower, green tea, grape seed, and horsetail; citrus and cranberry bioflavonoids; hyaluronic acid; zinc sulfate; and essential oils of lavender, rose geranium, and sweet lavender.

- Vita Synergy for Men from The Synergy Company. This is a combination nutritional supplement that contains a balanced blend of all major vitamins and minerals, trace elements, and a variety of herbal extracts used to support men's health.

- Wellness Formula from Source Naturals. This supplement is designed to support optimal health in cold weather. Its ingredients include vitamins A and C, beta-carotene, and bioflavonoids; the immune-boosting mineral zinc; bee propolis; and the herbs angelica, astragalus, boneset, cayenne, echinacea, garlic, goldenseal, hawthorn berry, horehound, mullein, pau d'arco, and Siberian ginseng.

Herbs

INTRODUCTION

The medicinal benefits of herbs have been known for centuries. Records of Native American, Roman, Egyptian, Persian, and Hebrew medical practices show that herbs were used extensively to treat practically every known illness.

Many herbs contain powerful ingredients that, if used correctly, can help heal the body. The pharmaceutical industry was originally based upon the ability to isolate these ingredients and make them available in a purer form. Herbalists, however, contend that nature provides other ingredients in the same herbs to balance the more powerful ingredients.

These other components, though they may be less potent, may help to act as buffers, synergists, or counterbalances working in harmony with the more powerful ingredients. Therefore, when you use herbs in their complete form, your body's healing process utilizes a balance of ingredients provided by nature.

In the United States, herbal remedies were used widely until the early 1900s, when what was to become the modern pharmaceutical industry began isolating individual active compounds and producing drugs based on them. American medicine became almost exclusively committed to a medical system some practitioners call *allopathy*, which seeks to treat illness by producing a condition in the body that does not allow the disease to live or thrive. Over the years, most Americans have become conditioned to rely on synthetic, commercial drugs for relief.

Today, however, scientists are taking a second look at herbal remedies. Particularly in the past twenty years, a growing body of research (much of it done in Europe) has pointed to the therapeutic potential of numerous herbs. And big pharmaceutical companies are always on the lookout for plants to help with a variety of diseases. But a lot of work remains to be done; less than 1 percent of the estimated plant species on earth have been investigated for possible medicinal uses. In 1978, the German Commission E monographs were created, which describe the safety and effectiveness of herbs. This is still considered the most authoritative modern work on the subject.

Today's renewed interest in herbs reflects increasing concern about the side effects of powerful synthetic drugs, as well as the desire of many people to take charge of their own health, rather than merely submitting themselves to a sometimes-impersonal health care system. We are also rediscovering the healthful benefits of tasty herbs for cooking and aromatic herbs for enhancing and helping to balance mental, spiritual, and physical health.

Nature's pharmacy is an abundant one. Many herbs are rich in compounds that have a beneficial effect on certain tissues and organs, and, therefore, can be used as medicines to treat, cure, or prevent disease. Herbal remedies can help nourish your immune system, stimulate the regeneration of damaged liver tissue, build the strength of the adrenal glands, counter the adverse side effects of chemotherapy, balance the endocrine system, stimulate milk production, and improve night vision, among other things.

Generally, medicinal herbs fall into two basic categories: *tonic* and *stimulating*.

Tonics help cells, tissues, and organs to maintain tone, or balance, throughout the body. Some tonics activate and invigorate bodily processes or parts. Other tonics supply important nutrients that cells, tissues, and organs need to function properly. Tonics ordinarily are taken regularly for three to nine months at a time to gently strengthen and improve overall health and/or certain organ functions.

Stimulating herbs have much stronger actions and are used to treat particular ailments. They should be taken in smaller doses than tonic herbs, and for shorter periods of time.

Just because an herb had an historical use doesn't necessarily mean it will work for your condition. There may be some trial and error with different herbs and herbal blends before you get satisfactory results. Today, some herbs have undergone processing to produce a standardized extract that targets specific conditions. Extracts are a good place to start if you have one of the targeted conditions because they have a known amount of the active compound, which is not the case with the herb itself.

PHYTOMEDICINALS: THE HEALING POWER OF HERBS

Ancient cultures had no idea why herbs worked—they simply knew that certain plants produced certain desired results.

Only in the last hundred years or so have chemists and pharmacists been isolating and purifying the beneficial chemical compounds in plants to produce reliable pharmaceutical drugs. About 25 percent of the prescription medicines sold today are (or were originally) derived from plants. For example:

- Morphine and codeine come from the opium poppy.

- Aspirin originated from willow bark.

- Digitalis, a heart muscle strengthener, is derived from the foxglove plant.

- Paclitaxel (Taxol), used in cancer chemotherapy, comes from the Pacific yew tree.

Phytomedicine, a recently coined term, refers to an herbal medicine that is a whole-plant preparation, rather than a single isolated chemical compound. (The prefix *phyto* comes from the Greek word *phyton,* meaning "plant.") The herbal preparation derived from a whole plant or plant part is considered the active entity, even though it may actually contain hundreds of individual active components. Phytomedicines are standardized, however—that is, they contain set percentages of specified active components—and their therapeutic values are backed by pharmacological and clinical studies and experience.

Phytomedicines are widely recognized in Europe, where they are categorized as plant-derived drugs. In Germany, for example, phytomedicines are considered "ethical drugs," and physicians prescribe them and pharmacists dispense them. In the United States, phytomedicines are sold as over-the-counter dietary supplements in health food stores and in some pharmacies. A few mainstream doctors, however, have begun prescribing herbal remedies along with standard drugs. Some health insurance companies cover the cost of herbal medicines when they are prescribed by health care professionals. The National Center for Complementary and Alternative Medicine (NCCAM), part of the National Institutes of Health, is funding research on herbal remedies (for more information, go to www.nccam.nih .gov). According to Dr. David Eisenberg at Harvard Medical School, more than 18 percent of the U.S. population, or 38 million adults, use herbal supplements.

Although herbal supplements are not subject to the same standards as are prescription and over-the-counter drugs, they are regulated by the FDA. In fact, in July 2008 the FDA applied a new set of regulations to supplements called Good Manufacturing Practices (GMP). These rules ensure that all supplements are manufactured in a uniform way and that what appears on the label is what is in the product.

OTHER HERBAL HEALING SYSTEMS

The World Health Organization estimates that 80 percent of the earth's population today depends on plants to treat common ailments. Herbalism is an essential part of Ayurvedic (Indian), traditional Asian, Native American, and naturopathic medicines. Many homeopathic remedies are derived from plants as well. Homeopathic remedies are regulated by the FDA, but are subject to slightly different rules than dietary supplements. This biggest difference is that unlike supplements, they can carry disease claims on the label. This means labels for homeopathic remedies used historically for cancer patients, for example, can say "helps prevent recurrence of cancer." Other supplements may not make such claims.

Oriental herbs are a recent addition to the American herb scene, with the influx of several popular Chinese herbs. The Chinese are today's foremost herbalists, drawing on thousands of years of experience in compounding and processing roots and herbs. In the Asian tradition, herbs are used to bring the whole body into balance and harmony. They are taken daily as a preventive measure, rather than as a treatment once illness has occurred. In the Orient, medicinal herbs often find their way into foods as seasoning and ingredients. Indeed, according to the late Chinese writer and scholar Lin Yutang, the Chinese view medicine and food as the same thing, believing that what is good for the body is medicine and at the same time is also food. Some of the Chinese herbs most readily found in U.S. herb and natural food stores include astragalus, Chinese ginseng, ginkgo biloba, gotu kola, licorice root, dong quai, ginger, and schizandra.

Every Native American nation has its own herbal medicine tradition based on the plants growing in the geographic area where it lives. Common among all Native American cultures is the spirituality attached to the gathering and use of herbs, and many peoples use the same herbs both medicinally and ceremonially. For the Navajos, for example, herbalism is a complex and specialized religion, in which the Navajo healer serves as both doctor and priest. Before plants are collected, prayers and offerings are made to the earth and the plant spirit. Herbs used in healing ceremonies are not thrown away, but are reverently placed back into the earth. Much like the Asian approach, Native American herbalism aims to achieve balance within the total person. Medicinal and ceremonial herbs commonly used by Native American cultures include American ginseng, yarrow, black cohosh, boneset, echinacea, goldenseal, nettles, juniper, wild buckwheat, and dogwood.

As they have for centuries, indigenous rainforest tribes around the world rely on the forests for virtually all their medicines. They too have incorporated herbs into their religions and everyday lives. Researchers estimate that the world's rainforests contain literally thousands of potentially useful medicinal plants. Rainforests exist on every continent, though most research attention is currently directed at the rainforests of South America, particularly in the Amazon, and of the South Pacific Islands. Out of this rich storehouse of natural remedies, only a handful are now commonly found in health food stores, among them pau d'arco, boldo, cat's claw, kava, yerba maté, suma, yohimbe (not recommended), guarana, and passionflower. More and more rainforest remedies are becoming available.

USING MEDICINAL HERBS

Commercial herbal preparations are available in several different forms, including bulk herbs, medicinal herb blends, teas, oils, tinctures, fluid extracts, and tablets or capsules. Following are some of the ways in which herbal remedies can be used.

Essential Oils

Essential oils are highly concentrated extracts—typically obtained either by steam distillation or cold pressing—from the flowers, leaves, roots, berries, stems, seeds, gums, needles, bark, or resins of numerous plants. They contain natural hormones, vitamins, antibiotics, and antiseptics. Essential oils typically come from anise, thyme, ginger, and chamomile. Some of these oils, and especially chamomile, appear to inhibit herpes simplex virus in a petri dish.

Known also as *volatile oils* because they evaporate easily in air, essential oils are soluble in vegetable oil, partially soluble in alcohol, and not soluble in water. Because they are so concentrated, they are likely to irritate mucous membranes and the stomach lining if taken internally. It is therefore best to use essential oils externally only, such as in poultices, inhalants, or bathwater, or on the skin (a few drops). The therapeutic properties of essential oils can help to remedy ailments ranging from insomnia to respiratory disorders to impotence to arthritis.

Extracts

An extract is a concentrate that results when crude herb is mixed with a suitable solvent, such as alcohol and/or water. Of the different herbal forms, extracts are generally the most effective because their active ingredients are more highly concentrated, and they can be standardized to a guaranteed potency. Extracts also have longer shelf lives than other herbal preparations. Fresh herbal extracts retain almost all of the original plant's benefits.

Alcohol-free extracts are available. When administered sublingually (drops are placed under the tongue), herbal extracts can be absorbed by the body quickly. This is an especially effective way for older adults and people with absorption problems to use herbs.

Plasters, Compresses, and Poultices

These are ways of applying herbal remedies directly to the skin. Plasters and compresses are cotton bandages soaked in infusions or decoctions and wrapped around the affected area or held on with pressure. Compresses are also warm. Poultices are made by moistening herbs, placing them on the skin, and holding them there with a bandage. Moistened and warmed herbal tea bags also help soothe and heal. Try using chamomile tea bags to relieve the itching and inflammation of insect bites and eczema.

Powders

Powders are dried herbs ground to a fine consistency. You can sprinkle them over food, stir them into a liquid such as juice or water for tonics, or add them to soup stocks. You also can take them in capsule or tablet form.

Salves, Ointments, and Creams

These preparations combine a medicinal herb with an oily base for external use. Creams are light and slightly oily, to blend with the skin's secretions and allow the active ingredients to penetrate the skin. The heavier and oilier salves and ointments apply protective remedies to the skin surface.

Syrups

Syrups are used to improve the taste of bitter herbal formulas and to administer soothing cough or throat medicines. Herbs often taken in syrup form include wild cherry, marshmallow root, and licorice.

Teas, Infusions, and Decoctions

People have been consuming herbal teas for as long as they have known how to heat water—since well before recorded history. Unlike green, black, and oolong teas, herbal teas can be made from virtually any plant, and from any part of the plant, including the roots, flowers, seeds, berries, or bark. There are some herbs, such as echinacea, ginkgo leaf, saw palmetto, and milk thistle, that are not effective at healing when taken in tea form because their active components are not water soluble, and the concentration needed for medicinal potency is so high it can be obtained only from an extract, pill, or capsule.

Different herbal teas, which sometimes contain thousands of beneficial active compounds, have their own distinctive healing uses. The late botanical expert Varro Tyler, Ph.D., formerly professor emeritus of pharmacognosy (the study of natural drug properties) at Purdue University, taught that herbal teas are very good for relieving mild to moderate ailments such as upset stomach, sore throat, coughs, stuffy nose, and insomnia.

Many herbal teas are available in tea bag form. They can also be prepared from the raw herb. To make an herbal tea, gently crumble leaves and flowers and break roots and bark into pieces (cutting the herbs causes the essential oils to dissipate) and place them in a ceramic or glass container. Cover the herb parts with boiling water (do not bring the herbs themselves to a boil), and allow them to steep. Most herbs should be steeped for four to six minutes, although some herbal teas, such as chamomile, need to be steeped for fifteen to twenty minutes in a covered container in order to deliver their full therapeutic effect. Other herbs, such as ginseng roots, can be boiled. Astragalus can be lightly simmered for several hours. In fact, in Asia, ginseng root, astragalus, dong quai, and other herbs are added to chicken broth to make a tonic soup that is both food and medicine.

Infusion is simply another term for tea. This is the easiest way to take herbal remedies. To make an infusion, you simply boil water and add leaves, stems, flowers, or powdered herbs—plant material whose active ingredients dissolve readily in hot water—then steep, strain, and drink the mixture as a tea.

A decoction is a tea made from thicker plant parts, such as bark, roots, seeds, or berries. These also contain lignin, a substance that is difficult to dissolve in water. Thus, decoctions require a more vigorous extraction method than infusions.

Tinctures

Plant components that are either insoluble or only partially soluble in water can be extracted with solvents such as alcohol or glycerol. The herb is soaked in the solvent for a period of time, then pressed to render the tincture. Tinctures can preserve extracted ingredients for twelve months or more.

Vinegars

Herbal vinegars can serve as both medicines and salad dressings. To make an herbal vinegar, add the herb or herbs of your choice to raw apple cider vinegar, balsamic vinegar, rice vinegar, or malt vinegar. Allow the herbs to steep for four days (agitate the container daily), strain, and then press through a straining cloth and bottle in a dark glass container.

Wines

Steeping herbs in wine is a novel and pleasant way to use them medicinally. Wine does not keep as long as the stronger alcohols, so refrigeration is a good idea.

TIPS AND PRECAUTIONS

However they are used, most herbs act gently and subtly. They do not produce the kind of dramatic, immediate results we expect from prescription drugs. Basically, herbs are balancers that work with the body to help it heal and regulate itself. They work better together than they do singly because the effect of one herb is usually supported and reinforced when combined with others.

While most herbs aren't likely to be harmful, keep in mind that "natural" isn't a synonym for "safe." Like synthetic drugs, herbal preparations may be toxic, cause allergic reactions, or affect your response to other medications.

Common sense, care, and forethought are needed when using herbs for either food or medicine. Here are some essential guidelines for herbal self-care:

- Use herbal self-care for minor ailments only, not for serious or life-threatening conditions.
- Use only recommended amounts for recommended periods of time.
- Use the correct herb. Buy your herbal remedies from a reputable company. If you collect or grow herbs on your own, be absolutely positive in your identification.
- Use the correct part of the plant. For instance, don't substitute roots for leaves. When buying fresh herbs, check to be sure which part of the herb is required for a remedy—the whole herb, flowers, fruit, leaves, stems, or roots.
- When using an herbal remedy for the first time, start with a small amount to test for possible allergic reactions.
- Don't take certain herbs if you are pregnant or planning to become pregnant.
- Don't take herbal remedies if you are nursing a baby.
- Don't give medicinal amounts of herbs to children without first consulting with your health care practitioner.

Buying Herbal Remedies

When choosing herbal remedies, it is important to select quality products from a reliable source. How do you know whether a manufacturer or supplier is reliable? Start by making a phone call to the manufacturer. Ask how long the company has been in business, if they are following the GMP guidelines from the FDA, and how they determine the identity and potency of the herbs they sell. Membership in trade groups such as the American Herbal Products Association (www.ahpa.org), while not a stamp of approval, does indicate the company's recognition of industry standards. The American Botanical Council provides regular updates on new science related to herbs (www.herbalgram.org). We recommend purchasing herbs sold by reputable companies that have been in the herb business for at least ten years. A number of manufacturers and distributors specializing in herbal products, including herbal combinations for management of certain disorders, are listed under Manufacturer and Distributor Information in the Appendix.

If you wish to buy organically grown herbs, look for the "certified organic" label on the product. More than half of U.S. states have certification programs for organic farms and products. Federal standards are now implemented through a nationwide certification system under the USDA National Organic Program. More information on the regulations governing these producers can be found at www.ams.usda.gov/nop.

Finally, look for herbal products that are standardized to contain a specific percentage of active ingredients extracted from the specific herb part known to be effective.

HERBS AND THEIR USES

The following table describes some of the most commonly used medicinal herbs, including which parts of each herb are used, its chemical and nutrient content, and its various uses.

Herb (Scientific Name)	Part(s) Used	Phytochemical and Nutrient Content	Actions and Uses	Comments
Acerola (*Malpighia glabra*)	Fruit.	Phytochemicals: Beta-carotene. Nutrients: Calcium, iron, magnesium, phosphorus, potassium, vitamins A, B_1, B_2, B_3, B_5, B_6, and C.	Has antioxidant, antifungal, and astringent properties. Helps to support the liver and hydrate the skin. Useful for diarrhea and fever.	A rainforest herb similar to the cherry. One of the richest natural sources of vitamin C; found in numerous multivitamin supplements.
Alfalfa (*Medicago sativa*)	Flowers, leaves, petals, sprouted seeds.	Phytochemicals: Alpha-carotene, beta-carotene, beta-sitosterol, chlorophyll, coumarin, cryptoxanthin, daidzein, fumaric acid, genistein, limonene, lutein, saponin, stigmasterol, zeaxanthin. Nutrients: Calcium, copper, folate, iron, magnesium, manganese, phosphorus, potassium, silicon, zinc, vitamins A, B_1, B_2, B_3, B_5, B_6, C, D, E, and K.	Alkalizes and detoxifies the body. Acts as a diuretic, anti-inflammatory, and antifungal. Lowers cholesterol, balances blood sugar and hormones, and promotes pituitary gland function. Good for anemia, arthritis, ulcers, bleeding-related disorders, and disorders of the bones and joints, digestive system, and skin.	Must be used in fresh, raw form to provide all nutrients. Sprouts are especially effective (be sure to rinse them thoroughly before use to remove mold and bacteria).
Aloe (*Aloe vera*)	Pulp from insides of succulent leaves.	Phytochemicals: Acemannan, beta-carotene, beta-sitosterol, campesterol, cinnamic acid, coumarin, lignins, p-coumaric acid, saponins. Nutrients: Amino acids, calcium, folate, iron, magnesium, phosphorus, potassium, zinc, vitamins A, B_1, B_2, B_3, C, and E.	Acts as an astringent, emollient, antifungal, antibacterial, and antiviral. Applied topically, heals mouth sores and stimulates cell regeneration. Ingested, helps to lower cholesterol, reduces inflammation resulting from radiation therapy, increases blood vessel generation in lower extremities of people with poor circulation, soothes stomach irritation, aids healing, and acts as a laxative. May be good for patients with AIDS and for skin. It supports a healthy digestive system probably by increasing short-chain fatty acid production from the friendly bacteria in the colon.	Allergic reactions, though rare, may occur in susceptible persons. Before using, apply a small amount behind the ear or on the underarm. If stinging or rash occurs, do not use. *Caution:* Should not be taken internally during pregnancy.
Anise (*Pimpinella anisum*)	Seeds, seed oil.	Phytochemicals: Alpha-pinene, apigenin, bergapten, caffeic acid, chlorogenic acid, eugenol, limonene, linalool, myristicin, rutin, scopoletin, squalene, stigmasterol, umbelliferone. Nutrients: Calcium, iron, magnesium, manganese, phosphorus, potassium, zinc, vitamins A, B_1, B_2, B_3, B_5, B_6, C, and E.	Aids digestion, clears mucus from air passages, combats infection, and promotes milk production in nursing mothers. Good for indigestion and for respiratory infections such as sinusitis. Also helpful for menopausal symptoms.	Used in many popular products as a fragrance and flavoring.
Annatto (*Bixa orellana*)	Leaves, roots, seeds.	Phytochemicals: Beta-carotene, bixin, cyanidin, ellagic acid, salicylic acid, saponin, tannins. Nutrients: Amino acids, calcium, iron, phosphorus, vitamins B_2, B_3, and C.	Has diuretic, antioxidant, antibacterial, anti-inflammatory, and expectorant properties. Helps to protect the liver and kidneys. May reduce blood sugar levels. Useful for indigestion, fever, coughs, burns, skin problems, and weight loss.	A rainforest herb used in skin care products as an emollient, and as an orange-yellow food coloring.

Herb (Scientific Name)	Part(s) Used	Phytochemical and Nutrient Content	Actions and Uses	Comments
Ashwagandha (Withania somnifera)	Roots.	Phytochemicals: Alkaloids, beta-sitosterol, chlorogenic acid, scopoletin, withaferin. Nutrients: Amino acids, choline.	Rejuvenates and energizes the nervous system. Helps prevent stress-related disorders and stress-related depletion of vitamin C and cortisol. Increases physical endurance and improves sexual function. Has anti-inflammatory and antiaging effects. In laboratory studies, has modulated and stimulated immune function.	An Ayurvedic herb also known as Indian ginseng and winter cherry. An important herb in Ayurvedic medicine.
Astragalus (Astragalus membranaceus)	Roots.	Phytochemicals: Betaine, beta-sitosterol, formononetin, isoliquiritigenin. Nutrients: Calcium, choline, copper, essential fatty acids, iron, magnesium, manganese, potassium, zinc.	Acts as a tonic to protect the immune system. Aids adrenal gland function and digestion. Increases metabolism, produces spontaneous sweating, promotes healing, and provides energy to combat fatigue and prolonged stress. Increases stamina. Good for colds, flu, and immune deficiency–related problems, including AIDS, cancer, and tumors. Effective for chronic lung weakness.	Also called huang qi. *Caution:* Do not use if fever is present.
Barberry (Berberis vulgaris)	Bark, berries, roots.	Phytochemicals: Berbamine, berberine, beta-carotene, caffeic acid, kaempferol, lutein, quercetin, sinapic acid, zeaxanthin. Nutrients: Calcium, iron, magnesium, manganese, phosphorus, potassium, selenium, silicon, zinc, vitamins B_1, B_2, B_3, and C.	Decreases heart rate, slows breathing, reduces bronchial constriction. Kills bacteria on the skin and stimulates intestinal movement.	*Caution:* Should not be used during pregnancy.
Bayberry (Myrica cerifera)	Root bark.	Phytochemicals: Beta-carotene, gallic acid, myristic acid, phenol. Nutrients: Calcium, iron, magnesium, manganese, phosphorus, potassium, selenium, silicon, zinc, vitamins B_1, B_2, B_3, and C.	Acts as a decongestant and astringent. Aids circulation, reduces fever. Helps stop bleeding. Good for circulatory disorders, fever, hypothyroidism, and ulcers. Also good for the eyes and the immune system.	The wax of the berries is used to make fragrant candles. *Caution:* Should not be used at high dosages or for prolonged periods. May temporarily irritate sensitive stomachs.
Bilberry (Vaccinium myrtillus)	Entire plant.	Phytochemicals: Anthocyanosides, beta-carotene, caffeic acid, caryophyllene, catechin, chlorogenic acid, ferulic acid, gallic acid, hyperoside, lutein, quercetin, quercitrin, ursolic acid, vanillic acid. Nutrients: Calcium, inositol, magnesium, manganese, phosphorus, potassium, selenium, silicon, sulfur, zinc, vitamins B_1, B_2, B_3, and C.	Acts as an antioxidant, diuretic, and urinary tract antiseptic. Keeps blood vessels flexible, allowing increased blood flow. Helps control insulin levels and strengthen connective tissue. Supports and strengthens collagen structures, inhibits the growth of bacteria, and has antiaging and anticarcinogenic effects. Useful for hypoglycemia, inflammation, stress, anxiety, night blindness, and cataracts. May help halt or prevent macular degeneration.	Also known as European blueberry. Related to the American blueberry. *Caution:* Interferes with iron absorption when taken internally. Should not be used by people with diabetes except under the supervision of a knowledgeable health professional.
Birch (Betula alba)	Bark, leaves, sap.	Phytochemicals: Betulin, betulinic acid, hyperoside, luteolin and quercetin glycosides, methyl salicylate.	Acts as a diuretic, anti-inflammatory, and pain reliever. Good for joint pain and urinary tract infections. Applied topically, good for boils and sores.	Betulinic acid in birch bark has been found to kill cancer cells.

Herb (Scientific Name)	Part(s) Used	Phytochemical and Nutrient Content	Actions and Uses	Comments
Black cohosh (*Cimicifuga racemosa*)	Rhizomes, roots.	Phytochemicals: Beta-carotene, cimicifugin, formononetin, gallic acid, phytosterols, salicylic acid, tannic acid, tannin. Nutrients: Calcium, chromium, iron, magnesium, manganese, phosphorus, potassium, selenium, silicon, zinc, vitamins B_1, B_2, B_3, and C.	Lowers blood pressure and cholesterol levels. Reduces mucus production. Helps cardiovascular and circulatory disorders. Induces labor and aids in childbirth (many herbalists recommend taking small amounts two weeks before expected delivery). Relieves menopausal symptoms, menstrual cramps with back pain, morning sickness, and pain. Helpful for poisonous snake bites. Good for arthritis.	Also known as black snakeroot. *Caution:* Do not use during pregnancy or in the presence of chronic disease. There have been reports of liver problems associated with the use of this herb in certain individuals. Some products contain Asian Actaea and not black cohosh. Buy from a reputable company.
Black walnut (*Juglans nigra*)	Husks, inner bark, leaves, nuts.	Phytochemicals: Beta-carotene, ellagic acid, juglone, myricetin, tannin. Nutrients: Calcium, iron, magnesium, manganese, phosphorus, potassium, selenium, silicon, zinc, vitamins B_1, B_2, B_3, and C.	Aids digestion and acts as a laxative. Helps heal mouth and throat sores. Cleanses the body of some types of parasites. Good for bruising, fungal infection, herpes, poison ivy, and warts. May help lower blood pressure and cholesterol levels.	When boiled, the hulls produce a dye that is used to color wool.
Blessed thistle (*Cnicus benedictus*)	Flowers, leaves, stems.	Phytochemicals: Beta-carotene, beta-sitosterol, cnicin, ferulic acid, kaempferol, luteolin, oleanolic acid, stigmasterol. Nutrients: Calcium, essential fatty acids, iron, magnesium, manganese, phosphorus, potassium, selenium, silicon, zinc, vitamins B_1, B_2, B_3, and C.	Stimulates the appetite and stomach secretions. Heals the liver. Lessens inflammation, improves circulation, cleanses the blood, and strengthens the heart. May act as brain food. Good for female disorders and increases milk flow in nursing mothers.	Also called St. Benedict thistle, holy thistle. *Caution:* Should be handled with care to avoid toxic skin effects.
Blue cohosh (*Caulophyllum thalictroides*)	Roots.	Phytochemicals: Anagyrine, beta-carotene, caulophylline, caulophyllosaponin, caulosaponin, hederagenin, phytosterols, saponin. Nutrients: Calcium, iron, magnesium, manganese, phosphorus, potassium, selenium, zinc, vitamins B_1, B_2, B_3, and C.	Eases muscle spasms and stimulates uterine contractions for childbirth. Useful for memory problems, menstrual disorders, and nervous disorders.	*Caution:* Should not be used during the first two trimesters of pregnancy.
Boldo (*Peumus boldus*)	Leaves.	Phytochemicals: Alpha-pinene, ascaridole, benzaldehyde, beta-pinene, boldin, boldine, camphor, coumarin, eugenol, farnesol, kaempferol, limonene, linalool, 1,8-cineole. Nutrients: Choline.	Acts as a diuretic, laxative, antibiotic, liver tonic, and anti-inflammatory. Aids in the excretion of uric acid and stimulates digestion.	Used by indigenous peoples of Chile and Peru for liver ailments and gallstones.
Boneset (*Eupatorium perfoliatum*)	Flower petals, leaves.	Phytochemicals: Astragalin, gallic acid, eufoliatin, eufoliatorin, eupatorin, euperfolin, euperfolitin, gallic acid, hyperoside, kaempferol, quercetin, rutin, tannic acid.	Acts as a decongestant, laxative, anti-inflammatory, and diuretic. Loosens phlegm, reduces fever, increases perspiration, calms the body. Useful for colds, flu, bronchitis, and fever-induced aches and pains.	Also called white snakeroot. *Caution:* Do not use on a daily basis for more than one week as long-term use can lead to toxicity.
Borage (*Borago officinalis*)	Leaves, seeds.	Phytochemicals: Beta-carotene, rosmarinic acid, silicic acid, tannin. Nutrients: Calcium, choline, essential fatty acids, iron, magnesium, phosphorus, potassium, zinc, vitamins B_1, B_2, B_3, and C.	Acts as an adrenal tonic and gland balancer. Contains valuable minerals and essential fatty acids needed for proper cardiovascular function and healthy skin and nails.	The flowers of the borage plant are edible.

Herb (Scientific Name)	Part(s) Used	Phytochemical and Nutrient Content	Actions and Uses	Comments
Boswellia (*Boswellia serrata*)	Gum resin.	Phytochemicals: Borneol, boswellic acids, carvone, caryophyllene, farnesol, geraniol, limonene.	Acts as an anti-inflammatory, antiarthritic, antifungal, and antibacterial. Used topically for pain relief. Lowers cholesterol, protects the liver. Useful for arthritis, gout, low back pain, myositis, and fibromyalgia. Helps repair blood vessels damaged by inflammation. Traditionally used as a remedy for obesity, diarrhea, dysentery, pulmonary diseases, ringworm, and boils.	An Ayurvedic herb also known as Indian frankincense. An important herb in Ayurvedic medicine.
Buchu (*Barosma betulina*)	Leaves.	Phytochemicals: Alpha-pinene, alpha-terpinene, barosma-camphor, diosphenol, hesperidin, limonene, menthone, pulegone, quercetin, quercetrin, rutin. Nutrients: Calcium, iron, magnesium, manganese, phosphorus, potassium, selenium, silicon, zinc, vitamins B_1, B_2, and B_3.	Lessens inflammation of the colon, gums, mucous membranes, prostate, sinuses, and vagina. Acts as a diuretic. Helps control bladder and kidney problems, diabetes, digestive disorders, fluid retention, and prostate disorders. A specific for bladder infections.	Do not boil buchu leaves.
Burdock (*Arctium lappa*)	Plant, roots, seeds.	Phytochemicals: Acetic acid, arctigenin, arctiin, beta-carotene, butyric acid, caffeic acid, chlorogenic acid, costic acid, inulin, isovaleric acid, lauric acid, lignin, myristic acid, propionic acid, sitosterol, stigmasterol. Nutrients: Amino acids, calcium, chromium, copper, iron, magnesium, manganese, phosphorus, potassium, selenium, silicon, zinc, vitamins B_1, B_2, B_3, and C.	Acts as an antioxidant. May help to protect against cancer by helping control cell mutation. Aids elimination of excess fluid, uric acid, and toxins. Has antibacterial and antifungal properties. Purifies the blood, restores liver and gallbladder function, and stimulates the digestive and immune systems. Helps skin disorders such as boils and carbuncles, and relieves gout and menopausal symptoms. Burdock root used as a hair rinse promotes scalp and hair health.	Also called bardana, beggar's buttons, clotbur, gobo, lappa, and thorny burr. *Caution:* Interferes with iron absorption when taken internally. Should not be used by pregnant or breast-feeding women, people with diabetes, or those with heart or cardiovascular conditions.
Butcher's broom (*Ruscus aculeatus*)	Plant, roots, seeds.	Phytochemicals: Beta-carotene, chrysophanic acid, glycolic acid, neoruscogenin, rutin, saponin. Nutrients: Calcium, chromium, iron, magnesium, manganese, phosphorus, potassium, selenium, silicon, zinc, vitamins B_1, B_2, B_3, and C.	Reduces inflammation. Useful for carpal tunnel syndrome, circulatory disorders, edema, Ménière's disease, obesity, Raynaud's phenomenon, thrombophlebitis, varicose veins, and vertigo. Also good for the bladder and kidneys.	More effective if taken with vitamin C.
Calendula (*Calendula officinalis*)	Flower petals.	Phytochemicals: Alpha-amyrin, beta-amyrin, beta-sitosterol, caffeic acid, campesterol, caryophyllene, chlorogenic acid, faradiol, galactose, gentisic acid, kaempferol, lutein, lycopene, malic acid, myristic acid, oleanolic acid, p-coumaric acid, phytofluene, quercetin, rutin, salicylic acid, saponin, stigmasterol, syringic acid, taraxasterol vanillic acid, zeta-carotene. Nutrients: Calcium, coenzyme Q_{10}, vitamins C and E.	Reduces inflammation and is soothing to the skin. Helps regulate the menstrual cycle and lower fever. Useful for skin disorders, such as rashes and sunburn, as well as for neuritis and toothache. Good for diaper rash and other skin problems in small children.	Also called pot marigold. Usually nonirritating when used externally.

Herb (Scientific Name)	Part(s) Used	Phytochemical and Nutrient Content	Actions and Uses	Comments
Cascara sagrada (*Frangula purshiana*)	Bark.	Phytochemicals: Aloe-emodin, anthraquinones, barbaloin, beta-carotene, casanthranol, chrysophanic acid, chrysophanol, frangulin, malic acid, myristic acid. Nutrients: Calcium, iron, linoleic acid, magnesium, manganese, phosphorus, potassium, selenium, silicon, zinc, vitamins B_1, B_2, B_3, and C.	Acts as a colon cleanser and laxative. Effective for colon disorders, constipation, and parasitic infestation.	Tastes very bitter taken as a tea.
Catnip (*Nepeta cataria*)	Leaves.	Phytochemicals: Alpha-humulene, beta-elemene, camphor, carvacrol, caryophyllene, citral, citronellal, geraniol, myrcene, nepetalactone, piperitone, pulegone, rosmarinic acid, thymol. Nutrients: Calcium, chromium, iron, magnesium, manganese, phosphorus, potassium, selenium, silicon, zinc.	Lowers fever (catnip tea enemas reduce fever quickly). Dispels gas and aids digestion and sleep; relieves stress; stimulates the appetite. Good for anxiety, colds and flu, inflammation, pain, and stress.	Can be given to children.
Cat's claw (*Uncaria tomentosa*)	Inner bark, roots.	Phytochemicals: Alloisopteropodine, allopteropodine, isomitraphylline, isopteropodine, mitraphylline, oleanolic acid, pteropodine, rhynchophylline, ursolic acid.	Acts as an antioxidant and anti-inflammatory. It may help with the management of arthritis. Stimulates the immune system. Cleanses the intestinal tract and enhances the action of white blood cells. Good for intestinal problems and viral infections. May help people with AIDS symptoms, arthritis, cancer, tumors, or ulcers.	Also called uña de gato. According to USDA research, cat's claw seeds contain an enzyme instrumental in converting saturated fats to unsaturated fats. *Caution:* Do not use during pregnancy.
Cayenne (*Capsicum frutescens* or *C. annum*)	Berries.	Phytochemicals: Alpha-carotene, beta-carotene, beta-ionone, caffeic acid, campesterol, capsaicin, carvone, caryophyllene, chlorogenic acid, citric acid, cryptoxanthin, hesperidin, kaempferol, limonene, lutein, myristic acid, 1,8-cineole, p-coumaric acid, quercetin, scopoletin, stigmasterol, zeaxanthin. Nutrients: Amino acids, calcium, essential fatty acids, folate, iron, magnesium, phosphorus, potassium, zinc, vitamins B_1, B_2, B_3, B_5, B_6, C, and E.	Aids digestion, improves circulation, weight loss, and stops bleeding from ulcers. Acts as a catalyst for other herbs. Good for the heart, kidneys, lungs, pancreas, spleen, and stomach. Useful for arthritis and rheumatism. Helps to ward off colds, sinus infections, and sore throats. Good for pain when applied topically. Used with lobelia for nerves.	Also called capsicum, hot pepper, red pepper. *Caution:* Avoid contact with the eyes.
Cedar (*Cedrus libani*)	Leaves, tops.	Phytochemicals: Dorncol, quinic acid.	Acts as an antiviral, antifungal, expectorant, lymphatic cleanser, and urinary antiseptic. Stimulates the immune system. Increases venous blood flow. Can be used externally for warts.	

Herb (Scientific Name)	Part(s) Used	Phytochemical and Nutrient Content	Actions and Uses	Comments
Celery (Apium graveolens)	Plant, roots, seeds.	Phytochemicals: Alpha-pinene, apigenin, bergapten, beta-carotene, caffeic acid, carvone, chlorogenic acid, coumarin, eugenol, ferulic acid, isoquercitrin, limonene, linalool, luteolin, mannitol, myristic acid, myristicin, p-coumaric acid, rutin, scopoletin, shikimic acid, thymol. Nutrients: Amino acids, boron, calcium, choline, essential fatty acids, folate, inositol, iron, magnesium, manganese, phosphorus, potassium, selenium, sulfur, zinc, vitamins A, B_1, B_2, B_3, B_5, B_6, C, E, and K.	Reduces blood pressure, relieves muscle spasms, and improves appetite. Good for arthritis, gout, and kidney problems. Acts as a diuretic, antioxidant, and sedative.	*Caution:* Do not use large amounts. Do not eat the seeds if you are pregnant.
Chamomile (Matricaria recutita or M. chamomilla)	Flowers, plant.	Phytochemicals: Alpha-bisabolol, apigenin, azulene, borneol, caffeic acid, chlorogenic acid, farnesol, gentisic acid, geraniol, hyperoside, kaempferol, luteolin, p-coumaric acid, perillyl alcohol, quercetin, rutin, salicylic acid, sinapic acid, tannin, umbelliferone. Nutrients: Choline, vitamins B_1, B_3, and C.	Reduces inflammation, stimulates the appetite, and aids digestion and sleep. Acts as a diuretic and nerve tonic. Helpful for colitis, diverticulosis, fever, headaches, and pain. Good for menstrual cramps. A traditional remedy for stress and anxiety, indigestion, and insomnia. Useful as a mouthwash for minor mouth and gum infections.	Also called German chamomile, wild chamomile. Roman chamomile (*Chamaemelum nobile*) is also available, but is less common. *Caution:* Do not use it if allergic to ragweed. Do not use during pregnancy or nursing. It may interact with warfarin or cyclosporine, so patients taking these drugs should avoid it.
Chanca piedra (Phyllanthus niruri)	Entire plant.	Phytochemicals: Limonene, lupeol, methyl salicylate, quercetin, quercitrin, rutin, saponins.	Fights inflammation and bacterial and viral infection. Acts as a diuretic. Useful for kidney stones, gallstones, colds, flu, digestion, asthma, bronchitis, diarrhea, pain relief, fever, sexually transmitted diseases, and muscle spasms.	A rainforest herb whose name means "stone crusher." Also known as seed-on-the-leaf.
Chaste tree (Vitex agnus-castus)	Fruit, leaf.	Phytochemicals: Alpha-pinene, alpha-terpineol, chrysosplenol, flavonoids, limonene, linalool, myrcene, 1,8-cineole, pinene, progesterone, testosterone.	Has a calming and soothing effect. Relieves muscle cramps. Regulates and normalizes hormone levels and menstrual cycles. Good for symptoms of PMS and menopause.	Also called chasteberry, vitex. *Caution:* Should not be used during pregnancy. Should not be given to children.
Chickweed (Stellaria media)	Leaves, stems.	Phytochemicals: Beta-carotene, genistein, rutin. Nutrients: Calcium, essential fatty acids, iron, magnesium, manganese, phosphorus, potassium, selenium, silicon, sulfur, zinc, vitamins B_1, B_2, B_3, C, and E.	Relieves nasal congestion. May lower blood lipids. Useful for bronchitis, circulatory problems, colds, coughs, skin diseases, and warts (applied topically). A good source of vitamin C and other nutrients.	Also called starweed.

Herb (Scientific Name)	Part(s) Used	Phytochemical and Nutrient Content	Actions and Uses	Comments
Chuchuhuasi (*Maytenus krukoviti*)	Bark, root, leaves.	Phytochemicals: Anthocyanidins, catechin, maytensine, nocotinyl, sesquiterpenes, triterpenes, tannins.	Fights inflammation and stimulates the immune system. Supports the adrenal system and balances and regulates menstrual cycles. Good for arthritis, rheumatism, back pain, muscle spasms, fever, skin tumors, bronchitis, diarrhea.	Also called chucchu huashu, chuchuasi, chuchasha, chuchuhuasha. Peruvian Amazon native name means "trembling back" for its value as an antiarthritic drug. This rainforest herb also used traditionally to stimulate sexual desire and give energy.
Cinnamon (*Cinnamomum verum*)	Bark, plant.	Phytochemicals: Alpha-pinene, benzaldehyde, beta-carotene, beta-pinene, borneol, camphor, caryophyllene, cinnamaldehyde, coumarin, cuminaldehyde, eugenol, farnesol, geraniol, limonene, linalool, mannitol, mucilage, 1,8-cineole, phellandrene, tannin, terpinolene, vanillin. Nutrients: Calcium, chromium, copper, iodine, iron, manganese, phosphorus, potassium, zinc, vitamins A, B_1, B_2, B_3, and C.	Relieves diarrhea and nausea; counteracts congestion; aids peripheral circulation. Warms the body and enhances digestion, especially the metabolism of fats. Also fights fungal infection. Useful for diabetes, weight loss, yeast infection, and uterine hemorrhaging.	*Cinnamon cassia* is used for diabetes management but with varying degrees of success. *Caution:* Should not be used in large amounts during pregnancy.
Clove (*Syzygium aromaticum*)	Flower buds, essential oil.	Phytochemicals: Beta-carotene, beta-pinene, beta-sitosterol, campesterol, carvone, caryophyllene, chavicol, cinnamaldehyde, ellagic acid, eugenol, gallic acid, kaempferol, linalool, methyleugenol, methylsalicylate, mucilage, oleanolic acid, stigmasterol, tannin, vanillin. Nutrients: Calcium, iron, magnesium, manganese, phosphorus, potassium, zinc, vitamins A, B_1, B_2, and C.	Has antiseptic and antiparasitic properties, and acts as a digestive aid. Essential oil is applied topically for relief of toothache and mouth pain.	*Caution:* Clove oil is very strong and can cause irritation if used in its pure form. Diluting the oil in olive oil or distilled water is recommended. Essential oil should not be taken internally except under the careful supervision of a health care professional.
Comfrey (*Symphytum officinale*)	Leaves, roots.	Phytochemicals: Allantoin, beta-carotene, caffeic acid, chlorogenic acid, rosmarinic acid, sitosterol, stigmasterol. Nutrients: Calcium, iron, magnesium, manganese, phosphorus, potassium, selenium, zinc, vitamins B_1, B_2, B_3, and C.	Speeds healing of wounds and many skin conditions. Beneficial for bedsores, bites and stings, bruises, inflamed bunions, dermatitis, dry skin, bleeding hemorrhoids, leg ulcers, nosebleeds, psoriasis, scabies, skin rashes, and sunburn.	Also called knitbone. *Caution:* Recommended for external use only.
Corn silk (*Zea mays*)	Styles, stigmas ("tassels").	Phytochemicals: Benzaldehyde, beta-carotene, betaine, beta-sitosterol, caffeic acid, campesterol, carvacrol, caryophyllene, dioxycinnamic acid, geraniol, glycolic acid, limonene, 1,8-cineole, saponin, thymol, vitexin. Nutrients: Calcium, chromium, iron, magnesium, manganese, phosphorus, potassium, vitamins B_1, B_3, and C.	Acts as a diuretic. Aids the bladder, kidney, and small intestine. Lessens the incidence of bed-wetting when taken several hours before bedtime. Good for carpal tunnel syndrome, edema, obesity, premenstrual syndrome, and prostate disorders. Used in combination with other "kidney herbs," opens the urinary tract and removes mucus from the urine.	

Herb (Scientific Name)	Part(s) Used	Phytochemical and Nutrient Content	Actions and Uses	Comments
Cramp bark (*Viburnum opulus*)	Bark, root.	Phytochemicals: Esculetin, scopoletin, valerianic acid. Nutrients: Calcium, iron, magnesium, manganese, phosphorus, potassium, selenium, zinc.	Relieves muscle spasms and pain. Good for menstrual cramps. Useful for lower back and leg spasms.	Also called guelder rose. Closely related to black haw, which has the same medicinal properties. *Caution:* Should be avoided during pregnancy.
Cranberry (*Vaccinium macrocarpon*)	Fruit.	Phytochemicals: Alpha-terpineol, anthocyanosides, benzaldehyde, benzoic acid, beta-carotene, chlorogenic acid, ellagic acid, eugenol, ferulic acid, lutein, malic acid, quercetin. Nutrients: Calcium, folate, iron, magnesium, manganese, phosphorus, potassium, selenium, sulfur, zinc, vitamins A, B_1, B_2, B_3, B_5, C, and E.	Acidifies the urine and prevents bacteria from adhering to bladder cells. Good for the kidneys, bladder, and skin. Has anticancer properties. Helpful for infections of the urinary tract. Shown to improve memory in older people (sixty years and older).	A good source of vitamin C. Cranberry juice cocktail products that contain sugar should be *avoided.*
Damiana (*Turnera diffusa*)	Leaves.	Phytochemicals: Alpha-pinene, beta-carotene, beta-pinene, beta-sitosterol, 1,8-cineole, tannins, thymol. Nutrients: Calcium, iron, magnesium, manganese, phosphorus, potassium, selenium, zinc, vitamins B_1, B_2, B_3, and C.	Stimulates muscular contractions of the intestinal tract and delivery of oxygen to the genital area. Used as an energy tonic and aphrodisiac, and to remedy sexual and hormonal problems. A "sexuality tonic" for women.	*Caution:* Interferes with iron absorption when taken internally.
Dandelion (*Taraxacum officinale*)	Flowers, leaves, roots, tops.	Phytochemicals: Beta-carotene, beta-sitosterol, caffeic acid, cryptoxanthin, lutein, mannitol, p-coumaric acid, saponin, stigmasterol. Nutrients: Calcium, iron, magnesium, manganese, phosphorus, potassium, selenium, zinc, vitamins B_1, B_2, B_3, and C.	Acts as a diuretic. Cleanses the blood and liver, and increases bile production. Reduces serum cholesterol and uric acid levels. Improves functioning of the kidneys, pancreas, spleen, and stomach. Relieves menopausal symptoms. Useful for abscesses, anemia, boils, breast tumors, cirrhosis of the liver, constipation, fluid retention, hepatitis, jaundice, and rheumatism. Believed to help prevent age spots and breast cancer.	Leaves can be boiled and eaten like spinach (young leaves can be used in salads). *Caution:* Should not be combined with prescription diuretics. Not recommended for people with gallstones or biliary tract obstruction.
Devil's claw (*Harpagophytum procumbens*)	Rhizome.	Phytochemicals: Chlorogenic acid, cinnamic acid, harpagide, harpagoside, kaempferol, luteolin, oleanolic acid. Nutrients: Calcium, iron, magnesium, manganese, phosphorus, potassium, selenium, zinc.	Relieves pain and reduces inflammation. Acts as a diuretic, sedative, and digestive stimulant. Good for back pain, arthritis, rheumatism, diabetes, allergies, liver, gallbladder and kidney disorders, arteriosclerosis, lumbago, gout, and menopausal symptoms. For backache, taking devil's claw allowed for a reduction in the use of rescue medications (i.e., pharmaceuticals for pain). When used by patients with arthritis there was less need for other medications. Migraine sufferers had a decreased number of headaches after one month.	Also called grapple plant, wood spider. *Caution:* Should not be used during pregnancy. Based on twenty studies, 3 percent of people reported side effects. Of that number, there were only a few cases—usually concerning gastrointestinal problems—that were severe enough to stop the use of the herb.

Herb (Scientific Name)	Part(s) Used	Phytochemical and Nutrient Content	Actions and Uses	Comments
Dong quai (Angelica sinensis)	Roots.	Phytochemicals: Alpha-pinene, bergapten, beta-carotene, beta-sitosterol, carvacrol, falcarinol, ferulic acid, ligustilide, myristic acid, p-cymene, scopoletin, umbelliferone, vanillic acid. Nutrients: Calcium, folate, iron, magnesium, manganese, phosphorus, potassium, selenium, zinc, vitamins B_1, B_2, B_5, and C.	Acts as a mild sedative, laxative, diuretic, antispasmodic, and pain reliever. Improves the blood. Strengthens the reproductive system. Assists the body in using hormones. Used to treat female problems such as hot flashes and other menopausal symptoms, premenstrual syndrome, and vaginal dryness.	Also known as Chinese angelica. *Caution:* Should not be used during pregnancy. Should not be used by people who have diabetes or are light-sensitive. Dong quai enhances the action of the blood-thinner warfarin, so the two should not be used together.
Echinacea (Echinacea species)	Leaves, roots.	Phytochemicals: Alpha-pinene, apigenin, arabinogalactan, beta-carotene, beta-sitosterol, betaine, borneol, caffeic acid, caryophyllene, chlorogenic acid, cichoric acid, cynarin, echinacoside, ferulic acid, kaempferol, luteolin, quercetin, rutin, stigmasterol, vanillin, verbascoside. Nutrients: Calcium, iron, magnesium, manganese, phosphorus, potassium, selenium, zinc, vitamins B_1, B_2, B_3, and C.	Fights inflammation and bacterial and viral infection. Stimulates certain white blood cells. Good for the immune system and the lymphatic system. Useful for allergies, colic, colds, flu, and other infectious illnesses. Results summarized from 234 studies showed that echinacea extracts were effective in preventing symptoms of the common cold compared to a placebo.	For internal use, a freeze-dried form or alcohol-free extract is recommended. *Caution:* Do not take for longer than three weeks. Should not be used by people who are allergic to ragwood.
Elder (Sambucus nigra)	Flowers, fruit, inner bark, leaves, roots.	Phytochemicals: Alpha-amyrin, astragalin, beta-carotene, beta-sitosterol, betulin, caffeic acid, campesterol, chlorogenic acid, cycloartenol, ferulic acid, isoquercitrin, kaempferol, lupeol, malic acid, myristic acid, oleanolic acid, p-coumaric acid, pectin, quercetin, rutin, shikimic acid, stigmasterol, ursolic acid. Nutrients: Calcium, essential fatty acids, vitamins A, B_1, B_2, B_3, and C.	Combats free radicals and inflammation. Relieves coughs and congestion. Builds the blood, cleanses the system, eases constipation. Enhances immune system function. Increases perspiration, lowers fever, soothes the respiratory tract, and stimulates circulation. Effective against flu viruses. The flowers are used to soothe skin irritations.	Also called black elder, black elderberry, European elder. *Caution:* Should not be used during pregnancy. The stems of this plant should be *avoided*. They contain cyanide, and can be very toxic.
Ephedra (Ephedra sinica)	Stems.	Phytochemicals: Beta-carotene, d-norpseudoephedrine, ellagic acid, ephedrine, gallic acid. Nutrients: Calcium, iron, magnesium, manganese, phosphorus, potassium, selenium, zinc, vitamins B_1, B_2, B_3, and C.		On February 6, 2004, the U.S. Food and Drug Administration (FDA) issued a final rule prohibiting the sale of dietary supplements containing ephedrine alkaloids (ephedra) because such supplements present an unreasonable risk of illness or injury. The ban was challenged in court in 2005, but it was ultimately upheld by a federal appellate court in 2006 and the U.S. Supreme Court refused to hear the case. As a result the FDA ban is still in effect in the U.S.

Herb (Scientific Name)	Part(s) Used	Phytochemical and Nutrient Content	Actions and Uses	Comments
Eucalyptus (*Eucalyptus globulus*)	Bark, essential oil, leaves.	Phytochemicals: Alpha-pinene, beta-pinene, caffeic acid, carvone, chlorogenic acid, ellagic acid, ferulic acid, gallic acid, gentisic acid, hyperoside, 1,8-cineole, p-cymene, protocatechuic acid, quercetin, quercitrin, rutin.	Acts as a decongestant and mild antiseptic. Reduces swelling by helping to increase blood flow. Relaxes tired and sore muscles. Good for colds, coughs, and other respiratory disorders. Inhaling vapor from a few drops of the oil helps to break up mucus.	Recommended for external use only. Should not be used on broken skin or open cuts or wounds.
Eyebright (*Euphrasia officinalis*)	Entire plant, except the root.	Phytochemicals: Beta-carotene, caffeic acid, ferulic acid, tannins. Nutrients: Calcium, chromium, iron, magnesium, manganese, phosphorus, potassium, selenium, zinc, vitamins B₁, B₂, B₃, and C.	Prevents secretion of fluids and relieves discomfort from eyestrain or minor irritation. Used as an eyewash. Good for allergies, itchy and/or watery eyes, and runny nose. Combats hay fever.	
False unicorn root (*Chamaelirium luteum*)	Roots.	Phytochemicals: Chamaelirin, helonin, saponins.	Balances sex hormones. Helps treat infertility, menstrual irregularities and pain, premenstrual syndrome, and prostrate disorders. May help prevent miscarriage.	Also called helonias.
Fennel (*Foeniculum vulgare*)	Fruit, roots, leaves, stems.	Phytochemicals: Alpha-pinene, benzoic acid, bergapten, beta-carotene, beta-phellandrene, beta-sitosterol, caffeic acid, camphor, cinnamic acid, cynarin, ferulic acid, fumaric acid, isopimpinellin, isoquercitrin, kaempferol, limonene, linalool, myristicin, 1,8-cineole, p-coumaric acid, pectin, protocatechuic acid, psoralen, quercetin, rutin, scopoletin, sinapic acid, stigmasterol, umbelliferone, vanillic acid, vanillin, xanthotoxin. Nutrients: Amino acids, calcium, choline, essential fatty acids, iron, magnesium, manganese, phosphorus, potassium, selenium, vitamins B₁, B₂, B₃, C, and E.	Used as an appetite suppressant and as an eyewash. Promotes the functioning of the kidneys, liver, and spleen, and also clears the lungs. Relieves abdominal pain, colon disorders, gas, and gastrointestinal tract spasms. Useful for acid stomach. Good after chemotherapy and/or radiation treatments for cancer.	The powdered plant can be used as a flea repellent.
Fenugreek (*Trigonella foenum-graecum*)	Seeds.	Phytochemicals: Beta-carotene, beta-sitosterol, coumarin, diosgenin, kaempferol, luteolin, p-coumaric acid, quercetin, rutin, saponin, trigonelline, vitexin. Nutrients: Amino acids, calcium, essential fatty acids, folate, iron, magnesium, manganese, phosphorus, potassium, selenium, zinc, vitamins B₁, B₂, B₃, and C.	Acts as a laxative, lubricates the intestines, and reduces fever. Helps lower cholesterol and blood sugar levels. Helps asthma and sinus problems by reducing mucus. Good for the eyes and for inflammation and lung disorders.	Oil of fenugreek has a maplelike flavor.

Herb (Scientific Name)	Part(s) Used	Phytochemical and Nutrient Content	Actions and Uses	Comments
Feverfew (*Chrysanthemum parthenium*)	Bark, dried flowers, leaves.	Phytochemicals: Beta-carotene, parthenolide, santamarin. Nutrients: Calcium, iron, magnesium, manganese, phosphorus, potassium, selenium, zinc, vitamins B_1, B_2, B_3, and C.	Combats inflammation and muscle spasms. Increases fluidity of lung and bronchial tube mucus, promotes menses, stimulates the appetite, and stimulates uterine contractions. Relieves nausea and vomiting. Good for arthritis, colitis, fever, headaches, mild and transient migraines, menstrual problems, muscle tension, and pain.	Chewing the leaves is a folk remedy, but this may cause mouth sores. Also called featherfew, featherfoil. *Caution:* Do not use when pregnant or nursing. People who take prescription blood-thinning medications or who regularly take over-the-counter painkillers should consult a health care provider before using feverfew, as the combination can result in internal bleeding.
Flax (*Linum usitatissimum*)	Seeds, seed oil.	Phytochemicals: Apigenin, beta-carotene, beta-sitosterol, campesterol, chlorogenic acid, cycloartenol, lecithin, luteolin, myristic acid, squalene, stigmasterol, vitexin. Nutrients: Amino acids, calcium, essential fatty acids, iron, magnesium, manganese, phosphorus, potassium, sulfur, vanadium, zinc, vitamins B_1, B_2, B_3, B_5, and E.	Promotes strong bones, nails, and teeth, as well as healthy skin. Useful for colon problems, female disorders, and inflammation.	The seeds are an excellent addition to a diet that is low in fiber. Flaxseed has the highest concentration of the phytoestrogen lignans of any other food. The lignans are removed during conversion to oil, so seeds are the only true source.
Garlic (*Allium sativa*)	Bulb.	Phytochemicals: Allicin, beta-carotene, beta-sitosterol, caffeic acid, chlorogenic acid, diallyl-disulfide, ferulic acid, geraniol, kaempferol, linalool, oleanolic acid, p-coumaric acid, phloroglucinol, phytic acid, quercetin, rutin, s-allyl-cysteine, saponin, sinapic acid, stigmasterol. Nutrients: Calcium, folate, iron, magnesium, manganese, phosphorus, potassium, selenium, zinc, vitamins B_1, B_2, B_3, and C.	Detoxifies the body and protects against infection by enhancing immune function. Lowers blood pressure and improves circulation. Lowers blood lipid levels. Helps stabilize blood sugar levels. Aids in the treatment of arteriosclerosis, arthritis, asthma, cancer, circulatory problems, colds and flu, digestive problems, heart disorders, insomnia, liver disease, sinusitis, ulcers, and yeast infections. May prevent ulcers by inhibiting growth of *Helicobacter pylori,* the ulcer-causing bacterium. Good for virtually any disease or infection.	Garlic contains many sulfur compounds, which give it its healing properties. Odorless garlic supplements are available. Aged garlic extract (such as Kyolic) is good. *Caution:* Not recommended for people who take anticoagulants, as garlic has blood-thinning actions.
Gentian (*Gentiana lutea*)	Leaves, roots.	Phytochemicals: Caffeic acid, carvacrol, gentiopicrin, limonene, linalool, mangiferin, sinapic acid, swertiamarin. Nutrients: Calcium, iron, magnesium, manganese, phosphorus, potassium, selenium, zinc, vitamins B_1, B_2, B_3, and C.	Aids digestion, stimulates appetite, and boosts circulation. Kills plasmodia (organisms that cause malaria) and worms. Good for circulatory problems and pancreatitis.	

Herb (Scientific Name)	Part(s) Used	Phytochemical and Nutrient Content	Actions and Uses	Comments
Ginger (*Zingiber officinale*)	Rhizomes, roots.	Phytochemicals: Alpha-pinene, beta-carotene, beta-ionone, beta-sitosterol, caffeic acid, camphor, capsaicin, caryophyllene, chlorogenic acid, citral, curcumin, farnesol, ferulic acid, geraniol, gingerols, lecithin, 1,8-cineole, zingerone. Nutrients: Amino acids, calcium, essential fatty acids, iron, magnesium, manganese, phosphorus, potassium, selenium, zinc, vitamins B_1, B_2, B_3, B_6, and C. Ground ginger also contains vitamin A.	Fights inflammation, cleanses the colon, reduces spasms and cramps, and stimulates circulation. A strong antioxidant and effective antimicrobial agent for sores and wounds. Protects the liver and stomach. Useful for bowel disorders, circulatory problems, arthritis, fever, headache, hot flashes, indigestion, morning sickness, motion sickness, muscle pain, nausea, and vomiting.	Can cause stomach distress if taken in large quantities. *Caution:* Not recommended for people who take anticoagulants or have gallstones. Not recommended for extended use during pregnancy.
Ginkgo (*Ginkgo biloba*)	Leaves, seed.	Phytochemicals: Amentoflavone, apigenin, beta-carotene, bilobalide, ginkgetin, isorhamnetin, kaempferol, luteolin, myristic acid, p-coumaric acid, procyanidin, quercetin, shikimic acid, stigmasterol, tannin, thymol. Nutrients: Amino acids, calcium, iron, magnesium, manganese, phosphorus, potassium, zinc, vitamins A, B_1, B_2, B_3, B_5, and C.	Improves brain functioning by increasing cerebral and peripheral circulation and tissue oxygenation. Has antioxidant properties. May slow the progression of Alzheimer's disease, and may relieve leg cramps by improving circulation. Beneficial for asthma, dementia, depression, eczema, headaches, heart and kidney disorders, memory loss, and tinnitis (ringing in the ears). Shows promise as a treatment for vascular-related impotence.	Can take at least two weeks to see results. *Caution:* Should not be used by people who have bleeding disorders, or who are scheduled for surgery or a dental procedure.
Ginseng (*Panax quinquefolius*) [American ginseng], (*P. ginseng*) [Chinese or Korean ginseng]	Roots.	Phytochemicals: Beta-sitosterol, campesterols, caryophyllene, cinnamic acid, escin (*P. quinquefolius*), ferulic acid, fumaric acid, ginsenosides, kaempferol, oleanolic acid, panaxic acid, panaxin, saponin, stigmasterol, vanillic acid. Nutrients: Calcium, choline, fiber, folate, iron, magnesium, manganese, phosphorus, potassium, silicon, zinc, vitamins B_1, B_2, B_3, B_5, and C.	Strengthens the adrenal and reproductive glands. Enhances immune function, promotes lung functioning, and stimulates the appetite. Useful for bronchitis, circulatory problems, diabetes, infertility, lack of energy, and stress; to ease withdrawal from cocaine; and to protect against the effects of radiation exposure. In a laboratory study, enhanced breast-cancer-cell suppression in combination with standard treatment. Used by athletes for overall body strengthening. May help improve drug- or alcohol-induced liver dysfunction in older adults.	Siberian ginseng (*Eleutherococcus senticosus*) belongs to a different botanical family than American and Korean ginseng, but its properties are similar, and all are commonly referred to simply as ginseng. *Caution:* Should not be used by people who have high blood pressure, are pregnant, or are nursing.

Herb (Scientific Name)	Part(s) Used	Phytochemical and Nutrient Content	Actions and Uses	Comments
Goldenseal (*Hydrastis canadensis*)	Rhizomes, roots.	Phytochemicals: Berberine, beta-carotene, canadine, chlorogenic acid. Nutrients: Calcium, iron, magnesium, manganese, phosphorus, potassium, selenium, zinc, vitamins B_1, B_2, B_3, and C.	Fights infection and inflammation. Cleanses the body. Increases the effectiveness of insulin and strengthens the immune system, colon, liver, pancreas, spleen, and lymphatic and respiratory systems. Improves digestion, regulates menses, decreases uterine bleeding, and stimulates the central nervous system. Good for allergies, ulcers, and disorders affecting the bladder, prostate, stomach, and vagina. Used at the first sign of possible symptoms, can stop a cold, flu, or sore throat from developing.	Alternating with echinacea or other herbs is recommended. Alcohol-free extract is the best form. *Caution:* Do not take goldenseal internally on a daily basis for more than one week at a time. Do not use it during pregnancy or if you are breast-feeding, and use with caution if you are allergic to ragweed. If you have a history of cardiovascular disease, diabetes, or glaucoma, use it only under a doctor's supervision.
Gotu kola (*Centella asiatica*)	Nuts, roots, seeds.	Phytochemicals: Beta-carotene, beta-sitosterol, campesterol, camphor, kaempferol, saponin, stigmasterol. Nutrients: Calcium, iron, magnesium, manganese, phosphorus, potassium, selenium, zinc, vitamins B_1, B_2, B_3, and C.	Helps eliminate excess fluids, decreases fatigue and depression, increases sex drive, shrinks tissues, and stimulates the central nervous system. May neutralize blood acids and lower body temperature. Promotes wound healing, and is good for varicose veins and for heart and liver function. Useful for cardiovascular and circulatory disorders, fatigue, connective tissue disorders, kidney stones, poor appetite, and sleep disorders.	May cause dermatitis if applied topically.
Gravel root (*Eupatorium purpureum*)	Flowers, root.	Phytochemicals: Euparin, eupatorin, resin.	Acts as a diuretic and urinary tract tonic. Combats prostate disorders, kidney stones, and problems related to fluid retention.	Also called joe-pye weed, queen-of-the-meadow.
Green tea (*Camellia sinensis*)	Leaves.	Phytochemicals: Apigenin, astragalin, benzaldehyde, beta-carotene, beta-ionone, beta-sitosterol, caffeic acid, caffeine, carvacrol, catechins, chlorogenic acid, cinnamic acid, cryptoxanthin, epicatechin, epigallocatechin, eugenol, farnesol, gallic acid, geraniol, hyperoside, indole, isoquercitrin, kaempferol, lutein, lycopene, myrcene, myricetin, myristic acid, naringenin, polyphenols, procyanidins, quercetin, quercitrin, rutin, salicylic acid, tannic acid, thymol, vitexin, zeaxanthin. Nutrients: Amino acids, calcium, iron, magnesium, manganese, phosphorus, potassium, zinc, vitamins B_1, B_2, B_3, B_5, and C.	Acts as an antioxidant and helps to protect against cancer. Lowers cholesterol levels, reduces the clotting tendency of the blood, stimulates the immune system, fights tooth decay, helps regulate blood sugar and insulin levels, combats mental fatigue, and may delay the onset of atherosclerosis. Good for asthma. Studies show promise as a weight-loss aid, but the green tea must not be decaffeinated. May help prevent enlarged prostate.	To get green tea's antioxidant benefits, drink it without milk (milk may bind with the beneficial compounds, making them unavailable to the body). *Caution:* Contains a small amount of caffeine. Should not be used in large quantities by pregnant women or nursing mothers. Persons with anxiety disorder or irregular heartbeat should limit their intake to no more than 2 cups daily.

Herb (Scientific Name)	Part(s) Used	Phytochemical and Nutrient Content	Actions and Uses	Comments
Guarana (Paullinia cupana)	Seeds.	Phytochemicals: Adenine, caffeine, D-catechin, saponin, tannins, theobromine, theophylline.	Acts as a general tonic, stimulant, and intestinal cleanser. Increases mental alertness as well as speed and accuracy when reading. Improves stamina and endurance. Reduces fatigue. Useful for headaches, urinary tract irritation, diarrhea. Also shown to improve mood.	Also called Brazilian cocoa, uabano. *Caution:* Due to guarana's caffeine content, taking more than 600 mg a day is not recommended. Not recommended for people with high blood pressure or heart conditions.
Hawthorn (Crataegus laevigata)	Flowers, fruit, leaves.	Phytochemicals: Acetylcholine, adenine, adenosine, anthocyanidins, beta-carotene, beta-sitosterol, caffeic acid, catechin, chlorogenic acid, epicatechin, esculin, hyperoside, pectin, quercitrin, rutin, ursolic acid, vitexin. Nutrients: Amino acids, calcium, choline, chromium, essential fatty acids, iron, magnesium, manganese, phosphorus, potassium, selenium, silicon, zinc, vitamins B_1, B_2, B_3, and C.	Dilates the coronary blood vessels, lowers blood pressure and cholesterol levels, and restores heart muscle. Decreases fat deposit levels. Increases intracellular vitamin C levels. Useful for anemia, cardiovascular and circulatory disorders, high cholesterol, and lowered immunity. Patients with diabetes who were already using blood pressure medicine experienced a greater drop in blood pressure with hawthorn.	*Caution:* Do not use if you take medication for heart disease.
Hops (Humulus lupulus)	Flowers, fruit, leaves.	Phytochemicals: Alpha-pinene, alpha-terpineol, beta-carotene, beta-eudesmol, beta-sitosterol, caffeic acid, campesterol, catechin, chlorogenic acid, citral, eugenol, ferulic acid, limonene, p-cymene, piperidine, procyanidins, quercetin, tannins. Nutrients: Amino acids, calcium, chromium, magnesium, potassium, selenium, silicon, zinc, vitamins B_1, B_3, and C.	Relieves anxiety. Stimulates the appetite. Useful for cardiovascular disorders, hyperactivity, insomnia, nervousness, pain, restlessness, shock, stress, toothaches, and ulcers.	Placed inside a pillowcase, aids sleep. *Caution:* Should not be used by people who take antidepressants.
Horehound (Marrubium vulgare)	Flowers, leaves.	Phytochemicals: Alpha-pinene, apigenin, beta-sitosterol, caffeic acid, gallic acid, limonene, luteolin, pectin, tannic acid, tannins, ursolic acid. Nutrients: B-complex vitamins, iron, potassium, vitamins A, C, and E.	Decreases thickness and increases fluidity of mucus in the bronchial tubes and lungs. Boosts the immune system. Useful for indigestion, loss of appetite, bloating, and hay fever, sinusitis, and other respiratory disorders.	*Caution:* Large doses may cause irregular heart rhythms.
Horse chestnut (Aesculus hippocastanum)	Bark, leaves, oil, seeds.	Phytochemicals: Allantoin, citric acid, epicatechin, escin, esculetin, esculin, fraxetin, fraxin, isoquercitrin, kaempferol, leucocyanidin, myricetin, quercetin, quercitrin, rutin, saponin, scopoletin, tannin.	Protects against vascular damage, makes capillary walls less porous, shields against UV radiation damage. Good for varicose veins, reducing excess tissue fluids, and easing nighttime muscle spasms in the legs. For chronic venous insufficiency, horse chestnut was effective at reducing leg pain and allowed for less blood to pool in the lower limbs. Used topically, reduces pain and swelling, and prevents bruising.	
Hydrangea (Hydrangea arborescens)	Rhizomes, roots.	Phytochemicals: Kaempferol, quercetin, rutin, saponin. Nutrients: Calcium, iron, magnesium, manganese, phosphorus, potassium, selenium, zinc.	Stimulates the kidneys and acts as a diuretic. Good for bladder infection, kidney disease, obesity, and prostate disorders. Combined with gravel root, good for kidney stones.	*Caution:* The leaves of this plant should *not* be consumed. They contain cyanide and can be toxic.

Herb (Scientific Name)	Part(s) Used	Phytochemical and Nutrient Content	Actions and Uses	Comments
Hyssop (*Hyssopus officinalis*)	Flowers, leaves, shoots.	Phytochemicals: Alpha-pinene, benzaldehyde, beta-ionone, beta-sitosterol, borneol, caffeic acid, camphor, carvacrol, eugenol, ferulic acid, geraniol, hesperidin, limonene, linalool, marrubiin, oleanolic acid, 1,8-cineole, rosmarinic acid, thymol, ursolic acid. Nutrients: Choline.	Promotes expulsion of mucus from the respiratory tract, relieves congestion, regulates blood pressure, and dispels gas. Used externally, helpful for wound healing. Good for circulatory problems, epilepsy, fever, gout, and weight problems. Poultices made from fresh green hyssop help heal cuts.	*Caution:* Should not be used during pregnancy.
Irish moss (*Chondrus crispus*)	Entire plant.	Phytochemicals: Beta-carotene. Nutrients: Calcium, iron, magnesium, manganese, phosphorus, potassium, selenium, zinc, vitamins B_1, B_2, B_3, and C.	Acts as an expectorant and aids in the formation of stools. Good for bronchitis and many intestinal disorders. Also used in skin lotions and in hair rinses for dry hair.	
Jaborandi (*Pilocarpus jaborandi*)	Leaves.	Phytochemicals: Alpha-pinene, limonene, myrcene, pilocarpine.	Fights inflammation and acts as a diuretic. Helps stimulate milk production and flow in nursing mothers. Beneficial for fever, colds and flu, bronchitis, colon disorders, and edema. Topically, useful for baldness and for promoting circulation in the capillaries.	A rainforest herb whose active compound, pilocarpine, has been used for over 120 years to relieve intraocular pressure in glaucoma.
Jatoba (*Hymenaea courbaril*)	Bark, leaves, fruit.	Phytochemicals: Beta-sitosterol, caryophyllene, delta-cadinene, epicatechin.	Fights inflammation, free radicals, and bacterial and fungal infection. Increases energy. Beneficial for asthma, bronchitis, bursitis, bladder infection, candida and other fungal infections, arthritis, and prostatitis.	A rainforest herb with a wide range of traditional uses.
Juniper (*Juniperus communis*)	Fruit.	Phytochemicals: Alpha-pinene, beta-carotene, beta-pinene, betulin, borneol, camphor, caryophyllene, catechin, farnesol, epicatechin, glycolic acid, limonene, linalool, menthol, rutin, tannins, umbelliferone. Nutrients: Calcium, chromium, iron, magnesium, manganese, phosphorus, potassium, selenium, zinc, vitamins B_1, B_2, B_3, and C.	Acts as a diuretic, anti-inflammatory, and decongestant. Helps regulate blood sugar levels. Helpful in treatment of asthma, bladder infection, fluid retention, gout, obesity, and prostate disorders.	*Caution:* May interfere with absorption of iron and other minerals when taken internally. Should not be used during pregnancy. Should not be used by persons with kidney disease.

Herb (Scientific Name)	Part(s) Used	Phytochemical and Nutrient Content	Actions and Uses	Comments
Kava kava (*Piper methysticum*)	Roots.	Phytochemicals: Cinnamic acid, kavalactones (including kawain, dihydrokawain, methysticin, dihydromethysticin, and yangonin).	Induces physical and mental relaxation. Acts as a diuretic, genitourinary antiseptic, and gastrointestinal tonic. Relieves muscle spasms and eases pain. Helpful for anxiety and anxiety disorders, insomnia, stress-related disorders, menopausal symptoms, and urinary tract infections. It has been shown to be an analgesic and an anticonvulsive, and protects the nervous system. Usually begins working within two hours, but multiple (about three times a day) dosing is needed to maintain blood levels.	Also called kava. *Caution:* Can cause drowsiness. If this occurs, discontinue use or reduce the dosage. Should not be combined with alcohol. Not recommended for persons under the age of eighteen, pregnant women, nursing mothers, individuals who suffer from depression or take certain prescription drugs, especially antianxiety drugs, or those with liver or skin diseases. Kava taken in large amounts for extended periods of time may worsen liver function tests.
Kudzu (*Pueraria lobata*)	Leaves, roots, shoots.	Phytochemicals: Daidzein, daidzin, genistein, p-coumaric acid, puerarin, quercetin. Nutrients: Calcium, iron, magnesium, phosphorus, potassium, vitamin B_2.	Suppresses alcohol cravings. Lowers blood pressure and relieves headache, stiff neck, vertigo, and tinnitus. Useful for treating alcoholism, colds, flu, and gastrointestinal problems.	In China and Japan, kudzu has been used as a food starch and medicine for centuries. The Chinese use kudzu extract to treat angina pectoris.
Lady's mantle (*Achillea millefolium*)	Entire plant, except the root.	Phytochemicals: Achilleine, alpha-pinene, apigenin, azulene, beta-carotene, betaine, beta-pinene, beta-sitosterol, betonicine, borneol, caffeic acid, camphor, caryophyllene, chamazulene, coumarins, eugenol, guaiazulene, isorhamnetin, limonene, luteolin, mannitol, menthol, myrcene, myristic acid, 1,8-cineole, p-cymene, quercetin, quercitrin, rutin, salicylic acid, stigmasterol, tannin, thujone. Nutrients: Amino acids, calcium, essential fatty acids, folate, iron, magnesium, manganese, phosphorus, potassium, selenium, zinc, vitamins B_1, B_2, B_3, and C.	Wound dressing. Has anti-inflammatory, diuretic, and antiviral effects. Helps to heal mucous membranes, improve blood clotting, and increase perspiration. Helps to regulate menstruation, reduce excessive bleeding, and ease cramps. Useful for muscle spasms, fever, gastrointestinal disorders, inflammatory disorders, and viral infections. Applied topically, stops bleeding and promotes healing. Good as a douche for vaginal irritation.	Also called milfoil, old man's pepper, soldier's woundwort, knight's milfoil, herbe militaris, thousand weed, nose bleed, carpenter's weed, bloodwort, staunchweed, devil's nettle, devil's plaything, bad man's plaything, yarroway. *Caution:* Interferes with iron absorption and other minerals. Topical use may cause irritation. Individuals who are sun sensitive should avoid it. Not to be used by pregnant women.
Lavender (*Lavandula angustifolia*)	Flowers.	Phytochemicals: Alpha-pinene, beta-pinene, beta-santalene, borneol, camphor, caryophyllene, coumarin, geraniol, limonene, linalool, luteolin, 1,8-cineole, rosmarinic acid, tannin, umbelliferone, ursolic acid.	Relieves stress and depression. Beneficial for the skin. Good for headaches, psoriasis, and other skin problems.	Essential oil of lavender is very popular in aromatherapy. *Caution:* Should not be used during pregnancy. Lavender oil should not be taken internally.

Herb (Scientific Name)	Part(s) Used	Phytochemical and Nutrient Content	Actions and Uses	Comments
Lemongrass (*Cymbopogon citratus*)	Leaves, stems.	Phytochemicals: Alpha-pinene, beta-pinene, beta-santalene, borneol, camphor, caryophyllene, coumarin, geraniol, limonene, linalool, luteolin, 1,8-cineole, rosmarinic acid, tannin, umbelliferone, ursolic acid. Phytochemicals: Alpha-pinene, beta-sitosterol, caryophyllene, citral, farnesol, geraniol, limonene, luteolin, myrcene, 1,8-cineole, quercetin, rutin, saponin, triacontanol. Nutrients: Calcium, iron, magnesium, manganese, phosphorus, potassium, selenium, zinc.	Acts as an astringent, tonic, and digestive aid. Good for the skin and nails. Useful for fever, flu, headaches, and intestinal irritations.	Used in perfumes and other products as a fragrance.
Licorice (*Glycyrrhiza glabra*)	Roots.	Phytochemicals: Apigenin, benzaldehyde, beta-carotene, beta-sitosterol, betaine, camphor, carvacrol, estriol, eugenol, ferulic acid, formononetin, geraniol, glabrene, glabridin, glabrol, glycyrrhetinic acid, glycyrrhizin, isoliquiritigenin, isoliquiritin, isoquercitrin, lignin, mannitol, phenol, quercetin, salicylic acid, sinapic acid, stigmasterol, thymol, umbelliferone, vitexin. Nutrients: Calcium, choline, iron, magnesium, manganese, phosphorus, potassium, selenium, silicon, zinc, vitamins B_1, B_2, B_3, and C.	Fights inflammation and viral, bacterial, and parasitic infection. Stimulates the production of interferon and may help inhibit replication of HIV. Cleanses the colon. Reduces muscle spasms, increases fluidity of mucus in the lungs and bronchial tubes, and promotes adrenal gland function. Has estrogen- and progesterone-like effects; may change the pitch of the voice. Helps to inhibit the formation of plaque and prevent bacteria from sticking to tooth enamel. Beneficial for allergies, asthma, chronic fatigue syndrome, depression, emphysema, enlarged prostate, fever, herpesvirus infection, hypoglycemia, glandular functions, inflammatory bowel disorders, premenstrual syndrome, menopausal symptoms, and upper respiratory infections. May prevent hepatitis C from causing liver cancer and cirrhosis and protect against atherosclerosis. Deglycyrrhizinated licorice may stimulate natural defense mechanisms that prevent the occurrence of ulcers by increasing the number of mucus-secreting cells in the digestive tract. This improves the quality of mucus, lengthens intestinal cell life, and enhances microcirculation in the gastrointestinal lining. Cancer patients who took licorice and a soup containing tonic vegetables had less pain. The plant has been shown to have anticancer properties.	Licorice derivatives have been recommended as a standard support for ulcer sufferers in Europe. Licorice-flavored candy does not work for medicinal purposes because it is mostly made with anise, not licorice. *Caution:* Should not be used during pregnancy, nor by persons with diabetes, glaucoma, heart disease, high blood pressure, severe menstrual problems, or a history of stroke.

Herb (Scientific Name)	Part(s) Used	Phytochemical and Nutrient Content	Actions and Uses	Comments
Maca (*Lepidium meyenii*)	Roots.	Phytochemicals: Beta-sitosterol, saponin, stigmasterol, tannins. Nutrients: Amino acids, calcium, iron, magnesium, phosphorus, zinc, vitamins B_1, B_2, B_{12}, C, and E.	Increases energy and supports the immune system. Good for anemia, chronic fatigue syndrome, impotence, fertility, menopausal symptoms, and menstrual problems.	A rainforest herb that is a member of the potato family. An important food in the diet of native Peruvians for over 2,000 years, it is rich in amino acids and high in protein. *Caution*: People with liver or heart disease should avoid high doses, as it has been shown to worsen liver blood tests and raise blood pressure.
Macela (*Achyrocline satureoides*)	Aerial parts.	Phytochemicals: Alpha-pinene, caffeic acid, caryophyllene, chlorogenic acid, coumarin, delta-cadinene, galangin, luteolin, 1,8-cineole, quercetagetin, quercetin, scoparone.	Acts as an anti-inflammatory, antiseptic, antiviral, and antiparasitic. Stimulates and supports the immune system. Good for gastrointestinal and respiratory disorders. Useful in treating cancer, Crohn's disease, colds and flu, diabetes, menstrual problems and menopausal symptoms, and muscle aches and spasms.	A rainforest herb that has been found to have potential anti-HIV properties.
Marshmallow (*Althaea officinalis*)	Flowers, leaves, roots.	Phytochemicals: Beta-carotene, betaine, caffeic acid, chlorogenic acid, ferulic acid, kaempferol, mucilage, paraffin, p-coumaric acid, pectin, phytosterols, quercetin, salicylic acid, scopoletin, sorbitol, tannins, vanillic acid. Nutrients: Amino acids, calcium, iron, magnesium, manganese, phosphorus, potassium, selenium, zinc, vitamins B_1, B_2, B_3, and C.	Aids the body in expelling excess fluid and mucus. Soothes and heals skin, mucous membranes, and other tissues, externally and internally. Good for bladder infection, digestive upsets, fluid retention, headache, intestinal disorders, kidney problems, sinusitis, and sore throat.	Often used as a filler in the compounding of pills.
Meadowsweet (*Filipendula ulmaria*)	Leaves, flower tops.	Phytochemicals: Anthocyanidin, avicularin, coumarin, hyperoside, methyl salicylate, quercetin, rutin, salicin, salicylic acid, vanillin.	Tightens tissues and promotes elimination of excess fluid. Reduces inflammation and strengthens and tones the system. Good for colds, flu, nausea, digestive disorders, muscle cramps and aches, and diarrhea.	The word *aspirin* is derived from an old name for this plant, *spirea*. *Caution:* Because this plant contains compounds related to aspirin, it should not be used by pregnant women, and it should not be given to children with fever due to cold, flu, measles, chickenpox, or any other viral infection, as this increases the risk of Reye's syndrome, a dangerous complication that can alter or damage the liver, brain, and heart.

Herb (Scientific Name)	Part(s) Used	Phytochemical and Nutrient Content	Actions and Uses	Comments
Milk thistle (Silybum marianum)	Fruit, leaves, seeds.	Phytochemicals: Apigenin, beta-carotene, fumaric acid, kaempferol, naringenin, quercetin, silandrin, silybin, silychristin, silydianin, silymarin, silymonin, taxifolin. Nutrients: Calcium, essential fatty acids, iron, magnesium, manganese, phosphorus, potassium, selenium, zinc.	Protects the liver from toxins and pollutants by preventing free radical damage and stimulates the production of new liver cells. People with liver disease who used silymarin had fewer liver-related symptoms and better quality-of-life scores. Also protects the kidneys. Good for gallbladder and adrenal disorders, inflammatory bowel disorders, psoriasis, weakened immune system, and all liver disorders. Has shown anticancer effects against prostate cancer and breast cancer. Silymarin inhibits COX-2 formation.	Also called Mary thistle or wild artichoke. Because milk thistle has poor water solubility, it is not effective as a tea. A concentrated capsule or extract form is best.
Motherwort (Leonurus cardiaca)	Leaves, flowers, stems.	Phytochemicals: Alpha-pinene, benzaldehyde, caryophyllene, catechin, hyperoside, isoquercitrin, limonene, linalool, marrubiin, oleanolic acid, quercetin, quercitrin, rutin, saponin, stachydrine, tannin, ursolic acid. Nutrients: Vitamin C.	Traditionally used to relieve childbirth pain and as a tranquilizer. Helpful for menstrual disorders, menopausal symptoms, vaginitis, thyroid and rheumatic problems. Has a tonic effect on the heart. Useful for headache, insomnia, and vertigo.	*Caution:* Should not be used during pregnancy (until the onset of labor), as it can stimulate uterine contractions. Check with your health care provider before using it during the birthing process. Not recommended for persons with clotting disorders, high blood pressure, or heart disease.
Muira puama (Ptychopetalum olacoides)	Bark, roots.	Phytochemicals: Beta-sitosterol, campesterol, coumarin, lupeol.	Helps relieve pain, acts as a mild laxative and detoxifier, and supports the heart. Has a general tonic effect and balances sex hormones. Beneficial in treating nervous system disorders, impotence, depression, stress, rheumatism, hair loss, asthma, and menopausal and menstrual problems.	An alcohol-based extract is believed to be the best form of this rainforest herb, as the active constituents are neither water soluble nor broken down in the digestive process.
Mullein (Verbascum thapsus)	Leaves.	Phytochemicals: Beta-carotene, beta-sitosterol, coumarin, hesperidin, saponins. Nutrients: Calcium, iron, magnesium, manganese, phosphorus, potassium, selenium, zinc, vitamins B_1, B_2, B_3, and C.	Acts as a laxative, painkiller, and sleep aid. Taken internally, aids in getting rid of warts. Clears congestion. Useful for asthma, bronchitis, difficulty breathing, earache, hay fever, and swollen glands. Used in kidney formulas to soothe inflammation.	
Mustard (Brassica nigra)	Seeds.	Phytochemicals: Allyl isothiocyanate, caffeic acid, chlorogenic acid, ferulic acid, p-coumaric acid, protocatechuic acid, sinapic acid, vanillic acid.	Improves digestion and aids in the metabolism of fat. Applied externally, helpful for chest congestion, inflammation, injuries, and joint pain.	*Caution:* Can be irritating when applied directly to the skin. Not recommended for use on children under the age of six.

Herb (Scientific Name)	Part(s) Used	Phytochemical and Nutrient Content	Actions and Uses	Comments
Myrrh (*Commiphora myrrha*)	Resin from stems.	Phytochemicals: Acetic acid, beta-sitosterol, campesterol, cinnamaldehyde, cuminaldehyde, dipentene, eugenol, limonene, m-cresol.	Acts as an antiseptic, disinfectant, expectorant, and deodorizer. Stimulates the immune system and gastric secretions. Tones and stimulates mucous tissue. Helps to fight harmful bacteria in the mouth. Good for bad breath, periodontal disease, skin disorders, asthma, bronchitis, colds, flu, sinusitis, sore throat, herpes simplex, and ulcers. Topically, useful for abscesses, boils, sores, and wounds.	Used in many perfumes and in incense for its aromatic properties. Guggul, the standardized extract of the Indian mukul myrrh tree, lowers both cholesterol and triglyceride levels.
Nettle (*Urtica dioica*)	Flowers, leaves, roots.	Phytochemicals: Acetic acid, beta-carotene, betaine, caffeic acid, ferulic acid, lecithin, lycopene, p-coumaric acid, scopoletin. Nutrients: Calcium, copper, essential fatty acids, folate, iron, magnesium, manganese, phosphorus, potassium, selenium, sulfur, zinc, vitamins B_1, B_2, B_3, B_5, C, and E.	Acts as a diuretic, expectorant, pain reliever, and tonic. Good for benign prostatic hyperplasia, anemia, arthritis, rheumatism, hay fever, and other allergic disorders, kidney problems, and malabsorption syndrome. Improves goiter, inflammatory conditions, and mucous conditions of the lungs. Used in hair care products, helps stimulate hair follicles and regulate scalp oil buildup.	Also called stinging nettle.
Oat straw (*Avena sativa*)	Whole plant.	Phytochemicals: Benzaldehyde, beta-carotene, beta-ionone, beta-sitosterol, betaine, caffeic acid, campesterol, caryophyllene, chlorophyll, ferulic acid, lignin, limonene, p-coumaric acid, quercetin, scopoletin, sinapic acid, stigmasterol, vanillic acid, vanillin. Nutrients: Calcium, folate, iron, magnesium, manganese, phosphorus, potassium, selenium, zinc, vitamins A, B_1, B_2, B_3, B_5, B_6, and E.	Acts as an antidepressant and restorative nerve tonic. Increases perspiration. Helps to ease insomnia. Good for bed-wetting, depression, stress, and skin disorders.	
Olive leaf (*Olea europaea*)	Extract from leaves.	Phytochemicals: Apigenin, beta-sitosterol glucoside, cinchonidine, esculetin, kaempferol, luteolin, mannitol, maslinic acid, oleanic acid, oleuropein, quercetin, rutin, tannins. Nutrients: Calcium.	Fights all types of bacteria, viruses, fungi, and parasites. Helps stave off colds and flu. May have antioxidant properties. Has shown potential for lowering high blood pressure. Good for virtually any infectious disease, as well as for chronic fatigue syndrome, diarrheal diseases, inflammatory arthritis, and psoriasis.	
Oregon grape (*Mahonia aquifolia*)	Roots.	Phytochemicals: Berberine, tannins.	Purifies the blood and cleanses the liver. Acts as a laxative. Good for many skin conditions, from acne to psoriasis.	Has actions similar to those of goldenseal and barberry.
Papaya (*Carica papaya*)	Fruit, leaves.	Phytochemicals: Benzaldehyde, beta-carotene, caryophyllene, linalool, lycopene, malic acid, methyl salicylate, myristic acid, papain, phytofluene, zeaxanthin. Nutrients: Calcium, iron, magnesium, manganese, phosphorus, potassium, zinc, vitamins B_1, B_2, B_3, B_5, and C.	Stimulates the appetite and aids digestion. Good for heartburn, indigestion, and inflammatory bowel disorders.	The leaves can be used to tenderize meat.

Herb (Scientific Name)	Part(s) Used	Phytochemical and Nutrient Content	Actions and Uses	Comments
Parsley (*Petroselinum crispum*)	Fruit, leaves, roots, stems.	Phytochemicals: Alpha-pinene, apigenin, apiole, benzaldehyde, bergapten, beta-carotene, caffeic acid, chlorogenic acid, geraniol, glycolic acid, kaempferol, limonene, linalool, lutein, myristic acid, myristicin, naringenin, p-coumaric acid, psoralen, quercetin, rosmarinic acid, rutin, xanthotoxin. Nutrients: Calcium, folate, iron, magnesium, manganese, phosphorus, potassium, selenium, zinc, vitamins A, B_1, B_2, B_3, B_5, C, and E.	Contains a substance that prevents the multiplication of tumor cells. Expels worms, relieves gas, stimulates normal activity of the digestive system, and freshens breath. Helps bladder, kidney, liver, lung, stomach, and thyroid function. Good for bed-wetting, fluid retention, gas, halitosis, high blood pressure, indigestion, kidney disease, obesity, and prostate disorders.	Contains more vitamin C than oranges by weight.
Passionflower (*Passiflora incarnata*)	Flowers, leaves, shoots, stems.	Phytochemicals: Apigenin, flavonoids, harmaline, kaempferol, luteolin, maltol, quercetin, rutin, scopoletin, stigmasterol, umbelliferone, vitexin. Nutrients: Amino acids, calcium.	Has a gentle sedative effect and helps lower blood pressure. Helpful for anxiety, hyperactivity, insomnia, neuritis, and stress-related disorders.	Also called maypop. *Caution:* Should not be used during pregnancy, as it may stimulate the uterus.
Pau d'arco (*Tabebuia heptaphylla*)	Inner bark.	Phytochemicals: Beta-carotene, beta-sitosterol, lapachol.	Fights bacterial and viral infection. Cleanses the blood. Good for candidiasis, smoker's cough, warts, and all types of infection. Helpful for AIDS symptoms, allergies, cancer, cardiovascular problems, inflammatory bowel disease, rheumatism, tumors, and ulcers. Another species, *Tabebuia avellanedae*, may help restore skin after exposure to fungi and yeasts.	Also called lapacho and taheebo and was first used by the ancient Paraguayans.
Peppermint (*Mentha piperita*)	Flowering tops, oil, leaves.	Phytochemicals: Acetic acid, alpha-carotene, alpha-pinene, azulene, beta-carotene, beta-ionone, betaine, caffeic acid, carvacrol, carvone, chlorogenic acid, coumarin, eugenol, hesperetin, limonene, linalool, luteolin, menthol, 1,8-cineole, p-coumaric acid, pectin, rosmarinic acid, rutin, tannin, thymol, vanillin. Nutrients: Calcium, choline, iron, magnesium, manganese, phosphorus, potassium, selenium, zinc, vitamins B_1, B_2, B_3, and E.	Increases stomach acidity, aiding digestion. Slightly anesthetizes mucous membranes and the gastrointestinal tract. Useful for chills, colic, diarrhea, headache, heart trouble, indigestion, irritable bowel syndrome, nausea, poor appetite, rheumatism, and spasms. Patients with irritable bowel syndrome who took peppermint had less abdominal pain, flatulence, and diarrhea.	*Caution:* May interfere with iron absorption. Should not be used by pregnant or nursing women. Do not ingest pure menthol or pure peppermint leaves.
Plantain (*Plantago major*)	Leaves.	Phytochemicals: Adenine, allantoin, aucubin, apigenin, benzoic acid, caffeic acid, chlorogenic acid, cinnamic acid, ferulic acid, fiber, luteolin, oleanolic acid, p-coumaric acid, salicylic acid, tannin, ursolic acid, vanillic acid. Nutrients: Potassium, vitamin A.	Acts as a diuretic and is soothing to the lungs and urinary tract. May slow the growth of tuberculosis bacteria. Has a healing, antibiotic, and styptic effect when used topically for sores and wounds. Useful for indigestion and heartburn. Applied in a poultice, good for bee stings and any kind of bite.	This is not the bananalike fruit. Young leaves are tasty and can be eaten in salads. *Caution:* Do not mistake plantain for foxglove (*Digitalis lanata*), which has a similar appearance.
Pleurisy root (*Asclepias tuberosa*)	Rhizome.	Phytochemicals: Alpha-amyrin, asclepiadin, beta-amyrin, isorhamnetin, kaempferol, lupeol, quercetin, rutin, viburnitol.	Reduces inflammation of the pleural membranes of the lungs, enhances secretion of healthy lung fluids, and stimulates the lymphatic system. Has antispasmodic properties. Induces sweating and aids expectoration. Beneficial for pleurisy, pneumonia, bronchitis, flu, and coughs.	Also called butterfly weed.

Herb (Scientific Name)	Part(s) Used	Phytochemical and Nutrient Content	Actions and Uses	Comments
Primrose (Oenothera biennis)	Seed oil.	Phytochemicals: Beta-sitosterol, caffeic acid, campesterol, ellagic acid, gallic acid, kaempferol, lignin, p-coumaric acid, phytosterols, quercetin, tannin. Nutrients: Amino acids, calcium, essential fatty acids, iron, magnesium, manganese, phosphorus, potassium, zinc, vitamin E.	Promotes cardiovascular health. Aids in weight loss and reduces high blood pressure. Acts as a natural estrogen promoter. Helpful in treating alcoholism, arthritis, hot flashes, menstrual problems such as cramps and heavy bleeding, multiple sclerosis, and skin disorders.	Also called evening primrose. *Caution:* Primrose *root* should not be used during pregnancy.
Pumpkin (Cucurbita pepo)	Flesh, seed.	Phytochemicals: Astragalin, beta-carotene, beta-sitosterol, caffeic acid, chlorogenin, cryptoxanthin, diosgenin, ferulic acid, gitogenin, kaempferol, lutein, mannitol, myristic acid, phytosterols, quercetin, ruscogenin, salicylic acid, zeaxanthin. Nutrients: Amino acids, calcium, essential fatty acids, iron, magnesium, manganese, phosphorus, potassium, selenium, zinc, vitamins A, C, and E.	Useful for prostate disorders and irritable bladder.	
Puncture vine (Tribulus terrestris)	Flowers, fruit, leaves, stems.	Phytochemicals: Astragalin, beta-sitosterol, campesterol, chlorogenin, diosgenin, gitogenin, kaempferol, quercetin, ruscogenin, rutin, stigmasterol. Nutrients: Amino acids, calcium, essential fatty acids, iron, phosphorus, potassium, vitamin C.	Improves sex drive. Eases menopausal symptoms. Stimulates production of and balances male and female hormones. Enhances the immune system. Helps build muscles and increase stamina and endurance. Has antifungal, antibacterial, and antiinflammatory actions. Useful as a general tonic and revitalizer for the liver, kidneys, and urinary tract.	Also called caltrop.
Pygeum (Pygeum africanum)	Bark.	Phytochemicals: Beta-sitosterol, oleanic acid, ursolic acid.	Reduces inflammation and congestion. Lowers levels of inflammatory compounds in the prostate. Effective in reducing prostate enlargement and symptoms associated with benign prostatic hyperplasia such as urinary hesitancy, weak urine flow, nighttime urination, and recurrent urinary infections.	Used clinically in Europe to treat benign prostatic hyperplasia. (BPH).
Red clover (Trifolium pratense)	Flowers.	Phytochemicals: Beta-carotene, beta-sitosterol, biochanin, caffeic acid, campesterol, chlorogenic acid, coumarin, coumestrol, daidzein, eugenol, formononetin, genistein, isorhamnetin, methyl salicylate, myricetin, p-coumaric acid, salicylic acid. Nutrients: Calcium, iron, magnesium, manganese, phosphorus, potassium, selenium, zinc, vitamins B_3, C, and E.	Fights infection, suppresses appetite, and purifies the blood. Has expectorant, antispasmodic, and relaxing effects. Relieves menopausal symptoms such as hot flashes. Good for bacterial infections, coughs, bronchitis, inflamed lungs, inflammatory bowel disorders, kidney problems, liver disease, skin disorders, and weakened immune system.	

Herb (Scientific Name)	Part(s) Used	Phytochemical and Nutrient Content	Actions and Uses	Comments
Red raspberry (*Rubus idaeus*)	Bark, leaves, roots.	Phytochemicals: Alpha-carotene, benzaldehyde, beta-carotene, beta-ionone, caffeic acid, ellagic acid, farnesol, ferulic acid, gallic acid, geraniol, lutein, tannin. Nutrients: Calcium, iron, magnesium, manganese, phosphorus, potassium, selenium, silicon, zinc, vitamins B_1, B_2, B_3, C, and E.	Reduces menstrual bleeding, relaxes uterine and intestinal spasms, and strengthens uterine walls. Promotes healthy nails, bones, teeth, and skin. Good for diarrhea and for female disorders such as morning sickness, hot flashes, and menstrual cramps. Also heals canker sores. Combined with peppermint, good for morning sickness.	
Rhubarb (*Rheum rhabarbarum*)	Roots, stalks.	Phytochemicals: Acetic acid, beta-carotene, caffeic acid, chrysophanol, emodin, epicatechin, ferulic acid, fumaric acid, gallic acid, isoquercitrin, lutein, p-coumaric acid, protocatechuic acid, rutin, sinapic acid, vanillic acid. Nutrients: Calcium, iron, magnesium, manganese, phosphorus, potassium, selenium, sulfur, zinc, vitamins B_1, B_2, B_3, B_5, C, and E.	Fights infection and eliminates worms. Enhances gallbladder function and promotes healing of duodenal ulcers. Good for constipation, malabsorption, and disorders of the colon, spleen, and liver.	*Caution:* Should not be used during pregnancy.
Rose (*Rosa canina*)	Fruit (hips).	Phytochemicals: Beta-carotene, betulin, catechin, epicatechin, flavonoids, isoquercitrin, lycopene, malic acid, pectin, tannin, vanillin, zeaxanthin. Nutrients: Calcium, iron, magnesium, manganese, phosphorus, potassium, selenium, zinc, vitamins B_1, B_2, B_3, C, and E.	Good for bladder problems and all infections. A good source of vitamin C when used fresh. Rose hip tea is good for diarrhea.	Many vitamins and other supplements are derived from rose hips.
Rosemary (*Rosmarinus officinalis*)	Leaves.	Phytochemicals: Alpha-pinene, apigenin, beta-carotene, beta-sitosterol, betulinic acid, borneol, caffeic acid, camphor, carnosol, carvacrol, carvone, caryophyllene, chlorogenic acid, diosmin, genkwanin, geraniol, hesperidin, limonene, linalool, luteolin, oleanolic acid, 1,8-cineole, phytosterols, rosmanol, rosmarinic acid, salicylates, squalene, tannin, thymol, ursolic acid. Nutrients: Calcium, iron, magnesium, manganese, phosphorus, potassium, zinc, vitamins B_1, B_0, and C.	Fights free radicals, inflammation (COX-2 enzyme), bacteria, and fungi. Relaxes the stomach, stimulates circulation and digestion, and acts as an astringent and decongestant. Improves circulation to the brain. Also helps detoxify the liver, and has anticancer and antitumor properties. Good for headaches, high and low blood pressure, circulatory problems, and menstrual cramps. Can be used as an antiseptic gargle. Rosemary oil impedes the growth of food-borne bacteria and fungi, and someday may be used to prolong the shelf life of foods.	Makes a good food preservative. *Caution:* Should not be used during pregnancy.

Herb (Scientific Name)	Part(s) Used	Phytochemical and Nutrient Content	Actions and Uses	Comments
Sage (*Salvia officinalis*)	Leaves.	Phytochemicals: Alpha-amyrin, alpha-pinene, alpha-terpineol, apigenin, beta-carotene, beta-sitosterol, betulin, borneol, caffeic acid, campesterol, camphene, camphor, carnosolic acid, caryophyllene, catechin, chlorogenic acid, citral, farnesol, ferulic acid, gallic acid, genkwanin, geraniol, hispidulin, limonene, linalool, luteolin, maslinic acid, oleanolic acid, 1,8-cineole, p-coumaric acid, pinene, rosmarinic acid, saponin, stigmasterol, tannins, terpineol, thymol, ursolic acid, vanillic acid. Nutrients: Boron, calcium, iron, magnesium, manganese, phosphorus, potassium, selenium, zinc, vitamins B_1, B_2, B_3, B_5, and C.	Stimulates the central nervous system and digestive tract, and has estrogenic effects on the body. Reduces sweating and salivation. Good for hot flashes and other symptoms of estrogen deficiency, whether in menopause or following hysterectomy. Beneficial for disorders affecting the mouth and throat, such as tonsillitis. In tea form, can be used as a hair rinse to promote shine (especially for dark hair) and hair growth. Also used to dry up milk when women wish to stop nursing.	*Caution:* Interferes with the absorption of iron and other minerals when taken internally, and decreases milk supply in nursing mothers. Should not be taken by individuals with seizure disorders or high blood pressure. Should not be taken during pregnancy or while nursing.
St. John's wort (*Hypericum perforatum*)	Flowers, leaves, stems, oil.	Phytochemicals: Carotenoids, caryophyllene, chlorophyll, flavonoids, hyperoside, isoquercitrin, limonene, lutein, mannitol, myristic acid, phenol, phloroglucinol, phytosterols, quercetin, quercitrin, rutin, saponin, tannins. Nutrients: Vitamin C.	Good for depression and nerve pain. It has been shown to help patients with mild depression get over an acute episode and recover. Helps control stress. In laboratory studies, protects bone marrow and intestinal mucosa from x-ray damage. Applied topically, the oil aids wound healing. It has not been shown to be effective for children with ADHD (attention-deficit/hyperactivity disorder).	*Caution:* May increase sensitivity to sunlight. It may also produce anxiety, gastrointestinal symptoms, and headaches. It can interact with some drugs including antidepressants, birth control pills, and anticoagulants.
Sangre de grado (*Croton lechleri*)	Bark, resin.	Phytochemicals: Alpha-pinene, betaine, beta-pinene, borneol, camphene, dipentene, eugenol, gamma-terpinene, lignin, linalool, myrcene, p-cymene, tannins, taspine, vanillin.	Fights free radicals, inflammation, and bacterial, viral, and fungal infection. Helps heal wounds and stop bleeding. Good for respiratory and skin disorders, mouth and skin ulcers, sore throat, colds and flu, candida, psoriasis, herpes, and vaginitis.	A rainforest herb whose name means "dragon's blood."
Sarsaparilla (*Smilax species*)	Roots, rhizomes.	Phytochemicals: Beta-sitosterol, saponin, stigmasterol. Nutrients: Iron, magnesium, manganese, phosphorus, potassium, selenium, zinc.	Promotes excretion of fluids, increases energy, protects against harm from radiation exposure, and regulates hormones. Useful for female sexual dysfunction, hives, impotence, infertility, nervous system disorders, premenstrual syndrome, psoriasis, rheumatoid arthritis, and disorders caused by blood impurities.	Also called Chinese root, small spikenard.
Saw palmetto (*Serenoa repens*)	Berries, seeds.	Phytochemicals: Beta-carotene, beta-sitosterol, ferulic acid, mannitol, myristic acid, tannins, vanillic acid, vanillin.	Acts as a diuretic, urinary antiseptic, and appetite stimulant. Inhibits production of dihydrotestosterone, a form of testosterone that contributes to enlargement of the prostate. Shown to improve lower urinary tract symptoms in men with benign prostatic hyperplasia. May also enhance sexual functioning and sexual desire.	Used clinically in Europe to treat benign prostatic hyperplasia (BPH). Can be combined with nettle root.

Herb (Scientific Name)	Part(s) Used	Phytochemical and Nutrient Content	Actions and Uses	Comments
Skullcap (*Scutellaria laterfolia*)	Leaves, shoots.	Phytochemicals: Beta-carotene, lignin, tannins. Nutrients: Calcium, iron, magnesium, manganese, phosphorus, potassium, selenium, zinc, vitamins B_1, B_2, B_3, and C.	Aids sleep, improves circulation, and strengthens the heart muscle. Relieves muscle cramps, pain, spasms, and stress. Good for anxiety, fatigue, cardiovascular disease, headache, hyperactivity, nervous disorders, and rheumatism. Useful in treating barbiturate addiction and drug withdrawal.	*Caution:* Should not be given to children under six.
Slippery elm (*Ulmus rubra*)	Inner bark.	Phytochemicals: Beta-carotene, campesterol, mucilage, starch, tannin. Nutrients: Calcium, iron, magnesium, manganese, phosphorus, potassium, selenium, zinc, vitamins B_1, B_2, B_3, and C.	Soothes inflamed mucous membranes of the bowels, stomach, and urinary tract. Good for diarrhea and ulcers and for treatment of colds, flu, and sore throat. Beneficial for Crohn's disease, ulcerative colitis, diverticulosis, diverticulitis, and gastritis.	Also called moose elm, red elm.
Squawvine (*Mitchella repens*)	Leaves, stems.	Phytochemicals: Alkaloids, glycosides, mucilage, saponins, tannins.	Relieves pelvic congestion and soothes the nervous system. Good for menstrual cramps.	Also called partridgeberry.
Stone root (*Collinsonia canadensis*)	Whole plant, fresh root.	Phytochemicals: Alpha-pinene, caffeic acid, caryophyllene, limonene. Nutrients: Magnesium.	Acts as a diuretic, sedative, antispasmodic, astringent, and tonic. Good for the urinary tract. Breaks up mucus. Helpful for bronchitis, headache, cramps, indigestion, and hemorrhoids.	Also known as heal-all, horse balm, knob root, and rich weed.
Suma (*Pfaffia paniculata*)	Bark, berries, leaves, roots.	Phytochemicals: Beta-sitosterol, saponin, stigmasterol. Nutrients: Iron, magnesium, zinc, vitamins A, B_1, B_2, B_5, E, and K.	Fights inflammation, boosts the immune system, and combats anemia, fatigue, and stress. Good for, arthritis, cancer, liver disease, menopausal symptoms, high blood pressure, Epstein-Barr virus, and weakened immune system.	Also known as Brazilian ginseng.
Tea tree (*Melaleuca alternifolia*)	Essential oil.	Phytochemicals: Alpha-pinene, alpha-terpineol, aromadendrene, beta-pinene, camphor, caryophyllene, limonene, linalool, 1,8-cineole, p-cymene, terpinenes, terpinolene.	Used topically, disinfects wounds and heals virtually all skin conditions, including acne, athlete's foot, boils, cuts and scrapes, earache, fungal infections, hair and scalp problems, herpes outbreaks, insect and spider bites, scabies, and warts. Added to water, can be used as a douche for vaginitis and a gargle for colds, sore throats, and mouth sores (do not swallow it, however).	*Caution:* Should not be taken internally; can be toxic. If irritation occurs, discontinue use or dilute with distilled water, vegetable oil, primrose oil, or vitamin E oil. If irritation persists after dilution, discontinue use.

Herb (Scientific Name)	Part(s) Used	Phytochemical and Nutrient Content	Actions and Uses	Comments
Thyme (*Thymus vulgaris*)	Berries, flowers, leaves.	Phytochemicals: Alpha-pinene, apigenin, beta-carotene, borneol, caffeic acid, camphor, caprylic acid, carvacrol, carvone, chlorogenic acid, cinnamic acid, citral, eugenol, ferulic acid, gallic acid, geraniol, kaempferol, lauric acid, limonene, linalool, luteolin, myristic acid, naringenin, oleanolic acid, p-coumaric acid, p-cymene, phytosterols, rosmarinic acid, salicylates, tannin, thymol, ursolic acid, vanillic acid. Nutrients: Amino acids, calcium, essential fatty acids, iron, magnesium, manganese, phosphorus, potassium, selenium, zinc, vitamins B_1, B_2, B_3, and C.	Eliminates gas and reduces fever, headache, and mucus. Has strong antiseptic properties. Lowers cholesterol levels. Good for asthma, bronchitis, croup and other respiratory problems, and for fever, headache, and liver disease. Eliminates scalp itching and flaking.	
Turmeric (*Curcuma longa*)	Rhizomes.	Phytochemicals: Alpha-pinene, alpha-terpineol, azulene, beta-carotene, borneol, caffeic acid, caryophyllene, cinnamic acid, curcumin, eugenol, guaiacol, limonene, linalool, 1,8-cineole, p-coumaric acid, p-cymene, turmerone, vanillic acid. Nutrients: Calcium, iron, manganese, phosphorus, potassium, zinc, vitamins B_1, B_2, B_3, and C.	Curcumin, the yellow pigment in turmeric, is the active ingredient. Fights free radicals, protects the liver against toxins, inhibits platelet aggregation, aids circulation, lowers cholesterol levels, and improves blood vessel health. Has antibiotic, anticancer, and anti-inflammatory (COX-2 enzyme) properties. Good for all arthritic conditions. Curcumin has been shown to stop the proliferation of rapidly dividing cancer cells. Under investigation for treating pancreatic and other cancers, psoriasis, and Alzheimer's disease.	Used as a seasoning and the main ingredient in curry powder. Has inhibited the spread of HIV in laboratory tests. *Caution:* Extended use can result in stomach distress. Not recommended for persons with biliary tract obstruction, as curcumin stimulates bile secretion.
Uva ursi (*Arctostaphylos uva-ursi*)	Leaves.	Phytochemicals: Arbutin, beta-carotene, beta-sitosterol, ellagic acid, gallic acid, hyperin, isoquercitrin, myricetin, oleanolic acid, quercetin, quercitrin, ursolic acid. Nutrients: Calcium, iron, magnesium, manganese, phosphorus, potassium, selenium, zinc, vitamins B_1, B_2, B_3, and C.	Promotes excretion of fluids, fights bacteria, and strengthens heart muscle. Good for disorders of the spleen, liver, pancreas, and small intestine. Useful for bladder and kidney infections, diabetes, and prostate disorders.	Also called bearberry. *Caution:* Not recommended for women who are pregnant or nursing, or for children under twelve.
Valerian (*Valeriana officinalis*)	Rhizomes, roots.	Phytochemicals: Azulene, beta-carotene, beta-ionone, beta-sitosterol, borneol, bornyl acetate, caffeic acid, caryophyllene, chlorogenic acid, isovaleric acid, kaempferol, limonene, p-coumaric acid, quercetin, valepotriates, valerenic acid, valerenone, valeric acid. Nutrients: Calcium, choline, essential fatty acids, iron, magnesium, manganese, phosphorus, potassium, selenium, zinc, vitamins B_1, B_2, B_3, and C.	Acts as a sedative, improves circulation, and reduces mucus from colds. Good for anxiety, fatigue, high blood pressure, insomnia, irritable bowel syndrome, menstrual and muscle cramps, nervousness, pain, spasms, stress, and ulcers. Shown to promote better sleep quality and longer sleeping periods, and reduce the number of times people get up at night. Combining valerian with hops can also promote a better quality of sleep and induce deeper sleep.	A water-soluble extract form is best. *Caution:* Should not be combined with alcohol.

Herb (Scientific Name)	Part(s) Used	Phytochemical and Nutrient Content	Actions and Uses	Comments
Vervain (Verbena officinalis)	Flowers, leaves, shoots, stems.	Phytochemicals: Adenosine, aucubin, beta-carotene, caffeic acid, citral, tannin, ursolic acid, verbenalin, verbenin.	Strengthens the nervous system. Promotes liver and gallbladder health. Reduces tension and stress. Induces sweating. Promotes menstruation and increases mother's milk. Useful for mild depression, insomnia, headache, toothache, wounds, colds, and fever.	Caution: Should not be used during pregnancy, as it stimulates uterine contractions.
White oak (Quercus alba)	Bark.	Phytochemicals: Beta-carotene, beta-sitosterol, catechin, gallic acid, pectin, quercetin, quercitrin, tannin. Nutrients: Calcium, iron, magnesium, manganese, phosphorus, potassium, selenium, zinc, vitamins B$_1$, B$_2$, B$_3$, and C.	Acts as an antiseptic. Good for skin wounds, bee stings, burns, diarrhea, fevers and cold, bronchitis, nosebleed, poison ivy, and varicose veins. Also good for the teeth. Can be used in enemas and douches.	
White willow (Salix alba)	Bark.	Phytochemicals: Apigenin, beta-carotene, catechin, isoquercitrin, lignin, p-coumaric acid, quercetin, rutin, salicin, salicylic acid, tannin. Nutrients: Calcium, iron, magnesium, manganese, phosphorus, potassium, selenium, zinc, vitamins B$_1$, B$_2$, B$_3$, and C.	Relieves pain. Good for allergies, headache, backache, nerve pain, joint pain, inflammation, menstrual cramps, toothache, and injuries. For backache, use of white willow allowed for a reduction in the use of medications such as for pain.	Contains compounds from which aspirin was derived. Caution: Not recommended for use during pregnancy. May interfere with absorption of iron and other minerals when taken internally. Should not be used by people who are allergic to aspirin.
Wild cherry (Prunus serotina)	Inner bark, root bark.	Phytochemicals: Benzaldehyde, caffeic acid, kaempferol, p-coumaric acid, quercetin, scopoletin, tannin, ursolic acid. Nutrients: Calcium, iron, magnesium, phosphorus, potassium, zinc.	Acts as an expectorant and mild sedative. Good for coughs, colds, bronchitis, asthma, digestive disorders, and diarrhea.	Also called chokecherry, wild black cherry, Virginia prune. Caution: Wild cherry bark should not be used during pregnancy. Also, the leaves, bark, and fruit pits contain hydrocyanic acid, which can be poisonous. A commercially prepared syrup or tincture is best.
Wild oregano (Origanum vulgare)	Leaves, shoots, stems.	Phytochemicals: Alpha-pinene, apigenin, beta-carotene, borneol, caffeic acid, camphor, capric acid, carvacrol, caryophyllene, catechol, chlorogenic acid, cinnamic acid, eriodictyol, eugenol, geraniol, kaempferol, limonene, linalool, luteolin, myristic acid, naringenin, naringin, oleanolic acid, 1,8-cineole, p-coumaric acid, phytosterols, quercetin, rosmarinic acid, rutin, tannins, thymol, ursolic acid, vanillic acid, vitexin. Nutrients: Calcium, essential fatty acids, iron, magnesium, manganese, phosphorus, potassium, zinc, vitamins A, B$_1$, B$_3$, and C.	Fights free radicals, inflammation, and bacterial, viral, and fungal infection. Boosts the immune system. Useful for acne, allergies, animal bites, arthritis, asthma, athlete's foot, bee stings, bronchitis, chronic infections, cold, cough, diarrhea, digestive problems, earache, eczema, fatigue, gum disease, headache, menstrual irregularities, muscle pain, parasitic infections, psoriasis, sinusitis, skin infections, urinary tract disorders, and wounds.	Oregano sold in supermarkets is usually a combination of several oregano species, and does not have the medicinal benefits of Origanum vulgare.

Herb (Scientific Name)	Part(s) Used	Phytochemical and Nutrient Content	Actions and Uses	Comments
Wild yam (*Dioscorea villosa*)	Rhizomes, roots.	Phytochemicals: Beta-carotene, diosgenin. Nutrients: Calcium, chromium, iron, magnesium, manganese, phosphorus, potassium, selenium, zinc, vitamins B_1, B_2, B_3, and C.	Relaxes muscle spasms, reduces inflammation, and promotes perspiration. Contains compounds similar to the hormone progesterone. Good for colic, gallbladder disorders, hypoglycemia, irritable bowel syndrome, kidney stones, neuralgia, rheumatism, and female disorders, including premenstrual syndrome and menopause-related symptoms. In one study, postmenopausal women who consumed yam experienced an improvement in the levels of sex hormones, blood lipids, and antioxidants.	Many yam-based products are extracted from plants treated with fertilizers and pesticides, which may end up in the final products. The selection, cleansing, and processing of the raw materials is very important. *Caution:* Should not be used during pregnancy and lactation. For use in children, check with your pediatrician.
Wintergreen (*Gaultheria procumbens*)	Leaves, roots, stems.	Phytochemicals: Caffeic acid, ferulic acid, gallic acid, p-coumaric acid, methyl salicylate, tannin, vanillic acid.	Relieves pain and reduces inflammation. Stimulates circulation. Good for arthritis, headache, toothache, muscle pain, and rheumatic complaints.	Oil distilled from the leaves is used in perfumes and as a flavoring. Contains a compound composed of 90 percent methyl salicylate, a substance similar to aspirin.
Witch hazel (*Hamamelis virginiana*)	Bark, leaves, twigs.	Phytochemials: Beta-ionone, gallic acid, isoquercitrin, kaempferol, leucodelphinidin, myrcetin, phenol, quercetin, quercetrin, saponins, tannins.	Applied topically, has astringent and healing properties, and relieves itching. Good for hemorrhoids, mouth and skin inflammation, and phlebitis. Very useful in skin care.	
Wood betony (*Stachys officinalis*)	Leaves.	Phytochemicals: Betaine, caffeic acid, chlorogenic acid, rosmarinic acid, stachydrine, tannin. Nutrients: Choline, magnesium, manganese, phosphorus.	Stimulates the heart and relaxes muscles. Improves digestion and appreciation of food. Good for cardiovascular disorders, hyperactivity, nerve pain, headaches, and anxiety attacks.	Also called betony. *Caution:* Should not be used during pregnancy.
Wormwood (*Artemisia absinthium*)	Leaves, tops.	Phytochemicals: Beta-carotene, chamazulene, chlorogenic acid, isoquercitrin, p-coumaric acid, rutin, salicylic acid, tannins, vanillic acid. Nutrients: Vitamin C.	Acts as a mild sedative, eliminates worms, increases stomach acidity, and lowers fever. Useful for loss of appetite and for liver, gallbladder, gastric, and vascular disorders, including migraines. Applied topically, good for healing wounds, skin ulcers and blemishes, and insect bites.	Ingredient of absinthe liquor, banned in many countries. Often used with black walnut for removal of parasites. *Caution:* Do not use in high doses or for extended periods because it contains the chemical component thujune that can be poisonous. Should not be used by those who suffer from any type of seizure disorder, or who are pregnant or nursing.

Herb (Scientific Name)	Part(s) Used	Phytochemical and Nutrient Content	Actions and Uses	Comments
Yellow dock (*Rumex crispus*)	Roots.	Phytochemicals: Beta-carotene, hyperoside, quercetin, quercitrin, rutin, tannin. Nutrients: Calcium, iron, magnesium, manganese, phosphorus, potassium, selenium, zinc, vitamins B_1, B_2, B_3, and C.	Acts as a blood purifier and cleanser, and as a general tonic. Improves colon and liver function. Good for inflammation of the nasal passages and respiratory tract, anemia, liver disease, and skin disorders such as eczema, hives, psoriasis, and rashes. Combined with sarsaparilla, makes a tea for chronic skin disorders.	Also called curled dock. *Caution:* Yellow dock leaves should not be consumed in soups or salads. They are high in oxalates and may cause oxalic acid poisoning.
Yerba maté (*Ilex paraguariensis*)	Leaves.	Phytochemicals: Caffeine, chlorogenic acid, chlorophyll, rutin, tannin, theobromine, theophylline, ursolic acid, vanillin. Nutrients: Choline, inositol, nicotinic acid, pyridoxine, trace minerals, vitamins B_3, B_5, B_6, C, and E.	Fights free radicals, cleanses the blood, and suppresses appetite. Fights aging, stimulates the mind, stimulates the production of cortisone, and tones the nervous system. Enhances the healing powers of other herbs. When combined with guarana, it was useful at slowing the rate that food left the stomach, thereby promoting a longer sense of fullness. This led to a signficant weight loss compared to a control group. Useful for allergies, constipation, and inflammatory bowel disorders.	Also called maté, Paraguay tea, South American holly. *Caution:* Should not be used by people who suffer from insomnia.
Yohimbe (*Pausinystalia yohimbe*)	Bark.	Phytochemicals: Ajmaline, corynantheine, corynanthine, tannin, yohimbine.	Increases libido and blood flow to erectile tissue. May increase testosterone levels.	Yohimbine, a key component of this herb, is sold as a prescription medication. Available in a wide variety of bodybuilding and sexual aid supplements. *Caution:* Yohimbe should not be used by women who are pregnant or nursing. Do not use yohimbe if you have high blood pressure, heart disease, stomach ulcers, depression, or other psychiatric conditions. There have been cases of people dying from taking too much yohimbe.
Yucca (*Yucca baccata*)	Roots.	Phytochemicals: Beta-carotene, sarsapogenin, tannin. Nutrients: Calcium, iron, magnesium, manganese, phosphorus, potassium, selenium, zinc, vitamins B_1, B_2, B_3, and C.	Purifies the blood. Beneficial in treating arthritis, osteoporosis, and inflammatory disorders.	Routinely prescribed for arthritis in some clinics. Can be cut up, added to water (1 cup of yucca in 2 cups of water), and used as a soap or shampoo substitute. Can be added to shampoo also.

Medicinal Herbs by Actions and Targets in the Body

Different medicinal herbs have different types of effects and tend to exert their activities on different body systems and organs. The following table classifies some of the best-known herbs according to their actions and areas of prime activity.

Action(s)	Herbs
Antibacterial/antiviral	Aloe, anise, annatto, astragalus, black walnut, boneset, boswellia, burdock, catnip, cat's claw, cayenne, cedar, chanca piedra, chickweed, echinacea, elder, eucalyptus, garlic, goldenseal, jaborandi, jatoba, kudzu, lady's mantle, lemongrass, licorice, macela, meadowsweet, myrrh, olive leaf, pau d'arco, pleurisy root, puncture vine, red clover, rose, rosemary, sangre de grado, slippery elm, suma, tea tree, turmeric, uva ursi, valerian, white oak, wild oregano.
Anticancer/antitumor	Astragalus, birch, burdock, cat's claw, chuchuhuasi, cranberry, dandelion, fennel, garlic, green tea, licorice, macela, milk thistle, parsley, pau d'arco, rosemary, suma, turmeric.
Antifungal	Acerola, alfalfa, aloe, black walnut, boswellia, burdock, cedar, cinnamon, jatoba, puncture vine, rosemary, sangre de grado, tea tree, wild oregano.
Anti-inflammatory	Alfalfa, aloe, annatto, ashwagandha, bilberry, birch, blessed thistle, boldo, boneset, boswellia, buchu, butcher's broom, calendula, catnip, cat's claw, chamomile, chanca piedra, chuchuhuasi, devil's claw, echinacea, elder, fenugreek, feverfew, flax, ginger, goldenseal, jaborandi, jatoba, juniper, lady's mantle, licorice, macela, meadowsweet, mullein, mustard, pleurisy root, puncture vine, pygeum, rosemary, sangre de grado, suma, turmeric, white willow, wild oregano, wild yam, wintergreen, witch hazel, yellow dock.
Antioxidant	Acerola, annatto, bilberry, burdock, cat's claw, celery, elder, ginger, ginkgo, green tea, jatoba, milk thistle, olive leaf, rosemary, sangre de grado, turmeric, wild oregano, yerba maté.
Cleanser/detoxifier	Alfalfa, black walnut, blessed thistle, cascara sagrada, cat's claw, cedar, dandelion, elder, garlic, ginger, goldenseal, guarana, licorice, muira puama, Oregon grape, pau d'arco, rosemary, yellow dock, yerba maté.
Bones/joints	Alfalfa, black cohosh, boswellia, cat's claw, cayenne, celery, chuchuhuasi, dandelion, devil's claw, feverfew, flax, garlic, ginger, jatoba, muira puama, nettle, olive leaf, pau d'arco, peppermint, primrose, red raspberry, St. John's wort, sarsaparilla, skullcap, suma, wild oregano, wild yam, wintergreen, yucca.
Brain/nervous system	Ashwagandha, astragalus, bayberry, bilberry, blessed thistle, blue cohosh, catnip, celery, chamomile, chaste tree, devil's claw, dong quai, eyebright, fennel, fenugreek, feverfew, ginger, ginseng, goldenseal, gotu kola, guarana, hops, jaborandi, kava kava, kudzu, lavender, lemongrass, licorice, marshmallow, motherwort, muira puama, oat straw, passionflower, peppermint, plantain, rosemary, sage, St. John's wort, sarsaparilla, skullcap, squawvine, stone root, suma, thyme, valerian, vervain, white willow, wild cherry, wild oregano, wintergreen, wood betony, wormwood, yerba maté.
Circulatory/cardiovascular systems	Aloe, barberry, bayberry, bilberry, black cohosh, black walnut, blessed thistle, borage, boswellia, butcher's broom, cayenne, celery, chickweed, cinnamon, devil's claw, elder, garlic, gentian, ginger, ginkgo, ginseng, gotu kola, green tea, hawthorn, hops, horse chestnut, hyssop, jaborandi, kudzu, licorice, motherwort, muira puama, olive leaf, parsley, passionflower, pau d'arco, peppermint, primrose, rosemary, skullcap, suma, uva ursi, valerian, white oak, wintergreen, wood betony.
Gastrointestinal/digestive systems	Acerola, alfalfa, aloe, anise, annatto, bilberry, black walnut, blessed thistle, boldo, boswellia, buchu, burdock, cascara sagrada, catnip, cayenne, chamomile, chanca piedra, chuchuhuasi, cinnamon, clove, dandelion, devil's claw, fennel, fenugreek, flax, garlic, gentian, ginger, ginseng, goldenseal, gotu kola, green tea, guarana, horehound, jaborandi, juniper, kava kava, kudzu, lady's mantle, lemongrass, licorice, macela, marshmallow, meadowsweet, muira puama, mustard, olive leaf, Oregon grape, papaya, parsley, pau d'arco, peppermint, plantain, puncture vine, red clover, red raspberry, rosemary, sage, slippery elm, stone root, suma, thyme, turmeric, uva ursi, valerian, vervain, white oak, wild cherry, wild oregano, wood betony, wormwood, yellow dock, yerba maté.
Hair/nails/teeth	Borage, burdock, clove, hops, Irish moss, lemongrass, muira puama, nettle, red raspberry, sage, tea tree, vervain, white willow, wintergreen.
Immune system	Ashwagandha, astragalus, bayberry, burdock, cat's claw, cedar, chuchuhuasi, devil's claw, echinacea, eyebright, elder, garlic, ginseng, goldenseal, green tea, horehound, licorice, maca, macela, milk thistle, myrrh, pau d'arco, puncture vine, red clover, suma, white willow, wild oregano, yerba maté.

Muscles	Blue cohosh, celery, chanca piedra, chuchuhuasi, eucalyptus, feverfew, ginger, hawthorn, horse chestnut, kava kava, lady's mantle, licorice, macela, meadowsweet, puncture vine, skullcap, uva ursi, valerian, wild oregano, wild yam, wintergreen, wood betony.
Reproductive system	*Menopause:* Chaste tree, dandelion, devil's claw, kava kava, licorice, motherwort, puncture vine, sage, suma, wild yam.
	Menstruation: Black cohosh, blue cohosh, calendula, chamomile, chaste tree, chuchuhuasi, corn silk, crampbark, dong quai, false unicorn root, feverfew, licorice, maca, macela, motherwort, muira puama, primrose, red raspberry, rosemary, sarsaparilla, squawvine, valerian, white willow, wild oregano, wild yam.
	Prostate: Buchu, goldenseal, gravel root, hydrangea, juniper, licorice, milk thistle, parsley, pumpkin, pygeum, saw palmetto, uva ursi.
	Sexual function/hormones: Alfalfa, ashwagandha, chaste tree, chuchuhuasi, damiana, dong quai, false unicorn root, gotu kola, muira puama, puncture vine, sarsaparilla, saw palmetto, yohimbe (not recommended).
Respiratory tract	Anise, astragalus, boneset, boswellia, catnip, cayenne, chanca piedra, chuchuhuasi, chickweed, elder, eucalyptus, fennel, fenugreek, feverfew, garlic, ginkgo, ginseng, goldenseal, green tea, horehound, Irish moss, jaborandi, jatoba, juniper, licorice, macela, muira puama, mullein, mustard, myrrh, nettle, parsley, plantain, pleurisy root, red clover, stone root, thyme, white oak, wild cherry, wild oregano, yellow dock.
Skin	Acerola, alfalfa, aloe, annatto, barberry, borage, boswellia, calendula, chickweed, chuchuhuasi, comfrey, cranberry, elder, flax, green tea, Irish moss, lavender, lemongrass, marshmallow, milk thistle, myrrh, oat straw, olive leaf, Oregon grape, primrose, red clover, red raspberry, sangre de grado, sarsaparilla, tea tree, white oak, wild oregano, witch hazel, wormwood, yellow dock.
Urinary tract	Annatto, bilberry, birch, buchu, butcher's broom, cayenne, cedar, celery, chanca piedra, corn silk, cranberry, dandelion, devil's claw, fennel, ginkgo, goldenseal, gotu kola, gravel root, guarana, hydrangea, jatoba, juniper, kava kava, marshmallow, milk thistle, mullein, nettle, parsley, plantain, puncture vine, pumpkin, rose, red clover, saw palmetto, slippery elm, stone root, uva ursi, wild oregano, wild yam.

Drug Interactions

INTRODUCTION

Mixing two or more drugs together in the body can sometimes create havoc, and instead of a health benefit the patient suffers a setback. Worse, you may be confronted with a health crisis. Most people think these unintended effects apply only to prescription drugs. However, dietary supplements and even the food we eat can interact with each other, or with over-the-counter (OTC) or prescription drugs, to cause problems. Herbs and vitamins, while not drugs in the strictest sense, are still complex organic chemicals that react with each other and with other chemicals in the body. This is, of course, how they work.

Types of drug interactions that you need to be concerned with can basically be summarized as follows:

- *Drugs interacting with drugs.* Both prescription and over-the-counter medications are included in this category. For instance, taking OTC antacids during a course of the antibiotic ciprofloxacin (Cipro) lowers the effectiveness of the antibiotic. If you take birth control pills, you should know that the antibiotic rifampin could lower their effectiveness. Miconazole (the active ingredient in Monistat and other products), an OTC drug for yeast infections, should not be used with warfarin (Coumadin) or bleeding and bruising could occur. Sildenafil (Viagra) should not be mixed with nitrates (such as nitroglycerin) used to treat heart disease, and certain antidepressants can interfere with blood pressure medicine.

- *Drugs interacting with dietary supplements.* There are many documented cases of herbs and vitamins interacting with prescription and OTC drugs. It was recently discovered that St. John's wort can interfere with the action of irinotecan, a standard chemotherapy drug. St. John's wort also acts with the blood-thinner warfarin and the heart medicine digitalis (Digoxin, Lanoxin), making them less effective. St. John's wort also lowers levels of theophylline, an asthma drug. Taking large doses of vitamin K can nullify the action of any blood-thinning medication a person might be taking. The list goes on and on. The five most common natural products with potential interaction are garlic, valerian, kava, ginkgo, and St. John's wort, according to a study at the Mayo Clinic. Children and adults can experience problems with dietary supplements. In one study, which tracked the adverse drug reaction (ADR) calls to the California Poison Control System, 28 percent were for children.

The most common products involved with ADRs were zinc, echinacea, chromium picolinate, and witch hazel. As of 2009, all dietary supplement labels include a company name to report any adverse events. This information is logged by the company and shared with the FDA if the problem is serious.

- *Drugs interacting with food and beverages.* Taking ciprofloxacin with coffee, chocolate, or even a cola drink that contains caffeine may cause excess nervousness or manic behavior. If foods containing tyramine, such as cheese or soy sauce, are mixed with some MAO inhibitors (a class of medication most often prescribed for mood disorders), there can be a fatal increase in blood pressure. Do not drink grapefruit juice along with blood pressure medications or cyclosporine (a transplant drug); doing this may increase the effect of these drugs. It was discovered in 1991 that grapefruit juice has the ability to inhibit an enzyme that metabolizes many drugs, thus allowing levels of the drugs to build up in the body. Older adults may have a special susceptibility to this reaction.

The U.S. Food and Drug Administration (FDA) has been trying to understand more about drug interactions, particularly in the past fifteen years or so, and has been developing laboratory testing programs to reveal possible problems early in the game. Because clinical trials with humans are generally based on small numbers of people, the safety profile of a proposed drug is not close to complete until the drug actually gets to market and a larger number of people get to try it under real-life conditions. A problem that is relatively rare in nature might not become apparent until several hundred thousand people have taken the drug. While there is a lot of emotion attached to this issue, it is simply impossible to predict beforehand every possible drug reaction and interaction. If people demand that kind of perfection, they have unrealistic expectations. Development costs, already unreasonably high, would certainly skyrocket, and development of new drugs that would benefit millions might be delayed indefinitely or even curtailed.

WHY ARE THERE DRUG INTERACTIONS?

In recent years, researchers have learned that there is a class of enzymes, called the CYP family of enzymes, that plays an essential role in the metabolism and detoxification of drugs. These enzymes act primarily in the liver, but also in the intestinal tract and other areas. For instance, there is a single enzyme (of the five known CYP enzymes) that plays a key role in metabolizing over half the drugs prescribed today. It is called CYP3A4 (or cytochrome P450). So, any substance—no matter whether it is another prescription drug, a common food, an OTC product, or an herbal or vitamin supplement—that either inhibits the action of this enzyme (or, conversely, increases its activity) will have a significant effect on how drugs are metabolized in the body. If more enzymes are produced, the drug is removed from the body too quickly and its effectiveness is lessened. If fewer enzymes are produced, the drug may build up in the body to toxic levels.

Further, it is important to know that many drugs operate within a fairly narrow "window" of concentration. That is, there must be enough of the drug to be effective, but only a little bit more can be toxic to the body.

Now that we know about these five enzymes, drugs can be tested by simply seeing if the drug interacts with each of the enzymes in a test tube. Knowing which enzyme actually metabolizes the new drug, researchers can then compare the drug with other drugs metabolized by the same enzyme and eventually build up a list of possible interactions. If two drugs use the same enzyme, it is possible that together there might be a conflict.

Test-tube studies certainly cannot tell the whole story, but they do point the way for targeted trials that might shed more light on possible problems before a new drug gets to market. There are race, gender, age, and other issues involved, too. Members of some ethnic groups may tend to produce very little of one enzyme but lots of the others. That means certain people might not be able to metabolize a new drug, and they can be tentatively identified beforehand.

Herbs and Drug Interactions

We have already noted that St. John's wort has the capacity to affect the activity of certain drugs. It does so notably through its potential to affect the enzyme CYP3A4. What about other herbs? We know that herbs are not routinely tested like prescription drugs. There are no FDA Phase 1, Phase 2, or Phase 3 trials for herbal remedies.

Additional investigations have found that kava kava extract made from *Piper methysticum* showed the ability to affect CYP3A4, and certain kavalactone compounds additionally affected CYP3A23. Kava also worsens the side effects of certain anesthetics, as does valerian. The plant sterol guggulsterone from the herb guggul (*Commiphora mukul*) and echinacea (*Echinacea purpurea*) appear to have some effect on one or more of the metabolizing enzymes. Echinacea may reverse the effects of certain steroids. Caffeine, a phytochemical found in a number of plants, certainly has a proven effect. Obviously, much more research is needed to see how herbs might interact with other substances and with prescription drugs.

Mineral and Drug Interactions

Minerals can form complexes, or chelates, with some drugs. This creates insoluble structures that the body cannot absorb. Antibiotics and calcium are a known interactive pair. Calcium-fortified orange juice has caused chelation with ciprofloxacin (Cipro), gatifloxacin (Tequin), and levofloxacin (Levaquin). These antibiotics were made less effective by the calcium, as was the antibiotic tetracycline. Tetracyclines also bind with aluminum and magnesium, among others.

Calcium carbonate, as used in common antacids, binds with the thyroid hormone levothyroxine. Calcium carbonate should be taken at least four hours before taking the medication.

Iron forms complexes with ciprofloxacin, as well as with the quinolone antibiotics nalidixic acid and norfloxacin. Iron also binds with the Parkinson's disease medication levodopa (L-dopa). This binding reduces the effectiveness of all these drugs. Copper, manganese, magnesium, and zinc have similar effects on the quinolone antibiotics. Magnesium hydroxide appears to enhance the activity of ibuprofen (found in Advil, Motrin, and other over-the-counter and prescription products), possibly by increasing the gastric pH and creating an environment conducive to absorption. Caution should be used when combining ibuprofen and magnesium hydroxide, as prolonged use has been shown to increase the risk of gastrointestinal irritation.

Vitamin and Drug Interactions

Interaction between vitamins and prescription and OTC drugs is a wide-open field that needs to be explored. We have already noted that vitamin K counteracts the effects of the blood-thinner warfarin. It is also known that vitamin B_6 (pyridoxine) reduces blood levels of the Parkinson's disease drug levodopa. Vitamin A supplements, although not at levels typically found in multivitamins, may react badly with isotretinoin (Accutane), an acne medication.

Dietary Supplements and Drug Interactions

Several interactions have been reported between dietary supplements and prescription medications. Work in rats showed that policosanol increased the anti-ulcer effects of cimetidine (Tagamet). Use of conjugated linoleic acid (CLA) may interfere with hepatic enzyme function and tamoxifen (a breast cancer drug). Some drugs, propranolol and tricyclic antidepressants, for example, lower coenzyme Q_{10} levels.

Several drugs have been shown to lower carnitine levels, including sodium valproate, pivampicillin, and isotretinoin. Some patients using these drugs benefit from supplements of carnitine. Melatonin has been reported to interact with a number of prescription drugs. For example, serum melatonin levels increase faster taking fluvoxamine, reducing CYP3A4 enzyme activity. Melatonin interacts with nifedipine, increasing blood pressure and heart rate.

Chondroitin may provoke autoimmune dysfunction and interact with the drug warfarin, increasing the time it takes your blood to clot.

Foods and Drug Activity

As has been noted throughout this book, supplemental fiber products can significantly delay the absorption of drugs and nutrients (vitamins and minerals). Psyllium-based products used in bulk laxatives, for example, should be taken at least two hours before or after taking medication or nutrients. Some products, such as bran fiber, bulk laxatives, and pectin-containing foods such as apples and pears, should not be consumed along with the heart drug digoxin. These lower the effect of the drug by binding with it and lowering its concentration.

There are many recent articles that have been written about the effects of grapefruit juice. Because drinking grapefruit juice is so common in the United States, especially among dieters, we have cut right to the chase. In short, it has been found that grapefruit juice increases the bioavailability of many drugs (makes their concentration higher in the body) by inhibiting the CYP3A4 enzyme in the small intestine. Some drugs that appear to be affected are:

- Cholesterol-lowering drugs: lovastatin (Mevacor), atorvastatin (Lipitor), simvastatin (Zocor)

- Antihistamines: ebastine (Kestine)

- Calcium channel blockers (blood pressure drugs): nimodipine (Nimotop), felodipine (Plendil), nisoldipine (Sular)

- Psychiatric medications: buspirone (Buspar), triazolam (Halcion), diazepam (Valium), midazolam (Versed), sertraline (Zoloft)

- Immune suppressants: cyclosporine (Neoral)

- Pain medications: methadone (Methadose)

- Anti-HIV medicine: saquinavir (Invirase)

- Antiarrhythmics: amiodarone (Cordarone)

- Antiseizure medications: carbamazepine (Carbatrol, Tegretol)

Reducing Your Risk of Interactions

There are many things you, as a consumer, can do to reduce your risk. First of all, be aware that drug interactions do exist, and that nutrients and vitamins, along with food and beverages, must be included in the equation. Second, always read labels carefully on both your prescription drugs and any over-the-counter products you buy. Learn about any warnings that apply to drugs you are taking. These warnings are available in the drug packaging, on the labels in abbreviated form, and on the Internet.

There are programs on the Internet that will allow you to check for drug interactions by typing in the names of the drugs you are going to take and letting the computer find any adverse interactions. One example of such a program can be found at www.drugdigest.org.

Do not trust any verbal advice unless it comes from a pharmacist or other health care practitioner. What worked for your friend or neighbor might not be best for *you*. Your doctor is a good source of information, but your pharmacist frankly knows more about the actions of drugs and might be a better source.

Before even filling a prescription, make sure your medical record is updated with everything you normally take, and ensure that your doctor is aware of any over-the-counter medications you normally use *plus* any herbal, vitamin, or mineral supplements.

Keep good records of all your medications and their dosages, such as how many milligrams or capsules and how often you take them. Be sure to include the name of the manufacturer. Make a list and keep it in your wallet. You may also want to keep a copy in your home. It's a good idea to let another family member know where you keep these "drug lists."

Ask your doctor if there are any foods, beverages, or supplements you should avoid when getting new medication prescribed. When your doctor writes a new prescription for you, be sure to mention the other drugs you are now taking (or show your list to the doctor). Don't forget to mention any OTC drugs you are taking.

If possible, it's best to use only one pharmacy to get all of your prescriptions. Pharmacies have computer-assisted drug interaction programs that will raise a red flag if they punch in a new prescription and it will interact badly with your other drugs already in the computer. But all of your drugs have to be on the same computer network for this to work properly.

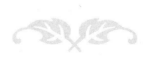

PART TWO

the
Disorders

Introduction

Part One explored the nutritional and dietary needs of the body. In order to be well, the parts of the body must be fueled properly so that breakdown does not occur. With the growing number of stressors in the environment today, the body must obtain the proper nourishment in order to maintain a healthy immune system. If the immune system weakens, the body becomes susceptible to a number of harmful conditions.

Your health care provider may recommend that certain diagnostic tests be performed to help in making a diagnosis. Some tests, such as amniocentesis or surgical biopsy, are invasive; others, such as urinalysis, are not. Many diagnostic tests—especially newer ones such as magnetic resonance imaging (MRI) and computerized tomography (CAT) scans—can be quite expensive. Always be sure you understand exactly what a test involves before agreeing to it—how it is done, what it will show, why it is necessary in your case, what the potential risks are, how much it will cost, and anything else you need to know to feel confident in making a choice. You should also inform your health care provider about all medications, including natural remedies, over-the-counter medications, and supplements you take regularly to avoid potential interactions; any known allergies to foods, medications, anesthetics, X-ray materi-als, and/or other substances; pregnancy, if applicable; and any other special concerns you may have.

Once a diagnosis has been confirmed, refer to the appropriate dietary guidelines, recommendations, and supplementation program in this book to help speed your recovery. Always be sure to learn as much as possible about the use of any supplement you take. (*See* Part One for more detailed supplement information.) Most of the suggestions in Part Two can be utilized either alone or in conjunction with other therapies. However, if you have any questions about any suggested nutrients or any other therapy, speak to your physician.

From time to time, we recommend specific products by brand name or specific manufacturer. These recommendations may appear on their own or in parentheses following the generic term for the substance in question. This should not be taken to mean that these are the only such products available, or that they are the only ones that will work. There are many good supplements and other nutritional products available from many different manufacturers, and new products are being introduced to the market all the time. However, we occasionally choose to make specific recommendations for particular products because we have found them to be effective and of good quality.

Troubleshooting for Disorders

Some symptoms are indicative of a variety of illnesses. The following table lists some of the more common disorders that are associated with particular symptoms. It is not meant to serve as a substitute for professional diagnosis. Although you may experience one or more of the symptoms below, you may or may not have one of the illnesses cited. Your body is simply sending a message that something is wrong. Listening to your body can help stop a problem before it becomes serious. The illnesses listed are in alphabetical order. Their inclusion in this sequence does not reflect your chances of having any of them. If you have symptoms, consult with your health care provider. Before contacting your health care provider, write down your symptoms, how frequently you have them, how severe they are, and how long you have experienced them. This information will help you to have a more productive conversation.

Symptom	Possible Cause
Abdominal pain, cramping	Across the abdomen: bladder or kidney disorder; pelvic inflammatory disease; premenstrual syndrome; uterine prolapse.
	Around the navel: appendicitis; constipation; gas.
	Lower left side: colitis; Crohn's disease; diarrhea; diverticulitis; lactose intolerance; ovarian cyst; regional enteritis; uterine fibroids or polyps.
	Lower right side: acute appendicitis; colitis; Crohn's disease; uterine fibroids or polyps.
	Upper left side: food allergies; heartburn, hiatal hernia; irritable bowel syndrome; peptic ulcer.
	Upper right side of rib cage: liver or gallbladder problems.
	Any location: endometriosis; food poisoning; indigestion; internal injury; miscarriage; stress.
Anal bleeding, itching, pain, swelling	Abscess; allergies; anal fissure; bruising; cancer; candidiasis; Crohn's disease; cysts; diverticulitis; food poisoning; genital warts; hemorrhoids; infection; muscle spasms; pinworms; polyps; sexually transmitted diseases; tumor; ulcers; ulcerative colitis.
Back pain	Aortic aneurysm; arthritis; awkward sleeping/sitting position; cancer; disk disease; endometriosis; gallbladder disorders; heart attack; improper lifting; injury; kidney disease; lack of exercise; menstrual cramps; muscle spasms; obesity; osteoporosis; Paget's disease of bone; pelvic inflammatory disease; peptic ulcer; pneumonia; poor posture; pregnancy; scoliosis; spinal tumor; sprain; strained muscle and/or ligament; urinary tract infection; uterine fibroids.
Bad breath	Abscessed tooth; bulimia; constipation; diabetes; dry mouth; gum disease; indigestion; infection (especially sinus and lung infection); liver disease; lung disease; mouth ulcers; mouth-breathing; kidney failure; liver malfunction; periodontal disease; poor oral hygiene; disorders of the metabolism; sinusitis; tooth decay.
Bleeding, menstrual, heavy or irregular	Blood-clotting disorders; cancer; endocrine disorders; endometriosis; hormonal imbalance; menopause; miscarriage; obesity; overzealous dieting or exercise; thyroid disorder; urinary tract infection; use of improper oral contraceptives; uterine polyps or fibroids; vaginal infection; weight loss or gain.
Blinking, frequent	Anxiety; dry eyes; foreign body in the eye; injury; mimic spasm or tic (may occur in Tourette syndrome); Parkinson's disease; stroke; use of contact lenses.
Bloating	Adrenal disorders; allergies; appendicitis; bowel or kidney obstruction; diverticulitis; edema; gallbladder disorders; heart failure; irritable bowel syndrome; kidney disease; lactose intolerance; menstruation; overeating; peptic ulcer; tumor.
Blood in sputum, vomit, urine, stools, or from vagina or penis	Blood clots and swelling of lung tissue; cancer of colon, bladder, etc.; hemorrhoids; infection; peptic ulcer; polyps; prostate cancer; prostatitis; ruptured blood vessel; sexually transmitted disease; tumor.
Body aches	Arthritis; infection; influenza; lupus; Lyme disease; overexertion.
Body odor	Constipation; diabetes; excess toxins; gastrointestinal abnormalities; indigestion; infection; liver dysfunction; poor hygiene.
Breast lumps	Boils; cancer; cysts; fibrocystic disease; infected milk duct; infected sweat gland or lymph node; injury; premenstrual syndrome.
Breast tenderness	Blood clots in veins of breast; breast-feeding-related problems; cancer; estrogen therapy, excessive consumption of fat, salt, and/or caffeine; fibrocystic breast disease; hormonal imbalance; menopause; pregnancy; premenstrual syndrome; stress.

Symptom	Possible Cause
Breath, shortness of	Asthma; cardiovascular disease (especially in women); chronic bronchitis; cystic fibrosis; emphysema; obesity; panic attacks; pneumonia.
Bruising, easy	AIDS; anemia; cancer; Cushing's syndrome; drug reaction; hemophilia; liver or kidney disorder; vitamin C or vitamin K deficiency; weakened immune system.
Chest pain	Angina; anxiety; bruised or broken rib; carditis (inflammation of the muscles of the heart); coronary artery disease; gas; heart attack; heartburn; hiatal hernia; hyperventilation; pleurisy; pneumonia; strained muscle; stress.
Chills	Acute infection; anemia; exposure to cold; fever; hypothermia; shock.
Cold sweats	AIDS; cancer; diabetes; food poisoning; influenza; menopause; mononucleosis; severe heart or circulatory disease; shock; tuberculosis.
Cough, persistent	Allergies; asthma; cancer; chronic bronchitis; emphysema; pneumonia; postnasal drip; tuberculosis.
Delirium	Alcohol abuse; appendicitis; diabetes; drug overdose; drug reaction; epilepsy; high fever; manic episode; stroke.
Disorientation	Acute anxiety (panic attack); alcohol abuse; Alzheimer's disease; anemia; drug reaction or overdose; hypoglycemia; poor circulation; schizophrenia; seizure; stroke; transient ischemic attack (TIA, temporary interference with blood flow to the brain).
Dizziness, light-headedness	Acute anxiety (panic attack); allergies; anemia; brain tumor; inhaling chemical products; dehydration; diabetes; drug reaction; heart disease; high blood pressure; hypoglycemia; infection; low blood pressure; Ménière's disease; motion sickness; stress; stroke or impending stroke; vertigo.
Double vision	Cataracts; concussion; excessive alcohol consumption; eye disorders; hyperthyroidism.
Drooling	Drug withdrawal; ill-fitting dentures; Parkinson's disease; pregnancy-related problems; salivary gland disorders; seizure; stroke.
Drowsiness	Acute kidney failure; allergies; caffeine withdrawal; drug reaction or overdose; encephalitis; narcolepsy; skull fracture; sleep disorders.
Dry mouth	Aging; breathing through the mouth; dehydration; diabetes; drug reactions; Sjögren's syndrome.
Ear discharge	Clogged eustachian tube; earwax buildup; immune system dysfunction; infection; middle-ear infection; ruptured eardrum; severe head injury; tumor.
Eye, bulging	Aneurysm; blood clot or hemorrhage; glaucoma; hyperthyroidism; infection.
Eyelid, drooping	Botulism; diabetes; head or eyelid injury; hypothyroidism; muscle weakness; stroke.
Fever, persistent	AIDS; autoimmune diseases; cancer (especially kidney cancer, leukemia, lymphoma); chronic bronchitis; chronic infection; diabetes; hepatitis; influenza; mononucleosis; rheumatic disorders.
Flushing	Alcohol consumption; anxiety; dehydration; diabetes; heart disease; high blood pressure; hyperthyroidism; menopause; pregnancy; rosacea; use of high doses of niacin or of cholesterol-lowering medications.
Gas, frequent burping	Allergies; candidiasis; digestive problems; gallbladder disorders; gluten intolerance; intestinal obstruction; intestinal parasites; irritable bowel syndrome; lactose intolerance; stomach acid deficiency; swallowing air; ulcer.
Hands and/or feet, cold	Circulatory problems; exposure to cold; Raynaud's phenomenon; stress.
Headaches, persistent	Allergies; asthma; brain tumor; cluster headaches; drug reaction; eyestrain; glaucoma; high blood pressure; migraine; sinusitis; stress; vitamin deficiency.
Heartbeat, irregular or rapid	Anemia; anxiety; arteriosclerosis; asthma; caffeine, alcohol, or tobacco consumption; calcium, magnesium, and/or potassium deficiency; cancer; cardiovascular disease; drug reaction; fever; heart attack; high blood pressure; hormonal imbalance; low blood pressure; obesity; overeating; overzealous exercising.
Hot sweats, then chills	Acute infection; excessive alcohol or sugar consumption; fever; hypoglycemia; thyroid disorders; tuberculosis (mainly night sweats).
Incontinence (urinary)	Advanced neurological disease; Alzheimer's disease; atrophic vaginitis; bladder infection; diabetes; excessive liquid consumption; loss of muscle tone; multiple sclerosis; prostatitis; psychological problems; restricted mobility; spinal cord trauma; stroke; urinary tract infection.
Intercourse, painful	Endometriosis; inflammation or infection of the vulva; muscle spasms; unaccustomed position during sex; urinary tract infection; vaginal dryness.

Symptom	Possible Cause
Irritability, mood swings	Alcohol or drug abuse; Alzheimer's disease; anxiety; brain tumor; depression; diabetes; drug reactions; excessive sugar intake; food allergies; hormonal imbalance; hyperthyroidism; hypoglycemia; hypothyroidism; menopause; nutritional deficiencies; premenstrual syndrome; schizophrenia; stress; stroke; virtually any chronic or disabling illness.
Joint pain, swelling	Arthritis; bone cancer; bone fracture; bone spur; bursitis; carpal tunnel syndrome; chronic overuse; cirrhosis of the liver; diabetes; edema; gout; hemophilia; hepatitis; hormonal imbalance; infection; injury; kidney disease; lupus; Lyme disease; neuritis; Paget's disease of bone; rheumatic fever; sprain; strained muscle and/or ligament; tendinitis.
Leg pain	Arteriosclerosis; bone fracture; cancer; fibromyalgia; improper footwear; injury; Lyme disease; obesity; osteomalacia; overuse; Paget's disease of bone; peripheral artery disease; rickets; sciatica; tendinitis; thrombophlebitis; tumor or infection in intervertebral disk or spinal canal.
Lymph nodes, swollen	AIDS; any acute or chronic infection; cancer; lymphoma; metal toxicity.
Mouth sores	Allergies; cancer; canker sores; chickenpox; consumption of overly acidic foods or liquids; denture wearing; herpes; local trauma; lupus; measles; oral herpes; oral thrush; use of tobacco or aspirin.
Muscle control, loss of	Alcohol and/or drug abuse; extreme exhaustion; fibromyalgia; head injury; multiple sclerosis; muscular dystrophy; narcolepsy; overuse; Parkinson's disease; seizure; stroke.
Muscle cramps	Arthritis; calcium, magnesium, and/or potassium deficiency; dehydration; diabetes; hypothyroidism; injury; overuse; poor circulation.
Muscle pain, weakness	Anemia; arthritis; chronic fatigue syndrome; dehydration; diabetes; drug reaction; fever; fibromyalgia; infection; injury; lupus; multiple sclerosis; overuse.
Nausea	AIDS; alcohol consumption; allergies; anxiety; cancer; celiac disease; cirrhosis of the liver; copper toxicity; dehydration; drug side effect; drug withdrawal; endometriosis; extreme fatigue; food poisoning; gallbladder disorders; heart attack; hepatitis; hormonal imbalance; indigestion; influenza; kidney disease; kidney stones; Ménière's disease; migraine; morning sickness (pregnancy); motion sickness; pancreatitis; poisoning; sinusitis; stress; ulcerative colitis.
Neck pain, stiffness	Allergies; awkward sleeping position; disk disease; fibromyalgia; injury; meningitis; strained muscle and/or ligament; stress.
Night sweats	AIDS; anxiety; autoimmune disorders; bowel disease; cancer; cardiovascular disease; fever; hepatitis; menopause; sleep apnea; stress; tuberculosis; weakened immune system.
Numbness	Carpal tunnel syndrome; diabetes; hyperventilation; multiple sclerosis; pinched nerve; poor circulation; rheumatoid arthritis; stroke; transient ischemic attack.
Pulse, weak	Blood loss; dehydration; drug reaction; heart attack; low blood pressure; malnutrition; shock; trauma; vomiting.
Seizure	Alcoholism; Alzheimer's disease; drug abuse; drug reaction; encephalitis; epilepsy; head injury; high fever; meningitis; stroke; tumor.
Swallowing, difficulty	Bulimia; cancer; dehydration; dry mouth; hiatal hernia; stress; tumor.
Sweating, excessive	Alcohol consumption; anxiety; cardiovascular disease; consumption of hot and/or spicy foods; cystic fibrosis; fever; food allergies; hormonal imbalance; hyperthyroidism; infection; kidney disease; liver disease; lymphoma; malaria; menopause; overexertion; pneumonia; stress.
Swelling of ankles, feet, legs, hands, abdomen	Arthritis; bursitis; cardiovascular disease; chronic overuse; cirrhosis of the liver; diabetes; drug reaction; edema; food allergies; gout; improper footwear; joint infection; kidney disease; lupus; lymphatic disorders; poor circulation; pregnancy; premenstrual syndrome; sprain; strained muscle and/or ligament; varicose veins.
Thirst, excessive	Dehydration; diabetes; diarrhea; drug reaction; fever; menopause-related problems; any viral or bacterial infection.
Tremors	Alcoholism; anxiety; caffeine consumption; drug reaction; hyperthyroidism; multiple sclerosis; muscle fatigue; Parkinson's disease; stress; stroke; tumor; withdrawal from drugs or alcohol.
Urination, frequent	Alcohol or caffeine consumption; bladder infection; cancer; Cushing's syndrome; diabetes; drug reaction; excessive liquid intake; kidney or bladder stones; pregnancy; prostatitis.
Vaginal discharge, itching	Allergies; cancer; chlamydia; genital herpes; pelvic inflammatory disease; polyps; sexually transmitted diseases; urinary tract infection; vaginitis; yeast infection.
Weight gain	Aging; congestive heart failure; depression; diabetes; drug reaction; edema; hormonal imbalance; hypothyroidism; kidney disease; lack of exercise; overeating; poor diet.

Symptom	Possible Cause
Weight loss	Aging; AIDS; Alzheimer's disease; anorexia nervosa; cancer; chronic infection; depression; diabetes; hepatitis; hyperthyroidism; malabsorption syndrome; mononucleosis; Parkinson's disease; stress; tuberculosis.
Wheezing	Allergies; asthma; bronchitis; cardiovascular disease; chronic bronchitis; croup; emphysema; lung cancer; pneumonia; tobacco; upper respiratory infection.

ABSCESS

An abscess is formed when pus accumulates in a tissue, organ, or confined space in the body due to infection. Abscesses may be located externally or internally, and may result from an injury or a lowered resistance to infection. An abscess can form in the brain, lungs, teeth, gums, underarms, abdominal wall, gastrointestinal tract, ears, tonsils, sinuses, bones, breasts, kidneys, prostate gland, rectum, scrotum, or almost any other body part. Infections are the most common human disorders and can be produced by bacteria, viruses, parasites, and fungi. A boil is an external (skin) abscess. (*See* BOIL in Part Two.)

The affected area may become swollen, inflamed, hot, red, and tender. The individual may also experience fatigue, loss of appetite, weight loss, and alternating bouts of fever and chills. In severe cases, bacteremia (blood infection) and/or rupture of the abscess can occur. The material inside an abscess consists of living and dead white blood cells, dead tissue, bacteria, and/or toxins—all of which need to be discarded from the body.

An abscess that appears suddenly (in a matter of a few hours or overnight) is said to be acute. If an abscess has been present for a period of days or weeks, it is termed chronic.

Chronic abscesses are more resistant to treatment because the damage is more severe and/or widespread. Acute abscesses are less extensive and generally respond to treatment within a matter of days.

An abscess, if treated, should begin to heal in a few days. Usually there is complete healing in a week or two. An abscess that does not show any signs of healing within this time can be an indication of problems within the immune system. Complications, although rare, can include bleeding or recurrence of the abscess.

Inflamed, red, and tender gums can characterize acute dental abscesses. The affected tooth may be sensitive or loose, and a dull pain is often present. A periodontal abscess can cause an overall sick feeling accompanied by fever and swollen lymph glands. However, chronic dental abscesses often produce no symptoms and are harder to treat than acute abscesses, as they have been present longer and have had the chance to do more extensive damage.

Basically, an abscess is a sign that the body is trying to rid itself of impurities. The impurities may be half-starved cells, deficient in nutrients such as sulfur, or toxins that accumulate because of a failure of the normal eliminative processes. Such a situation often stems from poor diet and exposure to environmental pollutants, chemicals, and other harmful substances. Eating junk food not only clutters the system with foods lacking in nutrients, but also prevents the cellular wastes from being eliminated efficiently by causing such problems as constipation and sluggish liver, spleen, and kidney function. Eating a diet rich in fruits and vegetables, which contain antioxidants and other nutrients, helps clean wastes and toxins from the body.

Unless otherwise specified, the dosages recommended here are for adults. For a child between the ages of twelve and seventeen, reduce the dose to three-quarters of the recommended amount. For a child between six and twelve, use one-half the recommended dose.

NUTRIENTS

SUPPLEMENT	SUGGESTED DOSAGE	COMMENTS
Very Important		
Zinc	80 mg daily, in divided doses. Do not exceed a total of 100 mg daily from all supplements.	Powerful immune system stimulant. Necessary for T lymphocyte function, which is needed to fight infection. Needed for all skin disorders.
Important		
Coenzyme A from Coenzyme-A Technologies	As directed on label.	Supports the immune system's detoxification of many dangerous substances.
Colloidal silver	Apply topically as directed on label.	Acts as a natural antibiotic and disinfectant. Destroys bacteria, viruses, fungi, and parasites.
Garlic (Kyolic)	2 capsules 3 times daily, with meals.	Acts as a natural antibiotic and stimulates the immune system, and contains sulfur, needed for skin tissue repair.
Methylsulfonyl-methane (MSM)	As directed on label.	Naturally occurring organic sulfur compound.
Superoxide dismutase (SOD) or	As directed on label.	A potent antioxidant. Use a sublingual form for best absorption.
Cell Guard from Biotec Foods	As directed on label.	An antioxidant complex that contains SOD.
Vitamin A	50,000 IU daily for 5 days, then 25,000 IU daily for 5 days, then reduce to 15,000 IU daily. If you are pregnant, do not exceed 10,000 IU daily.	Strengthens cell walls to protect against invasion by bacteria and promote tissue repair. Essential to the immune system. Use an emulsion form for easier assimilation and greater safety at high doses.
plus natural carotenoid complex (Betatene)	As directed on label.	Powerful antioxidants that promote healing.

Vitamin B complex	50 mg of each major B vitamin daily (amounts of individual vitamins in a complex will vary). Take with meals.	For repair and replacement of lost nutrients; aids in healing.
Vitamin C with bioflavonoids	5,000–20,000 mg daily, in divided doses. (*See* ASCORBIC ACID FLUSH in Part Three.)	Essential in immune function and tissue repair.
Vitamin E	200 IU daily. You can also open a capsule and apply it directly to the affected area.	Important in circulation and tissue oxygenation. Enhances the immune system and promotes healing. Use d-alpha-tocopherol form.
Helpful		
Bromelain	500 mg 3 times a day.	Reduces inflammation and swelling; speeds healing.
Multivitamin and mineral complex	As directed on label.	All nutrients are needed for healing.
Proteolytic enzymes or Inf-zyme Forte from American Biologics or Intenzyme Forte from Biotics Research	As directed on label. Take between meals. As directed on label. As directed on label.	To aid in cleanup of the abscess. Powerful free radical scavengers.

Herbs

❏ The following herbs are beneficial for healing abscesses and cleansing the blood: burdock root, cayenne (capsicum), dandelion root, red clover, and yellow dock root.

❏ Chamomile tea is good for treating dental abscesses. Drink a cup three or four times daily. If your face is swollen from the infection, chamomile can be prepared as a poultice and applied to the outside of the cheek once or twice a day for five to ten minutes until the infection is gone.

Caution: Do not use chamomile if you are allergic to ragweed. Do not use during pregnancy or nursing. It may interact with warfarin or cyclosporine, so patients using these drugs should avoid it.

❏ Consuming distilled water with fresh lemon juice, plus 3 cups of echinacea, goldenseal, and astragalus or suma tea every day is helpful. Goldenseal can also be made into a poultice and applied directly to the abscess. (*See* USING A POULTICE in Part Three.) Or, apply alcohol-free goldenseal extract to sterile gauze and place the gauze over the abscess.

Cautions: Do not use astragalus in the presence of a fever. Do not take echinacea for longer than three months. It should not be used by people who are allergic to ragweed. Do not take goldenseal internally on a daily basis for more than one week at a time. Do not use it during pregnancy or if you are breast-feeding, and use with caution if you are allergic to ragweed. If you have a history of cardiovascular disease, diabetes, or glaucoma, use it only under a doctor's supervision.

❏ Echinacea tea or extract in warm water can be used as a mouthwash for dental abscesses. Be sure to prepare it warm and rinse your mouth with it every two hours.

Caution: Do not take echinacea for longer than three months. It should not be used by people who are allergic to ragweed.

❏ A poultice that combines lobelia and slippery elm bark is soothing and fights infection. (*See* USING A POULTICE in Part Three.)

❏ Milk thistle, taken in capsule form, is good for the liver and aids in cleansing the bloodstream.

❏ Tea tree oil, applied externally, is a potent natural antiseptic that kills infectious organisms without harming healthy cells. Mix 1 part tea tree oil with 4 parts water and apply the mixture with a cotton ball three times a day. This will destroy the bacteria, hasten healing, and prevent the infection from spreading.

Recommendations

❏ Eat fresh pineapple daily. Pineapple contains bromelain, an enzyme that fights inflammation and aids healing.

❏ Include garlic and onions in your diet. They are high in sulfur and can help to both prevent and cure abscesses.

❏ Add kelp to the diet for beneficial minerals.

❏ Perform a liquid fast using fresh juices for twenty-four to forty-eight hours. (*See* FASTING in Part Three.)

❏ For an external abscess, apply honey to the affected area. Honey destroys bacteria and viruses, apparently by drawing all the moisture out of them.

❏ To cleanse the affected area, apply chlorophyll liquid mixed with water several times a day.

❏ If you must take antibiotics, supplement your diet with the B vitamins and products containing "friendly" bacteria, such as acidophilus and yogurt.

❏ If pain, redness, swelling, bleeding, or discharge increases or continues for more than a week, call your doctor.

Considerations

❏ For very mild external abscesses, the application of heat from a warm-water soak, along with improved nutrition, can usually provide sufficient treatment. Most abscesses, however, require treatment with antibiotics or herbs. Taking acidophilus and B vitamins and increasing your intake of liquids can often aid in the healing process. In some cases, the abscess may have to be lanced (pierced), drained, deep cleaned, and treated with antibiotics.

❏ To heal an abscess, you may have to get plenty of bed rest, drink plenty of fluids, and use warm-water packs, ice packs, hot baths, a heating pad, or a heat lamp to alleviate the pain.

❑ To aid healing, the blood must be cleansed, and vitamin deficiencies that accompany skin eruptions must be corrected.

❑ Abscesses do not usually interfere with normal bathing or showering, but you should remove bandages first so the wound may be gently washed with surgical, antibacterial, or other mild, unscented soap. Afterward, apply a new bandage.

❑ If an abscess breaks open and drains without assistance, your doctor may still need to make sure the entire area is sufficiently clean to prevent recurrence. This minor surgery involves making an incision across and through the abscess so it can be opened enough to ensure that all pockets of pus are opened and thoroughly drained. Sterile gauze may be provided to absorb any additional fluids that may appear. This also allows healing to begin from the base up.

❑ If an abscess spreads to the blood, it may jeopardize the health of the rest of the system, and immediate treatment by a health care professional is necessary.

❑ Deep abscesses must be watched to ensure that they are not affecting or obstructing the function of deeper tissues and organs.

❑ Good hygiene and careful cleansing of the skin to prevent a wound or injury from becoming infected may prevent some abscesses.

❑ Appropriate treatment for a dental abscess depends on the type of abscess. Most often, the pus is drained from the infected area, antibiotics are prescribed, and deep cleaning is necessary. In other cases, a tooth may have to be extracted or root-canal surgery performed. (See PERIODONTAL DISEASE in Part Two.)

❑ Good dental hygiene can help prevent dental abscesses. This includes regular brushing and flossing, as well as regular dental checkups.

ACID/ALKALI IMBALANCE

Acidity and alkalinity are measured according to the pH (potential of hydrogen) scale. Water, with a pH of 7.0, is considered neutral—neither acid nor alkaline. Any substance with a pH below 7.0 is acidic, while anything with a pH above 7.0 is alkaline. The ideal pH range for the human body is between 7.35 and 7.45 (the human body is naturally mildly alkaline). For the body, values below pH 7.35 are considered on the acidic side. Values above pH 7.45 are on the alkaline side.

Acid and Alkaline Self-Test

This test will determine whether your body fluids are either too acidic or too alkaline. Purchase litmus paper, which is available at most drugstores, and apply saliva and/or urine to the paper. The paper will change color to indicate whether your system is overly acidic or alkaline.

Red litmus paper turns blue in an alkaline medium and blue litmus paper turns red in an acid medium. Always perform the test either before eating or at least one hour after eating. If your test indicates that your body is too acidic, consult the recommendations under Acidosis, below. If your body is too alkaline, see Alkalosis on page 146. If you take a blood test for alkalinity or acidity, you may receive a normal result but still experience symptoms. This is because small changes in the body's pH can have a considerable impact on the body. Over the past twenty years, the pH of the human body is becoming more acidic due to poor diet.

Acidosis

Acidosis is a condition in which body chemistry becomes imbalanced and overly acidic. Symptoms associated with acidosis include frequent sighing, insomnia, water retention, recessed eyes, arthritis, migraine headaches, abnormally low blood pressure, acidic or strong perspiration, dry hard stools, foul-smelling stools accompanied by a burning sensation in the anus, alternating constipation and diarrhea, difficulty swallowing, halitosis, a burning sensation in the mouth and/or under the tongue, sensitivity of the teeth to vinegar and acidic fruits, and bumps on the tongue or the roof of the mouth.

There are two classifications of acidosis: respiratory and metabolic. Respiratory acidosis is caused by an interruption of the acid control of the body, resulting in an overabundance of acidic fluids or the depletion of alkali (base) fluids. Simply, it occurs if the lungs are unable to remove carbon dioxide. Respiratory acidosis can be a result of asthma, bronchitis, or obstruction of the airway. It can be either mild or severe.

Metabolic acidosis occurs when chemical changes in the body disturb the body's acid-base balance, creating an excessive amount of acid in the body fluids. Diabetes mellitus, kidney failure, the use of unusually large amounts of aspirin, and metabolic diseases are some of the conditions that can deplete the body's alkaline base. Other contributing factors can include liver and adrenal disorders, stomach ulcers, improper diet, malnutrition, obesity, ketosis, anger, stress, fear, anorexia, toxemia, fever, and the consumption of excessive amounts of niacin and vitamin C.

NUTRIENTS

SUPPLEMENT	SUGGESTED DOSAGE	COMMENTS
Very Important		
Tri-Salts from Ecological Formulas	As directed on label.	For acid-alkaline balance.
Helpful		
Buffer pH by Växa International, Inc.	As directed on label.	Helps to reduce the acidity in the body to normal.
Coenzyme A from Coenzyme-A Technologies	As directed on label.	Supports the immune system's detoxification of many dangerous substances.

Kelp	1,000–1,500 mg daily.	Reduces acid in the body. Aids in maintaining a proper balance of minerals.
Multi-Zyme from FoodScience of Vermont	As directed on label.	Contains HCl. Beneficial if you have too little stomach acid.
Oxy-Caps or Oxy-Max from Earth's Bounty	As directed on label. As directed on label.	Increases stamina and vitality. Nourishes the body's cells with added oxygen while reducing high acid content in the body. Has unique antiviral, antibacterial, and antifungal properties that help normalize friendly bacteria and keep the acid/alkali balance in check.
Phosphorus	As directed on label.	A mineral that helps in the conversion of food to energy.
Potassium	99 mg daily.	Increases metabolism. Aids in balancing the pH in the blood.
S-Adenosyl-methionine (SAMe)	As directed on label.	Helps reduce stress. Promotes a sense of well-being. *Caution:* Do not use if you have bipolar mood disorder or take prescription antidepressants. Do not give to a child under twelve.
Vitamin A	50,000 IU daily for one month, then reduce to 25,000 IU daily. If you are pregnant, do not exceed 10,000 IU daily.	Helps to protect mucous membranes.
Vitamin B complex	100 mg of each major B vitamin twice daily (amounts of individual vitamins in a complex will vary).	Needed for proper digestion.

Herbs

❑ Use elder bark, hops, and willow for acidosis.

❑ Externally, apply ginger compresses to the kidney area.

Recommendations

❑ Eat a diet of 50 percent raw foods. Raw foods not only maintain the correct acid/alkaline balance within the body, but they are also richer in nutrients that are easily assimilated into the body. Recommended foods include apples, avocados, bananas, bilberries, blackberries, grapefruit, grapes, lemons, pears, pineapples, strawberries, and all vegetables. Fresh fruits (especially citrus fruits) and vegetables reduce acidosis. Start with small amounts of citrus fruits and gradually add larger amounts. If you don't want to adopt a strict raw diet, eating lots of fruits and vegetables of any kind prepared in any way will help your pH to become more alkaline. In addition, limiting protein intake to no more than 80 grams a day and grains to 8 servings also will help reduce blood acidity.

❑ Chew your food slowly, and do not overindulge. Make sure food is mixed well with saliva to form a liquid consistency before swallowing. Do not drink fluids during meals.

❑ Prepare cooked foods with care. Maintain clean working surfaces and wash vegetables and fruit. Keep meat and vegetables separate—you can contaminate vegetables with bacteria from raw meat. Do not overcook vegetables, as this makes them lose not only their flavor, but also their nutritional value. Eat processed foods in moderation only. They are low in nutrients and overexert the digestive system. Both cooked and processed foods tend to make the body more acid. Also avoid eating late at night, as this makes the body work more on digestion and less on restoration.

❑ Drink potato broth every day. (*See* THERAPEUTIC LIQUIDS in Part Three for the recipe.)

❑ Avoid animal protein (especially beef and pork), as it leads to acidity.

❑ Since excess vitamin C may lead to acidosis, reduce your intake of vitamin C for a few weeks. When taking vitamin C, use a non-acid-forming (buffered) variety.

❑ Heartburn and indigestion can be the result of food digesting poorly. If you suffer from heartburn, taking small swallows of a teaspoon or two of natural cider vinegar in a glass of water may be of some help. It may cause a burning sensation when you swallow it, but then, in approximately twenty minutes, you should feel relief. If the cider vinegar method works, this may indicate that you lack sufficient acid in your stomach and the cider vinegar compensated for this insufficiency. In this case, consider taking digestive enzyme supplements containing hydrochloric acid (HCl). Stomach acid is important for breaking down food, and also prevents germs from irritating the intestines.

❑ Practice deep breathing.

❑ Check your urine pH daily using pH paper. See the inset on page 147 for a list of acid-forming foods to avoid until your pH is corrected.

Considerations

❑ Phosphorus and sulfur act as buffers to maintain pH. Sulfur can be taken in supplement form, and phosphorus is also found in dairy products.

❑ Umeboshi plums contain many alkaline minerals that aid in treating acidosis. You can eat one plum every four hours (four plums per day) for three days, then reduce your intake to one per day.

Alkalosis

Alkalosis is the inverse of acidosis—it is a condition in which the body is too alkaline. Alkalosis is less common than acidosis and produces overexcitation of the nervous system. The peripheral nerves are affected first. The symptoms may be manifested as a highly nervous condition, including hyperventilation and even seizures. Other symptoms can include sore muscles, creaking joints, bursitis, drowsiness, protruding eyes, hypertension, hypothermia, seizures, edema, allergies, night cramps, asthma, chronic indigestion, night coughs, vomiting, too-rapid blood clotting and thick blood, menstrual problems, dry hard stools, prostatitis, and thickening of the skin, with burning, itching sensations. Alkalosis may cause calcium to build up in the body, as in bone or heel spurs.

Alkalosis is often the result of excessive intake of alkaline drugs such as sodium bicarbonate for the treatment of gastritis or peptic ulcers. It can also result from excessive vomiting, high cholesterol, endocrine imbalance, poor diet, diarrhea, and osteoarthritis.

Unless otherwise specified, the dosages recommended here are for adults. For children between the ages of twelve and seventeen, reduce the dose to three-quarters of the recommended amount. For children between six and twelve, use one-half the recommended dose.

NUTRIENTS

SUPPLEMENT	SUGGESTED DOSAGE	COMMENTS
Helpful		
Alfalfa		*See under* Herbs, below.
Betaine hydro-chloride (HCl)	As directed on label.	A digestive enzyme that releases acid in the digestive tract.
Coenzyme A from Coenzyme-A Technologies	As directed on label.	Supports the immune system's detoxification of many dangerous substances.
L-cysteine	500 mg twice daily, on an empty stomach. Take with water or juice. Do not take with milk. Take with 50 mg vitamin B_6 and 100 mg vitamin C for better absorption.	Needed to produce glutathione, a major detoxifying chemical. Also aids in making the tissues more acid. (*See* AMINO ACIDS in Part One.)

Acid- and Alkaline-Forming Foods

A basic rule of thumb to follow to achieve and maintain pH balance is to eat 80 percent alkaline-forming foods and drinks and 20 percent acid-forming foods and drinks each day. If a pH test indicates that your body is too acidic, you should eat more alkaline-forming foods and omit acid-forming foods from your diet until another pH test shows you have returned to normal. Conversely, if your body is too alkaline, eat more acid-forming foods and omit alkaline-forming foods. Use the list below as a guide to which foods are acid-forming and which are alkaline-forming. Low-level acid-forming and low-level alkaline-forming foods are almost neutral.

Litmus paper may also be called nitrazine paper. It can be purchased at most local pharmacies. If your local pharmacy does not carry it or urine test strips for pH, check with a medical supply company (listed under *Medical Equipment, Supplies and Repair* in the yellow pages) or a hospital pharmacy. Or contact TriMedica or Växa, listed under Manufacturer and Distributor Information in the Appendix.

Acid-Forming Foods
Alcohol
Beans
Buckwheat
Catsup
Chickpeas
Cocoa
Coffee
Cornstarch
Cranberries
Eggs
Fish
Flour, flour-based products
Legumes
Lentils
Meat
Milk
Mustard
Noodles
Oatmeal
Olives
Organ meats
Pasta
Pepper
Poultry
Prunes
Sauerkraut
Shellfish
Soft drinks
Sugar, all foods with sugar
  added
Tea
Vinegar
 Aspirin, tobacco, and most
  drugs are also acid-
  forming.

Low-Level
Acid-Forming Foods
Butter
Canned or glazed fruit
Cheeses
Dried coconut
Dried or sulfured fruit (most)

Grains (most)
Ice cream
Ice milk
Lamb's quarters
Nuts and seeds (most)
Soy products

Alkaline-Forming Foods
Avocados
Corn
Dates
Fresh coconut
Fresh fruits (most)
Fresh vegetables (onions,
  potatoes, rutabagas)
Honey
Horseradish
Maple syrup
Molasses
Mushrooms
Onions
Raisins

Sprouts
Umeboshi plums
Watercress
   Note: All vegetables, especially raw vegetables, balance the acidity and alkali levels in the blood. Although it might seem that citrus fruits would have an acidifying effect on the body, the citric acid they contain actually has an alkalinizing effect in the system.

Low-Level Alkaline-
Forming Foods
Almonds
Blackstrap molasses
Brazil nuts
Chestnuts
Lima beans
Millet
Soured dairy products

Methylsulfonyl-methane (MSM)	As directed on label.	An acid-forming mineral that helps to correct pH balance.
Raw kidney glandular	500 mg daily.	Stimulates kidney function.
S-Adenosyl-methionine (SAMe)	As directed on label.	Good for the nervous system and chronic fatigue. *Caution:* Do not use if you have bipolar mood disorder or take prescription antidepressants. Do not give to a child under twelve.
Selenium	200 mcg daily. If you are pregnant, do not exceed 40 mcg daily.	Protects against free radicals produced in alkalosis.
Vitamin B complex	100 mg of each major B vitamin daily (amounts of individual vitamins in a complex will vary).	Essential for stable and normal pH.
plus extra vitamin B$_6$ (pyridoxine)	50 mg 3 times daily.	Needed for hydrochloric acid (HCl) production. Also relieves fluid retention.
Vitamin C with rose hips and citrus bioflavonoids	3,000–6,000 mg daily, in divided doses.	A potent antioxidant and free radical scavenger.
Vitamin D	400 IU daily.	Necessary for the absorption and utilization of calcium and phosphorus by the intestinal tract.
Vitamin E	As directed on label.	A powerful antioxidant. Use d-alpha-tocopherol form.

Herbs

❑ Alfalfa is beneficial for the digestive tract. It is a good source of vitamin K and other nutrients. Use supplements plus natural sources, such as alfalfa sprouts.

Recommendations

❑ Adopt a diet that consists of 80 percent whole grains and includes beans, breads, brown rice, crackers, lentils, macaroni, nuts, soy sauce, and whole-grain cereals. The other 20 percent of the diet should include fresh fruits, vegetables, fish, chicken, eggs, and natural cheese.

❑ Do not use antacids or mineral supplements, except those mentioned above, for two weeks.

❑ Avoid sodium.

❑ Cut back on megadoses of vitamins and minerals for two weeks.

❑ Check your urine pH daily using litmus paper. See the inset on page 147 for a list of alkaline-forming foods to avoid until your pH is corrected.

Considerations

❑ Your breathing can affect the acid-alkali balance of your body. Prolonged hyperventilation may cause tempo-

rary alkalosis, resulting in anxiety and a feeling that one cannot get enough air, despite the fact that breathing itself is not actually restricted in any way. If this happens, breathe into a paper bag and rebreathe the air from the bag. This often helps to correct the chemical imbalance.

ACIDOSIS

See under ACID/ALKALI IMBALANCE.

ACNE

Acne is an inflammatory skin disorder characterized by pimples, blackheads, and whiteheads. To some degree, it affects about 80 percent of all Americans between the ages of twelve and forty-four. According to the American Academy of Dermatology, acne is one of the most common skin abnormalities. For those who suffer from acne, it is not merely a cosmetic problem. The consequences include emotional stress that can have a strong impact on one's self-esteem.

Acne often arises at puberty, when the body dramatically increases its production of androgens (male sex hormones). These hormones stimulate the production of keratin (a type of protein) and sebum (an oily skin lubricant). If sebum is secreted faster than it can move through the pores, a blemish arises. The excess oil makes the pores sticky, allowing bacteria to become trapped inside. Blackheads form when sebum combines with skin pigments and plugs the pores. If scales below the surface of the skin become filled with sebum, whiteheads appear. In severe cases, whiteheads build up, spread under the skin, and rupture, which eventually spreads the inflammation. Although proper skin care is important in the treatment of acne, acne is not caused by uncleanliness, but is more likely to be a result of overactive oil glands.

Although more than 20 million teenagers suffer from this disorder, acne is not just affecting kids anymore—it is also affecting increasing numbers of adults. While teenage acne most commonly occurs on the face and/or upper body, adult acne is usually limited to the chin and jawline, and involves fewer, but possibly more painful, blemishes.

Many women suffer premenstrual acne flare-ups prompted by the release of progesterone after ovulation. Oral contraceptives high in progesterone can cause breakouts, too. The presence of candidiasis can also cause hormonal changes that encourage the liver to produce the wrong substances for healthy sebum. (*See* CANDIDIASIS in Part Two.)

Factors that can contribute to acne include heredity, oily skin, hormonal imbalance, monthly menstrual cycles, and candidiasis. Other possible contributing factors are allergies, stress, and the use of certain types of drugs, such as steroids, lithium, oral contraceptives, and some anti-epileptic drugs. Nutritional deficiencies and/or a diet high in saturated fats, hydrogenated fats, and animal products can also be involved. Exposure to industrial pollutants such as machine oils, coal tar derivatives, and chlorinated hydrocarbons are some environmental factors that can have an adverse effect on the condition. A body pH that is too acidic or too alkaline also fosters the nesting and breeding of acne-causing bacteria. (*See* ACID/ALKALI IMBALANCE in Part Two.)

The skin is the largest organ of the body. One of its functions is to eliminate a portion of the body's toxic waste products through sweating. If the body contains more toxins than the kidneys and liver can effectively discharge, the skin takes over. In fact, some doctors call the skin the "third kidney." As toxins escape through the skin, the skin's healthy integrity is disrupted. This is a key factor behind many skin disorders, including acne.

The skin also "breathes." If the pores become clogged, the microbes that are involved in causing acne flourish because they are protected against the bacteriostatic action of sunshine. Dirt, dust, oils, and grime from pollution clog the pores, but this can be eliminated by cleansing the skin properly, and with the proper products.

Unless otherwise specified, the dosages recommended here are for adults. For a child between the ages of twelve and seventeen, reduce the dose to three-quarters of the recommended amount. For a child between six and twelve, use one-half the recommended dose.

NUTRIENTS

SUPPLEMENT	SUGGESTED DOSAGE	COMMENTS
Very Important		
Acidophilus	As directed on label.	Replenishes essential bacteria to reduce outbreaks.
Acneadvance (Futurebiotics)	As directed on label.	Clinically tested ingredient from milk to reduce redness and heal skin.
Chromium picolinate	As directed on label.	Aids in reducing infections of the skin.
Essential fatty acids (flaxseed oil and primrose oil are good sources)	As directed on label.	To supply essential gamma-linolenic acid. Needed to keep the skin smooth and soft, repair tissues, and dissolve fatty deposits that block pores. Also aids in healing.
Potassium	99 mg daily.	Deficiency has been associated with acne.
Vitamin A	25,000 IU daily until healed. Then reduce to 5,000 IU daily. If you are pregnant, do not exceed 10,000 IU daily.	To strengthen the protective epithelial (skin) tissue. Use an emulsion form for easier assimilation.
with natural carotenoid complex (Betatene)	As directed on label.	Antioxidant and precursor of vitamin A.
Vitamin B complex	100 mg of each major B vitamin 3 times daily (amounts of individual vitamins in a complex will vary).	Important for healthy skin tone. The antistress vitamin.
plus extra vitamin B₃ (niacinamide)	100 mg 3 times daily. Do not exceed this amount.	Improves blood flow to the surface of the skin. Deficiencies have been associated with acne.

Caution: Do not substitute niacin for niacinamide. Do not take additional niacinamide if you have a liver disorder, gout, or high blood pressure.

Vitamin C with bioflavonoids	1,000–1,600 mg 3 times daily.	Promotes immune function and reduces inflammation. Needed for collagen repair of the skin tissue. Use a buffered type.
Vitamin D	400 IU daily.	Promotes healing and tissue repair.
Vitamin E	400 IU daily.	An antioxidant that enhances healing and tissue repair. Use d-alpha-tocopherol form.
Zinc	30–80 mg daily. Do not exceed a total of 100 mg daily from all supplements.	Aids in healing of tissue and helps to prevent scarring. A necessary element in the oil-producing glands of the skin.
Important		
Garlic (Kyolic) from Wakunaga)	2 capsules 3 times daily, with meals.	Destroys bacteria and enhances immune function.
Helpful		
Chlorophyll	As directed on label.	Aids in cleansing the blood, preventing infections. Also supplies needed nutrients.
Clear Skin Image from Coenzyme-A Technologies	As directed on label.	A nutrient formula that supports healthy skin by correcting imbalances to address deficiencies in fatty acid metabolism and balance production of adrenal and sex hormones.
Herpanacine from Diamond-Herpanacine Associates	As directed on label.	Contains antioxidants, amino acids, and herbs that promote overall skin health.
L-cysteine	500 mg daily, on an empty stomach. Take with water or juice.	Contains sulfur, needed for healthy skin. (*See* AMINO ACIDS in Part One.) Do not take with milk. Take with 50 mg vitamin B₆ and 100 mg vitamin C for better absorption.
Lecithin granules or capsules	1 tbsp 3 times daily, before meals. 1,200 mg 3 times daily, before meals.	Needed for better absorption of the essential fatty acids.
Methylsulfonyl-methane (MSM) (MSM Capsules from Aerobic Life Industries)	As directed on label.	Makes cell walls permeable, allowing water and nutrients to freely flow into cells, and wastes and toxins to properly flow out.
Multienzyme complex with hydrochloric acid (HCl)	As directed on label. Take with meals.	To aid digestion. *Caution:* Do not use HCl if you have a history of ulcers.
O₂ Spray from Earth's Bounty	As directed on label.	A skin cleanser with antibacterial and antifungal properties that aids in healing blemishes.
Oxy-Caps from Earth's Bounty	As directed on label.	Provides essential oxygen that allows cells to function at their optimum.

Proteolytic enzymes	As directed on label. Take with meals or between meals.	Free radical scavengers. Aid in breaking down undigested food particles in the colon.
Selenium	200 mcg daily. If you are pregnant, do not exceed 40 mcg daily.	Encourages tissue elasticity and is a powerful antioxidant.
Tretinoin (Retin-A)	As prescribed by physician.	Acts as a gradual chemical peel; speeds up sloughing off of top layers of skin, leaving new, smoother skin. Available by prescription only. Takes around 6 months to show results.

Herbs

❑ Burdock root, dandelion leaves, milk thistle, and red clover are good for acne. Burdock root and red clover are powerful blood cleansers. Milk thistle aids the liver in cleansing the blood. A good place to begin an acne program is herbal cleansing of the blood. Both burdock and dandelion can help cleanse the liver. A liver that is not performing at its best can worsen acne because it cannot break down and clear excess hormones from the body as it should. Burdock and dandelion also contain inulin, which can improve the quality of skin by removing bacteria.

❑ A poultice using dandelion and yellow dock root can be applied directly to the areas of skin with acne. (*See* USING A POULTICE in Part Three.)

❑ Chaste tree berry (*Vitex agnus-castus*) extract can aid in preventing premenstrual breakouts. Take it each morning as directed on the product label.

❑ Lavender, red clover, and strawberry leaves can be used as a steam sauna for the face. Lavender kills germs and stimulates new cell growth. Using a glass or enamel pot, simmer a total of 2 to 4 tablespoons of dried or fresh herbs in 2 quarts of water. When the pot is steaming, place it on top of a thick potholder on a table, and sit with your face at a comfortable distance over the steam for fifteen minutes. You can use a towel to trap the steam if you wish. After fifteen minutes, splash your face with cold water. Allow your skin to air-dry or pat it dry with a towel. If desired, you may follow this treatment with the use of a clay mask: Blend 1 teaspoon of green clay powder (available in health food stores) with 1 teaspoon raw honey, and apply the mixture to your face, avoiding the eye area. Leave it on for fifteen minutes, then rinse with lukewarm water.

Caution: If acne is extensive or badly inflamed, do not use steam treatments, as this may worsen the condition.

❑ Lavender essential oil is a good antibiotic and antiseptic that can be applied directly to individual blemishes.

❑ Tea tree oil is a natural antibiotic and antiseptic. Dab full-strength tea tree oil (sparingly) on blemishes three times a day, or add 1 dropper of tea tree oil to ¼ cup warm water and pat it on the affected area with a clean cotton ball (be sure to use 100 percent cotton). Tea tree oil soap also works well. Discontinue it if a rash appears.

❑ Other beneficial herbs include alfalfa, cayenne (capsicum), echinacea, and yellow dock root.

Caution: Do not take echinacea for longer than three months. It should not be used by people who are allergic to ragweed.

Recommendations

❑ Adopt a low-glycemic-load diet that is rich in fruits and vegetables and low in processed grains. Following this diet for twelve weeks has been shown to significantly reduce the number of acne lesions.

❑ Eat a high-fiber diet. This is important for keeping the colon clean and ridding the body of toxins.

❑ Increase your intake of raw foods. The more natural raw foods consumed, the faster the skin will clear and heal. Especially include raw foods that contain oxalic acid, including almonds, beets, cashews, and Swiss chard. Exceptions are spinach and rhubarb; these contain oxalic acid, but should be consumed in small amounts only.

❑ Eat a lot of fruits. This is always good for the skin because of the nutritional value and water content of fruit. You can also use certain fruits as a tonic on the surface of the skin. Grapes, strawberries, and pineapple are rich in alpha-hydroxy acids (AHAs). These acids help to exfoliate the skin by removing the dead skin cells that can clog the oil glands.

❑ Eat more foods rich in zinc, including shellfish, soybeans, whole grains, sunflower seeds, and a small amount of raw nuts daily. Zinc is an antibacterial agent and a necessary element in the oil-producing glands of the skin. A diet low in zinc may promote flare-ups.

❑ Be sure your diet contains vitamins A, C, E, and essential fatty acids. Supplements of these vitamins can prove to be beneficial for acne sufferers. Although vitamin A is important in fighting acne, you must be sure not to take too much. Vitamin E can help regulate vitamin A levels and can also aid in scar prevention.

❑ Drink at least eight glasses of quality water per day.

❑ Avoid alcohol, butter, caffeine, cheese, chocolate, cocoa, cream, eggs, fat, fish, fried foods, hot and spicy foods, hydrogenated oils and shortenings, margarine, meat, poultry, wheat, soft drinks, and foods containing brominated vegetable oils.

❑ Try eliminating dairy products from your diet for one month. Acne may develop due to an allergic reaction to dairy products, and the fat content of the dairy products can worsen the condition. Modern dairy and other animal products often contain hormones and steroids that can upset the body's natural hormonal balance. In the case of children, substitute soy milk for dairy products.

❑ If you are not allergic to dairy products, eat plenty of soured products, such as low-fat yogurt, to maintain healthy intestinal flora.

❑ Avoid all forms of sugar. Sugar impairs immune function. In addition, biopsies of individuals with acne have shown their tissues' glucose tolerance to be seriously flawed. One researcher calls this condition "skin diabetes." Sugar also promotes the growth of candida, which may be a contributing factor to acne. (*See* CANDIDIASIS in Part Two.)

❑ Eliminate all processed foods from the diet, and do not use iodized salt. Enzymes induce the nutrients in food to be used to construct muscle tissue, nerve cells, bone, skin, and glandular tissue. Because processed foods contain so few enzymes, they can result in damage to the skin and its collagen. Processed foods also contain high levels of iodine, which is known to worsen acne. For the same reason, avoid fish, kelp, and onions.

❑ Follow a fasting program. (*See* FASTING in Part Three.)

❑ Use cleansing enemas to remove toxic buildup in the system and promote faster healing. (*See* ENEMAS in Part Three.)

❑ Keep the affected area as free of oil as possible. Shampoo your hair frequently. Use an all-natural soap with sulfur that is designed for acne (available at health food stores). Wash your skin thoroughly but gently no more than twice daily; never rub hard. Overwashing, vigorous scrubbing, and repeated touching of the skin can make acne worse by overstimulating the sebaceous glands, causing them to produce excessive amounts of sebum.

❑ Avoid wearing makeup. If you feel you must use cosmetics, use only natural, water-based products. Do not use any oil-based formulas, and avoid any products containing harsh chemicals, dyes, or oils. Wash and dip makeup applicator brushes and sponges in alcohol after each use to avoid contamination.

❑ Use a mixture of organic apple cider vinegar and quality water to balance the skin's pH. Mix 1 part apple cider vinegar with 10 parts quality water, and apply the mixture on the affected area.

❑ Friction makes pimples more likely to rupture, so avoid wearing tight clothing like turtlenecks. Carefully adjust straps on sports equipment such as bicycle or football helmets. Even using the telephone can exacerbate inflammation if you hold the receiver against your cheek for long periods. Keep your hair away from your face to prevent excess oil and bacteria from being deposited on the skin.

❑ If you must shave an area of skin affected by acne, using an electric razor may be beneficial. When shaving with a blade, use a single-edge blade razor and always shave in the direction of hair growth.

❑ As much as possible, avoid stress. Stress can promote hormonal changes and cause flare-ups. Many dermatologists also recommend fifteen minutes of sunshine each day, regular exercise, and sufficient sleep for people with acne.

❑ Avoid the use of oral or topical steroids, which can aggravate acne.

❑ Do not squeeze the blemishes. To do so is to risk increasing the inflammation by causing breaks in the skin in which harmful bacteria can lodge. Do not touch the affected area unless your hands have been thoroughly cleaned.

Considerations

❑ Acne is a message that something may be wrong with your body chemistry, diet, and/or skin care routine. Proper diet, nutritional supplements, and finding the right skin care products may be all that is needed to correct the problem.

❑ For severe acne, the drug isotretinoin (Accutane) has been the only reliable treatment. It disrupts plug formation, shrinks the sebaceous glands, and reduces the amount of sebum within the glands. Isotretinoin cures or greatly reduces acne in about 90 percent of the people who use it, but it can cause side effects like dry skin, nosebleeds, headaches, and joint and muscle pain. The most dangerous side effect of isotretinoin is that it can cause serious birth defects, such as fetal brain deformities, if taken during pregnancy. It can even cause birth defects if a woman becomes pregnant up to two months after it is discontinued. If a woman with acne is in her childbearing years, isotretinoin is not recommended unless she is using effective birth control. There have also been isolated cases of depression and other mental disorders among people using this drug, and a study published in the *Archives of Dermatology* found that it might cause a loss of bone density, raising questions regarding its effect on the risk of developing osteoporosis later in life.

❑ For severe acne, a treatment that is much safer than Accutane has been developed. It is called Levulan PDT, or the "Blue Light Treatment," and it is ideal for patients of all ages, including teens. During a painless, in-office treatment, the face is first given a mild microdermabrasion (sanding) to remove the surface layer of dead skin, then Levulan (5-aminole-vulinic acid) is applied to the face. This application makes acne bacteria more sensitive to light. After about thirty minutes, the Levulan is washed off and up to ten minutes of a special high-intensity blue light (not ultraviolet) is used to kill the bacteria. Some people require more than one session. Skin is more sensitive to sunlight right after treatment, and SPF 45 sunscreen is recommended for at least twenty-four hours.

❑ The weapon of choice against moderate cases of acne is topical tretinoin (Retin-A). It helps to keep the pores from becoming clogged by increasing the rate at which dead surface skin cells are shed. Like isotretinoin, tretinoin should not be used during pregnancy. Use it with caution, because it renders the skin extremely vulnerable to sun damage. In addition, the safety of long-term use of tretinoin has not been established. Some "sibling" forms of tretinoin are being studied in the hope that they may not be as drying to the skin.

❑ Research is being conducted on the development and use of androgen-blocking drugs to stop the oil glands from being turned on by hormonal functions.

❑ An antibiotic cream or an oral antibiotic, such as tetracycline, erythromycin, or clindamycin, is sometimes prescribed for acne. If these drugs are not effective, minocycline may be prescribed. Be aware that this drug can have such side effects as shortness of breath and joint pain. Antibiotics have been known to cause yeast infections (candidiasis) in some people, leading to worsened acne. If you must take antibiotics, it is wise to take some form of acidophilus because antibiotics kill "friendly" bacteria along with "unfriendly" bacteria.

❑ Benzoyl peroxide is the active ingredient in many over-the-counter acne products. It can be helpful, particularly in mild cases, but it is extremely drying and can cause allergic reactions. It should not be applied around the eyes or mouth.

❑ A study conducted by the Department of Dermatology of the Royal Prince Alfred Hospital in New South Wales, Australia, found that a 5 percent solution of tea tree oil was as effective as a 5 percent solution of benzoyl peroxide for most cases of acne, without the irritating side effects.

❑ Blackheads should be removed only with a specially designed instrument, a procedure best done by a professional. Picking, squeezing, or scratching the blemishes may cause scarring, according to dermatologists.

❑ Niacinamide is a major nutrient in the repair of any skin condition because it aids circulation. This increases the supply of fresh, healthy blood to the surface of the skin, which supplies the skin with blood and nutrients.

❑ Dimethylsulfoxide (DMSO), a by-product of wood processing, can be applied to acne lesions to reduce inflammation and promote healing. If used regularly, it may also help minimize scarring from severe cystic acne.

Caution: Only pure DMSO from a health food store should be used. Commercial-grade DMSO such as that found in hardware stores is not suitable for healing purposes. Any contaminants on the skin or in the product can be taken into the tissues by action of the DMSO.

Note: The use of DMSO may result in a garlicky body odor. This is temporary, and is not a cause for concern.

❑ An acne treatment program called Derma-Klear from Enzymatic Therapy may be helpful.

❑ In rare cases, acne may be a sign of a potentially serious hormonal disorder caused by tumors in the adrenal glands or ovaries. Other symptoms of such problems include irregular menstrual periods and excess facial hair. If such symptoms develop, consult your health care provider.

❑ *See also* OILY SKIN and ROSACEA, both in Part Two.

ACQUIRED IMMUNODEFICIENCY SYNDROME

See AIDS.

ACUTE DISSEMINATED ENCEPHALOMYELITIS

See under RARE DISORDERS.

ADRENOLEUKODYSTROPHY

See LEUKODYSTROPHIES *under* RARE DISORDERS.

ADDISON'S DISEASE

See under ADRENAL DISORDERS.

ADRENAL DISORDERS

The adrenal glands are a pair of triangular-shaped organs that rest on top of the kidneys. Each gland normally weighs about 5 grams (slightly less than 1/5 ounce) and is composed of two parts. The cortex, or outer section, is responsible for the production of the hormones cortisone, cortisol, aldosterone, androstenedione, and dehydroepiandrosterone (DHEA). The medulla, or central section, secretes another hormone, adrenaline (also called epinephrine), and norepinephrine, which functions as both a hormone and a neurotransmitter.

Adrenaline, cortisol, DHEA, and norepinephrine are the body's four major stress hormones. The highest levels of these hormones are released in the morning and the lowest at night. Cortisol is also involved in the metabolism of carbohydrates and the regulation of blood sugar. Aldosterone helps to maintain electrolyte (salt) and water balance in the body. Androstenedione and DHEA are androgens, hormones that are similar to—and that can be converted into—testosterone. DHEA has been promoted as a cure-all for aging. However, very little is known about the action of DHEA in the body, and while it is available from numerous sources, it is a steroidal hormone and it should be used with caution, preferably under a doctor's supervision. The long-term effects of using DHEA are unknown. (*See* DHEA THERAPY in Part Three.) Adrenaline speeds up the rate of metabolism and produces other physiologic changes designed to help the body cope with danger. It is produced when the body is under stress. Under circumstances of extreme stress, large amounts of cortisol are released, which can lead to a host of health problems.

Disorders that are directly related to the adrenal glands include reduced adrenal function, usually referred to as *low adrenal reserve*. The adrenals still produce enough hormones to maintain a relatively normal state of health, but stressful situations increase the need for hormones that the malfunctioning adrenals cannot produce, leading to anything from fatigue to total collapse. Symptoms of reduced adrenal function can include weakness, lethargy, fatigue, recurrent infections, dizziness, low blood pressure when first standing, headaches, memory problems, food cravings, allergies, and blood sugar disorders.

If the adrenal cortex is seriously underactive, a rare condition called Addison's disease may develop. Symptoms include fatigue, loss of appetite, dizziness or fainting, low blood pressure, nausea, diarrhea, depression, craving for salty foods, moodiness, a decrease in the amount of body hair, and an inability to cope with stress. The individual may also constantly complain about feeling cold. Discoloration and darkening of the skin is common in people with Addison's disease; discoloration of knees, elbows, scars, skin folds, and creases in the palms are more noticeable when these body parts are exposed to the sun. The mouth, the vagina, and freckles may appear darker. This disease is also characterized by the development of bands of pigment running the length of the nails and by darkening of the hair. The most common type of this disorder is autoimmune Addison's disease. This comes about when the immune system mistakenly attacks the tissue of the adrenal glands, destroying them. It may be associated with other autoimmune diseases that affect other endocrine glands. The most common of these is hypothyroidism (an underactive thyroid). Addison's disease that coexists with hypothyroidism is known as Schmidt's syndrome. Less commonly, Addison's disease occurs together with insulin-dependent diabetes mellitus, another autoimmune disease; or insufficiencies of the parathyroid glands and/or gonads; or with pernicious anemia. Addison's disease is a chronic condition that requires lifelong treatment. Fortunately, people with Addison's disease can have a normal life expectancy if they stay on the proper medication as prescribed by an endocrinologist (a specialist in hormonal diseases).

Cushing's syndrome is a rare disorder caused by excessive production of cortisol or by excessive use of cortisol or similar glucocorticoid (steroid) hormones. Persons with Cushing's syndrome take on a characteristic appearance: They generally are heavy in the abdomen and buttocks but have very thin limbs, and they have rounded "moon" faces. Muscular weakness and wasting of muscles are also characteristic of this syndrome. Round, red marks mimicking acne may appear on the face, and the eyelids may appear swollen. An increased growth of body hair is common, and women may grow mustaches and beards. People with Cushing's syndrome generally are more susceptible to illness and have trouble healing properly. Thinning of the skin from Cushing's syndrome often leads to stretch marks and bruising. Other symptoms include fatigue, mood swings, depression, increased thirst and urination, and, in women, absence of menstrual periods. If untreated, Cushing's syndrome may cause extreme muscle weakness, poor skin healing, weakening of the bones that results in osteoporosis, and increased susceptibility to serious infections such as pneumonia and tuberculosis.

Adrenal problems that crop up in later life can be due to heredity. In addition, refined carbohydrates in the diet, such as sugar and white flour, deplete many of the nutrients required for adrenal support, especially the B vitamins. Adrenal enzyme deficiency, vascular spasm, degeneration, trauma, nutritional deficiencies, pituitary disease, tuberculosis, toxic chemical attack, or even exposure to electromagnetic fields can affect the adrenals. Organic chlorine and carbonates are suspected agents. Dioxin and fire ant poisons are known agents. Other chemicals that might be involved include tobacco, alcohol, street drugs, heavy metals, coffee, sugar, pesticides, herbicides, and fungicides.

The functioning ability of the adrenal glands can be impaired as a result of the extensive use of cortisone therapy for nonendocrine diseases, such as arthritis and asthma. The long-term use of cortisone drugs often causes the adrenal glands to shrink in size.

Unless otherwise specified, the dosages recommended in this section are for adults. For children between the ages of twelve and seventeen, reduce the dose to three-quarters of the recommended amount. For children between six and twelve, use one-half the recommended dose, and for children under the age of six, use one-quarter of the recommended amount.

Adrenal Function Self-Test

Normally, systolic blood pressure (the first number in the measurement of blood pressure—120/80) is approximately 10 points higher when you are standing than when you are lying down. If the adrenal glands are not functioning properly, however, this may not be the case.

Take and compare two blood pressure readings—one while lying down and one while standing. First, lie down and rest for five minutes. Then take your blood pressure. Then stand up and immediately take your blood pressure again.

If your blood pressure reading is lower after you stand up, suspect reduced adrenal gland function. The degree to which the blood pressure drops upon standing is often proportionate to the degree of hypoadrenalism. However, practice a bit with the blood pressure cuff, as readings can vary a lot, especially with beginners. Or use a digital blood pressure measuring device to avoid errors.

NUTRIENTS

SUPPLEMENT	SUGGESTED DOSAGE	COMMENTS
Essential		
Vitamin B complex	100 mg of each major B vitamin twice daily (amounts of individual vitamins in a complex will vary).	All B vitamins are necessary for adrenal function.
plus extra pantothenic acid (vitamin B₅)	100 mg 3 times daily.	The adrenal glands do not function adequately without pantothenic acid.
Vitamin C with bioflavonoids	4,000–10,000 mg daily, in divided doses.	Vital for proper functioning of the adrenal glands.

Very Important		
Coenzyme A from Coenzyme-A Technologies	As directed on label.	Needed for proper functioning of the adrenal glands. Reduces stress.
L-tyrosine	500 mg daily, on an empty stomach. Take with water or juice. Do not take with milk. Take with 50 mg vitamin B_6 and 100 mg vitamin C for better absorption.	Aids adrenal gland function and relieves excess stress put on the glands. (See AMINO ACIDS in Part One.) Caution: Do not take tyrosine if you are taking an MAO inhibitor drug.

Important		
Raw adrenal glandular and raw adrenal cortex glandular	As directed on label. As directed on label.	Protein derived from this adrenal gland substance helps to rebuild and repair the adrenal glands. (See GLANDULAR THERAPY in Part Three.)
Chlorophyll	As directed on label.	Cleanses the bloodstream.
Coenzyme Q_{10}	60 mg daily.	Carries oxygen to all glands.
Multivitamin and mineral complex with calcium and magnesium plus natural beta-carotene and copper and potassium and zinc	1,500 mg daily. 750 mg daily. 15,000 IU daily. 3 mg daily. 200 mg daily. 50 mg daily. Do not exceed a total of 100 mg daily from all supplements.	All nutrients are needed to support proper adrenal function. Use a high-potency formula. If you have diabetes, use a formula without beta-carotene. Needed to balance with sodium. Potassium is depleted with this disorder. Boosts immune function.
Raw liver extract	As directed on label.	Supplies natural B vitamins, iron, and enzymes.
Raw spleen glandular and raw pituitary glandulars	As directed on label.	Boosts immune function and aids healing process. (See GLANDULAR THERAPY in Part Three.)
S-adenosylmethionine (SAMe) (SAMe Rx-Mood from Nature's Plus)	As directed on label.	Helps reduce stress and depression. Gives a sense of well-being. Caution: Do not use if you have bipolar mood disorder or take prescription antidepressants. Do not give to a child under twelve.

Herbs

❑ The herb astragalus improves adrenal gland function and aids in stress reduction.

Caution: Do not use this herb in the presence of a fever.

❑ China Gold from Aerobic Life Industries is a liquid herbal combination formula that helps to stimulate adrenal function and combat fatigue. It contains ten different varieties of ginseng plus twenty-six other valuable herbs.

Caution: Do not use ginseng if you have high blood pressure, or are pregnant or nursing.

❑ Using echinacea can increase white blood cell production and protect tissues from bacterial invasion.

Caution: Do not take echinacea for longer than three months. It should not be used by people who are allergic to ragweed.

❑ Milk thistle extract aids liver function, which in turn helps adrenal function.

❑ Calming herbs such as kava kava, St. John's wort, and valerian are good stress reducers.

Cautions: Kava kava can cause drowsiness. It is not recommended for pregnant women or nursing mothers, and it should not be taken with other substances that act on the central nervous system, such as alcohol, barbiturates, antidepressants, and antipsychotic drugs. St. John's wort may cause increased sensitivity to sunlight. It may also produce anxiety, gastrointestinal symptoms, and headaches. It can interact with some drugs, including antidepressants, birth control pills, and anticoagulants.

❑ Siberian ginseng is an herb that helps the adrenal gland prepare the body for stressful situations. The best dosage is 1 to 2 grams (1,000 to 2,000 milligrams) per day, taken in divided doses. Use a ninety-day course for ginseng, alternating with licorice derivatives.

Cautions: Do not use Siberian ginseng if you have hypoglycemia, high blood pressure, or a heart disorder. Licorice root should not be used during pregnancy or nursing. It should not be used by persons with diabetes, glaucoma, heart disease, high blood pressure, or a history of stroke.

❑ Ashwagandha (*Withania somnifera*), also known as winter cherry, may be helpful.

Recommendations

❑ Consume plenty of fresh fruits and vegetables—particularly green leafy ones. Brewer's yeast, brown rice, legumes, nuts, olive and safflower oils, seeds, wheat germ, and whole grains are healthy additions to the diet as well.

Caution: Brewer's yeast can cause an allergic reaction in some individuals. Start with a small amount at first, and discontinue use if any allergic symptoms occur.

❑ Eat deepwater ocean fish, salmon, or tuna at least three times a week. Limit tuna to once a week.

❑ Include in the diet garlic, onions, shiitake mushrooms, and pearl barley. These foods contain germanium, a powerful stimulant for the immune system.

❑ Avoid alcohol, caffeine, and tobacco, as these substances are highly toxic to the adrenal and other glands.

❑ Stay away from fats, fried foods, ham, pork, highly processed foods, red meat, sodas, sugar, and white flour. These foods put unnecessary stress on the adrenal glands.

❑ Get regular, moderate exercise (at least three hours per week). This stimulates the adrenal glands and also helps relieve stress.

❏ Measure your waist circumference at the smallest width. Women should be less than 35 inches and men less than 40 inches. If you are over this number, you may be chronically overproducing cortisol, which forces body fat to appear on the abdomen. Following a low-glycemic-load diet can help maintain healthy adrenal function.

❏ Decrease your consumption of caffeine and alcohol, as well as your intake of fats, salt, and sugar.

❏ If you smoke, stop.

❏ As much as possible, avoid stress. Continuous and prolonged stress from a troubled marriage, job-related problems, illness, or feelings of low self-esteem or loneliness can be detrimental to the adrenal glands. Take positive action to relieve stressful situations. (*See* STRESS in Part Two.)

Considerations

❏ A person with Addison's disease must take medication as prescribed and pay careful attention to diet. Nutritional supplements are recommended. Patients with Cushing's syndrome need regular physician monitoring.

❏ Treatment of steroid excess involves management of high blood sugar with diet and medication, replacement of potassium, treatment of high blood pressure, early treatment of any infections, adequate calcium intake, and appropriate adjustments in steroid dosages at times of acute illness, surgery, or injury.

❏ Adrenocorticotropic hormone (ACTH), a hormone released by the pituitary gland when under stress, sets a sequence of biochemical events in motion, resulting in the activation of substances that raise blood pressure. The presence of this hormone leads to sodium retention and potassium excretion. As a result of this mechanism, stress not only puts strain on the adrenal glands, but may also cause the body to retain water, which can lead to hypertension.

❏ Unresolved stress is the most important factor in "adrenal burnout," with all its manifestations, including immune deficiency and degenerative diseases. Professional help to deal with anger and rage, and to deal with psychological or spiritual issues will help reduce cortisol levels. Any stress-reduction technique that works for you should be pursued.

AGE SPOTS

Age spots are flat brown spots that can appear anywhere on the body as it ages. They are also called liver spots. Most age spots appear on the face, neck, and hands. These brown spots are harmless, but they can be a sign of more serious underlying problems. They are the result of a buildup of wastes known as lipofuscin accumulation, a by-product of free radical damage in skin cells. (*See* FREE RADICALS under ANTIOXIDANTS in Part One.) These spots are actually signs that the cells are full of the type of accumulated wastes that slowly destroy the body's cells, including brain and liver cells. In other words, they are a surface sign of free radical intoxication of the body that may affect many internal structures as well, including the heart muscle and the retina.

Factors leading to the formation of age spots include poor diet, lack of exercise, smoking, poor liver function, the ingestion of oxidized oils over a period of time, and, above all, excessive sun exposure. Exposure to the sun causes the development of free radicals that may damage the skin. Most people who have significant numbers of age spots live in sunny climates or have had excessive sun exposure.

The formation of lipofuscin is associated with a deficiency of a number of important nutrients, including vitamin E, selenium, glutathione, chromium, and dimethylaminoethanol (DMAE). Consuming alcohol increases lipofuscin formation.

Unless otherwise specified, the dosages recommended in this section are for adults.

NUTRIENTS

SUPPLEMENT	SUGGESTED DOSAGE	COMMENTS
Very Important		
Zinc	80 mg daily, in divided doses. Do not exceed a total of 100 mg daily from all supplements.	Powerful immune system stimulant. Necessary for T lymphocyte function, which is needed to fight infection. Needed for all skin disorders.
ACES + Zn from Carlson Labs	As directed on label.	A combination of powerful antioxidants. Helps to protect against free radical damage.
Ageless Beauty from Biotec Foods	As directed on label.	A free radical destroyer.
Kyolic Formula 105 from Wakunaga	As directed on label.	Supplies an array of antioxidants that are potent cell protectors.
Vitamin B complex	100 mg of each major B vitamin 3 times daily. (amounts of individual vitamins in a complex will vary).	Needed by older adults for proper assimilation of all nutrients.
plus extra pantothenic acid (vitamin B$_5$)	50 mg 3 times daily.	Supports adrenal gland function.
Vitamin C with bioflavonoids	3,000–6,000 mg daily, in divided doses.	A powerful antioxidant and free radical scavenger necessary for tissue repair.
Important		
Kyo-Dophilus	As directed on label.	Aids in liver regeneration and digestion.
Vitamin E	200 IU daily.	A powerful antioxidant. Fights cellular aging by protecting cell membranes. Improves circulation and prolongs the life of red blood cells. Use d-alpha-tocopherol form.

Helpful		
Calcium and magnesium and vitamin D₃	1,500–2,000 mg daily. 750–1,000 mg daily. 400 IU daily.	Older adults need these nutrients. Asporotate or chelate forms are best.
Coenzyme A from Coenzyme-A Technologies	As directed on label.	Supports the immune system's detoxification of many dangerous substances.
Grape seed extract	As directed on label.	A powerful antioxidant that helps prevent age spots.
Herpanacine from Diamond-Herpanacine Associates	As directed on label.	To provide antioxidants, amino acids, and herbs that promote overall skin health.
L-carnitine	As directed on label. Take between meals.	Aids in breaking up fat in the bloodstream so it can be removed from the body.
Lecithin granules or capsules	1 tbsp 3 times daily, with meals. 1,200 mg 3 times daily, with meals.	Needed for proper brain function and healthy cell membranes. Works well as an antioxidant when taken with vitamin E.
Superoxide dismutase (SOD) plus selenium	As directed on label. As directed on label.	A powerful antioxidant. Good for reducing brown age spots. A powerful antioxidant.
Tretinoin (Retin-A)	As directed by physician.	Acts as a gradual chemical peel; speeds up sloughing off of top layers of skin. Also removes fine wrinkles. Available by prescription only. Takes around six months to show results.

Herbs

❏ Burdock, milk thistle, and red clover aid in cleansing the bloodstream.

❏ Ginkgo biloba improves circulation and is a potent antioxidant.

Caution: Do not take ginkgo biloba if you have a bleeding disorder, or are scheduled for surgery or a dental procedure.

❏ Emu oil has shown good results on brown spots.

❏ Other herbs beneficial for age spots include ginseng, green tea, and licorice.

Caution: Do not use ginseng if you have high blood pressure, or are pregnant or nursing. Green tea contains vitamin K, which can make anticoagulant medications less effective. Consult your health care professional if you are using them. The caffeine in green tea could cause insomnia, anxiety, upset stomach, nausea, or diarrhea. Licorice root should not be used during pregnancy or nursing. It should not be used by persons with diabetes, glaucoma, heart disease, high blood pressure, or a history of stroke.

Recommendations

❏ Eat a diet that is high in vegetable protein and that consists of 50 percent raw fruits and vegetables, plus fresh grains, cereals, seeds, and nuts. Be aware that seeds and nuts become rancid quickly when subjected to heat and/or exposed to the air. Purchase only raw nuts and seeds that have been vacuum-sealed; keep tightly sealed once opened.

❏ Omit all animal protein from the diet for one month.

❏ Avoid caffeine, fried foods, saturated fats, red meat, processed foods, sugar, and tobacco.

❏ Follow a fasting program to cleanse the liver and rid the body of toxins. A properly functioning liver and a clean colon are important. Use black radish extract or dandelion root and beet juice along with three days of fasting a month with distilled water and fresh lemon, fruit, and vegetable juices. (*See* FASTING in Part Three.) Use cleansing enemas while fasting. (*See* ENEMAS in Part Three.)

❏ Limit sun exposure.

❏ Do not use cleansing creams, especially hydrogenated, hardened creams. Cleanse your skin with pure olive oil and a warm wet washcloth, then rinse with lemon juice and water.

❏ This has worked for some people: At night, saturate a cotton ball with pure lemon juice and put it over the spots (but do not apply it near the eyes). There may be some tingling, but only for a few minutes. If there is no sign of irritation, apply morning and night.

Considerations

❏ The prescription drug tretinoin (retinoic acid or Retin-A) is being used for age spots with good results.

❏ Freezing brown or yellow spots off can usually eliminate them. During a painless in-office procedure, the doctor brushes liquid nitrogen on the spots with a cotton swab. In two seconds the cells freeze, and within five days, cells flake away, and the spots disappear. Alternatively, a doctor can burn the spots off with acid applied directly to the spots, or remove them using laser light. With this process, there is no lightening of the skin after removal is completed.

❏ *See* AGING in Part Two.

AGING

Aging is not an illness, but it does make the body more vulnerable to disease. There are many theories on aging and its causes. Some of the more prominent ones are as follows:

- *DNA/genetic theory.* The DNA in our bodies contains a genetic blueprint, which we inherit from our parents and ancestors. This is a unique code, which determines a number of factors affecting aging. Things that happen during our lifetime that damage the DNA, such as exposure to pollutants, toxins, radiation, our diet, and many other environmental and lifestyle factors, can affect the ability of our body to repair damage. This genetic damage can cause the production of abnormal proteins and sugar-protein complexes, which leads to defective cell repair, loss of cell elasticity, and other symptoms of the aging process.

- *Neuroendocrine theory.* The pituitary gland and hypothalamus (a structure in the brain) regulate the release of key hormones to influence cell metabolism, protein synthesis, immune function, and the biochemical functioning of all bodily cells. The theory is that the hypothalamus over time loses its ability to regulate all these functions. The secretion of hormones gradually decreases over time, and this deterioration in the regulatory and hormone production process leads to aging. For instance, the decline in the polypeptide hormone insulin-like growth factor 1, or IGF-1, is linked to a decline in cell activity. IGF-1 is a liver-produced product of human growth factor (HGH) that is secreted by the pituitary gland. Research has shown that IGF-1 increases insulin sensitivity, increases lean body mass, reduces fat, and builds bone, muscle, and nerves. One of IGF-1's greatest feats is the ability to repair peripheral nerve tissue that has been damaged.

- *Free radical or oxidation theory.* This theory asserts that unrepaired cumulative cell damage caused by free radicals, generated by normal metabolism, and contributed to by outside sources, is the cause for aging. Outside factors in the environment, such as exposure to toxins, pollutants, radiation, alcohol, and tobacco, as well as diet, cause highly reactive cell by-products called free radicals to be formed. These free radicals are molecules or portions of molecules capable of independent existence. Because they have odd numbers of electrons (electrons normally occur in pairs), they are unstable and react quickly with other compounds, trying to capture a needed electron to gain stability. When an attacked molecule loses an electron to a free radical, it becomes a free radical itself. This process can cascade to cause disruption to living cells. Only when two free radicals react together do they eliminate each other and stop the process. Of special interest in aging are the oxygen free radicals, which often take an electron away from another molecule to pair with their single free electron. This process is called *oxidation*. Toxic metabolites can accumulate that interfere with the function of the cell membranes, protein synthesis, and the cellular DNA/RNA itself. Cell energy production is adversely affected, which accelerates the aging process. The vitamins C and E, among many other antioxidants, are thought to protect against the destructive effects of free radicals by donating one of their electrons to end the cascading reaction. These nutrients are stable even in this state. In effect, they act as scavengers, helping to protect against

cell and tissue damage. Denham Harman, M.D., Ph.D., Professor Emeritus at the University of Nebraska, is considered the founder of the free radical theory of aging. He postulated that many of the degenerative disorders we associate with aging, including cancer and hardening of the arteries, are not inevitable results of the passage of time, but rather are the result of the breakdown of nucleic acids, proteins, and cell structures caused by the presence of free radicals. (*See* ANTIOXIDANTS in Part One.) One study showed that oxidation to DNA can be mitigated in elderly subjects who take one multivitamin each day. This indicates that the regular diet does not always supply the right mix of nutrients to reduce oxidative damage, and that supplementation, especially in the elderly, is warranted.

- *Cross-linking theory.* During normal metabolism, sugars such as glucose or fructose and reactive compounds known as aldehydes and ketones may attach to free amino groups on proteins. This process is called *glycation* and the protein is then saddled with sugar molecules. This protein then can react, or "cross-link," with other proteins to cause a bond between the two. The resulting so-called carbonyl groups act as a glue to attach the two proteins. Carbonyls are formed when either a sugar or free radical (or an aldehyde or ketone) reacts with amino acids on a protein. It is possible to have not only protein-protein cross-linking, but also protein-lipid and protein-DNA cross-linking. This cross-linking results in large aggregates of damaged proteins within the tissues, called advanced glycosylation end products (AGEs). These may go on to react with free radicals to cause tissue damage through oxidation, they inhibit certain cellular processes, they can be mutagenic (cancer-causing), and they stimulate cells to produce even more damaging free radicals. AGEs also act to accelerate cell death. Thus, treatment to both inhibit cross-linking and to reverse it, if possible, should be beneficial in combating the aging process.

- *Immune theory.* The immune system gradually gets less effective as we age. For instance, the thymus gland, which is responsible for the production of thymic lymphoid, or T cells, can decrease its function by up to 80 percent as we reach our middle years. As we age, the immune system is less able to produce the antibodies, macrophages, natural killer (NK) cells, and others that the body needs to fight off infections and other assaults from the outside. There is also an increased tendency to produce antibodies against the body itself—the autoimmune response, which is responsible for a host of autoimmune diseases.

- *Telomere theory.* Cells in the body are replaced by means of cell division, and there is a limit to the number of times they may divide successfully. That is, most cells normally divide approximately fifty times before they stop dividing and die a natural death. It is theorized that the mechanism that controls this cell division lies with the telomere, which is a caplike structure on the end of each of the twenty-three pairs of chromosomes. Chromosomes are the helical structures of DNA that are found in all cell nuclei that carry our genetic code. Every time a cell divides, the telomere shortens up a bit. This constant shortening of the telomere means that after a certain number of divisions the telomere disappears, and the end of the chromosome begins to fray and stop dividing. This leads eventually to the death of the cell. Over time, this cumulative cell death leads to aging. However, an enzyme called telomerase has been discovered. This enzyme acts to repair damage to the telomere, and helps to maintain its length and stability. The theory is that by using telomerase, we may be able to prolong cell life and slow down or even reverse the aging process. For now, we know that certain controllable factors—smoking, obesity, low vitamin D levels, and stress—hasten telomere attrition. Diseases such as heart disease and diabetes also speed up telomere shortening, but this process is slowed with good medical management such as by keeping blood cholesterol and blood sugar close to normal levels.

- *Stem cell theory.* This theory holds that as we age, we begin losing stem cells from the reserve we are granted at birth. This also means that the body's ability to repair and generate tissues is diminished, and we accumulate more and more dysfunctional cells as time passes. Aging is simply the accumulation of these dysfunctional cells, and the damage they cause to skin, organs, the immune system, the muscles, and every other system in the body can only be undone by the addition of new stem cells.

- *Cell metabolic theory.* Nutrition has an effect on the rate at which cells divide (*see* Telomere Theory, above). Caloric restriction has been shown in one animal study to increase life span by affecting the cell division rate. In another study, it was concluded that caloric restriction primarily slowed the aging process by an associated decrease in oxygen free radicals produced by the mitochondria (the energy-generating structures within the cells). No human studies have been conducted to date, but cultural/anthropological data indicates a possible link.

Whatever theory of aging ultimately proves to be correct, and probably there are a number of factors which, in combination, will eventually be found to have a profound effect, it is unquestionably true that a significant number of problems faced by people over the age of sixty may also be attributable to nutritional deficiencies. Many elderly people have malabsorption problems, in which the nutrients in food are not properly absorbed from the gastrointestinal tract. In addition, as we age, our bodies do not assimilate nutrients as well as they once did. At the same time, as the body ages, its systems slow down and become less efficient, so the correct nutrients are more important than ever for the support, repair, and regeneration of the cells.

There are many disorders associated with an inability to absorb nutrients successfully. One study of older people living in an urban area found that 90 percent of those examined had an inadequate intake of vitamins B_1 (thiamine) and B_6 (pyridoxine), and 30 to 40 percent demonstrated deficiencies of vitamin A, vitamin B_3 (niacin), vitamin B_{12}, vitamin C, calcium, and iron. Low blood levels of selenium and total carotenoids such as beta-carotene predicted early death. Only 10 percent of the subjects consumed adequate amounts of protein. Many Americans in nursing homes and other confined environments are deprived of sunlight, making them deficient in vitamin D. A diet that lacks essential nutrients over a long period of time leads to a greater risk of degenerative disease, heart disease, and some forms of cancer.

Vitamin B_{12} deficiency is a particular problem. A lack of vitamin B_{12} can lead to the development of neurological symptoms ranging from tingling sensations, inability to coordinate muscular movements, weakened limbs, and lack of balance to memory loss, mood changes, disorientation, and psychiatric disorders. Symptoms of vitamin B_{12} deficiency can easily be misinterpreted as signs of senility. Folic acid is also related to the level of cognition in the elderly. Low folate levels were indicators of cognitive decline with aging and could contribute to the development of Alzheimer's disease. Vitamin E is an important nutrient, but in one study, at doses of 300 IU per day, it did not have an effect on memory in elderly women. It is possible that this amount was too low to create a benefit.

Many older people become deficient in vitamin B_{12} because they do not produce adequate amounts of stomach acid for proper digestion. This creates a perfect environment for the overgrowth of certain bacteria that steal whatever vitamin B_{12} is extracted from protein in the digestive tract. Other people do not produce enough of a substance called intrinsic factor, without which vitamin B_{12} cannot travel from the stomach to the rest of the body, even if nothing else is standing in its way.

One can have vitality and a zest for living at any age. You should not assume that pain and illness are inevitable parts of aging. You can feel better at sixty than you did at thirty by making healthy changes in your diet and lifestyle.

Adding the right supplements should give you the added power needed to boost immunity and prevent or cure most disorders—not to mention making you able to work or play longer than people much younger than you are. Looking youthful for your age is an added bonus. But remember: It takes years for these problems to develop, so it usually takes some time to resolve them as well. There are no silver bullets or magic potions, only the simple fact that if you give your body the correct fuel, it will perform for you and ward off illness. Supplements work best in combination with a nutrient-rich diet that contains plenty of protein and regular exercise. Elderly people have been shown to benefit from including pomegranate juice in their diet instead of apple juice for better antioxidant protection. In addition, those who included chocolate, wine, and tea performed better on tests of memory and cognition.

Most of the supplements listed below can be found in complexes containing many nutrients. Be sure to check the amounts of different nutrients in your multinutrient supplements, and either exclude individual nutrients or adjust the dosages, as appropriate. For best absorption of nutrients, use as many sublingual, liquid, and powdered supplements as possible. It makes sense for older adults to use nutrients in drink form, but there are many good supplements in powder and liquid forms as well.

Unless otherwise specified, the dosages recommended in this section are for adults.

NUTRIENTS

SUPPLEMENT	SUGGESTED DOSAGE	COMMENTS
Essential		
Alpha-lipoic acid	As directed on label.	A powerful antioxidant. Aids proper blood sugar balance (diabetes) and liver function.
Super Carnosine	500–1,000 mg daily, or per health care practitioner's advice	Offers protection against glycation (cross-linking) that creates AGEs. Also available in combination with vitamin B$_1$, benfotiamine, and luteolin from Life Extension.
Coenzyme A from Coenzyme-A Technologies	As directed on label.	Supports the immune system's detoxification of many dangerous substances.
Coenzyme Q$_{10}$	100 mg daily.	Aids circulation, improves cellular oxygenation, and protects the heart.
Dimethylglycine (DMG) (Aangamik DMG from Food Science of Vermont)	As directed on label.	Improves cellular oxygenation. Use a sublingual form.
Glutathione	500 mg daily, on an empty stomach.	A potent free radical scavenger and mental booster that acts as a mood elevator. Also destroys ammonia, which interferes with brain function.
Inositol hexaphosphate (IP$_6$) from Enzymatic Therapy or Jarrow Formulas	As directed on label.	A powerful antioxidant that has many benefits (*see under* NATURAL FOOD SUPPLEMENTS in Part One).
L-arginine and L-carnitine and L-lysine and L-methionine and L-ornithine and L-tyrosine plus	500 mg each twice daily, on an empty stomach. Take with water or juice. Do not take with milk. Take with 50 mg vitamin B$_6$ and 100 mg vitamin C for better absorption. It is best to take a complex containing all the amino acids as well (but separately).	*See* AMINO ACIDS in Part One for the benefits of amino acids. Do not take single amino acids for longer than 2 months at a time. To avoid creating imbalances, alternate taking them for a month and then stopping for a month. Protects the heart and liver; decreases blood triglycerides; enhances the effectiveness of antioxidants; improves muscle strength and brain function.
N-acetylcysteine	500 mg twice daily, on an empty stomach.	Attaches to heavy metals such as lead and mercury and removes them from the body. Also enhances brain function. Used by the body to produce glutathione, a powerful antioxidant and detoxifier.
Liquid Kyolic with B$_1$ and B$_{12}$ from Wakunaga	As directed on label.	An excellent cell protector. *See under* ANTIOXIDANTS and NATURAL FOOD SUPPLEMENTS in Part One for its many benefits.
Multivitamin and mineral complex with vitamin A and	15,000 IU daily.	All nutrients are needed. Use a high-potency formula with chelated trace minerals. Important antioxidants. Protect the lungs. Needed for growth and repair of body tissues. Promotes smooth skin.
natural beta-carotene and all the carotenoids and	25,000 IU daily.	
potassium and	99–200 mg daily.	Plays a role in cellular integrity and water balance. Prevents premature aging, boosts immunity, protects against cancer and heart disease.
selenium and	300 mcg daily.	
zinc	50 mg daily. Do not exceed a total of 100 mg daily from all supplements.	Needed for wound healing and healthy skin. Enhances immune function.
Omega-3 essential fatty acids (flaxseed oil, primrose oil, salmon oil, and Ultra Omega-3 Fish Oil from Health From The Sun are good sources)	As directed on label 3 times daily, with meals.	Plays an important role in cell formation. Essential for proper brain function. Protects the heart and helps keep plaque from adhering to the arteries.
Pycnogenol or grape seed extract	50 mg twice daily. As directed on label.	Possibly the most powerful free radical scavengers. They can pass through the blood-brain barrier to protect brain cells from free radical damage.
Superoxide dismutase (SOD) or	As directed on label.	A potent antioxidant that destroys free radicals, which damage body cells and cause premature aging. Consider injections (under a doctor's supervision).
Cell Guard from Biotec Foods	As directed on label.	An antioxidant complex containing SOD.
Taurine Plus from American Biologics	As directed on label.	A building block for all amino acids that improves white blood cell function. Use the sublingual form.
Vitamin B complex plus extra pantothenic acid (vitamin B$_5$) and choline and inositol and para-aminobenzoic acid (PABA)	50–100 mg of each major B vitamin 3 times daily, with meals (amounts of individual vitamins in a complex will vary). If you use sublingual forms, you need less. Follow label directions. 50 mg 3 times daily. 50 mg 3 times daily. 50 mg 3 times daily. 50 mg 3 times daily.	The B vitamins fight depression; aid in transforming proteins, fats, and carbohydrates into energy. Necessary for the formation of certain proteins and for the functioning of the nervous system. Essential for healthy red blood cells and the absorption of nutrients, including iron. Injections (under a doctor's supervision) are best. If injections are not available, use sublingual forms.

Vitamin B₃ (niacinamide)	50–100 mg 3 times daily.	Important in proper functioning of the nervous system. A vasodilator that protects the heart and body cells. *Caution:* Do not substitute niacin for niacinamide. Niacin can be toxic in such high doses.
Vitamin C with bioflavonoids	4,000–10,000 mg daily, in divided doses.	A powerful antioxidant and immune system enhancer that reduces allergies, protects the brain and spinal cord, keeps white blood cells healthy, fights fatigue, and increases energy.
Vitamin E	Start with 100 IU daily and slowly increase to 200 IU daily. If you take blood-thinning medication, consult your physician before increasing the dose.	A potent antioxidant that fights cellular aging by protecting cell membranes. Also improves circulation and prolongs the life of red blood cells. Use d-alpha-tocopherol form.

Very Important

Boron	3–6 mg daily. Do not exceed this amount.	Aids calcium absorption and brain function.
Calcium	1,500–2,000 mg daily.	Necessary to prevent bone loss and for normal heart function. Use calcium chelate or calcium asporotate form.
and magnesium	750 mg daily.	Needed to balance with calcium for correct muscle and heart function.
and vitamin D or	600–1,000 mg daily.	Enhances calcium absorption and bone formation.
Bone Defense from KAL	As directed on label.	Contains calcium, magnesium, phosphorus, and other valuable bone-reinforcing nutrients.
Chromium picolinate	400–1,000 mcg daily.	Improves insulin efficiency, which maintains the health of the glands that control aging.
5-Hydroxy L-tryptophan (5-HTP) (Natural Balance is a good source)	As directed on label.	An important neurotransmitter.
Free form amino acid (Amino Balance from Anabol Naturals)	As directed on label 3 times daily. Take with 50 mg vitamin B₆ and 100 mg vitamin C for better absorption.	To supply needed protein. Older adults often have difficulty assimilating dietary protein, and so are likely to have amino acid deficiencies.
Lecithin granules or capsules	1 tbsp 3 times daily, with meals. 1,200 mg 3 times daily, with meals.	Improves brain function and memory. Protects nervous system cells. A fat emulsifier.
Phosphatidylserine	1,000 mg 3 times daily.	Improves brain function.
RNA and DNA	As directed on label.	Good for healthy cell reproduction. Use a sublingual form. *Caution:* Do not take this supplement if you have gout.

Helpful

Acidophilus	As directed on label.	To improve liver function and aid in digestion by replacing bowel flora.
Benfotiamine	150–600 mg daily, or as recommended by health care practitioner.	Protects against diabetic neuropathy or retinopathy. This fat-soluble form of

		vitamin B₁ lasts longer in the body and is less toxic than the water-soluble form. Blocks absorption of excess glucose into cells. *Caution:* Do not use if you are pregnant or nursing.
Dehydroepiandrosterone (DHEA)	As directed on label. Women should not take more than 15 mg daily except under medical supervision.	Studies show it slows the aging process. (*See under* NATURAL FOOD SUPPLEMENTS in Part One.)
Dimethylglycine (DMG)	As directed on label.	Boosts mental energy, enhances the immune system. (*See under* NATURAL FOOD SUPPLEMENTS in Part One.)
Glucosamine sulfate or N-Acetylglucosamine (N-A-G from Source Naturals) plus chondroitin	As directed on label. As directed on label. As directed on label.	Important for the formation of bones, skin, nails, connective tissues, and heart valves; also plays a role in the mucous secretions of the digestive, respiratory, and urinary tracts.
Lutein	As directed on label.	Protects the retinas from macular degeneration, the leading cause of blindness in older adults.
Melatonin or	1.5–5 mg daily, taken 2 hours or less before bedtime.	Delays the aging process and improves sleep. Good for many disorders associated with aging.
ChronoSet from Allergy Research Group	As directed on label.	Contains melatonin.
Multienzyme complex with pancreatin and ox bile (Digestive Aid #34 from Carlson Labs)	As directed on label, after meals.	To aid digestion. Most older adults lack sufficient digestive enzymes. *Caution:* If you have a history of ulcers, do not use a formula containing HCl.
Raw thymus glandular	500 mg daily.	Enhances the immune system.
S-adenosylmethionine (SAMe)	As directed on label.	Aids in reducing stress and depression, giving a sense of well-being. *Caution:* Do not use if you have bipolar mood disorder or take prescription antidepressants.
Silica (Jarrosil from Jarrow Formulas or Body Essential Silica from NatureWorks)	As directed on label.	Protects connective tissues and cells; keeps skin, bones, hair, nails, and other tissues youthful.
Zinc plus copper	50 mg daily. Do not exceed a total of 100 mg daily from all supplements. 3 mg daily.	Increases antibodies and protects the eyes against macular degeneration and vision loss. Very important for the prostate. Needed to balance with zinc.

Herbs

❑ Astragalus and echinacea help to boost the immune system.

Cautions: Do not use astragalus in the presence of a fever. Do not take echinacea for longer than three months. It should not be used by people who are allergic to ragweed.

❑ Bilberry and ginseng are good for giving extra energy, improving brain function, increasing circulation, and promoting better blood flow to supply oxygen to the cells. Bilberry also protects the eyes.

Caution: Do not use ginseng if you have high blood pressure, or are pregnant or nursing.

❑ Burdock root and red clover cleanse the bloodstream. They can be used separately or in combination.

❑ Dandelion and milk thistle promote good liver function and bile flow.

❑ Garlic helps immune function and protects the heart.

❑ Ginkgo biloba has powerful antioxidant properties and increases the supply of oxygen to the brain cells, enhancing brain function.

Caution: Do not take ginkgo biloba if you have a bleeding disorder, or are scheduled for surgery or a dental procedure.

❑ Green tea aids in cancer prevention and is a powerful antioxidant.

Caution: Green tea contains vitamin K, which can make anticoagulant medications less effective. Consult your health care professional if you are using them. The caffeine in green tea could cause insomnia, anxiety, upset stomach, nausea, or diarrhea.

❑ Noni (*Morinda citrifolia*) is a plant that grows in Hawaii. Its fruit has many health benefits and has been used for thousands of years to ease pain and inflammation, relieve joint problems, promote cellular regeneration, boost the immune system, and improve digestion. Earth's Bounty NONI is a good source of this herb.

❑ Kava kava, St. John's wort, and valerian root are valuable as sleep aids and tranquilizers. St. John's wort is also a natural antidepressant.

Cautions: Kava kava can cause drowsiness. It is not recommended for pregnant women or nursing mothers, and it should not be taken together with other substances that act on the central nervous system, such as alcohol, barbiturates, antidepressants, and antipsychotic drugs. St. John's wort may cause increased sensitivity to sunlight. It may also produce anxiety, gastrointestinal symptoms, and headaches. It can interact with some drugs including antidepressants, birth control pills, and anticoagulants.

❑ Licorice root is an effective anti-inflammatory and antiallergenic agent that supports the organ systems.

Caution: Licorice root should not be used during pregnancy or nursing. It should not be used by persons with diabetes, glaucoma, heart disease, high blood pressure, or a history of stroke.

❑ Nettle is full of vital minerals and is good for hypoglycemia, allergies, arthritis, depression, prostate and urinary tract disorders, and a host of other problems.

❑ Saw palmetto aids in preventing cancer and, for men, in improving benign (noncancerous) prostate enlargement. It inhibits the production of dihydrotestosterone, a hormone that contributes to enlargement of the prostate.

❑ Wild yam contains natural steroids that have a rejuvenating effect. Steroids are what help exercise to melt off more weight and build muscle. This hormone is found in the human body as dehydroepiandrosterone (DHEA). Take larger amounts—2,400 mg daily, dropping to 1,600 mg daily—for two weeks, then stop for two weeks.

Recommendations

❑ Eat a balanced diet that includes raw vegetables, fruits, grains, seeds, nuts, and quality protein such as fish and soy foods. Consume less animal protein. Include in your diet broccoli, cabbage, cauliflower, spinach, kale, fish, fruits, whole grains, nuts, oats, seeds, and soybeans. Avoid processed foods.

❑ Eat dark-skinned fruits such as red apples and nectarines, which are good sources of bioflavonoids. The skin contains the bioflavonoids, so leave it on. Red Delicious and McIntosh apples have the most bioflavonoids in the skin, the Northern Spy has the most in its flesh. Fuji apples have the highest overall.

❑ Eat blueberries, raspberries, and blackberries regularly. Wild blueberries contain more bioflavonoids than domestic varieties. Bioflavonoids found in most fruits and vegetables keep free radicals from harming the brain and may help protect against Alzheimer's disease.

❑ Black, green, and orange pekoe teas all contain bioflavonoids called catechins. Green tea contains the most epigallocatechin-3-gallate, an antioxidant effective in preventing degenerative brain disease.

Caution: Green tea contains vitamin K, which can make anticoagulant medications less effective. Consult your health care professional if you are using them. The caffeine in green tea could cause insomnia, anxiety, upset stomach, nausea, or diarrhea.

❑ Eat 80 to 100 grams of protein a day, meting it out evenly at three meals and two to three snacks. Protein, along with exercise, is important to prevent muscle wasting. Sarcopenia is a disease of muscle wasting that leads to profound weakness and ennui, and affects elderly people who do not consume adequate protein or get enough exercise. Sarcopenia is becoming a more prevalent condition as people live longer.

❑ Consume four or five small meals daily.

❑ A low-calorie diet is best for maintaining good health as you age. Eat only when you are hungry, and consume foods that are fresh and cooked in a fashion that maintains their nutritional content. A diet too high in carbohydrates may increase glucose levels (*see* DIABETES in Part Two). Decrease your overall food consumption, but increase your intake of raw foods.

❑ Avoid gaining and losing weight, which can result in the loss of lean tissue (or muscle). The loss of lean muscle tissue in the elderly could precipitate sarcopenia. However, excess body fat increases the risk of heart disease and diabetes, especially in the elderly, and weight loss will reduce these risks. If you are over sixty years of age and are advised to trim down, lose no more than six to nine pounds over one to one and a third years to avoid losing too much lean body mass.

❑ Consume steam-distilled water. Drink even when you don't feel thirsty—your body needs plenty of water. Dehydration has been identified as one of the most frequent causes of hospitalization among people over the age of sixty-five, according to a recent study published in the *American Journal of Public Health.* Common symptoms of dehydration include fatigue; headache; dry nasal passages; dry, cracked lips; and overall discomfort.

❑ Include in your diet garlic, onions, shiitake mushrooms, and pearl barley. These foods are good sources of germanium, potassium, and many other nutrients that lessen free radical damage and act as catalysts in the supply of oxygen to oxygen-poor tissue.

❑ An occasional glass of red wine is good for the heart, but limit your alcohol consumption otherwise.

❑ Cut back on salt.

❑ Avoid saturated fats.

❑ Avoid caffeine, red meat, white flour, white sugar, chemical food additives, drugs, pesticides, and tap water.

❑ Get regular exercise. Exercise is most important in slowing the aging process because it increases the amount of oxygen available to body tissues, a key determinant of energy and stamina. Brisk walking and stretching exercises are good. Swimming is even better because it provides low-impact exercise and exerts no pressure on the joints. For those with arthritic conditions, swimming is the ideal way to exercise. Exercise can ward off conditions such as arthritis, cardiovascular disease, diabetes, and osteoporosis, and because it releases endorphins into the body, exercise can also help overcome depression. Our brains need exercise as much as our bodies do. Bodily exercise increases the supply of oxygen to the brain. Studies have found that no matter how old you are—whether you are in your sixties, seventies, eighties, or even in your nineties—you can rebuild muscle. Science has found that brain cells do not die as we age if we keep our minds active. Hobbies, reading, and acquiring new skills exercise the brain and help prevent memory loss. If you don't currently exercise, start walking and build up to thirty minutes a day. The goal is to eventually be getting one hour of moderate exercise a couple of times a week. Some elderly people have found that the dietary supplement creatine increases muscle mass when coupled with exercise. In one study, people taking 20 grams of creatine a day experienced increased strength, power, and lower-body motor function performance in just seven days. Others found that taking 20 grams of creatine improved long-term memory. Even small amounts—about 3 grams a day—helped build muscle.

❑ Improve your blood's oxygenation and circulation with deep breathing exercises. Try holding your breath for thirty seconds every half hour. Inhale and hold for thirty seconds, then place your tongue on the roof of your mouth where your teeth meet your gums and release the air slowly. Repeat this exercise every day.

❑ Keep the colon clean. This is crucial for warding off degenerative diseases and slowing the aging process. Eat a high-fiber diet and use a cleansing enema once weekly. (*See* ENEMAS in Part Three.) Get extra fiber by eating plenty of fresh vegetables, whole grains, bran, and oats. Consider retention enemas, a potent way to assure that your body will assimilate and use needed nutrients.

❑ Learn how to relax. Keep active and be enthusiastic about life. By keeping up your appearance, exercising every day, and being involved in hobbies and other activities, you can keep your mind active. This is most important.

❑ Allow yourself sufficient sleep. Proper rest is important.

❑ Do not use harsh soaps on your skin. Use olive, avocado, or almond oil to cleanse the skin. Pat the oil on, then wash it off with warm water and a soft cloth. Use a facial loofah occasionally with the oil and warm water to remove dead skin. Use liquid creams and lotions (not solid creams) that contain nutrients and natural ingredients to keep your skin from becoming too dry. Do not use cold creams, cleansing creams, or solid moisturizing creams. These are hardened saturated fats that become rancid rapidly and then create free radicals, which can cause premature wrinkles. Free radicals can cause the brownish spots on the skin known as age spots. (*See* AGE SPOTS in Part Two.) Exposing the skin to the sun also promotes free radicals. To halt wrinkles, stay out of the sun and use all-natural lotions or oils that contain nutrients and antioxidants.

❑ Don't smoke or overexpose yourself to harmful chemicals such as environmental pollutants.

Considerations

❑ Growing older is inevitable; however, we can try to slow the aging process and prolong our lives by taking measures to promote continuous cell division. If science could keep the cells from dying and doing bodily harm, the aging process could conceivably be suspended.

❑ Many older adults complain of sleep difficulties. One common cause is the consumption of sugar after dinner. Complex carbohydrates have a relaxing effect. A good nighttime snack is popcorn, or nut butter and crackers.

❏ Fatigue is a common, but not necessary, result of aging. Human growth hormone is available to increase muscle mass, which in turn boosts strength and energy. Published studies on the use of human growth hormone in elderly people have shown that there are too many side effects and not enough benefits to endorse its widespread use. However, if fatigue is a serious issue, some medical centers offer human growth hormone treatment. For natural management of fatigue, some elderly people have reported less physical and mental fatigue after taking acetyl L-carnitine—2 grams, twice a day.

❏ A burning sensation, mainly on the bottom of the feet, is not unusual among elderly people. A deficiency of the B vitamins, especially vitamin B_{12}, is often the cause. Since many older people have problems with absorption of the B vitamins, it is best to take supplements of these nutrients in a way that bypasses the digestive tract. Injections are best. Sublingual administration is also effective.

❏ The *American Journal of Clinical Nutrition* reported that up to 30 percent of people over the age of sixty-five are unable to absorb vitamin B_{12} and folic acid properly because they do not produce enough hydrochloric acid and/or they suffer from an overgrowth of bacteria in the intestinal tract.

❏ There are a number of substances available that have properties that make them "natural life extenders," such as the following:

• Coenzyme Q_{10} protects the heart, increases tissue oxygenation, and is vital for many bodily functions. The liver and heart muscle have the highest levels of coenzyme Q_{10} of tissue. Since the liver is the main detoxifying organ of the body, optimal liver function is vital for minimizing damage to all the body's tissues.

• Dimethylaminoethanol (DMAE) is beneficial for memory and mental ability, acting to increase alertness and focus. It may also enhance mood and vision.

• Dimethylglycine (DMG) is a derivative of the amino acid glycine. It boosts immune function and improves tissue oxygenation.

• Glutathione is an amino acid compound that is a valuable antioxidant and detoxifier. Cellular glutathione levels tend to drop by 30 to 35 percent with age; increasing glutathione, particularly in the liver, lungs, kidneys, and bone marrow, may have an antiaging effect. Glutathione can be taken in supplement form. Glutathione levels can also be increased by taking supplements of N-acetylcysteine, which is converted into glutathione in the body. (*See* AMINO ACIDS in Part One.)

• Human growth hormone (HGH or GH), also known as somatotropin, is the hormone that regulates growth. Administered to older adults, it rebuilds muscle mass and reduces the amount of fat tissue, reversing changes that occur with aging. It is available only under the supervision of a physician. (*See* GROWTH HORMONE THERAPY in Part Three.)

• Lipoic acid is critical in glycolysis and in the Kreb's cycle, two complex biochemical processes essential for the generation of cellular energy. The liver relies on these processes to meet its large energy demands. Lipoic acid is used extensively in Germany to enhance liver function and treat diabetes. It should be taken with acetyl L-carnitine for maximum effectiveness. Juvenon from Juvenon Inc. is a good source of both ingredients.

• Melatonin is a natural hormone that acts as an antioxidant. Early in life, the body produces an abundant supply, but as we age, production steadily declines. In one laboratory experiment, mice given melatonin lived almost one-third beyond normal life expectancy. Melatonin may also help prevent cancer, counteract insomnia, and boost immunity.

• Morel, reishi, shiitake, and maitake are mushrooms that were touted by the ancient Chinese as superior medicines that give eternal youth and longevity. They prevent high blood pressure and heart disease, lower cholesterol, prevent fatigue and viral infections, and much more. They are found in supplement form as well as fresh.

• Pantothenic acid (vitamin B_5) keeps hair healthy, with little graying, and prevents premature hair loss. It is also very important for normal adrenal and immune function.

• Para-aminobenzoic acid (PABA) is one of the B vitamins. It keeps skin healthy and delays wrinkles. In addition, the combination of PABA and dimethylaminoethanol (DMAE) has been found to enhance brain function, immunity, and cellular regeneration.

• Pregnenolone is a naturally occurring hormone that may improve brain function, enhancing mood, memory, and thinking ability. (*See under* NATURAL FOOD SUPPLEMENTS in Part One.)

• Pycnogenol is a powerful bioflavonoid and antioxidant.

• Superoxide dismutase (SOD) is an enzyme that is a powerful free radical scavenger that protects the cells.

• Vitamin B_{12} and vitamin D are nutrients essential for optimal health and brain function, but many elderly people are deficient in both. Unfortunately, they are not common in many foods, so supplementation is often needed. The elderly should have their blood levels tested.

❏ As people age falls are all too common. Older adults are more likely to have weak muscles, poor vision, weaker legs, decreased sensation, or other medical conditions that make them more likely to fall easily, and with more troublesome consequences. They are also more likely than younger people to take prescription medications, some of which can slow reflexes, decrease perception, and/or impair mobility—in so doing, increasing the danger of injury through an accidental fall. Physical injury is only one potential consequence of a fall for older adults, especially those who are frail to begin with. Recovery is often prolonged even after relatively minor falls, and this can lead to complications such as bedsores,

Selected Prevention and Screening Recommendations for Adults

One of the keys to staying healthy as we age is to practice preventive health care. In addition to adhering to a healthy diet and lifestyle, with appropriate nutritional supplementation, doctors recommend undergoing certain routine screening procedures. The following is a summary of recom-mendations for some of the most important medical tests. If you are at risk of any particular illness due to heredity or personal history, you should probably undergo testing more frequently to ensure that all is well. Ask your physician what he or she recommends in your particular case.

Test	Why It's Done	Who Should Be Tested	How Often
Blood cholesterol	To look for signs of cardiovascular disease.	Men and women forty and over.	Once every five years. If your tests show a high LDL (bad cholesterol) level, you may need more frequent testing. Also, a high triglyceride level may be predictive of future heart disease. Ask your physician.
Blood pressure	To check heart function.	Men and women over forty.	Every visit to the physician, or at least once a year.
Breast self-exam and physician breast exam and mammogram	To detect breast cancer.	Women thirty and over. Women thirty and over. Women forty and over (men can get breast cancer too, but it is so rare that routine screening is not done).	Once a month. Once a year.
Colonoscopy	To detect colorectal cancer.	Men and women fifty and over, earlier if there is a family history of the disease.	Once every three to five years after initial exam, or more often if recommended by physician.
Complete physical examination; may include complete blood count (CBC) and/or blood chemistry (Chem 7 [SMA7] or Chem 20 [SMA20])	To assess overall health. To check for anemia and leukemia. To check for liver dysfunction, thyroid problems, kidney function, and diabetes.	Men and women twenty and over.	From age twenty to thirty, once every five years. From age thirty to sixty, once every two years. Over age sixty, once annually.
Pap smear/pelvic examination	To test for cervical cancer and other reproductive problems.	Women eighteen and over, or younger if they become sexually active at an earlier age.	Once a year. After three consecutive negative tests, frequency may be decreased at physician's discretion.
PSA test and rectal examination	To look for signs of prostate cancer.	Men forty and over.	Once a year.
Stool guaiac test	To test for blood in the stool.	Men and women over forty.	Once a year.

In addition, doctors recommend that all adults receive a tetanus vaccine booster every ten years.

greater muscle weakness, and increased susceptibility to infection. Keeping physically active is important for maintaining strength and coordination, and is one of the best defenses against such accidental injuries. It is also important to discuss with your physician or pharmacist the possible side effects of any medications you are taking.

❑ Aging is not an illness, but it does increase one's chances of developing certain health problems. Constipation, depression, diarrhea, dizziness, heart palpitations, heartburn and indigestion, and weight gain are some of the more common complaints that accompany aging. Detailed information on the causes of and treatments for many problems that commonly affect older people may be found in the relevant sections of this book. *See* AGE SPOTS; ALZHEIMER'S DISEASE; APPETITE, POOR; ARTERIOSCLEROSIS/ATHEROSCLEROSIS; ARTHRITIS; BEDSORES; CANCER; CARDIOVASCULAR DISEASE; CIRCULATORY PROBLEMS; CONSTIPATION; DEPRESSION; DIABETES; EYE PROBLEMS; GLAUCOMA; HAIR LOSS; HEARING LOSS; HEART ATTACK; HIGH BLOOD PRESSURE; HIGH CHOLESTEROL; INDIGESTION; INSOMNIA; MEMORY PROBLEMS; MUSCLE CRAMPS; OBESITY; OSTEOPOROSIS; PROSTATITIS/ENLARGED PROSTATE; SENILITY; WEAKENED IMMUNE SYSTEM; and/or WRINKLES, all in Part Two.

❑ If you follow the suggestions in this section and do not feel a positive change in your energy level, *see* COLITIS; DIVERTICULITIS; and/or MALABSORPTION SYNDROME in Part Two.

AGNOSIA

See under RARE DISORDERS.

AIDS (ACQUIRED IMMUNODEFICIENCY SYNDROME)

AIDS is an immune system disorder in which the body's ability to defend itself is greatly diminished. When human immunodeficiency virus (HIV, the virus that causes AIDS) invades key white blood (immune) cells called T lymphocytes and multiplies, it causes a breakdown in the body's immune system, eventually leading to overwhelming infection and, ultimately, to death. AIDS used to be a series of various illnesses such as cancer, infections, and skin problems made possible by the initial HIV infection. Since the mid-1990s, medicines have become available to reduce the stress load of the virus, thereby reducing its affect on the body. Since its discovery in the early 1980s, AIDS has transformed from a death sentence to a chronic condition that requires regular medical management. Just about anything you want to know about AIDs and HIV is found on the National Institutes of Health (NIH) website (www.aidsinfo.nih.gov), and it is updated regularly. Worldwide, approximately 33 million people have HIV infection and AIDS, and 7,500 become infected each day. On average, life expectancy is shortened by twenty years, but people with less access to modern drug regimens have below average life spans, and those in wealthier nations, with greater access to medical care, live longer.

The origin of HIV is unknown, but it is closely related to a virus found in simians (monkeys). Whatever its origin, HIV is a type of virus known as a retrovirus that is spread primarily through sexual contact or blood-to-blood contact, such as occurs with the sharing of needles by intravenous drug users. It can also be spread by blood transfusion (now rare) or the use of blood products such as clotting factors, if the blood used for these purposes is infected. Hemophiliacs, who require a specific coagulation factor from blood concentrates, historically have been especially vulnerable to HIV. In the United States, as well as in many other parts of the world, blood is routinely screened for the presence of HIV antibodies, the warning sign of HIV infection. It is possible HIV-infected blood may occasionally pass through the careful screening processes. HIV antibodies may not appear in the blood for as many as three to six months after a person is infected, so their presence in blood taken from a person who contracted the virus recently may not be detectable. Blood products are now subjected to heat to destroy the virus, although some AIDS advocates raise concerns that this process may not be 100 percent effective. The chance of a blood donation having undetectable HIV is less than one in one million. You cannot get HIV from donating blood, as was once rumored.

It is possible for dentists and medical workers who come into close contact with the bodily fluids of infected persons to become infected under certain conditions. This is why paramedics, emergency medical technicians, dentists and dental hygienists, hospital and clinic employees, emergency room personnel, and law enforcement officers wear rubber gloves to prevent contact with blood products or saliva. The practice of wearing gloves and eyewear also protects patients.

Many people who are infected with HIV are not even aware that they have it. The U.S. Centers for Disease Control and Prevention (CDC) has estimated that one in five of the more than one million HIV-infected people in the United States are not aware that they are infected. While some people experience a mild flulike illness within two to four weeks of exposure to the virus, it may take at least two to five years before any symptoms of HIV infection appear. The virus does not lie dormant during this time, however. Instead, it immediately attacks the immune system.

The virus quickly begins producing a billion copies of itself each day, which in turn forces the human immune system to produce the same number of antibodies as an attempted defense against the intruders. Year after year, the body struggles to beat the virus until finally, its overworked immune system simply wears out and AIDS results. The novelty of the virus is that it lives in the immune cells called T cells, which are your body's only defense against the disease. When the T cells are compromised, it's nearly impossible for the body to fight off the virus.

In many cases, the first symptoms of HIV and AIDS are nonspecific and variable. One of the most common is a tongue coated with white bumps. This is oral thrush, or candidiasis. Candidiasis indicates a compromised immune system. Intestinal parasites are another common problem.

Other possible symptoms include:

- Prolonged, unexplained fatigue.

- Swollen glands (lymph nodes).

- Unexplained fever lasting more than ten days.

- Excessive sweating (especially at night).

- Mouth lesions, including thrush and painful, swollen gums.

- Sore throat.

- Cough.

- Shortness of breath.

- Changes in bowel habits, including constipation.

- Frequent diarrhea.

- Symptoms of a specific opportunistic infection.

- Tumor (Kaposi's sarcoma).

- Skin rashes or lesions of various types.

- Unintentional weight loss.

- General discomfort or uneasiness (malaise).

- Headache.

Additional symptoms that may be associated with HIV and/or AIDS include speech impairment, memory loss, joint swelling, joint pain, bone pain or tenderness, a lump or lumps in the groin, blurred vision, genital sores, muscle atrophy, decreasing intellectual function, joint stiffness, unusual or strange behavior, anxiety, stress, tension, pruritus (generalized itching), sensitivity to light, decreased vision or blindness, blind spots in the field of vision, and chest pain.

No one should assume he or she is infected with HIV just because he or she has one or more of the above symptoms, however. These symptoms can be related to many illnesses, so being tested for HIV is the only way to be sure. This can be done by a doctor or with a home HIV testing kit. Simple to perform, this test requires a very small blood sample, obtained by pricking a fingertip. The sample is mailed to a laboratory, which analyzes it and offers a diagnosis by telephone in a matter of days. Each test is identified by a code number (no personal information is attached to any sample), so the test and the results are completely confidential.

To date, the FDA has approved only one home test kit, the Express HIV-1 Test System from Home Access Health Corporation (*see* Manufacturer and Distributor Information in the Appendix). Beware of fraudulent or unproven home HIV test kits. Doctors say if a kit claims to provide "instant" test results through a visual indicator such as a colored dot on a piece of paper after saliva has been applied, the outcome may be unreliable. If you believe you have used a questionable test kit, contact your doctor for another test or use the approved test kit.

Further, testing HIV-positive does not mean that one has AIDS. Rather, it means that one has been exposed to HIV, as demonstrated by the presence in the blood of antibodies to the virus. However, a confirmed positive HIV test result is often the earliest indication that the person may eventually develop AIDS. The medical criteria for a diagnosis of full-blown AIDS are quite specific, requiring the presence of one or more opportunistic infections or cancers known to be associated with HIV infection. According to the CDC, these include:

- *Pneumoncystis carinii* pneumonia.

- Candidal esophagitis, esophagitis from herpes simplex, or cytomegalovirus.

- Cryptosporidiosis of the intestine for more than four weeks.

- Primary lymphoma of the central nervous system.

- Kaposi's sarcoma.

- Herpes simplex ulcers, extensive in location, lasting for more than one month.

- Toxoplasmosis of the brain.

The risk of developing AIDS is proportional to the degree of immune suppression and the amount and duration of exposure to HIV.

HIV is highly adaptable and capable of changing its form. According to scientists at Oxford University in England, this may be the key to its survival. They say that through subtle mutations, or changes in its genetic structure, HIV evades and ultimately defuses the body's mechanisms for the elimination of infected cells. As a result, it continues to survive despite the immune system's aggressive attacks. If you suspect you have HIV, get tested immediately and begin treatment at once if necessary, because the earlier treatment is started the longer the life expectancy with fewer complications.

In 2007 there were 3,792 children under thirteen years of age living with AIDS in the United States. The vast major-

Risk Factors for AIDS

Since the beginning of the epidemic in the 1980s, several health conditions and lifestyle factors have been identified that increase an individual's risk of contracting HIV and developing AIDS. The more factors present, the greater the risk. They include the following:

- Male to male sexual contact
- High-risk heterosexual contact
- Injection drug use.

Women and AIDS

Seventy-five percent of people with AIDS in the United States are male. Women account for one out of every four new cases, and of these newly infected women, about two out of three are African American. AIDS is now the leading cause of death for African American women age twenty-five to thirty-four, and they are more than twenty-one times as likely to die from HIV/AIDS as non-Hispanic white women. Most women contract HIV through sex with a man who is infected. Today, AIDS in the fifth leading cause of death for women age thirty-five to forty-four. The following are steps you can take to protect yourself:

- Use latex condoms anytime you have sex, whether vaginal, oral, or anal.
- If you use drugs and cannot or will not stop injecting drugs, use new, sterile syringes to prepare and inject drugs.
- If you are getting a tattoo or having your body pierced, ask what procedures they use to combat the spread of HIV. If they do not use new, sterilized, or disinfected equipment, go somewhere else.

ity of these children acquired the virus from their mothers during pregnancy, labor, delivery, or breast-feeding. A pregnant woman can take medicine to lower the chance of giving her baby HIV, but research shows that only 33 percent of pregnant women with HIV take the drugs.

The optimal treatment of AIDS is called HAART (Highly Active Antiretroviral Therapy). HAART is made up of a combination of several different kinds of medicines. It is an aggressive therapy used to suppress the replication of the HIV virus and the progression of HIV disease. The reason that there are so many drug options is that the virus has mutated over the years and has become stronger and more difficult to treat. Patients with HIV/AIDS may get any of a number of drug combinations depending upon the physician's assessment. The virus gets attacked in a variety of ways using HAART. Viral loads are a measure of how active an impact the virus has in the body. Basically, HAART tries to outsmart a very smart virus. The drugs that may be used in HAART are:

- Nucleoside reverse transcriptase inhibitors (NRTIs)
- Non-nucleoside reverse transcriptase inhibitors (NNRTIs)
- Protease inhibitors (PIs)
- Fusion inhibitors
- Integrase inhibitors
- Entry inhibitors
- Combination drugs

After being diagnosed, patients usually start off with one NNRTI and two NRTIs, or with PIs and two NRTIs, but it is best to leave it to a physician to choose the best drugs for your individual case. If you experience side effects from one of the drugs, such as stomach pain, diarrhea, or both, tell your doctor as soon as possible so that a new one can be substituted. Once you are on HAART, it is important to stay on the medications. Since HAART was introduced, the death rate from non-HIV-related causes exceeded those caused directly by AIDS. Non-AIDS-related deaths in those thirteen years of age and older increased by 33 percent, while AIDS-related deaths decreased by 60 percent. Now the major cause of death in the United States is heart disease, non-AIDS-related cancer, and substance abuse.

Before HAART, many HIV/AIDS patients had difficulty absorbing nutrients from food and supplements and often appeared malnourished. This is not a concern with HAART. Instead HAART often leads to obesity, an increased risk of heart disease, and diabetes. Patients taking the HAART medications are also at risk of developing metabolic syndrome, which is common in patients with diabetes and heart disease. Metabolic syndrome is defined by having three of the following conditions: high blood sugar, high insulin, high cholesterol levels, high blood pressure, and abdominal obesity. In a three-hundred-patient study conducted in the greater Boston area, 13 percent of men and 29 percent of women with AIDS were obese. These obese HIV patients had lower essential micronutrient intakes than those patients of normal weight. Thus, despite eating more calories, the nutrient content of those calories was poor. What is interesting is that calorie needs are greater for HIV-positive patients compared to those without the virus. Patients with the virus need about 100 more calories per day. However, the Boston study underscores the fact that the calories consumed should come from high-quality, nutrient-dense foods.

Many patients taking HAART develop HIV lipodystrophy, which is characterized by abdominal fat, regional areas around the body of fat pads, and profound metabolic abnormalities like low good cholesterol (HDL), high triglycerides, and malfunctioning insulin (or insulin resistance). These factors predispose HIV patients to heart disease.

Because of the issues discussed above, people with HIV/AIDS are good candidates for supplementation. Multivitamins have been shown to delay the progression of HIV disease. Many of the nutrients listed below can be found in combination formulas. A high-potency multivitamin and mineral supplement should be included as well. Be sure to check the amounts of different nutrients in the complex you choose against those in the table below. Make sure that the supplement contains at least the DRI for vitamin A with beta-carotene, a B-complex with folate, and vitamins C and E. In studies, these were most likely to reduce the progression of the disease. The treatment of HIV/AIDS has come a long way in recent years. In this new edition we have fine-tuned the list of supplements to create a complementary regimen for people who are responding well to the new treatment protocols.

Unless otherwise specified, the dosages recommended in this section are for adults. For a child between the ages of twelve and seventeen, reduce the dose to three-quarters the recommended amount. Adolescents especially have been shown to have poor nutrient intakes, especially of vitamins A, E, and C, and the minerals zinc and iron. For a child between six and twelve, use one-half the recommended dose, and for a child under the age of six, use one-quarter of the recommended amount.

All ingested substances pose a threat to the way HIV/AIDS drugs are tolerated. If you are having trouble with your medications, stop any herbal or supplement use until the issue is resolved. It is more important to take the medications than the herbs or supplements.

NUTRIENTS

SUPPLEMENT	SUGGESTED DOSAGE	COMMENTS
Very Important		
Acetyl-L-carnitine	As directed on label.	An energy carrier, metabolic facilitator, and cell membrane protector. Also protects the heart.
Body Language Super Antioxidant from OxyFresh	As directed on label.	Protects the body from free radical damage, environmental stresses, and pollutants.
Bone Support from Synergy Plus	As directed on label.	Contains minerals needed for better absorption of calcium.
Coenzyme Q10	100–200 mg daily.	Increases circulation and energy, and protects the heart. A powerful antioxidant and significant immune stimulant.
Garlic (Kyolic from Wakunaga)	2 capsules 3 times daily, with meals. Or place 1 dropperful of Kyolic liquid in a 6- to 8-ounce glass of distilled water.	A powerful immunostimulant that also aids in digestion, endurance, and strength. It is a natural antibiotic and is good for candida infections.
Glutathione	As directed on label, on an empty stomach.	Inhibits the formation of free radicals. Aids in red blood cell integrity and protects immune cells.
Kyo-Dophilus	As directed on label.	To supply essential friendly bacteria for the intestinal tract and liver function. Fights candida infection, often associated with HIV.
Kyo-Green from Wakunaga	As directed on label.	Supplies nutrients and chlorophyll needed for repair. Important in immune response.
Lycopene	As directed on label.	A strong cancer preventer.
Multivitamin/ Multimineral with trace elements including selenium, copper, chromium, and mangesium	As directed on label.	Nutrients are designed to support general health and wellness, in addition to supporting immune function. Use a high-potency, hypo-allergenic powdered form.
Natural carotenoid complex (Betatene)	As directed on label.	Powerful antioxidant, free radical scavenger, potential cancer fighter, and immune enhancer. Also protects against heart disease.
Pycnogenol and/or	As directed on label.	A unique bioflavonoid. A potent antioxidant and immune enhancer.
grape seed extract or	As directed on label.	One of the most potent antioxidants known. Protects the cells.
OPC Goldblend from Primary Source	As directed on label.	A combination of grape seed and pine bark extracts.
Quercetin plus	As directed on label.	Aids in preventing allergic reactions and increases immunity.
bromelain or	As directed on label. Take on an empty stomach.	Increases absorption of quercetin and aids in reducing inflammation.
Activated Quercetin from Source Naturals	As directed on label.	Contains quercetin plus bromelain and vitamin C.
S-adenosylmethio- nine (SAMe)	As directed on label.	Good for depression and chronic fatigue. *Caution:* Do not use if you have bipolar mood disorder or take prescription antidepressants. Do not give to a child under twelve.
Superoxide dismutase (SOD)	As directed on label.	Free radical scavenger needed for cell protection.
Taurine Plus from American Biologics	As directed on label.	An important antioxidant and immune regulator necessary for white blood cell activation and neurological function. Use liquid sublingual form.
Vitamin C	1,000–3,000 mg daily.	Strengthens the immune system. Use buffered powdered ascorbic acid or Ester-C with minerals.
Vitamin D	400 IU daily.	Necessary for proper immune function.
Vitamin E	600 IU daily.	A powerful antioxidant.
Helpful		
Acid-Ease from Enzymatic Therapy	As directed on label. Take with meals. Take between meals also if excess acid is a problem.	Contains pure plant enzymes that function in the breakdown and assimilation of foods.
Aerobic 07 from Aerobic Life Industries	9 drops in water 3 times daily.	For tissue oxygenation. Kills harmful bacteria and viruses.
Ultimate Oil from Nature's Secret	As directed on label.	Supplies essential fatty acids, a most important element of the diet.

Herbs

❑ Aloe vera contains carrisyn, which appears to inhibit the growth and spread of HIV. Take 2 cups twice daily. Use a pure, food-grade product. If diarrhea occurs, reduce the dosage.

❑ Astragalus boosts the immune system.

Caution: Do not use this herb if you have a fever.

❏ Black radish, dandelion root, and silymarin (milk thistle extract) protect and aid in repairing the liver, and also cleanse the bloodstream. The liver is the organ of detoxification and must function optimally. Use these extracts as directed on the product labels.

❏ Cat's claw enhances immune function, and has been shown to be helpful for people with AIDS and AIDS-related cancers. Cat's Claw Defense Complex from Source Naturals is a combination of cat's claw and other herbs, plus antioxidants such as beta-carotene, N-acetylcysteine, vitamin C, and zinc.

Caution: Do not use cat's claw during pregnancy.

❏ The seeds and peels of the Chinese cucumber inhibit cancer. The root is currently being used in AIDS research.

❏ ClearLungs from Ridgecrest Herbals is a Chinese herbal formula that is good for all lung disorders.

❏ Ginkgo biloba extract is good for the brain cells and circulation.

Caution: Do not take ginkgo biloba if you have a bleeding disorder, or are scheduled for surgery or a dental procedure.

❏ For mouth sores, place alcohol-free goldenseal extract on a piece of sterile gauze and apply the gauze between the lips and gums or to mouth sores before going to bed. Leave it on overnight. Sores and inflammation should heal in a few days with this treatment.

❏ Licorice and wild yam root are good for endocrine gland function.

Caution: Licorice root should not be used during pregnancy or nursing. It should not be used by persons with diabetes, glaucoma, heart disease, high blood pressure, or a history of stroke.

❏ Magnolia vine berries increase oxygen absorption and boost the immune system. They coordinate the activities of the internal organs and help control the balance of the body's physiological processes.

❏ Pau d'arco is a natural antibiotic and potentiates immune function. It is also a powerful antioxidant and is good for destroying candida in the colon.

❏ St. John's wort contains two substances, hypericin and pseudohypericin, that inhibit retroviral infections and could be useful in the treatment of AIDS.

Caution: St. John's wort may cause increased sensitivity to sunlight. It may also produce anxiety, gastrointestinal symptoms, and headaches. It can interact with some drugs including antidepressants, birth control pills, and anticoagulants.

❏ Siberian ginseng helps bronchial disorders and boosts energy.

Caution: Do not use this herb if you have hypoglycemia, high blood pressure, or a heart disorder.

❏ Echinacea is an immune stimulant, and should be avoided. In fact, it stimulates replication of T cells, which in turn enhances replication of the virus, according to Dr. Tieraona Low Dog, Director of the Fellowship at the Arizona Center for Integrative Medicine.

Caution: Do not take echinacea for longer than three months. It should not be used by people who are allergic to ragweed.

Recommendations

❏ If you test positive for HIV, arrange for repeat testing as soon as you can to rule out the possibility of a false-positive result. If the initial result is confirmed, immediately begin taking measures to boost your immune system. This is the single most important factor in disease prevention, and it is the best defense for the person with HIV. Your first step should be to obtain the necessary medications to reduce your viral load. In addition, correct diet, appropriate supplements, exercise, stress reduction, a proper environment, and a healthy mental outlook all play significant roles in keeping the immune system working adequately.

❏ Pay special attention to meeting your nutritional needs and requirements, and keep in mind that a higher than normal intake of nutrients will probably be necessary.

❏ Increase your intake of fresh fruits and vegetables. Eat a diet consisting of 75 percent raw foods, organically grown if possible (avoid foods that have been treated with pesticides and other sprays), plus lentils, beans, seeds, nuts, and whole grains, including brown rice and millet, and also non-acid-forming fruit such as bananas, all berries, peaches, apples, and melons. Raw foods are particularly important because cooking depletes foods of their vital enzymes.

❏ Eat plenty of cruciferous vegetables, such as broccoli, Brussels sprouts, cabbage, and cauliflower. Also consume yellow and deep-orange vegetables such as carrots, pumpkin, squash, and yams.

❏ Consume plenty of fresh live juices. Juicing is extremely beneficial for supplying nutrients. (*See* JUICING in Part Three.) "Green drinks" made from leafy greens such as kale, spinach, and beet greens, and carrot and beet root juice, should be consumed on a daily basis, with garlic and onion added. Kyo-Green from Wakunaga is an excellent "green drink" product that contains chlorophyll, protein, vitamins, minerals, and enzymes. Take this drink three times a day.

❏ Drink steam-distilled water only (not tap water), and lots of it—eight to ten 8-ounce glasses daily—to flush out toxins from the body. All cells and organ systems need water. Drink plenty of water even if you are not thirsty. The organs, and especially the brain, become dehydrated long before thirst develops.

❏ Eat onions and garlic, or take garlic in supplement form (*see under* Nutrients, above).

❏ Add shiitake, reishi, and maitake mushrooms to the diet, or take them in supplement form (*see under* Nutrients, above).

❑ Eliminate from your diet colas, foods with additives and colorings, junk foods, peanuts, processed refined foods, saturated fats, salt, sugar and sugar products, white flour, all animal protein, and anything containing caffeine.

❑ Take supplemental fiber daily. Alternate between psyllium husks and freshly ground flaxseeds. Take psyllium with a glass of water and drink it quickly before it thickens.

Note: Always take supplemental fiber separately from other supplements and medications.

❑ Exercise caution in your choice of foods so as to avoid exposure to foodborne illness. Food poisoning can be very dangerous for people with HIV or AIDS infection. (*See* FOODBORNE/WATERBORNE ILLNESS in Part Two.)

❑ Do not smoke, and stay away from secondhand smoke.

❑ Avoid alcohol, noxious chemicals, and anything else that can damage the liver.

❑ Obtain as much fresh air and rest as possible, and moderate amounts of sunshine.

❑ Determine what food sensitivities or allergies may be present. The best way to do this is to have yourself tested by a health care professional. It is important to eliminate allergenic foods from the diet because they wreak havoc in the body, causing damage to the immune system. (*See* ALLERGIES in Part Two.)

❑ Always use a condom (latex, not sheepskin) and spermicide (spermicide kills HIV) for any sexual contact. If you use a lubricant with a latex condom, use only a water-based lubricant such as K-Y jelly. Do not use petroleum jelly (Vaseline), vegetable shortening (Crisco), hand lotion, or baby oil, as these substances can break down latex in a matter of minutes. Be aware, however, that even the proper use of a condom is not a guarantee against the transmission of HIV.

❑ Seek out the care of a qualified health care provider—if possible, one who has a great deal of experience in treating people with HIV. Research shows that the length of survival of a person with AIDS is closely linked to how much his or her physician knows about treating the condition.

❑ Educate yourself. HIV and AIDS are complicated conditions, and treatment options are constantly changing and expanding. In order to stay well, it is vital to be as informed as possible.

Considerations

❑ Studies show that a modified form of bacteria normally present in the vagina may one day be used to protect women from AIDS. Researchers used a strain of *Lactobacillus jensenii,* generally abundant in mucus secreted by the mucous membrane lining a healthy vagina. The bacteria were modified to produce a protein called CD4, which binds to the HIV virus that causes AIDS. In laboratory tests, the enhanced bacteria reduced the rate of HIV infection in susceptible cells by at least half.

❑ Ever since the AIDS epidemic began, researchers have been looking for a "magic bullet"—a single miracle drug to combat the virus, or a vaccine to seek out and destroy the virus in the bloodstream and lymphatic system. Research into this field is promising, however, and existing therapies almost guarantee that people with AIDS will live much longer and have more productive lives than was once the case.

❑ For persons infected with HIV, the most logical approach to staying well is to eliminate all known causes of immune suppression and to implement the use of therapies that inhibit viral activity and stimulate immune function.

❑ Human growth hormone (HGH) therapy has been shown to help prevent and/or reverse wasting syndrome. This treatment must be given under a doctor's supervision. Human growth hormone also has been shown to reduce abdominal body fat and correct abnormal fats in the blood. (*See* GROWTH HORMONE THERAPY in Part Three.)

❑ Hyperbaric oxygen therapy is sometimes used, together with medications and other treatments, to help overcome opportunistic infections associated with AIDS. (*See* HYPERBARIC OXYGEN THERAPY in Part Three.)

❑ N-acetylcysteine and L-carnitine both show some promise in the ability to prevent and counteract the extreme weight loss common in people with AIDS.

❑ There are some AIDS survivors (epidemiologists call them long-term nonprogressors) who are free from all symptoms and lead absolutely normal lives years after being identified as HIV-positive. This is a rare subset of all those infected worldwide, and they are being studied intensively. A key to the AIDS cure may reside in these people, some of whom have had HIV for over ten years and who nevertheless remain healthy. Many thousands will continue to be HIV-positive but not manifest full-blown AIDS. And, unknown to the general public and many in the medical establishment, there are also people who are now antibody-negative though once diagnosed as HIV-positive. They apparently no longer have the virus present in their bodies. The same thing happened during the plague; not everyone who was exposed developed symptoms.

❑ *See also* SEXUALLY TRANSMITTED DISEASE in Part Two.

❑ For information about organizations that can provide information and assistance for people with HIV and AIDS, *see* Health and Medical Organizations in the Appendix.

ALCOHOLISM

With an estimated 64 percent of American adults over eighteen consuming alcohol, it is hardly a surprise that one out of ten people suffers adverse consequences of alcohol consumption.

Alcoholism is a chronic, progressive disease that can have fatal consequences. It is a condition marked by a dependence on ethanol (ethyl alcohol). This dependence can be physiological, psychological, social, or genetic. There are two separate classes of alcohol-related problems: alcohol abuse, or "problem drinking," and alcohol dependence, or alcoholism. Problem drinkers use alcohol on a regular basis, and although they may need a degree of support or guidance, they are not as physically and/or emotionally dependent on the drug as chronic drinkers, or alcoholics. We will use the term alcoholism loosely below for practical purposes, but it is important to remember this distinction.

According to the National Council on Alcoholism and Drug Dependence, some 18 million Americans abuse alcohol, and heavy drinking contributes to illness in each of the top three causes of death: heart disease, cancer, and stroke. Alcoholism affects approximately four times as many men as women, but the incidence of alcoholism among women is on the rise, as is the use of alcohol by children, adolescents, and college students.

Women are physiologically more sensitive to alcohol than men are. Because of their bodies' lower water content and higher fat content, alcohol becomes more concentrated in the bloodstream and is also retained in their bodies longer. Also, men produce more alcohol dehydrogenase, the enzyme in the stomach that breaks down alcohol before it reaches the bloodstream, than women do. Even after you adjust for body weight, women are still affected more than men by the same amount of alcohol. This may be why alcohol abuse seems to have more serious long-term consequences for women.

The overall rate of premature death related to alcohol abuse is 50 to 100 percent higher for women than for men. Women develop liver disease at lower levels of alcohol intake than do men, and they are at increased risk for osteoporosis.

Alcoholic women are more likely than alcoholic men to suffer from other psychiatric disorders, including depression, anxiety, and eating disorders. Often, these disorders existed prior to the onset of alcoholism, which means that these problems do not go away once the drinking stops; usually, independent treatment is required. Early treatment for these disorders, however, may help prevent alcohol abuse from occurring.

Alcohol affects everyone differently. Some become intoxicated with the first drink; others may be able to consume four or five drinks before showing any effects, often because they have built up a tolerance to the drug. In alcoholics, each drink triggers a craving for another. Alcoholism is a progressive disease that usually starts with acceptable social drinking. This leads to a drink for every mood: one to calm down, one to perk up, one to celebrate, one to "drown one's sorrows," and so on. The alcoholic soon needs no excuse to drink. In time, the alcoholic is completely controlled by his or her dependence on alcohol.

Overindulgence often leads to depression, anxiety, memory loss, and lack of coordination, and can exaggerate antisocial behaviors such as aggression and/or other personality disorders.

Intoxication also causes blood pressure and heart rates to be higher at first and then to decrease with prolonged consumption. Irregular, inefficient beating of the heart can lead to stroke. Respiration rates are lowered, and reflexes and reaction times slowed.

Alcoholics often become ashamed and angry at their compulsive behavior, leading them to further alcohol abuse.

The National Council on Alcoholism and Drug Dependence and the American Society of Addiction Medicine define alcoholism as ". . . a primary, chronic disease with genetic, psychosocial, and environmental factors influencing its development and manifestations." It is a complex disorder that is unique to each individual.

Some people drink moderate to heavy amounts of alcohol for years before becoming clinically dependent on it, while others may become addicted to alcohol the very first time they ever take a drink. It is known, however, that alcohol itself is not the only cause of alcoholism. There is considerable debate as to whether alcoholism is principally caused by genetic, environmental, or psychological factors. There are certain stress hormones that appear to be associated with alcoholism. Depression can lead some people to alcohol. A family history of alcoholism is common among both men and women with the disorder, and research has shown that heredity is involved almost 50 percent of the time. Certain genetic factors may cause a person to be vulnerable due to an imbalance of brain chemicals.

Excessive alcohol use can produce harmful effects on the brain and nervous system and can cause fatigue, short-term memory loss, and weakness of the eye muscles. More serious health effects include:

- *Liver disorders*. The liver processes 95 percent of alcohol ingested, at a rate of about ¼ to ½ ounce per hour. The repeated consumption of alcohol inhibits the liver's production of digestive enzymes, impairing the body's ability to absorb proteins, fats, and the fat-soluble vitamins (vitamins A, D, E, and K), as well as B-complex vitamins (especially vitamin B_1 [thiamine] and folic acid) and other water-soluble vitamins. It inhibits protein uptake, leading to amino acid deficiencies, and reduces the body's storage of zinc. Furthermore, many essential nutrients are not retained for use by the body; they are rapidly eliminated through the urine. Alcoholic hepatitis, an inflammation of the liver, can follow. Signs and symptoms include loss of appetite, nausea, vomiting, abdominal pain and tenderness, fever, jaundice (yellow skin), and mental confusion. Excessive amounts of fat accumulate in the liver, a result of alcohol's effect on the body's ability to digest fats properly. Hepatitis is a condition in which liver cells become inflamed and may die. The final, usually fatal, stage of alcoholic liver damage is cirrhosis of the liver, which affects one in five alcohol abusers and is a disease characterized by inflammation, hardening, and scarring of the liver. This prevents the normal passage of blood through the liver, inhibiting the organ's ability to filter out toxins and foreign substances. The liver is one of the most robust organs of the body. It is the only organ that has the ability to regenerate itself after certain types of damage. Up to 75 percent of the liver can be removed in patients without any underlying liver disease—in those with liver disease 60 percent can be removed. It takes four to six weeks for the liver to grow back to its original size. If cared for properly, it will function more than adequately for decades. Alcohol is one of the toxins that the liver doesn't handle as well as others. The liver cannot regenerate after being severely damaged by alcohol.

- *Gastrointestinal problems.* Gastritis, or inflammation of the stomach lining, can lead to tearing in the upper part of the stomach and lower esophagus. Peptic ulcers also can form.

- *Cardiovascular problems.* High blood pressure and cardiomyopathy (heart muscle damage) are possible. Problem drinkers may also experience visible dilation of blood vessels just beneath the skin's surface, as well as pathological enlargement of the heart that can progress to congestive heart failure.

- *Blood sugar problems.* Alcohol prevents release of glucose from the liver and can cause low blood sugar (hypoglycemia). If you have diabetes and are taking insulin, this can have serious consequences. The pancreas also can be involved (pancreatitis), which can affect production of insulin so as to cause diabetes. A diseased pancreas can also interfere with the production of glucagon, a hormone that helps increase the amount of glucose in the blood, which can cause metabolism problems and can affect production of certain digestive enzymes.

- *Sexual function or menstrual problems.* Alcohol abuse can cause reduced testosterone production and erectile dysfunction in men and can interrupt menstruation in women.

- *Birth defects.* A woman who drinks excessively during pregnancy runs the risk of having a child with fetal alcohol syndrome and increases the chance of miscarriage. In fact, any alcohol consumption during pregnancy can affect the fetus. Alcohol passes through the mother's placenta and into the fetal circulation. This toxic substance depresses the central nervous system of the fetus. Further, the fetal liver must try to metabolize the alcohol, but since the fetus's liver is not fully developed, the alcohol remains in the fetal circulation. Women who drink during pregnancy generally give birth to babies with lower birth weights. Their growth may be retarded or stunted; their brains may be smaller than normal; and they may be of lower than normal intelligence, or even suffer mental retardation. Limbs, joints, fingers, and facial features may be deformed. Heart and kidney defects, and abnormalities of the skin, may occur. Some children exposed to alcohol *in utero* become hyperactive at adolescence and exhibit learning disabilities. Every drink a pregnant woman consumes increases her child's risk of being born with fetal alcohol syndrome, and also increases the chance of miscarriage. Even moderate amounts of alcohol may be harmful, especially in the first three to four months of pregnancy.

- *Neurological problems.* The nervous system can be affected by excessive drinking, causing numbness of extremities, disordered thinking, and, eventually, dementia.

- *Cancer.* The risk of getting cancer of the esophagus, larynx, liver, and colon is much higher for those who are alcohol abusers than for the general population.

Alcoholism causes metabolic damage to every cell in the body and depresses the immune system. It may take years before the consequences of excessive drinking become evident, but if an alcoholic continues to drink, his or her life span may be shortened by ten to fifteen years or more. The social consequences of alcoholism can be very destructive as well. Alcohol abuse takes a tremendous toll on society through traffic and other accidents, poor job performance, and emotional damage to entire families. Alcoholism is currently the second major preventable cause of death in the United States, second only to cigarette smoking.

Most alcohol abusers enter treatment with great reluctance because they are in denial. They refuse to believe that they have a problem and often think there is a conspiracy against them by family, friends, or coworkers. Intervention must be handled carefully with professional advice. Treatment can vary with the individual. If the person to be treated is alcohol dependent, complete abstinence should be the goal. If a person isn't dependent on alcohol but is experiencing the adverse effects of drinking, reduction of the alcohol-related problems is required. Seek counseling or intervention. Intervention may involve alcohol-abuse specialists, and should involve some type of goal-setting and behavior modification, along with counseling and follow-up care. Resident treatment programs for serious alcoholics are often complex and usually involve a professional staff.

Dietary supplements, while important for everyone, are especially vital for alcoholics. Evidence has shown that some of the diseases associated with alcoholism can be avoided by improving the nutritional health of the body. The program that follows is designed to help recovering alcoholics to improve their nutritional condition.

There are also some supplements that help with the psychological aspects of recovery by decreasing the desire for alcohol. You should begin with a high-potency multivitamin and mineral complex, and then add the nutrients listed that are not included in the complex.

Unless otherwise specified, the dosages recommended in this section are for adults. For children between the ages

Signs and Symptoms of Alcohol Abuse and Alcoholism

While each case of alcohol abuse and alcoholism is in some ways unique to the individual, there are certain common features that can serve as warning signs. These include:

- Drinking alone or in secret.
- Not remembering commitments or conversations. Having blackouts.
- Ritualizing drinking at certain times, places, or events, and becoming agitated or annoyed if the ritual is changed or questioned.
- Not caring anymore about long-term hobbies, interests, and activities.
- Feeling an overwhelming need for a drink.

- Irritability and agitation increasing as normal drinking time nears, especially if alcohol is not available or cannot be available due to work or social commitment.
- Hiding alcohol at work, at home, or in the car.
- When drinking, gulping drinks, ordering "doubles" or setups.
- Getting intoxicated to feel normal.
- Having problems with finances, social interaction, relationships, or employment.
- Building up a tolerance to alcohol that requires "more of the same" to hit the same plateau of intoxication.
- Having physical withdrawal symptoms when you can't drink, such as sweating, shaking, or nausea.

of twelve and seventeen, reduce the dose to three-quarters the recommended amount.

NUTRIENTS

SUPPLEMENT	SUGGESTED DOSAGE	COMMENTS
Essential		
Free form amino acid plus extra L-cysteine or N-acetylcysteine	500 mg each 3 times daily, on an empty stomach. Take with 50 mg vitamin B_6 and 100 mg vitamin C for better absorption. Start with 500 mg daily and slowly work up to 1,000 mg daily.	Aids in withdrawal; needed for brain and liver function; necessary for regeneration of liver cells. (*See* AMINO ACIDS in Part One.)
Gamma-aminobutyric acid (GABA) plus inositol and niacinamide	750 mg once or twice daily, as needed. As directed on label. 500 mg once or twice daily, as needed.	To calm the body and prevent anxiety and stress. *Caution:* Do not substitute niacin for niacinamide. Niacin can be toxic in such high doses.
Glutathione and L-methionine	3,000 mg daily, on an empty stomach. 1,000 mg daily, on an empty stomach. Take with water or juice. Do not take with milk. Take with 25 mg vitamin B_6 and 100 mg vitamin C for better absorption.	Protects the liver and reduces craving for alcohol. Note: Do not take substitute glutamic acid for glutathione. Protects glutathione, making it available to the liver. (*See* AMINO ACIDS in Part One.)
Pantothenic acid (vitamin B_5)	100 mg 3 times daily.	Aids the body in alcohol detoxification. Needed to counteract stress.
Vitamin B complex injections or sublingual plus extra vitamin B_6	As prescribed by physician. 100 mg of each major B vitamin daily (amounts of individual vitamins in a complex will vary). As directed on label.	To correct deficiencies. Injections (under a doctor's supervision) are best. If injections are not available, use a sublingual form. Often deficient in alcoholics.
along with vitamin B_{12}	1,000 mcg 3 times daily.	Reduces water retention and helps to relieve anxiety, fear, and tension associated with recovery.
Vitamin B_1 (thiamine)	200 mg 3 times daily.	Alcoholics often are deficient in B vitamins, especially B_1.
Very Important		
Alpha-lipoic acid	100 mg 2 times daily.	Aids in protecting the liver and pancreas from alcohol damage. A powerful antioxidant.
Calcium and magnesium	2,000 mg daily, at bedtime. 1,000 mg daily, at bedtime.	A vital mineral that has a sedative effect. Works with calcium. Magnesium is depleted from the body with alcohol use.
Multienzyme complex plus proteolytic enzymes	As directed on label. As directed on label. Take between meals.	To aid digestion. Essential for assimilation of protein. *Caution:* Do not give these supplements to a child.
Primrose oil	1,000 mg 3 times daily, with meals.	Used successfully in Europe, this supplement is a good source of essential fatty acids. It may also help reduce withdrawal symptoms.
Pycnogenol or grape seed extract	30 mg 3 times daily. 30 mg 3 times daily.	Powerful antioxidants for the protection of the cells.
Vitamin C with bioflavonoids	3,000–10,000 mg daily, in divided doses.	Acts as a powerful antioxidant with healing potential, and promotes production of interferon, which helps the body resist infection, to which alcoholics are generally more susceptible.
Important		
Acidophilus	As directed on label. Take on an empty stomach.	Needed for proper digestion. Helps the damaged liver.
Coenzyme A from Coenzyme-A Technologies	As directed on label.	Supports the immune system's detoxification of many dangerous substances.

Inositol hexaphosphate (IP$_6$) (Cell Forté with IP-6 from Enzymatic Therapy)	As directed on label.	Enhances natural killer cell activity.
Lecithin granules or capsules	1 tbsp 3 times daily, before meals. 1,200 mg 3 times daily, before meals.	Good for brain function. Helps correct fatty liver degeneration. May protect against cirrhosis.
Liquid Kyolic with B$_1$ and B$_{12}$ from Wakunaga	As directed on label.	Protects liver and brain cells. Reduces stress.
Multivitamin and mineral complex with manganese and selenium	As directed on label. 200 mcg daily. Take separately from calcium. 200 mcg daily. If you are pregnant, do not exceed 40 mcg daily.	All nutrients are needed because of malabsorption problems. Important trace minerals that enhance immune function.
Helpful		
Choline complex or acetylcholine complex or phosphatidyl choline	As directed on label. As directed on label. As directed on label.	Effective combinations that reduce fatty liver changes, improving liver function.
Dimethylglycine (DMG) (Aangamik DMG from FoodScience of Vermont)	125 mg 3 times daily.	Carries oxygen to the cells.
Flaxseed oil	As directed on label.	Strengthens the brain's gray matter.
L-glutamine	500 mg twice daily, on an empty stomach. Take with water or juice. Do not take with milk. Take with 50 mg vitamin B$_6$ and 100 mg vitamin C for better absorption.	An amino acid that helps to stop cravings and balance blood sugar.
Lithium	As prescribed by physician.	A trace mineral that may help depression. Available by prescription only.
Raw liver extract and raw pancreas glandular	As directed on label. As directed on label.	A rich source of vitamins and minerals that aids in repairing the liver and in preventing anemia. (*See* GLANDULAR THERAPY in Part Three.) Helps prevent pancreatic damage; beneficial for people with diabetes associated with alcoholism.
S-adenosylmethionine (SAMe)	As directed on label.	Its antioxidant effects can improve the health of the liver. *Caution:* Do not use if you have bipolar mood disorder or take prescription antidepressants.
Vitamin A	25,000 IU daily. If you are pregnant, do not exceed 10,000 IU daily.	To counteract deficiencies. Vitamin A is poorly absorbed if the liver is damaged. Use emulsion forms for easier assimilation and greater safety at higher doses. Avoid capsule or tablet forms.
Vitamin E	200 IU daily.	A powerful antioxidant. Use d-alpha-tocopherol form.
Zinc	50 mg daily. Do not exceed a total of 100 mg daily from all supplements.	Deficiency can cause pathological changes in the stomach similar to those caused by alcohol.

Herbs

❑ Alfalfa is a good source of needed minerals.

❑ Burdock root and red clover cleanse the bloodstream.

❑ Dandelion root and silymarin (milk thistle extract) help to repair damage done to the liver. Silymarin acts as a powerful antioxidant.

❑ Valerian root has a calming effect. It is best taken at bedtime.

Recommendations

❑ Avoid all alcohol. Total abstinence is an absolute requirement for regaining control over your life. Even after years of sobriety, you cannot begin drinking again.

❑ Seek help from someone knowledgeable about this disorder. Alcoholics Anonymous has been doing wonderful work for many years in helping alcoholics achieve and maintain sobriety. Al-Anon and Alateen are similar groups that provide support for the friends and families of alcoholics. A strong support system can make behavioral changes much easier for everyone. The assistance and counseling services of these groups are available in nearly every city and town nationwide. Look in your local telephone directory for the group nearest you, or call your local mental health association for information.

❑ Some programs, such as Moderation Management, are available to help problem drinkers (not true alcoholics) reduce their drinking without completely stopping. This program entails a thirty-day abstinence period. After that, you may consume no more than four drinks a day and no more than fourteen drinks per week (for women, three per day and nine per week).

❑ If possible, consult a nutritionally oriented physician to determine your specific nutritional needs.

❑ Go on a ten-day live juice and cleansing fast to remove toxins from the body quickly; only do this if you are at or above normal weight. (*See* FASTING in Part Three.)

❑ Eat a nutrient-dense diet of fresh whole foods, organically grown if possible, and follow the nutritional supplement program outlined above. Your primary foods should be raw fruits and vegetables, whole grains, and legumes.

❑ Avoid saturated fats and fried foods, which put stress on the liver. For essential fatty acids, use primrose oil supplements plus small amounts of cold-pressed organic vegetable oils.

❏ Do not consume refined sugar or anything that contains it. Alcoholics often have disorders of sugar metabolism.

❏ Get plenty of rest, especially in the early weeks of recovery, to allow your body to cleanse and repair itself.

❏ Avoid people, things, and places that are associated with drinking. Make new friendships with people who do not drink. Taking up a hobby, becoming involved in sports, and exercising promote self-esteem and provide a productive outlet for energy.

❏ As much as possible, avoid stress. Cultivate patience; this will be needed for the long, slow road to recovery.

❏ Do not take any drugs except for those prescribed by your physician.

❏ If you suspect that someone you know may be abusing alcohol, encourage the person to seek professional care.

Considerations

❏ Depending on the individual, treatment for alcoholism may involve one or more of the following:

- *Detoxification and withdrawal.* This usually takes four to seven days and will probably involve medications to prevent delirium tremens or withdrawal seizures. Alcoholics who stop drinking often experience withdrawal symptoms, especially during the first week or so that they abstain from alcohol. Insomnia, visual and auditory hallucinations, convulsions, acute anxiety, a rapid pulse, profuse perspiration, and fever can occur. With time and appropriate supervision, these symptoms pass and the alcoholic is set free to begin the lifelong work of recovery.

- *Medical assessment and treatment.* This may entail examination and treatment for high blood pressure, liver disease, high blood sugar, and heart disease, among other problems.

- *Psychological support/psychiatric care.* This includes counseling and therapy to get at the underlying problems that may have led to alcohol abuse.

- *Acceptance/abstinence.* It is necessary to accept the situation (admit that one is a problem drinker or an alcoholic) and desire to abstain in order to be cured.

- *Drug treatment.* A drug called disulfiram (Antabuse) may be used to cause an aversion reaction to the consumption of alcohol. Those on this drug experience nausea, vomiting, severe headaches, blurred vision, and sometimes an impending feeling of death if they take even a small sip of alcohol. Naltrexone (ReVia) is an opiate blocker and is used to block the alcohol "high" and reduce the urge to drink. This is usually administered as a 50-milligram daily dose for twelve consecutive weeks. A nonaddictive drug, acamprosate calcium (Campral), has been approved for treating those who want to re-main alcohol-free after successfully stopping their drinking. Administered as two 355-milligram capsules three times a day with meals, it effectively eliminates the discomfort caused by alcohol withdrawal. Acamprosate calcium is thought to act on the brain pathways directly to reduce withdrawal symptoms.

- *Aftercare.* This is continued care to manage relapses and assist with lifestyle changes.

❏ Poor nutrition can enhance the adverse effects of ethanol. Alcoholics are at much greater risk of malnutrition than other people, since as much as 50 percent of their caloric intake may come from ethanol at the expense of nutritious foods. Alcoholics are commonly deficient in folic acid, and malabsorption due to pancreatic insufficiency is often a major problem.

❏ Long-term alcohol abuse can promote a zinc-deficient state, most likely because of increased fecal and urinary losses. Zinc plays a vital role in a variety of enzyme systems in the body, as well as in DNA and RNA production. It also helps to regulate copper levels in the brain, reducing anxiousness and paranoia. A deficiency of zinc can result in anorexia, impaired senses of smell and taste, growth retardation, disorders of the reproductive system, and impaired wound healing and immune function. Pathological changes in the stomach occur due to zinc deficiency. Alcohol-related zinc deficiency accelerates the poisoning of cells that come into contact with alcohol by altering the metabolism of fats, carbohydrates, and nutrients. This leads to malabsorption problems, a depressed metabolism, and nutritional deficiencies.

❏ A Department of Health and Human Services study showed that tobacco smokers and alcohol drinkers who regularly use high-alcohol mouthwash may be more likely than other people to get oral, pharyngeal (throat), and esophageal cancers.

❏ Alcohol is one of the most damaging substances to the stomach and the small intestine. It reduces the absorption of nutrients in the small intestine, and it is one of the few substances that can penetrate the lining of the stomach to cause damage. Gastric secretions increase with alcohol consumption, causing excess acidity and diluting digestive enzymes. This can lead to gastritis.

❏ Chronic alcohol consumption alters red blood cell membranes and causes various other types of cells, including gastrointestinal cells, to lose their normal flexibility.

❏ A recovering alcoholic who resumes drinking, even after years of sobriety, will damage his or her liver as though the drinking had never stopped in the first place.

❏ The drug naltrexone (ReVia) blocks the pleasurable effects of endogenous opioids, opiatelike substances released by the brain in response to alcohol, and may help problem drinkers remain sober by reducing the craving for alcohol. In two separate studies conducted at the University of Pennsylvania and the Yale University School of Medicine, people who took this drug were three times likelier than other patients to stick with their recovery programs. However, this drug is not suitable for people with liver disease.

❑ Alpha-lipoic acid, a powerful antioxidant, has been used successfully to treat alcohol-induced liver damage. It aids in protecting the liver and pancreas from alcoholic damage.

❑ In some countries, hyperbaric oxygen has been used successfully in the treatment of alcoholism. (See HYPERBARIC OXYGEN THERAPY in Part Three.)

❑ Binge drinking is a sign of severe alcoholism. The binge drinker will drink to the point of intoxication and stay that way for a few days, often without consuming many solid foods. The binge may end in vomiting, which is the body's way of getting rid of the excess alcohol, and then passing out. Frequently the person does not remember the events that happened during the binge. Binge drinkers consume larger quantities of alcohol on a regular basis and also experience more intoxication and alcohol-related problems than non-binge drinkers do. Binge drinking can cause dangerous cardiac arrhythmias.

❑ Research has found that children of alcoholics are more inclined than children of nonalcoholics to use drugs, including cocaine. These children are 400 times more likely to use drugs than those who do not have a family history of alcohol addiction.

❑ Studies conducted in Sweden revealed that the majority of babies of alcoholics who were adopted by nonalcoholic families eventually grew up to become alcoholics, indicating a correlation between chemical dependency and genetics.

❑ Limiting one's drinking to beer or wine does not protect against alcoholism or damage from alcohol. Twelve ounces of beer or 5 ounces of wine is comparable in alcohol content to 1.5 ounces of 80-proof liquor. Because it is more concentrated, straight liquor is absorbed into the bloodstream more quickly than beer and wine.

❑ Researchers have found that children who were diagnosed with ADHD (attention deficit hyperactivity disorder) are more likely than their peers to report alcohol-related problems, as well as drug and tobacco addictions, later in life. This study was reported in the *Journal of Abnormal Psychology*. Youngsters with severe inattention problems were five times more likely than others to have used an illegal drug other than alcohol or marijuana at an early age. This turned out to be a uniquely important variable even when the presence of oppositional defiant disorder (ODD) and conduct disorder (CD) were considered. The risk factor for inattention paralleled the importance of family history as a predictor.

❑ Alcohol enters the bloodstream relatively quickly, as it can be absorbed through both the stomach and small intes-tines (unlike food, which is absorbed through the intestines only). It takes nearly one hour for the body to break down one unit of alcohol in the bloodstream (for older people, it can take longer). The more drinks are consumed in an hour, the higher the alcohol content of the blood. Blood alcohol levels of 400 mg/dL (milligrams per tenth of a liter) can be life-threatening.

❑ Once alcohol is in the blood, there is *nothing* that can be done to hurry the process of removing it. The idea that cold showers, coffee, and/or eating can help you sober up is false.

❑ Although some people fall asleep faster when drinking, alcohol depresses REM (rapid eye movement) sleep. REM is an essential part of the healthy sleep cycle, and if disturbed, the result is usually a desire to sleep longer in the morning and a sluggish feeling that lasts throughout the day.

❑ "Hangovers" could be caused by a combination of factors, including dehydration, overeating, and disturbed sleep. Even small amounts of alcohol can sometimes cause unpleasant side effects the next morning in some individuals. Usually, the best remedy includes rest and rehydration. Drinking a large glass of water before retiring and another in the morning may help take the edge off "the morning after." Taking over-the-counter pain medication such as acetaminophen, ibuprofen, naproxin, or aspirin before hangover symptoms begin sometimes helps with the headache; however, extreme caution must be used. When combined with alcohol, these medications may irritate your stomach and can even be toxic to the liver. The liver is the central clearinghouse for medications, including over-the-counter types, and it is already working in overdrive to clear the alcohol from the system. This is why there is now a required warning label on over-the-counter painkillers, and medications that contain them, cautioning against using them if you consume more than three alcoholic drinks per day. Mixing alcohol with any medication is not recommended.

❑ Medications such as tranquilizers, antidepressants, codeine, morphine, phenobarbital, and even some antibiotics can form toxic combinations with alcohol. Combining alcohol with antihistamines can enhance depression of the central nervous system. Combining alcohol with sleeping aids can be deadly.

❑ In recovery from alcoholism, it is best to avoid tranquilizers, as there is a danger of substituting one drug addiction for another. Sobriety should be drug-free.

❑ Pregnant women should avoid all alcohol.

❑ Women in general should limit their alcohol intake. Women who have had breast cancer and drink alcohol are at increased risk of recurrence. Although alcohol seems to affect women with estrogen-positive breast tumors, all women at risk of breast cancer should consider abstaining from alcohol. The more alcohol a woman consumes and the more years she drinks increase the chances that her breast tissue will be adversely affected.

❑ Alcohol has been shown to affect older adults differently than other people. It is more likely to hinder the absorption of nutrients, and it can also pose a danger if mixed with many medications taken to control age-related or chronic illnesses. Unfortunately, alcoholism among elderly people is more common than one might think, and can often go unnoticed or without intervention. Some people tend to think that older people have "earned the right to drink." The truth is, however, that elders have just as much right to recovery as anyone else.

❑ Contrary to popular belief that alcohol heightens sexual arousal, it actually has the opposite effect—depression. It can cause sexual dysfunction in men and disrupt menstrual cycles in women.

❑ Various studies have shown that, in small amounts, alcohol can have protective effects against certain cardiovascular and cancerous diseases. The amount of alcohol shown to be protective has varied slightly from study to study. The accepted definition of moderate alcoholic intake according to the U.S. Department of Agriculture is one drink or less per day for women and two drinks or less per day for men (a "drink" being defined as 12 ounces of beer, 5 ounces of wine, or 1.5 ounces of 80-proof liquor). Nobody is suggesting that nondrinkers begin drinking to protect their hearts. Instead, they suggest less risky options such as regular light exercise, not smoking, and decreasing the amount of saturated fat in the diet.

❑ *See also* CIRRHOSIS OF THE LIVER and DRUG ADDICTION, both in Part Two.

❑ For information about organizations that can provide information and assistance for people dealing with alcoholism, *see* Health and Medical Organizations in the Appendix.

ALKALOSIS

See under ACID/ALKALI IMBALANCE.

ALLERGIC RHINITIS

See HAY FEVER.

ALLERGIES

An allergy is an inappropriate response by the body's immune system to a substance that is not normally harmful. The immune system is a highly complex defense mechanism that helps us to fight infections. It does this by identifying foreign invaders and mobilizing the body's white blood cells to fight them. In some people, the immune system wrongly identifies a nontoxic substance as an invader, and the white blood cells overreact, creating more damage to the body than the invader. Thus, the allergic response becomes a disease in itself.

Typical allergic responses are nasal congestion, coughing, wheezing, itching, shortness of breath, headache, fatigue, and hives and other skin rashes. Substances that provoke allergic responses are called allergens. Almost any substance can cause an allergic reaction in someone, somewhere in the world, but the most common allergens are pollen, dust, certain metals (especially nickel), some cosmetics, lanolin, dust mites, animal hair, insect venom, some common drugs (such as penicillin and aspirin), some food additives (such as benzoic acid and sulfur dioxide), animal dander, and chemicals found in soap, washing powder, cleaning supplies, and many other chemicals.

Many people are allergic to mold. Molds are microscopic living organisms, neither animal nor insect, that thrive where no other life form can. Molds live throughout the house—under the sink and in the bathroom, basement, refrigerator, and any other damp, dark place. They also flourish in the air, in soil, on dead leaves, and on other organic material. Molds can be both destructive and beneficial. Molds help to make cheese, fertilize gardens, and speed decaying of garbage and fallen leaves. Penicillin is made from molds. Molds can also provoke allergic reactions.

Mold spores are carried by the wind and predominate in the summer and early fall. They thrive year-round in warm climates. Cutting grass, harvesting crops, or walking through tall vegetation can provoke an allergic reaction. People who repair old furniture are also at risk because old wood often harbors mold spores.

Foods also can provoke allergic reactions. Some of the most common allergenic foods in adults are shrimp, lobster, crab, strawberries, chocolate, shellfish, peanuts, walnuts and other tree nuts, fish, and eggs. In children, eggs, milk, peanuts, soy, and wheat are the main culprits. Children typically outgrow allergies to milk, egg, soy, and wheat, but allergies to peanuts, tree nuts, fish, and shrimp persist. Adults do not normally lose an allergy once they have it.

There is a difference between food allergies and food intolerances. A person with food intolerance is unable to digest and process that food correctly, usually due to a lack of a certain enzyme or enzymes. Many such people have gas, bloating, or other unpleasant reactions to something they eat. Only about 1.5 percent of adults, and less than 6 percent of children younger than age three, in the United States have a true food allergy. A food allergy occurs when a person's immune system generates an antibody response to the ingested food. Milk is a good example of the distinction between an allergy and intolerance. Most people who can't drink milk are lactose intolerant, not allergic. In rare cases (less than 10 percent), a person may have a true milk allergy where their body mounts an immune response to milk proteins rather than to the lactose (or sugar). An estimated 150 Americans die each year from severe allergic reactions to food, according to Hugh A. Sampson, M.D., director of the Jaffe Food Allergy Institute at the Mount Sinai School of Medicine in New York City. Food intolerances can lead to allergies, however, if particles of undigested food manage to enter the bloodstream and cause a reaction known as leaky gut syndrome.

Food should not normally provoke a response from the immune system. When someone has a food allergy, the immune system responds inappropriately. First, an antibody called immunoglobulin E (or IgE) is produced that circulates in the blood. People who have food allergies typically inherit this tendency to form the IgE against a particular food. During digestion of the problem food, tiny protein fragments prompt certain cells to produce the specific IgE against that food. The IgE then circulates and attaches to the surfaces of the mast cells. Mast cells are found in all body tissue, but especially in the areas that are typical sites for allergic reaction, such as the nose, throat, lungs, skin, and gastrointestinal tract. The next time that food is eaten, the protein reacts with the specific IgE on the mast cells to trigger the release of chemicals, such as histamine. It is these chemicals that cause the symptoms of an allergic reaction.

If the mast cells release their chemicals in the nose and throat, the person may experience an itching tongue or mouth, and may have trouble breathing and swallowing. If mast cells in the gastrointestinal tract are involved, the person may experience diarrhea or abdominal pain. Activated mast cells in the skin can produce hives or intense itching.

The food protein fragments responsible for initiating the allergic reaction are not broken down by either cooking, stomach acids, or enzymes. These proteins can cross the gastrointestinal lining, travel through the bloodstream, and cause allergic reactions throughout the body. The onset of symptoms may occur anywhere from a few minutes to an hour or two after ingestion.

Cerebral allergies cause swelling of the lining of the brain. Entire food families can cause such allergic reactions in susceptible individuals. Recurrent headaches, or schizophrenic, violent, or aggressive reactions, can be an indicator of cerebral allergy. Foods such as corn, wheat, rice, milk, and chocolate, along with certain food additives, are the most common offenders.

Research indicates that the number of people with allergies is skyrocketing in both developed and developing countries, and will probably continue to grow. Dr. Sampson also cites recent studies that indicate that growing up in a large family or attending a day care center appears to *decrease* a child's risk of developing an allergy. This is attributed to the immune system's being too "busy" fighting off infections and other environmental factors to concentrate on allergens.

Currently, the only way to deal with food allergies is to avoid foods that trigger reactions. In 2004, Congress passed the Food Allergen Labeling and Consumer Protection Act. The law applies to both domestic and imported foods and dietary supplements. The labels clearly identify the source of all ingredients that are—or are derived from—the eight most common food allergens. These food labels will help allergic consumers identify foods or ingredients so they can avoid them. There are 160 foods that can cause allergic reactions; the law identifies 8, which account for 90 percent of allergic reactions to foods. These foods are: milk, eggs, fish (bass, flounder, cod), shellfish (crab, lobster, shrimp), tree nuts (almonds, walnuts, pecans), peanuts, wheat, and soybeans.

Those with food allergies severe enough to cause anaphylactic reactions (shortness of breath, pale blue color, hives or itching, and anxiousness) should wear medical alert bracelets or necklaces and carry a syringe of adrenaline (epinephrine) to use in emergencies (these are available only by prescription). Anaphylactic reactions can be fatal even if they begin with mild symptoms, such as tingling in the throat or gastrointestinal discomfort. Antihistamines and bronchodilators can be used to treat less severe symptoms.

For most people, allergies are no more than another frustrating fact of life. But for people with asthma, or for those who suffer severe allergic reactions, allergies can be life-threatening. In people with asthma, hypersensitivity to irritants results in mucus secretions and, in severe cases, inflammation, edema, and swelling of the bronchial tubes. (*See* ASTHMA in Part Two.) According to the National Institute of Allergy and Infectious Diseases, serious allergies affect more than 50 million Americans. Allergies affect one's quality of life and productivity at work or home, school studies, or athletic pursuits. They can also lead to secondary diseases like ear and sinus infections.

To make matters worse, due to the consistently warmer and wetter winters occurring in most parts of the world in recent years, seasonal allergy sufferers can count on longer periods of misery. Hay fever (acute seasonal allergic rhinitis) is the most common type of seasonal allergy. Its symptoms closely resemble those of the common cold, but there are some differences. Cold symptoms generally disappear in a week to ten days, but allergic rhinitis can linger miserably for weeks, or even months. The nasal discharge caused by a cold is generally watery at the very beginning, but then turns thick and yellow, while the allergic reaction produces a consistently thin and clear discharge from the nose, in addition to itchy eyes, mouth, and skin. While it is difficult to determine the cause of the common cold, in most cases the cause of an allergy can be identified. This is at least one heartening fact for allergy sufferers. No one knows why some people are allergic to certain substances. According to the Asthma and Allergy Foundation of America, some allergies have a genetic component.

If one parent has allergies, it is statistically likely that one in three of their children will have allergies. If both parents have allergies, the chance that their children will have allergies rises to seven in ten. It is also believed that babies who are not breast-fed are more likely to develop allergies. Although persons between the ages of fifteen and twenty-five are the most allergy-prone, allergies can strike at any age. Emotional factors such as stress and anger may aggravate allergies, especially if the immune system is not functioning properly.

Food Allergy Self-Test

If you suspect that you are allergic to a certain food, a simple test can help you determine if you are correct. By recording your pulse rate after consuming the food in question, you can reveal if you are having an allergic reaction.

Using a watch with a second hand, sit down and relax for a few minutes. When completely relaxed, take your pulse at the wrist. Count the number of beats in a sixty-second period. Normal pulse readings, by age, are as follows:

- Newborn infants: 100 to 160 beats per minute

- Children 1 to 10 years: 70 to 120 beats per minute

- Children over 10: 60 to 100 beats per minute

- Adults: 60 to 100 beats per minute

- Well-trained athletes: 40 to 60 beats per minute

After taking your pulse, consume the food that you are testing for an allergic reaction. Wait twenty minutes and take your pulse again. If your pulse rate has increased more than ten beats per minute, omit this food from your diet for one month, and then retest yourself.

For the purposes of this test, it is best to use the purest form of the suspected food available. For example, if you are testing yourself for an allergy to wheat, it is better to use a bit of plain cream of wheat cereal than to use wheat bread, which contains other ingredients besides wheat. This way you will know that if you observe a reaction, it is the wheat that is responsible.

When choosing supplements such as the ones listed below, develop a plan. Consider introducing one new supplement at a time. Many people with allergies don't know the cause, and bombarding the system with too many new ingredients at once could set off an attack. If you find a company whose supplements seem to work for you, stick with that company when choosing other supplements; companies use different ingredients and some may cause allergic reactions. At the very least, include a multivitamin and calcium/magnesium supplement, especially if you are avoiding dairy or another major food group. Deficiencies can arise quickly, and treating allergies should not lead to malnutrition. If you are losing weight, contact your health care provider to help with dietary management.

Unless otherwise specified, the dosages recommended in this section are for adults. For children between the ages of twelve and seventeen, reduce the dose to three-quarters of the recommended amount. For children between six and twelve, use one-half of the recommended dose, and for children under the age of six, use one-quarter of the recommended amount.

NUTRIENTS

SUPPLEMENT	SUGGESTED DOSAGE	COMMENTS
Very Important		
Acidophilus	As directed on label.	Powerful immune enhancer with digestive enzymes for improved digestion.
Anti-Allergy formula from Freeda Vitamins	As directed on label.	A combination of quercetin, calcium pantothenate, and calcium ascorbate (vitamin C).
Calcium and magnesium	1,500–2,000 mg daily. 750 mg daily.	Needed to help reduce stress. Use calcium chelate form. Needed to balance with calcium.
Inositol hexaphosphate (IP₆) (Cell Forté from Enzymatic Therapy)	As directed on label.	Supports the immune system.
Kyolic Formula 102 from Wakunaga	50 mg 3 times daily.	Powerful immune enhancer with digestive enzymes. For improved digestion.
Methylsulfonylmethane (MSM)	As directed on label.	Has antiallergic properties equal to or better than those of antihistamines.
Multienzyme complex or pancreatin	As directed on label. Take with meals.	For improved digestion. *Caution:* If you have a history of ulcers, do not use a formula containing HCl.
Quercetin (Quercitin-C from Ecological Formulas) plus bromelain or	500 mg twice daily. 100 mg twice daily.	Increases immunity and decreases reactions to certain foods, pollens, and other allergens. Enhances absorption of quercetin and reduces inflammation.
Activated Quercetin from Source Naturals	As directed on label.	Contains quercetin plus bromelain and vitamin C.
Raw adrenal glandular and raw spleen glandular and raw thymus glandular	500 mg each twice daily.	To stimulate proper immune function. Raw adrenal is very important to prevent adrenal exhaustion.
Vitamin B complex plus extra pantothenic acid (vitamin B₅) and vitamin B₁₂ and Vitamin B₆	100 mg of each major B vitamin daily (amounts of individual vitamins in a complex will vary). 100 mg 3 times daily. 300–1,000 mcg 3 times daily. 50 mg 3 times daily.	Needed for proper digestion and nerve function. Use a high-stress formula. Consider injections. The antistress vitamin. Use a lozenge or sublingual form. Needed for proper assimilation of nutrients. Use a lozenge or sublingual form. Helps to relieve wheezing and allergy attacks.
Vitamin C with bioflavonoids	5,000–20,000 mg daily, in divided doses. (*See* ASCORBIC ACID FLUSH in Part Three.)	Protects the body from allergens and moderates the inflammatory response.
Important		
Liquid Kyolic with B₁ and B₁₂ from Wakunaga	As directed on label.	An excellent cell protector.
Natural carotenoid complex (Betatene)	As directed on label.	Free radical scavengers that inhibit allergic reactions.
Proteolytic enzymes	As directed on label. Take between meals on an empty stomach.	To aid digestion and destroy free radicals. *Caution:* Do not give these supplements to a child.

Helpful		
Aller Bee-Gone from CC Pollen	As directed on label.	A combination of herbs, enzymes, and nutrients designed to fight acute allergy attacks.
Bee pollen	Start with a few granules at a time and work up to 2 tsp daily.	Strengthens the immune system. Use raw crude pollen, preferably produced within 10 miles of your home. *Caution:* Bee pollen may cause an allergic reaction in some individuals. Discontinue use if a rash, wheezing, discomfort, or other symptoms occur.
Coenzyme A from Coenzyme-A Technologies	As directed on label.	Supports the immune system's detoxification of many dangerous substances.
Coenzyme Q$_{10}$	100 mg daily.	Improves cellular oxygenation and immune function.
Free form amino acid	As directed on label.	Supplies protein in a form that is rapidly absorbed and assimilated. Use a sublingual form.
Grape seed extract	As directed on label.	A powerful antioxidant to prevent free radical damage.
Glucosamine sulfate or N-acetylglucosamine (N-A-G from Source Naturals)	As directed on label. As directed on label.	Important for regulating the mucous secretions of the respiratory system.
L-cysteine and L-tyrosine	500 mg each daily, on empty stomach. Take with water or juice, not milk. Take with 50 mg vitamin B$_6$ and 100 mg vitamin C for better absorption.	Promotes healing from respiratory disorders. Helpful for stress and allergic disorders. (*See* AMINO ACIDS in Part One.)
Manganese	4 mg daily for 3 months. Take separately from calcium.	An important component in many of the body's enzyme systems. Use manganese chelate form.
Multivitamin and mineral complex with calcium and magnesium and vitamin D$_3$	As directed on label. 400 IU daily.	All nutrients are needed in balance. Use a hypoallergenic formula. Three nutrients necessary for proper immune function.
Potassium	00 mg daily.	Necessary for adrenal gland function. Use potassium protinate or potassium chelate form.
Proteolytic enzymes or Inf-zyme Forte from American Biologics	As directed on label. As directed on label. Take between meals, on an empty stomach.	To aid digestion and destroy free radicals. *Caution:* Do not give these supplements to a child.
Vitamin A and vitamin E and zinc	10,000 IU daily. 200 IU daily. 50 mg daily. Do not exceed a total of 100 mg daily from all supplements.	Three nutrients necessary for proper immune function. Use d-alpha-tocopherol form.

Herbs

❑ Herbs have the potential to create allergic effects, so introduce them slowly and systematically at the beginning.

❑ Boswellia (*Boswellia serrata,* also known as Indian frankincense) works at the cellular level to reduce inflammatory and allergic responses.

❑ Decongest Herbal Formula from ZAND is also a good allergy-fighting product.

❑ Eucalyptus and/or thyme leaves can be used to ease congestion. Soak an ounce of either one in a cup of boiling water and inhale the steam.

❑ Eyebright tea has been noted to reduce hay fever symptoms such as watery eyes and runny nose in children.

❑ Goldenseal root aids the absorption of nutrients. A saline nasal spray that contains goldenseal has been used to wash out pollen and help prevent infection.

Caution: Do not take goldenseal internally on a daily basis for more than one week at a time. Do not use it during pregnancy or if you are breast-feeding, and use with caution if you are allergic to ragweed. If you have a history of cardiovascular disease, diabetes, or glaucoma, use it only under a doctor's supervision.

❑ Japanese researchers have found that licorice root can help allergy sufferers. It has been traditionally used in Japan to battle allergic inflammation. Licorice root produces a hormone that acts as an anti-inflammatory agent and helps restore normal breathing.

Caution: Licorice root should not be used during pregnancy or nursing. It should not be used by persons with diabetes, glaucoma, heart disease, high blood pressure, or a history of stroke.

❑ Nettle (also known as stinging nettle) reduces inflammation in the sinus cavities. It is also a powerful antioxidant that helps prevent free radical damage and aids in preventing allergy attacks.

❑ Wild yam stimulates the production of hormones that reduce inflammation caused by allergies. Wild yam is not for everyone, however (*see* HERBS in Part One).

❑ Yerba maté helps to relieve allergic symptoms. Take 2 to 3 teaspoons of yerba maté in 16 ounces of hot water on an empty stomach.

❑ The following Chinese herbs support sinus health:

• Magnolia flower (*Magnolia liliflora,* also known as xho yi hua) has been used for centuries in traditional Chinese medicine to open nasal passages and relieve headaches associated with sinus problems.

• Scutellaria (*Scutellaria baicalensis*) root contains powerful flavonoids and antioxidants that enhance the immune system. It inhibits the contraction of tissues in allergic reactions.

- Trichosanth (*Trichosanthes kirilowii*) has been used for centuries in traditional Chinese medicine to benefit the respiratory system.

- Wild angelica (*Angelica dahurica*, also known as aka bai zhi) is particularly useful for clearing sinus problems. It has been found to help relieve discomfort around the eyes that occurs when the sinuses above the eyes are blocked. It normalizes swelling, opens nasal passages, and promotes the discharge of pus often associated with sinus infections. Another important action of this herb is the balancing of histamine levels.

❏ Ayurveda is a body of medical knowledge originating in India. (*See* AYURVEDIC REMEDIES in Part Three.) According to this system, some allergic responses are created by the presence of ama, or toxins in the system that are the by-products of improperly digested food. The Ayurvedic herbs picrorrhiza (*Picrorrhiza kurrooa*) and phyllanthus (*Phyllanthus acidus*) are suggested for cooling and cleaning the blood, and helping the liver detoxify the body of ama. Trifala is a traditional Ayurvedic herbal combination formula that is sometimes recommended for allergies. It is said to act on vata, one of the three vital principles that govern the body (vata controls respiration, among other functions) in the intestines and keep it from aggravating and drying the upper respiratory system. Other Ayurvedic herbs suggested for allergies include amla (*Emblica officinalis*), guggul (*Commiphora mukul*), and mulethi (*Glycyrrhiza glabra*, better known in English as licorice).

Caution: Licorice root should not be used during pregnancy or nursing. It should not be used by persons with diabetes, glaucoma, heart disease, high blood pressure, or a history of stroke.

❏ Other herbs that can be beneficial for allergies include burdock, milk thistle, butterbur, dandelion, ginkgo, and horseradish.

Caution: Do not take ginkgo biloba if you have a bleeding disorder, or are scheduled for surgery or a dental procedure.

Recommendations

❏ Rotate your foods. (*See* Rotating Foods: Sample Daily Menus, at the end of this section.) Eat a different group of foods for each of four days and then repeat the cycle. You can select as many of the foods allowed on a specific day as you like but it is essential that no type of food be ingested more often than every four days.

❏ If you suffer from ragweed allergy (or other weed allergies) do not eat melon, cucumbers, bananas, sunflower seeds, chamomile, or any herbal preparation containing echinacea. These substances can add to the symptoms during an episode.

Cautions: Do not use chamomile if you are allergic to ragweed. Do not use during pregnancy or nursing. It may interact with warfarin or cyclosporine, so patients using these drugs should avoid it. Do not take echinacea for longer than three months. It should not be used by people who are allergic to ragweed.

❏ *See* Detecting Hidden Food Allergies on page 182 and fill out the Food Sensitivity Questionnaire. Then omit from your diet for thirty days any food you have listed as consumed four times per week or more.

❏ Adults may follow a fasting program. (*See* FASTING in Part Three.) After a fast, you can try adding back the "foods to avoid" (listed below) in very small amounts, such as one teaspoonful at a time. Record your reactions after eating. If you feel bloated or have a slight headache, an upset stomach, gas, diarrhea, a rapid pulse, or heart palpitations after eating certain foods, eliminate them from your diet for sixty days and try introducing them again in small amounts. If you experience a reaction again, eliminate them from your diet permanently.

❏ Avoid the following foods until it is determined you are not allergic to them: bananas, beef products, caffeine, chocolate, citrus fruits, corn, dairy products, eggs, oats, oysters, peanuts, processed and refined foods, salmon, strawberries, tomatoes, wheat, and white rice.

❏ Avoid mucus-producing foods, such as dairy products, sugar, wheat, and food additives (*see below*).

❏ Avoid any food products that contain artificial color, especially FD&C Yellow No. 5 dye. Many people are allergic to food colorings. Other food additives to avoid include vanillin, benzaldehyde, eucalyptol, monosodium glutamate, BHT-BHA, benzoates, and annatto. Read labels carefully.

❏ If you are allergic to ragweed, do not eat cantaloupe. It contains some of the same proteins as ragweed.

❏ Take the underarm temperature test to determine if you have an underactive thyroid. (*See* HYPOTHYROIDISM in Part Two.)

❏ Be sure to take only hypoallergenic supplements, as these do not contain potentially irritating substances.

❏ Keep rooms free from dust, keep windows shut (use the air conditioner whenever possible), and use a dehumidifier in the basement.

❏ Use mold-proof paint and a disinfectant on walls and furniture.

❏ Purchase an air filter with fine enough filtering capability, such as the HEPA filter, to clean pollen, molds, and dust from your home or office. Standard air filters sold in most stores do not filter pollen. Make sure any filter purchased states on its label that it is suitable for filtering pollen and mold spores.

Detecting Hidden Food Allergies

The first step in discovering hidden food allergies is to develop a list of suspect foods. Using the form below, keep track of how often you consume different foods.

Be careful to note each time you consume one of the foods listed below. Add up your weekly total for each food. Do this for a four-week period.

FOOD SENSITIVITY QUESTIONNAIRE

Type of Food	First Week	Second Week	Third Week	Fourth Week
Beans and Legumes				
Kidney beans	_____	_____	_____	_____
Lentils	_____	_____	_____	_____
Lima beans	_____	_____	_____	_____
Mung beans	_____	_____	_____	_____
Pinto beans	_____	_____	_____	_____
Soybeans	_____	_____	_____	_____
Soymilk	_____	_____	_____	_____
Tofu and tofu products	_____	_____	_____	_____
White beans	_____	_____	_____	_____
Condiments				
Catsup	_____	_____	_____	_____
Gravy	_____	_____	_____	_____
Jams and jellies	_____	_____	_____	_____
Mustard	_____	_____	_____	_____
Pepper	_____	_____	_____	_____
Pickles	_____	_____	_____	_____
Salsa	_____	_____	_____	_____
Salt	_____	_____	_____	_____
Soy sauce	_____	_____	_____	_____
Dairy Products				
Butter	_____	_____	_____	_____
Buttormilk	_____	_____	_____	_____
Cheese	_____	_____	_____	_____
Cottage cheese	_____	_____	_____	_____
Cow's milk	_____	_____	_____	_____
Cream cheese	_____	_____	_____	_____
Eggs	_____	_____	_____	_____
Goat's milk	_____	_____	_____	_____
Ice cream	_____	_____	_____	_____
Margarine	_____	_____	_____	_____
Milk shakes	_____	_____	_____	_____
Sour cream	_____	_____	_____	_____
Yogurt	_____	_____	_____	_____

Type of Food	First Week	Second Week	Third Week	Fourth Week
Fruits and Their Juices				
Apples	_____	_____	_____	_____
Apricots	_____	_____	_____	_____
Bananas	_____	_____	_____	_____
Blackberries	_____	_____	_____	_____
Blueberries	_____	_____	_____	_____
Cherries	_____	_____	_____	_____
Coconut	_____	_____	_____	_____
Cranberries	_____	_____	_____	_____
Dates	_____	_____	_____	_____
Dried fruits (most)	_____	_____	_____	_____
Figs	_____	_____	_____	_____
Grapefruit	_____	_____	_____	_____
Grapes	_____	_____	_____	_____
Lemons	_____	_____	_____	_____
Melons	_____	_____	_____	_____
Nectarines	_____	_____	_____	_____
Oranges	_____	_____	_____	_____
Papayas	_____	_____	_____	_____
Peaches	_____	_____	_____	_____
Pears	_____	_____	_____	_____
Pineapple	_____	_____	_____	_____
Plums	_____	_____	_____	_____
Prunes	_____	_____	_____	_____
Raisins	_____	_____	_____	_____
Raspberries	_____	_____	_____	_____
Strawberries	_____	_____	_____	_____
Tangerines	_____	_____	_____	_____
Grains and Grain Products				
Brown rice	_____	_____	_____	_____
Buckwheat	_____	_____	_____	_____
Cold cereal	_____	_____	_____	_____
Cornmeal	_____	_____	_____	_____
Millet	_____	_____	_____	_____
Oats	_____	_____	_____	_____
Pancakes	_____	_____	_____	_____
Pasta	_____	_____	_____	_____
Quinoa	_____	_____	_____	_____
Rye	_____	_____	_____	_____
Spelt	_____	_____	_____	_____
Tapioca	_____	_____	_____	_____
Wheat and whole wheat products	_____	_____	_____	_____
White flour products	_____	_____	_____	_____
White rice	_____	_____	_____	_____

Type of Food	First Week	Second Week	Third Week	Fourth Week
Meats, Poultry, and Fish				
Bacon	_____	_____	_____	_____
Beef	_____	_____	_____	_____
Bologna	_____	_____	_____	_____
Chicken	_____	_____	_____	_____
Fish	_____	_____	_____	_____
Ham	_____	_____	_____	_____
Lamb	_____	_____	_____	_____
Liver	_____	_____	_____	_____
Luncheon meat	_____	_____	_____	_____
Pork	_____	_____	_____	_____
Sausage	_____	_____	_____	_____
Shellfish	_____	_____	_____	_____
Turkey	_____	_____	_____	_____
Veal	_____	_____	_____	_____
Nuts and Seeds				
Almonds	_____	_____	_____	_____
Brazil nuts	_____	_____	_____	_____
Cashews	_____	_____	_____	_____
Chestnuts	_____	_____	_____	_____
Hazelnuts	_____	_____	_____	_____
Nut butters (other than peanut)	_____	_____	_____	_____
Nut milk	_____	_____	_____	_____
Peanut butter	_____	_____	_____	_____
Peanuts	_____	_____	_____	_____
Pecans	_____	_____	_____	_____
Pistachios	_____	_____	_____	_____
Sesame seeds	_____	_____	_____	_____
Sunflower seeds	_____	_____	_____	_____
Walnuts	_____	_____	_____	_____
Oils				
Canola oil	_____	_____	_____	_____
Corn oil	_____	_____	_____	_____
Cottonseed oil	_____	_____	_____	_____
Olive oil	_____	_____	_____	_____
Peanut oil	_____	_____	_____	_____
Safflower oil	_____	_____	_____	_____
Sesame oil	_____	_____	_____	_____
Soy oil	_____	_____	_____	_____

Type of Food	First Week	Second Week	Third Week	Fourth Week
Sweeteners				
Aspartame (NutraSweet)	_____	_____	_____	_____
Brown sugar	_____	_____	_____	_____
Corn syrup	_____	_____	_____	_____
Fructose	_____	_____	_____	_____
Honey	_____	_____	_____	_____
Maple syrup	_____	_____	_____	_____
Saccharin (Sweet'N Low)	_____	_____	_____	_____
Sucralose (Splenda)	_____	_____	_____	_____
White sugar	_____	_____	_____	_____
Vegetables				
Alfalfa sprouts	_____	_____	_____	_____
Artichokes	_____	_____	_____	_____
Asparagus	_____	_____	_____	_____
Avocados	_____	_____	_____	_____
Beets	_____	_____	_____	_____
Broccoli	_____	_____	_____	_____
Brussels sprouts	_____	_____	_____	_____
Cabbage	_____	_____	_____	_____
Carrots	_____	_____	_____	_____
Cauliflower	_____	_____	_____	_____
Celery	_____	_____	_____	_____
Corn	_____	_____	_____	_____
Cucumbers	_____	_____	_____	_____
Eggplant	_____	_____	_____	_____
Garlic	_____	_____	_____	_____
Green beans	_____	_____	_____	_____
Kale	_____	_____	_____	_____
Lettuce	_____	_____	_____	_____
Mushrooms	_____	_____	_____	_____
Okra	_____	_____	_____	_____
Olives	_____	_____	_____	_____
Onions	_____	_____	_____	_____
Parsley	_____	_____	_____	_____
Peas	_____	_____	_____	_____
Peppers	_____	_____	_____	_____
Potatoes	_____	_____	_____	_____
Radishes	_____	_____	_____	_____
Spinach	_____	_____	_____	_____
Summer squash	_____	_____	_____	_____
Sweet potatoes	_____	_____	_____	_____
Swiss chard	_____	_____	_____	_____
Tomatoes	_____	_____	_____	_____
Turnips	_____	_____	_____	_____
Winter squash	_____	_____	_____	_____
Zucchini	_____	_____	_____	_____

Type of Food	First Week	Second Week	Third Week	Fourth Week
Miscellaneous and Junk Foods				
Alcoholic beverages	_____	_____	_____	_____
Candy	_____	_____	_____	_____
Cheeseburger	_____	_____	_____	_____
Chewing gum	_____	_____	_____	_____
Chocolate	_____	_____	_____	_____
Coffee	_____	_____	_____	_____
Cola	_____	_____	_____	_____
Corn chips	_____	_____	_____	_____
Flavored gelatin	_____	_____	_____	_____
French fries	_____	_____	_____	_____
Fried foods	_____	_____	_____	_____
Hamburger	_____	_____	_____	_____
Pastry	_____	_____	_____	_____
Peppermint	_____	_____	_____	_____
Pizza	_____	_____	_____	_____
Popcorn	_____	_____	_____	_____
Potato chips	_____	_____	_____	_____
Pudding	_____	_____	_____	_____
Tea	_____	_____	_____	_____

Note any other snacks or other foods not listed above that you eat regularly. _____

After the one-month recording period, go through the form and compile a list of all the foods you ate four times a week or more. This is your list of suspect foods.

KEEPING A FOOD DIARY

Once you have your list of suspect foods, omit these foods from your diet for a period of thirty days to give your body a rest from them. Then reintroduce the suspect foods, one at a time. Add only one new food a day. As you add foods back to your diet, keep a diary of any symptoms you experience and monitor your reaction with the Food Allergy Self-Test (see page 170), as in the following sample:

Sample Food Diary

Date	Meal	Time	Foods Consumed	Symptoms
4/12	Breakfast	8:39 a.m.	milk, toast	gas, bloating
	Lunch	12:30 p.m.	pea soup, salad	no symptoms

If you note a reaction to any of the reintroduced foods, omit that food from your diet for another two months, then try a small amount of it again. If you have a reaction after the second reintroduction, eliminate that food from your diet permanently.

Use the form that follows to record your experiences as you reintroduce the banished foods into your diet. By first eliminating foods, then slowly adding them back into your diet, you will be able to pinpoint exactly which foods are giving you trouble.

Food Diary

Date	Meal	Time	Foods Consumed	Symptoms
_____	Breakfast Lunch Dinner Snack			
_____	Breakfast Lunch Dinner Snack			
_____	Breakfast Lunch Dinner Snack			
_____	Breakfast Lunch Dinner Snack			
_____	Breakfast Lunch Dinner Snack			
_____	Breakfast Lunch Dinner Snack			
_____	Breakfast Lunch Dinner Snack			

Medications: _____

_____

_____

Herbs: _____

_____

Miscellaneous: _____

_____

When monitoring your reactions to different foods, it is important to be aware that food allergies can manifest themselves in many ways, not all of them obvious. The following symptoms are the most common manifestations of food allergies:

- Acne, especially pimples on the chin or around the mouth.
- Arthritis.
- Asthma.
- Chest and shoulder pains.
- Colitis.
- Depression.
- Fatigue.
- Headaches.
- Hemorrhoids.
- Insomnia.
- Intestinal problems.
- Muscle disorders.
- Sinus problems.
- Ulcers.

Your health care provider may look also for the following signs and symptoms when trying to determine if you have an allergy:

- Acid/alkaline imbalance.
- Anemia.
- Bed-wetting.
- Conjunctivitis.

- Diarrhea.
- Dizzy spells and floating sensations.
- Excessive drooling.
- Dark circles under the eyes or puffy eyes.
- Eye pain, tearing.
- Fluid retention.
- Hearing loss.
- Hyperactivity.
- Learning disabilities.
- Nasal congestion or chronic runny nose.
- Noises in the ear.
- Periods of blurred vision.
- Phobias.
- Poor memory and concentration.
- Poor muscle coordination.
- Red circles on the cheeks (as if wearing rouge, even in children).
- Repeated colds or ear infections, especially in children.
- Sensitivity to light.
- Severe menstrual symptoms.
- Swollen fingers and cold hands.
- Unusual body odor.
- Watery, itchy, red eyes.
- Recurrence of any illness despite treatment.

The Rotation Diet

Although some people have a reaction soon after ingesting a particular food for the first time, food allergies often develop slowly. The reason for this is that if you consume the same foods daily, your body eventually develops an intolerance. Rather than nourishing the body, these foods provoke harmful reactions.

Once you have identified and avoided an allergenic food for sixty to ninety days, you can usually reintroduce it without any adverse reactions, as long as you maintain a rotation diet. If you have been diagnosed with a food allergy, check with your health care provider before reintroducing the offending food. The basic principle behind the rotation diet is that each type of food is to be consumed only on one out of every four days. For example, if you eat beans on Monday, you wouldn't eat beans

again on Tuesday, Wednesday, or Thursday. If you eat salmon on Friday, you would wait at least until Tuesday before consuming any other fish. Rotating foods in this way will not only make you feel better, it will also help to stabilize your weight.

Before starting the rotation diet, follow a fasting program to cleanse your system of offending foods and toxins. (See FASTING in Part Three.) After you have finished the program, consume only the following foods for the next two weeks: For children, confirm with the pediatrician that this is acceptable to support growth and normal development.

- Baked or broiled chicken or turkey.
- Broiled, boiled, or baked fish.
- Brown rice.

- Fresh, unsweetened fruit and vegetable juices.

- Fresh fruits (except oranges).

- Herbal teas.

- Raw, steamed, or broiled vegetables.

Although you may feel that this list of foods does not offer much variety, there are numerous fruits and vegetables available, in addition to a variety of fish. After two weeks on this cleansing diet, you can once again begin to eat a greater number of different foods, but on a rotating basis, eating each type of food on no more than one out of four days. Use the sample menus below as a guide to help you put together daily menus rotating among different foods. Of course, if you are sensitive to any of the foods listed, substitute a food that agrees with you.

Once you start following this program, you should start seeing an increase in your energy level in a week or less.

Rotating Foods: Sample Daily Menus

Breakfast	Lunch	Dinner	Snacks
Day 1			
Glass of distilled water	Tomato stuffed with tuna	Broiled whitefish or salmon	Celery sticks
Papaya juice with vitamin C	salad or tuna burger on	with dill	Pecans
Fresh papaya or peach	wheat-free bread with	Cole slaw or sprout salad	Fresh papaya or peach
Oatmeal or oat bran cereal	tomato, onion, alfalfa	with tomato, onion, celery,	
with 1 tbsp raw honey	sprouts, and eggless	and eggless mayonnaise	
Skim milk	mayonnaise	Steamed asparagus	
Rose hip tea	Fresh lemonade	Herbal tea or lemonade	
		Substitutions: Cauliflower,	
		Brussels sprouts, or sau-	
		erkraut can be substituted	
		for asparagus.	
Day 2			
Glass of distilled water	Home-cooked sliced turkey	Baked skinless turkey or	Apple
Apple juice with vitamin C	or chicken on whole wheat	chicken with lemon juice,	Walnuts
Fresh apple	bread with lettuce and	garlic, and onion powder	
Cream of wheat cereal with	mustard	Baked potato with 2 tsp ses-	*Substitutions:* Baked apple
2 tsp pure maple syrup	Potato soup and wheat	ame oil, chopped chives,	with pure maple syrup;
and soymilk	crackers (make soup with	and a dash of onion pow-	wheat crackers; sugar-free
Herbal tea	soymilk)	der	applesauce topped with
	Herbal tea or apple juice	Tossed salad with radishes,	walnuts.
		zucchini, yellow squash,	
	Substitutions: Soy burger or	kale, and soy oil dressing	
	eggless egg salad with	Herbal tea	
	eggless mayonnaise for		
	turkey or chicken; tofu	*Substitutions:* Cornish game	
	soup for potato soup.	hens for turkey or chicken;	
		vinaigrette dressing for	
		soy oil dressing.	

Day 3

Glass of distilled water
Cranberry juice with
  vitamin C
Sliced banana with almond
  milk
Cream of rice or puffed rice
  cereal
Herbal tea

½ avocado filled with cooked
  brown rice and fresh
  peas, water chestnuts,
  and a dash of herbal seasoning and lemon juice,
  topped with slivered almonds
Split pea soup with rice
  crackers (make soup with
  rice milk)

Stir-fried vegetables with
  broccoli, green peppers,
  leeks, pea pods, sweet
  red peppers, bean
  sprouts, bamboo shoots,
  and grated fresh ginger,
  served over cooked brown
  rice
Rice cakes with almond
  butter
Coffee substitute (from a
  health food store) or
  herbal tea

Raw almonds
Rice crackers with almond
  butter
Sliced bananas

Day 4

Glass of distilled water
Grape juice with vitamin C
Rye toast with sugar-free
  grape jam
2 poached or soft-boiled
  eggs or corn cereal
Herbal tea

Egg salad with chopped cucumber, green onions,
  black olives, and low-fat
  cottage cheese, topped
  with raisins
RyKrisp crackers with sugar-
  free grape jelly or jam
Lentil soup or cool lentil
  salad

Spinach-mushroom quiche
Fresh spinach salad with
  hard-boiled eggs, arti-
  choke, shredded raw
  beets, raisins, and olive oil
  and lemon dressing
Iced herbal tea flavored with
  grape juice

RyKrisp crackers with sugar-
  free grape jam or sesame
  butter and sesame seeds
Fresh grapes
Raisins
Hard-boiled eggs

Sulfite Allergies

Sulfites are common food additives used as sanitary agents and preservatives to prevent discoloration of foods. They are usually used in restaurant salad bars and are also present in many supermarket foods, including frozen foods, dried fruits, and certain fresh fruits and vegetables. Many people are allergic to sulfites. The types and severity of reactions to sulfites in sensitive individuals vary, and may include breathing difficulties, anaphylactic shock, severe headaches, abdominal pain, stuffy and/or runny nose, flushing of the face and a "hot flash" feeling, diarrhea, irritability, and/or feelings of anger. These symptoms tend to occur quickly, usually within twenty to thirty minutes after consuming sulfites.

Sulfites pose a greater danger to some people than to others. People with asthma, a history of allergies, or a deficiency of the liver enzyme sulfite oxidase can suffer great harm. It is not always easy to determine if a food product contains sulfites. Sulfiting agents appear in food ingredient lists in a variety of ways, including sodium sulfite, sodium bisulfite, sodium metabisulfite, potassium bisulfite, potassium metabisulfite, and sulfur dioxide. Any ingredient ending in -*sulfite* should be assumed to be a sulfiting agent. If you have ever suffered a reaction after ingesting a food you believe contained sulfites, you should beware of the foods and beverages listed in the table below, which often contain these substances. Sulfite-free forms of some of these foods may be found in health food stores.

FOODS AND BEVERAGES THAT OFTEN CONTAIN SULFITES

Fresh Fruits and Vegetables

Avocado dip (guacamole)	Grapes	Potatoes	Prepared cut fruit or
Cole slaw	Mushrooms		vegetable salads

Fish and Shellfish

Canned seafood soups	Dried fish	Frozen, canned, or dried	Oysters
Clams	Fresh shellfish,	shellfish	Scallops
Crabs	especially shrimp	Lobster	Shrimp

Prepared/Processed Foods

Beet sugars	Cornstarch	Horseradish	Sauerkraut
Breading mixes	Dietetic processed foods	Jams and jellies	Shredded coconut
Breakfast cereals	Dried or canned soups	Maraschino cherries	Trail mixes
Brown sugar	Dry salad dressing mixes	Noodle and rice mixes	Wine vinegar
Canned fruit pie fillings	Frozen, canned, or dried	Olives	
Canned mushrooms	fruits and vegetables	Onion relish	
Caramels	Frozen French fries	Pickles	
Corn, maple, and	Glazed fruits	Potato chips	
pancake syrups	Hard candies	Sauces and gravies	

Miscellaneous

Apple cider	Bottled, canned, or frozen	Cordials	Gelatin
Baked goods	vegetable juices	Cornmeal	Instant tea mixes
Beer	Cocktail mixes	Frozen doughs	Wines
Bottled, canned, or frozen	Colas	Fruit drinks	
fruit juices			

❏ For airborne particles that cause allergies, try using a stand-alone air purification device. Many brands are available, the electrostatic type being the lowest maintenance and the replaceable filter type being the highest. The Air Supply personal air purifier from Wein Products is a miniature unit that is worn around the neck. It sets up an invisible pure air shield against microorganisms (such as viruses, bacteria, and mold) and microparticles (including dust, pollen, and pollutants) in the air. It also eliminates vapors, smells, and harmful volatile compounds in the air.

❏ Depending on the severity of your allergies be sure to wear long pants and long-sleeved shirts when spending time outside. Change your clothes and shower as soon as you return indoors. For some, using a "high-efficiency" mask (available in drugstores and medical supply stores) may be advisable.

❏ Pollen counts in late summer are highest between 5:00 A.M. and 10:00 A.M., so schedule your gardening and other outdoor activities with this in mind. You can learn what trees and plants are pollinating around you and what the mold and pollen count is by contacting the National Allergy Bureau (www.aaaai.org/nab/index.cfm?p=pollen).

❏ If you are a chronic allergy sufferer, avoid exercising outdoors.

❏ On windy days, when more pollen is blown through the air, try to avoid going outside if your allergies are severe. The best time for you to be outdoors is after a rainstorm, when pollen levels drop significantly.

❏ Do not smoke, and avoid secondhand smoke.

❏ Avoid taking aspirin within three hours of eating.

Considerations

❏ Steroid nasal sprays can be very effective for allergies and are less expensive than many prescription medications. These sprays, however, do not relieve itchiness of the eyes. They generally need up to ten days to become effective, so it is advisable to begin taking them about a week prior to hay fever season. Be sure to check first with your doctor before using them, as recent studies suggest a possible link between steroid nasal sprays and the development of glaucoma—a concern for older adults. In 2009, the FDA warned consumers to stop using and discard three zinc-containing Zicam intranasal products because the products may cause a loss of sense of smell.

❏ Plants produce oxygen as a normal part of their growth and living process, and help to remove pollutants from indoor air. Some plants suggested for this purpose include areca palm, bamboo palm, Boston fern, dracaena, dwarf date palm, English ivy, ficus alii, lady palm, peace lily, rubber plant, and spider plant.

❏ Acupressure and acupuncture have had some success in relieving allergy symptoms. (*See* ACUPRESSURE and ACUPUNCTURE *under* PAIN CONTROL in Part Three.)

❏ *The British Medical Journal* reported that taking aspirin before consuming an allergenic food makes it possible for more of the allergy-provoking food to be absorbed. In contrast, taking ABC Aerobic Bulk Cleanse from Aerobic Life Industries combined with aloe vera juice may slow the absorption of foods that cause a reaction. Taking oat bran or guar gum in the morning works in the same way. Wheat bran is not recommended as a source of fiber for allergy-prone individuals because wheat is highly allergenic. (*See* NATURAL FOOD SUPPLEMENTS in Part One for a discussion of fiber.)

❏ Many allergy sufferers are turning to homeopathic remedies to combat allergy symptoms. They work with the body's natural functions to shut off the allergic response instead of masking symptoms. Combination remedies are often the easiest way to use homeopathy for allergies. BioAllers has a line of homeopathic combination remedies designed for specific allergies, including Animal Hair/ Dander, Grain/Dairy, Grass Pollen, Mold/Yeast/Dust, Pollen/Hayfever, Sinus & Allergy Nasal Spray, and Tree Pollen Allergy Relief formulas.

❏ Research is being conducted on the ability of coenzyme Q_{10} to counter histamine for asthma and allergy sufferers.

❏ Quercetin—found in apples, berries, grapefruit, onions, cabbage, tea, and red wine—is a potent flavonoid. Recently, researchers at the Nippon Medical School in Japan found seasonal allergy sufferers taking it had a 96 percent decrease in histamine release. Quercetin is better absorbed when taken with bromelain, an enzyme normally found in pineapple. For allergies, try taking one 500-milligram quercetin capsule along with one 100-milligram bromelain capsule and 500 milligrams vitamin C with meals, twice daily.

❏ To find useful products for allergy sufferers, go to www.allergybuyersclub.com.

❏ *See also* CHEMICAL ALLERGIES in Part Two and FASTING in Part Three.

❏ For information about organizations that can provide information and assistance for people with allergies, *see* Health and Medical Organizations in the Appendix.

ALOPECIA

See HAIR LOSS.

ALPHA-1 ANTITRYPSIN DEFICIENCY

See under RARE DISORDERS.

ALUMINUM TOXICITY

Aluminum is not a heavy metal, but it can be toxic if present in excessive amounts—even in small amounts, if it is deposited in the brain. Many of the symptoms of aluminum toxicity are similar to those of Alzheimer's disease and osteoporosis. Aluminum toxicity can lead to colic, rickets, gastrointestinal disturbances, poor calcium metabolism, extreme nervousness, anemia, headaches, decreased liver and kidney function, forgetfulness, speech disturbances, memory loss, softening of the bones, and weak, aching muscles.

Because aluminum is excreted through the kidneys, toxic amounts of aluminum may impair kidney function.

The accumulation of aluminum salts in the brain has been implicated in seizures and reduced mental faculties. To reach the brain, aluminum must pass the blood-brain barrier, an elaborate structure that filters the blood before it reaches this vital organ. Although elemental aluminum does not readily pass through this barrier, certain aluminum compounds will, such as aluminum fluoride. Many municipal water supplies are treated with both alum (aluminum sulfate) and fluoride, and these two chemicals readily combine with each other in the blood. Moreover, aluminum fluoride, once formed, is very poorly excreted in the urine.

Intestinal absorption of high levels of aluminum and silicon can result in the formation of compounds that accumulate in the cerebral cortex and prevent nerve impulses from being carried to and from the brain in the proper manner. Chronic calcium deficiency can aggravate the situation.

People who have worked in aluminum smelting plants for long periods have been known to experience dizziness, impaired coordination, and loss of balance and energy. The accumulation of aluminum in the brain has been cited as a possible cause for these symptoms. Perhaps most alarming, there is evidence to suggest that long-term accumulation of aluminum in the brain may contribute to the development of Alzheimer's disease.

It has been estimated that the average person ingests between 3 and 10 milligrams of aluminum a day. Aluminum is the most abundant metallic element in the earth's crust. It is absorbed into the body primarily through the digestive tract, but also through the lungs and skin, and is absorbed by and accumulates in body tissues. Because aluminum permeates our air, water, and soil, it is found naturally in varying amounts in nearly all food and water. Aluminum is also used to make cookware, cooking utensils, and foil.

Many other everyday products contain aluminum, including over-the-counter painkillers, anti-inflammatories, and douche preparations. Aluminum is an additive in most baking powders, is used in food processing, and is present in products ranging from antiperspirants and toothpaste to dental amalgams to bleached flour, grated cheese, table salt, and beer (especially when packaged in aluminum cans). One prominent source of aluminum is our municipal water supplies.

The excessive use of antacids is probably the most common cause of aluminum toxicity in this country, especially in people who have kidney problems. Many over-the-counter antacids contain amounts of aluminum hydroxide that may be too much for the kidneys to excrete successfully. Even antacids containing a mixture of aluminum and other ingredients may pose a problem; in some people, such products may cause the same reaction as products composed entirely of aluminum compounds. Moreover, the chemical solution (dialysate) used during kidney dialysis contains aluminum. It may be associated with "dialysis dementia" sometimes experienced by patients. There has been some study on the possible link between aluminum and Alzheimer's disease, but the results have been mixed. (*See* ALZHEIMER'S DISEASE in Part Two for a discussion of aluminum and Alzheimer's disease.)

NUTRIENTS

SUPPLEMENT	SUGGESTED DOSAGE	COMMENTS
Helpful		
Apple pectin	2 tbsp twice daily.	Binds with metals in the colon and excretes them from the body.
Calcium and magnesium	1,500 mg daily. 750 mg daily.	Minerals that bind with aluminum and eliminate it from the body. Use chelate forms. *Caution:* Men should check with a physician before taking calcium.
Coenzyme A from Coenzyme-A Technologies	As directed on label.	Supports the immune system's detoxification of many dangerous substances.
Garlic (Kyolic from Wakunaga)	2 capsules 3 times daily.	Acts as a detoxifier.
Kelp	2,000–3,000 mg daily.	Has a balanced mineral content. Acts as a detoxifier of excess metals.
Lecithin granules or capsules	1 tbsp 3 times daily, before meals. 1,200 mg 3 times daily, before meals.	Aids in healing of the brain and cell membranes.
L-glutathione	As directed on label.	Aids in blocking damage from toxic metals and radiation.
Multivitamin and mineral complex	As directed on label.	Basic for stabilizing vitamin and mineral imbalances in toxic conditions. Use a hypoallergenic high-potency formula.
Oxy-Cleanse from Earth's Bounty	As directed on label.	Helps remove heavy metals, other pollutants, and anaerobic pathogens from the body.
S-Adenosylmethionine (SAMe)	As directed on label.	Helps reduce stress and nervousness caused by excess aluminum. *Caution:* Do not use if you have bipolar mood disorder or take prescription antidepressants. Do not give to a child under twelve.
Vitamin B complex plus extra vitamin B_6 and vitamin B_{12}	100 mg of each major B vitamin 3 times daily (amounts of individual vitamins in a complex will vary). 50 mg 3 times daily. 300 mcg 3 times daily.	The B vitamins, especially B_6, are important in ridding the intestinal tract of excess metals and in removing them from the body. Sublingual forms are recommended for better absorption. Injections (under a doctor's supervision) may be necessary.
Vitamin E	200 IU daily.	A powerful antioxidant. Fights cellular aging by protecting cell membranes. Also improves circulation and prolongs the life of red blood cells. Use d-alpha-tocopherol form.

Herbs

❑ Burdock root, echinacea, fiber, ginkgo biloba and ginseng when taken regularly, are beneficial for blocking damage to the body by toxic heavy metals and radiation.

Cautions: Do not take echinacea for longer than three months. It should not be used by people who are allergic to ragweed. Do not take ginkgo biloba if you have a bleeding disorder, or are scheduled for surgery or a dental procedure. Do not use ginseng if you have high blood pressure, or are pregnant or nursing.

Recommendations

❑ Maintain a diet that is high in fiber and includes apple pectin.

❑ Use only stainless steel, glass, or iron cookware. Stainless steel is best.

❑ Beware of products containing aluminum. Read labels and avoid those that contain aluminum, or dihydroxyaluminum.

❑ Include bottled waters with silica in your diet.

Considerations

❑ A hair analysis can be used to determine levels of aluminum in the body. (*See* HAIR ANALYSIS in Part Three.)

❑ If you use chelation therapy, use oral chelating agents only. (*See* CHELATION THERAPY in Part Three). Many researchers believe aluminum cannot be chelated out of the body, as some metals can, but it can be displaced or moved.

❑ Some research indicates that the longer you cook food in aluminum pots, the more they corrode, and the more aluminum compounds migrate into food and are absorbed by the body. Aluminum is more readily dissolved by acid-forming foods, such as coffee, cheeses, meats, black and green tea, cabbage, cucumbers, tomatoes, turnips, spinach, and radishes.

❑ Acid rain leaches aluminum out of the soil and into drinking water.

❑ *See also* ALZHEIMER'S DISEASE below.

ALZHEIMER'S DISEASE

Alzheimer's disease is a common type of dementia, or decline in intellectual function. Once thought rare, Alzheimer's disease is now known to affect as many as 5.3 million people in the United States, according to the Alzheimer's Association. It afflicts 10 percent of Americans over sixty-five and as many as 50 percent of those over eighty-five. However, the disease does not affect only the elderly, but may strike when a person is in his or her forties.

This disorder was first identified in 1906 by a German neurologist named Alois Alzheimer. It is characterized by progressive mental deterioration to such a degree that it interferes with one's ability to function socially and at work. Memory and abstract thought processes are impaired. Alzheimer's disease is an irreversible, progressive disorder. Deterioration in critical areas of the brain may precede symptoms by as much as twenty to forty years. As Alzheimer's disease progresses, there is severe memory loss, particularly in short-term memory. The person may recall past events but be unable to remember a just-viewed television show. At this stage, disorientation usually begins as well. Dysphasia (the inability to find the right word) may occur, and mood swings can be unpredictable and sudden. In the final stage, Alzheimer's disease creates severe confusion and disorientation, and possibly hallucinations or delusions. Some people become violent and angry, while others may be docile and passive. It is in this later stage that people with Alzheimer's disease may wander without purpose, experience incontinence, and neglect personal hygiene. Since the behavioral symptoms of Alzheimer's disease result from changes in the brain, the person neither intends to nor can control this behavior.

Once considered a psychological phenomenon, Alzheimer's disease is now known to be a degenerative disorder that is characterized by a specific set of physiological changes in the brain. Nerve fibers surrounding the hippocampus, the brain's memory center, become tangled (neurofibrillary tangles), and information is no longer carried properly to or from the brain. New memories cannot be formed, and memories formed earlier cannot be retrieved. Characteristic plaques accumulate in the brain as well. These plaques are composed largely of a protein-containing substance called beta-amyloid. Scientists believe that the plaques accumulate in and damage nerve cells.

Many people worry that their forgetfulness is a sign of Alzheimer's disease. Most of us forget where we have put our keys or other everyday objects at one time or another, but this is not an indication of Alzheimer's disease. A good example of the difference between forgetfulness and dementia is the following: If you do not remember where you put your glasses, that is forgetfulness. If you do not remember that you wear glasses, that may be a sign of dementia.

Other disorders can cause symptoms similar to those of Alzheimer's disease. Dementia may result from arteriosclerosis (hardening of the arteries) that slowly cuts off the supply of blood to the brain. The death of brain tissue from a series of minor strokes, or from pressure exerted by an accumulation of fluid in the brain, may cause dementia.

The presence of small blood clots in vessels that supply the brain, a brain tumor, hypothyroidism, and advanced syphilis all can cause symptoms similar to those of Alzheimer's disease. In addition, the average person over the age of sixty-five is likely to be taking between eight and ten different prescription and over-the-counter drugs. Drug reactions, coupled with a nutrient-poor diet, often adversely affect people not only physically, but mentally as well.

The precise cause or causes of Alzheimer's disease are unknown, but research reveals a number of interesting clues. Many of them point to nutritional deficiencies. For example, people with Alzheimer's disease tend to have low levels of vitamin B_{12}, vitamin B_3, and zinc in their bodies. The B vitamins are important in cognitive functioning, and it is well known that the processed foods constituting so much of the modern diet have been stripped of these essential nutrients. Low levels of B_6, B_{12}, and folic acid coupled with high homocysteine levels predict cognitive decline with aging. In fact, 1 milligram of folic acid helped one medication, a cholinesterase inhibitor used for treating early Alzheimer's disease, work more effectively. The development of the neurofibrillary tangles and amyloid plaques in the brain that are characteristic of the disease have been associated with zinc deficiency. Malabsorption problems, which are common among elderly people, make them more prone than others to nutritional deficiencies. Alcohol and many medications further deplete crucial vitamins and minerals.

Levels of the antioxidant vitamins A and E and the carotenoids (including beta-carotene) are also low in people with Alzheimer's disease. These nutrients act as free radical scavengers; deficiencies may expose the brain cells to increased oxidative damage. However, some data indicates that taking vitamin E or C does not reduce the risk of developing Alzheimer's disease or overall dementia. In addition, deficiencies of boron, potassium, and selenium have been found in people with Alzheimer's disease.

Some research has drawn a connection between Alzheimer's disease and high concentrations of aluminum in the brain. Autopsies of people who have died of Alzheimer's disease reveal excessive amounts of aluminum in the hippocampus area and in the cerebral cortex, the external layer of gray matter responsible for higher brain functions such as abstract thinking, judgment, memory, and language.

It may be that exposure to excessive amounts of aluminum, especially if combined with a lack of essential vitamins, minerals, and antioxidants predisposes one to developing Alzheimer's disease. However, one study, published in *Archives of Neurology* in May 1998, showed no further correlation between the density of neurofibrillary tangles in the frontal and temporal lobes of the cortex and bulk aluminum concentration. This study further demonstrated that levels of aluminum are not elevated in the cerebrospinal fluid of patients with Alzheimer's disease.

In a more recent study, a single dose of aluminum given to patients with Alzheimer's disease had no effect on cognition. However, there is concern that the correct dose may not have been used and that the one-day study was not sufficient to rule out aluminum as a cause of Alzheimer's disease. One way to rid the body of aluminum is to consume silicic acid (silica), which is found in some bottled waters. Silicic acid binds to aluminum and reduces its bio-activity. In one study, Alzheimer's patients who consumed about one and a half quarts of water daily with silicic acid showed an increase in their excretion of silicic acid and a decrease in urinary aluminum. This translated into an overall reduction of aluminum in the body. In fact, the study showed that women who drink water with appreciable amounts of silica have a reduced risk of developing Alzheimer's disease.

Many people who develop Alzheimer's disease have a family history of the disorder, suggesting that heredity may be involved. By age ninety, the risk is at least 50 percent for those with a first-degree relative (father, mother, brother, sister) who has (or had) Alzheimer's disease. For twins, it is even higher—58 percent to 79 percent of Alzheimer's disease is hereditary. As with other brain disorders, such as schizophrenia and bipolar mood disorder, the hereditary pattern is complicated.

At least four gene variations are linked to Alzheimer's disease. All of them reduce the clearance, or increase the production, of beta-amyloid. A variation of a gene involved in the synthesis of beta-amyloid, located on chromosome 21, is associated with a rare type of Alzheimer's disease that typically begins between the ages of forty and fifty. Interestingly, people with Down syndrome, who carry an extra copy of chromosome 21, are prone to develop very early Alzheimer's disease, beginning in their thirties and forties. No one knows for sure when the disease actually begins, and the onset of the illness may predate clinical symptoms by years, or even decades.

Yet another possible culprit in the death of brain cells is the immune system. Many illnesses result from immune system malfunction causing it to attack the body's own tissues. Powerful immune system proteins called complement proteins have been found around the plaques and tangles in the brains of people who have died of Alzheimer's disease.

In animals, brain injury is known to result in an alteration in the genetic "instructions" for two kinds of complement proteins. Some experts theorize that complement proteins normally help clear away dead cells, but in Alzheimer's disease, they begin to attack healthy cells as well. Cell degeneration results in accumulations of amyloid. Many researchers believe that beta-amyloid is a key player in this memory-destroying disease. This substance is not unique to the brain, but is produced in virtually every cell in the body as a result of the degeneration of tissue. Many of the dangerous effects of beta-amyloid seem to arise from oxidative damage. Amyloid itself is not highly toxic, but it might possibly trigger dementia if a critical mass accumulates in the brain. Further evidence reveals that the presence of amyloid may trigger the release of a cascade of complement proteins, perhaps sparking a vicious cycle of inflammation and further plaque deposits. However, an immune system attack on brain cells may be a result, or may be merely one element, of Alzheimer's disease, rather than the cause. Other potential risk factors being studied are head injury, very high blood pressure, and low education levels.

Although all of these findings offer hope that Alzheimer's disease may one day be fully understood, and thereby prevented, science does not yet know what can be done to arrest the mental deterioration. Even diagnosis of the disease is not a precise science.

There are tests that can suggest a diagnosis of Alzheimer's disease and that can dismiss other problems as the cause of symptoms, but currently there is no single laboratory procedure or biochemical marker that can definitively confirm the disorder in a living person. A study conducted at the National Institute of Mental Health (NIMH) and reported in the *Journal of the American Medical Association* (*JAMA*) showed that testing spinal fluid for beta-amyloid and tau proteins (which make up the tangles) could help identify people at risk for the disease. It would first be necessary to establish a baseline measurement, then track the changes over time, but using these two biomarkers may signify some progress in the diagnosis of the disease. At present, physicians make a probable diagnosis by performing a comprehensive evaluation including a complete health history and physical examination, a mental status assessment, neurological tests, blood tests, urinalysis, an electrocardiogram (EKG), and X-rays. Additional tests may be conducted, such as a computerized tomography (CAT) scan, electroencephalogram (EEG, a recording of brain-wave patterns), and formal psychiatric assessment. These tests are necessary to rule out other possible causes of dementia symptoms, such as pernicious anemia, hypothyroidism, or tumors. Documenting symptoms over time, in a diary-like fashion, helps doctors to understand each individual case. Unfortunately, the diagnosis of Alzheimer's disease is often made long after the person has lost the ability to communicate and comprehend information. Milder signs of Alzheimer's disease may not be detected in the very old, and many people die before developing obvious symptoms. People with family members who have Alzheimer's disease are probably more able to detect the early signs than are doctors.

As more is learned about the contribution of genetic and other factors to Alzheimer's disease, the possibility of delaying the progression of the disease may become more real.

Nutrients may have a beneficial effect, and one study has shown that vitamin E slowed the progress of some components of the disease by up to seven months in those who already have Alzheimer's disease. Research also indicates that the herb ginkgo biloba, a natural remedy known for many years, may be helpful in treating some symptoms, although it should be used with caution as its use can sometimes lead to excessive bleeding, especially if it is used in conjunction with aspirin therapy.

A study done at the Rush Institute for Healthy Aging in Chicago indicated that people with low levels of niacin (vitamin B_3) were 70 percent more likely to get Alzheimer's disease than those who had higher levels in their diet. Niacin is required for cell respiration, helps release energy, and assists in metabolizing carbohydrates, fats, and proteins. The secretion of bile, functioning of the nervous system, synthesis of sex hormones, and many other processes require this vitamin. The study showed the protective effect began at 17 milligrams per day, about what a healthy male normally requires (females require 13 milligrams per day). Supplements are usually taken in 100-milligram increments, so benefits certainly can be expected at this level.

No one should accept a diagnosis of Alzheimer's disease without first undergoing a trial of intensive nutritional therapy, using zinc, vitamin B_3 (as described above), and vitamin B_{12}, perhaps as injections. Vitamin B_{12} functions in numerous metabolic processes affecting nerve tissue, including the synthesis of neurotransmitters and the formation of the insulating sheath surrounding many nerves, and it may play a role in the fight against Alzheimer's disease. Strange prickly or tingling sensations, loss of coordination, and dementia can be caused by B_{12} deficiency even if the person does not have pernicious anemia, the classic sign of that deficiency. If an individual responds to vitamin treatment, Alzheimer's disease can be ruled out.

NUTRIENTS

SUPPLEMENT	SUGGESTED DOSAGE	COMMENTS
Essential		
Acetylcholine	500 mg 3 times daily, on an empty stomach.	Deficiency has been implicated as possibly causing dementia.
Acetyl-L-carnitine	500 mg twice daily.	May enhance brain metabolism. Slows down deterioration of memory and reduces the production of free radicals.
Boron	3 mg daily. Do not exceed this amount.	Improves brain and memory function.
Coenzyme A from Coenzyme-A Technologies	As directed on label.	Supports the immune system's detoxification of many dangerous substances.
Coenzyme Q_{10}	100–200 mg daily.	Increases oxygenation of cells and is involved in the generation of cellular energy.
Folic acid	As directed on label.	To aid in controlling homocysteine levels. Studies have shown high levels of homocysteine in this disorder.
Iron	As directed by physician.	A deficiency may be present. *Caution:* Do not take iron unless prescribed by your physician.
Lecithin granules or capsules	1 tbsp 3 times daily, before meals. 1,200 mg 3 times daily, before meals.	Needed for improved memory. Contains choline.
Multivitamin and mineral complex with potassium	99 mg daily.	All nutrients are necessary in balance. Use a high-potency formula. Needed for proper electrolyte balance.
Phosphatidyl serine	300 mg 3 times daily.	Improves memory. However, this was from bovine sources, which are no longer available, and the efficacy of newer products has not been determined.
Pycnogenol or grape seed extract	60 mg three times daily. As directed on label.	Potent antioxidants that readily pass the blood-brain barrier to protect brain cells from free radical damage.
S-Adenosylmethionine (SAMe)	400 mg twice daily.	Lowers homocysteine levels. *Caution:* Do not use if you have bipolar mood disorder or take prescription antidepressants.
Selenium	200 mcg daily.	Powerful antioxidant for brain cell protection.
Trimethylglycine (TMG)	500–1,000 mg daily, in the morning.	Assists the body in utilizing vitamin B_{12}, folic acid, and vitamin B_6. It also helps to rid the body of toxic elements (such as homocysteine) and increases levels of the natural mood elevator S-adenosyl-methionine.
Vitamin A plus carotenoids (including beta-carotene) and	15,000 IU daily. 25,000 IU daily.	Deficiencies of antioxidants expose the brain to oxidative damage.
vitamin E	200 IU daily.	An antioxidant that helps in the transport of oxygen to the brain cells and protects them from free radical damage. Use d-alpha-tocopherol form. *Caution:* If you are taking blood-thinning medication, consult your physician before taking vitamin E.
Vitamin B complex injections plus extra	2 cc 3 times weekly or as prescribed by physician.	Needed for brain function; aids in the digestion of food.
vitamin B_6 (pyridoxine) and	½ cc once weekly or as prescribed by physician.	Deficiency can cause depression and mental difficulties.
vitamin B_{12}	1 cc 3 times weekly or as prescribed by physician.	Important for brain function. Deficient in people with Alzheimer's disease. Injections (under a doctor's supervision) are fast and produce good results.
or vitamin B complex	100 mg of each major B vitamin 3 times daily (amounts of individual vitamins in a complex will vary).	If injections are not available, use a sublingual form.
plus extra pantothenic acid (vitamin B_5)	100 mg 3 times daily.	Plays a role in converting choline into acetylcholine, needed for memory.
Zinc	80 mg daily, in divided doses. Do not exceed a total of 100 mg daily from all supplements.	Powerful immune system stimulant. Necessary for T lymphocyte function, which is needed to fight infection.

Important		
Apple pectin	As directed on label.	Aids in removing toxic metals such as mercury, which can contribute to dementia.
Calcium and magnesium	1,600 mg daily, at bedtime. 800 mg daily.	Has a calming effect and works with magnesium. Acts as a natural calcium channel blocker.
Free form amino acid	1,000–2,500 mg daily, 1 hour before meals. Take with 8 oz of fluid and a small amount of vitamins B$_6$ and C for better assimilation.	Needed for improved brain function and tissue repair. Use free form amino acids for best absorption.
Huperzine A	100 mcg daily.	Improves cognitive functions and may improve short-term memory.
Kelp	1,000–1,500 mg daily.	Supplies needed minerals and aids in thyroid function.
Melatonin	2–3 mg daily, taken 2 hours or less before bedtime.	Improves brain function and aids sleep. Reduces cell destruction in the brain and has antioxidant properties.
RNA and DNA	As directed on label.	These are the brain's cellular building blocks. Use a formula containing 200 mg RNA and 100 mg DNA per tablet. Caution: Do not take this supplement if you have gout.
Superoxide dismutase (SOD) plus copper	As directed on label. 3 mg daily.	A potent antioxidant that improves utilization of oxygen. SOD needs copper to function properly as an antioxidant.
Vitamin C with bioflavonoids	6,000–10,000 mg daily, in divided doses.	Enhances immune function and increases energy level; a powerful antioxidant. Use a buffered form.

Herbs

❑ Butcher's broom promotes healthy circulation.

❑ Curry consumption in nondemented patients seemed to improve cognitive performance. Whether it helps patients who already have Alzheimer's disease is unknown, but it is certainly reasonable to include it when cooking.

❑ Ginkgo biloba extract, taken in liquid or capsule form, acts as an antioxidant and increases blood flow to the brain. According to a report published in the October 22, 1977, edition of the *Journal of the American Medical Association* (*JAMA*), ginkgo biloba extract can stabilize and, in some cases, improve the mental functioning and social behavior of people with Alzheimer's disease. This was later confirmed in a 1997 study. Take 100 to 200 mg of ginkgo biloba extract three times daily.

Caution: Do not take ginkgo biloba if you have a bleeding disorder, or are scheduled for surgery or a dental procedure.

❑ Kava kava and St. John's wort help to calm people who anger easily.

Cautions: Kava kava can cause drowsiness. It is not recommended for pregnant women or nursing mothers, and it should not be taken together with other substances that act on the central nervous system, such as alcohol, barbiturates, antidepressants, and antipsychotic drugs. St. John's wort may cause increased sensitivity to sunlight. It may also produce anxiety, gastrointestinal symptoms, and headaches. It can interact with some drugs including antidepressants, birth control pills, and anticoagulants.

❑ Recent studies from Japan suggest that curcumin (a compound in turmeric) and rosmarinic acid inhibit the formation and extension of beta-amyloid fibrils, and destabilize existing beta-amyloid plaques. The recommended dosage for curcumin is 600 mg a day. Rosmarinic acid is a plant phenolic that is present in significant quantities in oregano, sanicle, gypsywort, rosemary, marjoram, the mints, and sage. Capsules commonly contain 35 milligrams of rosmarinic acid; four to six capsules (140 to 210 milligrams) a day is the normal dosage.

Cautions: Do not use sage if you suffer from any type of seizure disorder, or are pregnant or nursing.

❑ The Chinese herb qian ceng ta (*Huperzia serata*) increases memory retention. This is the same herb that is the source of huperzine A, and it is also known as club moss. Pure and standardized extracts of this herb have been shown to increase mental acuity, language ability, and memory in a significant percentage of subjects with Alzheimer's disease. It is a potent blocker of acetylcholinesterase, an enzyme that regulates the activity of acetylcholine, which is an important chemical of the brain that maintains healthy learning and memory functions.

❑ Valerian root improves sleep patterns when taken at bedtime.

Recommendations

❑ Keeping the brain busy may help slow down the progression of the disease. This means keeping active and intellectually involved, as well as getting plenty of exercise.

❑ Eat a well-balanced diet of natural foods and follow the supplementation program recommended above.

❑ Have a hair analysis to rule out the possibility of heavy metal intoxication as the cause of symptoms. (*See* HAIR ANALYSIS in Part Three.)

❑ Include plenty of fiber in your diet. Try oat bran or rice bran.

❑ Have allergy testing performed to rule out environmental and/or food allergies. (*See* ALLERGIES in Part Two.)

❑ Avoid alcohol, cigarette smoke, processed foods, and environmental toxins, especially metals such as aluminum and mercury. Smoking more than doubles the risk of developing dementia and Alzheimer's disease, according to a study published in the British medical journal *Lancet*. While recent studies have not substantiated a connection between aluminum and Alzheimer's disease, it is still wise to avoid aluminum intake as much as possible. All metals in excess are toxic to the body.

❏ Do not drink tap water, as it may contain aluminum. Consume steam-distilled water only and drink at least eight glasses a day. (*See* WATER in Part One.)

❏ If you are involved in caring for someone with Alzheimer's disease, seek counseling and support from the various agencies and groups, such as the Alzheimer's Association, that are trained to help. They can teach you how to handle such things as difficult behaviors. With aggressive behaviors, for example—whether name-calling, shouting, or physical aggression toward the caregiver—understanding why the behavior occurred is the key. Some tips from the Alzheimer's Association:

- Think about what happened just before the reaction that may have "triggered" the behavior.

- Look for the feelings behind the words.

- Be positive, reassuring, and speak slowly, with a soft tone.

- Use music, massage, and/or exercise to help soothe the person.

Memory loss and confusion can cause a person with Alzheimer's disease to become suspicious of those around him or her. If this occurs, try not to take offense or argue, but rather offer a simple answer or try to divert the person's attention to another activity. For all caregivers, take time to care for yourself. The aging process is shown to increase according to telomere measurements in the caregivers of spouses who have Alzheimer's disease. Make arrangements to leave your spouse to engage in things you like to do. Be sure to keep up your own diet and exercise regimen.

Considerations

❏ A test that measures electrical activity in the brain and stores the information on a computer disk for analysis can be used to help diagnose Alzheimer's disease.

❏ A skin test using lasers under development in Australia may provide earlier and more rapid diagnosis. Developed at the National Ageing Research Institute at the University of Melbourne, this test detects blood flow restrictions associated with Alzheimer's disease. The test involves the use of lasers along with a mild electrical current that activates a chemical useful in assessing blood flow. It is hoped that the test will become a public screening measure in the near future.

❏ Using your brain, remaining busy, writing, reading, and learning new things are important overall factors in staying sharp and preventing mental disorders.

❏ Carbamazepine (Tegretol), an antiseizure medication, can ease Alzheimer's disease–related anger and hostility, according to one study. Aggression was markedly reduced in three out of four of the Alzheimer's disease patients in the study.

❏ Recent studies show that the progression of Alzheimer's disease can be slowed or even reversed by reducing free radical accumulation through the use of antioxidants. Tests conducted in Switzerland over a twenty-two-year period produced evidence of significantly higher memory scores associated with antioxidant therapy.

❏ Omega-3 fatty acids were tested in patients with mild to moderate Alzheimer's disease to see whether they would help slow the progression of the disease. At the dose used (1.7 grams DHA and 0.6 grams EPA), after six months no effect was observed. However, patients still have a biological need for omega-3 supplementation, so include fish in the diet and fish oil capsules if desired.

❏ The herbs balm and sage are being researched for possible beneficial effects on brain chemistry. Balm appears to simulate the neurological receptors that bind acetylcholine. Sage contains compounds that are cholinesterase inhibitors. Current drugs used to treat Alzheimer's disease are typically cholinesterase inhibitors.

Cautions: Do not use sage if you suffer from any type of seizure disorder, or are pregnant or nursing.

❏ Preliminary studies performed on rats at the University of Washington in Seattle indicate that cat's claw, when mixed with other herbal extracts (such as ginkgo, gotu kola, and rosemary), inhibits the buildup of plaques in the brain.

Caution: Do not use cat's claw during pregnancy. Do not take ginkgo biloba if you have a bleeding disorder, or are scheduled for surgery or a dental procedure.

❏ Some experts distinguish between a rapidly progressing form of Alzheimer's disease that begins earlier in life (usually between the ages of thirty-six and forty-five) and a more gradual form that develops in people around the ages of sixty-five or seventy. For more information, consult *Complete Guide to Symptoms, Illness and Surgery for People Over 50* by H. Winter Griffith, M.D. (The Body Press/Perigee Books, 4th revised edition, 2000).

❏ The signs of alcohol abuse and the symptoms of Alzheimer's disease can be very similar. For example, actress Rita Hayworth, who had Alzheimer's disease, was at first thought to be an alcoholic.

❏ Research studies supported by the Alzheimer's Association and studies done at the Department of Research at Oakwood College in Huntsville, Alabama, found that liquid aged garlic extract (Kyolic) might prove to be useful in the improvement of Alzheimer's disease symptoms. Kyolic protected the cells from toxic effects of beta-amyloid.

❏ Homocysteine, an amino acid that forms as the result of the breakdown of another amino acid, methionine, is a biomarker for the development of dementia and Alzheimer's disease. Some scientists speculate that Alzheimer's disease might be avoided if people reduced the levels of homocysteine in their blood, although it has not yet been determined whether homocysteine itself actually contributes to Alzheimer's disease. A more likely explanation is that elevated homocysteine levels are an indication of a severe disruption of methylation (a type of biochemical process essential for the repair and maintenance of genetic material and the production of neurotransmitters, among other things) in the brains of people with Alzheimer's disease. Methylation deficiencies can result in severe damage to brain cells. Other researchers report that abnormal amino acid metabolism in Alzheimer's disease causes higher homocysteine levels. This may lead to the neurological damage that occurs as the disease advances.

❑ A decline in the sense of smell often occurs as much as two years prior to the beginning of mental decline in people with Alzheimer's disease. Scientists at the University of California–San Diego Medical Center found that people with Alzheimer's disease must be exposed to very strong concentrations of a substance before they can detect its odor. The rate at which the sense of smell is lost can predict how rapidly cognitive functioning is lost. Smoking can damage cells involved in the sense of smell, making this test less useful for smokers.

❑ Regular exercise throughout adulthood can reduce the chances of developing Alzheimer's disease. Activities associated with reduced risk include biking, walking, swimming, and golf. Two studies in major medical journals showed that walking three times a day improved cognitive function and reduced the risk of Alzheimer's disease. Those already with the disease should continue this sort of exercise program for as long as possible.

❑ Researchers at the University of California–Davis questioned the caregivers of eighty-eight elderly people, half of whom had either Alzheimer's disease or a related form of dementia, about their eating habits. Half of the people with Alzheimer's disease had such a strong desire for sweets that their access to these foods had to be restricted.

❑ No treatment can stop or reverse Alzheimer's disease. However, for people in the early and middle stages of the disease drug therapy using cholinesterase inhibitors such as donepezil (Aricept), rivastigmine (Exelon), or galantamine (Razadyne) may alleviate some symptoms for a limited period of time. These are the first line of defense for drug therapies. They prevent the breakdown of acetylcholine, a chemical messenger important for learning and memory. A new class of drug introduced in 2003, which is currently the only available neuroprotective therapy, is memantine (Namenda), which has been approved for treatment of moderate to severe cases. However, this drug does not appear to be the "silver bullet" everyone has been looking for and, indeed, might only offer some slight relief to those patients already in the last stages of the disease. This

drug regulates the activity of glutamate, a different messenger involved in learning and memory.

❑ There is some evidence that inflammation in the brain may contribute to damage caused by the disease. As a result, studies were being conducted on the effect of nonsteroidal anti-inflammatory drugs (NSAIDs) to see if they could slow its progression. But at this point, one study on rofecoxib (Vioxx) and naproxen sodium (Aleve) was inconclusive, and another on celecoxib (Celebrex) and naproxen sodium was discontinued. Rofecoxib has since been withdrawn from the market.

❑ Because the beta-amyloid plaques appear to be in large measure the culprits behind Alzheimer's disease damage, if a way could be developed to clear them out, or prevent their buildup altogether, the disease could be managed. Researchers at Lilly Research Laboratories and Elan Pharmaceuticals have discovered that certain monoclonal antibodies bind to beta-amyloid and clear it from the brain. In animal experiments, a treatment with monoclonal antibody M266 both cleared beta-amyloid from the brains of the subjects and reversed some existing memory problems. Meanwhile, a study published in the *Journal of Neuroscience* in March 2003 showed that levels of neprilysin, a beta-amyloid-degrading enzyme, could be boosted by means of gene therapy. This caused a reduction in the plaque found in the brains of the animal subjects. Another study, published in *Nature Medicine*, was conducted that pointed to astrocytes, naturally occurring cells that protect neurons, as mechanisms that counter beta-amyloid. Researchers theorize that defects in the ability of astrocytes to clear beta-amyloid could be a contributing factor in plaque development.

❑ A research study published in the *Proceedings of the National Academy of Sciences* has shown that mice modified to lack the enzyme insulysin (which degrades insulin) had did levels of beta-amyloid 1.5 times greater in their brains than did control mice. Because insulysin is so closely tied to insulin and glucose metabolism, and because there appears to be a link between diabetes and Alzheimer's disease, scientists hope that modifying insulysin activity or some other aspects of insulin metabolism may assist in management of the disease.

❑ Research reported in the journal *Biochemistry* indicated possible therapeutic potential of anti-beta-amyloid proteolytic antibody light chain fragments. These fragments are able to zero in on the beta-amyloid and reduce its toxicity, and they can be introduced into the parts of the brain that contain heavy concentrations of the plaque by nonintrusive methods.

❑ A Phase I safety trial has been run on humans with a proposed vaccinelike drug that showed a lot of promise in animal studies. As these trials showed no ill effects on the subjects, a Phase II trial was begun in 2001 with 360 participants. Unfortunately, the trial was halted due to some severe side effects, but the results even of the foreshortened trial showed great promise. The drug appears to have reduced the amount of beta-amyloid plaques in one patient, and a significant number of those treated did develop antibodies to beta-amyloid, and showed little or no cognitive decline as compared to those who failed to develop the antibodies. This study has encouraged researchers to try different approaches based on the underlying theory because there did appear to be a positive effect caused by the drug. This avenue, immune therapy, shows much promise, and may be a path to an effective treatment in the future.

❏ Preliminary trials suggest that nicotinamide adenine dinucleotide (NADH) may benefit those afflicted with Alzheimer's disease. In a study conducted by Austrian researcher and physician Dr. George Birkmayer and colleagues, seventeen patients with Alzheimer-type dementia were treated with NADH for eight to twelve weeks. The patients' cognitive function improved as measured by two standard tests, according to the Folstein Mini-Mental Status Examination and the Global Deterioration Scale. The patients reportedly did not suffer any adverse side effects.

❏ High doses of lecithin may be helpful for people with Alzheimer's disease. However, a double-blind controlled trial of high doses of lecithin reported in the *Journal of Neurology, Neurosurgery & Psychiatry* found that there may be a "therapeutic window" for the effects of lecithin on people with Alzheimer's disease, and that this may be more evident in older people.

❏ Women with Alzheimer's disease have been found to have lower estrogen levels than their healthy counterparts.

❏ Researchers at the Massachusetts Institute of Technology discovered that levels of choline and ethanolamine are significantly lower than normal in people suffering from Alzheimer's disease. Both choline and ethanolamine are used for the synthesis of phospholipids that are major components of the cell membranes of neurons in the brain.

❏ Scientists at the University of Kentucky found that levels of glutamine synthetase, an enzyme that controls the production of ammonia and glutamate, were higher in a group of people with Alzheimer's disease than in a healthy control group. Glutamate is vital to the brain in small amounts, but it can be poisonous in high concentrations. Abnormally high levels of glutamate have recently been associated with amyotrophic lateral sclerosis (ALS, also known as Lou Gehrig's disease) and glaucoma.

❏ An estimated 2 percent of Americans have two copies of a gene for the production of a substance called apolipoprotein E4, or APO-E4. APO-E4 transports cholesterol through the bloodstream and also changes the form of amyloid in the brain. People who inherit one copy of the gene for the production of APO-E4 have an increased chance of developing Alzheimer's disease; those who inherit two copies of the allele are at even greater risk.

❏ Experts say that it is in an individual's best interest to be told as soon as there is reason to suspect a diagnosis of Alzheimer's disease. Early warning cannot prevent the disease, but it gives people time to settle their affairs and make informed judgments about future care and other matters.

❏ People who tend to experience psychological distress appear to be more likely to develop Alzheimer's disease than those who are less prone to experience distress. In a study reported in the journal *Neurology,* people who most often experienced negative emotions such as depression and anxiety were twice as likely to develop the disease as those who were less prone to experience these negative emotions. However, more research is needed before across-the-board prescription of antidepressants is approved to prevent Alzheimer's disease.

❏ The omega-3 fat DHA (docosahexaenoic acid), which is found in many cold-water fish (such as salmon, tuna, and mackerel), is known to have cardioprotective effects. Researchers at the University of California–Los Angeles School of Medicine found that genetically engineered mice fed a diet rich in DHA were found to have less brain cell damage than those fed a diet which substituted safflower oil, which is low in omega-3 fatty acids. The American Heart Association recommends at least two meals a week of fish rich in omega-3 fatty acids. While this is for good cardiovascular health, it is possible that this diet can also favorably affect people who have Alzheimer's disease or who have a high risk of developing the disease. This is surely a case of "It can't hurt, and it might help."

❏ Anyone who cares for a person with Alzheimer's disease may eventually find the job overwhelming and need support. For many, adult day-care centers are a godsend. A good day-care center should be clean, safe (without glass doors, uneven or slippery floors, furniture with sharp corners, and so on), and have barriers at entrances and exits to protect wanderers without making them feel trapped. Food should be nutritious and appetizing. Staff members should be friendly, compassionate, and professionally trained to work with Alzheimer's disease patients. There should be psychologists or social workers on the staff to help patients cope with the ordinary frustrations of daily life and to assist them in coping with anger and depression. A quiet room should be available where an agitated or ill person can be separated from others. The availability of other specific services, such as physical therapy, help with hygiene, family counseling, or support groups for caregivers, as well as the usual activities of the center, should be suited to the particular needs of the individual and his or her family.

❏ The calming effect of watching fish swimming peacefully in an aquarium is found to help people with Alzheimer's disease eat better by helping them to concentrate long enough to eat well, according to Nancy Edwards, Ph.D., an associate professor of nursing at Purdue University.

❏ For names and addresses of organizations that can provide further information about this disorder, *see* Health and Medical Organizations in the Appendix.

AMBLYOPIA

See DIMNESS OR LOSS OF VISION under EYE PROBLEMS.

ANEMIA

Millions of Americans suffer from anemia, a reduction in either the number of red blood cells or the amount of hemoglobin in the blood. This results in a decrease in the amount of oxygen that the blood is able to carry. Anemia reduces the amount of oxygen available to the cells of the body. As a result, they have less energy available to perform their normal functions. Important processes, such as muscular activity and cell building and repair, slow down and become less efficient. When the brain lacks oxygen, dizziness may result, and mental faculties are less sharp.

Anemia is not a disease, but rather a symptom of various diseases. Anything that causes a deficiency in the formation or production of red blood cells, or that leads to the too-rapid destruction of red blood cells, can result in anemia. It is sometimes the first detectable sign of arthritis, infection, or certain major illnesses, including cancer. Drug use, hormonal disorders, chronic inflammation in the body, surgery, infections, peptic ulcers, hemorrhoids, diverticular disease, heavy menstrual bleeding, repeated pregnancies, liver damage, thyroid disorders, rheumatoid arthritis, bone marrow disease, and dietary deficiencies (especially deficiencies of iron, folic acid, and vitamins B_6 and B_{12}) can all lead to anemia. Anemia can also be caused by medications such as chemotherapy. Women who are postmenopausal should not be anemic. If you are eating a normal diet and are not a vegetarian, and you become anemic, consult your doctor. The body likes to maintain its iron status, so anemia is a signal that something isn't right.

There are also a number of hereditary disorders, such as sickle cell disease and thalassemia, that cause anemia.

Sickle cell anemia affects about 70,000 to 80,000 people (mostly of African-American and Mediterranean descent) in the United States. It is a rare, inherited blood disease that causes red blood cells to become brittle and crescent-shaped. Painful "crises" arise when affected cells become jammed in narrow blood vessels, producing painful swelling of the hands and feet accompanied by fever, fatigue, and pneumonia-like symptoms.

Pernicious anemia is a severe form of anemia that is due to vitamin B_{12} deficiency. Persons with this disorder cannot absorb any form of vitamin B_{12} from the gastrointestinal tract. Malabsorption can cause pernicious anemia, as can poor eating habits, gastrointestinal infection, Crohn's disease, gastric surgery, and sometimes even strict vegetarianism. If B_{12} levels fall too far, the result is lagging energy, depression, indigestion, diarrhea, and anemia. Ongoing vitamin B_{12} deficiency carries a risk of neurological damage.

The most common cause of anemia is iron deficiency. Iron is an important factor in anemia because this mineral is used to make hemoglobin, the component of red blood cells that attaches to oxygen and transports it. Red blood cells exist only to oxygenate the body, and have a life span of about 90 to 120 days. If a person lacks sufficient iron, the formation of red blood cells is impaired. Iron-deficiency anemia can be caused by insufficient iron intake and/or absorption, or by significant blood loss. The latter is commonly seen in women who suffer from menorrhagia (heavy or prolonged menstrual bleeding), which in turn may be caused by a hormonal imbalance, fibroid tumors, or uterine cancer. Women who use intrauterine devices for contraception are also at a higher risk of blood loss, as are those who overuse anti-inflammatory medications such as aspirin or ibuprofen, which can cause blood loss through irritation of the digestive tract. Excessive aspirin usage, particularly by elderly people, may cause internal bleeding.

Anemia's symptoms can easily go unrecognized. The first signs of developing anemia may be loss of appetite, constipation, headaches, irritability, and/or difficulty in concentrating.

Established anemia can produce such symptoms as weakness; fatigue; coldness of the extremities; depression; dizziness; overall pallor, most noticeable in pale and brittle nails; pale lips and eyelids; soreness in the mouth; and in women, cessation of menstruation. Anemia has also been linked to a loss of libido. Twelve percent of females age twelve to forty-nine and 7 percent of children age one to two are iron deficient.

Anemia should always be investigated and the cause determined. A complete blood count, or CBC, should be run by your doctor if anemia is suspected. This will measure both your red blood cell count and hemoglobin level. Hemoglobin normally should be between 12 and 18 grams per deciliter (g/dL). If you are anemic and your diet is ironclad, your physician can run a simple test called ESR (erythrocyte sedimentation rate) to detect any inflammation lurking in the body.

Unless otherwise specified, the dosages recommended in this section are for adults. For a child between the ages of twelve and seventeen, reduce the dose to three-quarters of the recommended amount. For a child between six and twelve, use one-half of the recommended dose, and for a child under the age of six, use one-quarter of the recommended amount.

NUTRIENTS

SUPPLEMENT	SUGGESTED DOSAGE	COMMENTS
Essential		
Iron or	As prescribed by physician. Take with 100 mg vitamin C for better absorption. 2 tsp twice daily.	To restore iron. Use a ferrous gluconate form. *Caution:* Do not take iron unless anemia is diagnosed.
Floradix Iron + Herbs from Salus Haus		Contains a readily absorbable form of iron that is nontoxic and from a natural source.

Raw liver extract	500 mg twice daily.	Contains all the elements needed for red blood cell production. Use liver from organically raised beef. Consider injections (under a doctor's supervision).
Very Important		
Blackstrap molasses	1 tbsp twice daily for adults; 1 tsp added to milk for children and infants.	Contains iron and essential B vitamins.
Folic acid plus biotin	800 mcg twice daily. 300 mcg twice daily.	Needed for red blood cell formation.
Vitamin B_{12} injections or vitamin B_{12}	2 cc once weekly or as prescribed by physician. 2,000 mcg 3 times daily.	Essential in red blood cell production and to break down and prepare protein for cellular use. Injections (under a doctor's supervision) are best. If injections are not available, use a lozenge or sublingual form for best absorption.
Important		
Vitamin B complex plus extra pantothenic acid (vitamin B_5) and vitamin B_6 (pyridoxine)	50 mg of each major B vitamin 3 times daily (amounts of individual vitamins in a complex will vary). 50 mg 3 times daily. 100 mg daily.	B vitamins work best when taken together. A sublingual form is recommended. Important in red blood cell production. Involved in cellular reproduction. Aids absorption of vitamin B_{12}.
Vitamin C plus bioflavonoids	3,000–10,000 mg daily.	Important in iron absorption.
Helpful		
Brewer's yeast	As directed on label.	Rich in basic nutrients and a good source of B vitamins.
Coenzyme A from Coenzyme-A Technologies	As directed on label.	Supports the immune system's detoxification of many dangerous substances.
Copper and zinc	2 mg daily. 30 mg daily. Do not exceed this amount.	Needed in red blood cell production. Note: If more zinc is used, increase copper proportionately. Needed to balance with copper.
Raw spleen glandular	As directed on label.	*See* GLANDULAR THERAPY in Part Three for its benefits.
S-Adenosylmethio-nine (SAMe)	As directed on label.	Helps reduce stress and depression. *Caution:* Do not use if you have bipolar mood disorder or take prescription antidepressants. Do not give to a child under twelve.
Vitamin A plus natural beta-carotene or carotenoid complex (Betatene)	10,000 IU daily. 15,000 IU daily. As directed on label.	Important antioxidants.
Vitamin E	200 IU daily. Take separately from iron supplements.	Important for red blood cell survival; prolongs the life span of these cells. Use an emulsion form for easier assimilation. Use d-alpha-tocopherol form.

Herbs

❑ Alfalfa, bilberry, cherry, dandelion, goldenseal, grape skins, hawthorn berry, mullein, nettle, Oregon grape root, pau d'arco, red raspberry, shepherd's purse, and yellow dock are good for anemia.

Cautions: Do not take goldenseal or Oregon grape root during pregnancy. Do not take goldenseal internally on a daily basis for more than one week at a time. Do not use it during pregnancy or if you are breast-feeding, and use with caution if you are allergic to ragweed. If you have a history of cardiovascular disease, diabetes, or glaucoma, use it only under a doctor's supervision.

❑ Herbalists consider nettle (*Urtica dioica*), a nutritious plant rich in iron, vitamin C, chlorophyll, and other minerals, an effective supplement in the treatment of iron-deficiency anemia.

Recommendations

❑ Have a complete blood test to determine if you have an iron deficiency before taking iron supplements. Excess iron can damage the liver, heart, pancreas, and immune cell activity, and has been linked to cancer. Use iron supplements only under the supervision of a qualified health care provider. Include in your diet foods such as meats, poultry, fish, and enriched cereals. Continue with regular blood testing to monitor the effect of iron. Taking too much or too little could be harmful.

❑ Also include the following in your diet: apples, apricots, asparagus, bananas, broccoli, egg yolks, kelp, leafy greens, okra, parsley, peas, plums, prunes, purple grapes, raisins, rice bran, squash, turnip greens, whole grains, and yams. Also eat foods high in vitamin C to enhance iron absorption.

❑ Consume at least 1 tablespoon of blackstrap molasses twice daily (for a child, use 1 teaspoon in a glass of milk or formula twice daily). Blackstrap molasses is a good source of iron and essential B vitamins.

❑ Eat foods containing oxalic acid in moderation or omit them from the diet. Oxalic acid interferes with iron absorption. Foods high in oxalic acid include almonds, cashews, chocolate, cocoa, kale, rhubarb, soda, sorrel, spinach, Swiss chard, and most nuts and beans.

❑ Avoid beer, candy bars, dairy products, ice cream, and soft drinks. Additives in these foods interfere with iron absorption. For the same reason, avoid coffee (which contains polyphenols) and tea (which contains tannins).

Because iron is removed through the stool, do not eat foods high in iron and/or iron supplements at the same time as fiber. Avoid using bran as a source of fiber.

If you are a strict vegetarian, watch your diet closely. Taking supplemental vitamin B_{12} is advised. (*See* VITAMINS in Part One.)

Do not smoke. Avoid secondhand smoke.

Minimize your exposure to lead and other toxic metals. (*See* ALUMINUM TOXICITY; CADMIUM TOXICITY; LEAD POISONING; and/or MERCURY TOXICITY for suggestions.)

Do not take calcium, vitamin E, zinc, or antacids at the same time as iron supplements. These can interfere with iron absorption.

Considerations

Iron from animals is in a heme form (from animals). All other foods containing iron are in a non-heme form (not from animals). As mammals, our bodies preferentially recognize and absorb the heme form better than the non-heme form. The fastest way to restore iron in the blood to normal is to consume meat (beef and poultry) and seafood and take an iron supplement as needed.

The following foods are among the highest in iron content, with over 5 milligrams of iron per average serving: kidney beans, pinto beans, liver (eat only liver from organically raised animals), blackstrap molasses, rice bran, raw beet greens (not the beets), mustard greens, lentils, dried peaches, and prune juice. Foods with a moderately high iron content (3 to 5 milligrams per average serving) include cooked dried apricots, cooked beet greens, dates, lean meat (lamb, turkey, and veal), lima beans, chili, cooked spinach, and dry and fresh peas.

Eating fish at the same time as vegetables containing iron increases iron absorption. Omitting all sugar from the diet increases iron absorption as well.

Iron-deficiency anemia should disappear when the underlying cause is corrected.

Physicians can sometimes detect vitamin B_{12} deficiency by measuring serum B_{12} levels, taking a complete blood cell count, and doing a blood test called the Schilling test, which evaluates B_{12} absorption. Persons with pernicious anemia must take vitamin B_{12} sublingually (dissolved under the tongue), by retention enema, or by injection. This treatment must be maintained for life, unless the underlying cause of the deficiency can be corrected.

Hydroxyuria (Droxia), a cancer drug, may be prescribed for people with sickle cell anemia who are over the age of eighteen and have experienced three or more crises in a one-year period. The drug eases symptoms, but is not a cure for the disease.

The American Academy of Pediatrics (AAP) recommends that children under one year old not drink cow's milk. Milk can cause anemia by interfering with iron absorption and possibly causing internal bleeding. The AAP published the results of a University of Iowa study that found the blood content in the stool of infants fed cow's milk was five times higher than in children fed infant formula. Researchers concluded the amount of iron lost was "nutritionally important."

ANGINA

See under CARDIOVASCULAR DISEASE.

ANKYLOSING SPONDYLITIS

See under ARTHRITIS.

ANOREXIA NERVOSA

The term anorexia nervosa was first coined in 1873. A doctor writing in the British medical journal *The Lancet* used the term to describe people who, although thin and weak, insisted that they needed to lose weight and would not eat a sufficient amount of food to remain alive.

Anorexia nervosa is a nervous, psychological eating disorder characterized by a refusal to eat, even to the point of starvation. Other symptoms include an intense fear of becoming fat that never goes away, no matter how thin the individual becomes; extreme overactivity and an obsession with working out; negative feelings about the way the body looks; deep feelings of shame; and problems with drug and/or alcohol abuse. Ninety-five percent of the people who suffer from this disorder are female. Anorexia typically appears during adolescence. The incidence of eating disorders, particularly among young women in the United States, has escalated dramatically during the past decade.

An estimated 8 million Americans (7 million women and 1 million men) struggle with anorexia, according to the National Association of Anorexia Nervosa and Associated Diseases (ANAD). Eating disorders are not limited to teenage girls. Women aged forty and older are also susceptible. Doctors suspect that low levels of serotonin, a neurotransmitter, may be the cause, producing psychological problems linked to anorexia and bulimia.

Some people with anorexia just quit eating; some make themselves vomit immediately after eating; some take laxatives after eating; and some do all three. Most people with anorexia have normal feelings of hunger at the onset of the disease but teach themselves to ignore them. Despite their refusal to eat, people with anorexia often become obsessed with food and may spend hours fantasizing about it, reading recipes, or even preparing elaborate meals for others.

Another characteristic feature of the disorder is that people with anorexia usually deny that there is anything wrong and claim that they simply "aren't hungry" and even insist that they need to lose more weight.

Many females who are anorexic are also bulimic. Bulimia nervosa is defined as the consumption of extremely large quantities of food in short periods of time (bingeing), followed by self-induced vomiting or the use of either diuretics or cathartics (purging). (*See* BULIMIA.) If anorexia and bulimia occur in the same individual, the disorder is called bulimarexia.

Anorexia can lead to underweight, extreme weakness, dizziness, cessation of menstruation, swelling of the neck, ulcers and erosion of the esophagus, erosion of the enamel of the back teeth from repeated vomiting, broken blood vessels in the face, and a low pulse rate and blood pressure. In some extreme cases, spoons or sticks used to induce vomiting have become stuck in the digestive tract and have had to be surgically removed. Systemic physiological changes in those suffering from anorexia include thyroid dysfunction, disturbances in the heartbeat, and irregularity in the secretion of growth hormone and the hormones cortisol, gonadotropin, and vasopressin.

Eventually, if anorexic behavior continues long enough, classic complications associated with starvation appear.

Electrolyte imbalances created by insufficient potassium and sodium levels cause dehydration, muscle spasms, and, ultimately, cardiac arrest. If laxatives are used, these further deplete the body of potassium. Hypokalemia (potassium deficiency) is a major problem for people with anorexia. Chronic hypokalemia can cause an irregular heartbeat, which can lead to heart failure and death. Patients may require intravenous nutrition to restore normal body mass (muscle) and weight. Because it takes a long time both to lose and to gain weight, this is a slow process.

Initially, anorexia nervosa was thought to be strictly a psychological problem. However, in the last few years, medical scientists and nutritionists have identified several physical components as well. For example, people with eating disorders have been found to have chemical imbalances similar to those found in individuals with clinical depression. Some cases of anorexia have been found to be caused by severe zinc deficiency.

Nevertheless, the psychological elements continue to be important. Teasing by peers or parents can play a role in making individuals obsessed with the idea that they are fat. In addition, many people who suffer from anorexia display great fear at the prospect of growing up, and girls often have difficult mother/daughter relationships.

Some may try to live up to images their parents set for them, but feel inadequate—that they are not as beautiful or intelligent as their parents want them to be. A girl with anorexia may then develop an inferiority complex, seeing herself as fat and/or ugly, and no amount of common sense or persuasion can alter her distorted mental image.

About 30 percent of all people with anorexia struggle with the disorder all their lives. Another 30 percent have at least one life-threatening bout with it, while the remaining 40 percent outgrow it. Even if an individual recovers fully from the acute phase of the disorder, serious damage may have been done to the body.

Unless otherwise specified, the dosages recommended in this section are for adults. For a child between the ages of twelve and seventeen, reduce the dose to three-quarters of the recommended amount.

NUTRIENTS

SUPPLEMENT	SUGGESTED DOSAGE	COMMENTS
Very Important		
Multivitamin and mineral complex with		All nutrients are needed and must be taken in extremely high doses because they are passed through the gastro-intestinal tract rapidly and are poorly assimilated.
natural beta-carotene and	25,000 IU daily.	
mixed carotenoids and	Amounts in a complex will vary.	
vitamin A and	10,000 IU daily.	
calcium and	1,500 mg daily.	
magnesium and	1,000 mg daily.	
potassium and	99–200 mg daily.	
selenium	200 mcg daily. If you are pregnant, do not exceed 40 mcg daily.	
Zinc	80 mg daily. Do not exceed a total of 100 mg daily from all supplements.	All enzymes important for increased appetite and taste require zinc and copper. Zinc and copper work together to prevent copper deficiency.
plus copper	3 mg daily.	
Important		
Acidophilus	As directed on label. Take on an empty stomach so that it passes quickly to the small intestine.	Needed to replace the "friendly" bacteria lost from use of laxatives and/or from vomiting.
Free form amino acid (Amino Balance from Anabol Naturals)	As directed on label.	To supply easily assimilable protein, needed for tissue repair.
5-Hydroxy L-tryptophan (5-HTP)	As directed on label.	Aids in treating depression and nervousness.
Gamma-aminobutyric acid (GABA)	As directed on label.	Low levels of this amino acid have been found in people who suffer from anxiety and depression.
or S-Adenosylmethio-nine (SAMe)	As directed on label.	Aids in reducing stress and depression, providing a sense of well-being. *Caution:* Do not use if you have bipolar mood disorder or take prescription antidepressants. Do not give to a child under twelve.
Liquid Kyolic with B_1 and B_{12} from Wakunaga	As directed on label.	Helps reduce stress and anxiety.
Primrose oil or	As directed on label.	Important for all body functions and cell repair and reduces inflammation in nerve cells.
flaxseed oil or	As directed on label.	
Kyolic-EPA from Wakunaga	As directed on label.	To calm the nervous system.

Vitamin B complex	100 mg of each major B vitamin 3 times daily (amounts of individual vitamins in a complex will vary).	Helps to prevent anemia and replaces lost B vitamins. The B vitamins are important for proper brain functioning and help increase the appetite. Use a sublingual form.
Vitamin B$_{12}$ injections	1 cc 3 times weekly or as prescribed by physician.	Increases appetite; prevents loss of hair and damage to many bodily functions. If injections are not available, use a lozenge or sublingual form.
plus liver extract injections	2 cc 3 times weekly or as prescribed by physician.	To supply B vitamins and other valuable nutrients.
Vitamin C with bioflavonoids	5,000 mg daily, in divided doses.	Needed for the impaired immune system and to alleviate stress on the adrenal glands.
Helpful		
Bio-Strath from Nature's Answer or	As directed on label 3 times daily.	An herbal and yeast-based tonic. A natural source of iron.
Floradix Iron + Herbs from Salus Haus	As directed on label 3 times daily.	Aids in increasing the appetite.
Brewer's yeast	Start with 1 tsp daily and work up to 1 tbsp daily.	Contains balanced amounts of the B vitamins.
Kelp	2,000–3,000 mg daily.	Needed for mineral replacement and thyroid function.
Proteolytic enzymes	As directed on label. Take between meals and with meals.	To aid in digestion and in rebuilding of tissue.
Vitamin D	600 IU daily.	Needed for calcium uptake and to prevent bone loss.
Vitamin E	200 IU daily.	Increases oxygen uptake in the body for healing and a powerful antioxidant. Use d-alpha-tocopherol form.

Herbs

❑ To rebuild the liver and cleanse the bloodstream, use dandelion, milk thistle, red clover, or wild yam.

❑ The following herbs are appetite stimulants: ginger root, ginseng, gotu kola, and peppermint.

Caution: Do not use ginseng if you have high blood pressure, or are pregnant or nursing.

❑ St. John's wort and kava kava calm the nervous system and aid in preventing depression.

Cautions: St. John's wort may cause increased sensitivity to sunlight. It may also produce anxiety, gastrointestinal symptoms, and headaches. It can interact with some drugs including antidepressants, birth control pills, and anticoagulants. Kava kava can cause drowsiness. It is not recommended for pregnant women or nursing mothers, and it should not be taken together with other substances that act on the central nervous system, such as alcohol, barbiturates, antidepressants, and antipsychotic drugs.

Recommendations

❑ While a normal eating pattern is being established, eat a well-balanced diet that is high in fiber. Eat plenty of fresh raw fruits and vegetables. These foods are cleansing to the system. When the body is cleansed, the appetite tends to return to normal.

❑ Be sure to eat adequate amounts of healthy protein foods, such as fish and soy protein. Quality protein is important for repairing body tissues and restoring lost muscle mass.

❑ Many people with this disease will not eat any food that contains fat because they think it will make them fat. Fat is an essential component in the diet and should be included at every meal.

❑ Consume no sugar, and avoid white flour products.

❑ Avoid processed and junk foods. The additives these foods contain tend to add to the aversion to eating.

❑ Seek out a practitioner or practitioners who specialize in the treatment of eating disorders and who can address the complex of physical and psychological elements involved. Some type of specialized counseling, in addition to nutritional counseling, is usually necessary for recovery.

❑ Women with low self-esteem tend to engage in self-destructive behaviors such as entering into abusive relationships, compulsive sexual behavior, and eating disorders. Cultivate relationships with people who make you feel important—people who are admiring and encouraging of your accomplishments and interests. As much as possible, remove from your life anything and anyone who makes you feel inadequate and "put-down." Consider counseling to help you learn to cope with those negative situations you cannot avoid.

Considerations

❑ If an individual shows any of the signs of anorexia, he or she should be seen by a physician.

❑ In many cases, a person with anorexia must be hospitalized and given intravenous nutrient feedings of potassium and multivitamins.

❑ Starvation tends to increase feelings of depression, anxiety, irritability, and anger. It may take up to a year or more for a person recovering from anorexia to improve his or her body image, to establish normal eating patterns, and to reverse the effects of starvation on mood and behavior.

❑ Some researchers believe that neurotransmitters—such as dopamine, serotonin, norepinephrine, and the endogenous opioids—play a role in anorexia.

❑ Researchers have found that zinc supplementation not only decreases depression and anxiety, but that anorexic women taking zinc gain twice as much weight, on average, as anorexic women who do not take the supplement. Zinc, whether as part of the diet or in supplemental form, has been successful in helping many individuals with anorexia to regain their normal appetite and weight. Zinc deficiency by itself, however, does not cause anorexia nervosa.

❏ The self-esteem problems typical of those with anorexia often begin at an early age. A child who is told that she is stupid, worthless, and/or unlovable is likely to come to believe it. In addition, recent research has shown that many (if not most) American girls undergo a severe loss of self-esteem in early adolescence, the very time that eating disorders are most likely to occur.

❏ An unexplained loss of five to ten pounds requires immediate medical attention. Significant weight loss is considered a 10 percent decrease; 40 percent weight loss is nearly always associated with death. Weight loss can also be a sign of something other than anorexia nervosa.

❏ For information on organizations that can help you learn more about eating disorders and treatments, *see* Health and Medical Organizations in the Appendix.

ANXIETY DISORDER

Anxiety disorder is a far more common problem than was once thought. It can affect people in their teenage years through middle age and later. Anxiety disorder appears to affect twice as many women as men, though there may not actually be that wide a disparity between the sexes. Psychologists believe that men are far less prone to report or even acknowledge having a problem of this nature.

Anxiety disorder can be either acute or chronic. Acute anxiety disorder manifests itself in episodes commonly known as panic attacks. A panic attack is an instance in which the body's natural "fight or flight" reaction occurs at the wrong time. This is a complex, involuntary physiological response in which the body prepares itself to deal with an emergency situation. Stress causes the body to produce more adrenal hormones, especially adrenaline. The increased production of adrenaline causes the body to step up its metabolism of proteins, fats, and carbohydrates to quickly produce energy for the body to use. In addition, the muscles tense, and heartbeat and breathing become more rapid. Even the composition of the blood changes slightly, making it more prone to clotting.

In the face of a threat such as an assault, an accident, or a natural disaster, this type of reaction is perfectly normal and helpful for survival. At other times, the symptoms caused by a surge in adrenaline can be distressing and frightening. A person having a panic attack often is overwhelmed by a sense of impending disaster or death, which makes it impossible to think clearly. Other feelings that can accompany a panic attack include shortness of breath; a smothering, claustrophobic sensation; heart palpitations; chest pain; dizziness; hot flashes and/or chills; trembling; numbness or tingling sensations in the extremities; sweating; nausea; a feeling of unreality; and a distorted perception of the passage of time. Eventually, the disorder can have other, cumulative effects, such as generalized aches and pains, muscular twitching and stiffness, depression, insomnia, nightmares and early waking, decreased libido, and abnormal feelings of tension with an accompanying inability to relax. Women may experience changes in the menstrual cycle and increased premenstrual symptoms.

Panic attacks are usually abrupt and intense. They can occur at any time of the day or night, lasting from several seconds up to half an hour. To the panic sufferer, it often feels as though they are much longer. A person having a panic attack often believes that he or she is experiencing a heart attack or a stroke. The attacks themselves are very unpredictable; some people experience one every few weeks, while others may have several a day. They are often triggered by stress (conscious or unconscious) or certain emotions, but may also occur in response to certain foods, drugs, or illness. Food allergies and hypoglycemia are both common among people with this disorder, and can promote panic attacks. An attack may follow ingestion or overindulgence in caffeine-based stimulants such as tea or coffee. Some attacks occur with no apparent cause. The unpredictability of the attacks makes them even more distressing.

Many people with acute anxiety disorder become fearful of being alone and of visiting public places because they fear having a panic attack. Of course this only adds to the level of anxiety and leads to their lives being abnormally restricted. Many psychologists believe that at least in some cases, panic attacks are self-induced; that is, the fear of a panic attack is the very thing that brings one about.

For years, panic attacks were dismissed as a psychosomatic phenomenon. However, repeated studies have shown that this disorder has a real, physical basis. Experts believe that panic attacks are caused principally by a malfunction in brain chemistry, wherein the brain sends and receives false "emergency signals." Researchers have recently identified a genetic factor that appears to influence anxiety in women. Combining DNA analysis, brain activity recordings, and psychological testing, investigators at the National Institute on Alcohol Abuse and Alcoholism (NIAAA) found that both Caucasian and Native American women with the same gene variant had similarly high scores on anxiety tests. These women also had similar electroencephalograms (EEGs), recordings of the brain's electrical activity that indicated tendencies toward an anxious temperament. This study was reported in the journal *Psychiatric Genetics*.

COMT is an acronym for a major enzyme responsible for the metabolism of certain neurotransmitters (chemical messengers of the nervous system), including norepinephrine, which affects anxiety. Other studies have confirmed a genetic link that might explain why more women than men experience anxiety disorders. In general, women have been found to have lower COMT levels than men. If the gene that encodes the COMT enzyme is faulty, the metabolism of these neurotransmitters is affected. Hyperactivity in certain areas of the brain causes the release of norepinephrine, which causes the pulse, blood pressure, and breathing to become more rapid, producing the classic symptoms of a panic attack.

According to Mayo Clinic researchers, between 10 and 20 percent of Americans will have a panic attack at some time in their lives. Panic attacks are now recognized as a potentially disabling but treatable condition.

Chronic anxiety is a milder, more generalized form of this disorder. Many sufferers feel a vague sense of anxiety much of the time, but the intensity of the feeling does not reach the levels of those in an actual panic attack. They may feel chronically uneasy, especially in the presence of other people, and tend to startle easily. Headaches and chronic fatigue are common among people with this form of the disorder.

Generalized anxiety disorder can begin at any age, but the onset typically occurs in one's twenties or thirties. Some people with chronic anxiety disorder also suffer from occasional panic attacks.

Anxiety disorder may be hereditary to some extent, as it seems to run in families. Some cases may be linked to a relatively harmless abnormality of heart function called mitral valve prolapse. Anxiety disorder manifests itself in different ways, but doctors agree that conflict, whether internal or interpersonal, promotes a state of anxiety.

Unless otherwise specified, the dosages recommended in this section are for adults. For a child between the ages of twelve and seventeen, reduce the dose to three-quarters of the recommended amount.

NUTRIENTS

SUPPLEMENT	SUGGESTED DOSAGE	COMMENTS
Very Important		
Calcium	2,000 mg daily.	A natural tranquilizer.
and magnesium	600–1,000 mg daily.	Helps relieve anxiety, tension, nervousness, muscular spasms, and tics. Best taken in combination with calcium.
Floradix Iron + Herbs from Salus Haus	As directed on label.	Have your physician check for iron deficiency before taking any iron supplement. Floradix is a natural source of iron.
Liquid Kyolic with B_1 and B_{12} from Wakunaga	As directed on label.	Helps reduce stress and anxiety.
Multivitamin and mineral complex with	As directed on label.	To provide all needed nutrients in balance.
potassium	99 mg daily.	Essential for proper functioning of the adrenal glands.
and selenium	100–200 mcg daily. If you are pregnant, do not exceed 40 mcg daily.	Low levels have been found in this disorder. A powerful antioxidant that protects the heart.
S-Adenosylmethionine (SAMe)	400 mg twice daily.	Important physiological agent involved in over forty biochemical reactions in the body. Is a natural antidepressant and has a calming effect. *Caution:* Do not use if you have bipolar mood disorder or take prescription antidepressants. Do not give to a child under twelve.
Vitamin B complex	As directed on label.	Helps maintain normal nervous system function.
plus extra vitamin B_1 (thiamine)	50 mg 3 times daily, with meals.	Helps reduce anxiety and has a calming effect on the nerves.
and vitamin B_6 (pyridoxine)	50 mg 3 times daily, with meals.	A known energizer that also exerts a calming effect.
and niacinamide	100 mg 3 times daily.	Important in the production of certain brain chemicals. In large doses, has a calming effect. *Caution:* Do not substitute niacin for niacinamide. Niacin can be toxic in such high doses.
Vitamin C	5,000–10,000 mg daily, in divided doses.	Necessary for proper function of adrenal glands and brain chemistry. In large doses, can have a powerful tranquilizing effect and is known to decrease anxiety. Vital for dealing with stress.
Vitamin E	As directed on label.	Helps transport oxygen to brain cells and protect them from free radical damage. Use d-alpha-tocopherol form.
Zinc	50–80 mg daily. Do not exceed a total of 100 mg daily from all supplements.	Can have a calming effect on the central nervous system.
Important		
Chromium picolinate	200 mcg daily.	Chromium deficiency can produce symptoms of anxiety.
DL-Phenylalanine (DLPA)	600–1,200 mg daily. Discontinue use if no improvement is seen in 1 week.	For chronic anxiety. Increases the brain's production of endorphins, which help relieve anxiety and stress. *Caution:* Do not take this supplement if you are pregnant or nursing, or suffer from panic attacks, diabetes, high blood pressure, or PKU.
L-glutamine	500 mg 3 times daily, on an empty stomach. Take with water or juice. Do not take with milk. Take with 50 mg vitamin B_6 and 100 mg vitamin C for better absorption.	Has a mild tranquilizing effect. (*See* AMINO ACIDS in Part One.)
and L-tyrosine	500 mg 3 times daily, on an empty stomach.	Important for anxiety and depression. *Caution:* Do not take this supplement if you are taking an MAO inhibitor drug.
plus L-glycine	500 mg 3 times daily, on an empty stomach.	Necessary for central nervous system function.

Helpful		
Coenzyme A from Coenzyme-A Technologies	As directed on label.	Supports the immune system's detoxification of many dangerous substances.
Essential fatty acids (flaxseed oil and Total EFA from Health From The Sun)	As directed on label.	Important for proper brain function.
Gamma-aminobutyric acid (GABA) plus inositol	750 mg twice daily. As directed on label.	Necessary for proper brain function. (*See* AMINO ACIDS in Part One.) Combined with inositol, has a tranquilizing effect.
Melatonin	Start with 2–3 mg daily, taken ½ hour before bedtime. If necessary, gradually increase the dosage until an effective level is reached.	A natural sleep aid. Helpful if symptoms include insomnia.

Herbs

❏ A body under stress is more vulnerable to free radical damage. Bilberry, ginkgo biloba, and milk thistle are rich in flavonoids that neutralize free radicals. Milk thistle also protects the liver.

Caution: Do not take ginkgo biloba if you have a bleeding disorder, or are scheduled for surgery or a dental procedure.

❏ Catnip, chamomile, cramp bark, hops, kava kava, linden flower, motherwort, passionflower, and skullcap promote relaxation and aid in preventing panic attacks.

Cautions: Do not use chamomile if you are allergic to ragweed. Do not use during pregnancy or nursing. It may interact with warfarin or cyclosporine, so patients using these drugs should avoid it. Kava kava can cause drowsiness. If this occurs, discontinue use or reduce the dosage. It is not recommended for pregnant women or nursing mothers, and it should not be taken together with other substances that act on the central nervous system, such as alcohol, barbiturates, antidepressants, and antipsychotic drugs.

❏ Fennel relieves anxiety-related gastrointestinal upsets, reduces flatulence and abdominal tension, and relaxes the large intestine. It is most effective when taken as a tea, before or after meals, and has no known side effects. Lemon balm and willow bark also soothe stomach distress.

❏ Feverfew, used to relieve migraines, can help with anxiety-induced headaches. Drinking meadowsweet tea or extract can also relieve headaches related to anxiety and stress, with no side effects.

Cautions: Do not use feverfew when pregnant or nursing. People who take prescription blood-thinning medications should consult a health care provider before using feverfew, as the combination can result in internal bleeding.

❏ St. John's wort can ease depression and restore emotional stability. Results in mood should be noticed in approximately two to four weeks.

Caution: St. John's wort may cause increased sensitivity to sunlight. It may also produce anxiety, gastrointestinal symptoms, and headaches. It can interact with some drugs including antidepressants, birth control pills, and anticoagulants.

❏ Skullcap and valerian root can be taken at bedtime to promote sleep and aid in preventing panic attacks at night.

❏ Mandarin oil can help alleviate the oppressive feelings of anxiety and depression. A member of the orange family, mandarin (*Citrus nobilis*) originated in China. Mandarin peels are pressed to produce a pleasant aromatic oil. It can be rubbed on the skin, added to bathwater, or used in massage or aromatherapy. Try diffusing 5 drops of mandarin oil along with 3 drops of bergamot oil in an aroma lamp to relieve stress.

Caution: If you rub mandarin oil on your skin, try to avoid exposure to the sun for six hours after application. Brown spotting on the skin can occur when the oil is exposed to the sun's rays.

Recommendations

❏ Include in the diet apricots, asparagus, avocados, bananas, blackstrap molasses, brewer's yeast, broccoli, brown rice, dried fruits, dulse, figs, fish (especially salmon), garlic, green leafy vegetables, legumes, raw nuts and seeds, soy products, whole grains, and yogurt. These foods supply valuable minerals such as calcium, magnesium, phosphorus, and potassium, which are depleted by stress.

Caution: Brewer's yeast can cause an allergic reaction in some individuals. Start with a small amount at first, and discontinue use if any allergic symptoms occur.

❏ Try eating small, frequent meals rather than the traditional three meals a day.

❏ Limit your intake of animal protein. Concentrate on meals high in complex carbohydrates and vegetable protein.

❏ Avoid foods containing refined sugar or other simple carbohydrates. For a nutritional treatment plan to have maximum benefits, the diet should contain no simple sugars, carbonated soft drinks, tobacco, or alcohol.

❏ Do not consume coffee, black tea, cola, chocolate, or anything else that contains caffeine.

❏ Keep a food diary to detect correlations between your attacks and the foods you eat. Food allergies and sensitivities may trigger panic or anxiety attacks. (*See* ALLERGIES in Part Two.)

❏ Learn relaxation techniques. Biofeedback and meditation can be very helpful.

❏ Get regular exercise. Any type of exercise will work—a brisk walk, bicycle riding, swimming, aerobics, or whatever fits your individual lifestyle. After a few weeks of regular exercise, most people notice an improvement in anxiety symptoms.

❑ Be sure to get adequate rest. If sleep is a problem, consult INSOMNIA in Part Two for suggestions.

❑ To help manage an acute attack, use breathing techniques.

• Inhale slowly through the nose for a count of four.

• Hold your breath for a count of four.

• Exhale from the mouth slowly for a count of four.

• Repeat this sequence until the attack subsides.

• Remind yourself that panic attacks last for a limited amount of time, and that the attack will pass after a few minutes. Although it is rare, some may last up to a few hours.

❑ Call a trusted friend or family member. Talking things over can diffuse anxiety.

❑ If the self-help recommendations in this section do not help, and particularly if panic or anxiety is interfering with your life, consult your health care provider. If an underlying physical problem is ruled out, expect to be referred to a mental health professional for evaluation and treatment.

Considerations

❑ People with anxiety disorder, especially those who experience acute attacks, often seek medical assistance in hospital emergency rooms only to be told they are just suffering from stress and that everything will be fine with rest. In one study, up to 70 percent of people who had panic attacks were found to have seen ten or more different physicians before being correctly diagnosed.

❑ Taking tricyclic antidepressants such as imipramine hydrochloride (Janimine, Tofranil) or imipramine pamoate (Tofranil-PM) in the presence of low serum levels of iron may increase the risk of developing anxiety and jitteriness.

❑ A type of cognitive-behavioral therapy called panic control is being used with promising, long-term results for many chronic sufferers of panic attacks. Therapists coach patients into re-creating the feeling of an attack and then teach them to deal with the sensations it produces. Often panic control is used in conjunction with antidepressant drugs or tranquilizers.

❑ Chromium deficiency can produce nervousness, shakiness, and other general symptoms of anxiety. Chromium deficiency is common among alcoholics and people who consume large amounts of refined sugars. Brewer's yeast is a rich source of this essential trace element.

Caution: Brewer's yeast can cause an allergic reaction in some individuals. Start with a small amount at first, and discontinue use if any allergic symptoms occur.

❑ There have been numerous reports on the benefits of DL-phenylalanine (DLPA) in treating anxiety and depression. DLPA is a supplement consisting of both D-phenylalanine and L-phenylalanine, and is much more potent than either of these amino acids taken alone. This should be used under the supervision of a nutritionally oriented physician. Doses of 75 to 200 milligrams per day were shown to be effective for depression and anxiety.

❑ Selenium has been shown to elevate mood and decrease anxiety. These effects were more noticeable in people who had lower levels of selenium in their diets to begin with.

❑ Biofeedback can aid in managing anxiety symptoms. (*See under* PAIN CONTROL in Part Three.)

❑ Music can be effective in reducing anxiety. (*See* MUSIC AND SOUND THERAPY in Part Three.) Color also can be used to induce relaxation and calm. (*See* COLOR THERAPY in Part Three.)

❑ A number of different drugs are used to block panic attacks. Their use must be carefully monitored by a physician. The effectiveness of any given drug varies from individual to individual, and all drugs used for this disorder can cause unpleasant side effects. Alprazolam (Xanax), one of the drugs most commonly used for this illness, has varying effectiveness and can cause drowsiness and lightheadedness. It also can be very addictive. The risk of dependence and its severity seem to be higher if this drug is taken in relatively high doses (more than 4 milligrams per day) and for more than eight weeks.

❑ Recreational drugs such as marijuana can cause anxiety attacks.

❑ A healthy diet plus appropriate nutritional supplementation can be of considerable benefit, reducing overall anxiety and even decreasing the frequency and intensity of panic attacks. If you are taking antianxiety medication, following the plan outlined in this section may make it possible to stop taking the medication, or at least to reduce the dosage. You should always consult with your physician before making any change in a prescription regimen, however. *See also* STRESS in Part Two.

APPENDICITIS

Appendicitis is inflammation of the appendix, a lymphoid organ that opens into the first part of the large intestine. For many years, the appendix was believed to be a vestigial organ that served no function, but that is no longer the belief. In the fetus, the appendix contains endocrine cells that manufacture hormones and other important body chemicals. In young adults, the appendix is believed to play a part in the functioning of the immune system. It is involved in the maturation of B lymphocytes (a type of white blood cell) and assists in producing an antibody called immunoglobulin A.

Appendicitis is primarily caused by improper diet. It can be either acute or chronic. Most cases involve a blockage of the large intestine resulting from a fiber-deficient diet. The blockage stops the natural flow of fluids, which facilitates the growth of harmful bacteria from the intestinal tract, resulting in inflammation of the appendix. Appendicitis is rare in children under the age of two. The incidence peaks between the ages of fifteen and twenty-four. The risk of developing appendicitis increases after a recent illness, especially a gastrointestinal infection or a roundworm infestation.

Symptoms include severe abdominal pain that begins close to the navel and migrates toward the right lower abdomen. Taking deep breaths, coughing, sneezing, moving, or being touched in this area worsens the pain. Frequently, nausea and vomiting accompany these symptoms, with the pain becoming persistent and well-localized. Other symptoms may include diarrhea, abdominal swelling (in late stages), mild fever (usually less than 102°F), an elevated white blood cell count, constipation, inability to pass gas, painful urination, and blood in the urine.

Acute appendicitis is the most common reason for abdominal surgery. Without prompt treatment, the likelihood increases that the inflamed appendix will burst, contaminating the abdominal cavity with fecal matter and causing peritonitis. Seek help immediately. It is better to be assessed and told it was nothing than to have an appendix burst. Today, surgical treatment is mainly done laparoscopically, so hospitalization and postoperative care is shorter compared to the open appendectomies of the past, where a larger incision was made into the abdomen.

Appendicitis is seldom found in older people. Since the symptoms are usually milder in this age group, however, there is a greater danger for rupture, with resulting peritonitis or the formation of abscesses. In addition, the symptoms can be difficult to diagnose because they are similar to those of bladder infections, kidney stones, and inflammations of the colon, stomach, and small bowel (and, in women, pelvic infections or ovarian cysts). Older adults in particular should be very aware of the symptoms of appendicitis.

The nutrients and herbs recommended in this section are intended to support recovery after surgery, if appropriate, has been performed. Unless otherwise stated, the dosages recommended here are for adults. For children between the ages of twelve and seventeen, reduce the dose to three-quarters of the recommended amount. For children between the ages of six and twelve, use one-half the recommended dose, and for children under six, use one-quarter of the recommended amount.

NUTRIENTS

SUPPLEMENT	SUGGESTED DOSAGE	COMMENTS
Essential		
Carotenoid complex with beta-carotene	25,000 IU 4 times daily.	Enhances immunity and protects against infection.
Coenzyme A from Coenzyme-A Technologies	As directed on label.	Supports the immune system's detoxification of many dangerous substances.
Liquid chlorophyll	In water three times daily as directed on the label.	Helps speed the cleansing of the bloodstream.
Vitamin B complex	100 mg of each major B vitamin 3 times daily (amounts of individual vitamins in a complex will vary).	Necessary for proper assimilation of all nutrients.
Very Important		
Vitamin C (Ester-C, vitamin C crystals, or capsules)	¼ tsp 4 times daily or as directed on label.	Helps detoxify the system, protects against infection, and enhances immunity.
Vitamin E	200 IU twice daily, with meals.	Promotes healing. A powerful antioxidant. Use d-alpha-tocopherol form.
Important		
Zinc	30 mg daily.	Strengthens immune system and accelerates healing. Use zinc picolinate form.

Herbs

❏ Alfalfa, agrimony, buckthorn, and slippery elm teas are soothing.

❏ Aloe (*Aloe vera*) juice, cold-pressed from the whole leaf, can help to reduce intestinal problems and is good for general colon health.

❏ Echinacea relieves discomfort and enhances the immune system.

Caution: Do not take echinacea for longer than three months. It should not be used by people who are allergic to ragweed.

Recommendations

❏ If you suspect appendicitis, do not take a laxative and do not use a heating pad, as these can provoke rupturing of the appendix. Also, avoid pain relievers, as they can lead to a misdiagnosis. Avoid eating and drinking. See your doctor immediately.

Considerations

❏ To lessen the risk of appendicitis, you should eat a diet high in soluble fiber, avoid refined and fried foods, and limit your intake of cooked animal proteins to one serving a day.

APPETITE, POOR

A poor appetite is not a disorder in itself, but usually a symptom of some other problem. Emotional factors such as depression, illness, stress, and trauma may cause a person's appetite to diminish noticeably. Certain controllable factors, such as the use of alcohol, tobacco, or other drugs, can also result in poor appetite. An undetected underlying illness, heavy metal poisoning, and/or nutritional deficiencies may also be involved. If you lose even five to ten pounds unintentionally, you should consult your health care provider.

Unless otherwise specified, the dosages recommended in this section are for adults. For a child between the ages of twelve and seventeen, reduce the dose to three-quarters of the recommended amount. For a child between six and twelve, use one-half of the recommended dose, and for a child under the age of six, use one-quarter of the recommended amount.

NUTRIENTS

SUPPLEMENT	SUGGESTED DOSAGE	COMMENTS
Very Important		
Bio-Strath from Nature's Answer	As directed on label.	A yeast and herb formula that aids in gaining back strength and energy.
Coenzyme A from Coenzyme-A Technologies	As directed on label.	Supports the immune system's detoxification of many dangerous substances.
Floradix Iron + Herbs from Salus Haus	As directed on label.	Helps digestion and stimulates appetite. *Caution:* Do not use iron without a physician's consent.
Multivitamin and mineral complex with vitamin A and calcium and magnesium	25,000 IU daily. If you are pregnant, do not exceed 10,000 IU daily. 1,500 mg daily. 750 mg daily.	All nutrients are needed in large amounts. Use a high-potency formula.
S-Adenosylmethionine (SAMe)	As directed on label.	Helps reduce stress and depression. Gives a sense of well-being. *Caution:* Do not use if you have bipolar mood disorder or take prescription antidepressants. Do not give to a child under twelve.
Vitamin B complex	100 mg or more of each major B vitamin daily, before meals (amount of individual vitamins in a complex will vary).	Increases the appetite. Use a high-stress formula. A sublingual form is recommended. Injections (under a doctor's supervision) may be necessary.
Vitamin E	200 IU daily.	To correct deficiencies. All nutrients are important for improving appetite. Use a d-alpha-tocopherol form.
Zinc plus copper	80 mg daily. Do not exceed a total of 100 mg daily from all supplements. 3 mg daily.	Enhances the sense of taste. Needed to balance with zinc.
Helpful		
Brewer's yeast	Start with 1/2 tsp daily and work up to 1 tbsp daily.	Rich in nutrients, especially the B vitamins. Improves the appetite.
Spiru-tein from Nature's Plus	As directed on label. Take between meals.	To supply protein, needed to build and repair tissue. Also acts as an appetite stimulant.

Herbs

❑ To stimulate a poor appetite, try using catnip, fennel seed, ginger root (*see below*), ginseng, gotu kola, papaya leaves, peppermint leaves, and/or saw palmetto berries.

Caution: Do not use ginseng if you have high blood pressure, or are pregnant or nursing.

❑ Ginger helps to stimulate the heart and circulatory system and promotes appetite and digestion. Its spicy components activate the flow of saliva and the production of digestive juices. It is said that the Chinese scholar Confucius had every dish he ate spiced with ginger. The main active ingredients of ginger root are oils containing zingiberene and bisabolene, as well as camphene, linalol, citral, and cineol. It also contains vitamins A and B, minerals, fats, protein, and roughage. Ginger can be grated and sprinkled over selected portions of a meal to enhance appetite. Ginger tea is made by pouring boiling water over 1 to 2 tablespoons of freshly grated or chopped ginger. Steep for ten to fifteen minutes, then strain. Mix with honey and a splash of lemon juice to relieve gas, bloating, and cramping. We suggest that this tea be taken after meals. Ginger is also a well-known remedy for nausea and motion sickness.

Recommendations

❑ To obtain needed protein and calories, drink three or more 8-ounce glasses a day of 2 percent milk or soymilk. Use a soy carob drink and yogurt fruit shakes. Eat only whole-grain bread, rolls, macaroni, crackers, and hot and cold cereals. Use cream soups (made with soymilk) as desired. These are usually higher in protein than broth soups.

❑ Between meals, snack on foods such as avocados, banana soy pudding, buttermilk, cheese, chicken or tuna, custard, fruit shakes, nuts and nut butters, whole-grain breads and cereals, turkey, and yogurt. In addition to promoting weight gain, these snacks are easy to digest, and are high in protein and essential fatty acids.

❑ Do not drink liquids before or during meals.

❑ Take supplemental B vitamins as outlined under "Nutrients," above. The B-complex vitamins increase appetite.

❑ Try eating small quantities of food at frequent intervals throughout the day rather than two or three large meals. The sight of large amounts of food can cause a person to lose his or her appetite. Frequent small meals may be better tolerated, with a gradual increase in the volume of food.

❑ Exercise if possible, but avoid strenuous exercise. Walking and/or moderate exercise can increase the appetite. Exercise also helps the body to better assimilate nutrients.

❑ If you smoke, quit. Smoking decreases the appetite. It is one of the main causes of loss of appetite.

❑ When trying to stimulate a poor appetite, consider whether the appearance and aroma of the foods are appealing, and whether the environment is conducive to eating.

❑ If you experience a significant loss of appetite, see your physician to rule out an underlying physical problem.

Considerations

❑ To stimulate a poor appetite, the diet must be individualized according to the person's tolerances and tastes.

❑ There are many products on the market that can be helpful for people with appetite and weight problems. They are often found in the "sports" sections of health food stores, and quite often in grocery stores. These liquid drinks can be quite tasty and are similar to milk shakes. They are not only for those who are into sports. Because they are usually fortified with vitamins and minerals, don't forget to include these in calculating your daily intake of nutrients to prevent overdosing.

❑ Megace (megestrol acetate) was a drug used in breast cancer patients, but it was found to increase appetite and body weight, especially as fat. If you are prescribed this drug, be sure to engage in moderate exercise and consume adequate protein to avoid gaining weight.

❑ *See* ANOREXIA NERVOSA and BULIMIA in Part Two. *See also* HYPOTHYROIDISM in Part Two for the self-test.

ARSENIC POISONING

Arsenic is a highly poisonous metallic element found at varying levels in a wide variety of sources, including pesticides, laundry aids, smog, tobacco smoke, bone meal, dolomite, kelp, table salt, beer, seafood, and even drinking water. When ingested, inorganic arsenic is deposited in the hair, skin, and nails. Once it makes its way into the hair follicles, its presence can be detected in the hair shaft for years.

Headaches, confusion, drowsiness, convulsions, and changes in fingernail pigmentation may occur with chronic arsenic poisoning. Symptoms of acute arsenic poisoning include vomiting, diarrhea, bloody urine, muscle cramps and/or weakness, fatigue, hair loss, dermatitis, gastrointestinal pain, and convulsions. Arsenic poisoning primarily affects the lungs, skin, kidneys, and liver. The accumulation of toxic levels of arsenic can result in coma and death.

Exposure to arsenic has also been implicated in the development of certain types of cancer. Workers involved in pesticide production, agricultural insecticide spraying, copper smelting, mining, sheep dipping, and metallurgical industries are at a high risk for skin cancer, scrotal cancer, a type of liver cancer, cancer of the lymphatic system, and lung cancer due to arsenic exposure. The toxic effects of arsenic are cumulative.

Unless otherwise specified, the dosages recommended in this section are for adults. For a child between the ages of twelve and seventeen, reduce the dose to three-quarters of the recommended amount. For a child between six and twelve, use one-half the recommended dose, and for a child under the age of six, use one-quarter of the recommended amount.

NUTRIENTS

SUPPLEMENT	SUGGESTED DOSAGE	COMMENTS
Very Important		
Garlic (Kyolic from Wakunaga)	2 tablets 3 times daily, with meals.	A potent detoxifier.
Superoxide dismutase (SOD) or	As directed on label.	A powerful detoxifying agent.
Cell Guard from Biotec Foods	As directed on label.	An antioxidant complex that contains SOD.
Vitamin C with bioflavonoids	5,000–20,000 mg daily, in divided doses. (*See* ASCORBIC ACID FLUSH in Part Three.)	A potent detoxifier. (Use a buffered form.)
Helpful		
L-cysteine and L-methionine	500 mg each daily, on an empty stomach. Take with water or juice. Do not take with milk. Take with 50 mg vitamin B$_6$ and 100 mg vitamin C for better absorption.	Potent detoxifiers of the liver. Cysteine contains sulfur, which eliminates arsenic. (*See* AMINO ACIDS in Part One.)
Pectin plus	As directed on label.	Aids in removing arsenic from the body.
antioxidant complex (ACES + Zn from Carlson Labs)	As directed on label.	To protect against free radical damage.
Selenium	200 mcg daily. If you are pregnant, do not exceed 40 mcg daily.	Helps to rid the body of arsenic.

Recommendations

❑ Sulfur helps eliminate arsenic from the body. Eat eggs, onions, beans, legumes, and garlic to obtain sulfur. You can also obtain sulfur from garlic supplements, and the amino acid cysteine provides sulfur. Sulfur can be purchased in tablet form as well.

❑ Supplement your diet with plenty of fiber daily.

Note: Always take supplemental fiber separately from other supplements and medications.

❑ If you have symptoms of chronic arsenic poisoning, have a hair analysis performed to determine the level of toxic metals in your body. (*See* HAIR ANALYSIS in Part Three.)

❑ In case of accidental arsenic ingestion, immediately take 5 charcoal tablets, and take 5 more every fifteen minutes until you reach your health care provider or the emergency room of the nearest hospital. Charcoal tablets should be kept on hand in every household in case of accidental overdose of drugs.

Considerations

❑ Chelation therapy removes toxic metals from the body. (*See* CHELATION THERAPY in Part Three.)

☐ *See also* CHEMICAL POISONING and ENVIRONMENTAL TOXICITY in Part Two.

ARTERIOSCLEROSIS/ATHEROSCLEROSIS

Arteriosclerosis and atherosclerosis involve the buildup of deposits on the insides of the artery walls, which causes thickening and hardening of the arteries. In arteriosclerosis, the deposits are composed largely of calcium; in atherosclerosis, the deposits consist of fatty substances, and artery walls lose elasticity and harden. Both conditions have about the same effect on circulation, causing high blood pressure and ultimately leading to angina (chest pain brought on by exertion), heart attack, stroke, and/or sudden cardiac death.

Although arteriosclerosis causes high blood pressure, high blood pressure can also cause arteriosclerosis. Calcium-based and fatty deposits typically form in areas of the arteries weakened by high blood pressure or strain. The consequent narrowing of the arteries then makes blood pressure even higher. As the arteries become less pliable and less permeable, cells may experience ischemia (oxygen starvation) due to insufficient circulation. The fatty plaques can be either stable or unstable. Unstable plaque allows particles to break away and cause further blockage downstream, in the smaller vessels, so it is of more immediate clinical importance.

If one of the coronary arteries becomes obstructed by accumulated deposits or by a blood clot that has either formed or snagged on the deposit, the heart muscle will be starved for oxygen and the individual will suffer a heart attack, also referred to as a myocardial infarction (MI) or coronary occlusion (a coronary). Older adults are at a greater risk for this kind of heart trouble. When arteriosclerosis occludes the arterial supply of blood to the brain, a cerebrovascular accident, or stroke, occurs.

Approximately eight million Americans suffer from peripheral arterial disease (PAD), also called peripheral vascular disease, and three out of four people aren't aware they have it, according to a study published in *Circulation: Journal of the American Heart Association*. This is a relatively common condition affecting as many as 20 percent of the American population aged sixty-five or older at a given time. Most of those affected have at least one of the major risk factors for atherosclerosis: smoking, family history, hypertension, diabetes, or abnormal cholesterol levels. Advancing age increases the likelihood of developing these diseases, as does atherosclerosis of the coronary or cerebral arteries.

Peripheral atherosclerosis, also called arteriosclerosis obliterans, is a type of peripheral vascular disease in which the lower limbs are affected. In the early stages, the major arteries carrying blood to the legs and feet become narrowed by fatty deposits. Atherosclerosis of the leg or foot can not only limit a person's mobility, but can also lead to loss of a limb. People who have diseased arteries in the leg or foot are likely to also have them elsewhere, mainly in the heart and brain. Early signs of peripheral atherosclerosis are aching muscles, fatigue, and cramping pains in the ankles and legs. Depending on which arteries are blocked, there may also be pain in the hips and thighs.

Pain in the legs (most often in the calf, but sometimes in the foot, thigh, hip, or buttocks) brought on by walking and quickly relieved by rest is called intermittent claudication. This is typically the first symptom of developing peripheral atherosclerosis. Additional symptoms include numbness, weakness, and a heavy feeling in the legs. These symptoms occur because the amount of oxygenated blood passing through the plaque-clogged arteries is insufficient to meet the needs of the exercising leg muscles. The closer the problem lies to the abdominal aorta—the central artery that branches into the legs—the more tissue affected and the more dangerous the condition.

Peripheral Artery Function Self-Test

A simple test can determine how well your blood flows through the arteries of your legs. There are three areas on the lower leg where a pulsating artery can be felt by lightly touching the skin covering the artery. One spot is the top of the foot, the second spot is the inner aspect of the ankle, and the third spot is behind the knee.

Apply pressure lightly to the skin on these spots. If you cannot find a pulse, this is an indication that the artery supplying the leg may be narrowed. Special studies may be needed and you should consider consulting your health care provider.

NUTRIENTS

SUPPLEMENT	SUGGESTED DOSAGE	COMMENTS
Very Important		
Calcium and magnesium plus vitamin D	1,500 mg daily, taken at bedtime. 750 mg daily, taken at bedtime. 400 mg daily.	Needed to maintain proper muscle tone in the blood vessels. Use chelate forms. Aids calcium uptake; enhances immune system.
Coenzyme Q$_{10}$	100 mg daily.	Improves tissue oxygenation.
Essential fatty acids (flaxseed oil, MaxEPA, or omega-3 oil complex)	As directed on label.	Reduces blood pressure, and helps to maintain proper elasticity of blood vessels. Be sure to use a product that contains vitamin E to keep the essential fatty acids from becoming rancid.
Garlic (Kyolic from Wakunaga)	As directed on label.	Has a lipid (fat) regulating effect.
Multivitamin and mineral complex	As directed on label.	All nutrients are needed for protection.
Vitamin C (Ester-C) with bioflavonoids	5,000–20,000 mg daily, in divided doses. (*See* ASCORBIC ACID FLUSH in Part Three.)	Antioxidant that acts as a free radical scavenger. Use a buffered form.

Important		
Choline or lecithin granules or capsules	As directed on label. 1 tbsp 3 times daily, with meals. 2,400 mg 3 times daily, with meals.	Aids in breaking down fat and expelling it from the body. Phosphatidylcholine is best. A good source of choline.
Dimethylglycine (DMG) (Aangamik DMG from FoodScience of Vermont)	125 mg 3 times daily.	Improves tissue oxygenation.
Melatonin	2–3 mg daily, taken 2 hours or less before bedtime.	A powerful antioxidant that also improves sleep.
Multiple enzyme complex	As directed on label. Take with meals.	Important for proper digestion.
Proteolytic enzymes	As directed on label. Take with meals.	Aids in destroying free radicals. Improves digestive function.
Pycnogenol or grape seed extract	50 mg twice daily. As directed on label.	Possibly the most powerful free radical scavengers. Also enhances and strengthens connective tissue, including that of the cardiovascular system.

Helpful		
L-cysteine and L-methionine plus L-carnitine	500 mg daily, on an empty stomach. Take with water or juice. Do not take with milk. Take with 50 mg vitamin B$_6$ and 100 mg vitamin C for better absorption. 500 mg daily, on an empty stomach. 500 mg daily, on an empty stomach.	Promotes the burning of fat and the building of muscle. Helps to prevent fatty buildup in the arteries. Protects the heart and lowers blood triglyceride levels.
Trimethylglycine (TMG) (anhydrous betaine)	1,000 mg per day in divided doses, with meals, for maintenance; up to 2,000 mg to lower homocysteine levels under guidance of a health care professional.	Methyl donor, required for reduction of homocysteine back to methionine and for accurate synthesis of DNA and RNA. Homocysteine is a toxic amino acid, and maintenance of normal levels is important to the health of the cardiovascular system.

Herbs

❑ The following herbs are helpful if you suffer from arteriosclerosis: cayenne (capsicum), chickweed, and hawthorn berries.

❑ Ginkgo biloba has been called "nature's circulation wonder." It can improve circulation, increasing oxygen and blood flow in the arms, brain, and heart.

Caution: Do not take ginkgo biloba if you have a bleeding disorder, or are scheduled for surgery or a dental procedure.

❑ Green tea lowers cholesterol and lipid levels, thus decreasing chances of atherosclerosis. Drink green tea (we suggest one to four cups each day) or take it in extract form. A recent Japanese study recommends not only green tea but also black tea to lower your rate of lipoprotein oxidation, a chemical reaction that makes fats in the blood more likely to be deposited in the arteries.

Caution: Green tea contains vitamin K, which can make anticoagulant medications less effective. Consult your health care professional if you are using them. The caffeine in green tea could cause insomnia, anxiety, upset stomach, nausea, or diarrhea.

Recommendations

❑ Eat high-fiber foods that are low in saturated fat and cholesterol. Fruits, vegetables, legumes, and grains should be your primary foods.

❑ Eat plenty of foods rich in vitamin E to improve circulation. Good choices include dark green leafy vegetables, legumes, nuts, seeds, soybeans, wheat germ, and whole grains.

❑ Use only pure cold-pressed olive oil or unrefined canola oil (in moderate amounts) as fats in the diet. These may aid in lowering cholesterol. Do not heat these oils.

❑ Drink steam-distilled water only.

❑ Do not eat any candies, chips, fried foods, gravies, high-cholesterol foods, junk foods, pies, processed foods, red meat, or saturated fats. Avoid egg yolks, ice cream, salt, and all foods containing white flour and/or sugar. Do not use stimulants such as coffee, colas, and tobacco. Also, eliminate alcohol and highly spiced foods.

❑ Maintain a healthy weight for your height. Obesity causes unfavorable changes in serum lipoprotein levels.

❑ Reduce stress and learn techniques to help you handle stress that cannot be avoided. (*See* STRESS in Part Two.)

❑ Get regular moderate exercise. A daily walk is good.

Caution: If you are over thirty-five and/or have been out of shape for some time, consult your health care provider before beginning any type of exercise program.

❑ Periodically monitor your blood pressure, and take steps to lower it if necessary. Control of high blood pressure is important. (*See* HIGH BLOOD PRESSURE in Part Two.)

❑ Do not smoke. Avoid exposure to secondhand smoke. Cigarette smoke contains large quantities of free radicals, many of which are known to oxidize low-density lipoproteins (LDL, the so-called bad cholesterol), making them more likely to be deposited on the walls of blood vessels. The free radical is one of the primary factors in the development of atherosclerosis. The effect of cigarette smoke may be due to the direct oxidation of lipids and proteins, and may also have indirect effects, such as the depletion of various antioxidant defenses, which then allows other cellular processes (inflammation, for example) to modify LDL. In addition, smoking increases levels of LDL, lowers levels of high-density lipoproteins (HDL, or good cholesterol), and increases the blood's tendency to form clots.

❑ Do not take any preparations containing shark cartilage unless specifically directed to do so by your health care provider.

Considerations

❑ Because of the large number of new cases of peripheral arterial disease (PAD), each year the Society of Interventional Radiology recommends more-intensive screening efforts through the use of the ankle-brachial index (ABI) test. This simple, painless procedure tests the blood pressure in the legs versus that in the arms. This indicates whether or not blood flow is within a tolerable range and whether additional testing is required.

❑ In the Lifestyle Heart Trial study, conducted over a period of six years at the California Pacific Medical Center, eighteen of twenty-two people (82 percent) who adopted a vegetarian diet that restricted fat intake to 10 percent of total calories showed a significant regression of advanced coronary artery disease after one year, and even greater benefits after five years. The diet also limited dietary cholesterol to no more than 5 milligrams per day. In the Lyon Diet Heart Study, changes in fat composition but not the quantity of fat in the diet led to a significant reduction in heart and artery problems. Most Americans consume 37 percent of their total calories as fats and 300 to 500 milligrams of dietary cholesterol each day.

❑ Dehydroepiandrosterone (DHEA) is a natural hormone that has been shown to help prevent hardening of the arteries. (*See* DHEA THERAPY in Part Three.)

❑ Chelation therapy can break up arterial plaque and improve circulation. Some two to three thousand doctors perform this type of therapy in the United States. (*See* CHELATION THERAPY in Part Three.)

❑ Hyperbaric oxygen is used in some countries to treat arteriosclerosis. (*See* HYPERBARIC OXYGEN THERAPY in Part Three.)

❑ Many doctors recommend angioplasty or bypass surgery for people with hardening of the arteries, particularly for those with disabling angina. Angioplasty is a procedure in which blocked vessels are reopened by flattening cholesterol and debris against artery walls. Bypass surgery involves taking healthy blood vessels from elsewhere in the body (usually the leg) and inserting them to detour around a diseased coronary artery. According to a recent study, having a bypass performed while the heart beats (rather than while connected to a heart-lung machine) leads to fewer problems immediately after surgery and a shorter hospital stay. However, unless people undergoing these procedures make significant nutritional and lifestyle changes the disease process (atherosclerosis) will continue, and it is only a matter of time before the fatty deposits begin to build up again.

❑ Anticoagulants such as aspirin are often prescribed to make the blood less prone to clotting. For this to be effective, supplemental vitamin K and foods rich in vitamin K must be avoided. (*See* CARDIOVASCULAR DISEASE in Part Two.)

❑ Erectile dysfunction can result from this disease. (*See* ERECTILE DYSFUNCTION in Part Two.)

❑ Omega-3 essential fatty acids (EFAs) can be beneficial for the cardiovascular system. They are precursors of prostaglandins that aid in reducing hypertension, migraine headaches, arthritis, and other conditions. Omega-3 EFAs are found in fresh deepwater fish, fish oil, canola oil, flaxseed oil, and walnut oil. The omega-3s from fish are more bioactive than those from plants; the plant omega-3s are only 10 percent as effective as the fish oils. Reports indicate that native Arctic peoples, whose diets are high in omega-3s, have very low rates of arteriosclerosis. In a recent double-blind study at the University of Southampton in England, test subjects were given omega-3 fatty acid capsules, omega-6 capsules, and capsules containing a mixture of oils common in the Western diet. Those getting the omega-3 capsules had a 50 percent increase in stable over unstable plaque. While plaque was not removed, it was converted into a safer, more stable form that did not shed fat particles as easily. This reduces the risk of sudden heart attack. The study was published in the British medical journal *Lancet*.

❑ Enhanced external counterpulsation therapy (EECP) may provide relief for sufferers of stable angina and other conditions caused by blocked vessels in the lower extremities. This painless, noninvasive outpatient procedure involves wrapping inflatable cuffs around the calves, thighs, and buttocks. The cuffs inflate and gently force blood from the lower extremities to the heart. In a course of five treatments a week for seven weeks, blood vessels are encouraged to branch out and form natural bypasses around blocked vessels, thus restoring blood flow to the heart.

ARTHRITIS

Arthritis is the inflammation of one or more joints. It is usually accompanied by pain and stiffness, especially in the morning or after exercise, as well as swelling, deformity, and/or a diminished range of motion. Bone growths or spurs may develop in the affected joints, increasing pain and decreasing mobility. Arthritic joints may make noise when they move. Joints affected by rheumatoid arthritis tend to make a sound like crinkling cellophane, whereas osteoarthritic joints make popping, clicking, and banging noises.

Although the term *arthritis* literally means "joint inflammation," arthritis really refers to a group of more than one hundred rheumatic diseases and conditions that can cause pain, stiffness, and swelling in the joints. Certain conditions can affect other parts of the body—such as the muscles, bones, and some internal organs—and can result in debilitating and sometimes life-threatening complications. If left undiagnosed and untreated, arthritis can cause irreversible damage to the joints. According to the Arthritis

Foundation, 46 million Americans suffer from osteoarthritis, rheumatoid arthritis, and related conditions, including fibromyalgia, gout, lupus, Lyme disease, juvenile arthritis, psoriatic arthritis, bursitis, scleroderma, Reiter's syndrome, infectious arthritis, Sjögren's syndrome, and ankylosing spondylitis. Indeed, arthritis and other diseases of the musculoskeletal system are the primary source of disability in the United States today.

Arthritis is not a modern ailment—it has been with us since the beginning of time. Archeologists have discovered evidence of the disorder in the skeletons of Neanderthals and other prehistoric mammals, and even dinosaurs. Still, as long as this disorder has plagued humankind, conventional medicine has not conclusively proven how it occurs.

These conditions affect the body's movable, or synovial, joints at the knees, wrists, elbows, fingers, toes, hips, and shoulders. The neck and back also have joints between the bones of the spine. There are six different types of synovial joints (hinge, ball-and-socket, and so on), but although the types of motion they allow are different, their underlying physiological structure is essentially the same: two or more adjoining movable bones, whose adjacent surfaces are covered with a layer of cartilage, surrounded by a fluid-filled capsule made up of ligaments (tough, fibrous tissue). Fluid is secreted by a thin membrane, the synovial membrane, that lines the inside of the joint capsule. Thanks to this viscous fluid, and to the smooth, rubbery, blue-white cartilage covering the ends of the bones, the bones within the joint normally glide smoothly past one another. In healthy joints, the synovial membrane is thin, the cartilage that covers the bones is smooth, and a thin layer of synovial fluid covers the bone surfaces. A problem in any of these areas can result in arthritis. Arthritis may appear suddenly or come on gradually. Some people feel a sharp burning or grinding pain. Others compare the pain to that of a toothache. Moving the joint usually hurts, although sometimes there is only stiffness. The swelling and deformity that takes place in arthritic joints can result from a thickening of the synovial membrane, an increase in the secretion of synovial fluid, enlargement of the bones, or some combination of these factors.

There are many different types of arthritis. Refer to Quick Reference Guide: Common Forms of Arthritis and Related Conditions on page 218 for a quick summary of many of them. In this section, we primarily discuss the most common forms, osteoarthritis (OA) and rheumatoid arthritis (RA). Ninety percent of people with arthritis have OA.

Osteoarthritis, also called degenerative joint disease, involves deterioration of the cartilage protecting the ends of the bones. It is sometimes caused by injury or an inherited defect in the protein that forms cartilage. More commonly, it is a result of the wear and tear of aging, diet, and lifestyle. The once-smooth surface of cartilage becomes rough, resulting in friction. The cartilage begins to break down, and the normally smooth sliding surfaces of the bones become pitted and irregular. Osteoarthritis not only affects the weight-bearing joints—the knees, hips, and back—severely, but also commonly affects the hands and the knuckles. The tendons, ligaments, and muscles holding the joint together become weaker, and the joint becomes deformed, painful, and stiff. There is usually some stiffness and pain (more stiffness than pain at first), but little or no swelling. Any resulting disability is most often minor. However, fractures become an increasing risk because osteoarthritis makes the bones brittle. As osteoarthritis advances, bony outgrowths called osteophytes tend to develop. Often referred to as "spurs," osteophytes can be detected by X-ray, and develop near degenerated cartilage in the neck or in the lower back. This condition does not change a person's appearance.

Many people with this condition use glucosamine, chondroitin, or both to get relief from symptoms. Numerous studies support their use, but not all. In a two-year study in over two hundred patients with hip osteoarthritis, taking 1,500 milligrams a day of glucosamine did not lessen symptoms or progression of the disease. In addition, a meta-analysis (summary of twenty clinical studies) with chonroitin use in osteoarthritis of the hip and knee revealed no symptomatic benefit. These two studies appeared in major medical journals that strongly influence physician preference. However, since these supplements have few side effects at the recommended doses, it seems prudent to try them. If you do not experience a benefit within two months, you are not likely to.

Rheumatoid arthritis (RA) is an autoimmune disorder, usually affecting women and girls. The body's immune system inaccurately identifies the synovial membrane as "foreign." Inflammation, pain, and eventual destruction of cartilage ensue. Damaged tissue is replaced by scar tissue and bones fuse together. During the course of the disease, symptoms include stiffness, swelling, anemia, weight loss, fatigue, fever, and crippling pain. In one study, taking 10 grams of cod liver oil allowed patients to use 39 percent less of the medication—nonsteroidal anti-inflammatory drugs (NSAIDs)—used to treat RA. These drugs have side effects (gastrointestinal toxicities, increased blood pressure, and risk of heart disease) and lose their effectiveness over time, so cod liver oil (or fish oil) may offer a safe and natural way to manage patients' symptoms.

Arthritis can also be caused by bacterial, viral, or fungal infection of a joint. The microorganisms most commonly involved in this type of the disorder are streptococci, staphylococci, gonococci, hemophilus, or tubercle bacilli, and fungi such as *Candida albicans*. Usually the infecting organism travels to the joint through the bloodstream from an infection elsewhere in the body, but injury or even surgery can result in joint infection as well. Symptoms include redness, swelling, pain, and tenderness in the affected joint, often accompanied by systemic symptoms of infection such as fever, chills, and body aches.

The spondyloarthropathies are a group of rheumatic disorders that tend to affect the spine. Ankylosing spondylitis (AS) is the most common of these. In this disorder, certain joints of the spine become inflamed, then stiffen and become rigid. If confined to the lower back, AS causes virtually no limitation of movement. In some cases, however, the entire spine may become rigid and bent. If the joints between the ribs and spine are affected, breathing problems may result as the chest wall's ability to expand becomes limited. Postural deformities are common. It is estimated that at least 500,000 adults in the United States have AS, according to the Spondylitis Association of America. Canadians appear to have the condition in almost the same overall numbers as Americans. Some investigators feel that populations living closer to the poles have a higher incidence of the condition. Fish oil taken at large doses (4.55 grams of omega-3s a day) was shown to reduce the symptoms of the disease, allowing patients to feel and function better.

Gout, an acute form of inflammatory arthritis, occurs most often in people who are overweight and/or who indulge regularly in rich foods and alcohol. It typically attacks the smaller joints of the feet and hands, especially the big toe. Deposits of crystallized uric acid salt in the joint cause swelling, redness, and a sensation of heat and extreme pain. Approximately 1 million Americans suffer from gout, and unlike most forms of arthritis, gout overwhelmingly affects men. Ninety percent of those who suffer from gout are male. (*See* GOUT in Part Two.)

Some forms of arthritis can be reversible, and in some cases curable, with proper diet and lifestyle changes. These simple changes can not only relieve the inflammation and pain but also stop degeneration and rejuvenate the affected joints. Most of the supplements listed in Nutrients can be found in multinutrient complexes.

NUTRIENTS

SUPPLEMENT	SUGGESTED DOSAGE	COMMENTS
Essential		
Bromelain	As directed on label 3 times daily.	An enzyme that helps to stimulate production of prostaglandins. Reduces inflammation when taken between meals. Helps digestion of protein when taken with meals.
Chondroitin sulfate	500–1,000 mg daily.	Nutritional support for strengthening joints, ligaments, and tendons.
Essential fatty acids (Total EFA from Health From The Sun, omega-3 and omega-6 oil complexes, salmon oil from Carlson Labs, Kyolic-EPA from Wakunaga, or Lyprinol)	As directed on label twice daily. Take with meals.	To supply essential fatty acids that increase production and activity of anti-inflammatory prostaglandins. Helps to control arthritis pain and inflammation.
Glucosamine sulfate (GS-500 from Enzymatic Therapy) or	As directed on label.	Very important for the formation of bones, tendons, ligaments, cartilage, and synovial (joint) fluid.

N-Acetylglucosamine (N-A-G from Source Naturals)	500–1,000 mg daily.	
Methylsulfonyl-methane (MSM)	500–1,000 mg 3 times daily.	A sulfur compound needed for reducing inflammation and for joint and tissue repair.
S-Adenosylmethio-nine (SAMe) (SAMe Rx-Mood from Nature's Plus)	400 mg twice daily.	A deficiency results in the inability to maintain cartilage properly. Aids in reducing pain and inflammation. *Caution:* Do not use if you have bipolar mood disorder or take prescription antidepressants.
Sea cucumber (bêche-de-mer)	As directed on label.	A rich source of specific lubricating compounds found abundantly in all connective tissues, especially the joints and joint fluid. It may take 3 to 6 weeks to note an improvement.
Silica	As directed on label.	Supplies silicon, important for formation of apatite crystal, the primary constituent in bone.
Superoxide dismutase (SOD) or	As directed on label.	An antioxidant that protects fluid in the joints from destruction by free radicals. A sublingual form is recommended. Consider injections (under a doctor's supervision).
Cell Guard from Biotec Foods	As directed on label.	An antioxidant complex that contains SOD.
Trimethylglycine (TMG)	500–1,000 mg in the morning.	Reduces homocysteine levels.
Vitamin E	200 IU daily.	A powerful antioxidant that protects the joints from damage by free radicals. Increases joint mobility. Low levels of vitamin E have been found in people with arthritis and lupus. Use d-alpha-tocopherol form. *Caution:* If you are taking blood-thinning medication, consult your physician before taking this supplement.
Very Important		
Boron	3 mg with each meal.	A trace mineral required for healthy bones and uptake of calcium. Also reduces COX-2 and LOX enzymes for anti-inflammatory value.
Calcium and	2,000 mg daily.	Needed to prevent bone loss. Use calcium chelate form.
magnesium plus	1,000 mg daily.	Needed to balance with calcium.
copper	3 mg daily.	A cofactor for lysyl oxidase, which strengthens connective tissue and bone formation. Needed for calcium uptake and bone formation.
and vitamin D and	800 IU daily.	Needed for bone growth. Often deficient in those with arthritis.
zinc	50 mg daily. Do not exceed a total of 100 mg daily from all supplements.	Use zinc picolinate form.

Quick Reference Guide: Common Forms of Arthritis and Related Conditions

Swollen, painful joints can have a variety of causes. The particular symptoms make different arthritic and related conditions distinguishable from one another. Here is an overview of different types of arthritic disorders and their characteristic features.

Juvenile Arthritis

This is a general term for all types of arthritis that occur in children. Juvenile rheumatoid arthritis is the most prevalent form in children, and there are three major types: polyarticular (affecting many joints), pauciarticular (affecting a few joints), and systemic (affecting the entire body). The signs and symptoms of juvenile rheumatoid arthritis vary from child to child. There is no single test that establishes conclusively a diagnosis of juvenile arthritis, and the condition must be present consistently for six or more consecutive weeks before a correct diagnosis can be made. Heredity is thought to play some part in the development of juvenile arthritis. However, the inherited trait alone does not cause the illness. Researchers think this trait, along with some other unknown factor (probably in the environment), triggers the disease. The Arthritis Foundation says that juvenile arthritis is even more prevalent than juvenile diabetes and cerebral palsy.

Gout

Gout is a disease that causes sudden, severe attacks of pain, tenderness, redness, warmth, and swelling in some joints. It usually affects one joint at a time, especially the joint of the big toe. Needle-shaped uric acid crystals that precipitate out of the blood are deposited in the joint and cause the pain and swelling associated with gout. In people with gout, the body does not produce enough of the digestive enzyme uricase, which oxidizes relatively insoluble uric acid into a highly soluble compound. Factors leading to increased levels of uric acid, and then gout, include obesity, improper diet, overeating, stress, surgery, joint injury, excessive alcohol intake, hypertension, kidney disease, and certain drugs. (More details can be found in GOUT in Part Two.)

Ankylosing Spondylitis

This is a chronic inflammatory disease of the spine that can fuse the vertebrae to produce a rigid spine. Spondylitis is a result of inflammation that usually starts in tissue outside the joint. The most common early symptoms of spondylitis are low back pain and stiffness that continues for months. Although the cause of spondylitis is unknown, scientists have discovered a strong genetic or family link, according to the Arthritis Foundation. Most people with spondylitis have a genetic marker known as HLA-B27. (Genetic markers are protein molecules located on the surface of white blood cells that act as a "name tag.") Having this genetic marker does not mean a person will develop spondylitis, but people with the marker are more likely to develop the disease. Ankylosing spondylitis usually affects men between the ages of sixteen and thirty-five, but it also affects women. Other joints besides the spine can be involved.

Systemic Lupus Erythematosus

Systemic lupus erythematosus is an autoimmune disease that can involve the skin, kidneys, blood vessels, joints, nervous system, heart, and other internal organs. Symptoms vary among those affected, but may include a skin rash, arthritis, fever, anemia, hair loss, ulcers in the mouth, and kidney sediment or function abnormalities. In most cases, the symptoms first appear in women of childbearing age; however, lupus can occur in young children or in older people. Studies suggest there is an inherited tendency to get lupus, and lupus affects women about nine to ten times as often as men. It is also more common in African-American women.

Bursitis, Tendinitis, and Myofascial Pain

Bursitis, tendinitis, and myofascial pain are localized, nonsystemic (not affecting the entire body) painful conditions. Bursitis is inflammation of the sac surrounding any joint that contains a lubricating fluid. Tendinitis is inflammation of a tendon, and myofascial pain is a problem that results from the strain or improper use of a muscle. These conditions may start suddenly and usually stop within a matter of days or weeks.

Carpal Tunnel Syndrome

This is a condition in which pressure on the median nerve at the wrist causes tingling and numbness in the fingers. It can begin suddenly or gradually and can be associated with another disease, such as rheumatoid arthritis, or it may be unrelated to any other condition. If untreated, it can result in permanent nerve and muscle damage. With early diagnosis and treatment there is an excellent chance of complete recovery.

Fibromyalgia Syndrome

Fibromyalgia syndrome is a condition characterized by generalized muscular pain, fatigue, and poor sleep. It is believed to affect approximately 2 percent of the U.S. population, or about 5 million people. The name *fibromyalgia* means "pain in the muscles, ligaments, and tendons." The condition mainly affects muscles and their attachments to bones. Although it may feel like a joint disease, the Arthritis Foundation says it is not a true form of arthritis and it does not cause deformities of the joints. It is, instead, a form of soft tissue and muscular rheumatism.

Infectious Arthritis

This is a form of joint inflammation that is caused by a bacterial, viral, or fungal infection. The diagnosis is made by culturing the organism from the joint. Infectious arthritis can be cured using antibiotic medications.

Osteoarthritis (OA)

Osteoarthritis rarely develops before the age of forty, but it affects nearly everyone past the age of sixty. Nearly three times as many women as men have it and, at present, 27 million Americans, most over the age of forty-five, are affected. Previously known as "degenerative joint disease," osteoarthritis results from the "wear and tear" of life. Other risk factors include joint trauma, obesity, and repetitive joint use. The simple effect of gravity causes physical damage to the joints and surrounding tissues, leading to pain, tenderness, swelling, and decreased function. Initially, osteoarthritis is non-inflammatory, and it may be so mild that a person is unaware of it until it appears on an X-ray. Usually, only one or two joints are affected, most often the knee, hip, and hand. Pain is the earliest symptom, usually exacerbated by repetitive use.

Psoriatic Arthritis

This condition is similar to rheumatoid arthritis. About 5 percent of people with psoriasis, a chronic skin disease, also develop psoriatic arthritis. (*See* PSORIASIS in Part Two.) With psoriatic arthritis there is joint inflammation and sometimes inflammation of the spine. Fewer joints may be involved than in rheumatoid arthritis, and there is no rheumatoid factor in the blood.

Reiter's Syndrome

Reiter's syndrome involves inflammation in the joints, and sometimes at the location where tendons attach to bones. This form of arthritis usually develops following an intestinal or a genital/urinary tract infection. People with Reiter's syndrome have arthritis and one or more of the following: urethritis, prostatitis, cervicitis, cystitis, eye problems, or skin sores.

Rheumatoid Arthritis (RA)

Rheumatoid arthritis, a type of inflammatory arthritis, is an autoimmune disorder that occurs when the body's own immune system mistakenly attacks the synovium (the cell lining inside the joint). An overactive immune system can be just as harmful as a weak one. As with other autoimmune disorders, rheumatoid arthritis is a "self-attacking-self" disease. In this case, the body's immune system improperly identifies the synovial membrane as *foreign*. The synovium becomes inflamed and thickened. Inflammation damages cartilage and tissues in and around the joints. Often, the bone surfaces are destroyed as well because inflammation in the joints triggers the production of enzymes that slowly digest adjacent tissue. The body replaces this damaged tissue with scar tissue, forcing normal spaces within the joints to become narrow and the bones to fuse together. Rheumatoid arthritis creates stiffness, swelling, fatigue, anemia, weight loss, fever, and, often, crippling pain. Rheumatoid arthritis frequently occurs in people under forty years of age. Currently, 1.3 million Americans have this disabling disorder, down from 2.1 million just a decade ago. Women are two to three times more likely than men to develop RA. Juvenile arthritis is a form of rheumatoid arthritis that strikes children under the age of eighteen. It affects nearly 300,000 young Americans, again most of them female. The onset of rheumatoid arthritis is associated with physical or emotional stress, poor nutrition, and bacterial infection. Rheumatologists have discovered that the blood of many people with rheumatoid arthritis contains antibodies called *rheumatoid factors,* a finding that can aid in the diagnosis of the condition. While osteoarthritis affects individual joints, rheumatoid arthritis affects all of the body's synovial joints.

Scleroderma

This is a disease of the body's connective tissue that causes thickening and hardening of the skin. It can also affect joints, blood vessels, and internal organs. There are two types of scleroderma: localized and generalized.

Supplement	Suggested Dosage	Comments
Cerasomal-cis-9-cetylmyristoleate (CMO)	300 mg morning and night daily.	An anti-inflammatory that reduces inflammation in the joints. *Caution:* Do not take this supplement if you are pregnant or nursing, or if you have liver problems.
Dimethylglycine (DMG) (Aangamik DMG from FoodScience of Vermont)	125 mg 3 times daily.	Helps to prevent further damage to joints.
Free form amino acid (Amino Balance from Anabol Naturals)	As directed on label.	To supply protein, needed for tissue repair. Protein is a major component of bone tissue.
Glucosamine/Chondroitin MSM Ultra Rx-Joint Cream from Nature's Plus	As directed on label.	Topical cream for relief of inflamed joints.
Kelp or alfalfa	As directed on label.	A rich source of minerals needed for good skeletal health. *See under* Herbs, below.
Multienzyme complex	As directed on label. Take with meals.	To aid digestion. *Caution:* If you have a history of ulcers, do not use a product containing HCl.
Selenium	200 mcg daily. If you are pregnant, do not exceed 40 mcg daily.	A powerful antioxidant.
Vitamin B complex with para-aminobenzoic acid (PABA)	50 mg of each major B vitamin 3 times daily (amounts of individual vitamins in a complex will vary).	B vitamins work best when taken together. Use a hypoallergenic formula. Good for swelling.
plus extra vitamin B$_3$ (niacin) or niacinamide	100 mg 3 times daily. Do not exceed this amount. As directed on label.	Increases blood flow by dilating small arteries. Good for knee pain. *Caution:* Do not take niacin if you have a liver disorder, gout, or high blood pressure. *Caution:* Do not substitute niacin for niacinamide. Niacin can be toxic in such high doses.
plus vitamin B$_5$ (pantothenic acid) and vitamin B$_6$ (pyridoxine)	500–1,000 mg daily. 50 mg daily.	Especially for rheumatoid arthritis; vital for the production of steroids in the adrenal gland. Reduces swelling in tissue.
Vitamin B$_{12}$ and folic acid	1,000 mcg daily. 400 mcg daily.	Needed for proper digestion, the formation of cells, and the production of myelin, and the protective coating surrounding the nerves. Prevents nerve damage.
Vitamin C plus bioflavonoids	3,000–10,000 mg daily, in divided doses. 500 mg daily.	Powerful free radical destroyer that also aids in pain relief because of its anti-inflammatory effect. Use a buffered form. Boosts the activity of vitamin C.
Vitamin K	As directed on label.	Helps deposit minerals into the bone matrix.

Helpful		
Bone Defense from KAL	As directed on label.	Contains calcium, magnesium, phosphorus, and other valuable bone-reinforcing nutrients.
DL-Phenylalanine (DLPA)	500 mg daily every other week.	Good for pain relief. *Caution:* Do not take this supplement if you are pregnant or nursing, or if you suffer from panic attacks, diabetes, high blood pressure, or PKU.
Garlic (Kyolic from Wakunaga)	2 capsules 3 times daily, with meals.	Inhibits the formation of free radicals, which can damage the joints.
Healthy Joint Image from Coenzyme-A Technologies	As directed on label.	Contains pantothenic acid, glucosamine sulfate, chondroitin sulfate, cerasomal-cis-9-cetylmyristoleate, methylsulfonylmethane (MSM), and other nutrients to support healthy bone, joint, ligament, and cartilage function.
L-cysteine	500 mg twice daily, on an empty stomach. Take with water or juice. Do not take with milk. Take with 50 mg vitamin B$_6$ and 100 mg vitamin C for better absorption.	A detoxifier essential for immune function; a source of sulfur and a component of collagenous tissue. (*See* AMINO ACIDS in Part One.)
L-histidine	As directed on label.	Aids in building joints and connective tissue.
MSM Lotion from Aerobic Life Industries	Apply topically as directed on label.	Good for stiffness and pain.
Multivitamin complex with vitamin A and natural beta-carotene	10,000 IU daily. 15,000 IU daily.	All nutrients are needed to aid in repairing tissues and cartilage.
Pregnenolone	As directed on label.	Good for pain and inflammation.
Proteolytic enzymes or Inf-zyme Forte from American Biologics	As directed on label. Take between meals. As directed on label.	To protect the joints from free radical damage.
Pycnogenol or grape seed extract	As directed on label. As directed on label.	Improves joint flexibility, repairs connective tissue by reducing the prostaglandins that cause inflammation, and inhibits histamine release responsible for tissue damage.
Shark cartilage	Start with 1 gram per 15 lbs of body weight daily, divided into 3 doses. When relief is achieved, reduce the dosage to 1 gm per 40 lbs of body weight daily.	Treats pain and inflammation. Aids in repairing joints and bones.

Herbs

❑ Alfalfa contains all the minerals essential for bone formation, and may be helpful for arthritis. It can be taken in capsules or in whole, natural form. Kelp also contains essential minerals and is good for thyroid function.

❏ Boswellia, an Ayurvedic herb, is important for reducing inflammation. It is made from frankincense (*Boswellia serrata*). It also helps to restore blood vessels around inflamed connective tissue. Choose a product standardized to contain 150 milligrams of boswellic acids per tablet or capsule. Boswellia can also be used topically, in cream form, to relieve pain.

❏ The boswellic acids, a group of acids associated with *Boswellia serrata* resin, work to inhibit an enzyme called 5-lipoxygenase (5-LOX), which is instrumental in the synthesis of leukotrienes. The herbal preparation 5-Loxin contains AKBA, the most potent of the boswellic acids. It is a potent anti-inflammatory agent used successfully in the treatment of arthritis pain.

❏ Cat's claw is helpful for relieving arthritis pain. Feverfew and ginger also are good for pain and soreness.

Caution: Do not use cat's claw during pregnancy. Do not use feverfew when pregnant or nursing. People who take prescription blood-thinning medications should consult a health care provider before using feverfew, as the combination can result in internal bleeding.

❏ Ginger is a powerful antioxidant that has anti-inflammatory effects. The active component is gingerol. Ginger inhibits pain-producing prostaglandins.

❏ The hot peppers known as cayenne (capsicum) contain a compound called capsaicin that relieves pain, apparently by inhibiting the release of substance P, a neurotransmitter responsible for communicating pain sensations. Capsaicin can be absorbed through the skin. Mix cayenne powder with enough wintergreen oil to make a paste and apply it to painful joints, or use cayenne peppers in a poultice. (*See* USING A POULTICE in Part Three.) This may cause a stinging sensation at first, but with repeated use, pain should diminish markedly. Cayenne can also be taken in capsule form (Cool Cayenne from Solaray is a good source).

❏ Du Huo Jisheng Wan is an herbal Chinese patent medicine that has proven to be beneficial for arthritis sufferers.

❏ Joint Care from Himalaya Herbal Healthcare is an Ayurvedic herbal combination formula designed to support joint health.

❏ Nettle leaf is used in Germany for its anti-inflammatory properties. Nettle leaf extract inhibits TNF-alpha and IL-1 beta, which are pro-inflammatory signaling molecules. TNF is prominent in triggering inflammation, and IL is involved in cartilage and bone destruction. The prescription drug etanercept (Enbrel), prescribed for rheumatoid arthritis, acts by suppressing the TNF-alpha.

❏ Nexrutine is an herbal extract of the phellodendron tree (*Phellodendron amurense*). This tree has been a resource in traditional Asian medicine for more than 1,500 years. Developed by Next Pharmaceuticals, Inc., Nexrutine is an anti-inflammatory used for natural pain management. It is

uniquely suited for the treatment of arthritis pain due to its operational mechanisms. The COX-2 enzyme is inhibited, thus blocking one of the main pain pathways at the source. Additionally, its use does not cause blood platelets to stick together, thus reducing the cardiovascular risk associated with popular COX-2 inhibitors. No stomach problems were observed in trials. The usual dosage is 250 to 500 milligrams three times daily.

Caution: Do not use Nexrutine while pregnant or lactating. It is not intended for use by children.

❏ Noni, known as "the sacred plant" to Polynesian peoples in the South Pacific, has been used for more than 2,000 years for pain, arthritis, and other health problems.

❏ Olive leaf extract is good for infectious arthritis. Used for thousands of years by people living in the Mediterranean, it is said to be nature's safe and effective antibiotic. Natural compounds such as oleuropein in the leaf act as powerful germ killers capable of destroying microbes that can cause arthritis. There are reportedly no adverse side effects.

❏ Turmeric contains curcumin, which has anti-inflammatory and pain-relieving properties. It is good for inflammatory conditions such as arthritis. The recommended dose is 600 milligrams daily.

❏ Willow bark is also good for pain and inflammation.

❏ Borage seed oil in a dosage of 1,800 milligrams per day may be effective in pain control. However, fish oil has a better mix of fatty acids to reduce TNF and COX-2.

❏ Other beneficial herbs include brigham tea, buchu leaves, burdock root, celery seed, corn silk, devil's claw tea, parsley tea, and yucca.

Recommendations

❏ Eat more sulfur-containing foods, such as asparagus, eggs, garlic, and onions. Sulfur is needed for the repair and rebuilding of bone, cartilage, and connective tissue, and it also aids in the absorption of calcium. Other beneficial foods include fresh vegetables (especially green leafy vegetables, which supply vitamin K), nonacidic fresh fruits, whole grains, oatmeal, brown rice, fish, soybean products, and avocados. Be sure to include these foods in your diet. Also, tart red cherries can relieve pain and inflammation. Eat about twenty cherries each day. If you can't find fresh cherries, the frozen variety is fine.

❏ Consume foods containing the amino acid histidine, including rice, wheat, and rye. Histidine is good for removing excess metals from the body. Many people with arthritis have high levels of copper and iron in their bodies.

❏ Eat fresh pineapple frequently. Bromelain, an enzyme found in pineapple, is excellent for reducing inflammation. To be effective, the pineapple must be fresh, as freezing and canning destroy enzymes.

❏ Eat some form of fiber, such as ground flaxseeds, oat bran, or rice bran, daily.

❑ Reduce the amount of fat in your diet. Do not consume milk, dairy products, or red meat. Also avoid caffeine, citrus fruits, paprika, salt, tobacco, and everything containing sugar.

❑ Avoid the nightshade vegetables (peppers, eggplant, tomatoes, white potatoes). These foods contain a substance called solanine, to which some people, particularly those suffering from arthritis, are highly sensitive. Solanine interferes with enzymes in the muscles, and may cause pain and discomfort.

❑ If you use ibuprofen or other nonsteroidal anti-inflammatory drugs (NSAIDs), avoid sodium (salt), which causes water retention. Spread doses of these medications throughout the day, take them only after eating, and take an antacid an hour after taking the drug. Ask your health care provider about a protective agent to take along with the NSAID, especially if you are over sixty-five or have had previous gastrointestinal bleeding.

❑ Do not take iron supplements, or a multivitamin containing iron. Iron supplementation is suspected of being involved in pain, swelling, and joint destruction. Consume iron in foods instead. Good sources include blackstrap molasses, broccoli, Brussels sprouts, cauliflower, fish, lima beans, and peas.

❑ Boron is important as a trace mineral. It can be found naturally in noncitrus fruits such as plums, red grapes, apples, pears, and avocados, as well as in legumes and nuts. It can also be found in red wine and coffee. Dried fruits contain a much higher amount of boron than do fresh fruits. For instance, fresh plums contain 0.45 milligrams per 100 grams, but the same weight in dried prunes (about a dozen) contains 2.15 mg of boron. The body's boron requirements may be as high as 9 to 12 milligrams per day although most people naturally consume only about 1 to 2 milligrams in the diet.

❑ For relief of pain, try using cold gel packs. These retain cold for long periods when frozen. Place them on inflamed joints. Alternate with applications of heat.

❑ Hot tubs and baths may provide relief. Raw lemon rubs and hot castor oil packs are also extremely beneficial. To make a hot castor oil pack: place castor oil in a pan and heat but do not boil it. Dip a piece of cheesecloth or other white cotton material into the oil until the cloth is saturated. Apply the cloth to the affected area and cover it with a piece of plastic that is larger in size than the cotton cloth. Place a heating pad over the plastic and use it to keep the pack warm. Keep the pack in place for one-half to two hours, as needed.

❑ In the morning, take a hot shower or a bath to help relieve morning stiffness.

❑ Take free form amino acids regularly to help repair tissue.

❑ Check for possible food allergies. Many sufferers of neck and shoulder pain have found relief when they eliminate certain foods. Allergies trigger inflammation and can aggravate arthritic symptoms, especially those of rheumatoid arthritis.

❑ Consider having a hair analysis to determine the levels of toxic metals in your body. Lead levels have been found to be higher than normal in some arthritis sufferers. (See HAIR ANALYSIS in Part Three.)

❑ Spend time outdoors for fresh air and sunshine. Exposure to the sun prompts the synthesis of vitamin D_3, which is needed for proper bone formation.

❑ Get regular moderate exercise. Exercise is essential for reducing pain and retarding joint deterioration. Regular activity that does not put stress on affected joints, but that strengthens surrounding bones, muscles, and ligaments, is valuable for many types of arthritis. Bicycle riding, walking, and water exercises are good choices. Avoid weight-bearing or impact exercises.

❑ If you are overweight, lose the excess pounds. Being overweight can cause and aggravate osteoarthritis.

Considerations

❑ If the blood is too acidic, the cartilage in the joints may dissolve. The joints lose their normal smooth sliding motion, bones rub together, and the joints become inflamed, causing pain. (See ACIDOSIS under ACID/ALKALI IMBALANCE in Part Two.)

❑ Etanercept (Enbrel) is a drug used to treat rheumatoid arthritis. It apparently blocks the action of tumor necrosis factor (TNF) alpha, an infection-fighting protein linked to inflammation. However, this drug does affect the immune system and has been tied to a number of cases of serious infection including tuberculosis. The drug's manufacturer, Amgen, now adds a warning to the packaging label informing doctors about the infections.

❑ Researchers at Jefferson Medical College in Philadelphia have identified a possible genetic component of osteoarthritis. They found that some individuals have a defect in the gene that instructs cartilage cells to manufacture collagen, an important protein in connective tissue. As a result, the collagen in these individuals' joints is more prone to wear down, depriving the bones of their protective cushion.

❑ In one study, people with rheumatoid arthritis were found to have lower blood levels of folic acid, protein, and zinc than healthy persons. The researchers concluded that drugs prescribed for arthritis had brought about biochemical changes in the subjects' bodies, increasing their need for certain nutrients.

❑ Eating deep-sea fish, which are rich in eicosapentaenoic acid (EPA) and docosahexaenoic acid (DHA), helped relieve the symptoms of rheumatoid arthritis in a study conducted by Charles Dinarello, M.D., of the Tufts University School of Medicine in the mid-1990s. Albany Medical College researcher Joel M. Kremer conducted a similar study published in the *American Journal of Clinical Nutrition*, in which people with rheumatoid arthritis were given daily doses of a fish oil concentrate and twenty were given a placebo. After fourteen weeks, the groups were switched. The people taking the fish oil reported only about half as many tender joints as the placebo group. The fish oil also slowed the onset of fatigue.

❑ Omega-3 essential fatty acids found in fish oil may alleviate symptoms of rheumatoid arthritis by suppressing the immune system reaction that causes joint inflammation. Numerous studies over the past ten years have shown that people with rheumatoid arthritis have fewer tender and swollen joints and less morning stiffness after several months of taking large doses of fish oil supplements (2.5 to 5 grams a day) with meals. Using 3 grams of omega-3s from fish oil combined with 9.6 grams (about 2 teaspoons) of olive oil was more effective than fish oil alone at relieving symptoms associated with rheumatoid arthritis. Patients experienced less stiffness in the morning, less joint pain throughout the day, and better right handgrip strength.

❑ Bromelain has been shown to improve recent mild knee pain. Patients had a greater sense of well-being and were more mobile. A dose of 400 milligrams a day of bromelain worked better than a dose of 200 milligrams per day.

❑ Gamma-linolenic acid (GLA), an omega-6 fatty acid, may ease symptoms of rheumatoid arthritis by suppressing the production of prostaglandins that trigger inflammation. Evening primrose oil and borage seed oil contain GLA.

❑ The immunosuppressant drug cyclosporine, which is used in transplant patients to prevent rejection of the transplanted organ, is being used as a treatment for a variety of autoimmune diseases, including rheumatoid arthritis. Using the ointment form of cyclosporine apparently lessens the potentially hazardous side effects this drug has when administered by mouth or by injection, such as kidney damage and reduced resistance to infection. It has been found that cyclosporine improves pain and inflammation for many people who use it.

❑ Chlamydia, the organism responsible for many cases of urethritis, has been linked to a form of arthritis that affects young women. In nearly half of the women with unexplained arthritis tested in one study, chlamydia was found in the joints. Seventy-five percent had elevated levels of antibodies to chlamydia in their blood.

❑ Most chiropractors and osteopaths advise women to avoid high-heeled shoes because they place a greater compressive pressure on the knees than flat or low-heeled shoes, which may eventually lead to arthritis of the knees. The higher the heel, the greater the force.

❑ Silicone gel breast implants and other silicone prostheses may cause arthritis-like symptoms, such as swelling of joints, contractures, fever, chronic fatigue, and pain. Silicone has also been known to trigger such severe autoimmune diseases as scleroderma and lupus. Some women have seen arthritic symptoms disappear after having the implants removed but this is not true in all cases.

❑ Women who breast-feed are less likely to develop rheumatoid arthritis than women who don't. Dr. Elizabeth Wood Karlson of Brigham and Women's Hospital in Boston used data from the Nurses' Health Study to explore the contribution of hormonal factors on subsequent development of arthritis. Women who breast-fed for a total of twelve to twenty-three months during their lifetime had a 30 percent risk reduction. Those who breast-fed for at least twenty-four months had a 50 percent risk reduction.

❑ In one laboratory study, injections of a protein called anti-TGF-B banished painful joint swelling in 75 percent of the subjects, according to Dr. David Pisetsky of the National Arthritis Foundation. This protein destroys TGF-B, a chemical produced by the body in response to infection that causes inflammation and triggers swelling in the hands and feet.

❑ Cosamin from Nutramax Laboratories may help the joints and ligaments. (*See* Manufacturer and Distributor Information in the Appendix.)

❑ Dimethylsulfoxide (DMSO), a by-product of wood processing, is a liquid that can be applied topically to relieve pain, reduce swelling, and promote healing.

Caution: Only pure DMSO from a health food store should be used for the treatment of arthritis. Commercial-grade DMSO such as that found in hardware stores is not suitable for healing purposes. Any contaminants on the skin or in the product can be taken into the tissues by action of the DMSO.

Note: The use of DMSO may result in a garlicky body odor. This is temporary, and is not a cause for concern.

❑ Arthritic pain and inflammation may respond to treatment with honeybee venom. The venom contains a powerful anti-inflammatory substance and also acts as an immune system stimulant. It is administered by injection.

Caution: You should not use this product if you are allergic to bee stings.

❑ Nonsteroidal anti-inflammatory drugs (NSAIDs) such as ibuprofen (found in Advil, Nuprin, and numerous other products), indomethacin (Indocin), and piroxicam (Feldene) are commonly prescribed for relief of arthritis pain. Unfortunately, these drugs also can have side effects. About 1 percent of people who take NSAIDs on a regular basis develop stomach ulcers or experience severe gastrointestinal bleeding. As many as 200,000 cases of gastrointestinal bleeding, including 10,000 to 20,000 deaths, could be occurring each year in the United States as a result of nonsteroidal anti-inflammatory drugs prescribed for arthritis. These drugs can also cause kidney or liver damage when used in large doses and when used long-term.

❑ Misoprostol (Cytotec) and ulcer drugs like ranitidine (Zantac) and sucralfate (Carafate) might help prevent the development of ulcers associated with NSAIDs.

❏ Diclofenac sodium (Voltaren), a drug often prescribed for arthritis, has many serious potential side effects and may cause liver problems in some cases. People who take it should be monitored very closely. If this medication is prescribed, the physician should perform a blood liver enzyme study.

❏ For some forms of arthritis, drugs such as hydroxy-chloroquine (Plaquenil) and gold compounds (Ridaura) may be prescribed.

❏ For some individuals, the ulcer drug sucralfate (Carafate) may give the same relief as aspirin and other anti-inflammatory drugs without damaging the stomach lining.

❏ Acetaminophen (sold as Tylenol, Datril, and others) may be a better medication for osteoarthritis than ibuprofen. Acetaminophen is relatively safe and inexpensive, although if it is taken in excessive amounts or in combination with alcohol, this drug can cause liver damage.

❏ Kawasaki syndrome is an infectious disease that can cause symptoms of arthritis in children, accompanied by conjunctivitis; fever; a red rash on the body; a swollen, red tongue; and/or red or purplish red discoloration and swelling of the palms of the hands and the soles of the feet. The cause of this disorder is not known. It primarily affects children under five years of age. Most children recover, but some, unfortunately, suffer permanent heart damage.

❏ Lyme disease can mimic arthritis, causing many of the same symptoms. (See LYME DISEASE in Part Two.)

❏ Another autoimmune disease that often manifests itself as arthritis is systemic lupus erythematosus (Lupus). For reasons unknown, the body produces antibodies that act against its own tissues. (See LUPUS in Part Two.)

❏ In its early stages, ulcerative colitis can cause symptoms like those of arthritis. Because this may occur before there are any abdominal symptoms, it can lead to misdiagnosis and delayed treatment. (See ULCERATIVE COLITIS in Part Two.)

❏ More information about arthritis is available from the Arthritis Foundation (www.arthritis.org). (See Health and Medical Organizations in the Appendix.)

❏ See also GOUT in Part Two and PAIN CONTROL in Part Three.

ASTHMA

Asthma is a lung disease that causes obstruction of the airways. It is an overreaction of the body's own immune system usually caused by exposure to an allergen, a substance that the body perceives as foreign and dangerous.

During an asthma attack, spasms in the muscles surrounding the bronchi (small airways in the lungs) constrict, impeding the outward passage of air. Asthma sufferers often describe this plight as "starving for air." Typical symptoms of an asthma attack are coughing, wheezing, a feeling of tightness in the chest, and difficulty breathing. An attack can last for a few minutes or several hours.

The spasms characterizing an acute attack are not the cause of the disorder, but a result of chronic inflammation and hypersensitivity of the airways to certain stimuli. An attack can be triggered if a susceptible individual is exposed to an allergen, but irritants, infection, stress, exercise, or use of aspirin, ibuprofen, naproxen sodium, or other NSAIDS—or even rapid changes in weather and humidity—can trigger an attack.

There are two forms of asthma: allergic and nonallergic, although the two often occur together. Common asthma-provoking allergens include animal dander, cockroach allergens, pollens, mold, chemicals, drugs, dust mites, environmental pollutants, feathers, food additives (such as monosodium glutamate or sulfites such as sodium metabisulfite), seafood, dairy products, nuts, yeast-based foods, fumes, mold, and tobacco smoke. But any kind of allergen can precipitate an asthma attack. Factors that can trigger nonallergic asthma attacks include adrenal disorders, anxiety, temperature changes, exercise, extremes of dryness or humidity, fear, laughing, low blood sugar, and stress. A respiratory infection such as bronchitis can also provoke an attack. Whatever the particular instigator, the bronchial tubes swell and become plugged with mucus. This inflammation further irritates the airways, resulting in even greater sensitivity. The attacks become more frequent and the inflammation more severe.

Asthma can be difficult to diagnose conclusively. Its symptoms may resemble those of other diseases, such as emphysema, bronchitis, and lower respiratory infections. To distinguish asthma from other conditions, a physician may recommend blood tests, chest X-rays, and spirometry (a procedure that measures air breathed into and out of the lungs). If not treated properly, bronchial asthma can lead to pulmonary emphysema. However, with prompt diagnosis and appropriate treatment, serious danger from asthma should be preventable.

Cardiac asthma is a condition that causes the same symptoms as other types of asthma, but is caused by heart failure. Intrinsic asthma, a less common form of the disease, which generally appears during adulthood, is often associated with other respiratory diseases such as bronchitis or sinusitis, and tends to appear during upper respiratory viral infections. People who suffer from intrinsic asthma are usually vulnerable to changes in weather, exercise, emotional stress, and other factors related to inner feelings. However, 10 percent of adults with asthma remain symptomatic despite treatment with high-dose inhaled steroids and long-acting beta2 agonists.

A hereditary link to asthma was discovered in late 1999 by two Berkeley, California, researchers who spliced human genes into mice and determined that asthmatic activity could be diminished by slowing the activity of two particular genes. The value of the research, they said, centered on the fact that scientists now have an opportunity to develop a medicine to prevent asthma, rather than merely treat its symptoms.

This genetic-based research milestone in asthma prevention arrived at an important juncture. Medical scientists are growing increasingly alarmed over what they consider to be an epidemic rise in the number of new asthma cases each year. Asthma now affects 16.2 million people, 6.7 million of whom are children, according to the Centers for Disease Control (CDC). Children under age sixteen, particularly those living in urban areas, and adults over the age of sixty-five are most likely to suffer from asthma. Eighty percent of children get their first asthma symptoms before age five. It is the third leading cause of hospitalization for children, and the number-one cause of school absenteeism. The cause of asthma's continued rise over the years has researchers scratching their heads and looking at a wide spectrum of possible causes, including pollution, global warming, food additives, genetics, toxins, and allergens. Recently it has been discovered that large increases in the number of asthma sufferers in the American Southwest, the Caribbean, and Central American regions seem to have been brought on by drought-caused sub-Saharan dust and mold spores being swept across the Atlantic by prevailing winds—winds that have recently changed due to the effects of global warming. Asthma specialists speculate that rising levels of environmental pollution also lead to higher incidences of asthma. Asthma epidemics related to atmospheric contamination—situations in which dust and chemical particles are abundant, especially in enclosed environments—are well known. Occupational exposure to certain substances, such as urethane and polyurethane, used in the adhesives and plastics industry, along with rubber epoxy resins from paint, textile cleaner fumes, dry-cleaning chemicals, and others also may be major risk factors. Obesity has recently been linked to the development and severity of asthma in adults and children.

The dosages recommended here are for adults. For children between the ages of twelve and seventeen, reduce the dose to three-quarters of the recommended amount. For children between the ages of six and twelve years old, reduce the dose to one-half the recommended amount. For children under six years old, use one-third of the recommended amount.

NUTRIENTS

SUPPLEMENT	SUGGESTED DOSAGE	COMMENTS
Essential		
Fish oil	1,000 mg twice daily, before meals.	A source of essential fatty acids needed for production of anti-inflammatory prostaglandins.
Pantothenic acid (vitamin B$_5$)	50 mg 3 times daily.	The antistress vitamin.
Selenium	100 mcg daily.	Blood levels are low in asthmatics.
Vitamin C with bioflavonoids	1,500 mg 3 times daily. *Caution:* If you have a history of kidney stones or hemochromatosis, do do not take vitamin C at this dosage level.	Needed to protect lung tissue and keep down infection. Also increases air flow and fights inflammation.
Zinc lozenges	Do not take over 100 mg daily.	Can shorten an attack or halt one before it becomes severe.
Very Important		
Betaine hydrochloride with pepsin	As directed on label, or as prescribed by physician.	Combats malabsorption problems leading to "leaky gut syndrome."
Coenzyme Q$_{10}$	100 mg daily.	Has the ability to counter histamine.
Magnesium plus calcium	750 mg daily. 1,500 mg daily.	May stop the acute asthmatic episode by increasing the vital capacity of the lungs. Has a dilating effect on the bronchial muscles. Use chelate or asporotate forms.
Multivitamin and mineral complex with selenium and vitamin B$_{12}$	As directed on label. 200 mcg daily. If you are pregnant, do not exceed 40 mcg daily. 2000 mcg daily	Necessary for enhanced immune function. Use a high-potency formula. A powerful destroyer of free radicals created from air pollutants.
Helpful		
Bee pollen	Start with a few granules at a time and slowly work up to 2 tsp daily.	Strengthens the immune system. Use raw crude pollen, preferably produced within 10 miles of your home. *Caution:* Bee pollen may cause an allergic reaction in some individuals. Discontinue use if a rash, wheezing, discomfort, or other symptom occurs.
Coenzyme A from Coenzyme-A Technologies	As directed on label.	Promotes detoxification of dangerous substances from the immune system.
Dimethylglycine (DMG) (Aangamik DMG from FoodScience of Vermont)	As directed on label twice daily.	Improves oxygenation in lung tissue.
Glucosamine sulfate or N-Acetylglucosamine (N-A-G from Source Naturals)	As directed on label. As directed on label.	Important for regulation of mucous secretions of the respiratory tract.
Kelp	2,000–3,000 mg daily for 21 days, then reduce to 1,000–1,500 mg daily.	For minerals in balanced amounts.
L-cysteine	500 mg twice daily, on an empty stomach. Take with water or juice. Do not take with milk. Take with 50 mg vitamin B$_6$ and 100 mg vitamin C for better absorption.	Repairs lung tissue and reduces inflammation. (*See* AMINO ACIDS in Part One.)
Pycnogenol or grape seed extract	As directed on label. As directed on label.	Powerful antioxidants and anti-inflammatories.

225

S-Adenosylmethio-nine (SAMe)	As directed on label.	Reduces stress and eases depression. Promotes a sense of well-being. *Caution:* Do not use if you have bipolar mood disorder or take prescription antidepressants. Do not give to a child under twelve.
Urban Air Defense from Source Naturals	As directed on label.	Contains many of the necessary nutrients listed in this table, including vitamins A, C, and E, plus herbs and minerals.
Vitamin D	600 IU daily.	Needed for repair of tissues.

Herbs

❑ Asthma-X5 from Olympian Labs is an herbal combination formula containing coleus forskohlii, feverfew, ginger, green tea, licorice root, lobelia, Mormon tea, schisandra berries, and skullcap. The recommended dosage is 500 to 1,000 milligrams, three times daily. For best results, use for about eight weeks.

Cautions: Do not use feverfew when pregnant or nursing. People who take prescription blood-thinning medications should consult a health care provider before using feverfew, as the combination can result in internal bleeding. Green tea contains vitamin K, which can make anticoagulant medications less effective. Consult your health care professional if you are using them. The caffeine in green tea could cause insomnia, anxiety, upset stomach, nausea, or diarrhea. Licorice root should not be used during pregnancy or nursing. It should not be used by persons with diabetes, glaucoma, heart disease, high blood pressure, or a history of stroke.

❑ ClearLungs from RidgeCrest Herbals is a Chinese herbal formula designed to reduce inflammation and mucus, opening up the airways to the lungs and promoting free breathing. Take 2 capsules twice daily.

❑ Lobelia extract is helpful during an asthma attack; it is a bronchial-soothing muscle relaxant and expectorant.

Caution: Lobelia is only to be taken under supervision of a health care professional as it is potentially toxic. People with high blood pressure, heart disease, liver disease, kidney disease, seizure disorders, or shortness of breath should not take lobelia. Pregnant and lactating women should avoid lobelia as well.

❑ Boswellia, an Indian herb (also known as frankincense), in studies was shown to reduce asthma symptoms and reduce the number of attacks.

❑ Mullein oil is said to be a powerful remedy for bronchial congestion. The oil stops coughs, unclogs bronchial tubes, and helps clear up asthma attacks. Users say that when they take it in tea or fruit juice, the effect is almost immediate.

❑ Pau d'arco acts as a natural antibiotic and reduces inflammation. Drink 3 cups of pau d'arco tea daily.

❑ Proponents of the East Indian mind-body-earth philosophy called Ayurveda recommend the following herbs for people with asthma: vasaka (*Adhatoda vasica*) relieves cough, bronchitis, and other asthmatic symptoms; boswellia (*Boswellia serrata*), to relieve pain and inflammation; and tylophora (*Tylophora indica*) for respiratory relief. Sabinsa Corporation is a good source of these Ayurvedic herbs.

❑ Other herbs beneficial for asthma include echinacea, licorice root, and slippery elm bark tablets. Licorice root, ginger root, and elderberry open up the respiratory tract.

Cautions. Do not take echinacea for longer than three months. It should not be used by people who are allergic to ragweed. Licorice root should not be used during pregnancy or nursing. It should not be used by persons with diabetes, glaucoma, heart disease, high blood pressure, or a history of stroke.

Recommendations

❑ Homeopathic uses of belladonna have been shown to relax the bronchioles in the lungs, which alleviates the wheezing symptoms in an asthma attack.

❑ Black cumin seed oil (*Nigella sativa*) has been a primary treatment for allergies in the Middle East. The best seeds come from Egypt. These seeds contain more than one hundred different chemicals, including essential fatty acids. The seeds can be used to make tea by simply pouring a cup of hot water over about 1 tablespoonful of the seeds and letting the mixture steep for about ten minutes, then straining. Keep the tea covered until you are ready to drink it so as not to lose the aroma. Capsules are also available that contain the cold-pressed oil.

Caution: Do not use this product if you are pregnant. Skin exposure to undiluted oil can cause irritation in sensitive individuals.

❑ Eat a diet consisting primarily of fresh fruits and vegetables, nuts, oatmeal, brown rice, and whole grains. The diet should be relatively high in protein, low in carbohydrates, and contain no sugar. (*See* HYPOGLYCEMIA in Part Two for suggestions.) A diet rich in whole grains and fish has been shown to protect against asthma in children. Consuming one component of soy—the isoflavone genistein—was associated with better lung function in patients with asthma. Soy-based foods such as soy milk and tofu would provide this nutrient, unless you suspect that it is worsening your symptoms.

❑ Include garlic and onions in your diet. These foods contain quercetin and mustard oils, which have been shown to inhibit an enzyme that aids in releasing inflammatory chemicals.

❑ Include "green drinks" in your program. Kyo-Green from Wakunaga is excellent. Take it three times a day, one-half hour before meals.

❑ Avoid gas-producing foods, such as beans, brassicas (broccoli, cauliflower, and cabbage) and large amounts of bran, or take an enzyme complex. Gas can irritate an asthmatic condition by putting pressure on the diaphragm.

❏ Do not eat ice cream or drink extremely cold liquids. Cold can shock the bronchial tubes into spasms.

❏ Use a juice fast, a fast using distilled water and lemon juice, or a combination of both for three days each month to help rid the body of toxins and mucus. Growing children should not fast. (*See* FASTING in Part Three.)

❏ Eat lightly—a large meal can cause shortness of breath by making the stomach put pressure on the diaphragm. If you are overweight, lose weight; symptoms should improve. Eating margarine, in particular, was associated with an increased risk for developing asthma as an adult. Margarine is rich in oleic acid, but it is not known why this may precipitate asthma. If you must use it, use it sparingly.

❏ Use an elimination diet to see if certain foods aggravate the asthmatic condition. Common culprits include alfalfa, corn, peanuts, soy, eggs, beets, carrots, colas, cold beverages (which may cause bronchial spasm), dairy products (including milk and ice cream), fish, red meat (especially pork), processed foods, salt, spinach, chicken and turkey, white flour, and white sugar. (*See* ALLERGIES in Part Two.) It is a common belief that milk increases mucus production in the upper and lower respiratory tract. This goes back to the twelfth century and was first proposed by Dr. Moses Maimonides. Traditional Chinese medicine also supports this notion. However, there is no evidence that milk exacerbates symptoms of asthma. And eliminating dairy products makes it hard to obtain adequate vitamin D, calcium, and magnesium without supplementation.

❏ We all need exercise to become and remain healthy. If you find exercise can induce an asthma attack, try taking 2,000 milligrams of vitamin C one hour before your workout. Recent studies showed that those who took vitamin C prior to their workouts suffered no coughing, wheezing, or shortness of breath. However, people at risk for kidney stones or hemochromatosis (an iron-absorption disorder) should not take vitamin C at this dosage level.

❏ If exercise produces an asthmatic response, check your salt intake. According to one report, people with asthma who eat high-sodium diets (4,000 milligrams daily) have more difficulty breathing while exercising and immediately afterward than those who habitually consume far less sodium (1,500 milligrams daily). Ask your doctor what sodium level is right for you.

❏ If you use aspirin or any other nonsteroidal anti-inflammatory drugs (NSAIDs), do so with caution. Painkillers such as aspirin, ibuprofen (Advil, Nuprin, and others), naproxen (Naprosyn and Aleve), and piroxicam (Feldene) account for over two-thirds of drug-related asthmatic reactions, with aspirin causing over half of these. Experts don't know why one can take these medicines and others cannot. Studies have shown that around 20 percent of adults are prone to drug-induced attacks. Chemotherapeutic agents and antibiotics also can induce asthma reactions.

❏ Keep an ongoing list of things that trigger your asthmatic responses and then avoid them as best as you can. Also, try keeping a diary of your symptoms, medications, and so on. It can be very helpful to you and your doctor in creating and maintaining your best asthma management program.

❏ Apply castor oil packs to the back and around the lung and kidney areas. To make a castor oil pack, place castor oil in a pan and heat but do not boil it. Dip a piece of cheesecloth or other white cotton material into the oil until the cloth is saturated. Apply the cloth to the affected area and cover it with a piece of plastic that is larger in size than the cotton cloth. Place a heating pad over the plastic and use it to keep the pack warm. Keep the pack in place for one-half to two hours, as needed.

❏ Practice methods to relieve stress. Stress and strong emotions like worry and fear can trigger an asthma attack. (*See* STRESS in Part Two.)

❏ Avoid furry animals, the food additives BHA and BHT, FD&C Yellow No. 5 food dye, tobacco and other types of smoke, and the amino acid tryptophan.

❏ If you suspect that dust mites are causing your asthma symptoms, try to get rid of the microscopic bugs. There are vacuum cleaners on the market that destroy these mites. An application of benzyl benzoate powder (such as X-MITE from AllerGuard) will eliminate mites for two to three months. One pound of this powder treats approximately 150 square feet of carpeting or fabric. If local pharmacies don't carry the powder, you can order it from AllerGuard Corporation. (*See* Manufacturer and Distributor Information in the Appendix.)

❏ Consider removing carpeting, at least in the bedroom, to help keep dust mites, germs, and bacteria from aggravating asthma. Covering mattresses in plastic casings and washing sheets in hot water at least once a week can be helpful, too.

Considerations

❏ Until relatively recently, even with a good nutritional plan, the only sure way to avoid an allergic attack was to avoid the irritant that caused it. Today, treatment for asthma includes the use of anti-inflammatory and bronchodilating medications. The anti-inflammatories can halt inflammation quickly, but only temporarily, and there are side effects to using these drugs over long periods. Most medications stimulate the sympathetic nervous system and can produce anxiety, nervousness, insomnia, and dry or cotton mouth. Additionally, they can cause blood pressure to rise and, over the long term, can contribute to kidney and liver damage.

❏ A treatment has been approved that differs completely from current asthma medications. Instead of treating the symptoms, the medication goes to the source of the problem—the allergic reaction itself. Omalizumab (Xolair) is a drug that is designed to bind to the circulating antibodies in the blood, which decreases the number of antibodies that are available to bind to mast cells. This ultimately inhibits the mast cell's release of the chemicals that cause the inflammatory response of asthma. Thus, the first preventive medication is available for those adults and adolescents (aged twelve and up) with moderate to severe persistent asthma, especially those whose symptoms have not been adequately controlled by the use of inhaled corticosteroids. This is not a replacement for existing corticosteroid treatment, and any such replacement must be done under a physician's control. However, it is surely a step in the right direction.

❏ Life-threatening cases of asthma diagnosed as *status asthmaticus* require immediate hospitalization, and sufferers may have to remain hospitalized for days.

❏ People with asthma may be deficient in certain nutrients, such as vitamin B_6 (pyridoxine), vitamin C, magnesium, manganese, and selenium, as well as in the enzyme glutathione peroxidase. People with asthma often have lower than normal levels of gastric hydrochloric acid, which is needed for proper digestion. Dr. Jonathan Wright, a noted nutritionist, claims excellent results using a combination of gastric acid replacement therapy (usually in the form of betaine hydrochloride) and supplementation with vitamin B_6, vitamin B_{12}, and magnesium for treatment of asthma.

❏ According to *Nutrition Health Review,* strong feelings of anger, anxiety, and depression may be an important cause of asthma attacks. Unfortunately, many of the drugs used to control and alleviate asthma cause jittery nerves, mood swings, and insomnia. Other usual triggers include stress, acid reflux, smoking, and respiratory infections.

❏ Many people with asthma are sensitive to the food additives known as sulfites. Many restaurants use sulfiting agents—including sodium bisulfite, potassium metabisulfite, potassium bisulfite, and sulfur dioxide—to prevent discoloration and bacterial growth in green salads, cut and sliced fruit, frozen shellfish, and other foods. (*See* Sulfite Allergies on page 190 for additional information.)

❏ Beta-blocking medications, used to treat high blood pressure, can constrict the bronchial muscles and cause life-threatening problems for a person with asthma.

❏ Ozone, sulfur dioxide, nitrogen dioxide, cigarette smoke, carbon monoxide, hydrocarbons, nitrogen oxide, and photochemical substances are air pollutants that can trigger asthma attacks.

❏ Inhaling a muscle-relaxing medication such as albuterol from a bronchodilator can relieve an acute asthma attack immediately by opening the bronchial tubes. Bronchodilators do not treat the underlying problem.

❏ The FDA has approved new versions of the albuterol sulfate HFA metered dose inhaler (MDI) for asthma and other obstructive lung diseases. Unlike the older version of Ventolin, the new inhaler uses an alternative propellant called hydrofluoroalkane (HFA) rather than the traditional ozone-reducing chlorofluorocarbons (CFCs) used previously. There are now four HFA-propelled inhalers (ProAir, Proventil, Ventolin, and Xopenex) approved for use in the United States. Proventil HFA was approved in 1996. Although they have all been shown to be effective, there are some differences among the products. Talk to your health care provider to find the right one for you.

❏ Researchers at Cornell University studied children aged four through sixteen years who were part of the Third National Health and Nutrition Survey. It was found that the antioxidants beta-carotene and vitamin C were associated with a very significant reduction in asthma prevalence. An increase in selenium intake also was associated with a similar decrease in asthma prevalence. In this study, it was found that vitamin E had little or no association with asthma.

❏ A corticosteroid has been approved for young children with asthma. Budesonide inhalation suspension (Pulmicort Respules), a synthetic hormone, is designed for use once or twice daily to prevent asthma attacks, but is not used to treat acute attacks. Acute attacks are still best handled by a fast-acting bronchodilator. The drug is generally well tolerated, but side effects can include respiratory infection, coughing, and congestion.

Caution: Inhaled corticosteroids can have an effect on growth in children, and the effect on eventual adult height is not known.

❏ A sustained-release form of the drug theophylline, sold under the brand name Theo-Dur Sprinkle, has been used with good results. For children, this medication can be administered by opening a capsule and sprinkling the contents on a soft food such as applesauce. Theophylline has side effects, such as producing a rapid heartbeat and/or insomnia in some users. Some doctors believe that inhaled drugs or topical treatments are safer than asthma pills because they are drawn directly into the bronchial tubes and lungs.

❏ Researchers at Harvard University and the U.S. Environmental Protection Agency (EPA) have discovered that people with asthma who drink coffee and other caffeine-containing drinks generally have one-third fewer symptoms than those who do not. This is most likely due to the action of the caffeine, which has a dilating effect on the bronchial airways.

❏ A study reported in the *Journal of Allergy and Clinical Immunology* suggested that taking salmon oil capsules before each meal and eating fish three times weekly may be beneficial for asthma.

❏ The Air Supply personal air purifier from Wein Products is a miniature unit that is worn around the neck. It sets up an invisible pure air shield against microorganisms (such as viruses, bacteria, and mold) and microparticles (including dust, pollen, and pollutants) in the air. It also eliminates vapors, smells, and harmful volatile compounds in the air.

❑ Regular exercise is beneficial, but exercise can also trigger an acute attack in some individuals. No one is sure why this is, but it has been speculated that inhaling lots of cool, dry air while working out aggravates the respiratory system. Running, for example, induces many more asthma attacks than swimming. One way to control exercise-induced asthma is to wear a mask that retains heat and moisture and limits the effects of breathing cold, dry air.

❑ Zanamivir (Relenza), an antiviral drug used for the treatment of influenza, can have a detrimental side effect on asthma sufferers. The U.S. Food and Drug Administration notes that it should be used with caution by anyone with asthma or chronic lung disease, and if a person with asthma does take this drug, he or she should have emergency bronchodilator therapy readily available. Interestingly, although the FDA granted clearance for the drug to be marketed, an FDA advisory panel voted against approval, noting that it considered the drug's overall effectiveness as negligible.

❑ A study conducted by North Dakota State University found that people with asthma and arthritis markedly improved their health simply by setting aside time to write. Of the seventy patients participating in the one-month study, 47 percent showed definite improvement, as opposed to only 24 percent who showed improvement without writing. The researchers concluded that putting your thoughts and observations on paper relieves stress and eases the mind.

❑ Children with asthma experience much more successful treatment through mind and body control training, according to numerous recent studies. Asthma specialist Richard Firshein, D.O., based in New York City, uses a technique in which children are taught not to panic when they realize an asthma attack is approaching. He calmly guides their thought processes to focus on images and smells that please them; like the warm sun, hot dogs, or a favorite pet. At the same time, he helps them bring their breathing under control. This helps them feel less helpless and afraid. Adults too can benefit from this calming technique.

❑ Goose feathers can cause and aggravate lung ailments.

❑ The NIOX Nitric Oxide Test System can measure how well anti-inflammatory drugs may be working. The test is administered by a doctor.

❑ For names and addresses of organizations that can provide further information about this disorder, *see* Health and Medical Organizations in the Appendix.

ATAXIA

See under RARE DISORDERS.

ATHEROSCLEROSIS

See ARTERIOSCLEROSIS/ATHEROSCLEROSIS.

ATHLETE'S FOOT

Athlete's foot (*tinea pedis*) is a common fungal infection that thrives in an environment of warmth and dampness. The fungi live off the dead skin cells and calluses of the feet, especially on the skin between the toes, but can get under the fingernails as well. Symptoms include inflammation, burning, itching, scaling, cracking, and blistering. Some people, such as those with compromised immune systems, seem more susceptible to developing it.

The fungus that causes athlete's foot spreads rapidly when antibiotics, drugs, or radiation destroy beneficial bacteria. It is especially prevalent and highly contagious in warm, damp places such as gyms and swimming pool locker rooms.

NUTRIENTS

SUPPLEMENT	SUGGESTED DOSAGE	COMMENTS
Essential		
Colloidal silver	Apply topically as directed on label.	A natural antibiotic and disinfectant. Destroys fungi, viruses, and bacteria. Promotes healing.
Kyo-Dophilus from Wakunaga	As directed on label.	Contains acidophilus and aged garlic extract. Beneficial in treating fungal disease.
Very Important		
Garlic (Kyolic from Wakunaga)	2 capsules 3 times daily.	Aids in destroying fungus.
Important		
Vitamin B complex	As directed on label.	Needed for healthy skin. Use a yeast-free, high-potency formula. A sublingual form is best.
Vitamin C plus bioflavonoids	3,000–10,000 mg 3 times daily, in divided doses.	Reduces stress and promotes immune function. Use a buffered form.
Zinc	50 mg daily. Do not exceed a total of 100 mg daily from all supplements.	Inhibits fungus and stimulates the immune system.
Helpful		
Aerobic 07 from Aerobic Life Industries	9 drops in a glass of water twice daily. Also apply a few drops directly on affected areas and let dry.	Supplies oxygen to the cells, killing germs and harmful bacteria.
Essential fatty acids (Ultimate Oil from Nature's Secret)	As directed on label.	Promotes healing of skin disorders.
Vitamin A plus beta-carotene	25,000 IU daily for a month, then reduce to 15,000 IU. If you are pregnant, do not exceed 10,000 IU daily.	Needed for healing of tissues and stimulation of the immune system.
Vitamin E	200 IU daily.	An antioxidant that promotes healthy skin. Use d-alpha-tocopherol form.

Herbs

❑ Drink 3 cups of pau d'arco tea daily. Pau d'arco tea also can be used topically. Prepare a strong pau d'arco tea, using 6 teabags to 2 quarts of warm water. Add 20 drops of Aerobic 07 from Aerobic Life Industries. Soak your feet in this mixture for fifteen minutes three times daily for quick relief.

❑ For a natural remedy, cut raw garlic into tiny pieces (or into slivers, wrapped in gauze) and wear them in your shoes for a few days. The garlic will be absorbed into the skin. Also dust your feet with garlic powder. There are effective non-prescription antifungal drugs available, but for those who want a natural remedy garlic works just as well.

❑ Bathe your feet daily in a half-and-half mixture of vinegar and water. Dry them thoroughly and apply pure, unprocessed oil, such as olive oil, to the infected area. Or, soak your feet in a solution of 2 teaspoons of salt in a pint of warm water for ten minutes. Repeat this treatment daily until the condition clears up.

❑ As an alternative footbath, add 20 drops of tea tree oil to a small tub of water, and use this to soak your feet for fifteen minutes three times daily. After soaking your feet, dry them thoroughly and dab a few drops of undiluted tea tree oil on the affected area. Tea tree oil is a powerful natural antifungal agent.

❑ To help ease the redness, cracking, and itching of athlete's foot, rub the oils of myrrh and lavender into your feet at bedtime. Be sure to wash your hands well afterward to avoid spreading the fungus to your fingernails.

❑ Olive leaf extract is an excellent, safe natural healer of microbial infections.

Recommendations

❑ Keep your feet dry. After bathing, dry carefully between your toes. Make sure to use each towel only once before laundering. Wear absorbent socks made of cotton.

❑ Air your shoes out and change socks daily. Wash socks, towels, and anything that comes into contact with the infected area in very hot water, with chlorine bleach added if possible.

❑ Take care to protect your feet from direct contact with floors in communal areas such as locker rooms. Wear shoes or slippers in such places. Do not share shoes, socks, towels, or anything else that comes into contact with the feet. Wear well-ventilated shoes such as sandals, leather shoes, or sneakers with holes that allow your feet to breathe. Do not wear shoes made of rubber or vinyl material. Try not to wear the same shoes every day, and be sure to change wet shoes immediately.

❑ If the condition doesn't clear up in four weeks, if there is pus in the blisters or in the cracked skin, if a fever develops, or if there is swelling in the foot or leg, see your health care provider. Severe cases may require medical attention.

Considerations

❑ Several over-the-counter antifungal drugs called azoles are considered among the best treatments for athlete's foot. These include clotrimazole (in Lotrimin AF), miconazole (Micatin, Zeabsorb-AF), and undecylenic acid (Cruex, Desenex). A newer antifungal medication called terbinafine (Lamisil) cream is also available and is completely effective.

❑ Athlete's foot can become complicated by a fungal toenail infection (*see* NAIL PROBLEMS in Part Two). Keep the toenails clean, but do not use a metal file, which can damage the nail and give the fungus a place to grow. If the toenails become thick and discolored, see a podiatrist.

❑ Those with recurrent fungal infections of the feet often have a fungal infection in the groin area. Both areas must be treated simultaneously. To prevent transmission of the foot fungus to the groin area, put clean socks on before putting on your underwear when dressing.

❑ *See also* CANDIDIASIS and FUNGAL INFECTION in Part Two.

ATTENTION DEFICIT DISORDER (ADD)/ATTENTION DEFICIT HYPERACTIVITY DISORDER (ADHD)

Attention deficit hyperactivity disorder (ADHD), or attention deficit disorder (ADD) with hyperactivity, is the newest name given to a group of disorders of certain mechanisms in the central nervous system. With the long list of names this disorder has been given over the years, it can be confusing as to exactly what the criteria are for a diagnosis of ADHD or ADD. In the fourth edition of its *Diagnostic and Statistical Manual of Mental Disorders* (DSM-IV), the American Psychiatric Association describes three different categories of ADHD—ADHD inattentive, ADHD hyperactive-impulsive, and a third category that is a combination of the two. For the sake of simplicity, we will use the term ADD when referring to the inattentive form without hyperactivity, and ADHD for the hyperactive-impulsive and combined forms.

According to the Centers for Disease Control and Prevention (CDC), about 7.8 percent of children between four and eighteen years of age were reported to have a history of ADHD and about 56 percent of those were taking medications for the disorder. Three times as many boys are diagnosed with ADHD, but the condition is increasingly being diagnosed in girls as well, according to Nora Galil, M.D., a psychiatrist in private practice in Washington, D.C.

Although primarily thought of as a childhood disorder, ADD/ADHD can be found in adults as well. Experts estimate that 4 percent of adults aged eighteen to forty years of age may be affected, but only 11 percent of them were treated. Medical experts continue to debate whether children can expect to outgrow the symptoms. Some studies have shown a significant decline in ADHD symptoms as a person ages. Others estimate that between 30 and 70 percent of children with ADHD will carry some symptoms into adulthood. According to Russell Barkley, Ph.D., a professor of psychiatry at SUNY Upstate Medical University, ADHD is a more complex disorder in adults. It manifests itself not so much as problems with the ability to pay attention or impulse control, but a problem of self-regulation. Without this self-control, an adult's ability to do tasks is impaired, because not only must the tasks be done, but they have to be scheduled, organized, and placed in proper perspective. The condition can lead to marital conflicts, substance abuse, and financial problems. Infidelity is common because ADHD adults easily become bored with things—including spouses.

The disorder causes a variety of learning and behavioral problems, often making it difficult not only for the affected individual, but for the entire family. Although the ADD/ADHD child is often labeled as having a learning disability, the child usually is of average or above-average intelligence and is also highly creative.

Factors that have been linked to the development of ADD/ADHD include anxiety, allergies, smoking during pregnancy, hyperinsulinemia, oxygen deprivation at birth, environmental stress or pollutants, artificial food additives, injury, infection, lead poisoning, and prenatal trauma. Recent research suggests that watching too much television, with its fast-paced visual images, may permanently rewire the developing brain and cause ADHD-like symptoms. This is especially true in the first two or three years of life. ADHD is also hereditary. Each sibling of a child with ADHD has about a 20 percent chance of having it too, and 15 to 20 percent of parents of affected children also have the disorder.

In recent years, more emphasis has been placed on the role of diet in ADD/ADHD. Many people with these conditions react to certain preservatives, dyes, and salicylates in foods. These items can throw off the balance in the chemistry of the brain, often producing undesirable changes in behavior. A low-protein diet may be a contributing factor. Though the topic has been hotly debated for decades, studies have definitively shown that food additives do play a major role in hyperactivity.

There is no single test to determine if a person has ADHD. A specialist makes the diagnosis by comparing a person's behavior pattern against a set of criteria established by the American Psychiatric Association. These criteria are as follows:

1. The person has either six inattention symptoms or six hyperactivity and impulsiveness symptoms.

   Symptoms of inattention include:

- Does not pay close attention to details or makes careless mistakes.
- Has trouble keeping attention on activities.
- Does not seem to listen when spoken to.
- Does not follow through on instructions and fails to finish tasks.
- Has difficulty organizing tasks and activities.
- Avoids, dislikes, or is reluctant to do tasks requiring sustained mental effort.
- Loses things necessary to do tasks or activities.
- Is easily distracted.
- Is forgetful in daily activities.

   Symptoms of hyperactivity and impulsiveness include:

- Fidgets with hands or feet or squirms in his or her seat.
- Leaves his or her seat at times when remaining seated is necessary.
- Feels restless or, as a child, inappropriately runs about or climbs excessively.
- Has difficulty taking part in leisure activities or quiet play.
- Is "on the go" or acts as if driven.
- Talks excessively.
- Blurts out answers before questions have been completed.
- Has difficulty awaiting his or her turn.
- Interrupts conversations or intrudes on others' activities.

2. Symptoms continue for at least six months and are more frequent and severe than normal.

3. Symptoms cause significant damage to social, academic, or work function.

4. Some damage to function occurs in at least two settings, such as home, work, or school.

5. Some damaging symptoms occur before age seven.

6. The symptoms are not due to another disorder.

The ADD child may be harder to diagnose than the ADHD child because the hyperactivity is more obvious than the inattentiveness. However, the procrastination, difficulty in concentrating, and inability to start or finish projects that are characteristic of the disorder can have damaging effects that can last through adulthood. ADHD produces hyperactive, restless, impatient, and impulsive behavior.

Despite this, children with ADHD can have the ability to pay attention and complete assignments, often spending hours doing things that interest them. Adults with ADHD seem to constantly be going and getting things done, but they often grow impatient easily and have a tendency to lose their tempers quickly. The combined form of ADD/ADHD can be the most debilitating. Children with this type of the disorder often have low self-esteem, are impatient, do not follow rules or act responsibly, are often clumsy, think that they are always right, do not want to accept change, and do not adapt well.

With the enormous increase in the number of recently diagnosed cases of ADD and ADHD, many researchers feel that it is being overdiagnosed. It is difficult to diagnose accurately because many of the symptoms appear in normal, healthy children at many times during childhood. In fact, more than 60 percent of parents suspect that their child has ADD or ADHD at some point during the child's upbringing.

What may merely be creativity or a high energy level can be misdiagnosed as ADD or ADHD. A diagnosis of ADD/ADHD should be made by a team of specialists who are experts in the disorder, and it is wise to get a second opinion if your child is diagnosed as having ADD or ADHD. Be careful about jumping to medications. While medications are certainly helpful, a study released in the *Journal of the American Medical Association* (*JAMA*) discussed safety concerns and the rising number of two- to four-year-old children who are now on medications.

A better approach would be to consider nutritional and dietary measures. However, if you or your child are responding to medication, then the supplements below should be used in addition. Unless otherwise specified, the dosages recommended here are for adults. For a child between the ages of twelve and seventeen, reduce the dose to three-quarters of the recommended amount. For a child between six and twelve, use one-half of the recommended dose, and for a child under the age of six, use one-quarter of the recommended amount.

NUTRIENTS

SUPPLEMENT	SUGGESTED DOSAGE	COMMENTS
Essential		
Calcium and magnesium	As directed on label, at bedtime.	Has a calming effect.
Kyolic EPA from Wakunaga	As directed on label.	Provides essential fatty acids and helps to maintain eye and brain function. Restores proper fatty acid balance.
Gamma-amino-butyric acid (GABA)	750 mg daily.	Calms the body much in the same way as some tranquilizers, without side effects or danger of addiction. (*See* AMINO ACIDS in Part One.)
Multivitamin and mineral complex	As directed on label.	All nutrients are needed for equilibrium within the body. Use a liquid form such as Nature's Plus gel-capsules for best absorption.
Pycnogenol or grape seed extract	As directed on label. As directed on label.	Powerful antioxidants offering cellular protection for the body and brain.
Quercetin	As directed on label.	Prevents allergies from aggravating symptoms.
S-Adenosylmethio-nine (SAMe)	As directed on label.	Aids in relieving stress and depression. *Caution:* Do not use if you have bipolar mood disorder or take prescription antidepressants. Do not give to a child under twelve.
Helpful		
Acetylcholine	As directed on label.	Can improve memory and ability to pay attention.
Attend from Växa International	As directed on label.	A nutritional combination designed to address the specific dietary and neurochemical deficiencies thought to occur in people with ADD/ADHD. Can be used by both children and adults.
Dimethylamino-ethanol (DMAE)	As directed on label.	Aids in concentration by improving nerve impulse transmission in the brain. May also produce antidepressant effects. *Caution:* This supplement should be used by adults only. Do not give it to a child.
L-cysteine	As directed on label, on an empty stomach. Take with water or juice. Do not take with milk. Take with 50 mg vitamin B_6 and 100 mg vitamin C for better absorption.	Take this amino acid if a hair analysis reveals high levels of metals. (*See* AMINO ACIDS in Part One.)
Pedia-Calm from Olympian Labs	As directed on label.	A combination formula for hyperactive children that includes phoshatidyl serine, phosphatidyl choline, cephalin, phosphoinositides, DMAE, and GABA. It can be taken in capsule form or sprinkled on food.
Phosphatidyl serine	As directed on label.	May aid in balancing neuro-transmitters in the brain; also may alleviate depression.
Vitamin C with bioflavonoids	Adults and children over twelve: 1,000 mg 3 times daily. Children under twelve: 500 mg 3 times daily.	An anti-stress vitamin.
Zinc	As directed on label.	Many ADHD children are zinc-deficient. Zinc is important for metabolism of relevant neurotransmitters, fatty acids, and melatonin, and indirectly affects dopamine metabolism, which is thought to be involved with ADHD. Take in addition to the multivitamin and mineral complex. Do not exceed a total of 100 mg daily (or, for children, the appropriate fraction of 100 mg) daily from all supplements.

Herbs

If you are giving herbs to a child, be sure to adjust the dosage for age as recommended by the manufacturer.

❏ Bacopin from Sabinsa Corporation, an extract of the Ayurvedic herb bacopa (*Bacopa monniera*), is a good memory enhancer.

❏ Ginkgo biloba is helpful for brain function and concentration.

Caution: Do not take ginkgo biloba if you have a bleeding disorder, or are scheduled for surgery or a dental procedure.

❏ Ginseng or mullein oil may be helpful for memory.

Caution: Do not use ginseng if you have high blood pressure, or are pregnant or nursing.

❑ Valerian root extract has been used for this disorder with dramatic results and no side effects. Mix the alcohol-free extract in juice (as directed on the product label according to age) and drink the mixture two to three times a day.

❑ Other herbs that may be beneficial for hyperactivity include catnip, chamomile, gotu kola, hops, kava kava, lemon balm, licorice, lobelia, oats, passionflower, skullcap, St. John's wort, thyme, and wood betony.

Cautions: Do not use chamomile if you are allergic to ragweed. Do not use during pregnancy or nursing. It may interact with warfarin or cyclosporine, so patients using these drugs should avoid it. Kava kava can cause drowsiness. It is not recommended for pregnant women or nursing mothers, and it should not be taken together with other substances that act on the central nervous system, such as alcohol, barbiturates, antidepressants, and antipsychotic drugs. Licorice root should not be used during pregnancy or nursing. It should not be used by persons with diabetes, glaucoma, heart disease, high blood pressure, or a history of stroke. Lobelia is only to be taken under supervision of a health care professional as it is potentially toxic. People with high blood pressure, heart disease, liver disease, kidney disease, seizure disorders, or shortness of breath should not take lobelia. Pregnant and lactating women should avoid lobelia as well. St. John's wort may cause increased sensitivity to sunlight. It may also produce anxiety, gastrointestinal symptoms, and headaches. It can interact with some drugs including antidepressants, birth control pills, and anticoagulants.

Recommendations

❑ Include in the diet all fruits and vegetables (except for those containing salicylates, listed on this page), plus breads, cereals, and crackers that contain only rice and oats.

❑ Include cold-water fish such as tuna (limit to one serving per week), salmon, and herring in your diet. These are all good sources of omega-3 fatty acids and docosahexaenoic acid (DHA), which is an essential fatty acid that is thought to be vital for brain development and is often deficient in those with ADD/ADHD. Another omega-3, eicosapentaenoic acid (EPA), is also effective. In one study, children who took a very large dose of EPA plus DHA (up to 16 grams a day) showed improved behavior and less hyperactivity and inattention. Another fat, evening primrose oil, may also improve behavior in children.

❑ Follow a high-protein diet, similar to the one prescribed for hypoglycemia. (*See* HYPOGLYCEMIA in Part Two.) Proteins are needed to supply the body with amino acids. Some researchers are studying the similarities between hypoglycemia and ADD/ADHD. It is possible that a large number of ADD/ADHD diagnoses are in actuality hypoglycemia in disguise. The symptoms are so similar it is difficult to separate them. A low-carbohydrate, high-protein diet, particularly at breakfast, should assist in reducing symptoms if it is truly hypoglycemia.

❑ Be sure that your child is getting his or her carbohydrates from foods that contain complex carbohydrates and cut down on simple carbohydrates. Complex carbohydrates can be found in fresh vegetables, fresh fruits, beans, and natural whole grains. They provide dietary fiber and have only a third of the calories found in fats and simple carbohydrates. Simple carbohydrates, such as glucose, fructose, and galactose, are found in all forms of sugars, some juices, and in processed and refined grains (not whole grains).

❑ Limit dairy products if you notice behavioral changes after they are consumed. Dairy foods have been known to cause behavioral problems in some ADHD/ADD sufferers. Make sure that growing children get calcium, magnesium, and vitamin D from other sources like soymilk or supplements.

❑ Remove from the diet all forms of refined sugar (simple carbohydrates) and any products that contain it. Also eliminate junk food and all foods that contain artificial colors, flavorings, monosodium glutamate (MSG), yeast, or preservatives; processed and manufactured foods; and foods that contain salicylates. Certain foods naturally contain salicylates. These include almonds, apples, apricots, all berries, cherries, cucumbers, currants, oranges, peaches, peppers, plums, prunes, and tomatoes. A group of investigators published results in a major medical journal showing that neither sugar nor aspartame (an artificial sweetener) has any effect on behavior in children with ADHD. However, others have found that food additives like artificial colors and the preservative sodium benzoate increase hyperactivity in children without ADHD. The implication is that food additives might also affect children with ADHD.

❑ Do not consume any of the following: apple cider vinegar, bacon, butter, candy, catsup, chocolate, colored cheeses, chili sauce, corn, ham, hot dogs, luncheon meat, margarine, meat loaf, milk, mustard, pork, salami, salt, sausage, soy sauce, tea, and wheat.

❑ Do not use antacid tablets, cough drops, perfume, throat lozenges, or commercial toothpaste. Use a natural toothpaste from a health food store.

❑ Avoid carbonated beverages, which contain large amounts of phosphates. Phosphate additives may be responsible for hyperkinesis (exaggerated muscle activity).

❑ High levels of phosphorus and very low calcium and magnesium levels (which can be revealed through a hair analysis) can indicate a potential for hyperactivity and seizures.

❑ Meat and fat also are high in phosphorus.

❑ Limit exposure to television, video and electronic games, and loud music. Instead, encourage outdoor physical activity or activities to expand creativity.

❏ Consider trying cognitive-behavioral therapy. This can often alleviate or eliminate many of the behavior problems caused by ADHD/ADD.

❏ Use an elimination diet to identify foods that may be causing or aggravating symptoms. (*See* ALLERGIES in Part Two.)

Considerations

❏ When you are dealing with this disorder, it is best to think of the diet as feeding the brain rather than the stomach. Many researchers believe that if the contributors are removed from the diets of the patients and the right nutritional supplements are added, numerous symptoms often disappear, and medications used to treat ADD/ADHD (some of which can cause serious side effects) can often be eliminated.

❏ Not every dietary supplement has been tested in children with ADHD. However, acetyl L-carnitine is one that has been tested and was shown to be of no benefit.

❏ A hair analysis to rule out heavy metal intoxication is important. Lead and copper have both been linked to behavioral problems. (*See* HAIR ANALYSIS in Part Three.)

❏ Family- or allergy-related problems can elicit ADD/ADHD-related behaviors. It is important to explore this possibility with your specialist.

❏ A strong link has been established between learning disabilities and juvenile crime.

❏ The prescription medication methylphenidate (Ritalin) has become the most commonly prescribed medication to ease hyperactivity. Researchers are discovering, however, that this medication has many potentially serious, long-term side effects including decreased appetite, weight loss, insomnia, slowed growth, increased heart rate, increased blood pressure, a period of increased irritability and intolerance at the onset of use, and the possibility of developing Parkinson's disease. Adverse reports have been released in recent years warning parents of the possible side effects of Ritalin—with some reports even comparing it to cocaine.

❏ Other prescription medications often prescribed include dextroamphetamine (Dexedrine, a stimulant that produces calming effects equivalent to Ritalin), pemoline (Cylert, a stimulant that has been restricted by the FDA to use as a secondary medication because it can cause liver failure), methamphetamine (Desoxyn), an amphetamine and dextroamphetamine combination (Adderall), and tricyclic antidepressants (if depression is suspected). Various side effects, some of them serious, have been reported with all of these medications. Some of these drugs are available in time-released versions to reduce side effects and increase efficacy.

❏ Due to the many potentially harmful side effects of the medications available for ADD/ADHD sufferers, a growing number of parents and health professionals are turning to all or a combination of the following as a way to reduce, and even possibly eliminate, the symptoms of ADD/ADHD: alteration of diet, vitamin and mineral supplementation, herbal remedies, counseling, and the love and support of family, teachers, and friends. Many believe that medicating the problem is merely masking the symptoms without getting to the root of the problem.

❏ Homeopathic remedies, taken in small doses, may be helpful in relieving certain symptoms of ADD/ADHD. *Gelsemium* can help to relieve anticipatory anxiety, and *Ignatia* can help to alleviate anger or temper tantrums.

❏ Researchers who performed five-hour oral glucose tolerance tests on 261 hyperactive children found that 74 percent displayed abnormal glucose tolerance curves, suggesting a connection between hyperactive behavior and the consumption of sugar.

❏ Some studies have found that many children with ADD/ADHD have high levels of toxic by-products of yeast and other harmful bacteria in their urine. The use of probiotics (supplements that add beneficial bacteria to the body, such as acidophilus) can help to alleviate this problem.

❏ Studies indicate that administration of gamma-amino butyric acid (GABA) decreases hyperactivity, as well as tendencies toward violence, epilepsy, mental retardation, and learning disabilities.

❏ More and more evidence is showing that those with ADD/ADHD are at greater risk for depression, alcoholism, restlessness, difficulties with careers and relationships, and antisocial behavior as adults.

❏ Parents of children with ADD or ADHD often have a very difficult time dealing with the behavioral problems of their children. These parents deserve a lot of credit. It is important to remember, though, that the children deserve a lot of credit, too. When things seem as though they are getting out of control, it can be helpful to remember that a child with ADD or ADHD is dealing with a physiological disability. Although they desire to please and want to be good, their minds can go in and out of overload without their control. Because of this, they often feel confused and ashamed, and they can eventually develop low self-esteem. When problems arise, it is important to explain to them what they did wrong, and why it was wrong, in a calm, one-on-one fashion whenever possible. These children need a great deal of love, support, and encouragement from everyone around them—but most of all, from their parents.

❏ Ask your health care provider to help you find a professional who specializes in treating people with attention deficit disorders, or seek a referral through one of the resource organizations that deal with these disorders. (*See* Health and Medical Organizations in the Appendix.)

AUTISM OR AUTISM SPECTRUM DISORDER

Autism is not a disease. It is a little-understood developmental brain disorder. Autism (sometimes called "classical autism") is the most common condition in a group of developmental disorders known as the autism spectrum disorders (ASDs). Autism is characterized by impaired social interaction, problems with verbal and nonverbal communication, and unusual, repetitive, or severely limited activities and interests. How autistic individuals are affected by the disorder varies widely. In fact, the variety of autistic-like disorders has necessitated the creation of the term Autism Spectrum Disorder, or ASD, to be used instead of the older term "autism," which really describes only the most severe form of the disorder. Other ASDs include Asperger's syndrome, Rett syndrome, childhood disintegrative disorder, and pervasive developmental disorder not otherwise specified (usually referred to as PDD-NOS). People with severe cases display self-injurious, aggressive, and unusual behaviors. The mildest forms may appear, at least to the layperson, to be a personality disorder, possibly associated with a learning disability. While experts estimate that only three to six children out of every thousand will have autism, ASD affects approximately 1 out of every 150 children in the United States, according to the Centers for Disease Control. Researchers estimate that as many as 560,000 individuals in the United States between the ages of zero and twenty-one have an ASD.

In spite of more than fifty years of research into the varying manifestations of autism and ASD and the families affected by it, the disorder continues to mystify doctors, psychologists, and scientists. It is clear that more children than ever before are being classified as having autism spectrum disorders (ASDs). But it is unclear how much of this increase is due to changes in how we identify and classify ASDs in people, and how much is due to a true increase in prevalence. By current standards, ASDs are the second most common serious developmental disability after mental retardation/intellectual impairment, but they are still less common than other conditions that affect children's development, such as speech and language impairments, learning disabilities, and attention deficit/hyperactivity disorder (ADHD).

Males are three times more likely to have the disorder than females. Recent studies suggest that some people have a genetic predisposition to ASD. It is estimated that families with one child with ASD have a 2 to 8 percent chance of having a second child with ASD.

Someone with ASD might at first appear to be mentally retarded or hard of hearing. But caregivers stress that it is important to distinguish ASD from other conditions. Physically, individuals with ASD do not appear different from others but exhibit marked differences in behavior from a very early age. ASD is usually diagnosed in early childhood (before the age of three) and is characterized by a marked unresponsiveness to other people and to the surrounding environment. While most babies love to be held and cuddled, infants with ASD may appear indifferent to love and affection, or may be overly agitated, crying most of the time they are awake. Children with ASD may not be able to form attachments to others in the way most children do and seem to withdraw into themselves. Many exhibit various unpredictable and unusual behaviors that can range from constant rocking, feet-pounding, or sitting for long periods of time in total silence. Some experience bursts of hyperactivity that include biting and pounding on their bodies.

According to the National Institute of Neurological Disorders and Stroke, the criteria used to diagnose ASD include the following:

- Absence or impairment of imaginative and social play.

- Impaired ability to make friends with peers.

- Impaired ability to initiate or sustain a conversation.

- Stereotyped, repetitive, or unusual use of language.

- Restricted patterns of interests that are abnormal in intensity or focus.

- Apparent inflexibility with regard to changes in routine or rituals.

- Preoccupation with parts of objects.

Many children with ASD have learning disabilities and are often mentally disabled. Speech development is usually delayed and in many cases is absent or limited to nonsensical rhyming or babbling. Some children with ASD appear to have lower than normal intelligence, others seem to fall into the normal range, while some are highly intelligent. Unlike those with other ASDs, children with Asperger's syndrome typically do not have problems with language or intellectual disability. To be accurately diagnosed with ASD, a child must be observed by a skilled professional, because diagnosis is difficult for a practitioner with limited training or exposure to ASD. Specialists suggest a multidisciplinary team that would include, for example, a neurologist, a psychologist, a developmental pediatrician, a speech/language therapist, and a learning consultant.

Individuals diagnosed as autistic savants attract a great deal of attention from the media and general public. Many movies, television reports, and newspaper articles highlight the extraordinary skills of these individuals, most particularly in the areas of mathematics, art, music, and memory. Such an individual might, for example, be able to multiply and divide large numbers or calculate square roots with little hesitation, paint like Rembrandt without ever having a drawing lesson, memorize an entire phone book, or be capable of reciting the birth date of every person he or she has ever met. Less than 1 percent of the general population is capable of such feats, but the incidence of such abilities is 10 percent in individuals who are autistic. No one knows why this occurs. One speculation is that autistic people have incredible concentration abilities and can focus complete attention on a specific area of interest.

The cause of ASD is unknown. Some experts believe that it is a result of a neurological imbalance or malfunction that renders the autistic individual painfully oversensitive to external stimuli. Many researchers believe that ASD may be the result of genetics and/or some environmental factors, such as certain viruses or chemicals. Researchers are also studying how brain function differs in autistic individuals.

Some theories suggest that brain development may have been interrupted in the early fetal stages in people who develop ASD. Other studies reveal a possible signaling problem within the brain. It is known that ASD is not caused by parental neglect or actions as was once believed.

At one time there was some concern that there was a link between the MMR (measles-mumps-rubella) vaccine or the vaccine preservative thimerosal (ethyl mercury) and the onset of ASD. A report released in May 2004 by the Institute of Medicine (IOM) Immunization Safety Review Committee has concluded that there is no such link. A group in Denmark found the same thing. It must be noted that the National Autism Association disagrees to this day and believes there is some type of link. Whatever the truth might be, since 1999 drug companies have either removed or reduced significantly the amount of thimerosal in their vaccines, just as a precautionary measure. Whether to vaccinate your child is a very personal decision. You need to weigh the unknown risks against the risks of contracting any of the communicable diseases covered by the vaccines. In addition, most public schools will not allow children who have not been immunized to attend school. In some communities, you can petition to allow your child to enter school without immunizations.

Research continues to try to find the biological basis for ASD. The emergence of brain-imaging tools such as computerized tomography (CAT), positron emission tomography (PET), single photon emission computed tomography (SPECT), and magnetic resonance imaging (MRI) has allowed researchers to examine, in detail, portions of the brain never before seen in living people. In fact, instead of being able to single out one area of the brain that is affected, it looks as if many major brain structures are implicated in ASD. These include the cerebellum, the cerebral cortex, the limbic system, the corpus callosum, the basal ganglia, and the brain stem. Other research has focused on neurotransmitters such as serotonin, dopamine, and epinephrine. Evidence now points to genetic factors as the cause of ASD, a theory that has been strengthened by twin and family studies, which suggest an underlying genetic vulnerability. Recent neuroimaging studies have shown that abnormal brain development, beginning in an infant's first months, appears to be a contributing cause. This has resulted in a "growth dysregulation hypothesis" that holds genetic defects in brain-growth factors to be responsible.

Unless otherwise specified, the following recommended dosages are for persons over the age of eighteen. For a child between twelve and seventeen years old, reduce the dose to three-quarters of the recommended amount. For a child between six and twelve, use one-half the recommended dose, and for a child under six years old, use one-quarter of the recommended amount.

NUTRIENTS

SUPPLEMENT	SUGGESTED DOSAGE	COMMENTS
Very Important		
Calcium and magnesium	1,500 mg daily. 1,000 mg daily.	Essential for normal brain and nervous system function.
Choline	500–2,000 mg daily.	Improves brain function and circulation to the brain. Use under professional supervision.
Coenzyme Q₁₀	As directed on label.	Improves brain function.
Dimethylglycine (DMG) (Aangamik DMG from FoodScience of Vermont)	100 mg daily.	An oxygen carrier to the brain. Important for normal brain and nervous system function.
Iron	Only with a physician's recommendation.	In one study, 77% of children with autism were iron deficient. Sleep improved with iron supplementation.
Kyolic Neuro Logic from Wakunaga	As directed on label.	Contains elements essential for quick assimilation of brain nutrients. Enhances neuron function.
S-Adenosylmethionine (SAMe) (SAMe Rx-Mood from Nature's Plus)	As directed on label.	Critical in the manufacture of many body components, especially brain chemicals. A natural antidepressant. *Caution:* Do not use if you have bipolar mood disorder or take prescription antidepressants. Do not give to a child under twelve.
Vitamin B complex	50 mg of each major B vitamin 3 times daily, with meals (amounts of individual vitamins in a complex will vary).	Essential for normal brain and nervous system function. A sublingual form is recommended.
plus extra vitamin B₃ (niacin)	50 mg 3 times daily. Do not exceed this amount.	Improves circulation. Helpful for many psychological disorders. *Caution:* Do not take niacin if you have a liver disorder, gout, or high blood pressure.
and niacinamide	300 mg daily.	Aids circulation. *Caution:* Do not substitute niacin for niacinamide. Niacin can be toxic in such high doses.
and pantothenic acid (vitamin B₅)	500 mg daily.	Helps reduce stress.
and vitamin B₆ (pyridoxine)	50 mg 3 times daily. Do not exceed this amount except at the direction of a physician.	Deficiencies have been linked to autism.
Vitamin C with bioflavonoids	5,000–20,000 mg daily, in divided doses. (*See* ASCORBIC ACID FLUSH in Part Three.)	A powerful free radical scavenger.
Helpful		
L-glutamine and	500 mg each daily, on an empty stomach. Take	Amino acids needed for normal brain function. (*See* AMINO

L-phenylalanine and L-tyrosine and taurine	with water or juice. Do not take with milk. Take with 50 mg vitamin B$_6$ and 100 mg vitamin C for better absorption.	ACIDS in Part One.) *Caution:* Do not take phenylalanine if you are pregnant or nursing, or suffer from panic attacks, diabetes, high blood pressure, or PKU.
Melatonin	2–3 mg daily for adults, 1 mg or less daily for children, taken 2 hours or less before bedtime. If this is not effective, gradually increase the dosage until an effective level is reached.	Helpful if symptoms include insomnia.
Methylsulfonyl-methane (MSM)	As directed on label.	Increases alertness, mental calmness, the ability to concentrate, and energy.
Multivitamin and mineral complex with	As directed on label.	All nutrients are needed in balance. Use a high-potency formula.
vitamin A and	15,000 IU daily. If you are pregnant, do not exceed 10,000 IU daily.	
natural beta-carotene and	25,000 IU daily.	
selenium and	200 mcg daily.	
zinc	50 mg daily. Do not exceed a total of 100 mg daily from all supplements.	
RNA and	200 mg daily.	To aid in repairing and building of new brain tissues.
DNA	100 mg daily.	*Caution:* Do not take this supplement if you have gout.
Vitamin D	400 IU daily.	Protects against muscle weakness and is involved in regulation of heartbeat.

Herbs

❑ Ginkgo biloba is a powerful free radical destroyer that protects the brain. It also improves brain function by increasing circulation to the brain. Take it in capsule or extract form as directed on the product label, three times daily.

Caution: Do not take ginkgo biloba if you have a bleeding disorder, or are scheduled for surgery or a dental procedure.

Recommendations

❑ Eat a high-fiber diet consisting of 50 to 75 percent raw foods, including large amounts of fruits and vegetables plus brown rice, lentils, and potatoes. For protein, eat beans and legumes, fish, raw nuts and seeds, skinless white turkey or white chicken breast, tofu, and low-fat yogurt.

❑ Eliminate alcohol, caffeine, canned and packaged foods, carbonated beverages, chocolate, all junk foods, refined and processed foods, salt, sugar, sweets, saturated fats, soft drinks, and white flour from the diet. Avoid foods that contain artificial colors or preservatives. Avoid fried and fatty foods such as bacon, cold cuts, gravies, ham, luncheon meats, sausage, and all dairy products except for low-fat soured products.

❑ Omit wheat and wheat products from the diet.

❑ Drink steam-distilled water.

❑ Get regular moderate exercise.

❑ Use an elimination diet to test for food allergies, which can aggravate the condition. (*See* ALLERGIES in Part Two.)

❑ Have a hair analysis test to rule out heavy metal poisoning. (*See* HAIR ANALYSIS in Part Three.)

❑ Try to improve blood oxygen supply to the brain with deep breathing exercises. Hold your breath for thirty seconds each half hour for a thirty-day period. This promotes deeper breathing and helps to increase oxygen levels in the tissues of the brain.

❑ Do not go without food. Eating frequent small meals daily is better than eating two or three large meals.

Considerations

❑ In the medical sense, there is no cure for the differences in the brain that result in ASD. However, researchers are finding better ways to understand the disorder and help people cope with the various symptoms. Some symptoms can lessen as the child ages and others disappear altogether. With appropriate intervention, many behaviors can be changed for the better, even to the point that the affected individual may, to the untrained eye, seem perfectly normal. The majority of people with ASD continue to display some symptoms throughout their lives.

❑ The onset of puberty can be a difficult time for autistic children. Many experience more frequent and severe behavioral problems, and about 25 percent of those afflicted begin to experience seizures during puberty. This is believed to be the result of hormonal changes.

❑ During adulthood, appropriate living arrangements for people with ASD vary depending on the severity of each individual case. While those who are only mildly affected may be able to live on their own, other options can include living in a group home or residential home, or living with parents. For those who are severely affected, an institutional setting may be the only choice. While some autistic adults are unable to adapt to a regular lifestyle, others graduate from college, have careers, form relationships, and marry.

❑ Allergies and food sensitivities are beginning to receive more attention than ever before, because research and case studies are beginning to suggest that they contribute to certain behaviors.

❑ Researchers have also detected the presence of abnormal protein levels in the urine of autistic individuals. It is thought this protein may be due to the body's inability to break down certain dietary proteins into amino acids. These proteins are gluten (found in wheat, barley, oats, and other foods) and casein (found in human and cow's milk). However, some argue that not all cow's milk is potentially harmful. In New Zealand, milk from a certain breed of cows with a genetic makeup called A2 seems to not exacerbate symptoms of autism. Many parents of autistic children have removed these foods from their children's diets and have, in many cases, observed positive changes in health and behavior. Research strongly suggests that many autistic people are sensitive to dairy products and certain foods eaten most often in the spring and summer. These foods include strawberries and citrus fruits, which can affect an autistic individual's sensitive immune system. Doctors have noted that a variety of problems—including headaches, nausea, bed-wetting, appearing "spaced out," stuttering, excessive whining and crying, aggression, and depression—can be magnified by these food products. Such a reaction can be almost immediate or appear up to thirty-six hours after the suspect food is eaten. Besides eliminating problem foods, increasing the amount of vitamins such as vitamin C may reduce allergy and sensitivity symptoms. (*See* ALLERGIES in Part Two.)

❑ Some children have benefited from a ketogenic diet. This is a diet that is very high in fat and nearly devoid of carbohydrate. Given that it is a tricky diet to follow, it must be done under a doctor's supervision. In one study, after six months children between the ages of four and ten improved in the standard rating tool used, called the Childhood Autism Rating Scale.

❑ Children may benefit from taking vitamin B$_6$ and magnesium, as well as other nutrients vital to biochemical reactions in the body. One theory is that these children may have leaky gut syndrome and are unable to absorb nutrients from their diets efficiently. In studies of autistic children, a significant number have been found to have gastrointestinal disorders, including celiac disease and other food intolerances. Allergy induced Autism (AiA), a British support group and charity for autism, notes that some children with autism in England are taking enzymes to help them digest food more easily. Gastrointestinal disturbances are common in autism, especially abnormal stool consistency. A group at the University of Pennsylvania found the incidence to be 54 percent in a group of children aged three to eight years. These children consumed adequate calories and carbohydrate and about twice the RDI for protein.

❑ Elevated serum and tissue copper levels may be a factor in autism and other mental problems, as may excessive exposure to lead and mercury. Even low-level lead exposure in young children has been associated with impaired intellectual development and behavior problems.

❑ Children aged five to seventeen years with autism benefited from 1.5 grams a day of the omega-3 fatty acids EPA and DHA, in an equal ratio. After six weeks, behavior improved for self-injuries, aggression, and tantrums.

❑ Infants and toddlers whose diets consist largely of processed baby foods need supplemental vitamins and minerals to ensure that all of their nutritional needs are met. Nutritional deficiencies are a factor in many psychological disorders.

❑ The prognosis for autistic children is difficult to predict. There have been documented cases of apparent recovery from autism, usually after adolescence. Some children seem to progress well only to inexplicably regress. Many become marginally self-sufficient and independent. However, most autistic individuals ultimately need lifelong care of some type.

❑ *See also* HYPOGLYCEMIA and HYPERACTIVITY in Part Two.

❑ For further information about autism, *see* Health and Medical Organizations in the Appendix.

BACKACHE

Nearly 80 percent of adults in the United States are affected by back pain at some point in their lives, most often in the lower back. It can be either acute or chronic. Acute pain starts suddenly and is usually the result of misusing the body in some way.

Chronic backache keeps recurring and can be brought on by almost any movement, for no particular reason. It is one of the most common reasons for hospitalization. A variety of problems in the muscles, tendons, bones, ligaments, or an underlying organ, such as the kidneys, may also cause backaches. Attempting to move or lift heavy objects is said to be the primary cause of back problems in the United States, sometimes because of damage done to a spinal disk.

For many years, it was assumed that most back pain was the result of spinal degeneration or injury, especially damage to the intervertebral disks. These structures are located between the vertebrae and act as cushions. Each disk consists of a tough, fibrous outer layer surrounding the soft interior, which provides the cushioning. With the ordinary wear and tear of living, the disks show signs of aging, and may be injured. When a disk begins to degenerate, a strain—even something as small as a sneeze—can cause the disk to rupture, or herniate, allowing the soft interior material to protrude out of the disk and press against the spinal cord. This situation is sometimes erroneously referred to as a slipped disk.

Herniated disk, prolapsed disk, and slipped disk are all names for the same problem, and are usually found in the lumbar region of the back (the lower back). A herniated disk can result in severe intermittent or constant back pain, particularly if it presses on the sciatic nerves and causes a condition known as sciatica. The sciatic nerves are responsible for transmitting all signals from the lower body. They are the longest nerves in the body, and any pressure on them, typically by a disk protruding from the vertebrae, results in a shooting pain, usually in the leg and foot. Some people experience a debilitating numbness that renders them almost incapable of walking; others experience only a tingling sensation in the toes or numbness in the foot or leg. Infrequently, if the lower part of the spinal cord is inflamed, people may experience loss of bladder or bowel control.

It is difficult to pinpoint disk disease as the cause of most cases of back pain. That is because many adults past the age of forty—whether they experience back pain or not—can be shown to have some degree of disk degeneration. Further, in many instances, disk degeneration and even herniation do not produce any symptoms.

Simple muscle strain is another leading cause of back pain. Although symptoms may come on suddenly and can be acutely painful, this is actually a problem that develops over a long period of time. When muscles contract, lactic and pyruvic acids are produced as by-products of muscular activity. It is the presence of lactic acid in the muscles that produces the familiar sensation of muscle fatigue following strenuous activity. If high levels of these acidic by-products accumulate in the muscles, they cause irritation that can eventually turn into pain and interfere with the normal conduction of electrical impulses in the muscle tissue. This results in a phenomenon called delayed-onset muscle soreness (DOMS).

Fibrositis, a rather ill-defined soreness of the neck, trunk, and shoulders caused by inflammation of connective tissue, may also account for a number of backaches. This usually happens in older people, and is thought more likely to occur because of stress, tension, allergies, or fibromyalgia rather than from any particular injury.

Lumbago is a traditional term for muscle pain in the lower back, near the pelvis.

Backaches during pregnancy are commonplace. The abdominal muscles stretch because the uterus is getting bigger and the back muscles are becoming shorter and tighter. Coupled with this, your spine has to support additional weight, so your posture may change and backaches can result.

Most cases of back pain also have an important psychological component, usually a deep-seated emotional or stress-related problem. Other contributors can include poor posture, improper footwear and walking habits, improper lifting, straining, calcium deficiency, slouching when sitting, and sleeping on a mattress that is too soft. Kidney, bladder, and prostate problems, female pelvic disorders, and even constipation may produce back pain. Chronic conditions that can cause back pain include arthritis, rheumatism, bone disease, and abnormal curvature of the spine. Fractures are rarely the cause of back pain. The two biggest factors are likely being overweight and living a sedentary lifestyle.

Because the great majority of back pain cannot be explained—and is not due to protruding disks, arthritis, osteoporosis, poor posture, or any other discernible illness—it is always advisable to take back problems seriously and have them checked out.

NUTRIENTS

SUPPLEMENT	SUGGESTED DOSAGE	COMMENTS
Very Important		
Calcium

and | 1,500–2,000 mg daily. | Needed for strong bones. To assure absorption, use a mixture of 3 different forms: calcium carbonate, calcium chelate, and calcium asporotate. |
| magnesium

and

vitamin D | 700–1,000 mg daily.

400 IU daily. | Works with calcium. Use magnesium chelate form. Aids absorption of calcium and magnesium. |
| DL-Phenylalanine (DLPA) | Take daily every other week, as directed on label. | This natural amino acid helps to alleviate pain. *Caution:* Do not take this supplement if you are pregnant or nursing, or suffer from panic attacks, diabetes, high blood pressure, or PKU. |
| Multivitamin and mineral complex with vitamin A

and

natural beta-carotene | 15,000 IU daily. If you are pregnant, do not exceed 10,000 IU daily.

15,000 IU daily. | To supply a balance of nutrients important in formation and metabolism of bone and connective tissue, and needed for healing. |
| Silica | As directed on label, 3 times daily. | Supplies silicon, which improves calcium uptake. |
| Vitamin B$_{12}$

or

vitamin B$_{12}$ injections | 2,000 mcg daily.

As prescribed by physician. | Aids in calcium absorption and digestion. Use a lozenge or sublingual form. Requires visit to doctor. |
| Zinc

plus

copper | 50 mg daily. Do not exceed a total of 100 mg daily from all supplements.

3 mg daily. | Required for protein synthesis and collagen formation. Promotes a healthy immune system. Works in balance with zinc and vitamin C to form elastin, and is needed for healthy nerves. |
| *Important* | | |
| Boron | 3 mg daily. Do not exceed this amount. | Improves calcium uptake. Take boron only until healed, unless you are over age fifty. |
| Chondroitin sulfate (CS)

and

bovine cartilage

or

shark cartilage

and

glucosamine sulfate | As directed on label.

As directed on label.

As directed on label.

As directed on label. | Studies have shown these are important components of many body tissues, including bones and connective tissue. |
Free form amino acid	As directed on label.	Essential in bone and tissue repair.
L-proline	500 mg daily, on an empty stomach. Take with water or juice. Do not take with milk. Take with 50 mg vitamin B$_6$ and 100 mg vitamin C for better absorption.	Heals cartilage and strengthens muscles and tissues. (*See* AMINO ACIDS in Part One.)
Manganese	2–5 mg daily. Take separately from calcium.	Aids in healing cartilage and tissue in the neck and back. Use manganese gluconate form.
Methylsulfonyl-methane (MSM)	As directed on label.	Aids with inflammation.

S-Adenosylmethio-nine (SAMe)	As directed on label.	Methionine derivative. Eases arthritic pain. *Caution:* Do not use if you have bipolar mood disorder or take prescription antidepressants.
Helpful		
Essential fatty acids from fish oils	As directed on label. Take with meals.	Needed for repair and flexibility of muscles.
Glucosalage S04 (Extra Strength) from Olympian Labs	As directed on label.	To supply glucosamine, an important component of many body tissues, including bones and connective tissue. Contains several nutrients listed in this table plus enzymes. Children under twelve, see chart p. 232
Flex Able Chewable Wafers from Amerifit	As directed on label.	A chewable glucosamine and chondroitin formula that provides joint health.
Multienzyme complex with bromelain and pancreatin	As directed on label. Take with meals.	To aid digestion and relieve muscle tension and inflammation.
Vitamin B complex	As directed on label 3 times daily.	Needed for repair and to relieve stress in the back muscles. Use a high-stress formula high in vitamin B_6 (pyridoxine) and vitamin B_{12}.
Vitamin C with bioflavonoids	3,000–10,000 mg daily.	Essential for formation of collagen, which holds the tissues together. Needed for repair of tissues. Relieves tension in the back area.

Herbs

❑ Arth-X from Trace Minerals Research is a formula containing herbs, sea minerals, calcium, and other nutrients for the bones and joints.

❑ Other herbs recommended for backache include alfalfa, burdock, oat straw, slippery elm, and white willow bark. They can be taken in capsule, extract, or tea form. White willow bark, containing salicylic acid, is particularly helpful. Also, arnica, a homeopathic remedy, may prove useful as well.

Recommendations

❑ Avoid all meats and animal protein products until you are healed. Animal protein contains uric acid, which puts undue strain on the kidneys that can contribute to back pain. Do not eat gravies, oils, fats, sugar, or rich or highly processed foods.

❑ Follow a fasting program. (*See* FASTING in Part Three.)

❑ When pain hits, immediately drink two large glasses of water. This often gives relief within minutes. Muscle ache and back pain is frequently connected to dehydration. The body needs a minimum of ten 8-ounce glasses of water daily to keep acidic wastes from building up in muscles and other tissues.

❑ If pain follows an injury or sudden movement, apply ice for the first forty-eight hours, and then apply heat. Rest on a firm bed. When getting up, roll to your side, draw your knees up, push up to a sitting position, and stand by pushing up with your legs.

❑ To relieve back muscle pain, soak in a very warm bath or apply a heating pad directly to your back. Be careful not to set the heat too high, however.

❑ *Rhus toxicodendron,* a homeopathic remedy, is helpful in relieving stiffness. Take it as directed.

❑ Once the acute pain has subsided, doing exercises to strengthen the abdominal muscles may help to prevent recurrences; these muscles help to support the back. Sit-ups are good for this purpose. Always do sit-ups with your knees bent, not with your legs flat on the floor.

❑ When sitting, try to keep your knees a little higher than your hips and keep your feet flat on the floor. Placing your feet on a pillow or other support to hold this position might be helpful.

❑ When carrying things on your shoulder, switch the weight to the other side from time to time. Carrying heavy shoulder bags may produce neck, back, and shoulder pain.

❑ Learn to recognize and reduce stress. Relaxation techniques can be very helpful.

❑ Always push large objects; never pull them.

❑ Wear comfortable, well-made shoes. The higher the heels of your shoes, the greater the risk of backache.

❑ Move around. Do not sit in the same position for long periods of time.

❑ Never lean forward without bending your knees. Lift with your legs, arms, and abdomen—not with the muscles of the small of your back. Avoid lifting anything heavier than twenty pounds. If you must work close to the ground, squat down so that you avoid bending at the waist.

❑ Do not sleep on your stomach with your head raised on a pillow. Instead, rest your back by lying on your side with your legs bent, so that your knees are about an inch higher than your hips. Sleep on a firm mattress with your head supported on a pillow. If your mattress is not firm enough, place a board between the box spring and the mattress.

❑ Maintain a healthy weight and get regular moderate exercise. A lack of exercise can cause back pain. Activities that are good for the back include swimming, cycling, walking, and rowing. Find one that you like and commit to doing it regularly. Avoid the following activities if you have back problems:

• *Baseball, basketball, football.* The quick responses needed for these sports involve sudden twisting and jumping motions.

- *Bowling.* Lifting a heavy weight while bending and twisting puts strain on the back.

- *Golf.* The twisting motion involved in the swing, and the body's tendency to bend forward at the waist, are stressful to the lower back.

- *Tennis.* Playing tennis puts strain on the back due to the quick "stop-and-go" action of the game.

- *Weightlifting.* This sport is potentially the most damaging because it places great strain on the lower portion of the spine and back.

❏ If pain lasts longer than seventy-two hours, if pain radiates into the legs, or if other symptoms such as unexplained weight loss occur, consult your health care provider. If your backaches are chronic, look for a physician who specializes in backs—and who does not rush to recommend surgery. Get a second opinion if surgery is recommended.

❏ If your back pain also involves a high temperature or weight loss, or if you have a past history of cancer, bowel or bladder control problems, any numbness in the groin or lower back, or loss of feeling in the legs or feet, see your doctor.

❏ If you have pain in one side of the small of your back, feel sick, and have a fever, see your physician immediately.

❏ If pain follows an injury and is accompanied by sudden loss of bladder or bowel control, if you have difficulty moving any limb, or if you feel numbness, pain, or tingling in a limb, call for medical help immediately. You may have damaged your spinal cord.

Considerations

❏ People seeking professional advice about back pain face a bewildering array of generalists and specialists to choose from. Complex back problems are rapidly becoming a specialty. For alternative treatment of back pain, you can try any of the following types of therapy:

- Acupuncture has the backing of the World Health Organization for the treatment of back pain. (*See* PAIN CONTROL in Part Three.) However, new data questions its efficacy. In a large study of over six hundred patients with back pain, some patients were given an actual acupuncture treatment while others received a simulated one. Patients reported the same symptom relief regardless of which procedure they received.

- Chiropractic is conducted by professionals who are licensed to perform spinal manipulation and who may recommend nutritional and/or lifestyle changes. It primarily involves the use of high-velocity manipulations of the neck and back to correct problems. According to a 1994 report issued by the U.S. Agency for Health Care Policy and Research, spinal manipulation may be the most effective treatment for acute back pain. Chiropractors are not medical doctors and therefore cannot prescribe drugs or perform surgery. A good chiropractor should be willing to recommend a medical doctor if necessary.

- Kinesiology can sometimes alleviate back problems. By testing muscle response, practitioners can pinpoint the origin of the pain and use various methods, including gentle manipulation, to treat it.

- Magnet therapy is gaining ground in some quarters. A magnetic mattress pad has been developed, and some people have found relief from chronic back pain after sleeping on it for only a short time. Experiments have shown that magnet back support has proven useful for golfers.

- Massage therapy involves different techniques like muscle kneading and compression to lessen tension in the muscles. This increases circulation and helps the body flush out cellular debris, which speeds tissue repair and aids in healing back problems. (*See* MASSAGE THERAPY *under* PAIN CONTROL in Part Three.)

- Orthopedic surgery is performed by medical doctors who prescribe medication (painkillers, muscle relaxers, anti-inflammatory drugs), bed rest, and physical therapy for some cases of back pain. Since these doctors can perform surgery, they may be more likely to recommend it than other practitioners.

- Vertebroplasty, for vertebral compression fractures, has offered relief for some people. In this outpatient procedure, a needle inserted through the skin into the affected vertebra fills the vertebra with a cement-like substance called methylmethacrylate, and when this substance hardens (in about fifteen to twenty minutes), it offers support to an otherwise weak part of the backbone.

- Osteopathy, or osteopathic medicine, is based on the belief that most diseases are related to problems of the musculoskeletal system. The musculoskeletal system is made up of the nerves, muscles, and bones—all of which are interconnected and form the body's structure. Osteopaths (D.O.s) can prescribe drugs and perform surgery in many states, but because of their philosophy of treatment, they often try manipulation or physical therapy first.

- Physiatry is nonsurgical physical medicine and rehabilitation for patients who have been disabled as a result of a disease, disorder, or injury. Physiatrists, also known as doctors of physical rehabilitation medicine, are medical doctors who treat back pain by the use of various physical therapies, lifestyle changes, and back braces, which promote healing by reducing the load on the spine. Physiatrists are not licensed to perform surgery, and are less likely than other doctors to hospitalize their patients. They have a good record for treating back problems, including low back pain and herniated disks.

- Physical therapy focuses on improving joint and spine mobility and muscle strength. Physical therapists are not medical doctors, and are strictly limited to physical therapy.

❑ There is a theory that backache may be caused by repressed rage. This may be something to consider pursuing with a psychiatrist or other mental health professional.

❑ Bed rest makes little difference with sciatica. Both the long-term and short-term consequences of sciatica remain the same whether you observe complete rest or continue your usual routine.

❑ With signs of rapidly progressive nerve damage (increasing weakness in a leg, or loss of bladder or bowel function), back surgery moves high on the list of options. It must also be considered when pain is unremitting or getting worse. Surgery always entails a degree of risk; there is always the chance of permanent damage and impaired mobility.

❑ According to U.S. government data, only 1 percent of those who suffer from back pain appear to benefit from surgery. Back surgery is useful only for problems in four broad categories:

1. Disk displacement (a protruded or "slipped" disk).

2. Painful (and abnormal) motion of one vertebra in relation to another.

3. Narrowing of the spine around the spinal cord itself from overgrowth of bone (spinal stenosis).

4. Some cases in which misalignment of one vertebra with another (spondylolisthesis) leads to pain.

❑ In the past, removing a damaged disk and fusing a section of the spine was a major surgical procedure. Up to one year was required for recovery from this surgery. A procedure called minimal access spinal technologies (MAST) allows the operation to be performed through small incisions that do not even cut through muscle tissue. Someone who absolutely requires surgery should investigate this option. Recovery time is in the days-to-weeks range rather than months-to-years.

❑ X-rays are often considered a routine part of back pain diagnosis, yet only a few back conditions show up on X-rays. If muscle strain or a herniated disk causes the pain, an X-ray will do little to aid the diagnosis, since disks, muscles, and ligaments are all soft tissues. X-ray exposure bears special hazards for pregnant women.

❑ With imaging procedures such as computerized tomography (CAT) and magnetic resonance imaging (MRI), disks can be seen. However, Dr. Richard A. Deyo, of Oregon Health and Science University, notes that 20 to 30 percent of people with back pain have herniated disks that are not the source of their discomfort. If these disks show up during imaging procedures, a person may end up having surgery for a condition that, while present, is not really the cause of his or her pain.

❑ If pain comes after lifting something heavy, after coughing, or after unusually heavy exercise, and the pain prevents you from moving or shoots down one leg, you may have a herniated disk.

❑ Epidemiological studies in the United States, as well as studies of smoking and nonsmoking pairs of twins in Scandinavia, have shown that smoking aggravates problems in the disks.

❑ *See under* PREGNANCY-RELATED PROBLEMS in Part Two.

❑ *See also* PAIN CONTROL in Part Three.

BAD BREATH

See HALITOSIS.

BALDNESS

See HAIR LOSS.

BEDSORES

Bedsores, also known as pressure sores, are deep ulcers that form when pressure is exerted over bony areas of the body for long periods of time, restricting circulation and leading to the death of cells in the underlying tissue. They are most commonly found on the heels, buttocks, hips, sacrum, and shoulder blades.

As their name implies, they tend to occur during periods of prolonged bed rest, although wheelchair users also may develop bedsores. People who suffer from bedsores are usually deficient in many nutrients, especially protein, zinc, and vitamins A, E, B_2 (riboflavin), and C, and they often have a high bodily pH. (*See* ACID/ALKALI IMBALANCE in Part Two.)

Anyone who is confined to a bed, chair, or wheelchair due to illness is at risk for developing bedsores, which can range from mild to severe. Patients who are defined as being clinically malnourished (this is a physician diagnosis that you can ask about) are at greater risk of developing bedsores. Low scores on two important blood tests—cholesterol and albumin—are often indicative of who will develop bedsores. An area of reddening skin that doesn't go away, even after pressure is relieved, is an indication of a developing bedsore, as is local swelling and/or hardening of the tissue. Severe bedsores can require surgery for removal of dead tissue.

NUTRIENTS

SUPPLEMENT	SUGGESTED DOSAGE	COMMENTS
Very Important		
Essential fatty acids (flaxseed oil, primrose oil, and salmon oil) or	As directed on label.	Needed for proper cell reproduction.
Ultra Omega-3 Fish Oil from Health From The Sun	One or two capsules with each meal daily.	Prevents moisture loss and promotes healing.

Vitamin E	200 IU daily.	Improves circulation.
Zinc	50–80 mg daily. Do not exceed a total of 100 mg daily from all supplements.	Important in healing of tissues.
plus copper	3 mg daily.	Needed to balance with zinc.
Important		
Free form amino acid	As directed on label.	To supply protein needed for healing.
Vitamin B complex	100 mg of each major B vitamin twice daily, with meals (amounts of individual vitamins in a complex will vary).	Needed to reduce stress and for healing.
plus extra vitamin B$_{12}$	2,000 mcg twice daily.	Use a lozenge or sublingual form.
Vitamin C	3,000–10,000 mg daily, in divided doses.	Aids in healing, improves circulation, and enhances immune function.
Vitamin D	400–1,000 IU daily.	Essential for healing. Lack of exposure to sunshine increases the need for this nutrient.
Helpful		
Calcium and	2,000 mg daily.	Needed for the central nervous system and to keep bones from softening through disuse.
magnesium	1,000 mg daily.	
Carotenoid complex	As directed on label.	Repairs bedsores by improving skin tissue.
Colloidal silver	Apply topically as directed on label.	A natural antibiotic. Destroys bacteria, viruses, and fungi. Protects against infection and promotes healing.
Garlic (Kyolic from Wakunaga)	2 capsules 3 times daily, with meals.	Has a natural antibiotic effect; protects against infection.
Kelp	500–1,000 mg daily.	Provides necessary minerals.
Panoderm I from American Biologics	Apply topically as directed on label.	A natural antioxidant skin moisturizer and cleanser that contains squalene, an unsaturated carbohydrate from shark liver oil.
Vitamin A	50,000 IU daily for 1 month, then reduce to 15,000 IU daily. If you are pregnant, do not exceed 10,000 IU daily.	Needed for healing of skin tissue. Use an emulsion form for easier assimilation.

Herbs

❑ Herbal ointments should be applied to closed wounds only. Open wounds should always be treated by a qualified health care practitioner or physician.

❑ Aloe vera gel, ointment, or cream can be applied topically to bedsores.

❑ Calendula cream, gel, or ointment can be applied topically to an affected area. Use as directed on the label.

❑ Comfrey ointment or Calendula Ointment, from Nature-Works, can be used externally.

Note: Comfrey is recommended for external use only.

❑ Goldenseal, myrrh gum, pau d'arco, and suma, taken in tea or extract form, are beneficial for bedsores. Buckwheat tea and lime flower tea are also helpful.

Caution: Do not take goldenseal internally on a daily basis for more than one week at a time. Do not use it during pregnancy or if you are breast-feeding, and use with caution if you are allergic to ragweed. If you have a history of cardiovascular disease, diabetes, or glaucoma, use it only under a doctor's supervision.

Mix equal amounts of goldenseal powder or extract and vitamin E oil with a small amount of honey to make a paste, and apply the mixture to the sores as necessary. This mixture gives fast relief and helps the healing process. Alternate this with raw honey, vitamin E cream, and aloe vera gel.

Recommendations

❑ Eat a simple, well-balanced diet with plenty of raw, fresh fruits and green and yellow vegetables to ensure a good supply of vitamins, minerals, and phytonutrients. Patients usually don't get enough protein so it is important to focus on increasing its intake.

❑ Essential fatty acids (EFAs) have been shown to play an integral role in the health of the skin. Taken internally or applied externally as a lotion (only to closed, well-healed wounds), they help maintain the integrity and elasticity of the skin, as well as preventing a loss of moisture, which leads to dry and scaly skin. Excellent sources of EFAs are natural vegetable oils such as canola, corn, olive, safflower, and soy oils; wheat germ; edible seeds, such as pumpkin, sesame, and sunflower; and fish oils—especially cod-liver oil.

❑ Consume liquids around the clock, even if you are not thirsty. Use steam-distilled water, herbal teas, and sugar-free juices. Liquids are important in keeping the colon clean and the bladder functioning properly.

❑ Eliminate animal fats, fried foods, junk foods, processed foods, and sugar from the diet.

❑ Use ground flaxseeds, oat bran, psyllium husks, or Aerobic Bulk Cleanse (ABC) from Aerobic Life Industries to provide fiber. Fiber absorbs dangerous toxins and helps prevent constipation.

Note: Always take supplemental fiber separately from other supplements and medications.

❑ Make sure that the bowels move every day. On days when the bowels do not move, use an enema. (*See* ENEMAS in Part Three.)

❑ Give immediate attention to lowering the body's pH level to 5.5 or lower to prevent bacteria in the sores from multiplying. Place 2 to 3 teaspoons of apple cider vinegar in a glass of water, add a little honey, and sip this with meals. (*See* ALKALOSIS *under* ACID/ALKALI IMBALANCE in Part Two for additional suggestions.)

❑ Take the following measures to prevent development of bedsores:

- Prevention of bedsores is based on limiting the time an area of the body is subjected to pressure. Do not let an immobilized individual stay in one position for long—move him or her to alternate positions every two hours.

- Keep the skin dry, including thorough drying after bathing.

- Inspect pressure points daily for reddening or other signs that a sore may be developing.

- If the person can sit up, have him or her do so three to four times daily, or use pillows as a prop.

- Give a sponge bath daily using warm water and a mild herbal or vitamin E soap. Do not use harsh soaps.

- Gently but firmly massage pressure points and other affected areas once daily to increase circulation.

- Give frequent alcohol rubs to stimulate circulation and prevent blood vessels from closing up. Use isopropyl (rubbing) alcohol on cotton balls or sterile gauze to apply. As an alternative, witch hazel can be used.

- Allow as much light and fresh air into the bedridden person's room as he or she can tolerate.

- Have the individual wear loose-fitting clothing made from all-natural materials. Cotton is best because it allows air to penetrate to the skin. Pay attention to clothing construction as well. Avoid items with seams, gathers, or other features that may press on sensitive areas.

- Keep the bed clean, dry, and tidy. Lying on wrinkled bed linens can lead to bedsores.

Considerations

❑ A good diet is very important and makes bedsores less likely to develop. Maintaining adequate protein and calories is key.

❑ People who suffer from bedsores are usually seriously deficient in many nutrients, especially zinc and vitamins A, E, B$_2$ (riboflavin), and C. A good multivitamin and mineral supplement should be taken every day. A simple diet with plenty of fresh fruits is recommended. Vitamins A and E in moderation are useful in healing bedsores. Vitamin C acts as an anti-inflammatory and is generally good for the health of the skin and blood vessels.

❑ Although most bedsores can be prevented, once formed, they can be kept in check if you regularly examine the affected areas, keep the skin clean and dry, and relieve any pressure on sensitive areas. If mobility is limited, you can use special foam, gel, or air cushions to relieve this pressure. Also, make sure that anyone with limited mobility gets turned on a regular basis.

❑ Special air mattresses are available that help to decrease the pressure on sensitive areas when a person has to lie in one position for long periods of time. Anatomically shaped cushions can be used to help distribute the weight more evenly, along with special pads designed specifically for heels and elbows.

❑ Special absorbent foamlike bandages can be used for persistent bedsores to reduce the pressure on sensitive areas and help promote healing.

❑ Dimethylsulfoxide (DMSO) is also helpful for promoting healing. It is applied topically directly to the affected area once the skin has covered over the wound.

Caution: Only pure DMSO from a health food store should be used. Commercial-grade DMSO such as that found in hardware stores is not suitable for healing purposes. Any contaminants on the skin or in the product can be taken into the tissues by action of the DMSO.

Note: The use of DMSO may result in a garlicky body odor. This is temporary, and is not a cause for concern.

BED-WETTING

Bed-wetting, known in the medical community as enuresis, is the act of urinating in bed habitually and involuntarily at night when asleep. Bed-wetting is common in early childhood. It is uncommon in early adulthood but frequent among older adults. The causes are often unknown. The most popular theories center on the roles of behavioral disturbances, very sound sleeping, the consumption of too much liquid before bedtime, dreaming about using the rest room, food allergies, heredity, stress, nutritional deficiencies, and psychological problems (one of the most common factors in young adults).

In children under the age of five or so, the most common cause of bed-wetting is simply the size of the bladder; it is often too small to hold enough urine to last through the night every single night. This type of bed-wetting is usually outgrown. Occasional bed-wetting by older children usually stops spontaneously by the teenage years. An underlying illness such as a urinary tract infection or diabetes may also result in bed-wetting. It is wise to rule out the possibility of underlying medical problems before proceeding with any other form of treatment. Some children's hospitals have special clinics just to deal with this issue.

Unless otherwise specified, the following recommended doses are for those over the age of eighteen. For a child between twelve and seventeen years old, reduce the dose to three-quarters of the recommended amount. For a child between six and twelve years old, use one-half of the recommended dose, and for a child under six, use one-quarter of the recommended amount.

NUTRIENTS

SUPPLEMENT	SUGGESTED DOSAGE	COMMENTS
Very Important		
Free form amino acid	As directed on label.	Helps to strengthen bladder muscle. Use a product made from a vegetable source.

Important		
Calcium and magnesium	1,500 mg daily. 350 mg daily.	To aid in controlling bladder spasms.
Helpful		
Multivitamin and mineral complex with vitamin B complex with iron	As directed on label. Only with a physician's recommendation	Aids in relieving stress and supplies all needed nutrients.
Potassium	99 mg daily.	Aids in balancing sodium and potassium in the body.
Vitamin A or cod liver oil and vitamin E	As directed on label. If you are pregnant, do not exceed 10,000 IU daily. As directed on label. 200 IU daily.	To aid in normalizing bladder muscle function. Use d-alpha-tocopherol form.
Zinc	10 mg daily for children; 80 mg daily for adults. Do not exceed these amounts.	For improved bladder function. Also enhances the immune system.

Herbs

❑ For bed-wetting, try using buchu, corn silk, oat straw, parsley, and/or plantain. Take these herbs before 3:00 P.M. so that they have time to work before bedtime.

Recommendations

❑ Consume more foods that are high in vitamin B_2 (riboflavin) and vitamin B_5 (pantothenic acid), including bee pollen, brewer's yeast, soaked nuts, and spirulina.

Cautions: Both bee pollen and brewer's yeast can cause an allergic reaction in some individuals. Start with a small amount at first, and discontinue use if any allergic symptoms occur.

❑ Do not drink liquids within thirty minutes of bedtime.

❑ See your health care provider for food allergy testing. Bed-wetting is often caused by food allergies. Omit cow's milk, which is highly allergenic, from your diet. Also eliminate from the diet carbonated beverages, chocolate, cocoa, cooked spinach, refined carbohydrates (including junk food), rhubarb, and products containing caffeine or food coloring.

❑ Bed-wetting in children has been shown to cause low self-esteem, attention deficit, or behavioral problems and is best treated with sympathy and understanding. Do not spank or scold a child for bed-wetting. This only complicates the problem. Instead, give rewards for not wetting the bed.

Considerations

❑ We know of several cases of bed-wetting (among children and adults) that were relieved within a matter of days when supplements of certain nutrients were supplied. Among these were magnesium, vitamin B_2, and pantothenic acid. In addition, all allergy-causing foods were removed from the diet, and a protein supplement was added. Good supplements include soy powder, whey powder, and egg white powder.

❑ Supplemental magnesium is especially helpful for certain people. Magnesium citrate is one of the better forms to use, since the body can readily assimilate it. Too much magnesium produces diarrhea, so be careful when using it for children.

❑ Behavior modification techniques have proved useful in some cases, especially with children. One technique involves the use of an alarm that goes off as soon as the individual starts to wet the bed. Over time, this is believed to help a child respond to the body's cues and wake up when he or she needs to urinate during the night.

❑ The National Kidney Foundation hotline (888-925-3379) can provide information and a list of physicians in your area who are experienced in treating this condition.

BEE STING

There are numerous stinging insects in the United States, and not all of them are bees. Hornets, yellowjackets, wasps, spiders, and some species of ants can also inflict painful wounds. In some people, honeybee and yellowjacket stings can cause more serious reactions than the stings of hornets and wasps. When an insect stings, it injects venom through a stinger into the victim. Bees generally leave their stingers behind at the sting site; wasps most often do not. Usually, a stinging insect attacks because it is trying to protect itself, or its territory, from danger. This is why a person who stumbles on a beehive may end up receiving multiple stings from the hive's residents.

Most stings cause localized swelling, redness, and acute pain that may throb or burn. This is a reaction to the insect's venom. However, some people are highly allergic to insect venom, and if they are stung, a very severe reaction can occur. Symptoms of an allergic reaction include difficulty swallowing, hoarseness, labored breathing, weakness, confusion, severe swelling, and a feeling of impending disaster. People who are highly allergic to insect stings can experience anaphylactic shock, which can lead to unconsciousness and, in extreme circumstances, death. Anaphylactic shock can cause symptoms such as bluish skin; coughing; difficulty breathing; dizziness; hives; nausea; severely swollen eyes, lips, or tongue; stomach cramps; and wheezing.

Unless otherwise indicated, the following recommended dosages are for people over the age of eighteen. For a child between twelve and seventeen years old, reduce the dose to three-quarters of the recommended amount. For a child between six and twelve, use half of the recommended dose. Children under six years old should receive only one-quarter of the recommended amount.

NUTRIENTS

SUPPLEMENT	SUGGESTED DOSAGE	COMMENTS
Helpful		
Calcium	1,500 mg daily.	Helps relieve pain. Use calcium gluconate form.
O$_2$ Spray from Earth's Bounty	As directed on label.	Helps the healing process.
Pantothenic acid (vitamin B$_5$)	500 mg daily.	Acts to inhibit allergic response.
Vitamin C with bioflavonoids	10,000 mg within the first hour. Then 5,000–25,000 mg daily in divided doses. (*See* ASCORBIC ACID FLUSH in Part Three.)	Protects the body from allergens and moderates the inflammatory response.
Vitamin E	Slit capsule and apply oil topically to the sting site.	Promotes healing. Use d-alpha-tocopherol form.

Herbs

❑ Poultices made from comfrey and white oak bark and leaves can ease pain and promote healing. Lobelia poultices and plantain poultices or salve are also beneficial.

Note: Comfrey is recommended for external use only.

❑ Take echinacea and/or goldenseal in tea or capsule form to boost immune function. Goldenseal is a natural antibiotic and functions well as a poultice. It reduces inflammation and prevents infection.

Caution: Do not take echinacea for longer than three months. It should not be used by people who are allergic to ragweed. Do not take goldenseal internally on a daily basis for more than one week at a time. Do not use it during pregnancy or if you are breast-feeding, and use with caution if you are allergic to ragweed. If you have a history of cardiovascular disease, diabetes, or glaucoma, use it only under a doctor's supervision.

❑ Juniper tea cleanses the venom from your internal system, and can also make an excellent external poultice when the berries are crushed and applied to the sting.

❑ Drink as much yellow dock tea as you can, or take 2 capsules of yellow dock every hour until symptoms are relieved.

Recommendations

❑ If you are stung, immediately and carefully remove any stinger left in the skin. Do not pull the stinger out with your fingers or tweezers. Instead, gently scrape it out. A sterilized knife is best for this purpose, but you can use your fingernail or the edge of a credit card if nothing else is available. Be careful not to squeeze the stinger or the attached venom sac as this may inject more poison into the skin. Afterward, wash the area and rinse thoroughly. If you have ever had an allergic reaction to a sting in the past, seek emergency medical attention immediately. Life-threatening allergic reactions can come on suddenly and progress very quickly. If

you have no history of insect allergy, no medical treatment is needed, but do remain alert for symptoms of a developing allergic reaction. Reactions can occur within minutes or hours, and they can happen the first time or the thousandth time you are stung by a bee.

❑ If you are aware that you are highly allergic and prone to anaphylactic shock, carry an emergency kit containing a premeasured dose of epinephrine. You must obtain the kit by prescription, and your doctor should show you how to administer the epinephrine. Any allergic reaction to a sting should be taken seriously because, no matter how slight, the reaction may prove to be more serious in a second incident. Call 911 at once.

❑ If you are not highly allergic, once the stinger has been removed and the area cleansed, try one or more of the following home remedies to ease pain and swelling:

- Make a paste by adding a bit of cool water to baking soda, a crushed aspirin, or a crushed papaya enzyme tablet, and apply the mixture to the sting.

- Charcoal tablets, available in health food stores, can be used as a poultice. Empty 2 capsules, add 6 drops of liquid alcohol-free goldenseal extract to make a paste, then smooth on a sterile gauze pad and place on the sting area. This will absorb the poisons and prevent infection. Use only charcoal recommended for internal use.

- Apply an ice compress to the sting area a few minutes every two hours for the first day after you've been stung. Not only will you reduce the swelling and pain from the sting, but you will also be stopping the spread of venom.

- Apply lavender oil to the sting area to reduce inflammation and pain.

- Crush plantain leaves and squeeze out the juice. Apply this extract directly to the sting. Within thirty minutes, the pain and swelling should be greatly reduced.

- Other remedies to consider include: Rubbing toothpaste on the sting (its cooling effect can make the sting area feel better); applying calamine lotion to the area, or rubbing a meat tenderizer containing papain (an enzyme) on the sting can also ease the pain.

- If you have been stung on the foot or leg, elevate it for about half an hour after removing the stinger.

❑ Use *Apis mellifica,* a homeopathic remedy, to reduce inflammation and pain if the sting area is very swollen and red. *Ledum palustre,* a homeopathic remedy, reduces inflammation from stings, and is the most commonly used medication for insect stings and snakebite.

Considerations

❑ Aspirin or ibuprofen, taken every four hours, is helpful for pain and inflammation.

❏ Take an oral antihistamine and/or anti-itch medication, such as cortisone cream or Benadryl liquid, tablets, or cream to relieve itching caused by the sting.

❏ A venom extractor is available that fits inside a pocket or purse. If you get stung, it produces a vacuum that sucks the venom out within two minutes. The end of the extractor can also be used to remove a honeybee stinger.

❏ Taking large doses of vitamin C has been known to reduce the severity of bee stings.

❏ To avoid bee stings, wear plain, light-colored clothing. Also avoid wearing clothing that is flowered or dark colored; perfume, suntan lotion, hair spray, or anything scented; shiny jewelry; and open sandals or loose-fitting clothes.

❏ To protect yourself if you are highly allergic to bee stings, wear long-sleeved shirts and long pants when you are outdoors and near bees and wasps.

❏ When a yellowjacket is squashed, its body releases a chemical that causes other yellowjackets in the area to attack. If you are near a nest, hundreds of individuals can swarm you. It is better to leave the area fast than to swat at these insects.

❏ *See also* INSECT ALLERGY and INSECT BITE in Part Two.

BELL'S PALSY

See under RARE DISORDERS.

BENIGN PROSTATIC HYPERTROPHY

See under PROSTATITIS/ENLARGED PROSTATE.

BINSWANGER'S DISEASE

See under RARE DISORDERS.

BIPOLAR MOOD DISORDER (FORMERLY KNOWN AS MANIC-DEPRESSIVE DISORDER)

Bipolar mood disorder is a variant of classic depression. It typically begins as depression and then develops into alternating periods of depression and mania. A person with severe bipolar disorder may go from feeling unrealistically (and dangerously) invincible and elated to being overwhelmed with misery and despair, even suicidal. Some of the symptoms of bipolar disorder are changes in sleep pattern, withdrawal from society, extreme pessimism, a sudden loss of interest in and failure to finish projects that were started with enthusiasm, chronic irritability, sudden attacks of rage when crossed, loss of inhibition, and changes in sexual behavior that may range from a complete loss of sex drive to sexual excess. It is estimated that less than 2 percent of the population of the United States suffers from some form of this disorder.

The course of bipolar disorder is highly variable. Both mania and depression can vary in severity, and the length of the cycles, from depression to mania and back again, can occur over the course of a few days or over many months—even, in some cases, years. Low self-esteem and feelings of hopelessness characterize the depressive phase. A person experiencing depression may lack motivation to do anything, even to get out of bed. Some people simply sleep for weeks, withdraw from social activities, avoid relationships with others, and become unable to work. Others may seem to be living normal lives—going to work, interacting with others—but inwardly feel a deadening sadness and are unable to experience genuine pleasure.

The periods of mania often start suddenly and without warning. Some people experience what is called *hypomania,* excitement that does not necessarily appear to be a sign of mental illness—just great enthusiasm and energy. Others experience *full-blown manic psychosis,* in which they have seemingly boundless energy and are ceaselessly active and easily distracted. They may not want to rest or sleep for twenty-four hours or more. Mental activity is sharply accelerated, and delusions of grandeur, persecution, or invincibility are not uncommon. Most people in this condition seem to be utterly elated for no apparent reason, but some become unreasonably irritable and hostile. They may even have hallucinations. Despite all this, a person experiencing full-blown mania generally believes that he or she is functioning at peak efficiency.

The cause of this disorder is not well understood, but there are several theories as to its origin. It may be triggered by extreme stress. Heredity may be a factor in some cases. Some researchers believe that early experiences, such as the loss of a parent or other early childhood trauma, play an important role. Others believe that the manic phase is used (unconsciously) as a kind of psychological compensation for the depression that otherwise engulfs the individual. Biological factors are also possible. There is evidence that intracellular sodium increases during the mood swings of bipolar disorder, then returns to normal after recovery. It is also known that in depressed individuals, brain chemicals called monoamines are depleted.

The symptoms of some childhood psychological disorders such as attention deficit disorder (ADD), attention deficit hyperactivity disorder (ADHD), conduct disorder, and schizophrenia can be similar to those of mania, so a thorough examination is needed to avoid misdiagnosis. It is not uncommon for children who are diagnosed with psychotic depression to be diagnosed with bipolar disorder as adults.

Unless otherwise specified, the dosages recommended here are for adults. For children between the ages of twelve and seventeen, reduce the dose to three-quarters of the recommended dose. For children between six and twelve, use one-half of the recommended dose, and for children under the age of six, use one-quarter of the recommended amount.

NUTRIENTS

SUPPLEMENT	SUGGESTED DOSAGE	COMMENTS
Very Important		
Free form amino acid (Amino Balance from Anabol Naturals)	As directed on label twice daily, on an empty stomach.	To supply protein, needed for normal brain function and to combat depression.
L-tyrosine	500 mg twice during the day and again at bedtime. Take with water or juice on an empty stomach. Do not take with milk. Take with 50 mg vitamin B_6 and 100 mg vitamin C for better absorption.	Important in treating depression. Stabilizes mood swings. (*See* AMINO ACIDS in Part One.) *Caution:* Do not take this supplement if you are taking an MAO inhibitor drug.
Taurine	500 mg 3 times daily, on an empty stomach.	Deficiency can result in hyperactivity, anxiety, and poor brain function.
Vitamin B complex injections or	2 cc twice a week or as prescribed by physician.	To supply B vitamins essential for normal brain function and a healthy nervous system. All injectables can be combined in a single injection.
liver extract injections plus extra	As prescribed by physician.	
vitamin B_6 (pyridoxine) injections and	½ cc twice a week or as prescribed by physician.	
vitamin B_{12} injections or	1 cc twice a week or as prescribed by physician.	
vitamin B complex	100 mg of each major B vitamin 3 times daily (amounts of individual vitamins in a complex will vary).	Use a hypoallergenic formula. A sublingual form is best.
plus extra vitamin B_{12}	1,000–2,000 mcg daily, on an empty stomach.	Important in making myelin, the substance of which the sheaths covering the nerves are made. Use a lozenge or sublingual form.
Zinc	50 mg daily. Do not exceed a total of 100 mg daily from all supplements.	Protects the brain cells. Use zinc gluconate lozenges or OptiZinc for best absorption.
plus copper	3 mg daily.	Needed to balance with zinc.
Important		
Lithium	As prescribed by physician.	A trace mineral that alters the manic-depressive cycles, producing greater mood stability. Available by prescription only.
Helpful		
Essential fatty acids (Kyolic-EPA from Wakunaga)	As directed on label.	Important for improved cerebral circulation and blood pressure stability.
5-Hydroxytryptophan (5-HTP)	As directed on label.	Increases the body's production of serotonin. Note: Do not use this supplement with other antidepressants.
Multivitamin and mineral complex with	As directed on label.	Mineral imbalances may cause depression. Use a high-potency formula.
calcium and	1,500 mg daily.	
magnesium	750 mg daily.	Has a calming effect; enhances sleep if taken at bedtime.
Nicotinamide adenine dinucleotide (NADH)	As directed on label.	Enhances production of dopamine and serotonin.
Vitamin C with bioflavonoids	3,000–6,000 mg daily.	To aid in brain function and to protect the immune and nervous systems.

Recommendations

❑ Eat a diet consisting of vegetables, fruits, nuts, seeds, beans, and legumes. Whole grains and whole-grain products are recommended, except for those that contain gluten, which should be consumed in moderation only. (*See* CELIAC DISEASE for more information on a gluten-restricted diet.) Eat white fish and turkey twice a week.

❑ Eat fish that are high in omega-3 fatty acids. Tuna, salmon, mackerel, and herring are good choices. Omega-3 fatty acids may stabilize mood swings and have effects similar to those of the medication lithium.

❑ Consume no sugar or products containing sugar (read food product labels carefully). Also avoid alcohol, dairy products, caffeine, carbonated beverages, and all foods with colorings, flavorings, preservatives, and other additives.

❑ Be aware that food allergies may aggravate mood swings. Use an elimination diet to find which foods may be causing problems, and eliminate them from the diet. (*See* ALLERGIES in Part Two.)

❑ Take high doses of B-complex vitamins, approximately 100 mg of each major B vitamin three times daily (amounts of individual vitamins in a complex will vary). The B complex is very important for all mood disorders. Use injections (under a doctor's supervision) or a sublingual form for best absorption. Persons with bipolar disorder do not absorb the B-complex vitamins easily, and often have deficiencies of these vitamins.

❑ Avoid choline and the amino acids ornithine and arginine. These substances may make symptoms worse.

❑ Do not take any drugs except for those prescribed by your doctor.

❑ Establish and maintain a regular routine for your daily activities. A lack of sleep can trigger a relapse.

❑ As much as possible, avoid situations that cause stress, such as a turbulent relationship or a difficult working environment. Stress is a major contributor to serious problems for people with bipolar disorder.

Considerations

❑ Injections of vitamin B_{12} and megadoses of the B vitamins often bring about an improvement. The B vitamins have a lithium-like effect on the brain.

❑ Amino acids, especially taurine and tyrosine, are important in the treatment of this disorder.

❑ The trace minerals lithium carbonate and lithium citrate are known to alter the period of the rhythmic cycling of the brain, and help to even out the moods in persons with bipolar disorder. Lithium drugs' most important role is to prevent and decrease the occurrence of manic episodes. It is usually taken by mouth in capsule, tablet, or liquid form. The side effects of lithium drugs can include diarrhea, drowsiness, edema, frequent urination, kidney dysfunction, nausea, slight hand tremors, stomach cramps, thirst, thyroid enlargement, weight gain, and worsening of skin conditions such as acne and psoriasis. Toxic levels of lithium in the blood can cause blurred vision, confusion, muscle twitching and weakness, nausea, slurred speech, tremors, and vomiting. Lithium levels can be elevated to dangerous levels by changes in the diet, strenuous exercise, surgery, or illness, especially influenza. If you must take lithium drugs, try to keep your weight at a regular level and avoid crash dieting, as lithium levels are elevated by sudden weight loss. Keep your physician informed of any of the above-mentioned circumstances to avoid an imbalance in your dosage. Lithium drugs should not be taken by people with severely impaired kidney function. Make sure you take the drug with food and drink 10 to 12 glasses of water a day.

❑ Lithium orotate, a form of lithium, is also available.

❑ Food is known to increase the bioavailability of the antipsychotic drug ziprasidone (Geodon). In one study, researchers found that eating at least 500 calories per meal (but not as many as 1,000 calories) was sufficient to obtain maximum absorption of the drug. It didn't matter how much fat was included. This sort of diet made up of 500 to 600 calories per meal with 30 percent of the calories from fat is healthy and should help to avoid weight gain, which often happens with antipsychotic medications. In fact, weight gain is the second most common reason that people stop using antipsychotic drugs. In another study, patients taking the drug olanzapine (Zyprexa) ate 500 fewer calories each day and jogged 30 minutes three times a week, and were able to lose weight and reported that the drug remained effective. If you are not taking your medication for fear of weight gain, speak to your health care professional about seeing a dietitian to help you manage your weight.

❑ For those who cannot tolerate lithium, doctors may prescribe an anticonvulsant drug such as divalproex (Depakote). An antidepressant, such as Paroxetine (Paxil) or buproprion (Wellbutrin), may be prescribed for depressive episodes. To control acute manic episodes, the antipsychotic medications risperidone (Risperdal) and olanzapine (Zyprexa) are available. Other drugs include benzodiazepines such as diazepam (Valium) and MAOI antidepressants such as phenelzine sulfate (Nardil) and tranylcypromine sulfate (Parnate), but these aren't used as often because they are less effective. Electroconvulsive therapy (ECT) is sometimes used as a final choice to treat bipolar disorder. Today the treatment is much gentler than in the past and it is being recommended by some physicians.

❑ Psychotherapy and self-help support groups are very helpful in the treatment of bipolar mood disorder.

❑ According to an article in *The New England Journal of Medicine*, individuals with depression and bipolar disorder appear to be hypersensitive to the neurotransmitter acetylcholine. Therefore, choline should not be taken in a dose that exceeds the amount in a multiple vitamin.

❑ Bipolar mood disorder may be aggravated by an overgrowth of yeast in the intestinal tract and by nutritional deficiencies. Food allergies, such as an allergy to wheat products, and the consumption of large amounts of caffeine and/or refined sugar, can make symptoms worse.

❑ Certain systemic disorders can cause depression, including Alzheimer's disease, diabetes mellitus, encephalitis, hyper- and hypothyroidism, multiple sclerosis, and Parkinson's disease. Any depression diagnosis should be made only after a thorough physical examination to rule out an underlying illness.

❑ *See also* DEPRESSION in Part Two.

BITE

See BEE STING; DOG BITE; INSECT ALLERGY; SNAKEBITE; SPIDER BITES (AND SCORPION STINGS).

BITOT'S SPOTS

See under EYE PROBLEMS.

BLADDER INFECTION (CYSTITIS)

The kidneys, ureters, bladder, penis, and urethra all play a part in filtering and expelling waste material (urine) from the body. Cystitis (an infection of the bladder), urethritis (an infection of the urethra), and acute pyelonephritis (a kidney infection) are more common in women. All of these conditions can also occur in men, and may be a sign of serious underlying conditions such as problems with the prostate gland. Urethritis in the male is most often contracted as a result of sexual contact. Many conditions affecting the kidneys, bladder, or urethra are described as urinary tract infections, or UTIs, and most UTIs are concentrated in the bladder and urethra.

Bladder infections are characterized by an urgent desire to empty the bladder. Urination is typically frequent and painful; even after the bladder has been emptied, there may be a desire to urinate again. The urine often has a strong, unpleasant odor, and may appear cloudy. Children suffering from bladder infections often complain of lower abdominal pain and a painful burning sensation while urinating. There may be blood in the urine. While cystitis itself is usually more of an annoyance than a serious health problem, it can lead to kidney infection if left untreated.

Urinary tract infections are responsible for more than 8

million doctor visits each year. Between 80 percent and 90 percent of urinary tract infections are caused by *Escherichia coli*, a bacterium that is normally found in the intestines. Chlamydia may also cause bladder problems.

Both women and men suffer from bladder infections. In women, bacteria introduced by means of fecal contamination or from vaginal secretions can gain access to the bladder by traveling up through the urethra. Cystitis, pyelonephritis, and urethritis occur much more frequently in women than in men because of the close proximity of the anus, vagina, and urethra in females, and also because of the short length of the female urethra. This allows for relatively easy transmission of bacteria from the anus to the vagina and urethra, and thus to the bladder. In males, bacteria can reach the bladder either by ascending through the urethra or by migrating from an infected prostate gland. While bladder infections are relatively common in women, in men they may signal a more serious problem, such as prostatitis. Men should seek the advice of a physician to determine an exact diagnosis.

The possibility of developing a bladder infection can be increased by many factors, including pregnancy, sexual intercourse, the use of a diaphragm, and systemic disorders such as diabetes. The risk of cystitis is also increased if there is a structural abnormality or obstruction of the urinary tract resulting in restriction of the free flow of urine, or if past infections have resulted in a narrowing of the urethra. Bladder cancer, a condition more common among men than women, can often cause bladder infections. (*See under* CANCER in Part Two.)

Interstitial cystitis (IC) is a potentially debilitating disorder affecting 52 to 67 out of 100,000 women in the United States. Men can develop a similar condition called nonbacterial prostatitis or prostatodynia. IC is a chronic condition characterized by a combination of uncomfortable bladder pressure, bladder pain, and sometimes pain in your pelvis, which can range from mild burning or discomfort to severe pain. The severity of symptoms caused by IC often fluctuates, and some people may experience periods of remission. Because symptoms are similar to those of other disorders of the bladder and there is no definitive test to identify IC, doctors must rule out other treatable conditions before considering a diagnosis of IC. The most common of these diseases in both sexes are urinary tract infections and bladder cancer. Although there's no treatment that reliably eliminates interstitial cystitis, a variety of medications and other therapies offer relief.

Unless otherwise specified, the dosages recommended in this section are for adults. For a child between the ages of twelve and seventeen, reduce the dose to three-quarters of the recommended amount. For a child between six and twelve, use one-half of the recommended dose, and for a child under the age of six, use one-quarter of the recommended amount.

Urinary Tract Infection Self-Test

An FDA-approved home testing kit is available to help determine if you have a urinary tract infection. Bayer Multistix 7 and Multistix 10 SG reagent strips, and Roche Chemstrip 2LN, Chemstrip 6, 7, 8, 9, or 10SG are available in drugstores. All of the preceding test for the presence of leukocytes, or white blood cells (pus), which indicates infection. The pharmacist may have to order them if they are not in stock.

NUTRIENTS

SUPPLEMENT	SUGGESTED DOSAGE	COMMENTS
Very Important		
Garlic (Kyolic from Wakunaga)	2 capsules 3 times daily.	A natural antibiotic and immune enhancer.
Vitamin C plus bioflavonoids	4,000–5,000 mg daily, in divided doses. 1,000 mg daily.	Produces antibacterial effect through acidification of urine. Important in immune function.
Important		
Acidophilus (Kyo-Dophilus from Wakunaga)	As directed on label. Take on an empty stomach. Also use 1 tbsp in 1 qt warm water as a douche.	Needed to restore "friendly" bacteria. Especially important if antibiotics are prescribed.
Calcium and magnesium	1,500 mg daily. 750–1,000 mg daily.	Reduces bladder irritability. Aids in the stress response and works best when balanced with calcium. Use magnesium chelate form.
Multivitamin and mineral complex with vitamin A with carotenoids	10,000 IU daily. 15,000 IU daily.	Needed for essential balanced vitamins and minerals. Use a high-potency, hypoallergenic form.
N-acetylcysteine	500 mg twice daily, on an empty stomach.	A potent detoxifier that neutralizes free radicals.
Potassium	99 mg daily.	Replaces potassium lost as a result of frequent urination.
Vitamin B complex	50–100 mg of each major B vitamin twice daily, with meals (amounts of individual vitamins in a complex will vary).	Necessary for proper digestion. High doses are necessary if antibiotics are used.
Vitamin E	200 IU daily.	Combats infecting bacteria. Use d-alpha-tocopherol form.
Zinc plus copper	50 mg daily. Do not exceed a total of 100 mg daily from all supplements. 3 mg daily.	Important in tissue repair and immunity. Needed to balance with zinc.

Herbs

❏ Cranberry is one of the best herbal remedies for bladder infections. Quality cranberry juice produces hippuric acid in the urine, which acidifies the urine and inhibits bacterial growth. Other components in cranberry juice prevent bacteria from adhering to the lining of the bladder. Drink 1 quart of cranberry juice daily. Purchase pure, unsweetened juice from a health food store. If pure cranberry juice is not available, cranberry capsules can be substituted. Always take these with a large glass of water. Avoid commercial cranberry juice cocktail products. These contain relatively little pure cranberry juice (less than 30 percent in some cases) and have high-fructose corn syrup or other sweeteners added.

❑ Birch leaves are a natural diuretic and reduce some of the pain associated with bladder infections.

❑ Dandelion tea or extract acts as a diuretic and liver cleanser, and aids in relieving bladder discomfort.

❑ Hydrangea is good for stimulating the kidneys and flushing them clean.

❑ Diuretics help to cleanse the system. By promoting the release of fluids from the tissues, diuretics also help to relieve the false sensations of urgency that are characteristic of cystitis. Combinations of the herbs listed above are often most effective in flushing the kidneys and helping to reduce the urgent need to urinate.

❑ Fresh blueberries are a very effective antioxidant. Anthocyanidins are present in the blue pigment, and may prove as useful as cranberries in preventing urinary tract infections. The herb bilberry, a type of blueberry, is also good.

❑ Buchu is good for a bladder infection accompanied by a burning sensation upon urination.

❑ Goldenseal is good for bladder infections if there is bleeding, and is most effective as an herbal antimicrobial agent.

Caution: Do not take goldenseal internally on a daily basis for more than one week at a time. Do not use it during pregnancy or if you are breast-feeding, and use with caution if you are allergic to ragweed. If you have a history of cardiovascular disease, diabetes, or glaucoma, use it only under a doctor's supervision.

❑ Kidney Bladder formula from Nature's Way and Kidney Blend SP-6 from Solaray are herbal formulas that have a diuretic effect and reduce bladder spasms. Take 2 capsules twice daily.

❑ Marshmallow root increases the acidity of urine, inhibiting bacterial growth. Drink 1 quart of marshmallow root tea daily. It helps to strengthen and cleanse the bladder.

❑ Bearberry (*Uva ursi*, a type of cranberry), used in small amounts and diluted with other herbal teas, acts as a mild diuretic and antiseptic. It is effective against *E. coli*.

❑ Other beneficial herbs include burdock root, juniper berries, kava kava, echinacea flower root, stinging nettle, cleavers plant, yarrow, barley water, herbal teas, and rose hips.

Cautions: Kava kava can cause drowsiness. It is not recommended for pregnant women or nursing mothers, and it should not be taken together with other substances that act on the central nervous system, such as alcohol, barbiturates, antidepressants, and antipsychotic drugs. Do not take echinacea for longer than three months. It should not be used by people who are allergic to ragweed.

Recommendations

❑ Drink plenty of liquids, especially cranberry juice. (*See under* Herbs, above.) Drink at least one 8-ounce glass of water every hour. This is extremely beneficial for urinary tract infections. Steam-distilled water is preferable to tap water.

❑ Include celery, parsley, and watermelon in your diet. These foods act as natural diuretics and cleansers. Celery and parsley juice or extract can be purchased at a health food store or made fresh at home if you have a juicer.

❑ Avoid citrus fruits; these produce alkaline urine that encourages bacterial growth. Increasing the acid content in urine inhibits the growth of bacteria. (*See* ACIDOSIS *under* ACID/ALKALI IMBALANCE in Part Two for a list of acid-forming foods.)

❑ Stay away from alcohol, caffeine, carbonated beverages, coffee, chocolate, refined or processed foods, and simple sugars. Chemicals in food, drugs, and impure water have an adverse effect on the bladder.

❑ Perform a one- to three-day cleansing fast. (*See* FASTING in Part Three.)

❑ Take 2 teaspoonfuls of whey powder or 2 acidophilus tablets or capsules with each meal. This is especially important if antibiotic therapy is required.

❑ Take a twenty-minute hot sitz bath twice daily. Hot sitz baths help to relieve the pain associated with cystitis. Batherapy from Queen Helene, a product that can be found in health food stores or online, is excellent. Or you can add one cup of vinegar to a sitz bath (or to shallow bathwater) once a day. A woman should position her knees up and apart so that the water can enter the vagina. Alternate this with a bath made with two cloves of crushed garlic or an equivalent amount of garlic juice. (*See* SITZ BATH in Part Three.)

❑ Use acidophilus douches as recommended under Nutrients, above. If cystitis is associated with vaginitis, alternate this with apple cider vinegar douches.

❑ Avoid taking excess zinc and iron supplements until healed. Taking over 100 mg of zinc daily can depress the immune system; bacteria require iron for growth. If a bacterial infection is present, the body stores iron in the liver, spleen, and bone marrow in order to prevent further growth of the bacteria.

❑ Do not delay emptying the bladder. Making sure that you urinate every two to three waking hours—"voiding by the clock"—can help.

❑ Keep the genital and anal areas clean and dry. Women should wipe from front to back after emptying the bladder or bowels, should empty the bladder before and after exercise and sexual intercourse, and should wash the vagina after intercourse. Diaper wipes are soothing, sanitary options to clean oneself.

❑ Wear white cotton underwear; nylon underwear should be avoided.

❑ Change into dry clothes as soon as possible after swimming; avoid sitting around in a wet bathing suit.

❑ Do not use "feminine hygiene sprays," packaged douches, bubble baths, tampons, sanitary pads, or toilet paper containing fragrance. The chemicals these products contain are potentially irritating.

❑ If you suffer from frequent urinary tract infections, use sanitary pads rather than tampons.

❑ If urination is painful but harmful bacteria cannot be found, discontinue use of all types of soaps and use only water to cleanse the vaginal area. Some people are sensitive to soap; an all-natural soap from a health food store is recommended.

❑ If there is blood in the urine, consult your health care provider. This can be a sign of a more serious problem that warrants medical attention.

Considerations

❑ Optimal immune function is important in both fighting and preventing all bacterial disorders.

❑ Caffeine causes the muscles around the bladder neck to contract, and can produce painful bladder spasms.

❑ Habitually retaining the urine in the bladder for long periods increases a woman's risk of urinary tract infection, and may increase the risk of bladder cancer.

❑ Shrinkage of urethral and vaginal membranes, which most commonly occurs after menopause as a result of a reduction in the amount of estrogen in the body, can increase the tendency to develop bladder infections. Urethral dilation helps stretch a contracted urethra.

❑ Food allergies often cause symptoms that mimic bladder infections. Food allergy testing can determine which foods are causing the allergic reaction. (See ALLERGIES in Part Two.)

❑ Using aluminum cookware may cause cystitis symptoms.

❑ Cadmium, a toxic metal, may cause urinary problems.

❑ If you suffer from inconsistent bladder control, consider sacral nerve stimulation, a new implant designed to treat bladder problems. This small device sends electronic signals to the nerves connected to the bladder, which helps prevent incontinence and dramatically improves quality of life.

❑ Women who suffer from frequent urinary tract infections are forced to stay on a continued regimen of low-dose antibiotics to prevent recurrence. Researchers from the University of Michigan announced in 2009 that they had developed the first effective vaccine to prevent urinary tract infection (UTIs). Those who would benefit from a vaccine are people who are resistant to antibiotics, those who are allergic to antibiotics, or those who experience side effects that preclude them from using antibiotics for UTIs.

❑ Antibiotics and analgesics may be necessary treatments for cystitis, especially for persistent and/or painful infections. Beware of resorting to them too often, however. Antibiotics disturb the normal internal flora, and may actually promote recurrent infections by promoting the development of antibiotic-resistant strains of bacteria. In fact, because antibiotics have been widely prescribed over many years, there are many types of bacteria (estimates run from 50 to 80 percent) that are now resistant to common antibiotics, such as sulfa drugs and tetracycline. This forces doctors to resort to more powerful and potentially more dangerous antibiotics that pose a greater risk of adverse reactions and side effects. For most bladder infections, a natural approach to treatment is often effective, but if a severe condition persists beyond a day or two, consult your health care provider.

❑ Recurrent cystitis may be a sign of a more serious problem, such as bladder cancer, an anatomical anomaly, or immune deficiency. Cystoscopy, a simple visual examination of the bladder, is indicated.

❑ An oral medication, pentosan (Elmiron), is the only oral drug approved by the Food and Drug Administration specifically for interstitial cystitis (IC).

❑ In one study, one gram of quercetin improved symptoms of interstitial cystitis. In another study, 300 mg of quercetin helped women feel better and they scored better on a standardized test of symptoms. Both studies of quercetin used a blend of quercetin, condroitin sulfate, and sodium hyaluronate.

❑ See also KIDNEY DISEASE, PROSTATITIS, and VAGINITIS in Part Two.

❑ For sources of additional information about bladder infections, see Health and Medical Organizations in the Appendix.

BLEPHARITIS

See under EYE PROBLEMS.

BLOOD PRESSURE PROBLEMS

See HIGH BLOOD PRESSURE.

BLOOD SUGAR PROBLEMS

See DIABETES; HYPOGLYCEMIA.

BOIL

Boils, referred to as furuncles by medical professionals, are round pus-filled nodules on the skin that result from infection with *Staphylococcus aureus* bacteria. The infection begins in the deepest portion of a hair follicle, or in an oil-producing sebaceous gland, and works its way up to the skin's surface. Poor nutrition, illness that has depressed immune function, diabetes mellitus, poor hygiene, and the use of immunosuppressive drugs are common contributing factors.

This disorder is common, especially among children and adolescents. Boils often appear on the scalp, buttocks, face, or underarms. They are tender, red, and painful, and they appear suddenly. Symptoms that a boil may be forming include itching, mild pain, and localized swelling. Within twenty-four hours, the boil becomes red and filled with pus. Fever and swelling of the lymph glands nearest the boil may occur.

Boils are contagious. The pus that drains when a boil opens can contaminate nearby skin, causing new boils, or can enter the bloodstream and spread to other body parts.

A carbuncle is a cluster of boils that occurs when the infection spreads and other boils are formed. The formation of a carbuncle may be an indication of immune depression.

Without treatment, a boil usually comes to a head, opens, drains, and heals in ten to twenty-five days. With treatment, symptoms are less severe and new boils should not appear.

Unless otherwise specified, the following recommended doses are for those over the age of eighteen. For a child between twelve and seventeen years old, reduce the dose to three-quarters of the recommended amount. For a child between six and twelve, use one-half of the recommended dose, and for a child under six years old, use one-quarter of the recommended amount.

NUTRIENTS

SUPPLEMENT	SUGGESTED DOSAGE	COMMENTS
Essential		
Colloidal silver	Apply topically as directed on label.	A natural antibiotic and disinfectant. Destroys bacteria, viruses, and fungi. Promotes healing.
Garlic (Kyolic from Wakunaga)	2 capsules 3 times daily.	A natural antibiotic that potentiates immune function.
Kyo-Green from Wakunaga	As directed on label.	To aid in cleansing the bloodstream and reducing infection.
Very Important		
Proteolytic enzymes	As directed on label. Take on an empty stomach.	Speeds up cleansing process at infection sites.
Vitamin A and carotenoid complex	75,000 IU daily for 1 month, then reduce to 25,000 IU daily. If you are pregnant, do not exceed 10,000 IU daily. As directed on label.	Antioxidants necessary for proper immune system function. Use emulsion forms for easier assimilation and greater safety at high doses. *Caution:* Do not take this supplement if you are pregnant or nursing.
Vitamin C with bioflavonoids	3,000–8,000 mg daily, in divided doses.	Powerful anti-inflammatory and immune system stimulant.
Vitamin E	200 IU daily.	A powerful antioxidant. Use d-alpha-tocopherol form.
Zinc	50 mg daily	Aids in healing and enhances the immune system.
Helpful		
Coenzyme Q10 plus	60 mg daily.	Important for oxygen utilization and immune function.
Coenzyme A from Coenzyme-A Technologies	As directed on label.	Works well with coenzyme Q10 in ridding the body of impurities.
Kelp plus multimineral complex	2,000–3,000 mg daily, in divided doses. As directed on label.	To supply balanced minerals. Use a high-potency formula.
Raw thymus glandular	500 mg daily.	Stimulates the immune system. (*See* GLANDULAR THERAPY in Part Three.)
Silica or oat straw	As directed on label.	Supplies silicon, which reduces inflammatory reaction. *See under* Herbs, below.

Herbs

❑ Burdock root, goldenseal, olive oil extract, and pau d'arco are all natural antibiotics that help to rid the body of infections and toxins.

Caution: Do not take goldenseal internally on a daily basis for more than one week at a time. Do not use it during pregnancy or if you are breast-feeding, and use with caution if you are allergic to ragweed. If you have a history of cardiovascular disease, diabetes, or glaucoma, use it only under a doctor's supervision.

❑ Dandelion, burdock root, and milk thistle cleanse the bloodstream and the liver.

❑ Echinacea and goldenseal help to cleanse the lymph glands.

Cautions: Do not take echinacea for longer than three months. It should not be used by people who are allergic to ragweed. Do not take goldenseal internally on a daily basis for more than one week at a time. Do not use it during pregnancy or if you are breast-feeding, and use with caution if you are allergic to ragweed. If you have a history of cardiovascular disease, diabetes, or glaucoma, use it only under a doctor's supervision.

❑ Flax and fenugreek, simmered together and mashed into a pulp, can be used as a compress.

❑ Oat straw, taken in tea form, supplies silica, which has an anti-inflammatory effect.

❑ Onion poultices are good for boils. Apply pieces of onion wrapped in a piece of cloth—not directly to the area. (*See* USING A POULTICE in Part Three.)

❑ Red clover acts as a natural antibiotic and is good for bacterial infections. It cleanses the liver and the bloodstream.

❑ Suma boosts the immune system.

❑ Tea tree oil compresses act as an antiseptic. Add 9 to 10 drops of the oil to 1 quart of warm water. Soak a clean cloth in the warm liquid and apply to the boil. The tea tree oil can be left on the boil for thirty minutes or more, and may be applied three or four times a day.

Recommendations

❑ Use a cleansing fast to clear the system and rid the body of toxins that may cause boils. (*See* FASTING in Part Three.)

❑ To relieve pain and help to bring the boil to a head, apply moist heat three or four times a day. Wet a clean towel or sterile gauze pad with warm water and apply it to the boil. Place a heating pad or a hot water bottle on top. Do this for twenty minutes three or four times a day. Use a clean towel or fresh piece of gauze each time to prevent spreading the infection. Warm Epsom salts baths are also good.

❑ Do not cover a boil with an adhesive bandage, but do avoid irritation, injury, or trauma to the affected area. To avoid sweating, do not exercise or engage in strenuous activity until the boil heals.

❑ Keep the skin clean. Wash the infected area several times a day and swab it with antiseptic. You can also apply honey directly to the boil. Vitamin A and E emulsion, applied directly on boils, is helpful. Clay packs and/or chlorophyll are also good. Both of these can be found in health food stores. Apply them directly to the boil with a sterile gauze pad.

❑ Charcoal capsules made into a paste and applied to the boil will help draw out the infection. Break open 2 capsules of charcoal and mix with just enough water to make the paste.

❑ *Belladonna*, a homeopathic remedy, helps reduce swelling and inflammation. Another homeopathic remedy, *Calcarea sulphurica*, is useful if a boil has opened and is draining but is not healing properly.

❑ If a boil is very large, persistent, or recurrent, consult your physician. Surgical incision and drainage may be necessary. Severe cases may require bed rest.

Considerations

❑ Boils may be symptomatic of a more serious infection within the body. They should always be treated with care, especially if they are accompanied by other symptoms, such as a fever or a poor appetite.

❑ Boils should not be squeezed or punctured prematurely. In very serious cases, boils may need to be incised by a doctor.

❑ A doctor may prescribe an oral antibiotic. These drugs have side effects, however. It is best not to use them unless other measures fail.

❑ The area around a draining boil (especially on the face) may be protected with a prescribed antibiotic cream to help prevent complications such as septicemia or meningitis.

❑ Over-the-counter antibiotic ointments are ineffective for boils and should be avoided.

BREAST CANCER

The human breast is a gland that contains milk ducts, lobes, fatty tissue, and a network of lymphatic vessels. Cancerous tumors can arise in virtually any part of the breast and are most often detected when a woman feels a lump. In general, cancerous lumps are firm, never go away, and are usually (though not always) pain-free. The vast majority of breast lumps are not cancerous (many are cysts or fibroid masses), but there is no way to tell without a professional's examination. A lump that seems to be growing or that does not move when pushed may be cancerous or may simply be caused by normal fibrocystic changes during the menstrual cycle. A biopsy is required to identify the lump. Breast cancer can also cause a yellow, bloody, or clear discharge from the nipple.

People tend to think of breast cancer as a single entity, but there are actually different types of the disease. The most common types of breast cancer include the following:

- *Ductal carcinoma in situ* (DCIS). This is a condition that most doctors consider to be breast cancer at its earliest stage. DCIS is a cancer contained within the milk ducts. The rate of this type of cancer has increased dramatically over the past twenty-five years. Fortunately, the survival rate for DCIS is nearly 100 percent. However, having DCIS can increase the risk of developing invasive breast cancer.

- *Invasive ductal carcinoma (IDC)*. This is a cancer that arises in the lining of the milk ducts and infiltrates (invades) the surrounding breast tissue. Approximately 80 percent of all cases of breast cancer are infiltrating ductal carcinomas.

- *Lobular carcinoma in situ (LCIS)*. This condition begins in the milk-making glands but does not go through the wall of the lobules. Although not a true cancer, having LCIS increases a woman's risk of getting cancer later. For this reason, it's important that women with LCIS make sure they have regular mammograms.

- *Invasive lobular carcinoma (ILC)*. This cancer starts in the milk glands or lobules. It can spread to other parts of the body. About one out of ten invasive breast cancers is of this type.

- *Inflammatory Breast Cancer (IBC)*. A rare and aggressive form, it accounts for about 1 to 3 percent of all breast cancers. In this type of cancer, a tumor arises in the lining of the milk ducts and, as it grows, it plugs the lymphatic and blood vessels. The skin thickens and turns red, and the breast becomes extremely tender and looks infected. This type of cancer spreads very quickly due to the rich blood and lymph vessel supply associated with the inflammatory reaction.

Unusual types of breast cancer include phyllodes tumor, angiosarcoma, osteosarcoma, metaplastic breast cancer, adenoid cystic carcinoma, and Paget's disease of the breast. There are also rare subtypes of invasive ductal carcinoma—tubular, mucinous, medullary, and papillary.

Cancer of the breast is the most common cancer among women (other than skin cancer), and is the second leading cause of cancer death (following lung cancer) for women in the United States. The American Cancer Society estimates that in 2009 about 192,000 women were diagnosed as having breast cancer, and about 40,000 women die of it each year. The lifetime risk of developing breast cancer for American women is one in eight. The chance of dying from breast cancer is about one in thirty-five. Breast cancer death rates are going down, which is probably the result of finding the cancer earlier and improved treatment. Surveys suggest that it is the health problem most feared by women, but if breast cancer is detected early, the five-year-and-beyond survival rate is very high—about 95 percent. Right now there are about two and a half million breast cancer survivors in the United States.

There is probably no single answer as to what causes breast cancer. Researchers believe, however, that the female sex hormone estrogen is the most likely culprit in many cases of breast cancer. (Although not all breast cancers are related to estrogen.) Estrogen promotes cellular growth in the tissues of the breasts and reproductive organs, and cancer is a disorder of unrestrained cellular growth. Moreover, some of the known risk factors for breast cancer include onset of menstruation before age nine, menopause after age fifty-five, having a first child after age forty, and having no or few children. One thing all of these risk factors have in common is that they result in the breasts being exposed to more estrogen for longer periods.

Currently, research does not point clearly to environmental factors (such as exposure to pesticides and other pollutants) as a possible factor in the development of breast cancer. However, research on the effects of pesticides is ongoing, and there are many health care professionals who advise avoiding these substances as much as possible, as their effects may mimic those of estrogen in the body.

There may be a link between obesity and an increased risk of developing breast cancer, especially for women over fifty years of age. However, this is a complex issue. The risk appears to vary depending on whether a woman has been obese since childhood, or if she gained the excess weight during adulthood. A study reported in the journal *Cancer* found that women who gained more than twenty-two pounds since their teenage years doubled their chances of getting breast cancer. The increased risk posed by obesity may also be linked to estrogen. Obese women tend to have higher levels of estrogen in their bodies than thin women do. A study conducted in Mexico found that eating lots of carbohydrates raises the risk of getting breast cancer. In another study, the same was found for French women. The postmenopausal women who consumed more rapidly absorbed carbohydrates (high-glycemic-load carbohydrates) and who were overweight with a large waist circumference as a result of fat on the abdomen had a greater breast cancer risk.

There are conflicting reports as to whether eating a high-fat diet is linked to an increased risk of breast cancer. The largest study including nearly 50,000 postmenopausal women found no significant effect of dietary fat intake on the development of breast cancer. However, for women who already have breast cancer, a low-fat diet that results in weight loss has been shown to protect against a recurrence of the disease. The women in this study consumed about 22 percent of their calories from fat and lost about six pounds. Many physicians believe fat intake is among the highest risk factors. They argue that if a woman eats a diet high in fat and low in fiber her body produces more estrogen. Fiber from cereal and fruits appears to reduce the chances of getting breast cancer. Although it is possible for a woman to get breast cancer at any age, the disease is most common in women over forty, especially postmenopausal women.

Heredity is a factor in breast cancer as well; there are certain types of the disease that clearly run in families. Researchers estimate that only 5 to 10 percent of breast cancers occur in women with a clearly defined genetic predisposition for the disease. Hereditary cancers usually develop before the age of fifty. A Danish study of more than 100,000 women found that each 2.2-pound (1-kilogram) rise in birth weight was associated with an increase in breast cancer risk of some 9 percent. Another study showed that 10-pound babies had triple the incidence of breast cancer later in life than their peers who weighed in at between 5.5 and 7.7 pounds. Researchers theorize that faster growth in the womb might somehow "program" breast cells to multiply faster and raise the odds of having them turn cancerous.

Men also can get breast cancer, but they account for less than 1 percent of breast cancer cases. However, while it occurs less frequently, breast cancer in men usually is diagnosed at a later, and therefore more serious, stage because neither physicians nor their patients tend to suspect it. Every year in the United States fewer than 2,000 men are diagnosed with breast cancer—and 400 die from it. Cure rates are, in general, the same for men as they are for women.

It is important to detect breast cancer in its earliest and most curable stage. Making healthy changes in diet and lifestyle, examining your breasts regularly (*see* BREAST SELF-EXAMINATION, below), and having regular mammograms can increase your chances of avoiding or, if need be, overcoming breast cancer.

Breast Self-Examination

It is important to examine your breasts each month past age twenty, at the same point in your menstrual cycle, preferably the first week after your menstrual period ends. Do not examine them during your menstrual period. Before the period, a woman's breasts may swell and become tender or lumpy. This usually decreases after the period. The breasts also become larger and firmer during pregnancy, in preparation for breast-feeding. Familiarize yourself with the normal feel of your breasts so that you can detect any changes such as enlargement of a lump. A woman who is accustomed to the way her breasts feel is better able to notice subtle changes. Any changes in your breasts should be reported to your health care provider, and a professional should recheck you if you have any doubt concerning your examination. Since men also can get breast cancer, they can benefit from self-examination as well. The following is the recommended procedure for breast self-examination:

1. While standing and looking in the mirror, raise your hands over your head and press them together. Notice the shape of your breasts. Place your hands on your hips, apply pressure, and look for irritation or dimpling of the skin, nipples that seem to be out of position, one breast that looks different from the other, swelling in a portion of the breast, nipple pain, an inward curve of the nipple, a discharge from the nipple (other than breast milk), or red scaling or thickening of the skin and nipples.

2. Raise one arm above your head. With the other hand, firmly explore your breast. Beginning at the outer edge, using a circular motion, gradually work toward the nipple. Take your time when examining the area between the nipple and the armpit, and feel the armpit as well. You have lymph nodes in the armpit; they move freely and feel soft, and are not painful to the touch. Look for lumps that are hard and not mobile. Cancers are often attached to underlying muscle or the skin. When you have finished examining one breast, repeat this on the other side.

3. Lie down on your back and repeat step 2. Lumps may be more easily detected in this position. Also, squeeze each nipple gently to check for blood or a watery yellow or pink discharge.

In addition to monthly self-examination, the American Cancer Society recommends that women between the ages of twenty and thirty-nine have their breasts examined by a physician every one to three years. After age forty, the exam should be performed every year. Women should get their first mammogram by age forty, then have one every year along with their yearly exam.

The program recommended below is designed for women who have been diagnosed with breast cancer as well as for women who want to increase their odds of avoiding breast cancer.

NUTRIENTS

SUPPLEMENT	SUGGESTED DOSAGE	COMMENTS
Essential		
Coenzyme Q$_{10}$	100 mg daily.	Improves cellular oxygenation. There is mounting evidence supporting the theory that coenzyme Q$_{10}$ reduces the risk of breast cancer.
Colostrum (Colostrum Plus from Symbiotics or Colostrum Prime Life from Jarrow Formulas)	As directed on label.	Promotes accelerated healing and boosts the immune system.
Dimethylglycine (DMG) (Aangamik DMG from FoodScience of Vermont)	As directed on label.	Improves cellular oxygenation.
Essential fatty acids (Kyolic-EPA from Wakunaga, black currant seed oil, borage oil, flaxseed oil)	As directed on label.	Needed for proper cell reproduction.
Garlic (Kyolic from Wakunaga)	2 capsules 3 times daily.	Enhances immune function.
Germanium	200 mg daily.	A powerful immunostimulant that improves cellular oxygenation, deterring cancer growth.
Melatonin	3–50 mg at bedtime.	Blocks estrogen-receptor sites on breast cancer cells.
Multimineral complex with calcium and magnesium and potassium and zinc	2,000 mg daily. 1,000 mg daily. 99 mg daily. 50 mg daily.	Essential for normal cell division and function. Use a comprehensive formula that contains all major minerals and trace elements but that is iron-free. Good for strengthening immunity.
Multivitamin complex	As directed on label. Take with meals.	All nutrients are needed for nutritional balance. Do not use a sustained-release formula or a formula that contains iron.
Natural beta-carotene or carotenoid complex (Betatene)	10,000 IU daily. As directed on label.	A powerful antioxidant that destroys free radicals.
Proteolytic enzymes (Inf-zyme Forte from American Biologics) plus multiple enzyme complex	2 tablets between meals (to reduce inflammation) and 2 tablets with meals (to aid digestion). When taking them with meals, it is best to take them with protein foods. As directed on label.	Powerful free radical scavengers. Reduce inflammation. To aid in digestion.
Selenium	200–400 mcg daily. If you are pregnant, do not exceed 40 mcg daily.	Protects the immune system by preventing the formation of free radicals, which can damage the body. It has also been found to function as a preventive against the formation of certain types of tumors, including breast tumors.

Supplement	Suggested Dosage	Comments
Superoxide dismutase (SOD)	As directed on label.	Destroys free radicals. Consider injections (under a doctor's supervision).
Vitamin B complex	100 mg of each major B vitamin 3 times daily (amounts of individual vitamins in a complex will vary).	To improve circulation, build red blood cells, and aid liver function; necessary for normal cell division and function.
plus extra vitamin B$_3$ (niacin) and choline	100 mg daily. Do not exceed this amount.	Involved in the regulation of enzyme and hormone production. *Caution:* Do not take niacin if you have a liver disorder, gout, or high blood pressure.
plus vitamin B$_{12}$ and folic acid	2,000 mcg daily. 400–800 mcg daily.	To prevent anemia and aid in proper digestion and absorption of nutrients. Consider injections (under a doctor's supervision). If injections are not available, use a sublingual form such as Superior Source supplements from Continental Vitamin.
plus brewer's yeast	As directed on label.	Aids in reducing estrogen production. A source of B vitamins.
Vitamin C with bioflavonoids plus extra quercetin	5,000–20,000 mg daily, in divided doses. (*See* ASCORBIC ACID FLUSH in Part Three.) 400 mg 3 times daily or as directed on label.	Powerful anticancer agent.
Vitamin D	As directed on label.	Inhibits cell division and growth. Low levels of vitamin D have been linked to higher breast cancer rates.
Vitamin E	200 IU daily.	Deficiency has been linked to breast cancer. Also aids in hormone production and immune function. Use an emulsion form for easier assimilation and greater safety at higher doses. Blocks free-radical damage in fatty breast cells. Use d-alpha-tocopherol form.
Important		
Maitake	4,000–8,000 mg daily.	Inhibits the growth and spread of cancerous tumors. Also boosts immune response.
Helpful		
Acidophilus (Kyo-Dophilus from Wakunaga)	As directed on label.	To replenish "friendly" bacteria in the colon. Contains powerful anti-carcinogenic compounds. Breaks down metabolites of estrogen. Use a nondairy formula.
Aerobic 07 from Aerobic Life Industries	As directed on label.	Antimicrobial agents.
Kelp or seaweed	1,000–1,500 mg daily. As directed on label.	For mineral balance.
L-carnitine	As directed on label.	Protects the skin after mastectomy and/or radiation treatment. Use a form derived from fish liver (squalene).
L-cysteine and L-methionine and glutathione plus	As directed on label. As directed on label. Take with water or juice. Do not take with milk. Take with 50 mg vitamin B$_6$ and 100 mg vitamin C for better absorption	To detoxify harmful substances. (*See* AMINO ACIDS in Part One.)
Taurine Plus from American Biologics	As directed on label.	Functions as foundation for tissue and organ repair. Use the sublingual form.
Pycnogenol	As directed on label.	A powerful antioxidant.
Raw glandular complex plus raw thymus glandular and raw adrenal glandular	As directed on label. As directed on label. As directed on label.	To stimulate glandular function, especially the thymus, the site of T lymphocyte production. (*See* GLANDULAR THERAPY in Part Three.)
S-Adenosylmethio-nine (SAMe)	As directed on label.	Aids in stress-relief, relieves depression, eases pain, and produces antioxidant effects. Has been found to inhibit growth of breast cancer cells in laboratory tests. *Caution:* Do not use if you have bipolar mood disorder or take prescription antidepressants.

Herbs

❑ Astragalus root and echinacea enhance immune function. These herbs are best used in a rotating fashion, for no more than seven to ten days in a row.

Cautions: Do not use astragalus in the presence of a fever. Do not take echinacea for longer than three months. It should not be used by people who are allergic to ragweed.

❑ Drink herbal teas such as bilberry, burdock root, ginger, green tea, peppermint, and red clover instead of regular tea.

Caution: Green tea contains vitamin K, which can make anticoagulant medications less effective. Consult your health care professional if you are using them. The caffeine in green tea could cause insomnia, anxiety, upset stomach, nausea, or diarrhea.

❑ Black cohosh, chasteberry, red clover, and turmeric are herbs that are high in phytoestrogens. Phytoestrogens are forms of estrogen that are much weaker than the body's estrogens, but that are capable of blocking the stronger, more damaging estrogens (they can fit into the same receptors in breast cells that estrogens can, thus preventing the estrogen's ability to dock there). Phytoestrogens also expand the length of the menstrual cycle, possibly lowering the lifetime exposure to estrogen.

Caution: Do not use black cohosh if you are pregnant or have any type of chronic disease. Black cohosh should not be used by those with liver problems.

❑ Burdock root, dandelion root, milk thistle, and red clover all protect the liver and aid in cleansing the bloodstream.

❑ Red clover is often used to help with menopausal symptoms such as hot flashes. It contains isoflavones, which are hypothesized to protect against breast cancer. In one study, red clover did not increase mammographic breast density and had no effect on hormones, which are thought to promote breast cancer. Conventional hormone replacement increases breast density, so red clover may offer a natural alternative. However, other studies have found red clover to act like estrogen and therefore not be appropriate for women with some forms of breast cancer.

❑ Chaste tree berry (also known as vitex), ginseng, and soy extracts may inhibit the growth of breast cancer cells.

Caution: Do not use ginseng if you have high blood pressure, or are pregnant or nursing.

❑ Curcumin (the yellow pigment found in turmeric) is the chief ingredient of curry. It is a powerful anti-inflammatory and protects against inflammatory calcium loss from our bones.

❑ Calcium D-glucarate is a botanical extract found in grapefruit, apples, oranges, broccoli, and Brussels sprouts. Scientists are discovering that it appears to protect against cancer and other diseases via a different mechanism than antioxidants such as vitamin C, carotenoids, and folic acid. These vitamin antioxidants work by neutralizing toxic free radical damage in the body. There are, however, other mechanisms by which the human body can detoxify itself. Glucuronidation is a detoxification process that occurs when toxins or carcinogens are combined with water-soluble substances, thus making them more easily removed from the body. D-glucarate has been shown to support this process by inhibiting an enzyme called beta-glucuronidase.

❑ Rosemary extract is a powerful antioxidant that helps to remove estrogens and may inhibit breast cancer development.

❑ Lycopene may reduce the risk of breast cancer.

❑ Sulphoraphane, from broccoli sprout extract, has been shown to stimulate the body's production of detoxification enzymes that help eliminate xenoestrogens. It is also a powerful antioxidant.

❑ Green tea extract, which contains catechins and flavonoids, may be protective against estrogen-dominant breast cancer.

Caution: Green tea contains vitamin K, which can make anticoagulant medications less effective. Consult your health care professional if you are using them. The caffeine in green tea could cause insomnia, anxiety, upset stomach, nausea, or diarrhea.

❑ Garlic is known to be a cancer-preventing nutrient.

❑ Ginkgo biloba enhances circulation and brain function.

Caution: Do not take ginkgo biloba if you have a bleeding disorder, or are scheduled for surgery or a dental procedure.

❑ Licorice root aids in maintaining proper organ function.

Caution: Licorice root should not be used during pregnancy or nursing. It should not be used by persons with diabetes, glaucoma, heart disease, high blood pressure, or a history of stroke.

❑ Silymarin, an antioxidant extract of milk thistle, has shown promise for fighting breast cancer. It also protects the liver.

❑ The following combination of herbs was shown to have no effect on reducing breast cancer risk: *Curcuma longa, Cynara scolymus, Rosmarinus officinalis, Schisandra chinensis, Silybum mariunum,* and *Taraxacum officinalis.*

Recommendations

❑ Eat a high-fiber diet based on fresh fruits and vegetables, plus grains, legumes, raw nuts (except peanuts) and seeds, and soured products such as low-fat yogurt. Very important are the cruciferous vegetables, such as broccoli, Brussels sprouts, cabbage, and cauliflower, and yellow/orange vegetables, such as carrots, pumpkin, squash, sweet potatoes, and yams. Eat vegetables raw or lightly steamed. For grains, use unpolished brown rice, millet, oats, and wheat. Eat whole grains only. If at all possible, consume only organically grown foods. Pesticides and other chemicals have been linked to breast cancer (they may mimic the effect of estrogen on the body).

❑ Include soy foods in your diet. Diets high in fiber and soy foods are associated with a lowered risk of breast cancer. Some good sources of soy include fresh soybeans, tempeh, soymilk, soy nuts, tofu, and soy powder. However, if you have breast cancer check with your doctor before consuming soy because it may have a stimulating effect on breast tumors.

❑ Include in your diet fresh apples, cherries, grapes, plums, and all types of berries.

❑ Eat onions and garlic, or take garlic in supplement form.

❑ Lignins are a class of phytoestrogens (plant estrogens) that seem to reduce breast cancer risk. These substances are found in seeds (especially flax), whole grains, berries, fruits, vegetables (especially broccoli and sprouts), and nuts.

❑ Make sure your diet provides adequate amounts of essential fatty acids (EFAs). Omega-3 EFAs (found in fish and flaxseed) and omega-9 EFAs (found in olive oil) lower cancer risk. Eating salmon weekly and tuna three times a week will provide a good amount of EFAs. Processed fish oil supplements are also a good idea, but avoid cod liver oil, as its levels of vitamin A and D are too high. Fish oil has been reported to possibly slow tumor growth. Flaxseed oil or flaxseeds can be sprinkled onto food.

❑ Make a daily juice using a combination of fresh organic broccoli, cauliflower, carrots, kale, dark leafy greens, and an apple. These are high in phytochemicals such as indole-3-carbinol (I-3C) and help to combat breast cancer. The phytochemical I-3C has been shown to detoxify xenoestrogens via the liver and to even reverse abnormal Pap smears.

❑ Limit your intake of fatty, charred, or grilled foods, which have been linked with a higher risk of cancer.

❑ Drink spring or steam-distilled water only, never tap water. Also drink fresh homemade vegetable and fruit juices. Drink fruit juices in the morning and vegetable juices in the afternoon.

❑ If you consume meat, poultry, and dairy products, select organic, hormone-free products. These foods could contain residues of estrogenic hormones that are given to animals in order to promote growth. Well-done red meat has been linked to a higher risk for breast cancer in some studies. Unsweetened low-fat yogurt is an acceptable source of protein.

❑ Do not consume any alcohol, caffeine, junk foods, processed refined foods, saturated fats, salt, sugar, or white flour. Studies have shown that women who ate the most carbohydrates overall (62 percent or more of their total caloric intake) were more than twice as likely to have breast cancer as those eating fewer carbohydrates. Not all carbohydrates are necessarily bad, though. The greatest risk comes from sucrose (table sugar) and fructose (found in most nondiet soft drinks). Obviously, avoiding refined sugars and soft drinks will have a beneficial effect.

❑ Take extra fiber daily. Fiber keeps toxic wastes from being absorbed into the bloodstream. Psyllium husks are a recommended source. The colon must be kept clean, and the bowels must move daily for healing. (See COLON CLEANSING, ENEMAS, and FASTING in Part Three.)

Note: Always take supplemental fiber separately from other supplements and medications.

❑ Do not take supplements containing iron unless your doctor says you need it for anemia or other reasons. Iron may be used by tumors to promote their growth.

❑ If you experience itching, redness, and soreness of the nipples, especially if you are not currently breast-feeding, seek evaluation by a physician. These can be symptoms of Paget's disease.

❑ If you are undergoing treatment for breast cancer and find yourself feeling depressed or frightened, try to keep in mind that when medications (especially chemotherapy drugs) are stopped, you will probably start to feel better and look at things in a different light. Think about all the women, including many celebrities and public figures, who have had breast cancer and have gone on to have fulfilling lives and careers. Thousands of women who have had breast cancer are living happy, normal lives.

Considerations

❑ Mammograms can detect small tumors and breast abnormalities up to two years before they can be felt, when they are most treatable. A mammogram should be scheduled within the first fourteen days of your menstrual cycle, when the breasts are less likely to be swollen. You should not use any antiperspirant, deodorant, or powder on the day of the test, as it can interfere with the reading.

❑ Women, especially premenopausal women under age forty, who ate sport-caught fish had nearly double the risk of developing breast cancer than those who did not eat any sport-caught fish. Those women who ate Great Lakes–caught fish had a 74 percent greater risk. Carcinogens, which tend to concentrate in fish flesh, may be the cause. These carcinogens include halogenated hydrocarbons, such as PCBs, DDT, and PBDFs.

❑ Magnetic resonance imaging (MRI) with equipment specifically designed for imaging the breast can be used to evaluate a suspected rupture of a silicone gel–filled breast implant. Even though these are no longer being used, except in clinical studies, many thousands of women still have them. Physicians usually recommend removal of a ruptured implant, regardless of whether it is silicone-filled or a newer saline-filled type.

❑ A study showed that women who used aspirin at least four times a week for at least three months were almost 30 percent less likely to develop estrogen- or progesterone-related breast cancer than those who did not use aspirin. Published in the *Journal of the American Medical Association* in May 2004, the study was led by researcher Mary Beth Terry, Ph.D., and Alfred Neugut, M.D., Ph.D., of Columbia University. Researchers suspect aspirin works by interfering with estrogen production.

❑ One technique may cut down on unnecessary biopsies when dealing with implants, dense breast tissue, and high-cancer-risk patients. The alternative to the mammogram is the MRI, and this is used in most of the cases stated above because mammograms are more likely to miss cancer in these women. However, the MRI has a problem in that it "red flags" a lot of spots that turn out to be benign after biopsy. A newer version of MRI software, called CAD-stream, in conjunction with a dye injection, has shown promising results. In one study at the University of Washington School of Medicine, it missed no cancers and ruled out half of the "red flags" as benign, thus avoiding a biopsy in each case.

❑ There had been a great rise in the use of hormone-replacement therapy (HRT) in past years. This consists of a combination of synthetic estrogen and progestin, and was designed to help combat the symptoms of menopause (bone loss, night sweats, hot flashes, and so forth). A study reported in the *Journal of the American Medical Association* uncovered some serious problems with the use of this type of therapy. In fact, the study was ended after only five years (it had originally been scheduled to run 8.5 years) because women in the treatment group had a 26 percent increased risk of invasive breast cancer. The study also found that the women who took HRT were 29 percent more likely to have a heart attack and 41 percent more likely to have a stroke. The risk of getting gallbladder and liver disease was also higher, as was the risk of developing blood clots. There is enough clear evidence that the risks of HRT far outweigh any benefits. The millions of women who took or are taking HRT should consider using nutrients to detoxify their bodies of the cancer-causing estrogens and gradually weaning themselves off the therapy. However, some women can benefit from HRT to manage menopausal symptoms. The doses used today are lower and the hormones are prescribed for a limited time, making HRT much less risky today than it once was.

❑ Postmenopausal women who took the drug Letrozole experienced a reduction in breast cancer recurrence of 43 percent as opposed to 13 percent of women on a placebo. Letrozole is proposed as a drug to be used in conjunction with tamoxifen, which is the current post-cancer treatment. Tamoxifen blocks the production of estrogen, but becomes ineffective after five years or so. Letrozole, on the other hand, suppresses production of estrogen and is to be used after a period of tamoxifen treatment. The study results were so persuasive that the study was stopped early, which is a normal protocol, so that all participants could benefit from treatment with Letrozole. Studies on a similar drug, exemestane, showed similar results. Exemestane is sold under the brand name Aromasin.

❑ The connection between exercise and cancer is a fairly new area of research. Some studies suggest that getting regular exercise in youth might give lifelong protection against breast cancer. Even moderate physical activity as an adult may lower breast cancer risk. A study published in the *Journal of the American Medical Association* followed almost 75,000 women aged fifty to seventy-nine as part of the Women's Health Initiative Cohort Study. The study found that women who engaged in the equivalent of 1.25 to 2.5 hours of brisk walking per week had an 18 percent lower risk of getting breast cancer as compared to inactive women over the five-year study period. Women who engaged in up to 10 hours of similar exercise realized a small decrease in risk over and above the 1.25 to 2.5 hour group. Although not part of the study, outdoor exercise where you are getting some (but not too much) sun exposure also raises vitamin D levels.

❑ Most of the newest research on breast cancer focuses on the finding that low levels of vitamin D are associated with a greater risk. Some have proposed that very high doses of vitamin D (2,000 IU) and small amounts of sunlight exposure will reduce breast cancer risk by 50 percent. However, 2,000 IU exceeds the upper limit of safety set by the DRIs. During puberty, maintaining adequate vitamin D levels was shown to be important to protect against developing breast cancer later in life. The best sources of vitamin D are cow's milk, soymilk, and supplements. Some exposure to the sun with sunblock is also advised. Premenopausal women who had the highest intake of vitamin D and calcium had the lowest risk of breast cancer. Again, these women would benefit from cow's milk, soymilk, and calcium and vitamin D supplements.

❑ Relaxation techniques such as writing, meditation, yoga, or massage therapy can aid in battling breast cancer.

❑ There is a clear link between alcohol consumption and an increased risk of breast cancer. A study reported in *The New England Journal of Medicine* stated that consuming as few as three alcoholic drinks a week increases the potential for breast cancer by 50 percent. In a European study of more than 274,000 women, thirty-five to seventy-five years of age, recent (within six years) alcohol intake increased the risk of breast cancer. However, when the study looked at alcohol intake over a lifetime, it showed no effect on breast cancer risk. The American Cancer Society (ACS) estimates that those who have two to five drinks daily increase their risk to about 1.5 times that of women who drink no alcohol. The ACS recommends that you limit the amount you drink to two drinks, two times a week.

❑ A test from Genomic Health of Redwood City, California, could be helpful to patients who have early breast cancer and must make treatment decisions. The test looks at twenty-one different genes thought to play a role in developing cancerous cells, using them as predictors as to whether a tumor would return after initial treatment. The thrust of the test is to predict whether or not chemotherapy is necessary in individual cases. While it is a promising tool, many doctors are skeptical about trusting such an experimental procedure without further studies to confirm its value. The test is being marketed under the name OncotypeDX.

❑ There is great debate about whether or not fat intake has an effect on the risk of developing breast cancer. (For women who already have breast cancer, lowering fat intake seems to lessen the risk of recurrence of the disease.) The National Women's Health Network urges all women to cut their total fat intake to 20 percent of total calories. Saturated fats should account for no more than 5 percent of calories.

❑ The largest women's health study ever done, the Women's Health Initiative Cohort Study, had 162,000 participants. Some findings taken from the study that were recently presented at an American Society for Reproductive Medicine conference indicated that taking birth control pills during reproductive years was *not* as harmful as was once thought. In fact, the study indicated a lower risk for heart attack, stroke, high blood pressure, and other related cardiovascular disease (CVD) problems. The overall risk reduction for CVD was 8 percent, and a bonus was a risk reduction of 7 percent regarding any type of cancer. Researchers believe the type of hormones, and when they are taken in life, seems to be what makes them helpful at one point and harmful at another.

❑ Frequent exposure to medical X-rays has been linked to an increased risk for breast cancer.

❑ Early or prolonged use of permanent dark hair dyes has been linked to breast cancer.

❑ Testing methods for breast cancer are increasing the likelihood of catching it early. Minimally invasive breast biopsies (MIBBs) can be performed with virtually no recovery time. Ultrasounds and high-resolution ultrasounds offer a safer alternative to X-rays, and can provide sharp digital pictures. Magnetic resonance imaging can create a three-dimensional image and can be useful in detecting ruptures in silicone breast implants.

❑ A computerized mammogram scanner may increase the likelihood that a woman's cancer can be cured by calling a radiologist's attention to a suspicious area on a mammogram. The computer software analyzes the content of mammograms and highlights, or "red flags," suspicious areas on the images after the radiologist has done the initial evaluation. The device has been shown to improve a radiologist's detection rate from about 80 cancers out of 100 to 88 out of 100.

❑ For some women digital X-rays are better able to detect tumors than film mammography. The results of the Digital Mammographic Imaging Screening Trial (DMIST) indicate that only women who fit in any of the following three categories would benefit from digital mammography instead of film mammography: under age fifty (regardless of level of breast tissue density); of any age, with heterogeneously (very dense) or extremely dense breast tissue; or pre- or perimenopausal women of any age (defined as women who had a last menstrual period within twelve months of their mammograms). According to the results, women who fit all of the following three categories would *not* benefit from digital mammography instead of film mammography: over age fifty; those who do not have dense or heterogeneously (very dense) breast tissue; and those who are no longer menstruating.

❑ A method of detecting if cancer has spread to the lymph nodes, called sentinel node biopsy, allows doctors to pinpoint the first lymph node into which a tumor drains (the sentinel node), and remove only the nodes most likely to contain cancer cells.

❑ If you have a personal family history of breast cancer, you may want to consider genetic testing. Over half of women with certain genetic mutations develop breast cancer by the age of seventy. With the discovery of two "breast cancer genes" (BRCA1 and BRCA2), gene therapy is receiving more attention. This research is still in its infancy, and much more investigation in this area needs to be done. These genes are hereditary, so if one sister has the gene, other sisters and their mother might want to consider getting tested. A woman who has inherited a harmful mutation in BRCA1 or BRCA2 is about five times more likely to develop breast cancer than a woman who does not have such a mutation. Also, consider what you are going to do with the information. Some women opt to get prophylactic mastectomies after testing positive for a breast cancer gene even if they don't have cancer. Genetic testing can determine whether you have a genetic mutation, but it cannot predict whether you will develop breast cancer. Talk to your doctor if you are considering genetic testing. It is expensive, insurance companies do not always cover it, and if your results are positive, insurance companies may choose to deny you coverage.

❑ People with breast cancer have been found to have lower than normal levels of vitamin E and the mineral selenium, two important antioxidants that work together to neutralize free radicals. Selenium has been shown in lab studies to kill tumors and protect healthy tissue. Research has also shown that people with cancer of the lung, bladder, breast, colon, and skin all have lower than normal levels of vitamin A.

❑ It has been difficult to evaluate whether or not DHEA may prevent breast cancer because studies have yielded conflicting evidence on this point. A stronger, natural descendant of DHEA is 7-keto DHEA. Unlike DHEA itself, 7-keto DHEA is not converted into testosterone or estrogens in the body. It may be a safer alternative to DHEA in combating breast cancer.

❑ Low levels of vitamin B_{12} have been linked to an increased risk of breast cancer.

❑ Studies have shown that genistein, found in soy, inhibits new tumor growth, slowing the growth of existing cancer.

❑ Pro Fem progesterone cream from Life Extension Foundation is a natural progesterone cream that can be applied to the breast for direct absorption through the fat under the skin. Progesterone may help reduce the risk of breast cancer, but check with your physician first, as this is a bioactive substance and may interfere with other hormones in the body.

Caution: Pregnant women and nursing mothers should not use this product.

❑ Raloxifene (Evista), a drug similar to tamoxifen, has been found in two clinical trials to be at least as effective in the prevention of breast cancer, without the increased risk of uterine cancer linked to tamoxifen. In 2007, the FDA approved raloxifene for reducing the risk of invasive breast cancer in postmenopausal women with osteoporosis and in postmenopausal women at high risk for invasive breast cancer.

❑ Epirubicin (Ellence) is a chemotherapy drug that can be used to combat early-stage breast cancer that has spread to the lymph nodes.

❑ Capecitabine (Xeloda) is a drug approved for use in women with advanced breast cancer for which no acceptable alternative treatments are available. It was given accelerated approval, an early approval process applied to some drugs that are used to treat life-threatening conditions. This drug is specifically for patients whose tumors are resistant to other treatments. In studies, the drug measurably shrank some patients' tumors. Possible side effects include diarrhea, nausea, vomiting, fatigue, painful inflammation of the mouth, and painful rash and swelling of the hands and feet.

❑ Capecitabine (Xeloda), taken orally, and docetaxel (Taxotere), an intravenous drug, have been approved by the FDA to be used in combination to treat advanced cancer. This is to follow treatment with an anthracycline-containing therapy such as doxorubicin (Adriamycin). Doctors limit anthracycline-containing treatments to life-threatening situations. The FDA approved the drug combination after a study of 511 cancer patients demonstrated improvements in overall response rates, lengths of time before the disease worsened, and survival rates. Capecitabine and docetaxel individually are associated with side effects including gastrointestinal symptoms, nausea, vomiting, and painful inflammation of the mouth. If side effects occur it may be necessary to reduce dosages or to interrupt or discontinue treatment. Dosages also may have to be modified for people with impaired kidney function. Drug interaction between capecitabine and coumarin-derivative anticoagulants (Coumadin) may cause serious bleeding and must be carefully monitored.

❑ Doctors once believed that extensive surgery could control the spread of breast cancer. However, they now believe that cancer cells may break away from the primary tumor during surgery and spread through the bloodstream, even in the earliest stages of the disease. These cells cannot be felt by examination or seen on X-rays or other imaging methods, and they produce no symptoms. Adjuvant therapy—the use of drug treatment after surgery—can be used to kill these hidden cells. Your health care provider can make recommendations as to whether or not adjuvant therapy is needed in your individual situation. If surgery is recommended, get a second opinion. Drugs approved by the FDA to improve the chances of successfully treating breast cancer include:

- Paclitaxel (Taxol), which is used for both treatment of metastatic or advanced breast cancer and prevention of relapses and which a recent large study indicated was more beneficial when given once a week rather than once every three weeks (the previous standard treatment).

- Tamoxifen (Nolvadex).

- Trastuzumab (Herceptin), an immunotherapy regimen that can be used alone if other drugs have been unsuc-

cessful, or as a first-line treatment in combination with other drugs.

- Anastrozole (Arimidex) can be used in place of tamoxifen and it has fewer side effects. Anastrozole works by shutting down the hormone estrogen at the source.

- Lapatinib (Tykerb), which targets the HER2 protein and is approved for use in advanced breast cancer. Lapatinib is reserved for women who have already tried trastuzumab and their cancer has progressed.

- Bevacizumab (Avastin), which in 2008 was approved by the FDA as a treatment for late-stage breast cancer.

In addition, cyclophosphamide (Cytoxan) and doxorubicin (Adriamycin), with or without fluorouracil (Adrucil), may be used to treat breast cancer. Chemotherapy treatment is given in cycles, followed by recovery periods. Depending on how far the cancer has spread, treatments can last from three to six months.

❑ Fentanyl (Actiq) is a drug that may be prescribed for people in severe pain. It is a narcotic drug that is more potent than morphine and comes in a flavored sugar lozenge form.

❑ After surgery, analysis of the tumor is done to determine the type of cancer and to test for the presence of a substance called estrogen-receptor protein, to determine whether the cancer is estrogen-dependent. If the tumor is found to be estrogen-dependent, tamoxifen may be an alternative to conventional chemotherapy.

❑ Most women with breast cancer have some type of surgery, depending on the stage of the breast cancer. Options for the surgical treatment of breast cancer have expanded greatly in the past couple of decades. Surgical treatment now emphasizes breast conservation—preserving the breast when possible. Some of the treatment options in breast surgery include:

- *Lumpectomy,* also known as segmental mastectomy or tylectomy. The tumor and a small amount of surrounding tissue are removed. This is the least extensive type of breast cancer surgery. In most cases, a lumpectomy is followed by several weeks of radiation, which is an integral part of breast conserving treatment.

- *Quadrantectomy,* also known as partial mastectomy. The quadrant of the breast in which the tumor was found is removed, including some skin and the lining of the chest muscle below the tumor.

- *Simple mastectomy.* The entire breast is removed and a sample of the underarm lymph nodes is taken.

- *Modified radical mastectomy,* also known as total mastectomy. The entire breast and all underarm lymph nodes are removed. The lining over the chest muscles may also be removed.

- *Radical mastectomy,* also known as the Halsted radical mastectomy. The entire breast, all the axillary (underarm) lymph nodes, and the underlying chest muscle are removed. This procedure was once the standard in breast cancer surgery, but today, women with breast cancer rarely undergo this type of surgery because doctors believe that a modified radical mastectomy is just as effective.

- *Bilateral prophylactic mastectomy.* This type of surgery is done in a small percentage of women who are at particularly high risk for breast cancer. In this procedure, both healthy breasts are removed to prevent breast cancer from forming. This is most often performed on women who have an inherited genetic defect that increases their risk of getting breast cancer to 85 percent by the age of seventy. Researchers at the Mayo Clinic have found that this procedure may reduce the risk of developing the disease by almost 90 percent, and deaths due to breast cancer by over 80 percent.

No single procedure can be recommended as ideal for all individuals. A woman and her surgeon must base their decision on the patient's medical status and her particular concerns. Her choice may be influenced by emotional considerations, finances, access to care, body image, and personal beliefs. Depending on the type of surgery that is done, there is the option of having breast reconstruction later.

❏ A technique called rotating delivery of excitation off resonance (RODEO) MRI-guided laser lumpectomy soon may be available to treat breast cancer without surgery, radiation, or chemotherapy. The outpatient procedure uses magnetic resonance imaging with lasers that destroy early-stage cancers.

❏ In any type of breast cancer surgery, some or all of the underarm lymph nodes may be removed. This is done to check for possible spread of the cancer. If the cancer has spread to the lymph nodes, postoperative therapy may include radiation, chemotherapy, or hormonal therapy. Radiation is always required after a lumpectomy or quadrantectomy to ensure that no more cancer cells remain.

❏ After surgery, women are usually advised to avoid moving or carrying heavy objects, to wear loose-fitting clothes and gloves, and to avoid overexposure to the sun. Some women whose lymph nodes are removed during breast cancer surgery have a problem with swelling of the arm, or lymphedema, on that side due to an accumulation of lymphatic fluid. This is not unusual. It can develop just after surgery, or months or even years later, and can be brought on by an injury to (or overuse of) the arm or an infection. To reduce the risk of developing lymphedema, do not have any blood work, chemotherapy, or blood pressure work done on the affected arm. Certain arm exercises are usually prescribed to keep the arm from becoming stiff and to assist in healing. If there is any unusual swelling, redness, or pain in the hand or arm, this should be evaluated by a physician.

❏ Hospitals offer some women the opportunity to have a mastectomy on an outpatient basis. In one study, 4 percent of women who had outpatient surgery required later breast reconstruction, whereas 13 percent of women who had an inpatient procedure later required breast reconstruction. Only a surgeon can decide which method is best for you.

❏ Biopsies that are less invasive now can be done using a fine needle aspiration (removing cells from a breast lump) and stereotactic core biopsies (which uses a bigger needle that a computer guides to remove suspicious tissue seen on a mammogram).

❏ Combining an MRI with automatic tissue excision and collection (ATEC) allows for a nonsurgical biopsy for many women, particularly those with high-density tissue that masks suspicious lumps when taking a mammogram. This is basically a vacuum-assisted biopsy, and where the suspicious lump is under about 2 cm (about $^3/_4$ inch) it can be completely excised. Once the needle is removed, a simple Band-Aid is sufficient to cover the entry mark.

❏ Postmenopausal women who drink too much wine are at a higher risk for breast cancer. Moderate drinkers have a much lower (12 percent) risk of developing the disease. A study, conducted at Lund University in Sweden, found that the break point was only 1.5 glasses of wine per day. Moderate drinkers averaged less than that consumption per day.

❏ Even when treatment is initially successful, breast cancer returns in one out of three cases. New drugs, treatment regimens, and better diagnostic techniques have improved the outlook for many, and are responsible, according to the ACS, for a decline in breast cancer death rates.

❏ For agencies and organizations that can provide more information and services for people with breast cancer, *see* HEALTH AND MEDICAL ORGANIZATIONS in the Appendix.

BREAST-FEEDING-RELATED PROBLEMS

Breast-feeding, or lactation, is the natural way in which the mother of a newborn can feed her child instead of relying on cow's milk or artificial infant-formula preparations. A woman's breasts are ideally suited for the task of feeding a baby, and nursing provides many benefits to both mother and baby that bottles and formulas do not. For example, mother's milk is much easier to digest, prevents constipation, lowers the incidence of food allergies, and protects the baby from many infectious diseases. Nursing also promotes healthy oral development, satisfies suckling needs, and enhances bonding between mother and child. Breast-feeding is beneficial to the mother in that it reduces the chance of hemorrhaging from the placental site, gives the mother an opportunity to rest, and encourages the uterus to contract, returning it to its pre-pregnant size.

Women who breast-feed are less likely to develop rheumatoid arthritis than women who don't. Dr. Elizabeth Wood Karlson from Brigham and Women's Hospital in Boston used data from the Nurses' Health Study to explore the contribution of hormonal factors on subsequent development of arthritis. Women who breast-fed for a total of twelve to twenty-three months during their lifetime had a 30 percent risk reduction. Those who breast-fed for at least twenty-four months had a 50 percent risk reduction. Besides giving an infant more resistance to bacteria and illness and creating a closer bond between the mother and child, the benefits of breast-feeding include higher brain development.

Some studies have found breast-fed infants to have higher IQs as adults, on average, than formula-fed infants, and to have achieved higher academic levels in adult life. In an eighteen-year study conducted on 1,000 children, it was shown that polyunsaturated fatty acids, particularly the docosahexaenoic acid (DHA) contained in mother's milk, boosted intellectual (neural) development. DHA is considered essential for a baby's development. Formula-fed babies now receive DHA, and while the mother passes a large amount of DHA on to the infant in the last trimester of pregnancy, a baby fed with formula will continue to ingest this most important developmental nutrient. Data is conflicting as to the merits of supplementing DHA in infant formula during the first year of life. Early studies showed that babies were more alert early on, but that non-supplemented babies caught up by age four. Once infants begin eating regular foods they need the other important omega-3 fat, EPA. This comes from fish.

A study of 2,200 Australian children shows that infants who are breast-fed for at least the first four months of life are significantly less likely to develop asthma, wheezing, or respiratory allergies by the age of six. A mother's milk also prevents *Clostridium difficile*, the intestinal bacteria that causes serious colon inflammation and diarrhea in adults, from binding to the cells of the baby's intestinal walls.

Many infants are fed formulas, either for medical reasons or because the mother cannot or chooses not to breast-feed. No woman should feel inadequate or badly about not being able to breast-feed. Many more children today are born premature, which makes breast-feeding more difficult. Also, more multiple births are occurring, again limiting a mother's ability to successfully breast-feed.

In breast-feeding, as with anything else that is new and unfamiliar, problems may occur. This section offers explanations and solutions to the most common breast-feeding problems.

Engorgement

This is a temporary problem that most commonly occurs between two to five days after childbirth. It is caused by a combination of the increased blood supply to the breast and the pressure of the newly produced milk, resulting in the swelling of the tissues in the breast. A low-grade fever may be present; the breasts feel full, hard, tender, and tight; and the skin of the breasts is hot, shiny, and distended. You do not need engorgement in order to nurse. Seek medical attention immediately to determine if you have engorged breasts or mastitis (*see below*).

Recommendations

❏ Give your baby short, frequent feedings. A feeding schedule of every one and a half to two hours day and night should be maintained while engorgement lasts.

❏ Express milk between feedings to relieve pressure.

❏ Apply moist heat for thirty minutes preceding each feeding, and massage the breast during feedings to help get the milk flowing.

❏ Do not use nipple shields, as they can confuse the baby's sucking pattern, damage nipples, reduce stimulation of the breast, and decrease the milk supply.

❏ To prevent engorgement, feed your baby on demand and without delay, and allow unrestricted suckling time.

❏ Do not skip or delay feedings during the day or night. Do not give your baby any formula or sugar water, and allow the baby to empty each breast completely at each feeding.

❏ The American Academy of Pediatrics (AAP) recommends that newborns nurse eight to twelve times every twenty-four hours until the baby is satisfied, usually ten to fifteen minutes on each side.

Mastitis (Breast Infection)

If a plugged duct is not taken care of, mastitis can result. Acute mastitis is an infection and swelling of the breast, usually occurring as a result of bacteria (most often *Staphylococcus aureus*) entering the nursing mother's breast through cracks or fissures in the nipple. Mothers are most vulnerable to acute mastitis in the first few weeks of nursing because cracks in the nipple develop more often during this time. Soreness and redness in the breast; fever; yellow, puslike secretions from the nipple; general tiredness; and flulike symptoms are indicators of this problem. In fact, in a nursing mother, all flulike symptoms should be considered a breast infection until proven otherwise. A mother who has a high fever, in addition to the aforementioned symptoms, should see a doctor.

Recommendations

❏ Drink plenty of fluids.

❏ Get plenty of rest.

❏ Air-dry the nipples after nursing to prevent cracking. If the nipples do crack, you can coat them with breast milk, or apply aloe vera juice after they dry to help them heal. You can also apply heat with a hot water bottle or heating pad before and after nursing, or use a heat lamp with a regular 100-watt bulb for a few minutes after nursing in order to heal cracks and prevent infections. Place the lightbulb twelve to eighteen inches from the breast—not so close as to cause discomfort.

❏ Your doctor may advise you to stop breast-feeding until the infected breast heals. If so, use a breast pump to prevent the breast from becoming engorged.

❑ Remember to always wash your hands before and after breast-feeding to remove germs, and always wash the breast and nipple area afterward.

Considerations

❑ Most of the minor infections heal by themselves in a few days, but often the pain is significant and may get in the way of feeding your baby, so seeking medical help is best. More severe ones can heal in about a week if treated with antibiotics.

❑ Your health care provider may prescribe antibiotics that can be taken by a nursing mother.

❑ In rare cases, a breast infection results in a breast abscess, in which the sore breast fills with pus. An abscess may have to be incised to allow drainage. This procedure is performed in a physician's office. If an abscess develops, milk should be hand-expressed (massaged) from the infected breast and discarded. Breast-feeding should continue on the uninfected breast until the abscess is healed.

Plugged Duct

Incomplete emptying of the milk ducts by the baby, or wearing a tight bra, can cause a plugged duct. Soreness and a lump in one area of a breast is an indication of this problem.

Recommendations

❑ Check the nipple very carefully for any tiny dots of dried milk, and remove them by gentle cleansing. Together with frequent nursing on the affected breast, this should allow the duct to clear itself within twenty-four hours.

❑ Massage the breasts with firm pressure, from the chest wall toward the nipple, to stimulate milk flow.

❑ Alter the position of the baby on the nipple so all the ducts are drained.

❑ Make sure you offer the affected breast first, when the baby's sucking is strongest.

Sore Nipples

Sore nipples are usually caused by improper nursing positions and nursing schedules, or incorrect sucking by the baby. They can also be caused by infection, most commonly with the fungus *Candida albicans*.

Recommendations

❑ Nurse on the least sore side first. However, if both breasts are sore, hand-express (massage the breast) until letdown occurs and milk is readily available to the baby.

❑ Make sure that the baby's jaws exert pressure on the least tender spots. Do not pull away when the baby is about to begin feeding. Learn to relax.

❑ Massage your breasts from base to tip to prevent engorgement. Do this during the final weeks of your pregnancy and continue through postpartum.

❑ If cracked nipples accompany soreness, apply aloe vera gel to the nipples to alleviate pain and promote healing. Also, aloe vera (fresh), calendula, marshmallow, and slippery elm are soothing when used in paste form as a poultice, or as wet tea bags, and applied to sore nipples.

❑ Apply avocado oil, calendula ointment, lanolin, and olive oil (separately or in combination) to the breasts to help prevent soreness during pregnancy and while breast-feeding. Wash thoroughly before allowing the baby to breast-feed.

❑ To prevent sore nipples, feed your baby frequently to avoid having a baby who is overly hungry bite down roughly on the nipple. Be sure your baby's mouth takes in as much of the areola (the dark area of the nipple) as possible. The baby shouldn't make slurping noises when feeding.

❑ Change nursing positions often to rotate the pressure of the baby's mouth on the breast, and learn to break suction correctly. Between feedings, keep the nipples dry. Expose them to sunlight and air. Do not wash them with soap, alcohol, or petroleum-based products, which can wash away their natural protection. Instead, you can apply a little colostrum on the nipple and let it air dry.

❑ If the pain is severe and persists despite these measures, it may be a sign of a candida infection. (*See* FUNGAL INFECTION in Part Two.) Consult your health care provider.

Nutritional Health While Nursing

The following supplements are beneficial for nursing mothers. After a discussion with your health care provider, you may decide to supplement your diet with these vitamins and minerals.

NUTRIENTS

SUPPLEMENT	SUGGESTED DOSAGE	COMMENTS
Essential		
Free form amino acid (Amino Balance from Anabol Naturals)	As directed on label.	To supply needed protein. Soy protein and free-form amino acids are better sources than animal protein.
Helpful		
Bifido Factor from Natren	½ tsp daily, between meals.	For mother. Boosts immune system and provides necessary "friendly" bacteria. Use only unchilled water in preparation.
and LifeStart from Natren	¼ tsp daily, added to water or juice.	For babies over 6 months. Use only unchilled water in preparation.
Calcium and magnesium	1,000–1,500 mg daily. 500–750 mg daily.	Needed by both mother and baby. Use chelate forms. Do not use bone meal or dolomite, as these may contain lead.

Multivitamin and mineral complex with vitamin B complex plus extra	As directed on label.	All nutrients are needed by both mother and baby. Use a high-potency formula. Needed for production of milk and to relieve stress.
folic acid and	400 mcg daily.	Note: Do not take calcium and manganese together, as they compete for absorption.
vitamin C and	3,000 mg daily.	
vitamin D and	400 IU daily.	
iron and	As directed by physician.	
manganese	2 mg daily.	

Herbs

❏ Any of the following herbs can be beneficial for the nursing mother: alfalfa, blessed thistle, dandelion, fennel, and raspberry.

❏ Nettle leaf has a tonic effect and contains iron, in addition to many other nutrients.

❏ The following herbs decrease milk supply, and should be avoided until a woman is no longer nursing: black walnut, sage, and yarrow.

Caution: Do not use sage if you suffer from any type of seizure disorder, or are pregnant or nursing.

Recommendations

❏ Eat plenty of brewer's yeast, eggs, nuts and seeds, and whole grains. Raw foods should be plentiful in the diet.

Caution: Brewer's yeast can cause an allergic reaction in some individuals. Start with a small amount at first, and discontinue use if any allergic symptoms occur.

❏ A mother's milk is a nearly perfect food. However, it is low in vitamins A, D, and C. A nursing mother should maintain a balanced diet, but can also benefit from taking prenatal multivitamins and nutritional supplements like calcium, vitamin D, and fish oil. Discuss the need for supplements with your health care provider.

❏ Despite the conflicting data, if you need to supplement your infant's diet, use infant formula with DHA (docosahexaenoic acid) and ARA (arachidonic acid). Babies under six months should not have anything but water, breast milk, and infant formula—unless otherwise recommended by the child's pediatrician.

Considerations

❏ The UCLA Medical School has reported that mother's milk kills a tiny parasite (*Giardia lamblia*) that can cause intestinal disease in children.

❏ In recent studies, mothers who consumed garlic increased their babies' desire for milk, and the babies nursed longer. Garlic is good for both the mother and the infant. Kyolic from Wakunaga is an ideal way to consume garlic since it is odorless and is therefore more "sociable."

❏ Since breast milk is produced from protein drawn from either your diet or the protein stored in your body, you should consider increasing your protein intake, especially during postpartum weight loss. Studies show you will lose body fat, but not muscle. Make sure you get some exercise and do not overeat calories from fat and carbohydrate.

❏ The American Academy of Pediatrics (AAP) published a revised version of their 1998 guidelines urging women to breast-feed their infants. This restates their position that breast milk is the foundation of good infant nutrition. They recommend that newborns receive nothing other than breast milk for the first six months, meaning no juices, fluorides, iron, or vitamins. This will reduce the risk of obesity later in life. More information can be found at http://aap-policy.aappublications.org.

❏ Dr. Ruth Lawrence, author of *Breastfeeding: A Guide for the Medical Profession,* says that, depending on the mother's wishes, breast-feeding should continue for at least a year, along with other foods as they are introduced, and even longer if the mother feels it is best for her and her child.

❏ More than 90 percent of pregnant women take prescription or nonprescription drugs, or use social drugs (tobacco, alcohol) at some time during pregnancy. Some drugs are essential for health, but none should be used without consulting with your health care provider. Drugs can affect the fetus by causing direct damage such as abnormal development, altering placental function, and causing the uterus to contract prematurely. The FDA has classified drugs according to the degree of risk they pose for the fetus. Some are highly toxic and are never used (such as thalidomide). Sometimes safer drugs can be substituted for ones that are more toxic. For example, penicillin is a relatively safe antibiotic. Most antidepressants appear to be safe during pregnancy. Some drugs that cause the most problems during pregnancy include:

- antianxiety drugs (diazepam)

- antibiotics (chloramphenicol, kanamycin, nitrofurantoin, tetracycline)

- anticoagulants (heparin, warfarin)

- anticonvulsants (phenobarbital, phenytoin)

- antihypertensives (ACE inhibitors, beta-blockers, diuretics)

- mood-stablizing drugs (lithium)

- NSAIDS (aspirin, ibuprofren, naproxen)

- thyroid drugs (methimazole, radioactive iodine)

- vaccines with live virus (vaccine for German measles, and measles, mumps, polio). The H1N1 and regular flu shots are OK.

❏ In a study of new mothers, those who were trained and sent home from the hospital with a breast pump were found to breast-feed their infants longer than those who were given no pumps.

❑ Breast-fed babies may have a lower risk of becoming sick from several diseases later in life. For example, one study found breast-fed babies were less likely to get meningitis between the ages of five and ten. A Chinese study found that breast-feeding reduced the risk of lymphoma by 31 percent. Another study found that breast-feeding reduced the number of earaches in the first two years of life—even if the baby was only breast-fed for three months.

❑ Breast milk contains high amounts of inositol, a B vitamin that plays a crucial role in survival and infant development.

❑ Women who undergo reduction mammoplasty (breast-reduction surgery) and subsequently become pregnant can retain the ability to lactate and nurse. However, in one study, only 35 percent of such women breast-fed successfully, whereas 65 percent either did not breast-feed or discontinued nursing for various reasons. It was not disclosed whether any of these women were actually unable to secrete sufficient amounts of milk to nurse their babies. Women who are considering breast-reduction surgery should nevertheless consider this if they wish to have children later on and hope to breast-feed.

❑ Included among AAP recommendations to hospitals, pediatricians, and mothers are the following:

• Even if the baby and mother are hospitalized, breast-feeding should continue unless the mother is required to take a medication that could be harmful to the breast-feeding infant. If so, breast-feeding should only be stopped temporarily, until the mother's body no longer contains traces of the medication(s).

• Private areas for breast-feeding mothers should be provided by all hospitals.

• Breast pumps should be provided to breast-feeding mothers in hospitals.

• Insurance companies should be encouraged to provide breast-feeding services and supplies as part of coverage policies.

❑ There are resources available to help women learn to breast-feed successfully and overcome any problems that arise. Certified lactation consultants are practitioners who specialize in this area. Your health care provider or the facility where you give birth should be able to give you a referral.

❑ La Leche League is another valuable resource for the breast-feeding mother. This is an organization of nursing women that can serve as both an educational resource and a support group. Consult your local telephone directory for the chapter nearest you, or contact La Leche League International. (See Health and Medical Organizations in the Appendix.)

BRONCHITIS

The lungs are among the body's largest organs. The air we breathe enters our bodies through the trachea (windpipe), which connects with the bronchi, the breathing tubes that lead into the alveoli (air sacs) in the lungs. In the lungs, air is exchanged for carbon dioxide.

Doctors use the term chronic obstructive pulmonary disease (COPD) to describe lung damage caused by emphysema or chronic bronchitis. Emphysema hurts the lung's air sacs, while bronchitis injures the airway tubes. Both diseases make it hard for the lungs to take in enough oxygen. Oxidative stress worsens COPD, so antioxidants may help improve symptoms. However, in one study, use of a potent antioxidant, 600 milligrams of N-acetylcysteine, had no effect on preventing the deterioration of lung function and preventing exacerbation of symptoms in patients with COPD.

Bronchitis is an inflammation or obstruction in the bronchial tubes. This inflammation results in a buildup of mucus, along with coughing, fever, pain in the chest and/or back, fatigue, sore throat, difficulty breathing, and, often, sudden chills and shaking. Bronchitis occurs mostly in the winter and usually starts as a cold.

Bronchitis can be either acute or chronic. Acute bronchitis is usually caused by an infection, which can be bacterial, viral, chlamydial, mycoplasmal, or caused by a combination of agents. It typically follows an upper respiratory tract infection, such as a cold or influenza. Most cases of acute bronchitis are self-limiting, with full recovery in a matter of weeks. In some cases, however, the condition can lead to pneumonia. This is more likely to occur in those who also have a chronic respiratory disease or other debilitating health problem.

Chronic bronchitis results from frequent irritation of the lungs, such as from exposure to cigarette smoke, air pollutants, or other noxious fumes, rather than from infection.

Allergies may also be the cause of chronic bronchitis. As chronic bronchitis diminishes the exchange of oxygen and carbon dioxide in the lungs, the heart works harder in an attempt to compensate. Over time, this can lead to pulmonary hypertension, enlargement of the heart, and, ultimately, heart failure.

Chronic bronchitis is one of the most common diseases seen by allergists, otolaryngologists, and primary care physicians. Specialists in occupational medicine have long known that an adverse environment produces a vulnerability to respiratory infections. Climatic factors and epidemics of viral infections also increase the risk. Among people who live or work in unhealthy environments, shortness of breath is frequently aggravated by dampness and cold, exposure to dust, humid weather, or even minor respiratory infections.

More women than men develop chronic bronchitis. The disease is more prevalent in those age forty-five years and older. According to the Centers for Disease Control and

Prevention (CDC), in 2006 an estimated 740 Americans died from results of chronic and unspecified bronchitis. The COPD family of lung disorders is the fourth leading cause of death, and it is predicted that by the year 2020 COPD diseases will become the third leading cause of death.

Unless otherwise specified, the following recommended doses are for those over the age of eighteen. For a child between twelve and seventeen years old, reduce the dose to three-quarters of the recommended amount. For a child between six and twelve years old, use one-half of the recommended dose, and for a child under six, use one-quarter of the recommended amount.

NUTRIENTS

SUPPLEMENT	SUGGESTED DOSAGE	COMMENTS
Essential		
Pycnogenol	As directed on label.	Removes dangerous substances and protects the lungs. A powerful antioxidant.
Quercitin-C from Ecological Formulas or	500 mg 3 times daily.	For allergic bronchitis. Has an antihistaminic effect.
Activated Quercetin from Source Naturals	As directed on label.	Contains quercetin plus bromelain and vitamin C for increased absorption.
Vitamin A	20,000 IU twice daily for 1 month; then reduce to 15,000 IU daily. If you are pregnant, do not exceed 10,000 IU daily.	As directed on label. For healing and protection of all tissues.
plus natural beta-carotene or	50,000 IU daily.	Needed for protection and repair of lung tissue.
carotenoid complex (Betatene)	As directed on label.	
Vitamin C with bioflavonoids (including rutin)	3,000–10,000 mg daily, in divided doses.	Enhances immune function and reduces histamine levels. Use a buffered powder form.
Very Important		
Coenzyme Q10 plus	60 mg daily.	For improved circulation and breathing.
Coenzme A from Coenzyme-A Technologies	As directed on label.	Works well with coenzyme Q10 and removes dangerous substances from the body.
Methylsulfonyl-methane (MSM)	As directed on label.	Clinical tests have shown that this improves lung problems such as bronchitis, pneumonia, emphysema, cysts, or damage due to heavy smoking.
Proteolytic enzymes with bromelain	As directed on label. Take between meals.	Helps reduce inflammation.
Vitamin E	200 IU daily. Take with 50–100 mg vitamin C.	Powerful free radical scavenger and oxygen carrier. Needed for healing of tissues and improved breathing. Use d-alpha-tocopherol form.
Zinc lozenges	One 15-mg lozenge 5 times daily. Do not exceed a total of 100 mg daily from all supplements.	Needed for repair of all tissues.
Important		
Chlorophyll and	As directed on label, 3 times daily.	To improve circulation, and to keep tissues free of toxic substances. Use a liquid or tablet form.
"green drinks" (fresh wheatgrass juice or Kyo-Green from Wakunaga)	As directed on label.	To supply chlorophyll and important nutrients.
Garlic (Kyolic from Wakunaga)	2 tablets 3 times daily, with meals.	A natural antibiotic that reduces infection and detoxifies the body.
Vitamin B complex	100 mg of each major B vitamin 3 times daily (amounts of individual vitamins in a complex will vary).	Activates many enzymes needed for healing.
Helpful		
Magnesium plus	500 mg daily.	Acts as a bronchodilator. Use chelate or asporotate form.
calcium	1,000 mg daily.	Needed to balance with magnesium.
Maitake extract or	As directed on label.	Mushroom extracts that boost immunity and fight viral infection.
shiitake extract or	As directed on label.	
reishi extract	As directed on label.	
Multivitamin complex	As directed on label.	All nutrients are needed in balance for healing.
N-Acetylcysteine (NAC)	500 mg twice daily, on an empty stomach. Take with water or juice. Do not take with milk. Take with 50 mg vitamin B6 and 100 mg vitamin C for better absorption.	Protects and preserves the cells. A sulfur-bearing amino acid that lessens the viscosity of bronchial mucus, making it easier to expel. (*See* AMINO ACIDS in Part One.)
plus L-arginine and	500 mg twice daily, on an empty stomach.	Aids in liver detoxification.
L-lysine and	500 mg twice daily, on an empty stomach.	Needed for protein synthesis to aid in healing. Also aids in destroying serious viruses.
L-ornithine	500 mg twice daily, on an empty stomach.	Lowers blood ammonia levels, which can be increased by respiratory illness.
Raw thymus glandular	500 mg twice daily.	Needed to protect and enhance immune function. (*See* GLANDULAR THERAPY in Part Three.)
Silica	As directed on label.	Acts as an anti-inflammatory, reduces mucus flow, and reduces coughing.

Herbs

Herbal medicine has proven to be very effective in the treatment of bronchitis. The following treatment plans may be helpful in alleviating some of the symptoms common to bronchitis. Rather than using only one of the herbs listed below, alternate among several to get all of their healing benefits.

❑ American and Siberian ginseng are especially good for the lungs. They clear bronchial passages and reduce inflammation.

Cautions: Do not use American ginseng if you have high blood pressure, or are pregnant or nursing. Do not use Siberian ginseng if you have hypoglycemia, high blood pressure, or a heart disorder.

❑ Astragalus, myrrh, olive oil extract, and pau d'arco are natural antibiotics.

Caution: Do not use astragalus in the presence of a fever.

❑ Black radish, chickweed, elderberry, ginkgo biloba, lobelia, and mullein improve lung and bronchial congestion and circulation.

Cautions: Do not take ginkgo biloba if you have a bleeding disorder, or are scheduled for surgery or a dental procedure. Lobelia is only to be taken under supervision of a health care professional as it is potentially toxic. People with high blood pressure, heart disease, liver disease, kidney disease, seizure disorders, or shortness of breath should not take lobelia. Pregnant and lactating women should avoid lobelia as well.

❑ Boneset contains immunostimulatory polysaccharides that are good for inflammation of the mucous membranes.

Caution: Do not use boneset on a daily basis for more than one week, as long-term use can lead to toxicity.

❑ Boswellia, bromelain, cayenne, ginger, and peppermint can aid in reducing inflammation.

❑ Bronc-Ease from Nature's Herbs is an excellent herbal formula. It relieves congestion, coughing, and irritation.

❑ Expectorant herbs such as cayenne, elecampane, horehound, hyssop, and mullein have been effective in clearing congestion.

❑ Coltsfoot, slippery elm bark, and wild cherry bark soothe the throat and are good for a cough.

❑ Cordyceps is an herb used in Chinese medicine to restore the yin and yang connection between the lungs and the kidneys. It is said to contain inhibitor substances that attack damaged lung cells and may slow down the degeneration of the lung. Bai qian (*Cynanchum stautoni*), another Chinese herb, aids in coughing up the sputum obstructing the bronchial passageways.

❑ Echinacea, licorice, and Siberian ginseng are good for building up the immune system.

Cautions: Do not take echinacea for longer than three months. It should not be used by people who are allergic to ragweed. Licorice root should not be used during pregnancy or nursing. It should not be used by persons with diabetes, glaucoma, heart disease, high blood pressure, or a history of stroke. Do not use Siberian ginseng if you have hypoglycemia, high blood pressure, or a heart disorder.

❑ Echinacea and goldenseal help to fight viruses and bacteria and boost the immune system. At the first sign of illness, put ½ dropperful in your mouth. Hold it there for ten minutes, then swallow. Do this every three hours until symptoms are relieved (but not for longer than one week at a time). Be sure to use the alcohol-free extracts.

Cautions: Do not take echinacea for longer than three months. It should not be used by people who are allergic to ragweed. Do not take goldenseal internally on a daily basis for more than one week at a time. Do not use it during pregnancy or if you are breast-feeding, and use with caution if you are allergic to ragweed. If you have a history of cardiovascular disease, diabetes, or glaucoma, use it only under a doctor's supervision.

❑ Inhaling the vapors of eucalyptus leaves helps to relieve respiratory problems. To use eucalyptus as a steam inhaler, boil a quart of water, remove the boiling water from the stove, and add 6 to 8 drops of eucalyptus extract. Place a towel over your head and breathe in deeply through the nose, holding your breath for as long as is comfortable.

❑ Fenugreek is good for reducing the flow of mucus.

❑ Ginkgo biloba leaf is a free-radical fighter that is especially good for the lungs.

Caution: Do not take ginkgo biloba if you have a bleeding disorder, or are scheduled for surgery or a dental procedure.

❑ Goldenseal has antibiotic properties and is good for all conditions involving inflammation of the mucous membranes of the bronchial tubes, throat, nasal passages, and sinuses. In addition to taking goldenseal orally, you can place a cloth soaked with a strong goldenseal tea under a hot water bottle. Place 3 wet goldenseal tea bags on each lung under the soaked cloth.

Caution: Do not take goldenseal internally on a daily basis for more than one week at a time. Do not use it during pregnancy or if you are breast-feeding, and use with caution if you are allergic to ragweed. If you have a history of cardiovascular disease, diabetes, or glaucoma, use it only under a doctor's supervision.

❑ Gumplant (*Grindelia squarrosa*) is an expectorant and antispasmodic.

❑ Iceland moss is good for mucus congestion.

❑ A massage with essential oil of lavender is good for bronchitis. Also, to relieve congestion, put 4 drops of lavender oil, alone or combined with eucalyptus and lemon oils, in a pot of steaming water. Hold your head, covered with a towel, over the steaming pot and inhale the vapors.

Caution: Lavender oil is not to be taken internally.

❑ Lobelia may be rubbed directly on the chest to aid in breathing. It can also be used as an expectorant.

Caution: Use with caution, as too much may induce vomiting. Lobelia is only to be taken under supervision of a health care professional as it is potentially toxic. People with high blood pressure, heart disease, liver disease, kidney disease, seizure disorders, or shortness of breath should not take lobelia. Pregnant and lactating women should avoid lobelia as well.

❏ Lomatium (*Lomatium dissectum*) has been used by Native Americans to treat bronchitis. Lomatium acts in reducing mucus in the lungs and has an antibacterial effect.

❏ Lung Tonic from Herbs, Etc., is a combination of many organic herbs designed to support the lungs.

❏ Lungwort leaves are rich in vitamin C and quercetin and make an effective treatment for coughs and mucus.

❏ Thyme strengthens the lung tissue. It can be used for children with lung ailments.

❏ Omega-3 fatty acids are clearly associated with a reduction in chronic bronchitis.

Recommendations

❏ Include garlic and onions in your diet. These foods contain quercetin and mustard oils, which have been shown to inhibit lipoxygenase, an enzyme that aids in releasing an inflammatory chemical in the body. Garlic is also a natural antibiotic.

❏ Drink plenty of fluids. Pure water, herbal teas, and soups are all good choices.

❏ Avoid mucus-forming foods such as dairy products, processed foods, sugar, sweet fruits, and white flour; also avoid gas-producing foods such as beans, cabbage, cauliflower, and so on. Substitute soymilk for dairy foods to get adequate calcium and vitamin D. One epidemiological study showed the more vegetables eaten the less bronchitis.

❏ Do not smoke, and avoid secondhand smoke. Cigarette smoke is very harmful. If you have chronic bronchitis, little improvement can be expected unless the irritating substances that cause the mucus to clog the air passages are eliminated.

❏ It is not correct to assume that chronic bronchitis is a smoking-based disorder as commonly believed. *Helicobacter pylori* is an infection associated with chronic bronchitis.

❏ Add moisture to the air. Use a humidifier, a vaporizer, or even a pan of water placed on a radiator. Clean everything frequently to prevent the growth of bacteria.

❏ Rest in bed in the early stages, when fever is present. Once fever subsides and you are feeling better, alternate periods of rest with periods of moderate activity to prevent secretions from settling in the lungs.

❏ Apply warm, moist heat, or a hot water bottle over the chest and back before bedtime to aid in sleeping and reduce inflammation. It is also good to rub eucalyptus oil on your chest first.

❏ To aid recovery, blow up a balloon a few times daily.

❏ Supplement your diet with vitamin C.

❏ Do not use a cough suppressant if you have bronchitis.

❏ Do not swallow mucus.

❏ If persistent and/or severe coughing, difficulty breathing, high fever, lethargy, weakness, wheezing sounds, and/or chest pains develop, consult your health care provider. These may be signs of developing pneumonia. (*See* PNEUMONIA in Part Two.)

❏ If you are hospitalized, at first you will need to rest in bed, with a few pillows to keep you sitting up a little. This will help your breathing. Do not lie flat. You may also need oxygen at this time. It is administered either by a mask or nasal prongs. Blood will also be drawn to test for oxygen content.

Considerations

❏ Diet, nutrition, and environment all play important roles in any respiratory disease. A healthy household environment can make respiratory problems easier to control.

❏ Scientists have found many nutrients that make the lungs and bronchioles stronger and, therefore, better able to fight off infections. Many of these nutrients also make the lungs less sensitive to the air particles that can sometimes trigger bronchitis.

❏ For people who are unable to cough up sputum, bronchoscopy may be recommended. This is a procedure in which a flexible tube is inserted to examine the bronchial tree. It can be done simply for the sake of a visual examination, to suction out congestion, to remove foreign bodies, or even to biopsy (sample) tissue from the bronchial tubes for the purpose of identifying the infecting organism.

❏ If bronchitis does not clear up in a reasonable amount of time, a chest X-ray may be recommended to rule out lung cancer, emphysema, tuberculosis, or other conditions that can cause similar symptoms.

❏ It is not unusual for people with chronic respiratory disorders to be taking a variety of medications—inhalers, antianxiety medications, even diuretics—to help them breathe. Exercise is important; it helps one to breathe more efficiently and to tolerate daily activities.

❏ If bacteria are the cause of acute bronchitis, treatment with antibiotics may be necessary to cure the infection and to prevent pneumonia from developing.

❏ To prevent chronic lung disease in infants, doctors often prescribe the steroid dexamethasone to reduce inflammation.

Caution: A long-term study found that this common steroid treatment for premature babies can damage their brains and stunt their growth.

❏ A common treatment for bronchitis is a bronchodilator. If you use a bronchodilator, do not inhale more than the prescribed dose, as larger doses may cause side effects, including nervousness, restlessness, and trembling. Before using an inhaler, discuss with your doctor possible side effects and warning signs of dangerous reactions. Your doctor should be aware of any personal health concerns you have, such as a possible pregnancy; a medical problem, such as diabetes, hypothyroidism, or a seizure disorder; a history of drug use; adverse reactions to drugs; or current use of other over-the-counter or prescription drugs.

❑ The Air Supply personal air purifier from Wein Products is a small unit worn around the neck. It sets up an invisible pure air shield against microorganisms (such as viruses, bacteria, and mold) and microparticles (including dust, pollen, and pollutants) in the air. It also eliminates vapors, smells, and harmful volatile compounds in the air. The Air Supply is a very useful item when traveling, especially on a long flight when the air becomes stale.

❑ *See also* ASTHMA; EMPHYSEMA; HAY FEVER; PNEUMONIA; and SINUSITIS in Part Two.

BROWN-SEQUARD SYNDROME

See under RARE DISORDERS.

BRUISING

A bruise occurs when the tissues underlying the skin become injured. The skin is not broken, but the delicate capillaries (small blood vessels) below the skin's surface rupture, and blood drains out into the surrounding area.

The blood seeps into the layers of the skin, resulting in pain, swelling, and "black-and-blue marks"—discoloration that starts out red, then turns dark and bluish, and finally may become a yellowish color as the blood under the skin is absorbed.

Body parts often become bruised after banging into hard objects. This is normal. There are other factors that do not involve a trauma to the skin that can cause bruising.

People who do not eat enough fresh, uncooked foods to supply the body with needed nutrients are prone to easy bruising. Nutritional deficiencies, especially in vitamin C, or blood-clotting disorders can make the blood vessel walls very thin and delicate, causing them to rupture with even the slightest amount of pressure, such as leaning against a table or having someone grab you firmly with his or her hand. Unexplained or easy bruising can be related to heavy smoking or menstruation, or it can be an indication of an underlying health condition, including allergies, anemia, cancer, hemophilia, infections, obesity, myelocytic leukemia, and abnormal platelet function caused by a liver or kidney disorder. Any condition where blood platelet levels are too low may result in excess bruising. Most yearly physical exams should measure platelet number. If you are concerned, you can check with your doctor to learn what your number is.

Unless otherwise specified, the following recommended doses are for those over the age of eighteen. For a child between twelve and seventeen years old, reduce the dose to three-quarters the recommended amount. For a child between six and twelve years old, use one-half the recommended dose, and for a child under six, use one-quarter the recommended amount.

NUTRIENTS

SUPPLEMENT	SUGGESTED DOSAGE	COMMENTS
Very Important		
Multivitamin and mineral complex with zinc	As directed on label.	Needed to strengthen skin and reduce bruising.
Vitamin C with bioflavonoids	3,000–10,000 mg daily, in divided doses.	Helps to prevent bruising by supplying oxygen to the injured cells and strengthening capillary walls.
Vitamin K or alfalfa	As directed on label.	Necessary for blood clotting and healing. *See* under Herbs, below. *Caution:* Check with your physician first.
Important		
Inositol hexaphosphate (IP₆) (Cell Forté with IP-6 from Enzymatic Therapy or IP6 from Jarrow Formulas)	As directed on label.	A powerful antioxidant. Prevents blood clots.
Vitamin E	200 IU daily.	Powerful antioxidant. Also improves circulation in body tissues and prolongs the life of red blood cells. Fights cellular aging by protecting cell membranes. Use d-alpha-tocopherol form.
Helpful		
Coenzyme Q₁₀	60 mg daily.	Essential for construction and reconstruction of body cells.
Dimethylglycine (DMG) (Aangamik DMG from FoodScience of Vermont)	100 mg daily.	Improves oxygen metabolism in the cells and tissues.
Iron fumarate from (Floradix	As directed by physician. Take with 100 mg vitamin C for better absorption.	To correct deficiencies. *Caution:* Do not take iron unless anemia is diagnosed.
Iron + Herbs from Salus Haus)	As directed on label.	A natural iron supplement.
Multienzyme complex plus proteolytic enzymes	As directed on label. Take with meals. As directed on label. Take between meals.	To prevent inflammation in bruised areas.
Pycnogenol or grape seed extract	As directed on label.	Potent antioxidants for protecting skin tissue.
Vitamin B complex	100 mg of each major B vitamin twice daily (amounts of individual vitamins in a complex will vary).	Aids in protecting the tissues.
Vitamin D plus calcium and magnesium	400–800 IU daily. 2,000 mg daily. 1,000 mg daily.	To help protect the skin. Needed for blood cell formation.

Herbs

❑ Alfalfa supplies beneficial minerals and vitamin K, which is needed for healing. Take it in tablet form as directed on the product label.

❑ Bluebottle, buchu, and comfrey root have all been known to reduce the swelling, pain, and discoloration of bruising in some people. Make a tea from them and place a terry cloth towel that has been soaked in the tea over the bruised area for twenty minutes at a time, two or three times daily.

Caution: Comfrey is recommended for external use only.

❑ An ointment made by adding one part ground cayenne pepper to five parts melted Vaseline has been used successfully in China and Taiwan for treating bruises. Mix the combination well and cool. Apply it once every one or two days.

❑ Dandelion and yellow dock are good sources of iron.

❑ Oil of oregano, applied topically, has had some positive effects on healing bruises.

❑ Fresh parsley leaves, crushed and applied directly to the bruise, are known to ease discoloration within a few days.

❑ Wild pansy can be applied externally to treat a bruise.

❑ Other beneficial herbs include bilberry, black walnut, garlic extract, and rose hips.

Recommendations

❑ To minimize bruising, as soon as possible after an injury, place an ice pack on the bruised area and keep it in place for twenty to thirty minutes. This stops the bleeding by constricting the blood vessels. If the bruise is severe, you may wish to further treat the injured area with an ice pack every two to three waking hours for twenty-four to forty-eight hours, and then switch to fifteen minutes of heat, three times daily. The injured area should also be elevated above heart level, if possible, to allow blood to flow away from the injured area and minimize the bruise.

❑ If you have a bruise in an area of the body that requires a moldable ice pack, fill a plastic bag or a rubber surgical glove with a solution of two parts water and one part rubbing alcohol and put it in the freezer. The bag will be pliable and conform to your body, and it won't "sweat" like most ice packs do. This would be an ideal ice pack for a black eye. Another excellent ice pack for the eye, or any area, is a bag of frozen peas! They conform to any injured area and can be used over and over again. Be sure to set this bag of peas aside for use as an ice pack only; you should not consume the peas after they have been thawed and refrozen.

❑ To reduce the pain, swelling, and discoloration of a black eye, immediately apply cold compresses and an ice pack to the injury. Unfortunately, if the discoloration has set in before the ice bag has been applied, there will be little hope of lightening the bruise.

❑ Rub a sterile cotton ball soaked with distilled witch hazel on an injury to stop the swelling.

❑ To reduce discoloration and soreness, try applying shredded raw potato directly to the injury for about an hour.

❑ Eat a lot of fresh, uncooked foods—people who do not eat enough of these can be prone to easy bruising.

❑ Eat an abundance of dark green leafy vegetables, buckwheat, and fresh fruits. These foods are high in vitamin C and bioflavonoids, which help to prevent bruising. Dark leafy greens such as broccoli, Brussels sprouts, cabbage, kale, and spinach are also good sources of vitamin K, which is necessary for blood clotting and healing.

❑ Eat plenty of products rich in zinc, such as chicken, eggs, soybeans, and wheat germ. Zinc is important for strengthening blood vessel walls and aids in blood clotting.

❑ Try taking vitamin C with bioflavonoids if you find you are bruising very easily, as a deficiency in these often causes easy or unexplained bruising.

❑ Do not take aspirin or ibuprofen (Advil, Nuprin, and others) for pain, as these can worsen the discoloration due to their blood-thinning qualities. Instead, take acetaminophen (such as Tylenol) as directed on the label.

❑ Do not take any nonsteroidal anti-inflammatory drugs (NSAIDs). If bruising is frequent, consult your health care provider.

Considerations

❑ Bruising that is accompanied by swollen and/or bleeding gums can be an indication of a deficiency in vitamin C, folic acid, or riboflavin.

❑ Studies show that people with vitamin C deficiencies bruise more easily than others, probably because their blood vessels are generally weaker. Other studies have shown that vitamin C can actually reduce the time it takes for the discoloration to fade.

❑ A "black eye" is actually a bruise in the cheek, eyebrow, and/or eyelid area. An impact hard enough to cause a black eye can also cause damage to the eye itself. If your eye has swollen shut, it should not be forced open or pressed on in any way. Blurry vision or "seeing double" should prompt you to see an ophthalmologist, who may prescribe an antibiotic and/or an eye patch to protect the eye while healing.

❑ If a bruise does not begin to heal within a week, you may want to have your doctor examine it.

❑ Some people can bruise as a result of taking medications that can interfere with normal blood clotting, including local anesthetics, prescription anticoagulants, antidepressants, antihistamines, aspirin, cortisone, and penicillin. If you are taking any of these medications and find that bruises are appearing without any reason, you should contact your doctor, who may change or discontinue your medication.

❏ If you have bruising underneath the fingernails, this may be an early indication of skin melanoma. Consult your doctor.

BRUXISM

Bruxism, or bruxomania, is the medical term for tooth-grinding. This usually occurs during sleep, often without the person being aware of it (although family members may be). It can also occur when a person is awake, as a way of releasing tension. Over time, chronic tooth-grinding can result in loosened teeth with damage to the supporting bones in the jaw and receding gums. The teeth may be pushed out of line, and the bite may need adjusting. Eventually, tooth loss can occur. Long-term tooth-grinding can cause temporomandibular joint (TMJ) syndrome. This usually occurs in the muscles, joints, and disks of the jaw, and may cause pain while chewing. (*See* TMJ SYNDROME in Part Two.)

Bruxism can develop if the teeth are sensitive to heat and cold. Stress, allergies, and nutrient deficiencies are often the cause of tooth-grinding, which can also involve blood sugar levels.

NUTRIENTS

SUPPLEMENT	SUGGESTED DOSAGE	COMMENTS
Essential		
Calcium and magnesium	1,500–2,000 mg daily. 750 mg daily.	Deficiencies have been linked to tooth-grinding.
Vitamin B₅ (pantothenic acid)	500 mg twice daily.	Reduces stress.
Vitamin B complex	100 mg of each major B vitamin twice daily (amounts of individual vitamins in a complex will vary).	Necessary for proper nerve function. Use a high-stress formula.
Very Important		
Vitamin C with bioflavonoids	3,000–5,000 mg daily.	Potentiates adrenal function; acts as an antistress vitamin.
Helpful		
Chromium	200–400 mcg daily.	Helps to normalize blood sugar levels. Use chromium picolinate form. Hypoglycemia is often linked to this disorder.
L-tryosine	As directed on label.	An amino acid that reduces stress.
Melatonin	As directed on label.	Aids restful sleep and may reduce tooth-grinding. Not recommended for anyone under 30, or for long-term use.
Multivitamin and mineral complex plus	As directed on label.	All nutrients are needed to reduce stress.
raw adrenal glandular	As directed on label.	To support adrenal function. (*See* GLANDULAR THERAPY in Part Three.)
S-adenosylmethionine (SAMe)	As directed on label.	Reduces stress and acts as an antidepressant. *Caution:* Do not use if you have bipolar mood disorder or take prescription antidepressants. Don't give to a child under twelve.
Zinc	50 mg daily. Do not exceed a total of 100 mg daily from all supplements.	Helps to support the immune system and reduce stress.

Recommendations

❏ Adopt a hypoglycemic diet that is high in fiber and protein and includes plenty of fresh vegetables and high-fiber fruits, plus legumes, raw nuts and seeds, skinless white turkey or chicken, broiled fish, and whole grains. Consume starchy vegetables and very sweet fruits in moderation only. Eat six to eight small meals spread evenly throughout the day rather than two or three large meals. Hypoglycemia, related to low adrenal function, is often the cause of bruxism. (*See* HYPOGLYCEMIA in Part Two.)

❏ Do not consume alcoholic beverages. Alcohol often makes the problem worse.

❏ Avoid fast foods, fried foods, processed foods, red meat, refined sugar, saturated fats, and all dairy products except for yogurt, kefir, and raw cheese. Also avoid all foods with artificial flavors, colors, preservatives, and other chemicals.

❏ Do not eat anything sweet within six hours of going to bed. If you are hungry, have a light protein-and-fiber snack.

❏ As much as possible, avoid stress. Learn stress management and relaxation techniques. (*See* STRESS in Part Two.)

❏ Take supplemental calcium and pantothenic acid as directed under Nutrients, above. Calcium is often effective for treating involuntary movement of muscles.

❏ Consider having a hair analysis done to determine if you have any mineral imbalances, such as abnormal levels of sodium and potassium. (*See* HAIR ANALYSIS in Part Three.)

❏ *See* ALLERGIES in Part Two to rule out any food allergies that may be the problem.

Considerations

❏ Dentists sometimes recommend a type of plastic mouth guard that is worn over the teeth for people with bruxism. This does not cure the problem, but it can help to prevent future tooth damage.

❏ *Belladonna*, a homeopathic remedy, is known to be an effective treatment for this condition.

❏ Biofeedback is helpful for overcoming bruxism in some cases. (*See* BIOFEEDBACK *under* PAIN CONTROL in Part Three.)

BULIMIA

Bulimia nervosa is an eating disorder characterized by episodes of uncontrolled binge eating, often involving extremely large amounts of high-calorie foods, followed by one or more of the following: induced vomiting or the use of laxatives, diuretics, or enemas; and/or obsessive exercising to "purge" the body of the food eaten during the binge. The binge/purge episodes vary in frequency, from a few times a week to several times daily. The length of the bingeing can range from several minutes to an hour or two.

Usually the person doing the bingeing feels out of control—a sense of not being able to stop eating until he or she is completely full—then is so immediately overwhelmed and shamed by the sense of fullness that he or she feels the need to get rid of the food just consumed. The binge eating and purging are usually carried out in secret—an indication of a serious medical and psychological problem with potentially dangerous complications.

Some of the many serious problems bulimia can lead to include anemia, depletion of fluid balance, electrolyte imbalances, erratic heartbeat, hypoglycemia, infertility, internal bleeding, kidney or liver damage, malnutrition, cessation of the menstrual cycles, mental fuzziness, loss of muscle and bone mass, a low pulse rate and blood pressure, a ruptured stomach or esophagus, stones in the salivary glands, tooth and/or gum erosion, ulcers, and a weakened immune system. Also, if the fat content in a woman's body drops to too low a level, the body will not produce enough estrogen, which can result in destruction of bone tissue and an increased risk of osteoporosis. Due to extreme weight loss, extreme exercise, starvation, and/or lack of needed vitamins and minerals, the body can turn to using muscle mass as an energy source—a very serious side effect that few with eating disorders are aware of. Eventually, life-threatening problems can result, including cancers of the breast, bowel, esophagus, or reproductive organs; kidney or liver damage; and finally, cardiac arrest.

According to the National Association of Anorexia Nervosa and Associated Disorders, there are 8 million men and women with eating disorders in the United States, and this number is on the rise. Bulimia affects many more women than men (although the number of men with this disorder is increasing), and it does not discriminate on the basis of age, sex, or social status. In today's society, we are constantly bombarded with the message that the thinner you are, the better you look. Our role models are mostly actors/ actresses, musicians, and models who set standards of beauty that are difficult or impossible for most people to attain.

Although people may develop an eating disorder because they want to look and feel better about themselves, the opposite is usually the result. People with bulimia can become consumed with their weight, have a distorted image of their figures, and feel disgusted with themselves for not having what they think of as the "perfect body." Other typical psychological implications can include extreme anger at anyone they believe is trying to interfere, anxiety, depression, fear of being found out, isolation, loneliness, and obsessive-compulsive behavior. People with bulimia may also exhibit other extreme behavior, such as alcohol or drug abuse, credit card abuse, or shoplifting. They usually spend an exorbitant amount of money on food, sometimes using money meant for paying bills or other necessities to buy certain foods, and they may also bypass social or work-related obligations for an opportunity to binge.

Although there is no known cause of eating disorders, many believe that bulimia may result from one or a combination of psychological, biological, and societal factors.

Some studies of families and twins suggest that heredity may also play a role. Psychologically, food has offered us pleasure, comfort, solace, and security from the moment we are born. Episodes of bingeing are commonly stress-related, and they may be an attempt to manage emotions by focusing attention away from unpleasant or uncomfortable emotional problems. Many individuals who suffer from this disorder come from families in which they were subjected to physical or sexual abuse. In some families, substance abuse is also a factor. Many women started their first binge because of real or imagined male rejection. Others are perfectionists and overachievers with high standards, but low self-esteem.

In particular, if a woman's basic emotional needs were not met in childhood, she may come to believe that her problems would be resolved if only she were attractive (that is, thin) enough, and this obsession leads to bulimia.

There are indications of possible physiological elements in this disorder, as well. For example, people with eating disorders tend to have a type of chemical imbalance similar to one found in people with clinical depression. Both have high levels of adrenocorticotropic hormone (ACTH), produced by the pituitary gland, which inhibits T cell function and thereby depresses immunity. People who suffer from bulimia may also have low levels of the neurotransmitter serotonin, which can lead to cravings for simple carbohydrates—common binge foods. Some researchers have found bulimia to be associated with right temporal disturbance in the brain.

Unlike people with anorexia, whose self-starvation eventually becomes obvious, those with bulimia can hide the disorder for long periods, even years, because their weight is usually in the normal range (some are even overweight, depending on the frequency and length of the bingeing episodes) and the bingeing and purging are done in secret.

Physical signs of bulimia may be swollen glands in the face (resulting in a "chipmunk" appearance) and neck; erosion of the enamel of the back teeth; broken blood vessels in the eyes or face; constant sore throat; inflammation of the esophagus; and hiatal hernia. All of these are the consequences of induced vomiting. Sometimes emboweled spoons or sticks used to induce vomiting have to be surgically removed. If laxative abuse is part of the picture, damage to the bowel, rectal bleeding, and perpetual diarrhea may result. Laxative use also washes potassium and sodium from the body, which can result in electrolyte imbalances that may lead to dehydration, muscle spasms, and, eventually, cardiac arrest.

Other signs of bulimia can include bad dreams, bad breath, constantly cold feet and hands, dizziness, excess facial and body hair, fainting, hair loss, mental fuzziness, muscle fatigue, dry skin, yellowish or grayish skin, extreme weakness, and premature wrinkles.

People with bulimia often feel extremely guilty about their behavior, which is why they may successfully hide the disorder for years, even from their spouses and children. Trips to the bathroom after meals, the sudden disappearance of large quantities of food, frequent dental visits, scrapes and abrasions on the hands and knuckles, and mood changes may be hints that something is wrong.

Unless otherwise specified, the following recommended doses are for those over the age of eighteen. For a child between twelve and seventeen years old, reduce the dose to three-quarters the recommended amount. It is important for anyone with this condition to seek medical help.

NUTRIENTS

SUPPLEMENT	SUGGESTED DOSAGE	COMMENTS
Very Important		
Multivitamin and mineral complex with carotenoids and	As recommended by physician. Take with meals.	The bulimic syndrome results in severe vitamin and mineral deficiencies. Extremely high doses are needed because nutrients pass rapidly through the gastrointestinal system and are poorly assimilated. Do not use a sustained-release formula.
potassium and	99 mg daily.	
selenium	200 mcg daily. If you are pregnant, do not exceed 40 mcg daily.	
Zinc	50–100 mg daily. Do not exceed a total of 100 mg daily from all supplements.	Necessary in protein metabolism; aids the sense of taste and increases the appetite. May aid in easing depression and anxiety, and facilitating weight gain. Deficiencies are common in people with this disorder.
plus copper	3 mg daily.	Needed to balance with zinc.
Important		
Acidophilus	As directed on label. Take on an empty stomach so it can pass quickly to the small intestine.	Stabilizes intestinal bacteria. Protects the liver.
Calcium and magnesium	1,500 mg daily, at bedtime. 750 mg daily.	Has a calming effect and replaces lost calcium stores. Relaxes smooth muscles and has a bronchodilating effect.
Coenzyme A from Coenzyme-A Technologies and	As directed on label.	Can streamline metabolism, ease depression and fatigue, and increase energy. Supports adrenal glands, processes fats, and removes toxins from the body. Can also boost the immune system and improve overall physical and mental processes.
Coenzyme Q_{10}	60–100 mg daily.	Protects the heart muscle and aids in circulation.
Kyolic-EPA from Wakunaga	As directed on label.	Restores proper fatty acid balance. Needed by all bodily cells.
5-Hydroxy L-tryptophan (5-HTP from Solaray)	As directed on label.	Improves low levels of serotonin commonly associated with bulimia.
Free form amino acid (Amino Balance from Anabol Naturals)	As directed on label.	To counteract protein deficiency, a serious problem in bulimia. Free form amino acids are more readily available for use by the body than other protein forms.
Gamma-amino-butyric acid (GABA) compound plus	As directed on label.	Relieves stress and aids in nerve building.
Ester-C with bioflavonoids	3,000 mg daily.	Promotes healthy tissues and collagen growth.
Gamma-oryzonol (GO)	60 mg daily.	Aids in calorie use and muscle growth.
S-adenosylmethio-nine (SAMe)	As directed on label.	Aids in stress relief and depression, eases pain, and produces antioxidant effects. Do not use if you have bipolar mood disorder or take prescription antidepressants. Do not give to a child under twelve.
Vitamin B complex	100 mg of each major B vitamin 3 times daily (amounts of individual vitamins in a complex will vary).	Essential for all cellular functions.
Vitamin B_{12} injections or vitamin B_{12}	1 cc 3 times weekly or as prescribed by physician. As directed on label.	Needed for the digestion of foods and the assimilation of all nutrients, including iron. Injections (under a doctor's supervision) are best. If injections are not available, use a lozenge or sublingual form.
Vitamin C with bioflavonoids	5,000 mg daily, in divided doses.	Necessary for all cellular and glandular functions.
Helpful		
Bio-Strath from Nature's Answer or brewer's yeast	As directed on label 3 times daily. Start with 1 tsp daily and work up to the amount recommended on label.	For increased strength and energy. Aids in tissue repair and increases the appetite. Contains the B vitamins and other necessary nutrients. A good source of B vitamins. *Caution:* Discontinue use if any allergic reactions occur.
Iron (Floradix Iron + Herb from Salus Haus)	As directed on label, 3 times daily.	A natural source of iron that is easily assimilated. *Caution:* Do not take iron unless anemia is diagnosed.
Kelp	2,000–3,000 mg daily.	Supplies essential minerals, especially iodine.
Proteolytic enzymes or Inf-zyme Forte from American Biologics	As directed on label. Take with meals and between meals.	Important for proper digestion and absorption of nutrients.

Silica	As directed on label.	Aids in the growth of collagen and new body tissue.
Vitamin D	600 IU daily.	Needed to aid in calcium uptake and prevent bone loss, which can lead to tooth loss.
Vitamin E or ACES + Zn from Carlson Labs	200 IU daily. As directed on label.	Necessary for tissue repair and a powerful antioxidant. Use d-alpha-tocopherol form. To supply a combination of antioxidants.

Herbs

❑ Burdock root, milk thistle, and red clover are good for cleansing the bloodstream and protecting the liver.

❑ Ginger Dry Extract from Sabinsa Corporation helps in digestion.

❑ Licorice is good for glandular function.

Caution: Licorice root should not be used during pregnancy or nursing. It should not be used by persons with diabetes, glaucoma, heart disease, high blood pressure, or a history of stroke.

❑ A combination of high-potency royal jelly and angelica tea, taken once daily, has shown good results.

❑ St. John's wort is a good antidepressant and helps to reduce cravings.

Caution: St. John's wort may cause increased sensitivity to sunlight. It may also produce anxiety, gastrointestinal symptoms, and headaches. It can interact with some drugs including antidepressants, birth control pills, and anticoagulants.

Recommendations

❑ While healthier eating behaviors are being established, a well-balanced, high-fiber diet is essential. Eat as many vegetable proteins and complex carbohydrates as possible.

❑ Consume no sugar in any form. Avoid junk foods, heavy starches, and white flour products. Be aware that you may experience withdrawal symptoms such as anxiety, depression, fatigue, headache, insomnia, and/or irritability for a time after you eliminate sugar from the diet.

❑ Instead of the standard three meals a day, eat smaller, more frequent portions. It may help to control both feelings of fullness and hunger pains. Above all, don't go hungry. This only adds to your craving for food. Breakfast is especially important.

❑ Keep a variety of healthy snacks around you, both at work (or school) and at home, and make them readily available for when you feel a hunger pang.

❑ Chew your food slowly and well. Stop eating as soon as you feel uncomfortable or as if you might have to purge.

❑ Try keeping an eating journal with a price list of the foods you eat in it. This can sometimes help to break the bulimic chain. While seeing on paper what you have actually consumed will, no doubt, be overwhelming, it may make you realize exactly what you are doing and how much it is costing you financially. It can also help to note your surrounding circumstances (if you are alone, with someone, what you are doing at the time, and so forth) and how you feel before, during, and after you eat and/or purge. This will let you see how it happened, and how it made you feel. It can also help you to identify things that may trigger the pattern, such as certain foods, situations, or even people. Once these "trigger" elements have been identified, avoid them as much as possible.

❑ Taking 5-hydroxy L-tryptophan (5-HTP) improves serotonin levels and can be helpful if low serotonin levels are associated with bulimia. Several studies have also shown it can reduce caloric intake and curb hunger. Blood testing for eosinophil levels every three months is suggested if taking high doses of 5-HTP (greater than 300 mg per day). HTP.Calm from Natural Balance and L-5-HTP from Solaray are good sources of 5-HTP.

❑ Cravings can often trigger a binge. The first thing to remember is that cravings do not last long—from several seconds to ten or twenty minutes. When a craving hits you, you can do one of three things: grab a small, light snack (such as a carrot or grapefruit), distract yourself, or meet and defeat the craving head-on. To distract yourself, drink a full glass of water and then remove yourself from the area by taking a walk, going out somewhere, working on a hobby, or attacking a task that needs to be accomplished. After the task, reward yourself with a healthy snack.

❑ Practice control with other things you do in excess, whether it is alcohol consumption, exercising, shopping, or anything else. The key to a higher self-esteem is for you to be in control of your life, not for something else to be in control of you.

❑ Develop and maintain relationships with positive people who make you feel good about yourself and whom you admire. Anyone bad for your mental health is a waste of your time and feelings.

❑ Practicing stress management can greatly assist anyone fighting bulimia. Regular, moderate exercise, deep breathing, meditation, visualization, and yoga are all excellent ways to relieve stress. They are also good for easing depression.

Considerations

❑ It is wrong to categorize bulimia as "just a food addiction," as its roots are tied to many other factors that vary from case to case, including low self-esteem and psychological, biological, and societal factors.

❑ The most successful treatment plans for bulimia include a psychologist (who can help assess the psychological implications of the person's disorder) and a physician (to evaluate and monitor his or her physical state). Long-term treatment may be needed to improve self-esteem and ensure that the person is mentally and physically able to recover.

❑ Cognitive-behavioral therapy (CBT) and nutritional therapy are the preferred first treatments for bulimia. The drugs used for bulimia are typically antidepressants known as selective serotonin reuptake inhibitors (SSRIs). A combination of CBT and SSRIs is very effective if CBT is not effective alone.

❑ According to researchers at the National Institute of Mental Health (NIMH) and Duke University, lack of a hormone that controls appetite may be the reason those with bulimia fail to feel full. For these people, eating a meal apparently does not stimulate adequate production of the hormone cholecystokinin-pancreozymin (CCK), which is found in the small intestine and the brain. They have to keep eating, and bingeing, in order to feel satisfied. However, more research is needed to determine whether this is the cause behind the majority of cases of binge eating.

❑ According to an article published in *The Harvard Mental Health Letter,* women with diabetes who are bulimic often lose weight after a binge by reducing their doses of insulin. This can damage eye tissue and raise the risk of diabetic retinopathy, which can lead to blindness.

❑ A study conducted at the University of Iowa College of Medicine and the University of Wisconsin found that reducing weight as part of athletic training may lead to bulimia. A survey of seven hundred high school wrestlers found that 2 percent were involved with binge eating followed by vomiting, fasting, excessive exercise, or the use of laxatives to avoid weight gain.

❑ For sources of additional information about eating disorders and treatments, *see* Health and Medical Organizations in the Appendix.

BURNS

A serious burn on the skin is one of the most traumatic injuries that the body can sustain. The skin is the body's largest organ, and one of its most complex. Among other things, it helps to regulate temperature and it serves as the first line of defense against infection.

There are three basic classifications of burns on the skin, each varying in severity. First-degree burns affect only the outer layer of the skin, causing redness and sensitivity to the touch. Sunburn is usually a first-degree burn. Second-degree burns extend somewhat into underlying skin layers, and are characterized by redness, blistering, and acute pain. In third-degree burns, the entire thickness of the skin and possibly underlying tissues, such as muscle, are destroyed. The skin may be red, or it may be white or yellowish, or leathery and black. There is usually little or no pain because the nerves in the skin are severely damaged.

About 40,000 Americans are hospitalized for burn treatment each year, approximately 60 percent to the 125 specialized burn treatment centers, and 40 percent to the nation's other 5,000 hospitals. About 4,000 of these people die, according to the American Burn Association. As large as they are, these figures represent a significant decline in the number of incidents, and the severity of burn injuries, in the past twenty-five years, partly due to advances in treatment that lessen the initial shock and prevent fluid loss and infection. Doctors have also improved their techniques for surgically removing burned tissues from the wound as soon as possible and for subsequently transferring new skin grafts to the damaged area(s). In addition, specialized nutrition focusing on specific nutrients has been developed and shown to improve recovery and speed the healing process for both minor and serious burns.

The following nutrients are important for healing once appropriate local treatment has been administered. Choose a multivitamin that contains the trace minerals copper, selenium, and zinc to promote faster healing. Unless otherwise specified, the following recommended doses are for those over the age of eighteen. For a child between twelve and seventeen years old, reduce the dose to three-quarters the recommended amount. For a child between six and twelve years old, use one-half the recommended dose, and for a child under six, use one-quarter the recommended amount.

NUTRIENTS

SUPPLEMENT	SUGGESTED DOSAGE	COMMENTS
Very Important		
Colloidal silver	Apply topically as directed on label.	A natural antibiotic and disinfectant. Promotes healing. For severe burns, use spray form.
Free form amino acid	As directed on label.	Important in the healing of tissues.
Liquid Kyolic with B₁ and B₁₂ from Wakunaga	As directed on label.	Important for tissue repair. Promotes healing. Natural antibiotic.
Potassium	99 mg daily.	Needed to replace potassium lost from burns.
Vitamin A plus natural beta-carotene or carotenoid complex (Betatene)	100,000 IU daily for 1 month, then reduce to 50,000 IU daily. If you are pregnant, do not exceed 10,000 IU daily. 25,000 IU daily. As directed on label.	Needed for tissue repair. Use an emulsion form for easier assimilation and greater safety at high doses. An antioxidant and precursor of vitamin A.

Vitamin B complex	100 mg of each major B vitamin daily, with meals (amounts of individual vitamins in a complex will vary).	Important in the healing of skin tissue.
plus extra vitamin B$_{12}$	1,000 mcg twice daily.	Needed for protein synthesis and cell formation. Use a lozenge or sublingual form.
Vitamin C with bioflavonoids	10,000 mg immediately after a burn; 2,000 mg 3 times a day thereafter until healed.	An antioxidant that is essential in the formation of collagen; promotes the healing of burns.
Vitamin E	200 IU daily. Also open a capsule and apply the oil directly to the scar once healing has begun.	Needed for healing and to prevent scarring. Use d-alpha-tocopherol form.
Zinc	30 mg 3 times daily. Do not exceed a total of 100 mg daily from all supplements.	Needed for healing of tissues.
Important		
Essential fatty acids (Kyolic-EPA from Wakunaga, flaxseed oil, fish oil, or primrose oil)	As directed on label.	Omega-3 fats in fish oil have been shown to promote healing.
Selenium	200 mcg daily. If you are pregnant, do not exceed 40 mcg daily.	Needed for tissue elasticity. Provides antioxidant protection at the cellular level. Speeds healing.
Helpful		
Calcium and	1,500 mg daily.	Promotes healthy skin.
magnesium and	750 mg daily.	Loss of body fluids increases the need for magnesium.
vitamin D	400 IU daily.	Needed for calcium uptake.
Coenzyme Q$_{10}$	100 mg daily.	Helps circulation and healing of tissue.
Germanium	200 mg daily.	Enhances circulation and healing of tissue.
Inf-zyme Forte from American Biologics	As directed on label. Take between meals.	Reduces inflammation.

Herbs

❏ Aloe vera pulp, gel, or liquid can be applied to the burn as needed to relieve pain and to speed healing.

❏ Bayberry, black or green tea, blackberry leaves, sumac leaves, sweet gum, and white oak bark contain tannic acid, which has been used in clinics for surface burns that have begun to heal. These herbs can be used as teas and as wet compresses.

Caution: Green tea contains vitamin K, which can make anticoagulant medications less effective. Consult your health care professional if you are using them. The caffeine in green tea could cause insomnia, anxiety, upset stomach, nausea, or diarrhea.

❏ Calendula, applied topically to the burned area as a gel or ointment, is effective as an anti-inflammatory agent and antiseptic.

❏ An herbal compress made with comfrey leaf and wheat germ oil can be applied to the burn to help soothe the pain.

Caution: Comfrey is recommended for external use only.

❏ Apply fresh ginger juice or strong black tea to the burned area, using cotton balls or a compress.

❏ Goldenseal can be taken in pill or extract form, or used in a poultice and applied to the burned area. It is a natural antibiotic that helps to prevent infection.

Caution: Do not take goldenseal internally on a daily basis for more than one week at a time. Do not use it during pregnancy or if you are breast-feeding, and use with caution if you are allergic to ragweed. If you have a history of cardiovascular disease, diabetes, or glaucoma, use it only under a doctor's supervision.

❏ Tea tree oil is effective for minor burns, primarily as an antiseptic and to help soothe the burned area. It is safe for both children and adults. Apply topically to the burned area.

Recommendations

❏ If you suspect a third-degree burn, see your physician at once or go to the emergency room of the nearest hospital. Do not attempt to treat the injury, do not remove clothing that is stuck to the burned area, and do not put ice or water on the burn. A third-degree burn requires professional treatment.

❏ Cool a first- or second-degree burn at once to reduce pain and swelling. Immerse the area in cool running water, or use ice-filled bags and cool compresses for a minimum of ten minutes. While cooling the burn, remove rings, wristwatches, belts, or anything else that could constrict the injured area once it begins to swell. Also take away any loose clothing that has not adhered to the burned area.

❏ To remove hot tar, wax, or melted plastic from the skin, use ice water to harden the heated substance.

❏ After a minor burn has been cooled, apply aloe vera gel or a product such as Solarcaine Aloe Extra Burn Relief Gel, which contains aloe vera, to ease pain and promote healing.

Caution: Do not put oils, greasy ointments, or butter on burns. Do not break blisters.

❏ While your body is recovering from a burn—especially a second- or third-degree burn—change your diet to provide a high intake of protein (at least 100 grams) and vitamin- and mineral-rich foods, up to 2,500 calories per day. These are needed for tissue repair and healing. During convalescence you may not be as active as usual and will probably require about 500 fewer calories than usual. However, it is more important to focus on getting adequate protein and nutrient-dense foods rather than worry about calories.

❑ Watch for signs of infection, odor, pus, or extreme redness in the area of the burn. Protect the injury from exposure to sun. Stay away from soil and avoid digging in the garden or sitting on the grass until the skin is completely healed.

❑ Drink plenty of fluids throughout the healing phase. Potassium juice and green drinks are recommended for fast tissue repair. (*See* JUICING in Part Three.)

❑ Glutamine has been shown to hasten recovery after a burn injury by boosting immune function and strengthening the intestinal tract.

❑ Arginine may help hasten burn healing, especially when coupled with fish oil.

❑ Keep burn injuries elevated to minimize swelling and promote healing. This is especially important for burns on the hands, legs, or feet.

❑ Keep the burn lightly covered to minimize the chance of bacterial infection.

❑ After the burn has cooled down, try adding 1 tablespoon of powdered vitamin C to 1 quart of cool water and spraying it on the burn site. This has been found to enhance healing. Or try using cool clay poultices. (*See* USING A POULTICE in Part Three.)

❑ If infection starts to set in, see your physician.

Considerations

❑ Hygiene is very important when dealing with any type of burn.

❑ For third-degree burns, your doctor may prescribe silver sulfadiazine cream (Silvadene).

Caution: Reactions to silver sulfadiazine are rare, but they can occur.

❑ Severe burns are often preventable. Make sure that your home or apartment has working smoke alarms on each floor. If the home is large, you will need several around the house. Every January 1, change the batteries in each alarm. If the bedrooms are on the second floor, make sure there is a rope or rope ladder available near a window that can be used in case of a fast-moving fire. When staying at a hotel, locate the nearest fire exits.

❑ Don't ever smoke while pumping gas; if someone else is, urge them to put the cigarette out, tell the attendant, or leave immediately. Never use gasoline in place of kerosene or for removing head lice. Gasoline is extremely volatile and should never be used indoors.

❑ A medically supervised program for a more serious burn or for a burn in a sensitive location may include the use of antibiotics, debridement to remove dead tissue, hydrotherapy to loosen dead skin, and physical therapy or splinting to prevent contractures (permanent muscular contractions).

❑ Severe burns often need to be treated with skin grafts to help restore the damaged skin. Healthy upper-layer skin from another part of the body can be transplanted to the burned area, but people with large burns often do not have enough of their own skin for transplanting. There are several biotechnological companies that make an artificial skin from collagen, a fibrous protein, and this serves as a scaffold to help promote growth of new skin cells and blood vessels, and also to temporarily protect the wounded area. Cadaver skin can also be used as a temporary cover until you can grow more of your own skin to harvest.

❑ A study on the effects of high-dose vitamin C therapy for third-degree burns that was reported in the *Journal of Burn Care and Rehabilitation* concluded that people with serious burns should immediately begin taking vitamin C (*see under* Nutrients, above).

❑ *See* SUNBURN in Part Two.

❑ *See also* PAIN CONTROL in Part Three.

BURSITIS

Bursitis is an inflammation of a bursa. The bursae are small sacs filled with lubricating fluid that are located between tendons and bones in various places in the body. They help to promote muscular movement by cushioning against friction between bones and other tissues. An inflamed bursa causes pain, tenderness to the touch of the affected body part, and limitation of motion. There may be redness and swelling as well.

Bursitis can be caused by injury, chronic overuse, reactions to certain foods, airborne allergies, or calcium deposits. Tight muscles also may lead to bursitis.

Calcified bursitis occurs when scar tissue develops in the bursa because an original injury was left untreated. The bursae in the hip and shoulder joints are most often affected.

Epicondylitis or epitrochlear bursitis, affecting the arm, is often called "tennis elbow" or "frozen shoulder." Tennis elbow may start as a small tear in the tendon, and is more likely to occur in people whose jobs require repeated tight gripping of an object. Occupational bursitis is not uncommon and is known by old, familiar names such as "housemaid's knee," "policeman's heel," or the "beat knee" or "beat shoulder" of coal miners.

Trochanteric bursitis is inflammation of the bursa in the hip. This may be caused by continual physical activity, by standing for a long time, or by a displacement of the hip. An aching pain that may radiate down the leg normally accompanies it. One of the most common foot ailments, the bunion, is actually a form of bursitis caused by friction; a tight-fitting shoe causes a sac on the joint of the big toe to become inflamed.

Tendinitis is closely related to bursitis, and the two are often confused. Tendinitis is the inflammation of the tendons, usually caused by strain. It is found most commonly in the shoulders, hips, Achilles tendons, or hamstrings.

Bursitis can affect anyone, at any age. However, older people, especially athletes and those who are overweight, are more likely than others to get this ailment. Bursitis is usually characterized by a dull, persistent ache that increases with movement, whereas tendinitis typically causes sharp pain on movement, and rotation of the arm may be difficult if it is in the shoulder. This condition is often worse at night, and the pain usually extends from the top of the shoulder to just under the large shoulder muscle in the back. Tendinitis often affects people who routinely have to reach to perform certain activities, such as domestic workers and painters. Tendon inflammation may also result from calcium deposits that press against a tendon. Unlike tendinitis, bursitis is often accompanied by swelling and fluid accumulation.

Unless otherwise specified, the following recommended doses are for those over the age of eighteen. For children between twelve and seventeen years old, reduce the dose to three-quarters the recommended amount. For children between six and twelve years old, use one-half the recommended dose, and for children under six, use one-quarter the recommended amount.

NUTRIENTS

SUPPLEMENT	SUGGESTED DOSAGE	COMMENTS
Very Important		
Calcium and magnesium	1,500 mg daily.	Needed for repair of connective tissue.
	750 mg daily.	Needed to balance with calcium and for proper muscular function.
Free form amino acid	As directed on label. Take on an empty stomach.	Needed for healing of tendons and tissues.
Multienzyme complex with pancreatin	As directed on label. Take with meals.	To aid digestion. Use a formula with high amounts of pancreatin.
Proteolytic enzymes or Inf-zyme Forte from American Biologics	As directed on label. Take between meals. 2 tablets 2–3 times daily, between meals.	Contains a powerful anti-inflammatory substance.
Vitamin A	15,000 IU daily. If you are pregnant, do not exceed 10,000 IU daily.	Needed for tissue repair and immune function.
plus natural beta-carotene or carotenoid complex (Betatene)	25,000 IU daily. As directed on label.	Potent antioxidant and precursor of vitamin A.
plus selenium	200 mcg daily. If you are pregnant, do not exceed 40 mcg daily.	
Vitamin C with bioflavonoids	3,000–8,000 mg daily, in divided doses.	Reduces inflammation and potentiates immune function. Essential for the formation of collagen, a protein in connective tissue.
Vitamin E	200 IU daily.	An anti-inflammatory free-radical scavenger. Use d-alpha-tocopherol form.
Zinc plus copper	50 mg daily. Do not exceed a total of 100 mg daily from all supplements. 3 mg daily.	Important in all enzyme systems and tissue repair. Needed to balance with zinc.
Helpful		
Boron	3 mg daily. Do not exceed this amount.	For better calcium absorption.
Coenzyme Q10	60 mg daily.	Good for circulation.
Glucosamine sulfate or N-Acetylglucosamine (N-A-G from Source Naturals)	As directed on label. As directed on label.	Important for the formation of connective tissues.
Methylsulfonyl-methane (MSM)	As directed on label.	Has therapeutic properties. Aids in pain relief and immune function.
Multivitamin and mineral complex	As directed on label.	Needed for tissue repair.
Pycnogenol or grape seed extract	As directed on label. As directed on label.	Powerful antioxidants and anti-inflammatories.
Silica	As directed on label.	Supplies silicon, necessary for repair of connective tissues.
Vitamin B complex	100 mg of each major B vitamin twice daily (amounts of individual vitamins in a complex will vary).	Important in cellular repair.
Vitamin B12 injections or vitamin B complex	As prescribed by physician. As directed on label.	Needed for proper digestion and absorption of foods and for the repair of nerve damage. Injections (under a doctor's supervision) are best. If injections are not available, use a lozenge or sublingual form.

Herbs

❑ Boswellia and bromelain both reduce inflammation.

❑ Meadowsweet and willow bark, combined in equal measure and taken three times daily, help with inflammation.

Recommendations

❑ Go on a seven-day raw-food diet, followed by a three-day cleansing fast. (*See* FASTING in Part Three.)

❑ Eat no processed foods or any form of sugar.

❑ To relieve pain, use hot castor oil packs. Place castor oil in a pan and heat but do not boil it. Dip a piece of cheesecloth or other white cotton material into the oil until the cloth is saturated. Apply the cloth to the affected area and cover it with a piece of plastic that is larger in size than the cotton cloth. Place a heating pad over the plastic and use it to keep the pack warm. Keep the pack in place for one-half to two hours, as needed. Some physicians recommend ice packs.

❑ You may need to abstain from activity and get plenty of rest. When engaging in physical activity, do not push yourself too hard or too long. If you are in pain, stop. Try to find activities that don't exacerbate the pain, such as walking.

❏ If you are overweight, begin a weight loss program.

Considerations

❏ Treatment for bursitis involves removing the cause of the injury (controlled exercise of the affected area and/or immobilization and rest may be recommended for this), clearing up any underlying infection, and possibly surgically removing calcium deposits. Most treatment is dictated by the patient. If you are really in pain and can't stand it anymore, let your doctor know. Most doctors are waiting for a signal from you before they will advise more aggressive treatments.

❏ Applied topically, dimethylsulfoxide (DMSO), a by-product of wood processing, can relieve pain and reduce swelling. Always dilute 100 percent or 90 percent solutions down to 70 percent with water. The mixture will get hot, so allow it to cool first.

Caution: Only pure DMSO from a health food store should be used. Commercial-grade DMSO such as that found in hardware stores is not suitable for healing purposes. Any contaminants on the skin or in the product can be taken into the tissues by action of the DMSO.

Note: The use of DMSO may result in a garlicky body odor. This is temporary, and is not a cause for concern.

❏ *See also* PAIN CONTROL in Part Three.

CADMIUM TOXICITY

Cadmium is an inorganic metal that is naturally present in the environment. Like lead, cadmium accumulates in the body and has varying degrees of toxicity. Its half life is one to four decades in the human body, which means it's almost impossible to get rid of it once the body has absorbed it. Cadmium replaces the body's stores of the essential mineral zinc in the liver and kidneys. Not surprisingly, cadmium levels rise in people who have zinc deficiencies.

Cadmium is present in the environment in different chemical forms, such as cadmium sulfide, cadmium oxide, cadmium sulfate, cadmium carbonate, and cadmium chloride. It is used in the production of colored inks and dyes, as well as in many industrial applications, such as metal plating, engraving, and soldering. Cadmium is also used in plastics and in the production of nickel-cadmium (Ni-Cad) batteries, which are in widespread use in cell phones, portable computers, and in many toys. Trace amounts of cadmium are found in most foods. In shellfish, however, cadmium accumulates at a significantly higher level. Cadmium exposure from eating shellfish varies, depending on the origins of the shellfish. In other words, there is no way to know how much cadmium a specific clam or lobster

might have in its tissues. Other common sources of cadmium include drinking water, fertilizer, fungicides, pesticides, soil, air pollution, refined grains, rice, coffee, tea, and soft drinks. Dietary exposure to cadmium is estimated to be about 0.12 microgram to 0.49 microgram per kilogram (2.2 pounds) of body weight daily. This is *not* a recommendation, just the normal amount a person in modern society can expect to ingest. Intake of dietary cadmium should not exceed 7 micrograms per kilogram of body weight, per week, according to the World Health Organization. For a healthy male of about 80 kilograms (175 pounds) of body weight, that is only 560 micrograms per week, a very small amount indeed. (A microgram is one-millionth of a gram.)

Tobacco smoke also contains cadmium, and studies have shown that cigarette smokers have higher levels of cadmium in their bodies than nonsmokers. In one study, women who smoked were shown to have higher urinary cadmium levels than those who did not. Smoking a pack of cigarettes can add between 2 and 4 micrograms of cadmium to the body. You can also accumulate cadmium from secondhand smoke. Dangerous exposure to cadmium usually occurs through inhalation of fumes and dust. Cadmium in this form is extremely irritating to the lungs and can lead to such symptoms as headaches, chills, muscle aches, nausea, vomiting, and diarrhea. Cadmium is so hazardous the government has determined that for long-term workplace exposure to cadmium-contaminated dust and fumes, the level should be kept below 0.025 milligrams per cubic meter of air.

The human body can tolerate low levels of cadmium, but long-term chronic exposure can lead to serious health problems. In one study, lactating women with too much cadmium in their bodies were found to have low levels of calcium in their milk, which could impede the growth of the baby. Breast milk typically has very small amounts of cadmium—less than 1 microgram per liter—which is normal and has no impact on calcium absorption and thus no effect on the growth of the baby. Elevated levels of cadmium may result in hypertension (high blood pressure), a dulled sense of smell, anemia, yellow discoloration of the teeth, inflammation of the mucous membrane of the nose (rhinitis), joint soreness, hair loss, dry, scaly skin, and loss of appetite. Cadmium toxicity threatens the health of the body by weakening the immune system. It causes a decreased production of T lymphocytes (T cells), key white blood cells that protect the body by destroying foreign invaders and cancer cells.

Because cadmium is retained in the kidneys and liver (50 to 70 percent of accumulated cadmium is deposited in those organs), excessive exposure can lead to kidney disease and serious liver damage. Possible effects of intense cadmium exposure include emphysema, bone disorders such as osteoporosis and osteomalacia, cancer, and a shortened life span.

A blood test is the best method of determining acute cadmium toxicity. A urine test helps to determine the body's total burden of cadmium.

Unless otherwise specified, the dosages recommended here are for adults. For a child between the ages of twelve and seventeen, reduce the dose to three-quarters the recommended amount. For a child between six and twelve, use one-half the recommended dose, and for a child under the age of six, use one-quarter the recommended amount.

NUTRIENTS

SUPPLEMENT	SUGGESTED DOSAGE	COMMENTS
Important		
Alfalfa		See under Herbs, below.
Calcium and magnesium	2,000 mg daily. 1,000 mg daily.	Minerals that help rid the body of cadmium.
Coenzyme A from Coenzyme-A Technologies	As directed on label.	Aids in removing toxic substances from the body.
Garlic (Kyolic from Wakunaga)	2 capsules 3 times daily.	Helps to rid the body of cadmium. A potent detoxifier.
L-cysteine and L-lysine and L-methionine	500 mg each daily, on an empty stomach. Take with water or juice. Do not take with milk. Take with 50 mg vitamin B$_6$ and 100 mg vitamin C for better absorption.	These amino acids act as antioxidants; they protect the organs, especially the liver. (See AMINO ACIDS in Part One.)
Lecithin granules or capsules	2 tbsp 3 times daily, with meals. 2,400 mg 3 times daily, with meals. Take with vitamin E (see below) for better assimilation.	Protects all cells.
Rutin	200 mg 3 times daily. Take with 100 mg vitamin C.	Aids in removing high amounts of metals from the body.
Vitamin E	200 IU daily.	An antioxidant. Use d-alpha-tocopherol form, and use an emulsion form for easier assimilation.
Zinc	50–80 mg daily. Do not exceed a total of 100 mg daily from all supplements.	Needed to restore zinc displaced by cadmium and to prevent cadmium levels from rising.
Helpful		
Copper	3 mg daily.	Works with zinc to remove cadmium deposits.
Iron or	As directed by physician. Take with 100 mg vitamin C for better absorption.	To correct deficiency. Use ferrous fumarate form. *Caution:* Do not take iron unless anemia is diagnosed.
Floradix Iron + Herbs from Salus Haus	As directed on label.	Contains nontoxic, natural iron from food sources that is easily assimilated into the body.

Herbs

❏ Alfalfa contains chlorophyll and vitamin K, and helps to remove cadmium from the body. Take 2,000 to 3,000 milligrams in tablet form daily.

❏ Burdock root and red clover help to purify the bloodstream and stimulate the immune system.

❏ Milk thistle is very effective in protecting the liver. It also stimulates the production of new liver cells.

Recommendations

❏ Make sure that you include plenty of fiber and apple pectin in your diet. Eat pumpkin seeds and other foods that are high in zinc.

Considerations

❏ Chelation removes toxic metals from the body. (*See* CHELATION THERAPY in Part Three.)

❏ *See also* ENVIRONMENTAL TOXICITY in Part Two.

CANCER

The entire human body is made up of cells, each of which contains its own genetic material, or DNA—a long string of molecules that tells the cell what to do. In a healthy body, cells divide at a controlled rate so as to grow and repair damaged tissues and replace dying cells. This predetermined rate of cell division is what keeps our bodies healthy. If cells keep multiplying when new ones are not necessary, a mass of tissue called a growth, or tumor, is formed.

A tumor can be either benign or malignant. Benign tumors are not cancerous. They can occur anywhere in the body and generally do not pose a threat to health, do not metastasize (spread to other parts of the body), and do not grow back if removed. Malignant tumors are cancerous. They are usually serious and can be life-threatening. Malignant tumors grow uncontrollably, interfere with normal metabolic and organ functioning, and have the ability to metastasize and invade other tissues.

If a portion of a cell's DNA is damaged, the cell can become abnormal. When the abnormal cell divides, it forms new cells that contain a photocopy of the damaged genetic material. This is an ongoing process occurring constantly within our bodies. Most of the time, our bodies have the ability to destroy these abnormal cells and maintain a sort of cellular equilibrium. If a crucial portion of the DNA is destroyed, however, and the abnormal cells cannot be controlled any longer, cancer forms. All cancer cells have two things in common: they grow uncontrollably and they have the ability to metastasize. They can spread through the lymphatic system, the bloodstream, or avenues such as the cerebrospinal fluid (the watery cushion that protects the brain and spinal cord). The immune system generally does not recognize cancer cells as dangerous or foreign.

It is not known exactly what causes the cell damage that initiates the cancer process. The chain of events that leads to cancer is very complex, and each individual body reacts differently. A combination of genetic, behavioral, environmental, and lifestyle factors is believed to be involved in turning normal cells into abnormal cells, and abnormal cells into cancer. There are also factors called inhibitors (such as certain vitamins and nutrients found in fruits and vegetables) that are believed to slow the process, while other factors, called promoters (such as smoking or eating a high-fat diet), can speed up the process.

Possible contributors to the development and growth of cancer can be divided into three categories—external, internal, and lifestyle. External factors include unhealthy workplace environments and exposure to air and water pollution, chemicals, pesticides, and herbicides. Internal factors include both genetics (heredity) and infections. Lifestyle factors are those we personally can most readily control. These are also the factors scientists believe account for the largest proportion of cancers. They include diet, smoking, drinking, and sun exposure. For example, persons who do not smoke but are exposed to cigarette smoke have significantly higher rates of lung cancer than nonsmokers who are not. Regular alcohol consumption increases the risk of mouth and throat cancers. A diet that is high in fat and low in fiber is associated with a greater risk of colorectal cancer and is a factor in breast and prostate cancer as well.

Cancer death rates are falling steadily, according to the American Cancer Society's (ACS) annual cancer statistics report, *Cancer Facts & Figures* (2009). The drop is driven in large part by better prevention, increased use of early detection practices, and improved treatment for cancer. Still, ACS researchers estimate that there were about 1,479,350 new cancer cases and about 562,340 cancer deaths in 2009. External and lifestyle factors account for 80 percent of cancer deaths in the United States. The following are the major factors that researchers say can contribute to developing cancer:

- Growing older
- Tobacco.
- Sunlight.
- Ionizing radiation.
- Certain chemicals and other substances.
- Some viruses and bacteria.
- Certain hormones.
- Family history of cancer.
- Alcohol.
- Poor diet, lack of physical activity, being overweight.

Many experts believe that what these risk factors have in common is that they increase the body's exposure to free radicals. They theorize that damage from free radicals is an important factor in causing the uncontrolled cellular growth that is characteristic of cancer. (*See* FREE RADICALS *under* ANTIOXIDANTS in Part One.) Others believe that factors such as cigarette smoking and poor dietary habits increase the risk of cancer because they impair the immune system.

While most researchers do not think stress brings on cancer directly, they do believe that it weakens the immune system, impairing the body's ability to destroy precancerous cells before they develop into cancer. By making ourselves aware of all of the factors that may promote or inhibit the development and growth of cancer, and by taking appropriate action, we can reduce our cancer risk.

There are more than one hundred different varieties of cancer. They have different causes, cause different symptoms, and vary in aggressiveness (the speed at which they spread). However, most types of cancer fall into one of four broad categories:

1. Carcinomas—cancers that affect the skin, mucous membranes, glands, and internal organs.
2. Leukemias—cancers of blood-forming tissues.
3. Sarcomas—cancers that affect muscles, connective tissue, and bones.
4. Lymphomas—cancers that affect the lymphatic system.

The classic early warning signs of cancer are:

Unexplained weight loss.

Fever.

Fatigue.

Pain.

Skin changes.

For specific cancers:

Change in bowel habits.

Sores that do not heal.

White patches inside the mouth.

Unusual bleeding or discharge.

Thickening lump in the breast or anywhere in the body.

Indigestion or trouble swallowing.

Recent change in a wart or mole.

Nagging cough.

According to the American Cancer Society, 50 percent of all men and 33 percent of all women in the United States will develop some form of cancer at some point in their lives. The good news is that with the increasing information and treatment methods available today, millions of people are either living with, or have been cured of, cancer, and the risk of developing most types of cancer can be reduced by adopting a healthy lifestyle.

According to the Centers for Disease Control and Prevention (CDC), there are 11 million cancer survivors in the United States. A cancer survivor is defined as an individual who is still alive five years after his or her cancer diagnosis. Today, about 66 percent of cancer patients survive five

Types and Warning Signs of Cancer

Knowing the warning signs and factors that increase the risk of developing different forms of cancer can save your life. The American Cancer Society estimates that of the more than 500,000 cancer deaths that occur in the United States, about one-third can be attributed to dietary factors, with another third being caused by cigarette smoking. Healthy lifestyle choices at any stage of life are a major step toward cancer prevention. Following are descriptions of some of the major types of cancer, including information about who is affected, what the symptoms are, how these diseases can be detected and diagnosed, and what you can do to reduce your risk of contracting them.

Bladder Cancer

Bladder cancer is the fourth most common cancer in males, eighth most common in females, and fifth leading cause of cancer deaths in the United States. It is slightly more than three times as common in men than women and twice as common in Caucasians as in African-Americans. It is usually diagnosed later in life—nearly 90 percent of people with bladder cancer are over the age of fifty-five.

Causes and Risk Factors

The cause of bladder cancer is not known. Smoking is the number-one factor associated with bladder cancer. Also linked to bladder cancer are exposure to certain chemicals, such as benzidines, aniline dyes, and naphthalenes; radiation exposure; heredity; possibly extremely high consumption of saccharin; a history of schistosomiasis (a tropical disease); chronic urinary tract infections or inflammation; and working in the dye, chemical, rubber, and leather industries.

Signs and Symptoms

Often symptoms do not appear in the early stages. The first warning sign is usually blood in the urine. Other symptoms can be pain and burning with urination, increased frequency of urination, and difficulty urinating.

Detection and Diagnosis

Bladder cancer can be detected by examining the bladder through a cystoscope, examining cells in the urine, or having intravenous pyelography (IVP, a special kidney X-ray) performed. Sometimes a large tumor can be detected through a rectal or vaginal exam. Researchers are studying a new screening test that detects telomerase, an enzyme produced by bladder tumors.

Dietary and Nutritional Factors

Cruciferous vegetables such as broccoli, Brussels sprouts, cabbage, cauliflower, and kale have been credited with lowering the risk of bladder cancer due to their antioxidant and other cancer-fighting compounds. Eating the USDA-recommended number of servings of fruits such as apples, berries, cherries, oranges, pears, and tomatoes may reduce the risk of cancer. Drinking a lot of liquids, especially pure water, helps to dilute carcinogens and increase urination, lessening the time any carcinogens in the bladder have to do any damage.

Taking vitamin A, beta-carotene, vitamin C, and a multivitamin have shown reductions in the risk of getting bladder cancer. Eat a diet rich in vitamin E that includes nuts and olive oil. Dimethylsulfoxide (DMSO) is an FDA-approved, nontoxic solvent that has been shown to aid in treatment.

Caution: Only pure DMSO from a health food store should be used. Commercial-grade DMSO such as that found in hardware stores is not suitable for healing purposes. Any contaminants on the skin or in the product can be taken into the tissues by action of the DMSO.

Note: The use of DMSO may result in a garlicky body odor. This is temporary, and is not a cause for concern.

Breast Cancer

See BREAST CANCER in Part Two.

Cervical Cancer

The majority of cervical cancers grow gradually over several years with precancerous cells (dysplasia) existing previous to the cancer cells. If dysplasia is detected early enough and removed, cervical cancer can often be prevented. Cervical cancer was once one of the most common causes of cancer death for American women. However, the cervical cancer death rate declined by 74 percent between 1955 and 1992. The main reason for this change is the increased use of the Pap test. This screening procedure can find changes in the cervix before cancer develops. It can also find early cervical cancer in its most curable stage. The death rate from cervical cancer continues to decline by 4 percent a year.

A vaccine to prevent cervical cancer was made available in 2008 and is recommended for girls about the time they begin menstruation. The vaccine, Gardasil, has been approved by the FDA for use in the United States. There is a good chance that this cancer will be eradicated in the future if all women get vaccinated. However, use of the vaccine is associated with an unusually high rate of dizziness and blood clotting problems. More study is needed on the risks and benefits of this vaccine.

Causes and Risk Factors

Most cervical cancers are associated with infection with human papillomavirus (HPV), which can be transmitted sexually. Associated risk factors include having had more than five complete pregnancies; first intercourse before age eighteen; unprotected sex; sexually transmitted infections, including HIV, HPV, and genital herpes; early childbearing; multiple sex partners; infertility; low socioeconomic status; smoking; and nutritional deficiencies.

Signs and Symptoms

Cervical cancer usually causes no symptoms until it is advanced, which is why it is essential for women to have regular pelvic exams and Pap tests. It can cause bleeding between menstrual periods, bleeding after intercourse or douching, unusual discharge, painful menstrual periods, and heavy periods.

Detection and Diagnosis

The presence of abnormal cells can be detected by a Pap test, followed up with a biopsy. Women should begin having annual pelvic exams and Pap tests when sexual activity begins, or at age eighteen (after three or more normal exams, your doctor may recommend decreasing the frequency of the exams unless you have had dysplasia or are at increased risk for other reasons). Screening for HPV is a method of early detection.

Dietary and Nutritional Factors

A diet low in fatty meats (especially cold cuts), red meat, cheeses, and white bread, and high in soy products, fruits, dark green vegetables, tomatoes, whole grains, and yogurt offers the best dietary protection. Shiitake mushrooms are also a good source of protection.

If you do not consume three to five servings of fruits and vegetables daily, you should take vitamin C (500–1,000 milligrams daily), E, A, and beta-carotene (25,000–50,000 international units daily) in supplemental form. Folic acid, one of the B vitamins (400–800 micrograms daily), can not only aid in prevention, but it has been known to reverse precancerous changes in cervical cells.

Colorectal Cancer

The large intestine is made up of the colon (the upper five to six feet) and the rectum (the last six to eight inches). This is where the last stage of digestion occurs and where solid waste is held until it is released. Colorectal cancer is the third most common cancer (not including skin cancer) in men and women in the United States. Mostly credited to an increase in screening for and removal of polyps, the incidence has been declining during the past decade.

Colon polyps are found in 10 to 20 percent of people over fifty years of age. If left untreated, 8 to 12 percent of polyps will become cancerous. If allowed to grow, a tumor can invade nearby organs. Once the disease enters the lymph nodes or bloodstream, it most often spreads to the liver. The American Cancer Society estimates that more than 146,000 Americans will be diagnosed with colorectal cancer in a given year, and just under 50,000 will die from the disease. It strikes men and women nearly equally. Colorectal cancer develops over a ten- to fifteen-year period and produces no symptoms until it is advanced. If the disease is detected early enough and the tumor has not metastasized, the survival rate is quite high. Patients who get screened and have a tumor that is entirely localized to the bowel have the greatest chance of surviving. However, with tumors that have spread to the liver, the five-year survival rate is less than 5 percent.

High blood levels of a protein linked to heart attacks might also be an early warning sign of colon cancer. The substance, C-reactive protein, is produced in the liver in response to infection anywhere in the body.

Causes and Risk Factors

A genetic defect is connected with some forms of familial colon cancer. Other causes are not known. Risk factors associated with colorectal cancer include calcium deficiency; colorectal polyps; family history of colon cancer (Lynch syndrome); continued constipation and/or diarrhea; personal history of colon-related diseases or uterine or ovarian cancer, such as polyps, non-polyposis colon cancer, or inflammatory bowel disease; buildup of toxins in the colon; possibly diabetes; a diet high in saturated animal fat and low in fiber; high intake of charbroiled, burned, wood-smoked, or fried foods; obesity; smoking; alcohol consumption; and cancer in another part of the body. The consumption of white meat that has cooked at high temperatures and well-done red meat is associated with increased risk of rectal cancer among men. Many studies have shown that active people are not as likely to develop colon tumors as those who do not regularly engage in physical activity. Studies also show that women who eat diets high in beef, fats, desserts, and refined grains have an increased risk of colon cancer.

Signs and Symptoms

Symptoms of colorectal cancer can include rectal bleeding; blood in the stool; changes in bowel habits (persistent diarrhea, gas pains, and/or constipation); persistent abdominal pain or bloating; anemia or significant weight loss; unusual paleness or fatigue; and ulcerative colitis.

Detection and Diagnosis

Screening for colon cancer is the best way to detect polyps before they turn cancerous. During regular checkups (and annually after age forty), men and women should have a rectal exam. Beginning at age fifty, you also should have the first test listed below as well as either the second or third.

1. *Fecal occult blood test* (FOBT) and flexible sigmoidoscopy (if normal, repeat the FOBT yearly and the flexible sigmoidoscopy at 5-year intervals).

2. *Colonoscopy* (if normal, repeat at 10-year intervals).

3. *Virtual colonoscopy* is a computer-assisted method that allows doctors to visualize a person's colon in great detail. A small tube is inserted into the rectum and the colon is inflated with air. A CAT scan or MRI is then performed. A three-dimensional image of the colon is projected onto a computer screen and the physician analyzes the length of the colon looking for lumps that might be cancerous. The test is noninvasive, usually takes less than five minutes, and involves much less discomfort than conventional methods of examining the colon. Sedation is seldom required and the patient can go home immediately after the procedure.

In addition, a test kit for detecting blood in the stool can be purchased at most drugstores (*see* COLON CANCER SELF-TEST on page 292). For most people, polyps should never develop into colon cancer. Get regular colonoscopies so that precancerous polyps can be removed before they become cancer. If cancer develops, treatment is surgery and drugs such as chemotherapy with a long recuperation period.

Dietary and Nutritional Factors

It was once believed that a high-fiber diet protects the colon by reducing the time any harmful carcinogens that are present in the stool are in contact with the intestinal wall. There have since been conflicting reports on this, but most health professionals still recommend a high-fiber, low-fat diet. A high-fat diet has a strong link with colon cancer.

Either a vegetarian diet or a diet low in red meat, alcohol, and refined foods and high in vegetables, fruits, soy, fish, whole-grain breads, and cereals, as well as low- or nonfat dairy products and lots of fruit and vegetable juices offers optimum dietary protection. Garlic, broccoli, cabbage, cauliflower, Brussels sprouts, citrus fruits, melons, and dark green, red, and yellow vegetables are recommended for their antioxidant and sulfur compounds. Studies show that aged garlic slows the rate of progression of established colon cancer cells. Tomatoes may lower risk. Consumption of chlorinated water has been linked to a greater incidence of colon cancer. Coffee has been reported to have positive effects on reducing colon cancer risk. Drink milk. Studies show that drinking two 8-ounce glasses of milk daily may reduce the risk of developing colorectal cancer by as much as 15 percent.

Beta-carotene, calcium (1,200 milligrams daily), selenium, and vitamins C and E, and the long-term use of a multivitamin containing folic acid (above 400 micrograms daily) have been linked to a reduced risk of colon cancer.

Lutein and zeaxanthin, two of the carotenoids, help to protect against colon cancer. They are found in dark green leafy vegetables such as spinach, collard greens, kale, mustard greens, and turnip greens.

Probiotics (which can be found in yogurt and supplements) may inhibit colon cancer. Low levels of vitamin D and, possibly, excessive iron intake, have been associated with an increased risk of colon cancer. Quercetin has been shown to have anticancer properties with respect to colon cancer.

Endometrial Cancer

See under ENDOMETRIOSIS in Part Two.

Esophageal Cancer

Esophageal cancers are three to four times more common in men than in women, and now as common in African-Americans as in Caucasians. Tumors in the esophagus usually occur in the middle or lower half of the esophagus. Esophageal cancer is one of the deadliest forms of cancer in the United States because symptoms usually do not occur before it is in advanced stages when there is little chance of recovery. Still, survival rates have been going up in recent years.

Causes and Risk Factors

The cause or causes of esophageal cancer are not well understood. Risk factors include the use of tobacco and/or alcohol; age; personal history of Barrett's esophagus (a precancerous condition resulting from the reflux of stomach fluid into the bottom portion of the esophagus over an extended period of time), achalasia (constriction of the lower portion of the esophagus), tylosis (a very rare inherited disease that causes the overgrowth of skin on the palms of the hands and soles of the feet), or esophageal webs (small portions of tissue that stick out into the esophagus, often making it difficult to swallow); a high-fat diet; consumption of wood-smoked foods; previous ingestion of lye; and frequent heartburn. The risk generally rises with age. Those who smoke or drink heavily (or both) are at greatest risk. People with tylosis have nearly a 100 percent chance of developing esophageal cancer. Screening must begin at an early age for people with tylosis.

Signs and Symptoms

Usually there are no symptoms until the cancer is in the advanced stages. When they develop, symptoms may include progressive dysphagia (difficulty swallowing), often with a feeling of something being stuck in the throat or chest; vomiting and vomiting of blood; bringing up excess mucus; and unintended weight loss.

Detection and Diagnosis

See your doctor without delay if swallowing becomes even the slightest problem. Your doctor may use a barium X-ray and an endoscopic exam, or request a biopsy. A computerized tomography (CAT) scan or a newer procedure called an endoscopic ultrasound (an endoscope with an ultrasound probe) may also be ordered.

Dietary and Nutritional Factors

A diet high in fruits (including tomatoes) and vegetables may decrease the risk of this form of cancer. Fish, berries, mushrooms, and Brussels sprouts are all good sources of omega-3 fatty acids, which offer protection. The consumption of salted, pickled, or moldy foods has been associated with an increased risk. Another risk factor may be the consumption of extremely hot or cold foods that cause physical damage to the esophagus.

Green tea contains a mechanism that inhibits esophageal cancer. Vitamins A and C, selenium, and riboflavin may help protect against esophageal cancer. Spirulina has been found in several studies to inhibit the growth of oral tumors.

Laryngeal Cancer

The larynx (also known as the voice box) is the part of the respiratory tract between the pharynx and the trachea, containing the vocal cords. Cancer of the larynx affects more men than women. It usually strikes after the age of fifty. Most laryngeal cancers develop from squamous cells, the thin layer of cells that make up the lining of the larynx.

This type of laryngeal cancer usually begins as dysplasia and forms over a period of time—in fact, most of the precancerous cells go away on their own without treatment.

However, some of them form *carcinoma in situ* (CIS), the earliest form of cancer. Tumors located on the true vocal cords rarely spread because the connective tissues underneath do not contain lymph nodes, but tumors on other parts of the larynx are apt to spread early. Laryngeal cancer can be treated by radiation therapy, especially if diagnosed early, and by surgery to remove part or all of the larynx. If the larynx is completely removed, you must learn a new method of speech that involves the swallowing of air and bringing it up again. Some surgical techniques have been developed to reconstruct larynx tissue so that speaking can be returned to almost normal. One method that has worked for many people is the insertion of a prosthetic device.

Causes and Risk Factors

Most cases of laryngeal cancer are associated with the prolonged use of tobacco and/or alcohol. Associated risk factors include chronic inhalation of fumes; frequent laryngitis or vocal straining; and an inherited predisposition.

Signs and Symptoms

Possible symptoms of laryngeal cancer include a persistent cough; hoarse throat; swallowing difficulties, sometimes with a pain that radiates to the ear; persistent ear pain; chronic sore throat, sometimes so mild that it is hardly noticed; blood in saliva or sputum; unintended weight loss; and difficulty breathing.

Detection and Diagnosis

Persistent symptoms such as those listed above should be evaluated by a doctor who specializes in the head and neck area, or an otolaryngologist. Most voice changes are not a sign of cancer, but it is better to be safe and see a doctor if you are hoarse for more than two weeks. Diagnosis is made by laryngoscopy (visual examination of the larynx by means of a scope) plus biopsy.

Dietary and Nutritional Factors

The diet should be rich in fruits, vegetables, and foods containing vitamin A, the B vitamins, and retinoids. It is best to avoid alcohol.

If you are unable to acquire proper amounts of the above nutrients through diet alone, you should take supplements. Be sure that your total daily intake of vitamin A does not exceed 25,000 international units.

Leukemia

Leukemia is any of a variety of diseases of the blood-forming tissues (bone marrow, lymph system, or spleen).

Leukemia involves the production of abnormal white blood cells that do not function like normal cells, do not mature properly, and do not die off in a normal fashion. Leukemia affects both children and adults, although certain forms are most common in particular age groups. It is somewhat more common in Caucasians than in African-Americans.

According to the American Cancer Society, about 45,000 new cases of leukemia were diagnosed in the United States in 2008. There are four main types of leukemia:

1. *Acute lymphocytic leukemia* (ALL). ALL develops from cells in the bone marrow called *lymphocytes*. It accounts for slightly more than half of all cases of childhood leukemia. The most common type of cancer overall in children, it progresses rapidly.

2. *Acute myelogenous leukemia* (AML), also known as acute myeloid leukemia. AML develops from either granulocytes or monocytes (types of white blood cells). The chance of getting AML increases with age. However, children and adults of any age can develop AML. About one in five children with leukemia has AML. AML progresses rapidly.

3. *Chronic lymphocytic leukemia* (CLL). CLL develops from lymphocytes. The cells look mature but their function may not be normal. This disease occurs almost exclusively in adults, in whom it is the most common type of leukemia in adults. CLL progresses slowly.

4. *Chronic myelogenous leukemia* (CML). CML is another form of myeloid leukemia. It develops from granulocytes or monocytes. CML affects adults and is about half as common as CLL. It progresses slowly.

While there is no known cure, transfusions, chemotherapy, and bone marrow transplants are often effective treatments. Newer treatments include stem cell transplant, umbilical cord blood cell transplant, infusion of cell-specific antibodies, and biological therapy.

Causes and Risk Factors

No one knows exactly what causes leukemia, but suspected causal factors include genetics, viruses, and exposure to certain toxic chemicals. Known risk factors include heredity, radiation exposure, chronic viral infections, age, Down syndrome, having a sibling with leukemia, exposure to human T-cell lymphotropic virus 1 (HTVL-1), use of commercial hair dyes, alkylating agents, certain cancer therapies, and environmental exposure to benzene (found in unleaded gasoline) or radon.

Signs and Symptoms

Signs and symptoms of leukemia can include paleness; fatigue; shortness of breath when active; weight loss; repeated infections; excessive sweating; fever; easy bruising; slow-healing cuts; bone and joint pain; nosebleeds; swollen lymph nodes; increased susceptibility to infection; and an enlarged liver or spleen.

Detection and Diagnosis

Leukemia is usually diagnosed by means of blood tests and, possibly, bone marrow biopsy.

Dietary and Nutritional Factors

Soy products, which contain genistein and other isoflavones, may offer protection against leukemia. Good soy foods include tempeh, roasted soy nuts, soy powder protein, and miso. The bioflavonoid quercetin has been found in numerous studies to have anti-leukemia properties. Genistein has shown positive effects in destroying leukemia cells in laboratory tests. Low selenium levels have been associated with a greater risk.

Breast-fed babies have a reduced risk of contracting childhood leukemia than non-breast-fed babies.

Lung Cancer

Lung cancer is the most common cause of cancer-related death in both men and women. The average age at diagnosis is sixty. There are two general types of lung cancer: small cell (or oat cell) lung cancer, which accounts for approximately 13 percent of all lung cancers, and non-small-cell lung cancer, which accounts for approximately 87 percent of lung cancers. Small cell lung cancer grows very rapidly and has a tendency to spread early to other parts of the body. This type of lung cancer is commonly found in smokers.

There are three main types of non-small-cell lung cancer: squamous cell carcinoma (the most common form of lung cancer), adenocarcinoma, and large cell carcinoma.

More than 200,000 new cases of lung cancer are diagnosed each year, and nearly 160,000 people die of the disease. If caught before it has spread to the lymph nodes or other organs, lung cancer has about a 50 percent survival rate. However, most cancers are not caught at an early stage because they do not generally produce early symptoms, making the all-around survival rate for lung cancer relatively low—about 3 percent—although it has been improving thanks to new diagnostics and drugs.

Causes and Risk Factors

Smoking is the leading cause of lung cancer, and is thought to be responsible for 85 to 90 percent of cases. If you don't smoke, breathing in the smoke of others (called secondhand smoke) can increase your risk of developing lung cancer. A nonsmoker who lives with a smoker has a 20 to 30 percent greater risk of developing lung cancer, according to the American Cancer Society. Radon—a naturally occurring radioactive gas—is the second-leading cause of lung cancer, and the first among nonsmokers, according to the Environmental Protection Agency.

Other associated risk factors include marijuana use; exposure to asbestos, nickel, chromates, and radioactive materials; alcohol consumption; chronic bronchitis; history of tuberculosis; exposure to certain carcinogenic chemicals in the workplace, such as pesticides and herbicides; pollution; radon exposure; having had previous lung cancer; personal history of lung diseases caused by breathing certain minerals; tuberculosis; arsenic compounds; lung scarring from certain types of pneumonia; exposure to raw forms of talcum powders (not those found in household powders such as baby and facial powders); and deficiency (or excess) of vitamin A.

Signs and Symptoms

Lung cancer can cause a persistent cough; sputum with blood; chest pain; shortness of breath; fatigue; hoarseness; unintended weight loss; loss of appetite; recurring bronchitis or pneumonia; fever for an unknown reason; new onset of wheezing; and swelling of neck and face.

Detection and Diagnosis

If you have any persistent symptoms, see your doctor. Although many of these symptoms are often caused by other conditions, an examination is a crucial step in early detection. If your doctor does suspect lung cancer, he or she may order a series of imaging screenings, a study of a phlegm culture, a biopsy, a mediastinoscopy, a bronchoscopy, a bone marrow biopsy, and/or blood tests. There are also two diagnostic imaging tools that may be used in place of a biopsy: The Xillix LIFE-Lung Fluorescence Endoscopy System and Nofetumomab. Another imaging test, called NeoTect, may also aid in diagnosing cancer—possibly eliminating the need to have a biopsy done on a suspicious growth. A spiral CAT scan may eventually prove to be an effective lung cancer screening tool. However, it can trigger adverse side effects leading to decreased breathing function and death. Sixty percent of hospitals in the United States own spiral CAT machines, but for now they are mostly used *after* diagnosis for helping health care providers come up with a treatment plan. If you want to have this procedure, talk to your health care provider about the risks and benefits.

Dietary and Nutritional Factors

A diet high in fruits (including tomatoes) and vegetables is associated with a greatly reduced risk of lung cancer.

Shiitake mushrooms contain lentinan, which may also offer protection.

Genistein, an antioxidant found in soybeans, may have an inhibiting effect on the growth of lung cancer cells.

Alpha-carotene, beta-carotene, and other carotenoids are believed by many researchers to aid in reducing the risk of lung cancer, although there is some evidence that beta-carotene may be linked to a higher rate of lung cancer and mortality in smokers, former smokers, and those subjected to exposure to asbestos in their working environments.

Vitamins C and E and beta-carotene all work together, and when taken together, the potential adverse side effects are counteracted. Selenium, lycopene, lutein, and glutathione have been associated with a reduced risk of lung cancer.

The B vitamins have also been associated with a decreased risk of lung cancer.

Lymphoma

A key player in the body's immune system, the lymphatic system is made up of a circuitry of vessels that branch out and spread to all of the body's tissues—much like blood vessels do. Lymph nodes, found in the abdomen, chest, groin, neck, and underarms, are located along these vessels. Other parts of the lymph system include adenoids, bone marrow, the spleen, tonsils, and thymus gland. The intestines, skin, and stomach also contain lymphatic tissue. Lymph is a colorless fluid that contains lymphocytes, which fight infection.

Cancer that develops within the lymphatic system is categorized as either *Hodgkin's disease* or *non-Hodgkin's lymphoma* (all other forms of cancers in the lymph system). In non-Hodgkin's lymphoma (NHL), the body's ability to fight off infection is significantly decreased because fewer than normal white blood cells are produced. In addition, the cancer can spread through the lymphatic vessels to other parts of the body. NHL can be low-grade (slow-growing), intermediate-grade, or high-grade. Both intermediate-grade and high-grade NHL are fast-growing and can be deadly within one to two years if left untreated.

Non-Hodgkin's lymphoma is the seventh most common cancer in the United States. The actual number of new cases has increased, but the increase is also due in part to better methods of detection. Although this type of cancer can develop at any age, older adults are at highest risk.

A Danish study revealed a suspected link between mononucleosis and Hodgkin's disease. Those who contract mononucleosis may have a higher risk of developing Hodgkin's disease, and the increased risk appears to last for two decades.

Causes and Risk Factors

At least some cases of lymphoma are linked to a viral cause. In other cases, the cause is unknown. Risk factors include heredity; immune system dysfunction; exposure to herbicides, pesticides, or black hair dye; a diet high in red meat; AIDS; immune-depressing therapies; previous organ transplantation; benzene; and HTVL-1.

Signs and Symptoms

Symptoms of non-Hodgkin's lymphoma vary, depending on the area of cancer growth. If cancer is in the abdomen, it can cause nausea, vomiting, and abdominal pain or enlargement; in the chest—shortness of breath and cough; in the brain—headaches, vision changes, and seizures; in the bone marrow—anemia; in the thymus—shortness of breath or feeling of suffocation, and coughing.

Detection and Diagnosis

A biopsy can be done on lymphatic tissue to detect if there is any cancer present, and if so, what type. If any symptoms of non-Hodgkin's lymphoma are persistent, you should see your doctor for proper evaluation.

Dietary and Nutritional Factors

The diet should be low in animal protein and fat and high in fiber. Alcohol should be avoided.

Oral (Mouth) Cancer

Each year about 7,500 Americans die from oral cancer. It is twice as common in men as in women, although the incidence is rising in women.

Tumors in the oral cavity are not always malignant; however, some tumors can be precancerous. Oral leukoplakia is a precancerous condition of the mouth to which smokers and drinkers are particularly prone. People who have had cancer in the oral cavity are at greater risk of developing cancer in nearby areas and should have follow-up exams regularly throughout their lives.

Causes and Risk Factors

Smoking and the use of chewing tobacco are the primary causes of oral cancer. According to the American Cancer Society, 90 percent of people with mouth and throat cancers use tobacco, and the risk of developing these cancers increases with the amount smoked or chewed and the duration of the habit. Other risk factors include irritants inside the mouth, such as a broken tooth or ill-fitting or broken dentures; excessive alcohol intake; chronic use of a mouthwash with high alcohol content; poor oral and dental hygiene; ultraviolet light exposure to the lips; vitamin deficiency; Plummer-Vinson syndrome; HPV; and immune system depression.

Signs and Symptoms

While some oral cancers produce early symptoms, others do not until they are advanced. Symptoms may include a chronic sore of the mouth, tongue, or throat that does not heal; loss of feeling in the mouth or tongue; discolored patches in the mouth or throat area; swallowing difficulty or a feeling that something is stuck in the throat; mass in the cheek or neck; swelling or motion difficulty of the jaw; changes in the voice; and unintended weight loss. Cancer in the mouth has been known to disguise itself as another condition—even as a toothache.

Detection and Diagnosis

Cancer in the mouth can be found early through recommended regular exams by the dentist or doctor. If cancer is suspected, your doctor will refer you to an otolaryngologist (head and neck specialist). The doctor may perform a complete head and neck exam, which may or may not include a biopsy. If it is likely that cancer is present, a panendoscopy will be done, which includes a complete, thorough exam performed under anesthesia.

A mouthwash containing a dye that helps dentists to see very small suspicious sores and ulcers is available, and it may be useful for people with a high risk for oral cancer.

Dietary and Nutritional Factors

A diet low in fat and high in fruits (including tomatoes) and vegetables, with little or no alcohol consumption, is recommended. Omega-3 fatty acids, found in fish, berries, mushrooms, and Brussels sprouts, offer protection against oral cancer. Fiber-containing foods, soy, and other legumes may also reduce the risk. A study published in the journal *Archives of Otolaryngology—Head and Neck Surgery* suggests that taking beta-carotene supplements may reverse oral leukoplakia.

Vitamin deficiencies have been associated with oral cancer. Spirulina has been found in several studies to inhibit the growth of oral tumors.

Ovarian Cancer

Ovarian cancer is a deadly form of cancer—it kills more women than any other type of cancer of the reproductive system. If diagnosed and treated early, however, the survival rate is quite high—nine out of ten women treated will live longer than five years. Unfortunately, ovarian cancer is known as a silent disease—it produces no symptoms until it is in its later stages, so the death rate is also quite high. Of the 21,550 expected new cases in 2009, 14,600 women were expected to die.

Ovarian cancer is the second most common cancer of the female reproductive system. It affects approximately 1 in 71 American women at some point in their lives. The risk of developing ovarian cancer heightens past the age of forty and menopause further increases the risk.

Causes and Risk Factors

The cause or causes of ovarian cancer are not known. Risk factors include not having gone through pregnancy and childbirth; exposure to asbestos or radiation; high dietary fat intake; the use of talcum powder in the genital area; personal history of breast, uterine, colon, or nonpolyposis colon cancers; family history of breast or ovarian cancer; HPV infection; early onset and/or late cessation of menstruation; obesity; and a diet high in saturated animal fat and low in fiber. Taking birth control pills has been known to reduce the risk of ovarian cancer by 50 to 60 percent.

Signs and Symptoms

Often there are no obvious symptoms until the cancer is in its later stages of development. These symptoms may include enlargement of the abdomen, diarrhea or constipation, frequent urination, or in rare cases, vaginal bleeding.

Detection and Diagnosis

Any enlargement of the abdomen or persistent digestive disturbances that cannot be explained by any other condition should prompt you to see a gynecologist for an exam. Women who have a family history of ovarian cancer may want to be tested for genes with which it has been associated. Routine pelvic exams can detect a hardened or enlarged ovary or an ovarian growth, while Pap smears are not very useful in detecting this. A tumor may also show up on a transvaginal ultrasound. A biopsy is needed to confirm any suspicions. There are blood tests to detect ovarian and other gynecological cancers in women who are at high risk. However, in women with an average risk, these tests have not proven to lower the chance of dying from ovarian cancer. Levels of lysophosphatidic acid (LPA), a substance found in the blood, seem to rise consistently in women who have ovarian cancer. This may provide a basis for a blood test.

Dietary and Nutritional Factors

A diet that is high in fiber and low in saturated animal fats is a good defense against ovarian cancer. A diet high in folate intake may reduce the risk of ovarian cancer.

Quercetin has been found to have properties that protect against ovarian cancer. Low levels of selenium have been associated with a greater risk of ovarian cancer.

A study in Queensland, Australia, reported that women who drink more than one glass of red wine a day decrease their risk of developing ovarian cancer seven times over women who do not drink red wine.

Prostate Cancer

See PROSTATE CANCER in Part Two.

Skin Cancer

See SKIN CANCER in Part Two.

Stomach Cancer

There were an estimated 21,130 new cases of stomach cancer in the United States in 2009, and about 10,620 people died from it. It is nearly twice as common in men as in women, and is more common among lower-income people. The risk of stomach cancer increases past the age of forty.

Stomach cancer is more common in other countries including Japan, Chile, and Austria, while stomach cancer in the United States is on the decline. It may be that high intake of raw fish in Japan contributes to the high gastric cancer rates in that country.

The stomach is divided into five portions, and cancer can develop in any of them. Depending on the location where the cancer develops, stomach cancer can produce different symptoms and different outcomes. Most researchers agree that stomach cancer develops gradually and is often preceded by the development of precancerous cells. Stomach cancer has the ability to spread in several ways: through the stomach lining to surrounding organs, through the blood or lymphatic system, or by extending into the esophagus or small intestine.

Causes and Risk Factors

Some cases are probably a result of *Helicobacter pylori* (*H. pylori*) infection. In other cases, the cause is unknown.

Risk factors for stomach cancer include pernicious anemia; lack of hydrochloric acid and dietary fiber; high-fat diet; diet high in smoked, salted, or pickled foods; foods high in starch and low in fiber; tobacco and/or alcohol use; previous stomach surgery; chronic gastritis; stomach polyps; heredity; having type A blood; and a personal history of pernicious anemia or atrophic gastritis (a condition resulting in a reduction of gastric acid secretions).

Signs and Symptoms

There are often no symptoms in the early stages. When they develop, symptoms can include indigestion, pain, and bloating after eating; pain in the stomach that cannot be relieved by antacids; vomiting after eating or vomiting blood; black or tarry stools; anemia; fatigue; and unintended weight loss.

Detection and Diagnosis

If you are experiencing any of the symptoms listed above, it is important to see your doctor (especially if you are in a higher-risk category), even though many of the symptoms can be caused by other less-threatening conditions. If your doctor suspects stomach cancer, he or she may run several tests, including laboratory blood and fecal occult blood tests, an endoscopy, or a barium upper GI radiograph. A biopsy is needed for formal diagnosis. An endoscopic ultrasound is a newer method that can be used to see how far along the cancer is.

Dietary and Nutritional Factors

A diet high in fruits (including tomatoes), vegetables, rice, pasta, and beans, with limited amounts of meat products, is a good defense. Broccoli, onions, garlic, and pineapple are high in sulfur compounds, which offer protection against stomach cancer. Also, you should keep your consumption of smoked, barbecued, pickled, or salt-cured foods to a minimum, and avoid alcohol and tobacco products.

Antioxidants are a strong defense against free radicals that can damage cells and, possibly, make them turn cancerous. Vitamins C and E, alpha-carotene, beta-carotene, selenium, and lycopene are good sources of protection.

Testicular Cancer

Testicular cancer generally strikes men of younger ages—usually between the ages of twenty and thirty-five—and the chance of developing testicular cancer declines with age. It is more likely to occur in Caucasians than in African-Americans. The American Cancer Society estimates that about 8,400 new cases of testicular cancer will be diagnosed in the United States in 2009 and 380 men will die

from it. Because treatment is so successful, the risk of dying from testicular cancer is very low.

Tumors in the testicle tend to grow very rapidly—they can double in size in only twenty to thirty days. They can also spread quickly through the lymph nodes. For this reason, testicular cancer often spreads before diagnosis. The cure rate for testicular cancer is very high—over 95 percent—if it is detected early. Thankfully, new treatment methods can destroy even testicular cancers that have spread.

Causes and Risk Factors

The cause of testicular cancer is not known. It is known that cryptorchidism (undescended testicles) substantially increases the risk, even if the condition is corrected by surgery. Other risk factors include inguinal hernia during childhood and a personal history of mumps orchitis.

Signs and Symptoms

Symptoms of testicular cancer include a lump or lumps in a testicle; enlargement of a testicle; thickening of the scrotum; sudden collection of fluid in the scrotum; pain or discomfort in a testicle or in the scrotum; mild ache in the lower abdomen, back, or groin; enlargement or tenderness of the breasts; blood in the semen; and breast enlargement.

Detection and Diagnosis

A monthly self-exam is the best way to detect testicular cancer early (see TESTICULAR CANCER SELF-TEST on page 292), especially for boys and men between the ages of fifteen and forty. Yearly examinations by a physician are suggested as well. If cancer is suspected after examination of a mass, your physician will request a testicular ultrasound. Ultimately, a biopsy is needed for complete diagnosis.

Dietary and Nutritional Factors

A low-fat diet that includes generous helpings of fruits, vegetables, and grains is recommended. Tomatoes and watermelon are good sources of lycopene, which may protect against testicular cancer. Avoid high-fat foods and alcohol.

Vitamin E and other antioxidants may help reduce the risk. Some studies have suggested that vitamin A supplements may raise the risk.

years after being diagnosed, a rate that has been climbing since the 1970s, when only 50 percent lived that long. Sixty-one percent of survivors are age sixty-five and older. Seventy-five to eighty-five percent of childhood cancer survivors (90 percent with non-Hodgkin's lymphoma) are living five years after diagnosis.

Just as each of us looks different, each of our bodies has its own unique composition. What some of us react well to may cause an adverse reaction in others, which is why some treatments prove to be successful for some, but not

for others. This is why dietary wellness and prevention are so important. If we can keep our bodies healthy and avoid known cancer-causing agents, we have a good defense against ever getting cancer in the first place. And if you have cancer, it is imperative to maintain optimum health: If you go into battle unarmed, you don't stand much chance of winning; but if you go in with a full coat of armor, through the healthiest diet and nutrition, you have the best fighting chance to successfully conquer cancer.

The nutritional program and other recommendations

outlined in this section are designed for persons who have been diagnosed with cancer, as well as for those who wish to enhance their chances of avoiding this disease. In one survey, vitamin and mineral supplementation was found to be higher among patients with cancer or those who had recovered from it than the general population. About 50 percent of Americans use supplements, whereas 64 to 81 percent of cancer patients or survivors of cancer use them. If you take oral supplements, take them daily with meals (except for vitamin E, which should be taken before meals). Sometimes with certain cancers, such as of the intestines, where supplements are not adequately absorbed, it may be necessary to provide them intravenously. This should always be done under the supervision of a doctor.

CANCER SELF-TESTS

Breast Cancer Self-Test

See under BREAST CANCER in Part Two.

Colon Cancer Self-Test

A test kit can be purchased at most drugstores for detecting blood in the stool (an early sign of colon cancer). In one test, you simply drop a strip of chemically treated paper into the commode after a bowel movement. The paper will change to the color blue if blood is present in the stool.

If your test result is positive, take a second test in three days. If the second test is also positive, see your physician immediately. The presence of blood in the stool does not necessarily mean that you have cancer. The consumption of red meat or the presence of diverticulitis, hemorrhoids, polyps, ulcers, or an inflamed colon can all cause a positive test result. Only about 10 percent of those who test positive for blood in the stool have cancer. Women can get this test yearly at a gynecological examination; men can get it at their yearly physical exam. In any case, starting at age fifty, a colonoscopy is the best way to rule out colon cancer.

Testicular Cancer Self-Test

With the fingers of both hands, gently roll each testicle between the thumb and the fingers, checking for hard lumps or nodules. Be sure to include the epididymis (the ropelike portion) in your examination. Normally, testicles feel smooth and a little spongy. A mass will feel firm but not painful when pressed, unless there is bleeding inside the tumor. If you find a suspicious lump, see your physician. This test should be performed routinely by your physician at your yearly physical exam.

You will be better able to feel for lumps if you check for them after a warm bath or shower, when the scrotal skin is relaxed.

Unless otherwise specified, the doses recommended below are for persons over the age of eighteen. For children be-

tween twelve and seventeen years old, reduce the dose to three-quarters the recommended amount. For children between six and twelve, use one-half the recommended dose, and for a child under six years old, use one-quarter the recommended amount. The nutritional suggestions are intended to help support your body while you have cancer. Most nutrients are not preventive or curative, and they will not reduce the size or impact of the cancer, except where noted.

NUTRIENTS

SUPPLEMENT	SUGGESTED DOSAGE	COMMENTS
Essential		
Coenzyme Q₁₀ plus	90 mg daily.	Improves cellular oxygenation
Coenzyme A from Coenzyme-A Technologies	As directed on label.	Facilitates the repair of RNA and DNA. Supports the immune system's detoxification of many dangerous substances. Can streamline metabolism, ease depression and fatigue, and increase energy.
Colostrum (Plus Colostrum from Symbiotics [original and high-Ig formulas] or Colostrum Prime Life from Jarrow Formulas)	As directed on label.	Promotes accelerated healing and boosts the immune system.
Dimethylglycine (DMG) (Aangamik DMG from FoodScience of Vermont)	As directed on label.	Enhances oxygen utilization.
Garlic (Kyolic from Wakunaga)	2 capsules 3 times daily.	Enhances immune function.
Inositol hexaphosphate (IP₆)	As directed on label.	Has powerful anticancer properties; possesses natural killer cell activity.
Melatonin	2–3 mg daily, taken 2 hours or less before bedtime.	A powerful antioxidant that also aids sleep.
Methylsulfonylmethane (MSM)	As directed on label.	A powerful cancer prevention agent.
Selenium	200 mcg daily. Do not exceed a total daily intake of 800 mcg from all sources, including diet. If you are pregnant, do not exceed 40 mcg daily.	Powerful free radical scavenger and protector against cancer. Aids in protein digestion. *Caution:* Do not take supplemental selenium if you are pregnant or have heart, kidney, or liver disease.
7-Keto DHEA	As directed on label.	A metabolite of DHEA that possesses anticancer properties without being converted into testosterone or estrogens.
Superoxide dismutase (SOD)	As directed on label.	Destroys free radicals. Consider injections (under a doctor's supervision).

Supplement	Suggested Dosage	Comments
Vitamin A (Micellized Vitamin A and E from American Biologics)	50,000 IU daily for 10 days, then reduce to 25,000 IU daily. If you are pregnant, do not exceed 10,000 IU daily.	People with cancer require higher than normal amounts of this antioxidant. Use an emulsion form for easier assimilation and greater safety at higher doses. Capsule forms put more stress on the liver.
plus carotenoid complex with beta-carotene	As directed on label.	Enhances natural killer cell activity. Low beta-carotene levels have been especially associated with lung, bronchial, and stomach cancer. A powerful antioxidant
plus vitamin E	200 IU daily.	and cancer-fighter. Use d-alpha-tocopherol emulsion form for easier assimilation and greater safety at high doses.

Important

Supplement	Suggested Dosage	Comments
Grifron Maitake D-fraction from Maitake Products	As directed on label.	A mushroom extract that contains D-fraction form of isolated beta-1, 6-glucan, a substance that prevents carcinogenesis and inhibits the growth of cancerous tumors. Also helps the body adapt to the stress of cancer treatments such as chemotherapy.
Shiitake extract or reishi extract	As directed on label. As directed on label.	Mushroom extracts with valuable immune-boosting and antitumor properties.

Helpful

Supplement	Suggested Dosage	Comments
Acidophilus	As directed on label. Take on an empty stomach.	Has an antibacterial effect on the body. Use a nondairy formula.
Aerobic 07 from Aerobic Life Industries	As directed on label.	Contains antimicrobial agents.
Chromium picolinate	At least 600 mcg daily.	Helps to build and maintain muscle mass. Useful if muscle atrophy exists.
Grape seed extract	As directed on label.	A powerful antioxidant.
Kelp or seaweed	1,000–1,500 mg daily. As directed on label.	For mineral balance and to help the body avoid damage resulting from radiation therapy.
L-carnitine	As directed on label.	Protects against damage from free radicals and toxins. Use a form derived from fish liver (squalene).
Multienzyme complex	As directed on label, with meals.	To aid digestion. Caution: Do not give this supplement to a child.
Multimineral complex with calcium and magnesium and potassium plus vitamin D3	2,000 mg daily. 1,000 mg daily. 99 mg daily. 400–600 IU daily.	Essential for normal cell division and function. Use a comprehensive formula that contains all major minerals and trace elements except iron. Important for the prevention and/or treatment of several forms of cancer.
Multivitamin complex	As directed on label, with meals.	Do not use a sustained-release formula. Use a formula without iron.

Supplement	Suggested Dosage	Comments
N-Acetylcysteine (NAC)	As directed on label, on an empty stomach. Take with water or juice. Do not take with milk. Take with 50 mg vitamin B6 and 100 mg vitamin C for better absorption.	To detoxify harmful substances and protect the liver and other organs. Has shown preventive effects against cancer. (See AMINO ACIDS in Part One.)
plus glutathione and lipoic acid	As directed on label. As directed on label.	Essential for the functioning of the immune system. Found to be deficient in cancer patients. Can boost glutathione levels.
Omega-3 fatty acids (fish oil, flaxseed oil)	As directed on label.	Has antioxidant properties and may protect against, and prevent the spread of, cancer. Omega-3 fats from fish oil may attenuate muscle wasting (cancer cachexia).
Raw glandular complex plus raw thymus glandular and raw spleen glandular	As directed on label. As directed on label. As directed on label.	Stimulates glandular function, especially the thymus (site of T lymphocyte production). (See GLANDULAR THERAPY in Part Three.)
Taurine Plus from American Biologics	As directed on label.	Functions as foundation for tissue and organ repair. Necessary for white blood cell activation. Use the liquid or sublingual form.
Vitamin B complex plus extra vitamin B3 (niacin) and choline plus vitamin B12 and folic acid	50 mg of each major B vitamin 3 times (amounts of individual vitamins in a complex will vary). 100 mg daily. Do not exceed this amount. 500–1,000 mg daily. 1,000–2,000 mcg daily. 400–600 mcg daily.	B vitamins that improve circulation, build red blood cells, and aid liver function. Caution: Do not take niacin if you have a liver disorder, gout, or high blood pressure. To prevent anemia. Use a lozenge or sublingual form. Affects the repair of DNA. Has been linked to cancer protection.

Herbs

❑ Alternate the following in your cancer prevention or cancer therapy program: astragalus, birch, burdock root, cat's claw, chuchuhuasi (a rainforest herb), cranberry, dandelion, echinacea, fennel, green tea, licorice root, macela, milk thistle, parsley, pau d'arco, red clover, and suma.

Cautions: Do not use astragalus in the presence of a fever. Do not use cat's claw during pregnancy. Do not take echinacea for longer than three months. It should not be used by people who are allergic to ragweed. Green tea contains vitamin K, which can make anticoagulant medications less effective. Consult your health care professional if you are using them. The caffeine in green tea could cause insomnia, anxiety, upset stomach, nausea, or diarrhea. Licorice root should not be used during pregnancy or nursing. It should not be used by persons with diabetes, glaucoma, heart disease, high blood pressure, or a history of stroke.

❏ Spices such as cardamom, cayenne pepper, ginger, rosemary, sage, thyme, and turmeric have anticancer properties.

Caution: Do not use sage if you suffer from any type of seizure disorder, or are pregnant or nursing.

❏ Dozens of studies show that astragalus is a potent cancer fighter as well as a powerful immune booster that increases your body's production of T cells, macrophages, and natural killer cells. In one study astragalus was able to restore immune function in 90 percent of the cancer patients studied. Also, in two other studies, cancer patients who received astragalus had twice the survival rate of those who received standard therapy.

Caution: Do not use astragalus in the presence of a fever.

❏ Cat's claw enhances immune function and has antitumor properties. Cat's Claw Defense Complex from Source Naturals is a combination of cat's claw and other herbs, plus antioxidant nutrients such as beta-carotene, N-acetylcysteine, vitamin C, and zinc.

Caution: Do not use cat's claw during pregnancy.

❏ Many people with external cancers, such as skin cancers, have responded well to poultices made from comfrey, pau d'arco, ragwort, and wood sage. (*See* USING A POULTICE in Part Three.)

Caution: Comfrey is recommended for external use only.

❏ Curcumin, an extract from the spice turmeric, is gaining attention for its antioxidant properties and its ability to protect against cancer. Laboratory studies indicate that curcumin has the ability to guard against many carcinogenic substances, and that it may inhibit the rapid cell division characteristic of cancer cells.

❏ Green tea, which has gained a lot of attention for its cancer-fighting properties, contains a substance known as epigallocatechin-3-gallate (or EGCg), which has been found by a Swedish research team to cut off blood vessels that feed cancerous tumors.

Caution: Green tea contains vitamin K, which can make anticoagulant medications less effective. Consult your health care professional if you are using them. The caffeine in green tea could cause insomnia, anxiety, upset stomach, nausea, or diarrhea.

❏ Modified citrus pectin has been shown to substantially inhibit the growth of cancer cells and is especially effective in combating skin and prostate cancers.

❏ Noni is a fruit resembling the pineapple. Research suggests it may be effective not only in blocking tumor growth, but also in inducing cancer cells to return to normal. Studies also show that noni stimulates the immune system.

❏ Ojibwa Herbal Tea, a Native American Indian herbal tea composed of sheep sorrel, burdock root, slippery elm bark, and turkey rhubarb root, reportedly has healing powers for battling cancer.

❏ Olive leaf extract enhances the immune system and has shown good results in fighting cancer.

❏ Rosemary is currently being studied as a form of cancer therapy due to its antioxidant, anti-inflammatory, and carcinogen-blocking effects.

❏ Ayurvedic herbs said to protect against cancer include boswellia (*Boswellia serrata*), green tea (*Camellia sinensis*), and haldi (*Curcuma longa*, known in English as turmeric).

❏ The Chinese patent medicine Dang Gui Longhui Wan (a traditional mixture of eleven herbs that is customarily prescribed for chronic myelocytic leukemia) contains indirubin, which is currently under study for its possible ability to control the division of cancer cells.

Recommendations

❏ Eat a diet that includes grains, nuts, seeds, and unpolished brown rice. Millet cereal is a good source of protein. Eat wheat, oat, and bran.

❏ Eat plenty of cruciferous vegetables, such as broccoli, Brussels sprouts, cabbage, cauliflower, and spinach. Eat plenty of asparagus. Also consume yellow and deep-orange vegetables such as carrots, pumpkin, squash, and yams. Apples, berries (including blueberries, raspberries, and strawberries), Brazil nuts, cantaloupe, cherries, grapes, legumes (including chickpeas, lentils, and red beans), oranges, and plums all help to fight cancer. Most berries protect DNA from damage. Many of the plant pigments in red, yellow, orange, and blue fruits and vegetables are good sources of antioxidants. Green plants contain chlorophyll, which has been studied as a cancer fighter. Broccoli contains indole-3-carbinol (I-3-C), a compound known to eradicate many types of cancer cells on contact.

❏ Cook all sprouts slightly (except for alfalfa sprouts, which should be washed thoroughly and eaten raw).

❏ Eat onions and use garlic liberally, as it enhances the immune system and is a good cancer-fighter. Crushing garlic and then leaving it to rest for ten minutes before use seems to raise the levels of its cancer-fighting component, allyl sulfide. If you do not like the taste of garlic, take it in supplement form.

❏ Take ginger. Ginger suppresses nausea and therefore is an excellent treatment and preventive for the nausea and upset stomach that sometimes occurs with chemotherapy treatment. Ginger works best when taken with protein. In one study, the combination of the two resulted in a reduced use of medications for nausea and vomiting by cancer patients.

❏ Try to eat seven servings of whole-grain foods a day. Include at least five different types of grain foods in your diet each week.

❏ Eat ten raw almonds every day. They contain laetrile, which may have anticancer properties.

❏ Eat as many tomatoes and tomato-based products as you can. Lycopene, an antioxidant agent in tomatoes, protects

Alternative Cancer Therapies

A growing number of people with cancer are now turning to alternative means of cancer treatment. Some of the available alternative therapies provide help by strengthening the body and controlling the side effects of conventional treatments. Other approaches, because of their gentle, noninvasive nature, may in some cases be preferred over, or used in tandem with, more orthodox treatments.

Although there are a large number of different alternative therapies, most of them do have common themes. For instance, many of them are based on the belief that a truly healthy body is less vulnerable to cancer. They emphasize that cancer develops as the result of a problem with the immune system or an imbalance in the body, either or both of which may allow the cancer to develop. Thus, they try to reduce or eliminate the underlying problem that allowed the cancer to take hold, and to activate the body's own inherent healing processes so that the body can heal itself.

Usually, alternative treatments are holistic in approach. This means that the goal is to treat the whole body, rather than just the area seemingly affected by the cancer. Cancer is seen as a systemic disease and treatment is individualized, depending on the particular person. Many alternative approaches also aim to treat the individual on a number of different levels, including physical, mental, spiritual, and emotional.

Types of Alternative Treatments

Most of the alternative treatments used in cancer therapy fall into one of the following categories: biologic and pharmacological therapies, immunologic therapies, herbal therapies, metabolic therapies, mind-body therapies, and nutritional therapies. Although there is a certain amount of overlapping between categories—an immunologic therapy, for instance, may have nutritional components—these categories do serve to highlight the central focus of the many treatments and regimens that fall within them. Be aware, though, that the following discussion by no means mentions all of the individual therapies available. It is meant to familiarize you with the various approaches that may be used. Nor should this be seen as a recommendation for any of the following methods of treatment. The choice to seek alternative approaches of treatment for any illness must be made by the individual after a great deal of research and soul-searching. You may want to ask a conventional medical doctor and an alternative practitioner what the expected outcomes are based on the latest data. Do your research and find an experienced practitioner who can give you an informed and honest appraisal of your treatment.

Biologic and Pharmacological Therapies

Biologic and pharmacological treatments include the off-label use of prescription drugs, hormones, complex natural products (such as extracts), vaccines, and other biological interventions not yet accepted in mainstream medicine. These therapies use biologic substances or nontoxic phar-macological agents—nontoxic medications usually derived from biological sources, such as plants or human cells. Each of these treatments works in a different way.

Antineoplaston therapy, for instance, uses amino acid derivatives to inhibit the growth of cancer cells. Dr. Stanislaw Burzynski maintains that antineoplastons are part of the body's defense system and appear to be absent in people with cancer. He has been able to construct synthetic antineoplastons and administer them to cancer patients.

Another such treatment, shark cartilage therapy, is thought to work by blocking angiogenesis, the creation of new blood vessels required for tumor growth, and thus starve the tumor of needed nourishment.

Russian immunologist Dr. Valentin Govallo's VG–1000 theory, developed in the 1960s, is based on the belief that cancer results when a tumor evades and suppresses the immune system. Dr. Govallo believes that placenta extracts allow the immune system to readjust and attack the tumor that had escaped its attention in the first place. This method of treatment is called immuno-placental therapy.

The Revici method, developed by the late Dr. Emanuel Revici, is based on the premise that tumors are a result of an imbalance of lipids in the cells. After analysis of the tumor, the doctor delivers a compound into the tumor to establish the proper balance within the cells.

French physician Dr. Gaston Naessens developed a system of treatment known as 714-X treatment, which consists of injections of nitrogen-rich camphor and organic salts directly into the lymphatic system. The theory behind this treatment is that cancer cells excrete a poisonous compound that shuts down the immune system. The 714-X allows the immune system to reestablish itself and fight the cancer.

The National Institutes of Health's Office of Cancer Complementary and Alternative Medicine (OCCAM) also lists hydrazine sulfate, laetrile, and melatonin as pharmacological and biologic cancer treatments worth further study.

Herbal Therapies

In these therapies, herbal remedies—probably the oldest forms of treatment in the world—are used to strengthen the body's ability to eliminate cancer cells. Hoxsey therapy, for instance, first tested in the 1920s, employs internal and external herbal preparations, along with diet, vitamin and mineral supplements, and psychological counseling, to strengthen the body and fight the cancer. Hoxsey's treatment proved to be too controversial for America, however, and the Hoxsey formula is now used for cancer treatment more often in Mexico than in the United States.

Immunologic Therapies

Immunologic therapies are based on the belief that cancer develops because of a breakdown of the immune system. The aim of these therapies is to bolster those parts of the immune system that combat and destroy cancer cells. An example of the treatments in this category is that of the late

Dr. Josef Issels, who offered a comprehensive, nontoxic strategy for all types and stages of cancer to stimulate the body's immune system to attack cancer cells.

Metabolic Therapies

These therapies are based on the idea that many factors cause the occurrence of cancer and that a multifaceted healing approach is required to eliminate the disorder. The therapies use detoxification, including colon cleansing, to flush out toxins; anticancer diets based on whole foods; and vitamins, minerals, and enzymes that further cleanse the body, repair damaged tissues, and stimulate immune function.

Mind-Body Therapies

These treatments focus on the role that emotions, behavior, and faith play in recovery from illness. In the case of some therapies, counseling, hypnosis, biofeedback, or other techniques are used to promote greater emotional and spiritual well-being. In other therapies, the aim is to use mind-body techniques to actually change the course of the illness, possibly bringing the person into remission. For instance, Dr. O. Carl Simonton, with his Simonton Cancer Center, based in California, developed an imagery and visualization technique to help patients increase the effectiveness of their immune system. Yoga has become popular as part of this type of treatment. Dr. Barrie Cassileth of Memorial Sloan-Kettering Cancer Center in New York City has designed a series of complementary treatments for cancer patients. These include massage therapy, meditation, music therapy, imagery, and relaxation techniques. Dr. Herbert Benson at the Beth Israel Deaconess Medical Center in Boston has done the most research over thirty-five years on the mind-body connection in helping patients cope with disease including cancer.

Nutritional Therapies

Therapies that focus on nutrition are perhaps the most popular alternative approach to cancer, especially since research began showing the link between diet and health.

Almost every alternative therapy includes an emphasis on diet as an important component of both prevention and, possibly, cure. For instance, studies have indicated that a high-fat diet increases the risk of cancer, while a low-fat diet that is rich in fiber, fresh fruits and vegetables, and whole grains actually helps the body to fight cancer. Three of the therapies that fall into this category are wheatgrass therapy, a diet based on wheatgrass and other raw foods; the macrobiotic diet, a traditional Japanese diet high in whole grains and vegetables; and the Moerman regimen, a meatless high-fiber diet that includes nutritional supplements.

Choosing an Alternative Therapy

Unless you already have a specific therapy in mind, the first step in choosing one is to learn more about those that are available. By visiting libraries and bookstores and contacting health organizations that focus on cancer, you should be able to find a number of comprehensive, up-to-date books that provide additional information about alternative treatments.

Once you have a better idea of the therapy or therapies that would best serve your needs, contact educational organizations and patient-referral services that provide information on these treatments. (*See* Part Three, REMEDIES AND THERAPIES, for further information about alternative treatments.)

When researching a particular therapy, try to get information from other people who have used that treatment. Some information organizations and some alternative clinics will provide lists of recovered patients whom you can call or write to. Focus on those people who have the same kind of cancer you have, and ask them what specific treatments they found helpful.

When screening alternative practitioners and clinics, ask what their success has been in treating your specific form of cancer. Keep in mind that a therapy that is effective against one type of cancer will not necessarily be effective against another. Ask to see supportive studies, documented cases, and patients' testimonials, and view all information with a healthy dose of skepticism. As much as possible, pin the practitioner down regarding what you can expect from the treatment—short-term improvement or long-term survival, for instance. Finally, consider whether the therapy fits in with your lifestyle, personality, and belief system. Be honest with yourself. Some therapies require a degree of commitment that you may not be willing to make. Others may require too much time, too much travel, or too much money to truly be feasible. However, if you have the fortitude and resources to follow an alternative method of treatment to overcome an illness, the rewards are priceless. It is worth checking to see if your health insurance will cover any part of your alternative medicine. Conventional and alternative (or secondary) treatments may be used together—one method of treatment does not necessarily preclude the other.

To get started, why not explore those endorsed by the American Cancer Association. These have worked for many cancer patients already.

- Acupuncture
- Aromatherapy
- Art therapy
- Biofeedback
- Labyrinth walking
- Massage therapy
- Meditation
- Music therapy
- Prayer and spirituality
- Tai chi
- Yoga

cells from oxidants associated with cancer. Eating a diet that includes plenty of tomatoes cuts the risk of cervical, lung, stomach, and prostate cancers. Preliminary reports suggest it may also prevent breast, colorectal, esophagus, mouth, and pancreatic cancers.

❏ Eat a lot of tart cherries, both fresh and in pies, jams, and sugar-free juice. They contain anthocyanins, antioxidants that may help prevent cancer and heart disease.

❏ Drink beet juice (from roots and greens), carrot juice (a source of beta-carotene), fresh cabbage juice, and asparagus juice often. Grape, black cherry, and all dark-colored juices are good, as are black currants. Also beneficial is apple juice, if it is fresh. Fruit juices are best taken in the morning, vegetable juices in the afternoon.

❏ Drink spring or steam-distilled water only, not tap water. Increased levels of contaminants in public water have been associated with an increased rate of lung, bladder, and breast cancers, as well as leukemia.

❏ Limit your consumption of dairy products. A little yogurt, kefir, or raw cheese occasionally is okay, but make sure that you are getting enough calcium, magnesium, and vitamin D from other foods or supplements. Calcium and vitamin D at levels slightly above the DRI have been shown to reduce the risk of all cancers in postmenopausal women. Since it is difficult to obtain these nutrients from food alone, it makes sense to take daily supplements, especially if you are eliminating dairy from your diet.

❏ Do not consume any of the following: peanuts, junk foods, processed refined foods, saturated fats, salt, sugar, or white flour. Instead of table salt, use sea salt, kelp, or a potassium substitute. If necessary, a small amount of blackstrap molasses or pure maple syrup can be used as a natural sweetener in place of sugar. Use whole wheat or rye instead of white flour. Do not consume anything containing alcohol or caffeine.

❏ Limit your intake of luncheon meats, hot dogs, or smoked or cured meats. Broiled fish or poultry are better choices. Fish is particularly important because it has not been associated with an increased risk of cancer, as beef has.

❏ See FASTING in Part Three, and follow the program.

❏ A green drink that is a good master cleanser combines the juice of 2 organic lemons, 2 tablespoons pure maple syrup, ¼ teaspoon cayenne pepper, 1 ounce fresh wheatgrass juice, and 1 quart of distilled water. If fresh wheatgrass is not available, powdered Sweet Wheat from Sweet Wheat, Inc. is a good substitute.

❏ Take coffee enemas alternated with enemas made by adding 1 ounce of fresh wheatgrass juice to 1 cup of water. Do this daily to help the body eliminate toxins, if your gastrointestinal tract can handle it. Avoid enemas if you have colon cancer—an enema will hurt the inside lining of the GI tract. Wheatgrass enemas contain many nutrients and enzymes, and are used in many alternative clinics for cancer treatment. Also use cleansing enemas with lemon and water or garlic (Kyolic liquid) and water two or three times weekly. (See ENEMAS in Part Three.)

❏ Do not take supplemental iron, unless your doctor has told you that you are anemic or require it for other reasons. If you are not iron deficient, the body naturally withholds iron from cancer cells to inhibit their growth. People with excessive iron in their blood have an increased risk of developing cancer. Excess iron may suppress the cancer-killing action of macrophages (cells that engulf and devour bacteria and other foreign invaders) and interfere with the activity of lymphocytes.

❏ Use only glass or stainless steel cookware and wooden cooking utensils.

❏ Get regular exercise. Cancer is less prevalent in physically active people. Exercise also helps to stave off depression and promotes oxygenation of the tissues.

❏ Check the radon level in your home. Radon is a radioactive gas that occurs naturally within the earth's crust that has been classified by the Environmental Protection Agency (EPA) as a known carcinogen. Radon test kits are easy to find at hardware stores and are relatively inexpensive. If radon is found, sealing cracks and improving ventilation in the basement will usually improve the situation.

❏ Because of potential low-level radiation leakage, avoid microwave ovens. Do not sit close to television sets—sit at least eight feet away. Also avoid X-rays.

❏ Avoid chemicals such as hair sprays, cleaning compounds, waxes, fresh paints, and garden pesticides. Many chemicals promote the formation of free radicals in the body, which may lead to cancer. People with cancer can further weaken their immune systems by coming into contact with chemicals. The body then must expend energy trying to protect itself from the damaging chemicals instead of fighting the cancer.

❏ Use a shower head that removes the chlorine from your water. A product called Showerwise from Waterwise will do this. (See Manufacturer and Distributor Information in the Appendix.)

❏ Remove known and suspected carcinogens from your life and from your home. *Diet for a Poisoned Planet* by David Steinman (Running Press, 2006) provides information on the safety of our food, water, and the products we use every day.

❏ Do not take any drugs except for those prescribed by your physician.

❏ As much as possible, avoid stress. Learn relaxation and stress management techniques (such as meditation, visualization, deep breathing, and participation in support groups) to help you deal with those stresses you cannot avoid. (See STRESS in Part Two.)

Considerations

❑ Many people with cancer have achieved good results with a macrobiotic diet.

❑ Some oncologists dissuade their patients from using dietary supplements when they are undergoing chemotherapy, radiation, or both, because of possible interactions. However, in a review of fifty clinical, peer-reviewed articles, involving over 8,000 patients, those who took supplements consistently had no problem with interactions. The nutrients most used by the cancer patients in this study were vitamins A, B complex, C, D, E, and K, selenium, cysteine, and glutathione. In a subset of these studies, survival was increased in those using supplements.

❑ If weight loss and muscle wasting are significant, you may have cachexia, which is associated with a high mortality, so early treatment is advised. More than 5 million people with a variety of diseases including cancer have this condition. It may be treatable with aggressive nutritional therapies such as intravenous or tube-feeding formulas.

❑ High doses of L-carnitine (6 grams a day for four weeks) were shown to increase energy levels and quality of life in patients with cancer.

❑ In a recent study, red meat and processed meats were associated with modest increases in cancer deaths, as well as death by any cause and death from heart disease. These findings were published in the prestigious medical journal *Archives of Internal Medicine*. The safest amount of red meat or processed meat was an average of ½ ounce per day. Thus, you can eat a serving (3 to 4 ounces) of these once a week without increasing your risk of developing cancer.

❑ Linoleic acid was once thought to be anti-carcinogenic, but a recent study suggests it is not. However, if you have been advised to lose weight, conjugated linoleic acid may be helpful. It helps to burn fat and induce a slow weight loss.

❑ German physician and cancer specialist Dr. Hans Nieper used fresh raw cabbage and carrot juice with excellent results. Dr. Nieper also used Carnivora, a substance derived from a South American plant, to fight cancer.

❑ New York–based immunologist Dr. Nicholas Gonzalez developed a cancer treatment regimen that has been studied by the National Institutes of Health that incorporates changes in diet, nutritional supplementation, and toxin-removal systems, including coffee enemas.

❑ Various types of mushrooms can be good sources of vitamin D, B$_1$ (thiamine), B$_2$ (riboflavin), B3 (niacin), minerals, and amino acids. They have the ability to enhance the body's immune system T cells that seek and destroy cancer cells. Shiitake, zhu ling, enoki, reishi, and maitake mushrooms have all been reported to have anticancer properties.

❑ Exceptionally low cholesterol levels have been associated with an increased risk of dying from cancer, possibly because people with lower cholesterol levels tend to consume more polyunsaturated fats, which may increase cancer risk.

❑ The rates of breast cancer among some women of Asian-American descent, particularly Japanese Americans, may be approaching those of white women, according to new research. University of Southern California researchers examined the trends in Los Angeles County and reported their results in the *International Journal of Cancer*. Women living in Asian countries have some of the lowest breast cancer rates of any group in the world, in contrast to women in the United States, where rates are among the highest in the world. Much of this has been linked to differences in lifestyle factors such as diet, exercise, body weight, and choosing to have children later in life (or not at all). Ethnicity and national origin are among the strongest known predictors of breast cancer risk, the authors said. These factors are thought to affect a woman's risk even more than those associated with menstrual periods and childbearing. But breast cancer rates have risen sharply in recent years in some Asian countries such as Japan, where women have adopted more "Westernized" lifestyles. In fact, breast cancer is expected to soon become the most common cancer among women in Japan, the authors said.

❑ A daily dose of seven to ten servings of fruits and vegetables can reduce cancer risk by about 30 percent. Eating smaller amounts—5 servings a day—does not reduce the risk. In a study published in the *Journal of the American Medical Association*, women who had breast cancer and were in remission who ate 5 servings of fruits and vegetables a day did not have a reduced rate of recurrence of the disease. Still, many phytochemicals found in plant foods are currently being studied for anticancer properties, including:

- Lutein, one of the carotenoids, is under investigation as a possible anticancer nutrient. Good sources of lutein include dark, leafy greens and broccoli.

- Genistein and diadzein, two isoflavones found in soy, act as antioxidants and may protect against most forms of cancer, especially prostate cancer, breast cancer, leukemia, glioblastoma multiforme, and bladder cancer. Soy's soluble fiber reduces the risk of many digestive system cancers, such as colon and rectal cancer. The water-absorbing fiber may dilute intestinal carcinogens and usher them out of the body, as well as spur growth of bifidobacteria, the good bacteria that help prevent colon cancer. Mega Soy Formula from Prolongevity is a good supplement that contains a substantial amount of genistein and other isoflavones that help to fight cancer. Although they may reduce risk of cancer, because of their estrogen-like properties, isoflavones may actually increase the risk of some kinds of cancer. A new review says phytoestrogens may have both a protective role and a stimulatory role in breast cancer cell growth depending on several factors, including at what age they're consumed and whether they're consumed as food or as supplement. The report appeared in the September/October 2007 issue of *CA: A Cancer Journal for Clinicians*, a peer-reviewed journal of the American Cancer Society.

- D-glucaric acid, a phytochemical found in broccoli, Brussels sprouts, and cauliflower, has shown evidence in several clinical studies of reducing the incidence of cancers of the breast, lung, liver, and skin. D-glucaric acid is also available in supplement form combined with calcium (calcium D-glucarate).

❑ A four-year study conducted at the University of Illinois College of Medicine showed that high levels of antioxidants have a protective effect against cancerous tumors. However, there have been some mixed results from other studies. Alpha-tocopherol has been shown to protect against tumors, while in one study beta-carotene and vitamin A had no effect. In another study, large amounts of vitamin E had no significant effect, but seemed to trend toward *increasing* risk of prostate cancer.

❑ Calcium may prevent precancerous cells from becoming cancerous.

❑ Inositol hexaphosphate (IP_6), a form of the B vitamin inositol, is gaining attention for its ability to aid in the prevention and treatment of cancer. It is found naturally in whole grains, beans, lentils, pork, veal, citrus fruits, and nuts. Evidence has shown that it may not only shrink tumors, but also prevent tumor growth.

❑ Niacin may play a major role in the prevention and treatment of cancer.

❑ The lower the serum concentrations of the mineral selenium, the greater the associated risk of several types of cancer, including leukemia, esophageal, lung, colorectal, prostate, breast, and ovarian cancers. However, according to the National Institutes of Health's Office of Dietary Supplements, the tolerable upper level for adults is 400 micrograms (mcg) per day. Selenium supplementation should be discussed with a physician. Dietary sources of selenium include Brazil nuts, tuna, flounder, pork, turkey, pasta, pinto beans, and navy beans.

❑ Studies have shown that supplementation of vitamins A, C, and E can decrease the effect of lipid peroxidation, or the oxidation of body fats, which leads to the creation of free radicals in the body.

❑ Research is under way to determine the effects of vitamin D on cancer. Early findings suggest that daily exposure to a limited amount of sunlight (a good source of vitamin D) may reduce the risk of breast, colon, and prostate cancers. If sunlight is not available all year round, taking a vitamin D supplement is just as effective.

❑ Gamma E Tocopherol from Prolongevity is a vitamin E supplement containing gamma-tocopherol, delta-tocopherol, alpha-tocopherol, and beta-tocopherol—all natural forms of vitamin E. This product offers powerful protection against dangerous free radicals.

❑ Nutritional supplements and better dietary habits offer great support to cancer patients who are receiving chemotherapy and/or radiation, or who are in remission. Taking shark liver oil prior to radiation therapy has been shown to protect healthy tissue against injury from the procedure. Shark liver oil contains alkylglycerols (AKGs), vitamins A and E, omega-3 fatty acids, trace minerals, and squalene. A study published in the *European Journal of Cancer* in 1997 reported that glutamine can reduce adverse side effects associated with chemotherapy.

❑ Some types of cancer are treated with chemotherapy, which can apparently cause cancer to go into remission. Cancer chemotherapy is the administration of highly toxic medications meant to kill cancer cells. Most chemotherapy medications destroy normal cells in the process, causing adverse side effects including hair loss, extreme nausea, vomiting, fatigue, weakness, sterility, and damage to the kidneys and heart. Certain nutrients may help the body avoid some of the damage done by this treatment, among them vitamin B_6 (pyridoxine), coenzyme Q_{10}, glutathione, and vitamin C.

❑ In some cases, radiation therapy may be recommended. This involves aiming concentrated X-rays directly at a tumor to kill the cancerous cells. Radiation therapy too has unpleasant side effects, including fever, headache, nausea and vomiting, and loss of appetite.

❑ Moderate use of low-dosage aspirin may aid in killing tumor cells. *The New England Journal of Medicine* found that patients who had been treated for colorectal cancers had a lower rate of recurrence when they took a daily dose of aspirin and that aspirin reduces the growth of polyps in the colon that may lead to cancer. However, the Nurses' Health Study at Boston's Brigham and Women's Hospital came to the unexpected conclusion that women who take aspirin twice daily increased their risk of getting pancreatic cancer.

❑ Non-small-cell lung cancers, which account for most cases of lung cancer in the United States, may be treated with porfimer (Photofrin), gefitinib (Iressa), and gemcitabine (Gemzar) in combination with cisplatin. Paclitaxel (Taxol) taken in combination with the commonly used cancer drug cisplatin (Platinol) is still being investigated.

❑ Docetaxel (Taxotere) is a drug approved for treating non-small-cell lung cancer that does not respond to cisplatin-based chemotherapy.

❑ Doxorubicin (Adriamycin) is a potent chemotherapeutic drug used for treating many forms of cancer. Patients on this drug should avoid curcumin (turmeric).

❑ The genetically engineered virus ONYX-015 is designed to infect and kill cancer cells without harming healthy ones. It is under study. Other drugs undergoing testing as cancer therapies include:

- Angiostatin and endostatin, promising anticancer agents that stop the growth of new blood vessels to feed tumors.

- BR96-DOX, a drug that zeroes in on cancer cells, leaving the healthy cells alone. Its active ingredient is doxorubicin, a proven chemotherapy cancer-killing substance.

- Hydrazine sulfate is a monoamine oxidase (MAO) inhibitor available as a dietary supplement that may help offset the inability to eat, fatigue, weight loss, and muscle deterioration often associated with cancer. It also has been studied for over three decades as a treatment for cancer itself. Possible side effects include nausea and vomiting, tingling, loss of feeling, and inflammation of the nerves in the hands and feet, and irregularities in glucose level, alkaline phosphatase, and liver function tests have been reported. Dizziness, weakness, drowsiness, and itching may also occur.

• Interferon and interleukin-2 (IL-2) were the standard treatment for metastatic kidney disease. Now two drugs replace this therapy: sunitinib, which inhibits several cellular proteins that promote growth of blood vessels in tumors; and temsirolimus, which targets another cellular protein that regulates the growth of tumor cells.

❏ Two preventive vaccines have been approved for cancer. One prevents the hepatitis B virus, which can cause liver cancer. The other is a vaccine against the human papillomavirus (HPV) types 16 and 18, which are responsible for many cases of cervical cancer. Effective cancer treatment vaccines are under investigation, including one for non-Hodgkin's lymphoma and another for advanced non-small-cell lung cancer.

❏ Hyperthermia, a procedure in which body tissue is exposed to extremely high temperatures (up to 106°F), may be effective against tumor cells and can be used alone or in combination with radiation therapy and other therapies. Researchers believe that the heat may damage tumor cells or deprive them of the nutrients they need to live. It is important that hyperthermia is applied in a safe way under a physician's care.

❏ Conventional therapies (chemotherapy, radiation, and surgery) may not be as effective at fighting cancers of the lung, pancreas, liver, and bone, and advanced colon and breast cancers, as they are at fighting other types of cancer.

❏ The hormone dehydroepiandrosterone (DHEA) is believed by some to help prevent cancer by blocking an enzyme that promotes cancer cell growth. A form of DHEA, 7-keto DHEA, unlike DHEA itself, is not converted into testosterone or estrogens. It may be a better option for those at high risk for breast, endometrial, uterine, and prostate cancers. (See DHEA THERAPY in Part Three.) However, according to the American Cancer Society, available scientific evidence does not support claims that DHEA supplements are safe or effective for treating cancer. Caution is advised in their use in people who have cancer, especially types of cancer that respond to hormones, such as certain types of breast, prostate, and uterine cancer. People younger than thirty may run the risk of suppressing the body's natural production of DHEA if they take DHEA supplements.

❏ Studies have shown grape seed extract to not only enhance the development of normal cells, but also to inhibit abnormal cell growth.

❏ Research has shown hyperbaric oxygen therapy (HBOT) is effective when used in addition to conventional treatment for the prevention and treatment of osteoradionecrosis, a term for delayed bone damage caused by radiation therapy. There is also some evidence suggesting HBOT may be helpful as an additional treatment for soft tissue injury caused by radiation. However, there is no evidence that HBOT cures cancer. (See HYPERBARIC OXYGEN THERAPY in Part Three.)

❏ Research is ongoing regarding the anticancerous effects of the hormone melatonin, which is produced by the pineal gland. It has strong antioxidant effects and acts as a scavenger of free radicals that induce DNA damage. Melatonin may inhibit tumor growth by interaction with interleukin 2 (IL-2) and seems to have a beneficial effect particularly on endocrine tumors. The synthetic form is preferred since the natural form, recovered from animal pineal glands, could contain harmful viruses. Melatonin can be used to good effect on various types of tumors, under supervision of a physician. It seems to be effective in fighting cancers of the male and female reproductive system, breast, and prostate. Studies are still needed to determine the effects of long-term use of melatonin in supplement form. Some recent studies have found that people who work night shifts may be at increased risk for cancer, which could be linked to melatonin levels in the body. Study results regarding the effect of melatonin supplements on survival and quality of life in people with cancer have been mixed, and further research in this area is needed.

❏ In older studies shark cartilage has been shown to be helpful for certain types of cancer, including cancer of the breast, cervix, pancreas, and prostate, as well as Kaposi's sarcoma, a type of skin cancer. It suppresses angiogenesis (the development of new blood vessels), depriving cancerous tumors of nourishment and, often, causing them to shrink and die. Although some laboratory and animal studies have shown that some components in shark cartilage have the ability to slow the growth of new blood vessels, these effects have not been proven in humans. The few small clinical studies of shark cartilage products published more recently have not shown any benefit against cancer. Further clinical trials of the supplements and of a purified cartilage extract are currently under way.

❏ Shark liver oil is a rich source of alkylglycerols, chemicals that may have anticancer properties. Alkylglycerols are also found in human bone marrow and in breast milk. Other chemicals in shark liver oil being studied against cancer are squalamine and squalene.

❏ The single most avoidable cancer risk is smoking. Cigarette smoke is made up of more than 4,000 chemicals, including 43 that are known to cause cancer. It also contains the poisonous gases nitrogen oxide and carbon monoxide. Lung cancer was a rare disease until the twentieth century, when cigarette smoking became widespread. In 2009 there were an estimated 219,440 new lung cancer diagnoses and

159,390 deaths. Besides lung cancer, smoking can cause cancers of the cervix, kidney, pancreas, and stomach. The cancerous effects of smoking are multiplied by alcohol consumption, and the two are frequently used in combination. Research suggests that if you quit smoking when precancerous signs are found, damaged lung tissue may return to normal, oftentimes within five years. Statistics show that 1 out of 5 women diagnosed with lung cancer has never smoked, compared to 1 out of 10 men. Regular exposure to secondhand smoke can increase a nonsmoker's chance of getting cancer by 20 to 30 percent.

❑ There have been some claims that dairy products increase the risk of cancer. However, it is more likely that it is fat that is the problem, not milk. Almond, rice, and soy milk are good low-fat alternatives.

❑ A study published by the *American Journal of Epidemiology* has disproved suggestions that there is a link between lactose and/or galactose (sugars found in milk) and ovarian cancer.

❑ Obesity in men may cause or contribute to colon and rectal cancer; in women, it has been linked to gallbladder, cervical, uterine, and breast cancer. Overweight women are more likely to develop cancer of the uterine lining than other women and tend to do poorly if they develop breast cancer. Fat affects the level of sex hormones in the body. Hormones produced by the adrenal glands are converted into estrogen in fat tissue, so the greater the amount of fat present, the higher a woman's estrogen levels are likely to be. Estrogen stimulates cells in the breast and reproductive system to divide.

❑ Some people believe that fluoride (which is in toothpaste, tap water, and every product made with tap water) may be a risk factor for cancer.

❑ The incidence of leukemia among children who were breast-fed has been found to be significantly lower than that among bottle-fed children.

❑ A group of seventy-five Environmental Protection Agency (EPA) experts ranked pesticide residues among the top three environmental cancer risks.

❑ Men who undergo vasectomy do not increase their prostate cancer risk, according to researchers in the *Journal of the American Medical Association (JAMA)*. There had been some concern about vasectomies and prostate cancer because two 1990 studies reported an increased risk of prostate cancer after vasectomy.

❑ High-voltage power lines have been under study as a possible contributor to cancer. Researchers at the National Institute of Environmental Health Sciences (NIEHS) have reported that, while it is a possibility, it is not likely.

❑ Since women have been having Pap smears, the mortality rate for cervical cancer has dropped by more than 70 percent. However, Pap smears are not always accurate. Some tests show promise for improving the accuracy of Pap tests. AutoPap is a computerized screening test designed to improve the Pap test's accuracy. ThinPrep is another variation on the Pap test. It utilizes a different method of collecting the cells that can make it easier to detect cell abnormalities. The FDA has approved an HPV DNA test that can detect the presence of human papillomavirus (HPV), which is associated with cervical cancer. Women over age thirty and who are at higher risk for cervical cancer may want to discuss these tests with their doctors. Research on other types of tests to detect cervical cancer is ongoing.

❑ Irritable bowel syndrome does not increase the risk of colon cancer.

❑ Men who receive either of two kinds of treatment for testicular cancer appear to be at increased risk for leukemia. A recent study highlighted those getting radiation treatment and Cisplatin, a standard cancer chemotherapy agent. The study also noted that the higher the dosage, the greater the risk. Researchers are quick to point out that the benefits of both treatments far outweigh the small increased risk of leukemia.

❑ Most people are unfamiliar with head and neck cancer, yet worldwide more than 500,000 people are diagnosed with these cancers every year. According to the National Cancer Institute (NCI), men are three times more likely than women to be diagnosed with head and neck cancer and almost twice as likely to die from their disease. Patients with head and neck cancer suffer a high mortality rate. Head and neck cancer does not include brain tumors. Treatment includes radiation therapy, which is often implemented following surgery. However, radiation therapy can cause adverse, even lethal, side effects. Lethal radiation necrosis (tissue death) in the brain is one potential side effect of radiation therapy. Also, stroke rates increase by five times in people who have undergone radiation therapy for head and neck cancer. Stroke is the official cause of death among many people who have had head and neck cancer who later die after radiation therapy treatments. For this reason, cancer cure statistics can be misleading. Even though radiation therapy may cure cancer, nonrelated cancer deaths seem to be a long-term side effect of radiation. Although more people with cancer are now living beyond five years after diagnosis, premature death can be a direct result of toxic therapies used to eradicate cancer. We do not recommend that people with head and neck cancer refuse radiation therapy, as it often buys years of extra life. They should, though, take extra precautions to reduce their risk of stroke. (*See under* CARDIOVASCULAR DISEASE in Part Two.)

❑ A small portion of colorectal cancers are known to be caused by inherited gene mutations. Hereditary nonpolyposis colon cancer is caused by changes in genes that normally help a cell repair faulty DNA. Cells must make a new copy of their DNA each time they divide into two cells. Sometimes errors are made in copying the DNA code. Cells usually have DNA repair enzymes, but some mutations in these enzymes such as MLH1 may allow DNA errors to go uncorrected. These errors will sometimes affect growth-regulating genes, which may lead to cancer. Genetic tests are available that can detect gene mutations associated with some inherited gene mutations.

❑ Cancer has been reported to be badly underdiagnosed. In one autopsy review of those found with malignancies, over half of the deaths were caused by undiagnosed cancer.

❑ There are many hospitals, research centers, and treatment centers that specialize in cancer treatment. For a list of organizations that may be of assistance in obtaining information and/or treatment options, *see* Health and Medical Organizations in the Appendix.

❑ *See* BREAST CANCER; PROSTATE CANCER; SKIN CANCER; and TUMORS, all in Part Two.

❑ *See also* PAIN CONTROL in Part Three.

CANDIDIASIS

Candida albicans, a single-celled fungus, is always present in the genital and intestinal tracts. If it is present in disproportionate quantities, however, it can cause infection. Diaper rash, vaginitis, and thrush are some of the possible manifestations of candida infection.

Because candidiasis can affect various parts of the body—the most common being the mouth, ears, nose, toenails, fingernails, gastrointestinal tract, and vagina—it can be characterized by a wide array of symptoms. These include constipation, diarrhea, colitis, abdominal pain, headaches, bad breath, rectal itching, low libido, memory loss, mood swings, prostatitis, canker sores, persistent heartburn, muscle and joint pain, sore throat, congestion, nagging cough, numbness in the face or extremities, tingling sensations, acne, night sweats, severe itching, clogged sinuses, PMS, burning tongue, white spots on the tongue and in the mouth, extreme fatigue, vaginitis, kidney and bladder infections, arthritis, depression, hyperactivity, hypothyroidism, adrenal problems, and even diabetes. Symptoms often worsen in damp or moldy places, or after consumption of foods containing sugar and/or yeast. Because of its many and varied symptoms, this disorder is often misdiagnosed. Many of these symptoms can be related to other diseases, so a firm diagnosis is warranted.

When the candida fungus infects the mouth, it is called thrush. White sores form on the tongue and gums and inside the cheeks. In a baby, the white spots of oral thrush may resemble milk spots. Oral thrush in an infant can spread to the mother's nipples by breast-feeding, and can lead to a situation in which mother and baby continually reinfect each other. Thrush may also infect a baby's buttocks, appearing as diaper rash. Candida infection may also take the form of athlete's foot or jock itch. Systemic candidiasis is an overgrowth of candida everywhere, through-

out the body. In the most severe cases, candida can travel through the bloodstream to invade every organ system in the body, causing a type of blood poisoning called candida septicemia. This condition almost always occurs in persons with serious underlying illnesses, such as advanced cancer or following a severe burn injury.

Candidiasis may affect both men and women; however, it is rarely transmitted sexually. It is most common in babies (an infected mother may pass the fungal infection to her newborn) and in persons with compromised immune systems, and as it proliferates the fungus releases toxins that weaken the immune system further. Other factors that increase the chances of contracting a yeast infection include pregnancy and the use of corticosteroid drugs.

Very often, people with candida infections also have food allergies. Oral thrush, athlete's foot, ringworm, jock itch, fingernail or toenail fungus, and even diaper rash can develop as a result of the combination of food allergies and *C. albicans.* The symptoms of a food allergy or environmental sensitivity can also mimic those of candidiasis. To further complicate matters, some people with candidiasis go on to develop environmental sensitivities as well. Many cannot tolerate contact with rubber, petroleum products, tobacco, exhaust fumes, and chemical odors.

Yeasts, including candida, feed on sugar. If the body's pH balance is upset for any reason, the friendly bacteria (such as lactobacilli) that normally metabolize sugars cannot thrive and do their job properly, and there is a risk of *Candida albicans* flourishing in this sugar-rich environment.

Some women find they suffer more yeast infections when using oral contraceptives or during pregnancy. This is most probably due to an increase in the amount of sugar (glycogen) in the vagina induced by changing hormone levels. Antibiotics, which kill beneficial bacteria along with the harmful ones, are another common cause of yeast infections.

It is said that infections such as candidiasis rarely occur in people with robust immune systems who eat a healthy diet that is low in sugar and yeast. The debate continues as to whether candidiasis exists in the body as the result, or the cause, of some immunologic diseases.

Unless otherwise specified, the dosages recommended here are for adults. For a child between the ages of twelve and seventeen, reduce the dose to three-quarters of the recommended amount. For a child between six and twelve, use one-half of the recommended dose, and for a child under the age of six, use one-quarter of the recommended amount.

NUTRIENTS

SUPPLEMENT	SUGGESTED DOSAGE	COMMENTS
Very Important		
Acidophilus (Kyo-Dophilus from Wakunaga) or	As directed on label. Take on an empty stomach.	Fights candida infection. Use a nondairy formula.
Bio-Bifidus from American Biologics	As directed on label.	Enhances cell function to destroy candida.

Caprylic acid (Caprystatin from Ecological Formulas)	As directed on label.	An antifungal agent that destroys the candida organism.
Essential fatty acids (black currant seed oil and flaxseed oil)	As directed on label.	Important in healing candidiasis and preventing the fungus from destroying cells.
Garlic (Kyolic from Wakunaga)	2 capsules 3 times daily.	Inhibits the infecting organism. For candida vaginitis, use Kyolic vaginal suppositories as directed on label.
Quercetin plus bromelain or Activated Quercetin from Source Naturals	500 mg twice daily, 30 minutes before meals. 100 mg twice daily, 30 minutes before meals. As directed on label.	Speeds healing and reduces the effects of food allergies and inflammation. Improves absorption of quercetin. Contains quercetin plus bromelain and vitamin C for increased absorption.
Vitamin B complex plus extra biotin and vitamin B$_{12}$	100 mg of each major B vitamin 3 times daily (amounts of individual vitamins in a complex will vary). 50 mg 3 times daily. 1,000–2,000 mcg daily.	B vitamins are required for all bodily functions, resistance to infection, and all enzyme systems. Important for brain function. Use a yeast-free formula. Consider injections (under a doctor's supervision). Needed for healthy skin. Important for digestion. Needed for metabolism of carbohydrates, fats, and proteins. Use a lozenge or sublingual form.

Important

Calcium and magnesium and vitamin D	1,500 mg daily. 750–1,000 mg daily. 400 IU daily.	Often deficient in people with this disorder. Use calcium citrate form. Needed to balance with calcium. Enhances calcium absorption.

Helpful

Coenzyme A from Coenzyme-A Technologies and Coenzyme Q$_{10}$	As directed on label. 100 mg daily.	Removes toxins from the body. Improves tissue oxygenation.
Colostrum Plus from Symbiotics	As directed on label.	Powerful immune enhancer.
Colloidal silver	As directed on label.	Can aid in healing.
Free form amino acid (Amino Balance from Anabol Naturals)	As directed on label. Take between meals, on an empty stomach.	Rebuilds damaged tissue. Use a sublingual form for best absorption.
Glutathione	500 mg twice daily.	Needed for brain function. Candida may impair brain function.
Grapefruit seed extract	As directed on label. Always dilute before use.	Rids the body of potentially harmful microorganisms.
L-cysteine	500 mg twice daily, on an empty stomach. Take with water or juice. Do not take with milk. Take with 50 mg vitamin B$_6$ and 100 mg vitamin C for better absorption.	A potent antioxidant and free radical destroyer. (See AMINO ACIDS in Part One.)

Multivitamin and mineral complex with vitamin A and mixed carotenoids and selenium	25,000 IU daily. If you are pregnant, do not exceed 10,000 IU daily. 15,000 IU daily. 200 mcg daily. If you are pregnant, do not exceed 40 mcg daily.	All nutrients are needed for proper immune function and for repair of intestinal lining and all tissues; build resistance to infection. Choose a yeast-free formula that includes zinc and iron.
Orithrush from Ecological Formulas	Use as a mouth rinse or as a douche.	Aids in destroying candida.
Vitamin C with bioflavonoids	1,000 mg 3 times daily.	Builds up immunity and protects the body tissues from damage by the toxins released from candida. Use an esterified form.
Vitamin K	As directed on label.	To replace vitamin K balance upset by antibiotic use or overgrowth of bad candida.

Herbs

❑ Aloe vera juice has been shown to boost the white blood cells' ability to kill yeast cells.

❑ Kolorex Advanced Candida Care is a patented herbal formula from Forest Herbs Research (it is sold in the United States by Nature's Sources) containing extracts of the New Zealand herb horopito (*Pseudowintera colorata*) and aniseed. Horopito contains a strong antifungal agent called polygodial. Kolorex has been shown in laboratory experiments to be effective in controlling *Candida albicans*.

❑ Olive leaf extract with oleuropein is a powerful healer of microbial infections.

❑ Pau d'arco (also known as lapacho or taheebo) contains an antibacterial and antifungal agent; although it does have an alkaloid base, a small percentage of people may not benefit from its use. If you do not benefit from this tea, try clove tea instead. It is a good idea to alternate between the two, because clove tea has some benefits that pau d'arco does not have and vice versa. To make pau d'arco tea, boil 1 quart of distilled water with 2 tablespoons of herb for five minutes. Cool and store it in the refrigerator with the tea leaves in. Strain before drinking, if needed. Drink 3 to 6 cups daily.

❑ Some people who no longer respond to pau d'arco can benefit from maitake tea. It is a good alternative. While pau d'arco must be boiled, maitake is prepared as a regular tea. Resistant strains of candida develop rapidly due to genetic mutation. Rotating treatment programs is beneficial.

❑ Wild oregano oil is a potent antiseptic, powerful in killing a range of fungi.

Recommendations

❑ Eat vegetables, fish, and gluten-free grains such as brown rice and millet.

❏ Eat plain yogurt that contains live yogurt cultures. For vaginal candidiasis, apply natural unprocessed and unsweetened yogurt directly into the vagina or mix one small container of plain yogurt with an equal amount of water and use it as a douche once or twice daily until you see an improvement. You can also open two capsules of acidophilus and add the contents to a douche. This helps to inhibit the growth of the fungus. If symptoms persist, seek medical treatment.

❏ Take supplemental acidophilus or bifidus to help to restore the normal balance of flora in the bowel and vagina.

❏ Take some type of fiber daily. Oat bran or flaxseed is a good source.

❏ Drink distilled water only.

❏ Make sure your diet is fruit-free, sugar-free, and yeast-free. Candida thrives in a sugary environment, so your diet should be low in carbohydrates and contain no yeast products or sugar in any form.

❏ Avoid aged cheeses, alcohol, baked goods, chocolate, dried fruits, fermented foods, all grains containing gluten (wheat, oats, rye, and barley), ham, honey, nut butters, pickles, potatoes, raw mushrooms, soy sauce, sprouts, and vinegar.

❏ Eliminate citrus and acidic fruits such as oranges, grapefruit, lemons, tomatoes, pineapple, and limes from your diet for one month; then add back only a few twice weekly. Although they seem acidic, these fruits are actually alkaline-forming in the body, and candida thrives on them.

❏ Once a month, to replace "friendly" intestinal bacteria, use an *L. bifidus* retention enema until the infection is better. (*See* ENEMAS in Part Three.)

❏ Take only hypoallergenic supplements.

❏ To prevent infection, replace your toothbrush every thirty days. This is a good preventive measure against both fungal and bacterial infections of the mouth.

❏ Wear white cotton underwear, or at least make sure that the panty liner is cotton. Synthetic fibers lead to increased perspiration, which creates a hospitable environment for candida, and also trap bacteria, which can cause a secondary infection. Change underclothing daily.

❏ Do not use corticosteroids or oral contraceptives until your condition improves. Oral contraceptives can upset the balance of microorganisms in the body, leading to proliferation of *C. albicans*.

❏ Avoid household chemical products and cleaners, chlorinated water, mothballs, synthetic textiles, and damp and moldy places, such as basements.

❏ If you have chronic and/or unusually persistent candida infections, consult your health care provider. This may be a sign of an underlying illness such as diabetes or immune system dysfunction, which makes for an environment more conducive to the growth of yeast.

Considerations

❏ All persons on long-term antibiotics or chemotherapy are at high risk for severe cases of candidiasis. Taking antibiotics also can cause a deficiency of vitamin K, which is manufactured by the "good bacteria" in the intestines. Eating plenty of leafy greens, alfalfa, strawberries, whole grains, and yogurt can restore the vitamin K balance.

❏ If a breast-fed baby develops oral thrush or a nursing mother develops a thrush infection of the nipples, both mother and baby should be treated to eradicate the infection, even if only one of them seems to be affected.

❏ Because there is no simple, accurate test for candida, it is difficult to determine if it is the cause of a baby's diaper rash.

❏ Allergy testing is advised for anyone with symptoms of candida infection. (*See* ALLERGIES in Part Two.)

❏ Medical treatment for vulvo-vaginal candidiasis may involve the use of antifungal medications such as butoconazole cream, clotrimazole vaginal tablets, miconazole cream or suppositories, nystatin vaginal tablets, tioconazole ointment or cream, or fluconazole oral tablets. Most of these preparations are now available over the counter under various brand names. We recommend that only women who have been diagnosed with candidiasis use these preparations. Unfortunately, the use of these agents, especially if chronic or repeated, can lead to the development of stronger strains of yeast that are drug resistant. Higher dosages are then required, which in turn further weaken the immune system. Many doctors no longer use nystatin or antibiotics because they weaken the immune system and can damage certain organs. Others prescribe them for short-term treatment only. If you treat yourself with over-the-counter medications and symptoms continue or recur within two months, it would be wise to seek medical advice.

❏ High levels of mercury in the body can result in candidiasis. Mercury salts inhibit the growth of the necessary "friendly" bacteria in the intestines. You may want to have a hair analysis done to determine the levels of toxic metals. (*See* HAIR ANALYSIS in Part Three.)

❏ Candida Forte from Nature's Plus is good for mild cases.

❏ Candidiasis may be related to hypoglycemia. (*See* HYPOGLYCEMIA in Part Two.)

❏ *See also* FUNGAL INFECTION and YEAST INFECTION in Part Two.

CANKER SORES (APHTHOUS ULCERS)

Canker sores are small, white swellings that develop into ulcers. They can appear on the tongue, the lips, the gums, or the insides of the cheeks. A coagulated yellowish mixture of fluids, bacteria, and white blood cells then covers the ulcers. The development of a canker sore may be preceded by a burning and tingling sensation.

Canker sores do not form blisters as cold sores (fever blisters) do. The herpes simplex virus type 1 causes the cold sore, commonly confused with the canker sore. The canker sore, on the other hand, is an inflammation, rather than an infection.

Canker sores range in size from as small as a pinhead to as large as a quarter. They appear suddenly and often leave suddenly, usually lasting from four to twenty days. Some experts believe that these painful mouth ulcerations are contagious, but others disagree. Canker sores occur most often in females. They can be triggered by any of a number of factors, including poor dental hygiene, irritation from dental work, food allergies, nutritional deficiencies, hormonal imbalances, viral infection, an underlying immunologic disease (such as HIV infection), trauma (such as that caused by biting the inside of the cheek or using a hard-bristled toothbrush), stress, and/or fatigue. They may result from an abnormal immune response to normal bacteria in the mouth. Canker sores are occasionally associated with Crohn's disease, which affects the bowels. Deficiencies of iron, lysine, vitamin B_{12}, and folic acid have been linked to this disorder in some people.

Unless otherwise specified, the dosages recommended here are for adults. For a child between the ages of twelve and seventeen, reduce the dose to three-quarters the recommended amount. For a child between six and twelve, use one-half the recommended dose, and for a child under the age of six, use one-quarter the recommended amount.

NUTRIENTS

SUPPLEMENT	SUGGESTED DOSAGE	COMMENTS
Very Important		
Acidophilus	As directed on label. Take on an empty stomach.	Aids in maintaining healthy balance of intestinal flora ("friendly" bacteria). Use a high-potency powdered form.
L-lysine	500 mg 3 times daily, on an empty stomach. Take with water or juice. Do not take with milk. Take with 50 mg vitamin B_6 and 100 mg vitamin C for better absorption.	A deficiency may cause an outbreak of sores in and around the mouth. (See AMINO ACIDS in Part One.) Caution: Do not take lysine for longer than six months at a time.
Vitamin B complex	50 mg of each major B vitamin 3 times daily (amounts of individual vitamins in a complex will vary).	B vitamins are basic for immune function and healing.
plus extra vitamin B_3 (niacin)	50–100 mg 3 times daily. Do not exceed this amount.	Deficiencies have been linked to mouth sores. Caution: Do not take niacin if you have a liver disorder, gout, and/or high blood pressure.
and vitamin B_5 (pantothenic acid)	50–100 mg 3 times daily.	An antistress vitamin necessary for adrenal function.
and vitamin B_{12}	1,000–2,000 mcg daily, on an empty stomach.	Use a lozenge or sublingual form.
and folic acid	400 mcg daily.	Use a lozenge or sublingual form.
Vitamin C with bioflavonoids	3,000–8,000 mg daily, in divided doses.	Fights infection and boosts the immune system. Use a buffered form.
Important		
Zinc lozenges	1 15-mg lozenge every 3 waking hours for 2 days. Do not exceed a total of 100 mg daily.	Enhances immune function and aids healing.
Helpful		
Garlic (Kyolic from Wakunaga)	3 capsules 3 times daily.	Acts as a natural antibiotic and immunostimulant.
Iron	As prescribed by physician.	May be helpful if canker sores are related to iron deficiency. Caution: Do not take an iron supplement unless your physician finds that you are iron-deficient.
Multivitamin and mineral complex	As directed on label.	A balance of minerals is always important.
Vitamin A with mixed carotenoids	50,000 IU daily for 10 days, then reduce to 25,000 IU daily. If you are pregnant, do not exceed 10,000 IU daily. Also put a few drops of vitamin A oil directly on the affected area.	Speeds healing, especially of the mucous membranes. Use an emulsion form for easier assimilation.

Herbs

❑ Alfalfa, calendula, capsicum, comfrey, garlic, and peppermint are useful in the treatment of canker sores.

Caution: Comfrey is recommended for external use only. Do not take it internally.

❑ Use burdock, goldenseal, pau d'arco tea, and red clover to cleanse the bloodstream and decrease infection.

Cautions: Do not take goldenseal internally on a daily basis for more than one week at a time. Do not use it during pregnancy or if you are breast-feeding, and use with caution if you are allergic to ragweed. If you have a history of cardiovascular disease, diabetes, or glaucoma, use it only under a doctor's supervision.

❑ Goldenseal extract or tea tree oil, applied gently on the sore twice during the day and again at bedtime, helps to speed healing. To use these as mouthwashes, add 3 drops to 4 ounces of water. Add a drop or two to your toothpaste before brushing. Use alcohol-free goldenseal extract.

Caution: Do not take goldenseal internally on a daily basis for more than one week at a time. Do not use it during pregnancy or if you are breast-feeding, and use with caution if you are allergic to ragweed. If you have a history of cardiovascular disease, diabetes, or glaucoma, use it only under a doctor's supervision.

❑ Red raspberry tea contains valuable flavonoids and is very helpful.

❏ Rockrose, also known as sun rose, used as a mouthwash, both heals and eases the pain of mouth sores.

❏ Wintergreen mouthwash is a good antiseptic. Wintergreen oil can be rubbed into the sores for temporary relief.

Recommendations

❏ Eat plenty of salad with raw onions. Onions contain sulfur and have healing properties.

❏ Include in the diet yogurt and other soured products, such as kefir, cottage cheese, and buttermilk.

❏ Avoid sugar, citrus fruits, and processed and refined foods.

❏ Do not eat fish or meat of any kind for two weeks. The consumption of animal protein increases the body's acidity, which slows healing. Be sure to substitute vegetable proteins to meet your body's needs.

❏ Avoid chewing gum, lozenges, mouthwashes, tobacco, coffee, citrus fruits, and any other foods that you know trigger these sores.

❏ Consider trying the homeopathic remedies *Belladonna*, *Echinacea*, and *Borax*. These agents are commonly used in the treatment of canker sores.

Caution: Do not take echinacea for longer than three months. It should not be used by people who are allergic to ragweed.

❏ If you have repeated attacks of canker sores, check for nutritional deficiencies.

❏ To avoid getting canker sores, it is important to maintain a proper balance of minerals, acidity, and alkalinity in the body. (*See* ACID/ALKALI IMBALANCE in Part Two for the acid and alkaline self-test.) Have a hair analysis done to test for mineral levels. (*See* HAIR ANALYSIS in Part Three.)

❏ Do not take iron supplements unless your doctor prescribes them. Obtain iron from natural food sources.

❏ Consult your health care provider or dentist if you have a mouth sore that does not heal.

Considerations

❏ Stress and allergies are probably the most common causes of open sores in the mouth.

❏ Some doctors prescribe mouthwashes that contain tetracycline, an antibiotic, for canker sores.

❏ If you get recurrent canker sores, your toothpaste may be the culprit. Try toothpaste that does not contain the detergent sodium lauryl sulfate. This is a detergent that may cause the mucous surfaces in the mouth to dry out, leaving them vulnerable to attack from acidic foods. Also, do not use the same toothbrush for longer than one month. When canker sores on the gum are healing, it is best to use a very soft toothbrush.

❏ The drug Zilactin is a gel-like ointment that is applied directly to the ulcer. It sticks to the canker sore and gives relief from irritating foods.

❏ *See also* COLD SORES in Part Two.

CARDIOVASCULAR DISEASE

Cardiovascular disease (CVD) is a general term encompassing heart attack, stroke, and other disorders of the heart and blood vessel system. (Heart disease refers only to diseases of the heart and blood vessel system within the heart.) Cardiovascular disease is the leading health problem in the Western world. It is the number-one cause of death in the United States. An estimated 80 million Americans have heart and blood vessel disease, although many do not know it because they have no overt symptoms. Traditionally thought of as a disease primarily affecting men, cardiovascular disease is a growing problem for women. In fact, coronary heart disease, which causes heart attack, is the single leading cause of death for American women. It is responsible for the deaths of as many as 500,000 women a year in the United States. More women die from cardiovascular diseases than from all forms of cancer combined. Lower levels of estrogen during and after menopause are thought to increase a woman's risk for CVD. African-American woman are at greater risk than women of other ethnic backgrounds.

The arteries that supply blood to the heart are called the coronary arteries. If the heart's blood vessels narrow, the amount of blood they supply to the heart may be insufficient to provide the oxygen the heart needs. This oxygen deprivation is what causes a type of chest pain known as angina pectoris. A heavy, tight pain in the chest area characterizes angina, usually after some type of exertion. The pain usually recedes with rest.

If the coronary arteries that carry oxygen and nutrients to the heart muscle become obstructed, the flow of blood is cut off completely, and a heart attack, or myocardial infarction, can occur, resulting in damage to the heart muscle. Arteriosclerosis, or hardening of the arteries, and the presence of a thrombus, or clot, in a blood vessel are the most common causes of obstruction. Arteriosclerosis is responsible for most of the deaths resulting from heart attacks. Spasms of the coronary arteries can also result in a heart attack. A heart attack may feel as if someone is applying intense pressure to the chest. This pain may last for several minutes, often extending to the shoulder, arm, neck, or jaw. Other signs of heart attack include sweating, nausea, vomiting, shortness of breath, dizziness, fainting, feelings of anxiety, difficulty swallowing, sudden ringing in the ears, and loss of speech. The amount and type of chest pain vary from one person to another. Some people have intense pain, while others feel only mild discomfort. Many mistake the signs of a heart attack for indigestion. Some have no symptoms at all, a situation referred to as a "silent" heart attack.

Hypertension (high blood pressure) is often a precursor to heart problems. Hypertension is an extremely common form of cardiovascular disease. It usually results from a decrease in the elasticity or a reduction in the interior diameter of the arteries (or both), which may be caused by arteriosclerosis, defects in sodium metabolism, stress, nutritional deficiencies, and enzyme imbalances. Kidney disease, hyperthyroidism, disorders of the pituitary or adrenal glands, and heredity may be contributing factors. People considered to be at high risk are those with diabetes, those who smoke, or those who already have had a heart attack or stroke. Because it is essentially painless, especially in the early stages, many people don't even know they have it—hence the term "silent killer." By the time hypertension causes complications that result in symptoms (such as rapid pulse, shortness of breath, dizziness, headaches, and sweating), the disorder is more difficult to treat. Untreated hypertension is the leading cause of stroke and also greatly increases the risk of heart attack, heart failure, and kidney failure. Treatment seeks to lower blood pressure to less than 140 mm Hg (millimeters of Mercury) systolic and less than 90 mm Hg diastolic for most people. Treatment for those with diabetes and chronic kidney disease aims to lower blood pressure to less than 130 mm Hg systolic and less than 80 mm Hg diastolic. For people aged fifty and older, systolic blood pressure may be a more important cardiovascular risk factor than diastolic pressure.

Other types of cardiovascular disease include heart failure, arrhythmias, and valvular disease. While a heart attack occurs because of an interruption in blood flow to the heart, heart failure is characterized by inadequate blood flow from the heart—the heart fails to pump enough blood to meet the body's needs. Symptoms include fatigue, poor color, shortness of breath, and edema (swelling due to the accumulation of fluid in the body's tissues), especially around the ankles.

Arrhythmias are disturbances in the normal rhythm of the heartbeat. There are different kinds of arrhythmias. Some are quite dangerous—even immediately life-threatening—while others may be merely annoying (or scarcely noticeable), and pose no particular danger.

Valvular disease is a term for disorders that impair the functioning of one or more of the heart's valves. It may be caused by congenital defect, or it may be the consequence of illness such as rheumatic fever or endocarditis (infection of the heart muscle). Mitral valve proplapse (MVP) is a condition in which the mitral valve, which controls blood flow from the left atrium to the left ventricle (the heart's main pumping chamber), protrudes too far into the left atrium while it is pumping. In many cases, this causes no symptoms at all, although some people experience occasional fatigue, dizziness, palpitations, and/or vague chest pain. Mitral valve prolapse also causes a distinctive sound that a skilled physician can identify by means of a stethoscope. This condition is now known to be rarer than was once thought. And for most of those who do have MVP, it is not thought to lead to severe complications.

Syndrome X (now known as metabolic syndrome) is characterized by a number of signs of overall poor health. People with metabolic syndrome are more likely to suffer strokes than other people. About 50 million Americans are estimated to have metabolic syndrome. That means they have at least three of the five common conditions associated with the syndrome: abdominal obesity, high blood sugar, high triglyceride levels, high blood pressure, and low HDL ("good") cholesterol levels. While diabetes significantly increases the risk for stroke, it has been found that for people who have not been diagnosed with diabetes, having metabolic syndrome can be as powerful a risk factor. Some strokes could be prevented by correcting abnormalities associated with metabolic syndrome. The role of nutrition in achieving this is crucial.

Unfortunately, despite remarkable new technology for both diagnosis and treatment of heart-related conditions, the first sign of cardiovascular disease may be a life-threatening calamity. Disorders of the cardiovascular system are often far advanced before they become symptomatic. Some people who have heart attacks have no previous symptoms of heart trouble. According to a recent study, the blockages in arteries that can lead to a heart attack or sudden death appear to start forming early in life, in young adults and adolescents as young as age fifteen.

Cardiovascular disease is not an inevitable result of aging. Many preventive measures can be taken to avoid heart disease. Controllable factors that can contribute to heart disease include smoking, high blood pressure, excessive alcohol consumption, elevated serum cholesterol, stress, obesity, a sedentary lifestyle, and diabetes. Another big factor is not taking prescribed medications on a regular basis. You can alter your lifestyle to keep your heart healthy.

Heart Function Self-Test

Your heart is the most important muscle in your body. A simple pulse test can help you determine how well your heart is functioning. The best time to check your pulse is first thing in the morning. The heart rate should be between 60 and 100 beats per minute. To take your pulse, place the first two fingers of your right hand between the bone and tendon of your left wrist. Count the beats for fifteen seconds, and then multiply by four to find the beats per minute. If your pulse remains rapid, consult your health care provider to rule out problems. A chronically high pulse rate is often a precursor of hypertension. Taken daily, this pulse test can forewarn you of oncoming illness, but a high pulse also could be caused by other health issues including being out of shape. Check with your health care provider.

As the most active muscle in the body, the heart requires proper nutrition. Poor nourishment has a profound effect on the heart, and research has shown that as people age, their eating habits get worse, thus increasing their risk of cardiovascular disease.

Cardiovascular Risk Factors and Warning Signs

Following is a brief summary of known risk factors and warning signs of present or possible future cardiovascular problems, including stroke.

Risk Factors

- High blood pressure.
- Heart disease, especially a type of arrhythmia (irregular heartbeat) called atrial fibrillation (AF).
- Smoking.
- Diabetes.
- High blood cholesterol.
- Obesity/poor diet.

Warning Signs

- Numbness or weakness in face, arm, or leg.
- Difficulty speaking.
- Severe dizziness, loss of balance or coordination.
- Sudden dimness, loss of vision.
- Sudden intense headache.
- Brief loss of consciousness.

If any of the known risk factors apply to you, consult with your health care provider about ways to lower your risk. If you experience any of the warning signs listed above, seek medical attention at once.

NUTRIENTS

SUPPLEMENT	SUGGESTED DOSAGE	COMMENTS
Essential		
Coenzyme Q$_{10}$	50–100 mg 3 times daily.	Increases oxygenation of heart tissue. Has been shown to prevent recurrences in individuals who have had a heart attack.
plus Coenzyme A from Coenzyme-A Technologies	As directed on label.	Can streamline metabolism, increase energy, support adrenal glands, process fats, remove toxins from the body, boost the immune system, and improve overall physical and mental processes.
Kyolic-EPA from Wakunaga or	As directed on label.	Reduces triglyceride levels in the blood.
essential fatty acids (black currant seed oil, flaxseed oil, primrose oil, and salmon oil)	As directed on label.	Helps prevent hardening of the arteries. If you use a fish oil, use a product with vitamin E added to prevent rancidity.
L-arginine	As directed on label. Take with carbohydrates rather than protein, which inhibits absorption.	Improves blood flow.
Selenium	200 mcg daily. If you are pregnant, do not exceed 40 mcg daily.	Deficiency has been linked with heart disease. Destroys free radicals in the heart. Selenium supplements help reduce heart disease risk.
Vitamins B$_{12}$, B$_6$, and folic acid	400 mcg, 50 mg, 400 mg, respectively	These are needed for maintaining normal homocysteine and C-reactive protein levels and may help with cognition. C-reactive protein is a risk factor for developing diabetes.
Vitamin C with bioflavonoids and L-lysine	1,000 mg 3 times daily.	Extremely important as a regulator of high blood pressure.
Vitamin D	400–800 IU.	Do not exceed 1,000 IUs per day. Get your vitamin D levels in your blood checked. Reduces your risk of heart disease.
Very Important		
Calcium and magnesium	1,500–2,000 mg daily, in divided doses, after meals and at bedtime. 750–1,000 mg daily, in divided doses, after meals and at bedtime. Take with 50 mg vitamin B$_6$.	Important in the proper functioning of the cardiac muscle. Use chelate forms. Vital for a healthy heart. Connected to over 300 enzyme actions controlling glucose, proteins, and fats.
Cardio Logic from Wakunaga	As directed on label.	Increases the oxygenation of heart tissue.
Heart Science from Source Naturals	1 tablet 3 times daily, on an empty stomach.	Contains antioxidants, cholesterol fighters, herbs, and vitamins that work together to protect the heart and promote cardiovascular function.
L-carnitine	500 mg twice daily, on an empty stomach. Take with 50 mg vitamin B$_6$ and 100 mg vitamin C for better absorption.	Reduces fat and triglyceride levels in the blood. Increases oxygen uptake and stress tolerance.
Lecithin granules or capsules	1 tbsp 3 times daily, before meals. 2,400 mg 3 times daily, with meals. Take with vitamin E (see below).	Acts as a fat emulsifier.
Liquid Kyolic with B$_1$ and B$_{12}$ from Wakunaga and	2 capsules 3 times daily.	Lowers blood pressure and thins the blood.
Kyo-Green from Wakunaga	As directed on label.	Concentrated barley and wheatgrass juice; contains nutrients needed for healing and prevention of heart disease.
Lycopene plus lutein	As directed on label. As directed on label.	Carotenoids that lower LDL ("bad") cholesterol
Pantethine	As directed on label.	A derivative of pantothenic acid that reduces LDL cholesterol.

Phosphatidyl choline or lipotropic factors	As directed on label.	Reduces fat and triglyceride levels in the blood.
Pycnogenol	As directed on label.	Found to be more effective than aspirin in reducing buildup of plaques in the arteries, a major risk factor in heart disease.

Important		
Chitosan	As directed on label.	A polysaccharide derived from shellfish that has been shown to reduce blood cholesterol levels.
Dimethylglycine (DMG) (Aangamik DMG from FoodScience of Vermont)	50 mg 4 times daily.	Promotes the utilization of oxygen.
Kyolic Homocysteine from Wakunaga	As directed on label.	Contains aged garlic extract with vitamin B_6, vitamin B_{12}, folic acid, and betaine to support healthy homocysteine levels.
Lycopene	250 mg of tomato extract (Lyc-O-Mato)	Used to reduce blood pressure.
Potassium	99 mg daily.	Needed for electrolyte balance, especially if taking cortisone or blood pressure medication.
Red yeast rice (Cholestin from Pharmanex)	As directed on label.	Contains lovastatin, which has been proven to reduce cholesterol levels (synthetic lovastatin is often prescribed for this purpose).
Superoxide dismutase (SOD)	As directed on label.	A powerful antioxidant.
Taurine Plus from American Biologics	1,000 mg daily. Take with 50 mg vitamin B_6 and 100 mg vitamin C for better absorption.	Helps stabilize the heartbeat and correct cardiac arrhythmias. An important antioxidant and immune regulator, necessary for white blood cell activation and neurological function. Use the sublingual form.
Vitamin E	Start with 100 IU daily and increase slowly, adding 100 IU until daily dosage is 200 IU.	Strengthens the immune system and heart muscle, improves circulation, and destroys free radicals. Use d-alpha-tocopherol form. *Caution:* Use this supplement only under the supervision of a physician.

Helpful		
Copper	As directed by physician.	Deficiency may be linked to some heart problems.
Green tea extract	6 capsules a day (equal to 714 mg green tea poly-phenols).	May help reduce the risk of heart disease by lowering the ratio of the good cholesterol to total cholesterol (a marker of heart disease risk). *Caution:* Contains vitamin K, which can make anticoagulant medications less effective. Consult your health care professional if you are using them. The caffeine in green tea

		could cause insomnia, anxiety, upset stomach, nausea, or diarrhea.
Kelp	1,000–1,500 mg daily, with meals.	A rich source of important vitamins, minerals, and trace elements.
Melatonin	2–3 mg daily, taken 2 hours or less before bedtime.	A powerful antioxidant that may help prevent stroke and also aids sleep.
Multienzyme complex (Inf-zyme Forte from American Biologics) plus	As directed on label. Take between meals.	To aid digestion.
bromelain	300 mg daily.	
Octacosanol and/or wheat germ	As directed on label. As directed on label.	Improves endurance; relieves muscle pain.
Sea mussel	As directed on label.	A source of protein that aids in the functioning of the cardiovascular system.
Trimethylglycine (TMG)	As directed on label.	TMG converts homocysteine into methionine. SAMe is a by-product of this conversion.

Herbs

❑ Researchers have found that pomegranate juice not only seems to prevent hardening of the arteries by reducing blood vessel damage, but also may reverse the progression of atherosclerosis (plaque buildup). This may be due to the high antioxidant content of the juice, which is higher than that found in other fruit juices, including blueberry, cranberry, and orange. The results of this study appear in the *Proceedings of the National Academy of Sciences*.

❑ Cordyceps, a Chinese herb, can slow the heart rate, increase blood supply to the arteries and heart, and lower blood pressure.

❑ Ginkgo biloba can benefit the cardiovascular system by preventing the formation of free radicals. Take a ginkgo extract containing 24 percent ginkgo flavone glycosides.

Caution: Do not take ginkgo biloba if you have a bleeding disorder, or are scheduled for surgery or a dental procedure.

❑ Grape seed extract with oligomeric proanthocyanidins (OPCs) may lower high blood pressure, which can cause heart disease.

❑ Consuming ¼ cup of tomato sauce or three medium-sized tomatoes per day can have a beneficial effect due to lycopene, a natural antioxidant. Harvard University researchers found that middle-aged women who consumed that amount of lycopene were 30 percent less likely to de-

Healthy Cholesterol and Blood Pressure Levels

Two important measurements used in assessing cardio-vascular health are blood fat (including cholesterol and tri-glycerides) levels and blood pressure. The tables below are approximate guides to both cholesterol and blood pressure levels. Keep in mind that both levels vary from person to person, so it is always wise to have your blood pressure and cholesterol level checked by your physician on a regular ba-sis. Also note that the values here reflect recent revisions in desirable levels.

Cholesterol and Triglyceride Levels for People without Heart Disease (mg/dL)

Blood Lipid	Good	Borderline	High
Total cholesterol	200 or less	200–239	240 and above
LDL ("bad") cholesterol	100 or less	100–159	160 and above
Triglycerides	150 or less	150–199	200 and above

The desirable level of HDL cholesterol ("good" cholesterol) is 60 mg/dL or above.

Blood Pressure Levels for People without Heart Disease (HT=Hypertension)

Blood Pressure	Normal	Pre-HT	Stage 1 HT	Stage 2 HT
Systolic (when the heart contracts and pumps blood out)	120 or less	120–139	140–159	160 and higher
Diastolic (between beats, your heart fills with blood again)	80 or less	80–89	90–99	100 and higher

velop heart disease than women who got less lycopene. Patients with high blood pressure who were already taking medications to lower it achieved an even lower systolic (10 mmHg) and diastolic (5 mmHg) rate from a standardized tomato extract rich in lycopene.

❏ Hawthorn increases blood flow and lowers blood pressure.

❏ People with cardiovascular disease may benefit from suma tea. Take 3 cups of this herbal tea daily with ginkgo biloba extract as directed on the product label.

Caution: Do not take ginkgo biloba if you have a bleeding disorder, or are scheduled for surgery or a dental procedure.

❏ Other herbs and herbal products beneficial for cardiovascular disorders include barberry, black cohosh, butcher's broom, cayenne (capsicum), dandelion, ginseng, SP-8 Heart Blend from Solaray, and valerian root.

Cautions: Do not use barberry during pregnancy. Do not use black cohosh if you are pregnant or have any type of chronic disease. Black cohosh should not be used by those with liver problems. Do not use ginseng if you have high blood pressure, or are pregnant or nursing.

Recommendations

❏ If you experience any of the symptoms of a heart attack, call 911, and then contact your doctor or go immediately to the emergency room of the nearest hospital, even if symptoms last only a few minutes. Half of all heart attack deaths occur within three to four hours of the onset of the attack, so a person suffering from a heart attack requires immediate medical attention.

❏ Make sure your diet is well balanced and contains plenty of fiber. Some studies have found that among the sources of dietary fiber—cereal, vegetables, and fruits—the fiber from breakfast cereals appears to be the most beneficial.

❏ Eat fish several times a week. Fish is an extremely important food for those with heart disease. Eating fish has been shown to lower the risk of dying from heart disease by reducing arrhythmia in patients with the disease. It has also been shown to reduce the risk of developing heart disease in healthy people. If you don't have heart disease and eat 2 to 4 servings of fish a week, you have a 15 percent lower chance of developing it. If you don't like fish or don't want to eat it, take fish oil capsules; supplementation was shown to be as effective. Patients with heart disease who took 1 gram of omega-3s (1 gram capsules usually have about one-third omega-3s, so they took about three capsules)

Common Heart Problems and Procedures

If either you or a loved one has heart trouble, you can better understand and participate in treatment if you familiarize yourself with the following medical terms that may be used by your physician:

- **Aneurysm.** A spot in a blood vessel where the wall becomes thin and bulges outward as blood presses against it. If it ruptures, circulation is disrupted. Depending on the location of the aneurysm, the consequences of this can be grave. If detected in time, aneurysms can be repaired surgically in many cases.

- **Angina pectoris.** Pain or heavy pressure in the chest that is caused by an insufficient supply of oxygen to the heart tissue. This chest pain may be severe or mild and is usually associated with physical exertion and relieved by rest. It can be a warning sign of impending heart attack.

- **Angiogram.** A diagnostic picture produced by injecting into the heart and/or blood vessels a type of dye that is visible on X-ray. It may be done to diagnose valvular disease, blood vessel blockage, and other conditions.

- **Angioplasty.** A procedure in which a small balloon is inserted into a blocked or partially blocked artery and then inflated. This compresses the plaque on the vessel wall, widening the artery and allowing more blood to flow through it.

- **Aorta.** The main channel for arterial circulation; the large artery into which oxygenated blood is pumped by the heart.

- **Aortic atherosclerosis.** A systemic disease involving the heart, brain, aorta, and peripheral arteries. Blood tests have not traditionally been used to diagnose or to assess risk. Transesophageal echocardiography, a type of ultrasound test, and MRI (magnetic resonance imaging) have been used to identify plaque buildup. A blood test for the presence of C-reactive protein may be helpful. The C-reactive protein is a systemic biomarker for inflammation.

- **Aortic stenosis (AS).** A condition in which the aortic valve is narrowed, restricting blood flow from the heart into the aorta. It can result from congenital malformation of the valve or from damage, such as from rheumatic fever. Symptoms, which may begin in early childhood, include fainting, chest pain, and shortness of breath, especially with exertion.

- **Arrhythmia.** Disruption in the natural rhythm of the heartbeat caused by improper functioning of electrical system cells in the heart. There are different kinds of arrhythmias. Palpitations is a term that refers to the feeling of a pounding heartbeat, whether regular or irregular. Tachycardia is an abnormal increase in the resting heart rate; bradycardia is the opposite, an abnormally slow heart rate. Ectopic beats are premature beats (often felt as "skipped" beats). Flutter and fibrillation are situations in which the normal steady beating of the heart is converted by electrical error into a rapid twitching of the heart muscle. This ineffective functioning results in an insufficient supply of blood being carried to the body's tissues.

- **Cardiac arrest.** Cardiac arrest occurs when the heart stops beating. When this happens, the blood supply to the brain is cut off and the person loses consciousness. A person in apparent good health who experiences cardiac arrest usually has unsuspected coronary artery disease.

- **Cardiomegaly.** The medical term for enlargement of the heart. If the heart is unable to function effectively, as in heart failure, or if there is too much resistance to the normal pumping of blood through the blood vessels, as in high blood pressure, the body attempts to increase the strength of the heart by increasing its size. Cardiomegaly is characteristic of a number of different heart disorders. It is also known as cardiac hypertrophy.

- **Cardiomyopathy.** Any of a group of diseases of the heart muscle that result in impaired heart function and, ultimately, heart failure. Cardiomyopathies are classified according to characteristic physical changes in the heart, such as enlargement of the heart, dilation of one or more of the heart's chambers, or rigidity of the heart muscle. These disorders may be related to inherited defects or may be caused by any of a number of different diseases. Often, the cause is unknown.

- **Cardioversion.** A procedure used to correct arrhythmia, in which electrical current is applied to the heart to restore normal rhythm.

- **Carditis.** Inflammation of the heart muscle. This can result from infection or from an inflammatory response, as in rheumatic fever, and it can lead to permanent heart damage if not treated.

- **Carotid artery.** The major artery to the brain.

- **Catheterization.** A procedure sometimes used to diagnose the condition of the heart and/or circulatory system and, in some cases, to treat cardiovascular disease. A hollow, flexible tube called a catheter is inserted by means of a very fine flexible wire into a blood vessel somewhere in the body (usually the arm, neck, or leg), and from there is threaded through the blood vessel to the heart or other location being investigated. Catheterization can be used to detect (and in some cases to treat) arterial blockage, to discover malformations of the heart, and to study electrical conduction in the heart, among other things.

- **Claudication.** Cramplike pains in the legs as a result of poor circulation to the leg muscles. This usually occurs as a result of atherosclerosis.

- **Congenital heart defect.** A heart defect that is present at birth, though not necessarily inherited.

- **Congestive heart failure.** A condition of chronic heart failure that results in fluid accumulation in the lungs, labored breathing after even mild exertion, and edema (swelling) in the ankles and feet.

- **Coronary arteries.** The arteries that supply blood to the heart.

- **Coronary artery disease (CAD).** Atherosclerosis of the coronary arteries.

- **Echocardiogram.** A procedure in which ultrasound technology is used to form an image of the heart. It is used to detect structural and functional abnormalities, enlargement or inflammation of the heart, and other conditions.

- **Electrocardiogram (ECG or EKG).** A diagnostic test that tracks electrical impulses in the heart.

- **Embolism.** A circulatory condition in which a foreign object such as air, tissue, gas, or a piece of a tumor is transported around the body and becomes trapped in a blood vessel, obstructing the flow of blood.

- **Endoarteritis obliterans.** Inflammation of the arterial walls that narrows the passage and obstructs the flow of blood.

- **Endocarditis.** Inflammation of the endocardium, the membrane surrounding the heart muscle, usually as a result of bacterial infection. Endocarditis is not uncommon in persons with compromised immune systems, such as those with HIV and AIDS. It also can occur as a complication of surgery to replace defective heart valves. This disorder can result in permanent heart damage.

- **Fibrillation.** An irregular heartbeat characterized by a rapid twitching or vibrating of heart muscle rather than slow, steady beats. Atrial fibrillation can be episodic or chronic, even constant. Symptoms may include dizziness, light-headedness, and general weakness. Atrial fibrillation can cause blood to pool in the heart and subsequently shed clots, causing ischemic stroke. Ventricular fibrillation is a medical emergency that can lead rapidly to loss of consciousness and death. It most often is a complication of heart attack.

- **Gated blood pool scan.** A diagnostic test in which a small amount of radioactive tracer is injected to "tag" red blood cells, which are then tracked as they progress through the heart, creating a series of pictures that show the size and shape of the heart, the motion of the heart wall, and the heart's pumping efficiently. The test can be done while you are resting or during exercise. It is also known as multi-unit gated analysis (MUGA).

- **Heart attack.** The medical term for a heart attack is myocardial infarction (MI). This refers to the formation of infarcts (areas of local tissue death or decay) in the myocardium (heart muscle). Infarction occurs when the blood supply to an area of the heart is cut off, usually as a result of a blood clot that blocks a narrowed coronary artery. Depending on the size and location of the areas affected, a heart attack may be described as mild or severe, but it always involves some irreparable damage to the heart.

- **Heart failure.** This disorder occurs when a damaged heart becomes unable to pump effectively, depriving the body's tissues of adequate oxygen and nutrients to function properly. Heart failure can be either acute (short-term) or chronic, and has a variety of different causes.

- **Heart murmur.** A sound made by the heart that may or may not point to the existence of a heart condition. A diastolic murmur occurs between beats. A systolic murmur occurs during heart contractions.

- **Hematoma.** A collection of blood trapped in the skin, or in an organ, after a trauma or surgery.

- **Holter monitor.** A small device worn on the body that monitors the heart on a twenty-four-hour basis.

- **Hypertension.** High blood pressure.

- **Hypotension.** Low blood pressure.

- **Ischemic heart disease.** Ischemic heart disease is caused by obstruction of the blood flow to the heart, usually as a result of atherosclerosis. Ischemia (lack of sufficient oxygen) can lead to angina, cardiac arrhythmias, congestive heart failure, or a heart attack.

- **Magnetic resonance spectroscopy (MRS).** Used in conjunction with magnetic resonance imaging (MRI), an imaging test that can show areas of damaged heart muscle. It does this by measuring levels of creatine kinase MB, an enzyme that is severely depleted after a heart attack.

- **Mitral valve prolapse (MVP).** A condition in which the mitral valve, which controls blood flow from the left atrium and left ventricle, protrudes too far into the left atrium between beats. It may or may not cause symptoms, such as dizziness or palpitations. It is not considered dangerous. It may also be called Barlow's syndrome.

- **Pericarditis.** Inflammation of the sac that surrounds the heart.

- **Phlebitis (or thrombophlebitis).** Inflammation of a vein, most often accompanied by a clot. This condition may be caused by trauma to the vessel wall, clots forming in the blood, infection, or long periods of immobility.

- **Positron emission tomography (PET) scan.** A diagnostic test that can be used to assess blood flow through the arteries to the heart.

- **Pulmonary stenosis (PS).** A condition in which the pulmonic valve is narrowed, restricting the flow of blood from the heart to the pulmonary artery, which carries blood from the heart to the lungs. This is most often a congenital defect. It causes a distinctive murmur and may or may not cause symptoms.

- **Rheumatic heart disease.** Damage to the heart caused by rheumatic fever, a complication of infection with group A streptococcus bacteria, the bacteria that cause strep throat. It causes scarring and contracture of heart valves, and can lead to arrhythmias and heart failure.

- **Stress test.** A diagnostic test used to assess blood flow to the heart. The first part of the test involves the injection of a radioactive imaging agent into the arm. About an hour later, the heart is photographed. In the second part of the test, an intravenous line is placed in the arm and an EKG reading is taken as the patient walks on a treadmill. When the heart is working at its hardest, the first part of the test is repeated. Also known as a myocardial perfusion stress test.

- **Stroke.** Interruption of blood flow to the brain. A hemorrhagic stroke occurs when there is bleeding in the brain; an ischemic stroke, which is more common, is caused by a clot that forms in a blood vessel that supplies the brain, or a clot that moves from another part of the body to the brain.

- **Thrombosis.** The formation of a clot in a blood vessel.

- **Troponin T test.** A blood test that can detect damage to heart muscle from a heart attack. It assesses levels of the protein troponin T, which is released into the bloodstream after a heart attack. This test can detect even the mildest "silent" heart attack.

of equal EPA and DHA had fewer deaths and admissions to the hospital for treatment of their heart disease. This amount of fish oil is safe and well tolerated, and it seemed to slow the progression of heart disease. If you take just one supplement, fish oil is the one to take. If you are a vegetarian, flax and soy oil are good sources.

❑ Eat plenty of raw foods. For protein, eat broiled fish and skinless turkey and chicken, which are low in fat.

❑ Include garlic and onions in your diet. They contain compounds that help to reduce serum cholesterol levels.

❑ Eat plenty of fresh fruits and vegetables. An eight-year study of almost 40,000 men found that men who ate five or more servings of fruits and vegetables each day had a 39 percent lower risk of stroke than those who did not.

❑ Add raw nuts (except peanuts), olive oil, pink salmon, trout, tuna, Atlantic herring, and mackerel to your diet. These foods contain omega-3 essential fatty acids.

❑ Do not consume stimulants, such as coffee and black tea, that contain caffeine. Studies show that coffee increases stress hormones in the body, putting coffee drinkers at greater risk of heart disease. Also avoid tobacco, alcohol, chocolate, sugar, butter, red meat, fats (2 grams or less saturated fat per serving, particularly animal fats and hydrogenated oils), fried foods, processed and refined foods, soft drinks, spicy foods, and white flour products, such as white bread.

❑ Drink steam-distilled water only, and get at least ten 8-ounce glasses every day. It is recommended that you drink at least 80 ounces of water a day. One study found that men who drank at least five glasses of water every day had a 51 percent lower risk of heart disease than those who did not. For women, the risk of heart disease was 35 percent lower.

❑ Eliminate all known sources of sodium from your diet. Almost everything contains some sodium. Keeping consumption below 5 grams per day is a good target. Read all labels and avoid those food products that have "soda," "so-dium," or the symbol "Na" on the label. These indicate that the product contains sodium. Some foods and food additives that should be avoided on a salt-free diet include:

- Monosodium glutamate or MSG (flavor enhancers such as Accent).
- Baking soda.
- Canned vegetables.
- Commercially prepared foods.
- Diet soft drinks.
- Foods with mold inhibitors.
- Foods with preservatives.
- Meat tenderizers.
- Saccharin (found in Sweet'N Low) and products containing saccharin.
- Some medicines and dentifrices (toothcare products).
- Softened water.

❑ If you take an anticoagulant (blood-thinner) such as warfarin (Coumadin) or heparin, or even aspirin, limit your intake of foods high in vitamin K. Eating foods containing vitamin K increases the blood's tendency to clot, so they should be eaten only in small quantities. Foods that are rich in vitamin K include alfalfa, broccoli, cauliflower, egg yolks, liver, spinach, and all dark green vegetables. To enhance the effect of anticoagulants, eat more of the following: wheat germ, vitamin E, soybeans, and sunflower seeds.

❑ Learn everything about any drugs that have been prescribed for you. Know what to do in case of an emergency. Keep emergency and ambulance numbers easily accessible. If you have a heart condition, someone close to you should know what to do if cardiac arrest occurs. Make sure someone living with you knows how to do cardiopulmonary resuscitation (CPR) and mouth-to-mouth resuscitation. The American Red Cross and many local hospitals

Quick Reference Guide: The Top Ten Healthiest Foods for Your Heart

When it comes to promoting a healthy cardiovascular system, not all foods are created equal. Following is a list of the top ten foods for heart health.

1. *Fresh fruit.* Fruit contains fiber, antioxidants, vitamins, and minerals.

2. *Beans and legumes.* Beans and legumes contain fiber and plant proteins that help to lower LDL ("bad") cholesterol levels.

3. *Fish.* The omega-3 essential fatty acids in cold-water fish help to lower LDL levels.

4. *Dark leafy greens.* Spinach, mesclun, Swiss chard, arugula, and other greens help to reduce levels of a blood enzyme implicated in heart disease.

5. *Avocados.* Avocados are rich in potassium, which helps to regulate heart rhythm and blood pressure, and monounsaturated fats, which lower LDL levels.

6. *Whole grains.* Fiber and B vitamins are their greatest assets.

7. *Nuts.* A good source of monounsaturated fats and minerals.

8. *Soy foods.* These are useful in keeping correct blood fat levels and are rich in phytoestrogens.

9. *Spices and herbs.* Fat is better digested with the help of the antioxidants and phytochemicals available in many herbs.

10. *Wheat germ and flax meal.* These are good for boosting your intake of fiber, vitamin E, and omega-3 essential fatty acids. Flax in the form of meal, seeds, or oil coupled with a high-fiber diet from whole-grain cereals, fruits, vegetables, and added dietary fiber such as wheat bran is the best for reducing the risk of developing coronary heart disease. In fact, a diet such as this is extremely low in saturated fat, which means that you can safely indulge in an egg a couple of times a week, or an occasional serving of red meat.

offer training in these techniques. Eighty percent of heart attacks occur at home, according to the American Heart Association.

❏ Keep your weight down. Obesity is a risk factor for heart attacks and high blood pressure. Get regular moderate exercise. Because medical care has improved so much over the past thirty years, there is less of a chance of developing heart disease as a result of being overweight and obese. Compared to obese patients in 1960 to 1962, obese patients in 1999 to 2000 had 21 percent lower cholesterol levels and 18 percent lower blood pressure.

❏ When trying to lose weight, the so-called low-carb diets are easy to follow and produce fast weight loss, so many people like to use them to jump-start a weight reduction program. An important paper published in *The New England Journal of Medicine* showed that it is fine to follow a low-carb diet as long as the fat and protein come from vegetable sources. A low-carbohydrate diet naturally results in a low-glycemic-load diet as well. A high-glycemic-load diet nearly doubles the chances of developing heart disease.

❏ If you are over thirty-five and/or have been sedentary for some time, consult with your health care provider before beginning an exercise program.

❏ Avoid stress, and learn stress-management techniques. (*See* STRESS in Part Two.)

Considerations

❏ The so-called bad cholesterol, LDL, is commonly measured and is considered a key predictor of cardiovascular risk. A component in cholesterol called apolipoprotein B (aop B) may be more closely linked to heart disease risk factors, and measuring aop B rather than LDL levels eliminates errors that can be caused by the size of the LDL particles. Small, dense LDL particles are more harmful than larger ones; thus, it would be nice to know how many small particles there are in the mix. But current tests do not differentiate for particle size or number. Testing for aop B gives the actual number of LDL particles, and the number of small particles can then be calculated. Canada has instituted testing for aop B and is currently updating the guidelines for lipids and diabetes to include an aop B test.

❏ Both homocysteine and C-reactive protein are new markers of inflammation and are directly related to heart disease risk. Learn what your number is for each and get yearly testing. The numbers should be very low except for when inflammatory processes are occurring. Because the tests are new, your doctor might not routinely order them and insurance may not pay for them. Moreover, there is disagreement in the medical literature as to what added value they provide (especially for C-reactive protein) beyond the usual blood cholesterol tests.

❏ Eating a high choline and betaine diet seems to lower homocysteine levels and potentially reduces your risk of heart disease. Choline-rich foods include red meat, poultry, milk, eggs, fish, and potatoes. Betaine-rich foods are spinach, pasta, white breads, cold cereals, beets, and red meat. The effect of betaine is also immediate. In one study, within two hours, a single dose of betaine significantly lowered plasma homocysteine levels.

❏ Foods containing certain plant extracts that have been shown to reduce cholesterol levels now may be labeled as such. The FDA has given food manufacturers the go-ahead to put labels on foods containing plant sterol esters and plant stanol esters to indicate that they may reduce the risk of coronary artery disease. These work by blocking the absorption of cholesterol from the diet, and have been known for some time to reduce the blood cholesterol levels that are responsible for most heart attacks. Plant sterol esters can be found in soybean oil as well as in many fruits, vegetables, nuts, cereals, and other plants. Plant stanols occur naturally in smaller quantities in some of the same sources. In one study, people with heart disease who ate a diet rich in olive oil lowered their risk for further worsening of the disease. In another study, those who took a fish oil–plant sterol mixture lowered their bad cholesterol and triglycerides. Patients took about 5 grams of omega-3 fats and 3 to 4 grams of sterols a day.

❏ The best fiber appears to come from wheat bran, which was even better than whole-wheat products. In one study, including a lot of wheat bran in the diet (7 grams per day) reduced the risk of heart disease by 30 percent. Those who consumed about 3 servings of whole-grain foods per day had a reduced risk of heart disease of 18 percent. Wheat germ was not associated with a reduced risk of heart disease in this study, but because it is rich in a variety of micronutrients it may be beneficial to add it to your diet.

❏ An eight-year study that followed nearly 50,000 women who ate a very low-fat diet with only 20 percent of the calories from fat and about 5 servings of fruits and vegetables a day did not result in significant reductions in heart disease risk. It seems that these dietary adjustments were not enough and that added emphasis should be placed on lifestyle modifications such as incorporating more exercise and obtaining more fiber. Fiber can easily be added to your diet by upping your fruit and vegetable intake as well as consuming whole-grain foods. More recently, the Dietary Approaches to Stop Hypertension (DASH) diet study (funded by NIH), which included 36,000 women who followed a fiber-rich diet from fruits and vegetables and whole grains and made lifestyle changes such as increasing exercise, showed a 37 percent lower rate of heart failure.

❏ Erythromycin, an antibiotic that has been marketed for over fifty years, has been implicated in cardiac deaths. The problem appears to be interaction with some newer drugs that tend to increase its concentration in the blood. Although it has long been known that erythromycin could present problems when used intravenously, nobody suspected a problem with the pill form. Newer calcium channel blockers and perhaps other medications can slow the breakdown of erythromycin. The result is trapping of salt inside resting heart muscle cells, prolonging the time until the next heartbeat starts and sometimes triggering an abnormal, fatal rhythm.

❏ The Japanese traditional remedy natto, which comes from the popular food made from fermented soybeans, may be very helpful in both preventing and treating cardiovascular disease. It fights the buildup of fibrin (a protein that reduces circulation), breaks up clots, and restores blood circulation to diseased vessels. Studies have indicated that natto may be an effective replacement for warfarin (Coumadin). A side benefit was an approximate 10 percent lowering of both diastolic and systolic blood pressure. More research is taking place to develop physicians' guidelines for the use of this natural medication.

❏ A Taiwanese study reported in the *Archives of Internal Medicine* indicated that habitual tea drinkers may have a significantly reduced risk of hypertension as compared with non-tea-drinkers. Although the tea-drinking group was generally found to be more obese, consume more alcohol, exercise less, and smoke more than the non-tea-drinking group in the study, those habitual tea drinkers who consumed between 120 and 599 milliliters (about 4 to 19 fluid ounces) of tea daily exhibited a 46 percent reduction in hypertension compared with the other group. Those who ingested in excess of 600 milliliters of tea in a given day had a remarkable 65 percent reduction in hypertension. No mechanism has been proposed to explain these results; however, discussions regarding the effects of caffeine, the neurotransmitter theanine, and the antioxidant effects of tea polyphenols (all compounds found in tea) have been advanced. These may act to relax and dilate blood vessels.

❏ Defibrillators are devices used to restore a normal rhythm to the heart during a heart attack. Portable defibrillators are available, and are commonly used in aircraft and police cars during emergencies. The Philips HeartStart home defibrillator is available for use in the home. It costs approximately $1,200. Training on the proper use of defibrillators is conducted by both the American Red Cross and the American Heart Association.

❏ The use of a test called cardiokymography (CKG) together with electrocardiograms (ECGs) may help to detect "silent" heart disease. A comparison study revealed that electrocardiograms alone missed 39 percent of heart disease cases. When CKG was used along with ECGs, only 8 percent of cases were undetected.

❏ Nitroglycerin, which is sold in sublingual tablet, patch, and lingual spray forms, is commonly prescribed to relieve chest pain and to improve the oxygen supply to the heart. This drug is taken at the first sign of chest pain. If dry mouth prevents sublingual nitroglycerin tablets from dissolving, the spray form may be a better choice. Nitroglycerin has some side effects, including headache, weakness, and dizziness. These usually disappear with continued use.

❏ Some studies suggest that the hormone dehydroepiandrosterone (DHEA) may help to prevent cardiovascular disease in some people. One study showed that men with high DHEA levels were less likely to die of heart disease, but women with high DHEA levels were at greater risk of dying from heart disease. Another study found little relationship between DHEA levels in the blood and heart disease risk in either gender. (*See* DHEA THERAPY in Part Three.)

❏ When vitamin C was obtained from citrus bioflavonoids coupled with tocotrienols, people with high cholesterol levels saw significant improvements. These people experienced reductions in the bad cholesterol and triglycerides, and the good cholesterol level increased after twelve weeks.

❏ In two large-scale studies (1,400 women and 1,200 men), no effect was seen for vitamin C and E on reducing heart-related events in healthy individuals.

❏ Low levels of vitamin D have been associated with heart disease. Those with blood vitamin D levels below 15 nanograms/mL had a 60 percent greater chance of developing heart disease. Low vitamin D levels also are associated with high blood pressure, diabetes, obesity, and high triglyceride levels. Each of these is a risk factor for developing heart disease. The best blood levels of vitamin D in this study were equal to or greater than 37 nanograms/mL and the worst were less than 21 nanograms/mL.

❏ Selenium supplements help reduce heart disease risk. A meta-analysis of twenty-five studies on selenium supplementation compared persons with the lowest blood level of selenium to persons with the highest and found that persons with the highest levels of selenium in their blood had 15 to 57 percent less risk of heart disease. Make sure that you don't exceed 400 micrograms from all sources (diet and other supplements).

❏ In one study, after thirty days of taking coenzyme Q_{10}, patients with heart disease who had leg pain related to statin use experienced a 40 percent reduction in pain and reported being able to move more easily. It is thought that Coenzyme Q_{10} decreases with statin use, thereby impairing muscle energy metabolism.

❏ Policosanol, a product made from sugar cane wax, was thought to lower the bad cholesterol and raise the good cholesterol; however, several recent studies have not supported these beneficial findings.

❏ We cannot recommend that people take up drinking to prevent heart disease, but research has shown that having a small amount of beer, wine, or liquor occasionally may make it more likely that you will avoid heart disease.

❏ Current research indicates that soy isoflavones may enhance coronary blood flow and prevent blocked arteries.

❏ According to some studies, magnesium supplementation can correct some types of irregular heartbeat, and could save the lives of many people with heart trouble.

❏ The mechanisms responsible for omega-3 essential fatty acids' reduction of cardiovascular disease risk are still being studied. However, it appears that benefits include decreases in triglyceride levels and blood clots, lower risk of sudden death, improved arterial health, and lower blood pressure. In one study, when omega-3s were taken with statin medications, there was a decrease in triglycerides and an increase in the good cholesterol (HDL). Patients in this study took 4 grams of a concentrated fish oil (about 80 percent omega-3s). This is good news for patients who need statins to control their cholesterol, as they may be able to use less of the drugs if they also take fish oil. Certain patients with implantable defibrillators may do worse in terms of cardiac function with fish oil. It may induce arrhythmias, so it is always important to speak with a health care professional before using fish oil. Flaxseed did not seem to have the same benefits to the heart as fish oil even though it has omega-3s.

❏ Studies indicate that depression plays an important role in the occurrence of heart disease in patients who already have it and those who are at risk. People who took about 400 milligrams a day of omega-3s (about one 1-gram fish oil capsule) had the lowest level of depression.

❏ The largest women's health study ever done, the Women's Health Initiative, had 162,000 participants. Some findings taken from the study that were recently presented at an American Society for Reproductive Medicine conference indicated that taking birth control pills during reproductive years was *not* as harmful as was at one time thought. In fact, the study indicated a lower risk for heart attack, stroke, high blood pressure, and other related cardiovascular disease (CVD) problems. The overall risk reduction for CVD was 8 percent, and a bonus was a risk reduction of 7 percent regarding any type of cancer. Researchers believe the type of hormones, and when they are taken in life, seems to be what makes them helpful at one point and harmful at another.

❏ People who have had ischemic strokes and had a clot somewhere in the brain where it was impractical to remove had only one treatment possibility in the past, the clot-dissolving medication TPA. Use of TPA is a long shot by any definition, and not too many stroke patients ever receive it. A tiny experimental corkscrew-like device is now being tested that allows a surgeon to thread the device through a blood vessel in the leg to the clot in the brain, where it is used like a corkscrew to physically extract the clot. This is just like pulling the cork out of a wine bottle, according to Dr. Sidney Starkman at UCLA Stroke Center. Blood starts flowing again to the brain, and that, in the final analysis, is what it's all about.

❏ Catheters are also used to carry specialized tools and medicines to the heart, using the femoral artery. After removing the catheter, a titanium staple is often used to stop the bleeding by closing the hold in the artery.

❏ *Arnica montana*, *Arsenicum album*, *Magnesia phosphorica*, and *Spongia tosta* are homeopathic remedies often recommended for angina. They should be used only under the direction of a qualified homeopathic physician.

❏ Correcting potassium deficiencies before surgery can lessen the risks of coronary bypass surgery.

❏ Studies have shown a connection between heart disease and infection with *Chlamydia pneumoniae, Helicobacter pylori,* herpesviruses, and, possibly (but not conclusively) bacteria in dental plaque. The inflammatory response, which is associated with the body's defense mechanisms triggered by infection, may affect the arteries and ultimately lead to the deposition of plaque there. More alarming, researchers have found that some adenoviruses, which cause respiratory infections, may cause left ventricular dysfunction that can lead to sudden death. Because of the connection between infection and heart disease, research is being conducted on the use of antibiotics and prevention of heart attacks. Data published in the *Journal of the American Medical Association* indicates that people who had taken either tetracycline or quinolones in the three years preceding this research proved to be at a lower risk for heart attacks.

❏ Research is being conducted into the role of nitric oxide (NO) in the cardiovascular system. NO keeps the surface of blood vessels smooth so that platelets cannot bind together to form potentially dangerous clots. Researchers are aware that too much NO is toxic to the body, and studies are being conducted into controlling NO levels. Research has shown that by removing oxidants from the blood, vitamins C and E stabilize the NO and allow it to rise to higher levels. Additionally, L-arginine acts to increase the NO level, as does moderate exercise.

❏ Testosterone deficiency is a factor in causing heart disease, depression, and a host of aging-related ailments in men. This is a relatively new opinion, but it is supported by fact. Many people are leery of testosterone because of media hype concerning sports-related usage. But there is more than one type of testosterone, and one is beneficial. First of all, it is true that all the anabolic steroids are bad if taken over the long term. Their molecules resemble those of natural testosterone but are chemically different and do not react the same way in the body. The notorious methyltestosterone may be the worst of these steroids. In the body, natural testosterone is either bound (attached to a protein known as sex hormone binding globulin [SHBG]) or free. While the total amount in the body might be the same as a man ages, more and more of it is bound rather than free. A test might show no difference in overall testosterone levels, but the bound testosterone can no longer interact with testosterone receptors and therefore is in effect biologically inert. So the free testosterone available shrinks as men age. As it turns out, this free testosterone is important to cardiovascular health in many ways. Men with low free testosterone levels are more prone to high blood sugar, high blood cholesterol and triglycerides, high blood pressure, obesity in general and abdominal obesity in particular, high levels of clotting factors, and low levels of clotting inhibitors. There is data that suggests osteoporosis, which affects millions of men, and depression also are linked to low testosterone levels. Aside from testosterone therapy under a physician's care, an herbal product that can help the body produce testosterone naturally is the bioflavonoid chrysin (5,7-dihydroxyflavone), which is found in the passionflower plant (*Passiflora coerula*). Another useful herbal is an extract made from nettle root (*Urtica dioica*). The latter binds to SHBG better than testosterone, which helps increase the body's level of "free" testosterone. Make sure you use a product made from the root, not the stems and leaves.

Caution: Men with prostate cancer or possible prostate cancer should not take any herbal product that increases the supply of free testosterone because it can promote the growth of the cancer.

❏ Transmyocardial laser revascularization is a method of treating refractory angina. In this technique, a laser is used to create holes in the heart in order to increase the flow of blood to deprived areas of the heart.

❏ Substances known as thrombolytic agents, including streptokinase (Streptase) and alteplase (Activase, also known as tissue plasminogen activator [TPA]) have the ability to break up clots. When injected intravenously, they circulate through the arteries, locating and disintegrating blood clots. Studies have shown that thrombolytic therapy within the first six hours of the onset of a heart attack increases the chances of survival. However, this treatment probably should not be used by people who have peptic ulcers, extremely high blood pressure, a history of stroke, or recent head injury or abdominal surgery.

❏ It is important for women over the age of fifty-five, and women of any age who have gone through menopause, to consider heart disease as a possible cause of chest pain or discomfort. The chest pain may even be mild and less prominent than upper abdominal pain, shortness of breath, or nausea. Studies have shown that women are not as likely as men to receive drugs protecting them against heart disease; that they are less likely to undergo bypass surgery or angioplasty if they have cardiovascular disease; and that, when symptoms of heart trouble occur, they do not go to the hospital for treatment as quickly as men do. Because of these factors, women with cardiovascular disease are more likely to die from it than are men in comparable health.

❏ Research has shown that women with hypothyroidism (underactive thyroid) have a sharply increased risk of developing blockages in the aorta.

❏ The FDA asserts that taking one baby aspirin a day can reduce the risk of heart attack and/or stroke without side effects. You should consult with your physician first.

Caution: If you do use aspirin, keep in mind that it can cause internal bleeding and stomach ulceration.

❏ Allergies may be linked to some heart attacks. When a reaction in the walls of the arteries triggers a spasm in the coronary arteries, a heart attack may result. Allergies can also cause a temporarily rapid pulse. Your pulse rate may increase after you eat certain foods or when you come into contact with particular allergens. Allergy testing is recommended to determine whether you react to certain foods or other allergens. (*See* ALLERGIES in Part Two.)

❏ Being exposed to excessive noise for more than thirty minutes can increase blood pressure considerably.

❏ People who have had a heart attack that resulted in damage to the left ventricle have been shown to have a longer life expectancy if given the angiotensin-converting enzyme (ACE) inhibitor trandolapril (Mavik) for at least two years. ACE inhibitors are a type of drug most often used to treat high blood pressure. Other ACE inhibitors include enalapril (Vasotec) and ramipril (Altace). These drugs stop the formation of a natural chemical, angiotensin II, that narrows the blood vessels. (Angiotensin II inhibitors block the action, rather than the formation, of the same chemical.) Possible side effects are constipation, dry mouth, decreased sexual desire or erectile dysfunction, and a decrease in mental function.

❏ Other drugs often prescribed for people with high blood pressure include beta-blockers, calcium channel blockers, central-acting agents, and diuretics. Beta-blockers allow the heart to beat more slowly and with less force. Side effects can include a decrease in left ventricular function, a decrease in sexual desire in women, and erectile dysfunction in men. Calcium channel blockers, also known as calcium antagonists, relax the blood vessel muscle. Possible side effects are sexual dysfunction, dryness of the mouth, muscle pain, and heart arrhythmia. Central-acting agents (central adrenergic inhibitors) act on the brain, preventing the nervous system from increasing the heart rate and narrowing the blood vessels. Diuretics, also known as water pills, help the kidneys get rid of sodium and water, thus reducing the volume of blood coursing around the body. Possible side effects of diuretics include dehydration, diabetes, fainting spells, and possible heart and kidney malfunctions. Anticoagulant (blood-thinning) drugs, such as warfarin (Coumadin), are often prescribed for those in particular danger of developing blood clots, such as people who are bedridden, cancer patients (the formation of blood clots containing cancer cells that may colonize other parts of the body is a concern), and people with certain types of cardiac arrhythmias. Studies show that for those in peril of recurring clots, blood-thinning drugs should be taken for at least two years.

❏ A study reported in *The New England Journal of Medicine* indicated that for most people, aspirin works as well as warfarin in helping to prevent recurrent strokes. Although not found in this study, the author believes that baby aspirin should work as well as regular aspirin and pose less of a risk of internal bleeding. Vitamin E (200 IU a day) along with aspirin also makes an effective blood-thinning combination. However, you should never take warfarin and vitamin E at the same time (do not mix them), as this might cause severe bleeding.

❏ Men who take medication for hypertension can suffer from erectile dysfunction (ED) as a side effect. The anti-erectile-dysfunction drug sildenafil (Viagra), once thought to be dangerous for such individuals, may in fact be a viable option for those with high blood pressure, researchers say. It is advisable to consult your physician to determine if your medication for high blood pressure has lowered your blood pressure too much, and if any of your medications contain nitrates. The combination of nitrates and sildenafil can cause dangerously low blood pressure. Your doctor may also suggest a stress test before he or she makes a decision about prescribing sildenafil.

❏ For further information on cardiovascular disease, you can consult the American Heart Association or the National Heart, Lung, and Blood Institute. (*See* Health and Medical Organizations in the Appendix.)

❏ *See also* ARTERIOSCLEROSIS; CIRCULATORY PROBLEMS; HEART ATTACK; and HIGH BLOOD PRESSURE, all in Part Two, and CHELATION THERAPY in Part Three.

CARPAL TUNNEL SYNDROME

Almost unheard-of only a generation ago, carpal tunnel syndrome (CTS) has rapidly become a curse of modern existence. It is one of many injuries called repetitive strain injuries (RSIs), which include trigger finger, nerve spasms, and carpal tunnel syndrome. CTS is the term used to describe a set of symptoms that occur when the median nerve in the wrist is compressed or damaged. The median nerve controls the thumb muscles, and is also responsible for sensation felt in the thumb, the palm, and the first three fingers of the hand. The carpal (from the Greek word *karpos,* meaning "wrist") tunnel is a very small opening about one-quarter inch below the surface of the wrist through which the median nerve passes. The median nerve is vulnerable to compression or injury from a number of sources—swelling due to pregnancy or water retention, pressure from bone spurs, diabetes, bone dislocation or fracture, inflammatory arthritis, or even tendinitis.

CTS has been associated with repetitive wrist motion injury, which is linked to continuous rapid use of the fingers. Once considered an occupational hazard affecting only supermarket checkout clerks and bookkeepers, CTS did not become widely known until the 1980s, when personal computers came to dominate the workplace. Today, CTS is commonplace among people who use computers extensively. However, it must be noted that repetitive motion by itself has never conclusively been linked to increased pressure on the median nerve. Typing with the hand in an overextended, or "hyperflexed," position because the keyboard is too high or too low can cause an increase in symptoms that lead to CTS. In other words, the task itself doesn't cause the problem, but the position of the hands during the task does.

Carpal tunnel syndrome has also been linked to strong,

steady vibrations that shake the wrist for long periods (such as using a jackhammer or chain saw). Other people whose occupations have been associated with CTS include assembly line workers, athletes, drivers, hairstylists, musicians, restaurant servers, and writers. Although CTS affects both sexes, women between the ages of twenty-nine and sixty-two seem to be affected more than any other segment of the population. People with square wrists (wrists that are roughly as deep as they are wide) are said to be more disposed to getting CTS. Whatever the cause, an estimated 4 to 10 million Americans have CTS, according to the American College of Rheumatology. Factors that increase the risk of CTS include menopause, obesity, Raynaud's disease, pregnancy, hypothyroidism, and diabetes mellitus.

Symptoms of CTS can range from mild numbness and faint tingling to excruciating pain accompanied by a crippling atrophy of the muscles in the thumb. Most commonly, it is experienced as burning, tingling, or numbness in the thumb and the first three fingers. (The little finger is spared because it receives its nerve impulses from outside the carpal tunnel.) The tingling is often referred to as feeling similar to the "pins and needles" associated with a limb "falling asleep," and it also involves a gradual weakening of the thumb. In the beginning, symptoms are often intermittent, but they become persistent as the condition worsens.

CTS can affect one or both hands. Symptoms are often worse at night or in the morning, when circulation slows down. Pain may spread to the forearm and, in severe cases, to the shoulder. Carpal tunnel syndrome may have its genesis in either the neck, upper back, and/or shoulders. A visit to a chiropractor or osteopath may help in determining whether this is the case.

Not all nerve entrapment problems are in the carpal tunnel area. Though far less common, entrapment of the ulnar nerve, located in the elbow, produces symptoms almost identical to those of CTS. This condition can be very painful and disabling. It can also be misdiagnosed as myofascial dysfunction. Myofascial dysfunction stems from the overuse or misuse of muscles. It is not connected with nerve damage.

CTS Self-Test

A quick way to diagnose carpal tunnel syndrome is to perform a simple hand-flexing test called Phalen's maneuver. Place the backs of your hands together with the wrists bent at a 75-degree angle. If you experience tingling and numbness in your fingers after a few minutes, it may be CTS. If your job or hobby causes you to develop a burning sensation, numbness, or clumsiness affecting the first three fingers of one or both hands, chances are that CTS is the culprit.

This self-test is not foolproof, however. The only truly conclusive test for CTS is electromyography (EMG), which involves transmitting electrical impulses through the arm. The nerve impulses that direct motion are nothing more than a very low voltage current. Normal nerve impulse

transmission occurs at a speed of approximately 136 meters per second, which is fast enough to appear instantaneous to us. If nerves are damaged or entrapped by swollen tissue, however, they cannot transmit electrical neural impulses at the normal rate of speed. If you are found to have a neurotransmission speed of only 90 to 95 meters per second, nerve damage or compression is strongly suggested. A recent study suggests that sonography may be just as accurate as the preceding test to determine whether or not you have the prerequisites for CTS. Ultrasound images can show swelling within the carpal tunnel and how much space is available there for the nerve.

NUTRIENTS

SUPPLEMENT	SUGGESTED DOSAGE	COMMENTS
Essential		
Coenzyme Q10 plus Coenzyme A from Coenzyme-A Technologies	30–90 mg daily.	Improves tissue oxygenation.
Lecithin granules or capsules	1 tbsp 3 times daily, before meals. 1,200 mg 3 times daily, before meals.	Supplies choline and inositol for nerve function. A fat emulsifier.
Vitamin B complex	100 mg of each major B vitamin 3 times daily (amounts of individual vitamins in a complex will vary).	B vitamins are essential in nerve function.
plus extra vitamin B1 (thiamine) and	50 mg 3 times daily for 12 weeks.	Increases the uptake of vitamin B6 and improves tissue oxygenation.
vitamin B6 (pyridoxine)	100 mg twice daily for 12 weeks. Do not exceed this amount, or nerve damage may result.	A potent diuretic.
Zinc	50 mg daily. Do not exceed a total of 100 mg daily from all supplements.	Enhances healing. Use zinc gluconate lozenges or OptiZinc for best absorption.
Helpful		
Grape seed extract	As directed on label.	A powerful antioxidant and anti-inflammatory.
Kelp	As directed on label.	Beneficial to nerves.
Manganese	As directed on label. Take separately from calcium.	Helpful for nerve problems.
Multivitamin and mineral complex	As directed on label.	For general nutritional supplementation. Use a formula without iron.
Primrose oil or Kyolic-EPA from Wakunaga	As directed on label. As directed on label.	Contain essential fatty acids necessary for nerve function.
Vitamin A with mixed carotenoids	25,000 IU daily. If you are pregnant, do not exceed 10,000 IU daily.	Important antioxidants.
Vitamin C with bioflavonoids	1,000 mg 4 times daily.	Important in healing. A potent antioxidant. Aids in reducing swelling.
Vitamin E	200 IU daily.	An important antioxidant. Use d-alpha-tocopherol form.

Herbs

❏ Aloe vera, devil's claw, yarrow, and yucca are helpful for restoring flexibility and reducing inflammation.

❏ Bromelain and boswellia both reduce inflammation and swelling.

❏ Butcher's broom helps to relieve inflammation.

❏ Capsicum relieves pain and is a catalyst for other herbs.

❏ Corn silk and parsley are natural diuretics that help keep swelling down.

❏ Ginkgo biloba, taken in either tea or capsule form, is beneficial for improving circulation and also aids nerve function.

Caution: Do not take ginkgo biloba if you have a bleeding disorder, or are scheduled for surgery or a dental procedure.

❏ Gravel root tightens and soothes tissues and acts as an antiseptic.

❏ Marshmallow root soothes and softens tissues and promotes healing.

❏ *Rhus toxicodendron,* a homeopathic remedy, helps in any conditions where stiffness exists in a joint when it is first used. This substance is also helpful in soothing restlessness at night and in injuries caused by overuse of the joints.

❏ St. John's wort stimulates circulation and helps to restore local nerve impulse transmission.

Caution: St. John's wort may cause increased sensitivity to sunlight. It may also produce anxiety, gastrointestinal symptoms, and headaches. It can interact with some drugs including antidepressants, birth control pills, and anticoagulants.

❏ Skullcap relieves muscle spasms and pain.

❏ Venaforce from Bioforce, which contains a standardized extract of horse chestnut, helps improve circulation.

❏ Wintergreen oil aids in pain relief and circulation to the muscles.

❏ Zhen Gu Shi, a potent Chinese liniment for inflamed joints, is good for easing CTS symptoms. It is also sold in many Asian markets.

Recommendations

❏ Consume foods that contain or lead to the production of oxalic acid in moderation only. These include asparagus, beets, beet greens, eggs, fish, parsley, rhubarb, sorrel, spinach, Swiss chard, and vegetables of the cabbage family. Large amounts of oxalic acid can promote joint problems.

❏ Eat half of a fresh pineapple daily for one to three weeks, until relief is achieved. Pineapple contains bromelain, which reduces pain and swelling. Only fresh pineapple is effective. Bromelain is also available in supplement form.

❏ Eat foods high in vitamin B_6, such as bananas, avocados, potatoes, nuts, bluefin tuna, Atlantic salmon, chicken, whole grains, and sweet potatoes.

❏ Avoid salt and all foods containing sodium. They promote water retention and may aggravate carpal tunnel syndrome. They also counteract the effects of any diuretics that your physician may prescribe.

❏ If you engage in repetitive mechanical tasks, try to reduce the impact on your wrists and hands. *See* MINIMIZING THE RISK OF CARPAL TUNNEL SYNDROME, below.

❏ If possible, stop all repetitive finger movements for several days and see if any improvement occurs. If it does, try to rearrange your schedule so that you spend less time in CTS-stimulating activities. If possible, alternate tasks rather than performing a single task for long periods. Fortunately, employers have become more mindful of the possibility of repetitive motion injuries and are often more understanding than they might have been only a few years ago. Many now try to have their employees rotate the tasks they perform so that the risk of injury is reduced.

❏ Maintain ideal weight, and lose weight if necessary. Excess weight results in extra pressure on the carpal tunnel. Losing weight has brought relief to many people with CTS.

❏ Try using *Rhus toxicodendron,* a homeopathic remedy that helps in any conditions in which there is stiffness in a joint when it is first used. This substance is also helpful in soothing restlessness at night and in injuries caused by overuse of the joints.

❏ Use a splint to help prevent flare-ups. Splints are cloth-covered metal or plastic braces that attach to the forearm with an elastic bandage (an Ace bandage or the equivalent) or hook-and-loop fasteners (Velcro). These devices are available at medical supply houses and many pharmacies. If you cannot find one that fits properly, have one custom-made. Be sure to apply and wear the splint properly; if you don't, its effectiveness may be reduced or it may even aggravate the problem. Cock your wrist back slightly so that your thumb is parallel to your forearm. Your hand should be in approximately the same position as if it were holding a pen. This position keeps the carpal tunnel as open as possible. Wear the splint as much as possible for several days to see if your symptoms are reduced. Splinting is often very helpful for those who have suffered a repetitive motion injury that results in CTS.

❏ Keep your workplace warm and dry. Cool and/or damp conditions tend to aggravate CTS.

❏ Avoid taking supplements that contain iron. They are suspected of aggravating pain and swelling in joints.

Considerations

❏ If CTS develops as a result of the edema of pregnancy, it usually clears up of its own accord once the baby arrives and the excess fluid of pregnancy disappears.

Minimizing the Risk of Carpal Tunnel Syndrome

Carpal tunnel syndrome is an occupational hazard for anyone whose job involves making repetitive movements with the hands and/or fingers. In this age of computers, that means virtually anyone who works in an office, as well as assembly line workers, bookkeepers, cashiers, jackhammer operators, musicians, and many others. Spending a great deal of time engaging in a hobby such as knitting and needlework can also cause problems. No matter what your occupation, the following measures are recommended to help you reduce the risk of developing this painful and disabling condition:

- Use your whole hand and all of your fingers when you grip an object.

- Whenever possible, use a tool instead of flexing your wrists forcibly.

- Make sure your posture is correct. For keyboard tasks, sit straight in your chair with your body tilted slightly back. Raise or lower your chair so that your knees are bent at a right angle and your feet are flat on the floor. Your wrists and hands should be straight and your forearms parallel to the floor. Keep your wrists and hands consistently in a straight line.

- Keep your elbows bent. This lessens the load close to your body and reduces the amount of force required to do your job. Give yourself elbow room to allow you to use as much of your arm as you can while keeping your wrist straight. Use your whole arm while performing tasks in order to minimize the stress on your elbow.

- Adjust your computer screen so that it is about two feet away from you and just below your line of sight.

- Use armrests that attach to the chair to keep your wrists from flexing too much.

- If the relative positions of your desk, chair, and keyboard do not allow you to keep your wrists straight while keyboarding, the use of a "wrist rest" pad in front of the keyboard is highly recommended to alleviate pressure on the carpal tunnel.

- Slow your rhythm while varying wrist and hand movements.

- Take a break from handwork for a few minutes every hour.

- Shake out your hands periodically throughout the day.

- Resting one forearm on a table, grasp the fingertips of that hand and pull back gently. Hold this position for five seconds, then repeat the exercise with the other hand.

- Press the palms flat on a table, as if doing a push-up. Lean forward to stretch the forearm muscles and the wrists.

- Another recommended gentle exercise is done by rotating the wrist. Move your hands around in a circle for about two minutes, thoroughly stretching the muscles of the hand. This helps to restore circulation and improve the posture of the wrist.

- Do strengthening exercises. Place a rubber band around the fingers to provide resistance, and then open and close the fingers. Three times a day, do a set of ten repetitions with each hand.

❑ Physicians treat CTS in a variety of ways, most often with a combination of anti-inflammatory medications, splints, and the recommendation that you avoid any aggravating activity. Sometimes corticosteroid injections in the wrist are used. This treatment is controversial, however, and should not be used unless the pain from CTS is debilitating, since the injections themselves may produce discomfort.

❑ If weakness develops in the thumb, it is an indication that the median nerve has sustained some amount of damage, and surgical treatment may be recommended. This surgery involves cutting the transverse carpal ligament, a thick, fibrous band that covers part of the carpal tunnel. The surgeon can make either a small incision or a relatively large one. A small incision causes minimal scarring, but it affords the surgeon a very limited area view, which increases the risk of damage to other important structures in the wrist. A larger incision reduces the risk of peripheral damage, but a more prominent scar is usually the result,

and the scarring itself may cause some pain and disability. A splint or cast must be worn for two to four weeks following surgery. A less invasive type of surgery, called the endoscopic technique, has become popular. This procedure takes only ten minutes and the incision, made in the palm, is tiny. Most people return to work within a few days.

❑ Many doctors maintain that surgery for CTS is too often performed unnecessarily. A second opinion should always be obtained before surgery is agreed to. However, if the second doctor's opinion confirms that surgery is unavoidable, it is best not to put the operation off for too long, as delay may result in permanent nerve damage.

❑ The numbness, tingling, and pain of CTS usually subside within a few days after surgery, but some people find that it takes as much as two years for the symptoms to resolve. When this happens, it is often because the median nerve has sustained some damage and a long time is needed for any nerve regeneration to occur. If surgery is necessary and is put off for too long, the thumb may be left permanently weakened and the mobility of the affected hand may be diminished.

❏ A new treatment for CTS involves the use of a low-energy ("cold") laser to penetrate tissues, stimulate nerves, and increase microcirculation in the affected area.

❏ Additional information about repetitive strain injuries is available from the National Institute for Occupational Safety and Health. (*See* Health and Medical Organizations in the Appendix.)

❏ *See also* PAIN CONTROL in Part Three.

CATARACTS

See under EYE PROBLEMS.

CAVITIES

See TOOTH DECAY.

CELIAC DISEASE

Celiac disease (also called celiac sprue) is a chronic digestive disorder that is caused by a hereditary intolerance to gluten. Gluten is a protein component of wheat (including durum, semolina, and spelt), rye, oats, barley, and related grain hybrids such as triticale and kamut. The cause of celiac disease is unknown, although it is known to affect mostly Caucasians of European descent.

When a person with celiac disease consumes gluten, damage to the small intestine results. It is believed that the body responds to gluten as if it was an antigen, and launches an immune system attack when it is absorbed by the intestine. This, in turn, causes the lining of the small intestine to swell. As a result, tiny hairlike projections called villi suffer damage and destruction, which impairs the body's ability to absorb vital nutrients. Malabsorption becomes a serious problem, and the loss of vitamins, minerals, and calories results in malnutrition despite an adequate diet. Diarrhea compounds the problem. Because celiac disease impairs digestion, food allergies may also appear.

Celiac disease affects both adults and children, and it can appear at any age. It often appears when a child is first introduced to cereal foods, at around three or four months of age. In others, the disease can be triggered by emotional stress or physical trauma, such as a surgery or pregnancy.

The first signs are usually bloating, chronic diarrhea, pain, weight loss, and nutritional deficiencies. Other symptoms can include nausea; abdominal swelling; large, pale, light-yellow-colored stools that float; depression; fatigue; irritability; muscle cramps; wasting; and joint and/or bone pain. Infants and children may exhibit stunted growth, vomiting, an intense burning sensation in the skin, and a red, itchy skin rash called *dermatitis herpetiformis*. A baby with celiac disease may gain weight more slowly than normal or may lose weight. The infant may have a poor appetite, gas, and offensive-smelling bowel movements. The child is likely to have an anemic, undernourished appearance. Ulcers may develop in the mouth.

If left untreated, celiac disease can be quite serious, even life-threatening. Bone disease, such as osteoporosis, central and peripheral nervous system impairment, seizures caused by inadequate absorption of folic acid, internal hemorrhaging, pancreatic disease, infertility, miscarriages and birth defects, and gynecological disorders are just some of the long-term maladies that can affect those with celiac disease. There is also a risk of developing intestinal lymphoma and other intestinal malignancies. Certain autoimmune disorders also can be associated with celiac disease, including kidney disease (nephrosis), sarcoidosis (the formation of lesions in the lungs, bones, skin, and other places), insulin-dependent diabetes mellitus, systemic lupus erythematosus, thyroid disease, and, rarely, chronic active hepatitis, scleroderma, myasthenia gravis, Addison's disease, rheumatoid arthritis, and Sjögren's syndrome.

Celiac disease is often difficult to diagnose because the symptoms are similar to those of other diseases, such as irritable bowel syndrome, gastric ulcers, and anemia. The average time it takes for a person to be diagnosed is eleven years. Advances in blood testing have made it easier to detect celiac disease. A diagnosis based on a blood test can be followed up with a biopsy of intestinal tissue, which is usually an outpatient procedure. However, due to the fact that symptoms are so diverse, and that some people with celiac disease do not show obvious symptoms, many people go a long time before being diagnosed correctly. Because celiac disease is hereditary, if one family member is diagnosed with it, other family members should also be tested.

Celiac disease is much more prevalent in the population than was once believed, affecting at least 3 million Americans. Studies by the University of Chicago Celiac Disease Program indicate that as many as 1 in 133 apparently healthy people is affected. For those with related symptoms, the incidence may be as high as 1 in 56. (The incidence may be even higher in many areas of Europe.) Celiac disease affects 1 percent of the population worldwide. About 4 percent of patients diagnosed with inflammatory bowel disease have celiac disease. It is estimated that 97 percent of people living with the disease have not been diagnosed.

There is no known cure for celiac disease, but it can be controlled by lifelong adherence to a gluten-free diet.

Unless otherwise specified, the dosages recommended here are for adults. For a child between the ages of twelve and seventeen, reduce the dose to three-quarters of the recommended amount. For a child between six and twelve, use one-half of the recommended dose, and for a child under the age of six, use one-quarter of the recommended amount.

NUTRIENTS

SUPPLEMENT	SUGGESTED DOSAGE	COMMENTS
Essential		
Essential fatty acids (Kyolic-EPA from Wakunaga, flaxseed oil, or primrose oil)	As directed on label.	Needed for the villi in the intestines.
Free form amino acid	As directed on label.	To supply protein in a form readily available for use by the body.
Glutathione	500 mg 3 times daily.	An amino acid needed for repair of the intestinal tract.
Kyo-Dophilus from Wakunaga	As directed on label.	A dairy- and yeast-free probiotic formula to replace the friendly bacteria.
Liquid Kyolic with B_1 and B_{12} from Wakunaga	As directed on label.	Dramatically increases levels of vitamins B_1 and B_{12} for immune enhancement.
Multivitamin and mineral complex with		All nutrients are necessary in balance. Use a wheat- and yeast-free product only.
vitamin A	15,000 IU daily. If you are pregnant, do not exceed 10,000 IU daily.	
and mixed carotenoids and	10,000 IU daily.	
vitamin E	200 IU daily.	
Vitamin B complex injections plus extra	2 cc weekly, or as prescribed by physician.	Necessary for proper digestion. Injections (under a doctor's supervision) are best because they bypass the digestive system. If injections are not available, a sublingual form is recommended. Use a wheat- and yeast-free product.
vitamin B_6 (pyridoxine) or	1/2 cc weekly, or as prescribed by physician.	
vitamin B complex	As directed on label.	
Vitamin B_{12} and	1,000–2,000 mcg daily.	Malabsorption of vitamin B_{12} results from celiac disease. Injections may be necessary. If injections are not available, use a lozenge or sublingual form.
folic acid	400–800 mcg daily.	
Important		
L-carnitine	2 grams a day.	Shown to increase energy levels because it is involved with muscle energy production.
N-acetylglucosamine (N-A-G from Source Naturals)	As directed on label.	Forms the basis of complex molecular structures of the mucous membranes of the intestinal lining.
Vitamin K or alfalfa	As directed on label.	Fat-soluble vitamins are not absorbed well in this disorder. *See* under Herbs, below.
Zinc lozenges	1 15-mg lozenge 5 times daily. Do not exceed a total of 100 mg daily from all supplements.	Needed for immunity and healing.
plus copper	3 mg daily.	Needed to balance with zinc.
Helpful		
Magnesium	750 mg daily.	Helps maintain the body's normal pH balance. Deficiency is common in people with celiac disease.
plus calcium	1,500 mg daily.	Works with magnesium.
Proteolytic enzymes	As directed on label, 3 times daily. Take between meals, on an empty stomach.	Additional digestive enzymes may be needed to aid in breakdown and absorption of foods.
Psyllium seed or flaxseeds or ABC Aerobic Bulk Cleanse from Aerobic Life Industries	As directed on label. Take separately from other supplements and medications.	Fiber products not absorbed by the intestines. Drink large amounts of water because the fiber expands to several times its dry volume.
Vitamin C plus bioflavonoids	2,000–5,000 mg daily, in divided doses.	Boosts immune function.
Vitamin D_3	As directed on label.	Stimulates absorption of calcium. People with celiac disease frequently have calcium deficiencies.

Herbs

❑ Alfalfa supplies vitamin K, which is often deficient in those with celiac disease. Take 2,000 to 3,000 milligrams of alfalfa in tablet form daily.

❑ Olive leaf extract and/or goldenseal is helpful for keeping infection down.

Caution: Do not take goldenseal internally on a daily basis for more than one week at a time. Do not use it during pregnancy or if you are breast-feeding, and use with caution if you are allergic to ragweed. If you have a history of cardiovascular disease, diabetes, or glaucoma, use it only under a doctor's supervision.

Recommendations

❑ Avoid any and all foods that contain gluten. Do not eat any products that contain barley, oats, rye, or wheat. Rice and corn can be eaten. Substitute rice, potato, cornmeal, and soy flour for wheat flour. Read all labels carefully. Watch for "hidden" sources of gluten, such as hydrolyzed vegetable protein, textured vegetable protein, hydrolyzed plant protein, and all derivatives of wheat, rye, oats, and barley, including malt, modified food starch, some soy sauces, grain vinegars, binders, fillers, inert substances, and "natural flavorings." Do not consume hot dogs, gravies, luncheon meat, beer, mustard, catsup, nondairy creamer, white vinegar, curry powder, or seasonings. Gluten-free products are available at health food stores. Natural foods stores such as Whole Foods Market have a wide selection of gluten-free foods.

❑ Eat fresh vegetables, legumes (such as lentils, beans, and peas), rice bran, nuts, sunflower seeds, raisins, figs, and "seedy" fruits, such as strawberries, raspberries, and blackberries.

❑ Include in the diet blackstrap molasses, which is high in iron and the B vitamins. People with celiac disease need fiber and foods rich in iron and the B vitamins.

❑ Be sure to chew your foods thoroughly before swallowing. This improves the intake of nutrients.

❑ Do not eat sugary products, processed foods, dairy products, bouillon cubes, chocolate, and bottled salad dressings.

❑ Celiac disease causes malabsorption of the B vitamins and the fat-soluble vitamins (vitamins A, D, E, and K), so take these nutrients. Note that gluten is found in many nutritional supplements. Read labels carefully, and use supplements that are hypoallergenic, wheat-free, and yeast-free.

❑ If a child develops any of the symptoms of celiac disease, omit all gluten-containing foods from the child's diet and see if the problem clears up. Also eliminate milk, as lactose intolerance can occur with celiac disease. If you do this, be sure to offer another source of calcium, vitamin D, and magnesium. The disease can begin in the first few months of life, depending on the child's diet.

Considerations

❑ Any child who is not thriving could have celiac disease. The disease manifests itself differently with each person. Symptoms can include irritability, fatigue, and/or behavior changes; they do not always involve obvious digestive problems.

❑ A child who gets blisters and sores all over his or her body should be checked for celiac disease.

❑ If celiac disease is suspected, a blood test and then an intestinal biopsy should be performed to make a definitive diagnosis. Make a list of symptoms and foods that set off these symptoms for your child's health care provider. Growing children need a wide range of nutrients to grow and for their brains to develop. Don't restrict a child's diet before seeking medical help.

❑ Starting a gluten-free diet is challenging because gluten is present in so many foods, including most grains, pasta, cereals, and processed foods. However, people with celiac disease can still eat a varied, well-balanced diet that includes breads and pastas made from potato, rice, soy, or bean flour. Gluten-free products are available from many health food stores and specialty food companies. There are also many cookbooks available for those on a gluten-free diet. Grainaissance is an industry leader in providing wheat-, gluten-, and dairy-free products. Mochi bake-and-serve rice squares are wheat-, gluten-, and dairy-free, as are Amazake Rice Shakes. Enjoy Life Foods sells a number of foods that are ideal for a gluten-free diet, including breakfast cereals. Mrs. Leepers carries a line of organic rice pastas and corn pastas that are gluten-, wheat-, and casein-free. Rizopia rice pasta is gluten-free. Nature's Path carries a number of gluten-free products. U.S. Mills offers wheat- and gluten-free cereals under the Erewhon and New Morning brands.

❑ Several studies suggest that people with celiac disease can safely eat oats. However, since oats are frequently processed with other grains, it is difficult to determine whether oats are completely gluten-free. Follow your physician's or dietician's advice about including oats in a gluten-free diet. A clinical study in Finland showed that patients with celiac disease were able to tolerate both highly processed oats and those left in a more natural state, indicating that oats may be part of a gluten-free diet.

❑ It may be necessary to remove milk and milk products from the diet because of a secondary lactase deficiency. (See LACTOSE INTOLERANCE in Part Two.) Many lactose-free dairy substitute products are available (milk, ice cream, cheese), so if you enjoy dairy, there are ample healthy options.

❑ Vitamin K deficiency caused by celiac disease may lead to hypoprothrombinemia (a lack of clotting factors in the blood). "Friendly" bacteria in the intestines manufacture one form of vitamin K; another is present in certain foods, especially leafy greens, alfalfa, tomatoes, strawberries, whole grains, and yogurt. Bacteria such as those found in yogurt and acidophilus can also help to restore the intestinal flora necessary for vitamin K production.

❑ Martin F. Kagnoff, M.D., of the University of California–San Diego says that heredity is a vital factor in the development of this disease. He also says that celiac disease often develops in childhood but may trail off in adolescence; in some cases, reappearing in adults in their thirties and forties. Factors that may trigger the onset of celiac disease are emotional stress, physical trauma, a viral infection, pregnancy, or surgery.

❑ A report published in the British medical journal the *Lancet* pointed to a possible connection between celiac disease and epilepsy. Theories as to how the two might be linked include the possibility that endorphin-like substances may be created from wheat gluten and may affect brain metabolism; another possibility is that celiac disease increases intestinal permeability, which in turn allows the absorption of substances that may affect brain chemistry.

❑ Schizophrenia has been observed to occur more often in those with celiac disease. (See SCHIZOPHRENIA in Part Two.)

❑ For more information about celiac disease, you can contact the Celiac Disease Foundation. (See Health and Medical Organizations in the Appendix.) There are also good books available on this subject.

❑ See also ALLERGIES and MALABSORPTION SYNDROME in Part Two.

CHEMICAL ALLERGIES

When the body is exposed to certain foreign chemicals, it may respond by producing antibodies to defend itself against the foreign invaders. Virtually any substance can provoke a reaction in some individuals. Some of the environmental contaminants that frequently cause problems include air pollution; gas, oil, or coal fumes; formaldehyde; chlorine; phenol; carbolic acid; insecticides; disinfectants;

paint strippers; paint; hair sprays; household cleaning products; and metals such as nickel, mercury, chrome, and beryllium.

Chemical allergies often manifest themselves as skin reactions. Other possible allergic responses to foreign chemicals include watery eyes, ringing in the ears, stuffy nose, diarrhea, nausea, upset stomach, asthma, bronchitis, arthritis, fatigue, eczema, intestinal disorders, depression, and headache. Some people may have a reaction immediately after encountering a chemical allergen; others may not react for up to twenty-four hours. Seek medical help if the reaction is severe.

The following supplement program is designed to protect you from, and help you cope with, the effects of chemical allergies. Unless otherwise specified, the dosages recommended here are for adults. For a child between the ages of twelve and seventeen, reduce the dose to three-quarters the recommended amount. For a child between six and twelve, use one-half the recommended dose, and for a child under the age of six, use one-quarter the recommended amount.

NUTRIENTS

SUPPLEMENT	SUGGESTED DOSAGE	COMMENTS
Very Important		
Vitamin A plus carotenoid complex	50,000 IU daily for 10 days, then reduce to 25,000 IU daily. If you are pregnant, do not exceed 10,000 IU daily.	Powerful free radical scavengers and immune enhancers. Use emulsion forms for easier assimilation.
with beta-carotene plus	5,000–10,000 IU daily.	
vitamin E	200 IU daily.	A powerful antioxidant. Use d-alpha-tocopherol form.
Vitamin B complex	100–200 mg of each major B vitamin daily (amounts of individual vitamins in a complex will vary).	Allergies hinder absorption of B vitamins. Consider injections (under a doctor's supervision).
plus extra vitamin B$_6$ (pyridoxine)	100 mg 3 times daily.	A natural antihistamine. Also aids in detoxifying foreign substances and eliminating them through the kidneys.
plus niacinamide	500 mg 3 times daily.	Aids circulation. *Caution:* Do not substitute niacin for niacinamide, or toxicity may result.
Vitamin C with bioflavonoids	5,000–20,000 mg daily, in divided doses. (*See* ASCORBIC ACID FLUSH in Part Three.)	Protects the body from allergens and moderates the inflammatory response.
Important		
Coenzyme Q$_{10}$	60 mg daily.	Helps to counter histamine, a body chemical involved in allergic reactions.
plus Coenzyme A from Coenzyme-A Technologies	As directed on label.	Supports the immune system's detoxification of many dangerous substances. Removes toxins from the body.
Pycnogenol or grape seed extract	As directed on label. As directed on label.	Serves as a free radical scavenger and aids in protecting bodily cells from damage.
Selenium	200 mcg daily. If you are pregnant, do not exceed 40 mcg daily.	Essential in immune function and protection of cells.
Superoxide dismutase (SOD) or Cell Guard from Biotec Foods	As directed on label. As directed on label.	A potent free radical scavenger. An antioxidant complex that contains SOD.
Zinc plus copper	50 mg daily. Do not exceed a total of 100 mg daily from all supplements. 3 mg daily.	Important in proper immune function. Use zinc gluconate lozenges or OptiZinc for best absorption. Needed to balance with zinc. Copper is lost when high doses of vitamin C are taken.
Helpful		
Aller Bee-Gone from CC Pollen	As directed on label.	A combination of herbs, enzymes, and nutrients that fight allergic outbreaks.
Garlic (Kyolic from Wakunaga)	2 capsules 3 times daily.	A powerful immunostimulant.
L-cysteine and L-methionine plus L-glutamic acid	500 mg each daily. Take on an empty stomach with juice or water. Do not take with milk. Take with 50 mg vitamin C for better absorption.	Excellent detoxifiers, especially of the liver. (*See* AMINO ACIDS in Part One.)
Manganese	As directed on label. Take separately from calcium.	Interacts with zinc and copper. Use manganese chelate form.
Pancreatic enzymes and proteolytic enzymes	As directed on label 3 times daily, with meals. As directed on label 3 times daily, between meals.	Both pancreatic and proteolytic enzymes are needed for proper digestion and assimilation of necessary nutrients. Proteolytic enzymes also control inflammation.
Raw thymus glandular	As directed on label.	Important for immune function.
Taurine Plus from American Biologics	500 mg daily.	The most important antioxidant and immune regulator, necessary for white blood cell activation and neurological function. Use the sublingual form.

Herbs

❑ If you develop a skin rash from exposure to metal in watchbands, earrings, snaps, or other items that come in contact with the skin, try using Calendula Cream from NatureWorks. Calendula, chamomile, elder flower, and tea tree oil also can be used as a soothing wash on rashes.

Caution: Do not use chamomile if you are allergic to ragweed. Do not use during pregnancy or nursing. It may interact with warfarin or cyclosporine, so patients using these drugs should avoid it.

Recommendations

❑ The first step in managing chemical allergies is to determine which chemicals are provoking the allergic reaction, then to avoid coming in contact with them. If the source of the problem is not obvious, see an allergy specialist.

❑ Avoid foods that have been sprayed or that contain artificial colorings (found in some apples and oranges), ripening agents, or protective waxes (found on some apples, cucumbers, and other items). Avoid things containing FD&C Yellow No. 5 dye. Read all food product labels carefully.

❑ Supplement your diet with plenty of fiber. Oat bran is a good source of fiber. Apple pectin also can be a useful addition to your diet. It removes unwanted metals that may trigger allergic reactions.

Note: Always take supplemental fiber separately from other supplements and medications.

Considerations

❑ Mercury and silver in old dental fillings can cause allergic reactions as well as heavy metal poisoning. (*See* MERCURY TOXICITY in Part Two.)

❑ *See also* CHEMICAL POISONING below.

CHEMICAL POISONING

Like toxic metals, poisonous chemicals such as chlorine, disinfectants, heavy metals, herbicides, insecticides, petroleum products, and solvents can enter the body and decrease the functional capacity of its organs. This is chemical poisoning. Some chemicals are absorbed through the skin; others may be inhaled or ingested. The body's immune system is threatened by these chemicals and tries to cleanse the body of the poisons. Damage to internal organs, especially the liver, may occur.

Chronic chemical poisoning occurs most often in people who use or who are exposed to chemicals in their work environments, or who use excessive amounts of chemical sprays. People who live near landfills or certain industrial installations also may be chronically exposed to toxic chemicals.

Acute chemical poisoning can result from accidental ingestion of household chemicals (particularly by children) or taking improper or excessive medications.

Unless otherwise specified, the dosages recommended here are for adults. For a child between the ages of twelve and seventeen, reduce the dose to three-quarters the recommended amount. For a child between six and twelve, use one-half the recommended dose, and for a child under the age of six, use one-quarter the recommended amount.

NUTRIENTS

SUPPLEMENT	SUGGESTED DOSAGE	COMMENTS
Very Important		
Free form amino acid	As directed on label twice daily, on an empty stomach.	Helps liver function. Use a sublingual form.
Garlic (Kyolic from Wakunaga)	As directed on label.	Helps to detoxify and cleanse the bloodstream; chelates heavy metals.
Raw liver extract	As directed on label or as prescribed by physician.	Supplies needed B vitamins and iron, and detoxifies chemicals. For severe chemical poisoning, injections (under a doctor's supervision) are best.
Superoxide dismutase (SOD) or	As directed on label.	A powerful free radical destroyer.
Cell Guard from Biotec Foods	As directed on label.	An antioxidant complex that contains SOD.
Vitamin B complex injections	As prescribed by physician.	Protects the liver and bodily functions. Injections (under a doctor's supervision) are best. If injections are not available, use a sublingual form.
plus choline and inositol	50 mg 3 times daily, with meals. 50 mg 3 times daily, with meals.	
Vitamin C with bioflavonoids	5,000–20,000 mg daily, in divided doses. (*See* ASCORBIC ACID FLUSH in Part Three.)	Protects the body from pollutants and aids in the elimination of toxic substances.
Important		
Grape seed extract	As directed on label.	A powerful antioxidant.
L-cysteine and L-methionine	500 mg each daily, on an empty stomach. Take with water or juice. Do not take with milk. Take with 50 mg vitamin B₆ and 100 mg vitamin C for better absorption.	To remove toxins and rebuild the body. (*See* AMINO ACIDS in Part One.)
Selenium	200 mcg daily. If you are pregnant, do not exceed 40 mcg daily.	Works with vitamins C and E to detoxify the body.
Vitamin E	200 IU daily.	A powerful antioxidant. Use d-alpha-tocopherol form.
Helpful		
Coenzyme Q₁₀	30–60 mg daily.	Aids in rebuilding the immune system and providing oxygen to the tissues.
Multivitamin and mineral complex	As directed on label.	All nutrients are needed to aid in strengthening the immune system and lessening toxicity.

Recommendations

❑ To aid recovery, eat a well-balanced diet that is high in fiber. Fiber helps to cleanse the system. Recommended foods include almonds, apricots, bananas, barley, beans, beets, Brazil nuts, brown rice, carrots, dates, fish, garlic, grapes, hazelnuts, lemons, lentils, oatmeal, onions, spinach, and yogurt.

❏ If at all possible, eat only organically grown foods.

❏ Always wear protective clothing and rubber or latex gloves when handling chemicals, even commonly available products such as solvents, paint strippers, and paint thinners (most of which contain methylene chloride, xylene, acetone, toluene, benzene, and other extremely hazardous chemicals). One of the worst is the cleaning solvent used to prepare plastic pipe for the application of glue. It contains methylethylketone (MEK), a great solvent but a known carcinogen. Carefully follow the directions on the label of any product that contains chemicals. Avoid breathing the fumes, especially in a confined area.

❏ Avoid being outside during any aerial application of insecticides or pesticides.

❏ Drink steam-distilled water only. (*See* WATER in Part One.)

❏ Perform a cleansing fast for three days each month to help the body get rid of toxins. (*See* FASTING in Part Three.)

❏ Avoid chemicals whenever possible. Even getting gasoline on your hands while fueling the car or lawn mower is not a good idea.

Considerations

❏ *See also* CHEMICAL ALLERGIES and POISONING in Part Two.

CHICKENPOX

Chickenpox was once a very common and highly contagious disease. Most children now get a chickenpox vaccine, which can prevent chickenpox. About eight or nine out of ten people who get chickenpox vaccine will not get chickenpox. But if someone who has been vaccinated does get chickenpox, it is usually very mild. They will have fewer blisters, are less likely to have a fever, and will recover faster. Children who have never had chickenpox should get two doses of chickenpox vaccine at twelve to fifteen months and at four to six years of age. Anyone who is not fully vaccinated, and never had chickenpox, should receive one or two doses of chickenpox vaccine. The timing of these doses depends on the person's age. Ask your health care provider.

A vaccine, like any medicine, is capable of causing problems, such as severe allergic reactions. However, the risk of chickenpox vaccine causing serious harm, or death, is extremely small. Getting chickenpox vaccine is much safer than getting chickenpox disease. Most people who get chickenpox vaccine do not have any problems with it. But if they do, reactions are usually more likely after the first dose than after the second.

Before a vaccine was available approximately 4 million people contracted chickenpox, approximately 11,000 people were hospitalized, and approximately 100 died as a result of chickenpox in the United States every year. Once the vaccine was introduced, there was a 75 percent decrease in chickenpox in children aged one to four. Deaths from chickenpox went down 66 percent overall. These data are very compelling.

The same virus that causes chickenpox—*Varicella zoster*—can lie dormant for years, then resurface as shingles in adulthood. In 2006, the FDA approved a vaccine for shingles. The FDA advises that everyone over sixty years of age get vaccinated. (*See* SHINGLES in Part Two.)

The chickenpox virus is transmitted by direct contact with an infected person or through the air when an infected person coughs or sneezes. A person can also contract chickenpox (but not shingles) from direct contact with a person with the shingles rash. Outbreaks are common within families and in schools and day care facilities. Symptoms do not appear until after a person reaches the infectious stage, so it is difficult to isolate those who are contagious. Repeated exposures to the virus during the incubation period can result in worse symptoms. One bout with chickenpox generally affords lifetime immunity against the illness. Second attacks are possible but rare.

Most children contract chickenpox before the age of ten. It first manifests itself as a fever and headache, usually starting between seven and twenty-one days after exposure to the virus. Twenty-four to thirty-six hours later, small round "pimples" appear on the face and body. They are filled with fluid and look like water blisters. The fluid leaks from the swollen areas of the skin, forming a crust. These eruptions continue in cycles, lasting from three days to one week. The blisters and crusts are infectious and itchy, and scratching them can lead to bacterial infection and scarring. Once the scabs are gone, the individual is no longer infectious. Adults who contract the infection tend to have more severe cases than do children.

Chickenpox usually runs its course in two weeks or less for otherwise healthy children. Potentially serious complications can arise for some people, especially for newborns, adults, and those with weakened immune systems. Anyone with an impaired immune system, such as a person whose immune system is suppressed by drugs or who has a disorder such as AIDS, can develop pneumonia or encephalitis, an infection of the brain. A newborn baby also can develop complications from chickenpox, especially if infected prenatally or soon after birth.

Unless otherwise specified, the dosages recommended here are for adults. For children between the ages of twelve and seventeen, reduce the dose to three-quarters the recommended amount. For children between six and twelve, use one-half the recommended dose, and for children under the age of six, use one-quarter the recommended amount.

NUTRIENTS

SUPPLEMENT	SUGGESTED DOSAGE	COMMENTS
Essential		
Carotenoid complex with beta-carotene	15,000 IU daily.	Heals tissues and stimulates the immune system.
Vitamin A capsules or emulsion	20,000 IU daily for 1 month, then 15,000 IU daily for 1 week. 100,000 IU daily for 1 week, then 75,000 IU daily for 1 week. If you are pregnant, do not exceed 10,000 IU daily.	An immunostimulant that aids healing of tissues. Emulsion form is recommended for easier assimilation and greater safety at higher doses.
Vitamin C with bioflavonoids	1,000 mg 4 times daily.	Powerful immune stimulant that aids in keeping down fever.
Very Important		
Potassium and zinc	99 mg daily. 80 mg daily. Do not exceed a total of 100 mg daily from all supplements.	Helps reduce fever and speed healing. Enhances immune function. Use zinc gluconate lozenges or OptiZinc for best absorption.
Vitamin E	200 IU daily.	A powerful free radical scavenger that increases oxygenation and promotes healing. Use d-alpha-tocopherol form.
Helpful		
Maitake extract or shiitake extract or reishi extract	As directed on label. As directed on label. As directed on label.	Mushroom extracts with immune-stimulating and antiviral properties.
Multivitamin and mineral complex	As directed on label.	All nutrients help to speed the healing process.
Raw thymus glandular	As directed on label.	Stimulates the production of T lymphocytes by the thymus gland. Needed for immune function. (*See* GLANDULAR THERAPY in Part Three.)

Herbs

❏ Catnip tea sweetened with molasses is good for fever and can be given to infants and children as well as to adults. For a child over age two, catnip tea enemas can reduce fever.

❏ Other recommended herbs include burdock root, echinacea, ginger, goldenseal, pau d'arco, and St. John's wort.

Cautions: Do not take echinacea for longer than three months. It should not be used by people who are allergic to ragweed. Do not take goldenseal internally on a daily basis for more than one week at a time. Do not use it during pregnancy or if you are breast-feeding, and use with caution if you are allergic to ragweed. If you have a history of cardiovascular disease, diabetes, or glaucoma, use it only under a doctor's supervision. St. John's wort may cause increased sensitivity to sunlight. It may also produce anxi-

ety, gastrointestinal symptoms, and headaches. It can interact with some drugs including antidepressants, birth control pills, and anticoagulants.

Recommendations

❏ Drink freshly made juices with protein powder and brewer's yeast added. Also drink pure vegetable broth.

Caution: Brewer's yeast can cause an allergic reaction in some individuals. Start with a small amount at first, and discontinue use if any allergic symptoms occur.

❏ When the fever drops and the appetite returns, use a "starter diet" consisting of only mashed bananas, avocados, fresh raw applesauce, and/or yogurt. Do not use cooked or processed foods.

❏ Infants under one year of age need breast milk or infant formula, even when they have a fever. Give an older child lots of water or an electrolyte replacer such as Pedialyte to prevent dehydration.

❏ Consult a doctor immediately if symptoms include dizziness, a fever higher than 103°F, rapid heartbeat, shortness of breath, loss of muscle coordination, tremors, vomiting, and/or a stiff neck.

❏ Take warm baths with uncooked oatmeal or cornstarch added to the water to help relieve some of the itching caused by chickenpox.

❏ Stay out of bright sunlight and keep interior areas dimly lit. Do not expose the patient to bright lights until he or she is completely healed.

❏ Take care not to scratch the pocks. Keep a child's nails short and clean, and bathe the child often. Put mittens on a young child's hands if necessary. Use warm baths made with tea prepared with the recommended herbs, or ginger baths using cool water. Sponge the affected area with the tea. Wet compresses help to control the itching; use these often.

❏ Family members who have not had chickenpox should have limited contact with other family members who are known to be infected. Repeated exposure to the virus can worsen the effects. Keep an infected child away from elderly people, newborn babies, and pregnant women who have not had chickenpox.

❏ Never give aspirin to a child who has a fever. Studies have shown an increased risk of Reye's syndrome, a rare and potentially fatal disorder, in children given aspirin for fever. This is also true for those who have received a vaccination (Varivax; *see under* Considerations, below). (*See* REYE'S SYNDROME in Part Two.)

❏ If you are unlucky enough to contract chickenpox in adulthood, contact your health care provider. Use a fasting program to help speed healing. (*See* FASTING in Part Three.)

Considerations

❑ Fetal exposure to chickenpox has been associated with an increased risk of birth defects.

❑ If the sores become infected, an antibiotic ointment is usually prescribed.

❑ Acyclovir (Zovirax) is an antiviral medication that lessens the severity of symptoms and shortens the duration of rash formation. It is most often recommended for those at risk for severe chickenpox: premature babies, adolescents, and adults.

❑ A chickenpox vaccine called Varivax was approved by the FDA in 1995. This is an attenuated live-virus vaccine. No aspirin or other similar medication should be taken for at least six months after the vaccine is administered. (See REYE'S SYNDROME in Part Two)

❑ See also SHINGLES in Part Two.

CHLAMYDIA

According to the U.S. Centers for Disease Control and Prevention (CDC), sexually transmitted chlamydia infection accounts for the bulk of the sexually transmitted disease (STD) epidemic in the United States. *Chlamydia trachomatis* is believed to be twice as common as gonorrhea. This infection can be transmitted or contracted during anal, oral, or vaginal sex with an infected partner. In 2007, 1,108,374 cases of chlamydia were reported, a big jump from 1997 when only 537,904 cases were reported. It is estimated that the true number is 2.8 million cases, more than half of which are undiagnosed. About 4 percent of eighteen- to twenty-six-year-olds who were sexually active had chlamydia.

Symptoms of chlamydia include genital inflammation, vaginal or urethral discharge, difficulty in urinating and a burning sensation during urination, painful intercourse, and itching around the inflamed area. The symptoms appear within one to three weeks of contact with an infected partner. These symptoms can appear in both men and women. However, as many as 50 percent of the men and 75 percent of the women who have chlamydia experience no symptoms at all, or symptoms so mild that they do not seek treatment. This is unfortunate, as untreated chlamydia infection in women leads to sterility in an estimated 30 percent of cases. Pelvic inflammatory disease and irreparable damage to the reproductive system can occur, and a hysterectomy may be required. Also, women who have been infected with chlamydia may have three to five times the risk of becoming infected with HIV if they are exposed to it. Babies born to mothers with chlamydia may suffer from pneumonia or conjunctivitis (an eye infection). Both of those ailments require treatment with antibiotics.

In males, prostatitis and inflammation of the seminal vesicles may be caused by chlamydia. Symptoms of prostatitis include pain when urinating and a watery mucous discharge from the penis. Men may also notice pain and swelling in the testicles. Diagnosis of chlamydia infection is made on the basis of bacteriologic examination of urine or vaginal or urethral discharge. There are also a number of tests available today that can supplement or even replace the traditional culture.

NUTRIENTS

SUPPLEMENT	SUGGESTED DOSAGE	COMMENTS
Important		
Garlic (Kyolic from Wakunaga)	2 capsules 3 times daily.	Acts as a natural antibiotic and aids in healing.
Vitamin B complex	50–100 mg of each major B vitamin 3 times daily, with meals (amounts of individual vitamins in a complex will vary).	Needed for proper functioning of the liver and gastrointestinal tract.
Vitamin C	1,500 mg 4 times daily.	Immunostimulant that aids healing. Use a buffered form.
Vitamin E	200 IU daily. Can also be used directly on the inflamed site; cut open a capsule and apply.	Needed to protect red blood cells. Immune enhancer. Use d-alpha-tocopherol form.
Helpful		
Acidophilus	As directed on label. Take on an empty stomach.	Replenishes "friendly" bacteria destroyed by antibiotics. Use a nondairy formula.
Bio-Bifidus from American Biologics	Use as a vaginal douche as directed on label.	Replaces normal vaginal and bowel flora.
Coenzyme Q$_{10}$ plus Coenzyme A from Coenzyme-A Technologies	60 mg daily. As directed on label.	Aids in healing and is a powerful antioxidant and immune stimulant. Works with coenzyme Q$_{10}$ and aids in the detoxification of many dangerous substances.
Kelp	2,000–3,000 mg daily.	A rich source of minerals.
Multivitamin complex with mixed carotenoids	As directed on label.	Necessary for healing of all bodily tissues. Use a high-potency formula.
Zinc plus copper	50 mg daily. Do not exceed a total of 100 mg daily from all supplements. 3 mg daily.	Important for immune function and healing. Use zinc gluconate lozenges or OptiZinc for best absorption. Needed to balance with zinc.

Herbs

❑ Astragalus, echinacea, goldenseal, pau d'arco, and red clover aid in healing.

Cautions: Do not use astragalus in the presence of a fever. Do not take echinacea for longer than three months. It should not be used by people who are allergic to ragweed. Do not take goldenseal internally on a daily basis for more than one week at a time. Do not use it during pregnancy or if you are breast-feeding, and use with caution if you are allergic to ragweed. If you have a history of cardiovascular disease, diabetes, or glaucoma, use it only under a doctor's supervision.

Recommendations

❏ Eat a diet consisting mainly of fresh vegetables and fruits, plus brown rice, raw seeds and nuts, well-cooked poultry, white fish, and whole grains.

❏ Avoid highly processed, fried, and junk foods.

❏ Drink only steam-distilled water, sugar-free juices, and herbal teas.

❏ Take acidophilus to replenish the "friendly" bacteria destroyed by antibiotics.

❏ If you have symptoms of chlamydia infection, do not delay seeking treatment. The danger of complications increases as time passes.

Considerations

❏ If you are under thirty-five and have had more than one sexual partner, you should be tested for infection yearly.

❏ All partners must be treated for this disorder so that the disease is not transmitted back and forth. (Both sexes have similar discharges, and it is through this discharge that the disease is transmitted during sexual contact.) Antibiotics such as tetracycline and doxycycline (Doryx, Vibramycin, and others) kill chlamydia. Alternatively, a single 1-gram oral dose of azithromycin (Zithromax) may be used. This is relatively expensive (a single dose costs as much as a one-week regimen of doxycycline), but the convenience of single-dose treatment may be worth it.

❏ Chlamydia has been linked to a form of arthritis in young women. In one study, the microorganism was found in the joints of nearly half those with unexplained arthritis.

❏ There are currently three FDA-approved methods of testing for chlamydia:

1. *Nucleic acid amplification test (NAAT).* This method is based on amplification of the DNA that is present in *chlamydia trachomatis.* This is the best test and is widely used.

2. *Direct fluorescent antibody stain test (DFA).* In this method, a scientific technique called staining makes chlamydia antigens easier to detect under the microscope. A culture can be taken from the eye, cervix, or penis.

3. *DNA probe.* Looks for chlamydia DNA but is less sensitive than NAAT.

❏ *See also* SEXUALLY TRANSMITTED DISEASE (STD) in Part Two.

CHOLESTEROL PROBLEMS

See HIGH CHOLESTEROL.

CHRONIC FATIGUE SYNDROME

Chronic fatigue syndrome (CFS) is not a disease as such, but a characteristic and complex array of symptoms that may mimic other illnesses. The symptoms of this syndrome resemble those of flu and other viral infections, so it is often mistaken for other disorders. In fact, it is often misdiagnosed as hypochondria, psychosomatic illness, or depression because routine medical tests do not detect any problems. The symptoms of CFS may include aching muscles and joints, anxiety, depression, difficulty concentrating, poor memory, fever, headaches, low blood pressure, intestinal problems and pain, irritability, environmental sensitivities, jaundice, loss of appetite, mood swings, muscle spasms, recurrent upper respiratory tract infections, nasal congestion, candidiasis, sensitivity to light and heat, sleep disturbances, night sweats, sore throat, swollen glands (lymph nodes)—and most of all, extreme and often disabling mental and physical fatigue. Immunologic abnormalities that show up on various diagnostic tests are common as well.

The syndrome is three times more prevalent in women than in men, and primarily affects young adults between the ages of twenty and fifty. In all, there are about 500,000 cases of people in the United States who have a CFS-like condition.

The cause or causes of chronic fatigue syndrome are not well understood, but it may be related to defects in immune function, psychological problems, or neurological problems. Some experts believe it is linked to infection with the Epstein-Barr virus (EBV) and/or cytomegalovirus (CMV), members of the herpesvirus family that also cause mononucleosis and retinal and gastrointestinal infections. This belief is based in large part on the fact that many people with chronic fatigue syndrome have been found to have high levels of EBV antibodies in their blood, and that many people date the onset of symptoms to a prolonged bout with a viral infection. However, no connection between EBV and chronic fatigue syndrome has ever been proven conclusively. Moreover, it is now known that many people have high EBV antibody levels without any apparent ill effects on their health. Many cases of chronic fatigue syndrome occur without any known preceding infection. This has led researchers to look for other possible causes. Some suspect an immune system problem or a defect in the mechanisms that regulate blood pressure.

Other proposed causes of chronic fatigue syndrome include anemia, arthritis, chronic mercury poisoning from amalgam dental fillings, hypoglycemia, hypothyroidism, infection with the fungus *Candida albicans,* and sleep problems.

Fibromyalgia, a muscle disorder that causes muscle weakness and fatigue, has been found in many people with chronic fatigue syndrome. Intestinal parasites are also comparatively common in people with this condition. It is likely that poor diet, nutritional deficiencies, allergies, thyroid dysfunction, candida, anemia, and stress all compromise the immune system, and can contribute to CFS.

Even though chronic fatigue syndrome is not life-threatening, it cannot be cured, and it can result in serious damage to the immune system. Some people appear to recover spontaneously, but once you have had this condition, it can recur at any time, usually following a bout with another illness or during times of stress.

The major criterion used to distinguish chronic fatigue syndrome is:

- Persistent fatigue that does not resolve with bed rest and that is severe enough to reduce average daily activity by at least 50 percent for at least six months.

The presence of other chronic clinical conditions, including psychiatric disorders, should also be ruled out.

Chronic fatigue syndrome should not be confused with the results of overwork and stress. With CFS, a normal, active level of life is impossible to maintain and the symptoms exceed, by far, the normal lethargy or tiredness associated with a stressful and hardworking lifestyle. Medical treatments for CFS are numerous but have mixed outcomes because there are no standardized tests. Some people with CFS find lifestyle changes such as adopting a regular exercise routine can help. Certain over-the-counter medicines such as ibuprofen or antihistamines or prescribed medications such as antidepressants may also help to relieve some of the symptoms.

NUTRIENTS

SUPPLEMENT	SUGGESTED DOSAGE	COMMENTS
Essential		
Chromium polynicotinate	200–300 mg daily.	Aids in controlling hypoglycemia.
Coenzyme Q_{10}	75 mg daily.	Enhances the effectiveness of the immune system and protects the heart.
plus Coenzyme A from Coenzyme-A Technologies	As directed on label.	Works with coenzyme Q_{10} and aids in the removal of toxic substances from the body.
Kyolic-EPA from Wakunaga	As directed on label.	Supplies essential fatty acids.
L-carnitine	1,000 mg daily, on an empty stomach. Take with 50 mg vitamin B_6 and 100 mg vitamin C for better absorption.	Transports fatty acids into the mitochondria, where it is used to make ATP, thus increasing energy levels.
Lecithin granules or capsules	1 tbsp 3 times daily, with meals. 1,200 mg 3 times daily, with meals.	Promotes energy and enhances immunity.
Malic acid	As directed on label.	Involved in energy production in many cells of the body, including muscle cells. Needed for sugar metabolism. Deficiency has been linked to CFS.
and magnesium	500–1,000 mg daily.	Often deficient in people with CFS, magnesium is needed for ATP synthesis.
Manganese	5 mg daily.	Influences the metabolic rate by its involvement in endocrine function.

Nicotinamide adenine dinucleotide (NADH)	10–20 mg with water first thing in the morning, on an empty stomach.	Studies have shown that it increases energy levels and aids in preventing depression. May take 2–3 weeks to work.
Proteolytic enzymes or Inf-zyme Forte from American Biologics	As directed on label, 6 times daily, on an empty stomach. Take with meals, between meals, and at bedtime.	Reduces inflammation and improves absorption of nutrients, especially protein, which is needed for tissue repair.
Vitamin A with mixed carotenoids and vitamin E	25,000 IU daily for 1 month, then slowly reduce to 10,000 IU daily. If you are pregnant, do not exceed 10,000 IU daily. 200 IU daily for 1 month, then slowly reduce to 100 IU daily.	Powerful free radical scavengers that protect the cells and enhance immune function to fight viruses. Use emulsion forms for easier assimilation and greater safety at high doses. Use d-alpha-tocopherol form of vitamin E.
Vitamin C with bioflavonoids	5,000–10,000 mg daily.	Has a powerful antiviral effect and increases the energy level. Use a buffered form.
Very Important		
Dimethylglycine (DMG) (Aangamik DMG from FoodScience of Vermont)	50 mg 3 times daily.	Enhances oxygen utilization and destroys free radicals.
Free form amino acid (Amino Balance from Anabol Naturals)	As directed on label.	For tissue and organ repair. Use a formula containing all the essential amino acids.
Kyo-Green from Wakunaga	As directed on label.	To improve digestion and cleanse the bloodstream.
Liquid Kyolic with B_1 and B_{12} from Wakunaga	As directed on label.	Provides energy and builds red blood cells.
Vitamin B complex injections	2 cc twice weekly or as prescribed by physician.	B vitamins are essential for increased energy levels and normal brain function. Injections (under a doctor's supervision) are best. All injectables can be combined in a single syringe.
plus extra vitamin B_6 (pyridoxine) and	½ cc twice weekly or as prescribed by physician.	Aids in absorption of vitamin B_{12}.
vitamin B_{12} plus	1 cc twice weekly or as prescribed by physician.	A natural energy booster needed to prevent anemia.
liver extract injections or	2 cc twice weekly or as prescribed by physician.	A good source of B vitamins plus other valuable nutrients.
vitamin B complex	100 mg of each major B vitamin 3 times daily (amounts of individual vitamins in a complex will vary).	If injections are not available, a sublingual form is recommended for best results.
plus pantothenic acid	100 mg 3 times daily.	Needed for proper adrenal function.
Important		
D-ribose	5 grams, 3 times daily.	Ribose is a sugar needed by the mitochondria to produce energy for the cells. In one study, 66% of patients found that they had more energy.

Gamma-amino-butyric acid (GABA)	As directed on label, on an empty stomach. Take with water or juice. Do not take with milk. Take with 50 mg vitamin B_6 and 100 mg vitamin C for better absorption.	To maintain proper control of brain activity and to control anxiety. (See AMINO ACIDS in Part One.)
Multivitamin and mineral complex with		All nutrients are necessary in balance. Use a high-potency, hypoallergenic product.
calcium and	1,500 mg daily.	
potassium and	99 mg daily.	
selenium	200 mcg daily. If you are pregnant, do not exceed 40 mcg daily.	
and zinc	50 mg daily.	
Raw thymus glandular and	As directed on label.	To boost the immune system. (See GLANDULAR THERAPY in Part Three.)
spleen glandular plus	As directed on label.	
raw glandular complex	As directed on label.	
Shiitake extract or	As directed on label.	Help to combat fatigue, boost immunity, and fight viral infection.
reishi extract or	As directed on label.	
maitake extract	As directed on label.	
Helpful		
Acidophilus (Kyo-Dophilus from Wakunaga)	As directed on label.	To replace necessary "friendly" bacteria. Also fights candida infection. Chronic fatigue and candidiasis often occur together. Use a nondairy formula.
Melatonin	As directed on label, taken 2 hours or less before bedtime.	A natural sleep-regulating hormone that is helpful for promoting sound, restful sleep.

Herbs

❏ Astragalus and echinacea enhance immune function and are good for cold and flu symptoms.

Cautions: Do not use astragalus in the presence of a fever. Do not take echinacea for longer than three months. It should not be used by people who are allergic to ragweed.

❏ Fresh black walnut hulls, garlic, gentian root, fresh ginger root, neem leaves, quassia bark, and fresh wormwood all help to rid the body of parasites, a common problem for people with CFS.

Caution: Do not use wormwood in high doses or for extended periods because it contains the chemical compound thujone that can be poisonous. Do not use wormwood if you suffer from any type of seizure disorder or are pregnant.

❏ Teas brewed from burdock root, dandelion, and red clover promote healing by cleansing the blood and lymphatic system, as well as enhancing immune function.

Combine or alternate these herbal teas, and drink 4 to 6 cups daily.

❏ China Gold from Aerobic Life Industries is an herbal formula containing thirty-six different herbal extracts, including ten varieties of ginseng. It helps to enhance adrenal function and overcome fatigue.

❏ Use goldenseal to control infection. At the first signs of a sore throat, take a few drops of alcohol-free goldenseal extract, hold it in your mouth for a moment, then swallow.

Caution: Do not take goldenseal internally on a daily basis for more than one week at a time. Do not use it during pregnancy or if you are breast-feeding, and use with caution if you are allergic to ragweed. If you have a history of cardiovascular disease, diabetes, or glaucoma, use it only under a doctor's supervision.

❏ Ginkgo biloba improves circulation and brain function.

Caution: Do not take ginkgo biloba if you have a bleeding disorder, or are scheduled for surgery or a dental procedure.

❏ Kava kava, skullcap, and valerian root all improve sleep.

Caution: Kava kava can cause drowsiness. It is not recommended for pregnant women or nursing mothers, and it should not be taken together with other substances that act on the central nervous system, such as alcohol, barbiturates, antidepressants, and antipsychotic drugs.

❏ Licorice root supports the endocrine system and increases cortisol levels by blocking the action of an enzyme that breaks it down. Adrenal exhaustion leads to low production of cortisol, and licorice may prove to be beneficial for CFS sufferers.

Caution: Licorice root should not be used during pregnancy or nursing. It should not be used by persons with diabetes, glaucoma, heart disease, high blood pressure, or a history of stroke.

❏ Milk thistle protects the liver.

❏ Olive leaf extract has antibiotic and antiviral properties, and helps fight infections.

❏ Pau d'arco, taken in capsule or tea form, is good for treating candida infection.

❏ St. John's wort has antiviral properties and is a good antidepressant.

Caution: St. John's wort may cause increased sensitivity to sunlight. It may also produce anxiety, gastrointestinal symptoms, and headaches. It can interact with some drugs including antidepressants, birth control pills, and anticoagulants.

Recommendations

❏ Eat a well-balanced diet of 50 percent raw foods and fresh "live" juices. The diet should consist mostly of fruits, vegetables, and whole grains, plus raw nuts, seeds, skinless turkey, and some deepwater fish. These quality foods supply nutrients that renew energy and build immunity.

❑ Add some form of acidophilus to your diet, and regularly consume soured products such as yogurt and kefir. Many people with chronic fatigue syndrome also are infected with candida. Acidophilus helps to keep candida under control.

❑ Consume plenty of water—at least ten 8-ounce glasses a day—plus juices, preferably freshly made vegetable juices. Drink a full glass of water at least every two waking hours. Water flushes out toxins and aids in reducing muscle pain.

❑ Do not eat shellfish, fried foods, junk foods, processed foods; stimulants such as coffee, tea, and soft drinks; sugar; and products containing yeasts and/or white flour, such as bread and pasta. You may find this difficult—people with CFS generally have cravings for sugar and carbohydrate products, and could also develop a craving for alcohol—but it is important.

❑ Make sure that the bowels move daily, and add fiber to the diet. Give yourself occasional cleansing enemas. (*See* ENEMAS in Part Three.)

❑ Take chlorophyll in tablet form or obtain it from the liquid of vegetables, such as a "green drink" from leafy vegetables, wheatgrass, or Kyo-Green from Wakunaga.

❑ Take a protein supplement from a vegetable source—Spiru-tein from Nature's Plus is a good protein drink to take between meals.

❑ Get plenty of rest, and make sure that you do not overexert yourself. Moderate exercise may be helpful, however. Deep breathing exercises in particular are recommended. People with CFS tend to take shallow breaths, which can cause sleeping problems. (*See* BREATHING EXERCISES *under* PAIN CONTROL in Part Three.)

❑ Avoid chocolate, soft drinks, caffeine, and highly processed foods. These foods deplete the body of magnesium, which leads to fatigue. Magnesium is important for people with CFS.

❑ Do not smoke, and avoid secondhand smoke. This can make symptoms worse.

❑ Do not take aspirin. If a viral infection is present, Reye's syndrome may result.

❑ Get some exercise, but be careful not to overdo the duration of the activity or the intensity. Doing too much can lead to short-term pain and further fatigue.

❑ In one study, the use of Bo's abdominal acupuncture daily for two weeks improved general symptoms, especially on lassitude, anorexia, insomnia, amnesia, and general pain.

Considerations

❑ There are other health problems that can cause symptoms of chronic fatigue, including anemia, cardiovascular disease (especially in women), depression, fibromyalgia, hepatitis, and Lyme disease, among others. Anyone who experiences extreme fatigue that persists for longer than a week or two should consult a health care provider.

❑ In one study, adolescents with chronic fatigue benefited from cognitive behavioral therapy for as long as two years after treatment had finished. Children had increased physical functioning, better school attendance by 10 percent, and were less fatigued.

❑ In one study, adults around age forty to fifty years had less fatigue from a combination of behavioral therapy with or without the drug mirtazapine (15 milligrams).

❑ In one study, patients with chronic fatigue who followed a low-yeast, low-sugar (anti-candida) diet did not experience increased energy.

❑ In 2009, researchers at the Whittemore Peterson Institute in Nevada found that people with CFS were more likely to have the retrovirus XMRV in their blood; 67 percent of patients had the virus compared to only 4 percent in a healthy population. Researchers caution that this is an association, but does not prove that the virus causes chronic fatigue. However, this data is compelling enough to warrant further investigation.

❑ Some researchers believe that CFS may be hormone-related. Pregnenolone is a steroidal hormone that the body can metabolize into a variety of other vital hormones. It is a precursor hormone to DHEA and most of the other steroid hormones, such as progesterone, testosterone, the estrogens, and cortisol. The body naturally produces about 14 milligrams a day, but as we age this production drops. It has been found to be a hundred times more effective for memory enhancement than other steroids or precursors, and has been reported to reduce stress-induced fatigue. While it appears to be safe if the dosage is kept between 10 and 100 mg a day, it is recommended that any therapy involving its use be done under medical supervision with the appropriate pretherapy tests being given to ensure safety.

❑ If you are diagnosed as having chronic fatigue syndrome, it is wise to seek out a health care provider who has specific experience in the management and treatment of this complex condition.

❑ Taking regular cold showers may produce an improvement in CFS symptoms. Many also find improvement with taking hot baths or showers. However, people with heart or circulatory disorders or other serious health problems should not attempt cold or hot water treatment without first consulting their health care providers.

❑ Amino acids may be beneficial. These include tyrosine, leucine, isoleucine, and valine, as well as lysine and taurine. (*See* AMINO ACIDS in Part One.)

❑ A study at Johns Hopkins University Hospital in Baltimore identified a link between chronic fatigue and a problem in the body's mechanisms for regulating blood pressure.

In this study, twenty-two out of twenty-three subjects with chronic fatigue were found to have a syndrome in which the body responds inappropriately to periods of prolonged standing—the heart rate slows and blood pressure drops, resulting in light-headedness, followed by a feeling of weakness and exhaustion that can persist for days afterward. A significant percentage of those in the study experienced an improvement when they were treated for this blood pressure problem.

❏ Some research points to chemical and/or food sensitivities and hypoglycemia as possible contributors to chronic fatigue. People living in the past fifty years have been exposed to more different chemicals than all of the rest of humankind combined. (*See* CHEMICAL ALLERGIES in Part Two.)

❏ Evidence is pointing to exhausted adrenal glands and a disturbance in the hypothalmic-pituitary-adrenal axis (HPA axis, a complex of biochemical controls that coordinate certain basic metabolic activities) as a possible cause of this disorder.

❏ Parasites are common in people with chronic fatigue. Parasitin from Växa International is a supplement designed to rid the body of parasites.

❏ Family members, friends, and coworkers must understand the nature of the disorder and realize that the person suffering from it is not exaggerating or faking symptoms.

❏ Depression can be a major feature of this illness. To combat it, your physician may prescribe an antidepressant. Antidepressants commonly recommended for people with CFS include the following:

- Doxepin (Sinequan) is a tricyclic antidepressant that may relieve symptoms of general fatigue, nasal congestion, gastritis, muscle tension and tightness, and insomnia. Other tricyclic antidepressants such as amitriptyline (Elavil) may also be prescribed for people with CFS.

- Fluoxetine (Prozac) increases the amount of serotonin in the brain. Serotonin is a neurotransmitter, a natural chemical that transmits messages from one part of the brain to another. Prozac may help to give people more energy but will not help with sleeplessness.

❏ Gamma-globulin treatment uses a transfusion of a blood product to provide protective antibodies that may be absent in the person suffering from CFS. Some consider this treatment ineffective and in rare instances it may even produce adverse side effects such as anaphylactic shock.

❏ People with CFS often suffer from disturbing side effects from prescription drugs. If this is the case, S-adenosylmethionine (SAMe) and 5-hydroxy L-tryptophan (5-HTP) both work well as antidepressants, help to relax muscle tension, and prevent insomnia.

❏ The National Institute of Allergy and Infectious Diseases (NIAID), a part of the National Institutes of Health, provides current information on chronic fatigue syndrome (*See* Health and Medical Organizations in the Appendix.)

❏ A large review on CFS published in the *Journal of the American Medical Association (JAMA)* reported that people have found varying degrees of benefit from magnesium supplements, liver extracts, homeopathy, massage therapy, and having a buddy/mentor.

❏ *See also* CANDIDIASIS; FIBROMYALGIA; HYPOTHYROIDISM; and MONONUCLEOSIS, all in Part Two.

CIRCULATORY PROBLEMS

There are many disorders associated with circulatory problems, which exist when oxygenated blood cannot make the complete circuit of the body without restriction. There are many reasons why blood flow around the body may be inhibited.

Clots may form in the larger veins in the leg or pelvic area, travel to the lung, and become trapped in a pulmonary artery. This results in diminished blood flow and less oxygen getting pumped to the rest of the body. Pulmonary embolism, as this condition is called, is difficult to detect, but is usually accompanied by a sudden shortness of breath and can be life-threatening.

When plaque or fatty deposits form along the walls of the arteries, it causes them to harden and constrict. Hypertension, or high blood pressure, results because the blood exerts greater force against the walls of the narrowed and/or more rigid blood vessels. Hypertension can lead to stroke, angina pectoris (chest pain), kidney damage, and heart attack.

A circulatory disease that is brought on by chronic inflammation of the blood vessels in the extremities is thromboangiitis obliterans (Buerger's disease). This disease is most prevalent among people who smoke. It usually affects the foot or lower leg, but it can occur in the hand, arm, or thigh as well. Early signs of Buerger's disease are a tingling sensation (commonly referred to as "pins and needles") and a burning sensation in the fingers and toes. It can lead to ulceration and gangrene; in severe cases, amputation may be required.

Another serious circulatory condition is Raynaud's disease, which is characterized by constriction and spasm of the blood vessels in the extremities, such as in the fingers, toes, and tip of the nose. Cold, stress, smoking, and other factors may cause fingers and toes to become numb; extremities may appear colorless or bluish due to lack of circulation and arterial spasm. This disorder most commonly affects women between fifteen and fifty, and, although rare, it can lead to dry gangrene if tissue dies because of a lack of oxygen. In most cases, the cause of Raynaud's disease is not known. Raynaud's phenomenon, or secondary Raynaud's, is a condition with the same symptoms as Raynaud's disease, but it is brought on by another condition, such as surgery, injury, or frostbite. Raynaud's phenomenon may be provoked or aggravated by some heart medications and drugs taken for migraine, lupus, and rheumatoid arthritis. Primary Raynaud's is more common and tends to be less severe than secondary Raynaud's. (*See* RAYNAUD'S PHENOMENON in Part Two.)

Marfan's syndrome, a very rare condition, can also lead to serious circulatory problems. This syndrome is characterized by defects of the connective tissue in areas such as the skeletal system, eyes, and blood vessels, as well as such anatomical anomalies as unusually long toes and/or fingers, a high palate, an enlarged aorta, and/or taller than average height. This condition is hereditary.

Poor circulation can also result from varicose veins, which develop because of a loss of elasticity in the walls of the veins.

Impeded blood flow, from whatever cause, leads to ischemia, or oxygen deprivation and deficiency in the tissues. This, at the local level, results in tissue atrophy. Just fifteen seconds of ischemia turns off the mitochondria in the cells (the cellular energy-producing structures) and begins their programmed death spiral. In order to fight this, the blood must be kept from getting too viscous or sluggish, and to prevent platelets from clumping too rapidly. The various micronutrients in the table that follows—such as vitamins B_6 and B_{12} and folic acid—are not only good antioxidants but also are good anticoagulants. The nutrient dosages below are assumed to be for adults.

NUTRIENTS

SUPPLEMENT	SUGGESTED DOSAGE	COMMENTS
Essential		
L-carnitine	500 mg twice daily.	Helps to strengthen the heart muscle and to promote circulation by transporting long fatty acid chains.
Very Important		
Chlorophyll (Kyo-Green from Wakunaga and wheatgrass)	As directed on label.	Enhances circulation and helps build healthy cells. Use a liquid or tablet form. Also prepare fresh "green drinks" from green leafy vegetables.
Coenzyme Q_{10} plus	100 mg daily.	Improves tissue oxygenation.
Coenzyme A from Coenzyme-A Technologies	As directed on label.	Removes toxic substances from the body.
Lecithin granules or capsules	1 tbsp 3 times daily, before meals. 2,400 mg 3 times daily, before meals.	Emulsifies (breaks up) fats.
Liquid Kyolic with B_1 and B_{12} from Wakunaga	As directed on label.	Helps to build red blood cells and lower blood pressure.
Multienzyme complex	As directed on label. Take with meals.	To aid digestion and circulation and enhance oxygen use in all body tissues.
Vitamin B complex	50–100 mg of each major B vitamin 3 times daily (amounts of individual vitamins in a complex will vary).	Needed for metabolism of fat and cholesterol. Consider injections (under a doctor's supervision). If injections are not available, use a sublingual form.
plus extra vitamin B_1 (thiamine)	50 mg daily.	Enhances circulation and brain function.
and vitamin B_6 (pyridoxine)	50 mg daily.	A natural diuretic that protects the heart.
and vitamin B_{12}	1,000–2,000 mcg daily.	Prevents anemia and acts as a natural energy booster.
and folic acid	300 mcg daily.	Needed for the formation of oxygen-carrying red blood cells.
and para-aminobenzoic acid (PABA)	25 mg daily.	Assists in the formation of red blood cells.
Vitamin C with bioflavonoids	5,000–10,000 mg daily, in divided doses.	Helps prevent blood clotting.
Important		
Calcium and	1,500–2,000 mg daily, in divided doses, after meals and at bedtime.	Essential in normal blood viscosity.
magnesium and	750–1,000 mg daily, in divided doses, after meals and at bedtime.	Strengthens the heartbeat. Calcium and magnesium work together.
vitamin D	400 IU daily.	Important for utilization of calcium.
Dimethylglycine (DMG) (Aangamik DMG from FoodScience of Vermont)	50 mg twice daily.	Enhances tissue oxygenation.
Multivitamin and mineral complex	As directed on label.	To provide a balance of nutrients basic to good circulatory function.
Vinpocetine	As directed on label.	A derivative of vincamine (an extract of periwinkle) that helps with cerebral circulatory disorders.
Vitamin A with mixed carotenoids	25,000 IU daily. If you are pregnant, do not exceed 10,000 IU daily.	Aids in storage of fat and acts as an antioxidant. Use emulsion form for easier assimilation and greater safety at high doses.
and vitamin E	200 IU daily.	Inhibits the formation of free radicals. Use d-alpha-tocopherol form; use emulsion form for best absorption.
Helpful		
Choline and inositol plus	100 mg each 3 times daily, with meals.	Helps to remove fat deposits and improve circulation. Helps to lower cholesterol.
vitamin B_3 (niacin)	50 mg 3 times daily. Do not exceed a total of 300 mg daily from all supplements.	Helps to lower cholesterol. *Caution:* Do not take niacin if you have a liver disorder, gout, or high blood pressure.
L-cysteine and	500 mg each daily, on an empty stomach. Take with juice or water. Do not take with milk. Take with 50 mg vitamin B_6 and 100 mg vitamin C for better absorption.	Protects and preserves cells by detoxifying harmful toxins.
L-methionine		Prevents accumulation of fat both in the liver and in the arteries, where it may obstruct blood flow. (*See* AMINO ACIDS in Part One.)
Proteolytic enzymes	As directed on label. Take between meals.	To combat leaky gut syndrome.
Pycnogenol or grape seed extract	As directed on label. As directed on label.	Neutralize free radicals, enhance the action of vitamin C, and strengthen connective tissue, including that of the cardiovascular system.

Selenium	200 mcg daily. If you are pregnant, do not exceed 40 mcg daily.	Deficiency has been linked to heart disorders.
Shiitake extract or	As directed on label.	Helps to prevent high blood pressure and heart disease; lowers cholesterol levels.
reishi extract or	As directed on label.	
maitake extract	As directed on label.	
Zinc	50 mg daily. Do not exceed a total of 100 mg daily from all supplements.	Needed for immune function. Use zinc chelate form.
plus copper	3 mg daily.	Needed to balance with zinc.

Herbs

❑ The following herbs support the heart and circulatory system: black cohosh, butcher's broom, cayenne (capsicum), chickweed, gentian root, ginkgo biloba, goldenseal, hawthorn berries, horseradish, hyssop, licorice root, pleurisy root, rose hips, and wormwood. Cayenne increases the pulse rate, while black cohosh slows it. Ginkgo is being used for circulatory disorders in many clinics.

Cautions: Do not use black cohosh if you are pregnant or have any type of chronic disease. Black cohosh should not be used by those with liver problems. Do not take ginkgo biloba if you have a bleeding disorder, or are scheduled for surgery or a dental procedure. Do not take goldenseal internally on a daily basis for more than one week at a time. Do not use it during pregnancy or if you are breast-feeding, and use with caution if you are allergic to ragweed. If you have a history of cardiovascular disease, diabetes, or glaucoma, use it only under a doctor's supervision. Licorice root should not be used during pregnancy or nursing. It should not be used by persons with diabetes, glaucoma, heart disease, high blood pressure, or a history of stroke. Do not use wormwood in high doses or for extended periods because it contains the chemical compound thujone that can be poisonous. Do not use wormwood if you suffer from any type of seizure disorder or are pregnant.

Recommendations

❑ Make sure that your diet is high in fiber. Oat bran can help lower cholesterol levels.

❑ Include the following in your diet: bananas, brown rice, endive, garlic, lima beans, onions, pears, peas, and spinach.

❑ Drink steam-distilled water only.

❑ Eliminate animal protein and fatty foods (such as red meat), sugar, and white flour from your diet. Do not use stimulants such as coffee, colas, or tobacco, or eat foods with a lot of spices.

❑ Get regular exercise to help blood flow and to keep the arteries soft and unclogged.

Caution: If you are over thirty-five and/or have been sedentary for some time, consult your health care provider before beginning any type of exercise program.

❑ Keep your weight down.

❑ To boost circulation, give yourself a dry massage over your entire body using a loofah sponge or natural bath brush. Always massage toward the heart, even when massaging your legs. Also dip a towel in cold water and rub it briskly over parts of the body.

❑ If you have circulatory problems, do not take any preparations containing shark cartilage unless specifically directed to do so by your physician. Shark cartilage inhibits the formation of new blood vessels, the mechanism by which the body can increase circulatory capacity.

Considerations

❑ Blood-thinning drugs, such as warfarin (Coumadin), may be prescribed for people deemed to be in particular danger of developing blood clots, such as people who are bedridden or cancer patients. Studies show that, for those in danger of recurring clots, blood-thinning drugs should be taken for a while.

❑ Chelation therapy is helpful for improving circulation. (*See* CHELATION THERAPY in Part Three.)

❑ The simple fact of being pregnant places great strain on the circulatory system. Blood volume increases by up to 50 percent by the time a woman is nine months pregnant, and although most women with heart disease can safely have children, any such pregnancy should be closely monitored by both a cardiologist and an obstetrician.

❑ *See also* ARTERIOSCLEROSIS/ATHEROSCLEROSIS; CARDIOVASCULAR DISEASE; HIGH BLOOD PRESSURE; HIGH CHOLESTEROL; HYPOTHYROIDISM; RAYNAUD'S PHENOMENON; and VARICOSE VEINS, all in Part Two.

CIRRHOSIS OF THE LIVER

Cirrhosis of the liver is a degenerative inflammatory disease that results in hardening and scarring of liver cells. The liver becomes unable to function properly due to the scarred tissue, which prevents the normal passage of blood through the liver.

The most common cause of cirrhosis of the liver is excessive alcohol consumption. Liver disease resulting from alcohol intake is the fourth leading cause of death among people aged twenty-five to sixty-four in urban areas of the United States. A less frequent cause of cirrhosis is the hepatitis C virus (HCV). It is estimated that 3.2 million people in the United States have hepatitis C, and about 75 to 85 percent of those will go on to develop chronic liver disease, including cirrhosis. Blood transfusions given before routine testing for HCV are presumed to be the main cause of the rising number of people diagnosed as infected with HCV. Malnutrition and chronic inflammation can also lead to liver malfunction.

In the early stages, symptoms of cirrhosis of the liver may include constipation or diarrhea, fever, upset stomach, fatigue, weakness, poor appetite, generalized itching, weight loss, enlarged liver, vomiting, red palms, and swelling of the abdomen and legs. Those in the later stages of the disease may develop anemia, bruising due to bleeding under the skin, jaundice, and edema. People with alcoholic cirrhosis may experience no symptoms, or they may develop very slowly. Approximately 8,000 to 10,000 people die every year from hepatitis C–related liver disease.

Complications of cirrhosis are commonplace, and as the disease develops, the liver starts losing its ability to function. This can lead to:

- High blood pressure in the veins that connect the digestive system with the liver. This is called *portal hypertension.* It can cause thinning of the walls of the vessels, with possible rupture in the areas of the esophagus and stomach.

- Fluid buildup in the abdomen (called *ascites*), or in the legs or feet (called *edema*). Severe ascites can make breathing difficult by pressing on the diaphragm, and can lead to blood poisoning.

- Kidney failure, which often follows or is a result of liver disease.

- Encephalopathy, diseases of the brain, may develop because toxins that the liver usually removes are not removed. The toxins can then be carried to the brain to cause anything from anxiousness and drowsiness to disorientation and coma.

Cirrhosis is usually permanent once you have developed it, but its progress can be slowed by completely abstaining from alcohol, changing your diet to include fresh fruits and vegetables along with whole grains, and carefully checking to make sure any drugs you are taking are not toxic to the liver. Some drugs are more dangerous in combination with each other than individually for people with cirrhosis. Also, many supplements and herbals can have an effect on the liver and they also need to be considered in the mix. Check with your doctor or pharmacist regarding effects and possible harmful interactions. The liver is the clearinghouse for all of the substances listed below. Although each has been shown to be of benefit, don't take too many different supplements at once. Start with a good multivitamin/mineral mix. Add one or two supplements at a time and see if you notice a positive change. If not, try something else. Of course, if you have any adverse reactions, stop taking them immediately. For people with this disease, protecting the health of the liver is the primary goal. These are adult recommendations only.

NUTRIENTS

SUPPLEMENT	SUGGESTED DOSAGE	COMMENTS
Essential		
Liquid Kyolic with B_1 and B_{12} from Wakunaga	As directed on label.	An excellent liver detoxifier.
Phosphatidyl choline plus choline and inositol	As directed on label.

As directed on label. | For fatty liver. |
| Primrose oil or Total EFA from Health From The Sun | 500 mg twice daily, with meals. As directed on label. | To prevent an imbalance of fatty acids, found in cirrhosis of the liver. |
| Vitamin B complex

plus extra vitamin B_{12}

and folic acid | 100 mg of each major B vitamin 3 times daily (amounts of individual vitamins in a complex will vary).

1,000–2,000 mcg daily.

200 mcg daily. | The B vitamins are necessary for proper digestion, absorption of nutrients, and formation of red blood cells. Use a high-potency formula. Injections (under a doctor's supervision) may be necessary. To prevent anemia and protect against nerve damage. Use a lozenge or sublingual form. To correct deficiencies. |
| *Very Important* | | |
| Bifido Factor from Natren or Kyo-Dophilus from Wakunaga | As directed on label. Take on an empty stomach.

2 to 3 capsules 3 times daily. | Repairs liver cells and aids in healing.

Human-cultured flora from the small intestine, primarily to improve assimilation of nutrients. Detoxifies ammonia. |
| Garlic (Kyolic from Wakunaga) | 2 capsules 3 times daily, with meals. | Detoxifies the liver and bloodstream. |
| Inf-zyme Forte from American Biologics | As directed on label. | Balanced potent enzymes that act to inhibit inflammation. |
| L-arginine plus L-cysteine

and L-methionine plus L-carnitine plus glutathione | 500 mg each daily, on an empty stomach. Take with water or juice. Do not take with milk. Take with 50 mg vitamin B_6 and 100 mg vitamin C for better absorption. 500 mg daily, on an empty stomach. 500 mg daily, on an empty stomach. | Helps to detoxify ammonia, a by-product of protein digestion that can accumulate when the liver isn't functioning properly.

Helps detoxify harmful toxins.

Helps prevent accumulation of fat in the liver. A powerful antioxidant that protects against liver cancer. |
| Lecithin granules or capsules | 1 tbsp 3 times daily, with meals. 2,400 mg 3 times daily, with meals. | A powerful fat emulsifier. |
| Multienzyme complex with betaine and hydrochloric acid (HCl) plus ox bile extract | As directed on label. Take with each meal.

As directed on label. | Needed for digestion to lessen the strain on the liver.

Replaces the digestive enzymes normally produced by the gallbladder. |
| Colostrum Plus from Symbiotics | As directed on label. | Improves immune function and protects the liver. |
| Raw liver extract | As directed on label. | Prevents anemia and aids in building the liver. (*See* GLANDULAR THERAPY in Part Three.) |

S-Adenosylmethionine (SAMe)	As directed on label.	Provides antioxidant effects that improve the health of the liver. *Caution:* Do not use if you have bipolar mood disorder or take prescription antidepressants.
Taurine Plus from American Biologics	20 drops 3 times daily.	The most important antioxidant for health and stress from free radical damage. Use the sublingual form.
Important		
Alfalfa		*See* under Herbs, below.
Calcium and magnesium	1,500 mg daily, in divided doses, after meals and at bedtime. 750 mg daily.	To promote healing of tissue. Beneficial for the nervous system. Use chelate forms.
Dimethylglycine (DMG) (Aangamik DMG from FoodScience of Vermont)	As directed on label.	Supplies oxygen for healing.
Vitamin C with bioflavonoids	3,000–8,000 mg daily, in divided doses.	An important antioxidant. Use a buffered form.
Helpful		
Alpha-lipoic acid	400 mg daily	Acts as a powerful antioxidant and balances blood sugar levels.
Coenzyme Q_{10} plus	100 mg daily.	Promotes tissue oxygenation.
Coenzyme A from Coenzyme-A Technologies	As directed on label.	Works with coenzyme Q_{10} and removes toxic substances from the body.
Free form amino acid	As directed on label.	A good source of protein that is easy on the liver.
Grape seed extract or Pycnogenol	As directed on label.	Powerful antioxidant. Aids the liver in removing toxic substances from the body.
Inositol hexaphosphate (IP_6) (Cell Forté with IP-6 and Inositol from Enzymatic Therapy)	As directed on label.	Aids in reducing the buildup of fats in the liver.
Selenium	200 mcg daily. If you are pregnant, do not exceed 40 mcg daily.	A good detoxifier.
Vitamin A (Micellized Vitamin A from American Biologics) plus vitamin D and vitamin E	As directed on label. Do not exceed 10,000 IU daily. As directed on label. 200 IU daily. Do not exceed this amount.	Needed for healing. Use emulsion form for easier assimilation and greater safety at higher doses. *Caution:* Do not substitute pill forms of vitamin A for emulsion forms. Pills put extra stress on liver. To correct deficiencies. A potent antioxidant that aids circulation. Use d-alpha-tocopherol form.
Zinc	50 mg daily. Do not exceed a total of 100 mg daily from supplements.	Needed for the immune system and the healing process. Use zinc gluconate lozenges or OptiZinc for best absorption.

Herbs

❑ Alfalfa helps to build a healthy digestive tract and is a good source of vitamin K. It helps to prevent bleeding as a result of vitamin K deficiency, which is common with cirrhosis. It can be taken in tablet or liquid form.

❑ Aloe vera helps to cleanse and heal the digestive tract. Drink ¼ cup of aloe vera juice every morning and evening. George's Aloe Vera Juice from Warren Laboratories is a good product. It can be taken in a cup of herbal tea if you wish.

❑ Burdock root, dandelion, and red clover aid in liver repair by cleansing the bloodstream.

❑ Silymarin (milk thistle extract) has been shown in scientific studies to repair and rejuvenate the liver. Take 200 milligrams of silymarin three times daily. Liv-R-Actin from Nature's Plus is also a good source of milk thistle.

❑ Other herbs that can be beneficial for people with cirrhosis include barberry, black radish, celandine, echinacea, fennel, fringe tree, goldenseal, hops, Irish moss, rose hips, suma, thyme, and wild Oregon grape.

Cautions: Do not use barberry, celandine, goldenseal, or wild Oregon grape during pregnancy. Do not take echinacea for longer than three months. It should not be used by people who are allergic to ragweed. Do not take goldenseal internally on a daily basis for more than one week at a time. Do not use it during pregnancy or if you are breast-feeding, and use with caution if you are allergic to ragweed. If you have a history of cardiovascular disease, diabetes, or glaucoma, use it only under a doctor's supervision.

Recommendations

❑ A diet that is rich in carbohydrates is preferred for those with cirrhosis or for those at risk for it. Saturated fat from sources such as meat and dairy products has been shown to cause significant adverse effects when alcohol is consumed at the same time. Total fat intake should be around 60 to 80 grams per day, of which only one-third should be from saturated fats.

❑ Obtain protein from vegetable sources; do not eat foods containing animal protein.

❑ Eat a diet consisting of 75 percent raw foods. If cirrhosis is severe, consume only fresh vegetables and fruits and their juices for two weeks.

❑ Include the following in your diet: almonds, brewer's yeast, grains and seeds, raw goat's milk, and products derived from goat's milk. Nuts must be raw and from tightly sealed packages.

Caution: Brewer's yeast can cause an allergic reaction in some individuals. Start with a small amount at first, and discontinue use if any allergic symptoms occur.

❑ Increase your consumption of foods high in potassium, such as bananas, blackstrap molasses, brewer's yeast, dulse, kelp, prunes, raisins, and rice and wheat bran.

The Liver

Weighing about four pounds, the liver is the largest gland of the body and the only internal organ that will regenerate itself if part of it is damaged. Up to 75 percent of the liver can be removed in patients without any underlying liver disease—in those with liver disease 60 percent can be removed. It takes four to six weeks for the liver to grow back to its original size. If cared for properly, it will function more than adequately for decades. Alcohol is one of the toxins that the liver doesn't handle as well as others. The liver cannot regenerate after being severely damaged by alcohol.

The liver has many functions, perhaps the most important of which is the secretion of bile. This fluid is stored in the gallbladder and released as needed for digestion. Bile is necessary for the digestion of fats; it breaks fat down into small globules. Bile also assists in the absorption of the fat-soluble vitamins (A, D, E, and K) and helps to assimilate calcium. In addition, bile converts beta-carotene into vitamin A. It promotes intestinal peristalsis as well, which helps prevent constipation.

After nutrients have been absorbed into the bloodstream through the intestinal wall, they are transported by way of the hepatic portal system to the liver. In the liver, nutrients such as iron and vitamins A, B_{12}, and D are extracted from the bloodstream and stored for future use. These stored substances are utilized for everyday activities and in times of physical stress. The liver plays an important role in fat metabolism; in the synthesis of fatty acids from amino acids and sugars; in the production of lipoproteins, cholesterol, and phospholipids; and in the oxidation of fat to produce energy. The liver creates a substance called glucose tolerance factor (GTF) from chromium and glutathione. GTF acts with insulin to regulate blood sugar levels. Sugars not required for immediate energy production are converted into glycogen in the liver; the glycogen is stored in the liver and the muscles, and is converted back into sugar when needed for energy. Excess food is converted to fat in the liver, and the fat is then transported to the fatty tissues of the body for storage.

In addition to its important functions in digestion and energy production, the liver acts as a detoxifier. Protein digestion and bacterial fermentation of food in the intestines produce ammonia as a by-product; this ammonia is detoxified by the liver. The liver combines toxic substances (including metabolic waste products, insecticide residues, drugs, alcohol, and other harmful chemicals) with substances that are less toxic. These substances are then excreted via the kidneys and bowels. Thus, in order for the liver to function properly, you must also have proper kidney and bowel function.

Finally, the liver is responsible for regulating thyroid function by converting thyroxine (T4), a thyroid hormone, into its more active form, triiodothyronine (T3). Inadequate conversion of T4 into T3 by the liver may lead to hypothyroidism.

The liver also breaks down hormones like adrenaline, aldosterone, estrogen, and insulin after they have performed their needed functions.

Caution: Brewer's yeast can cause an allergic reaction in some individuals. Start with a small amount at first, and discontinue use if any allergic symptoms occur.

❏ Eat plenty of foods high in vitamin K. Persons with cirrhosis of the liver are often deficient in vitamin K. Good sources of vitamin K include alfalfa sprouts and green leafy vegetables.

❏ Include legumes (kidney beans, peas, and soybeans) and seeds in your diet. These foods contain the amino acid arginine, which helps to detoxify ammonia, a by-product of protein digestion.

❏ Drink fresh vegetable juices, such as beet, carrot, dandelion extract, and "green drinks."

❏ Drink steam-distilled water or sip barley water throughout the day. (*See* THERAPEUTIC LIQUIDS in Part Three.) When taking supplements, always take them with a full glass of water.

❏ Use only cold-pressed vegetable oils as sources of dietary fats. Consume oils in uncooked form only, such as in salad dressings.

❏ Limit your intake of fish to two servings a week, and do not eat raw or undercooked seafood. A damaged liver cannot handle the amount of vitamin A contained in these foods. Avoid cod liver oil.

❏ Keep the colon clean. Toxins accumulate in the liver and must be excreted via the colon and kidneys. (*See* COLON CLEANSING in Part Three.)

❏ Avoid constipating foods. The liver has to work twice as hard if you are constipated. Be sure your diet contains sufficient amounts of choline, inositol, and lecithin, as well as bulk and fiber.

❏ Do not use harsh laxatives to cleanse the system. Lemon enemas are preferred; take these twice weekly. You can also alternate wheatgrass enemas with coffee enemas for two weeks. Both of these detoxify the system. (*See* ENEMAS in Part Three.)

❏ Do not take any drugs (over-the-counter or prescription) except those prescribed by your doctor. Some over-the-counter products, including some medicines for children, contain alcohol in the form of propylene glycol.

This product may cause liver problems and a mild form of drunkenness.

❑ Consume no alcohol in any form. Also eliminate the following from your diet: animal products, candies, milk, pastries, pepper, salt, spices, stimulants of any kind (including caffeine and colas), white rice, products containing sugar and/or white flour, and spicy or fried foods. Virtually all commercially prepared foods contain some of the above.

❑ Read all food labels carefully, and avoid most fats. Do not eat any of the following: butter, margarine, vegetable shortening, and any other hardened fats; fried or fatty foods; melted or hard cheeses; nuts or oils that have been subjected to heat (either in processing or in cooking); potato chips; and all refined and processed foods. These overwork and damage the liver.

❑ Do not smoke, and avoid secondhand smoke.

Considerations

❑ If alcoholic cirrhosis is detected in the early stages and the individual stops consuming alcohol, it may be possible to halt the damage to the liver.

❑ In one study, people with cirrhosis of the liver were found to have an imbalance of essential fatty acids, which are needed for cell protection. After taking 10 capsules of primrose oil daily for three weeks, these individuals showed a marked improvement in the balance of their fatty acids.

❑ Animal studies indicate that the typical American diet is damaging to the liver. Improper diet results in allergies, digestive disorders, a low energy level, and an inability to detoxify harmful substances.

❑ The four basic reasons for poor liver function are:

1. *The presence of cumulative poisons.* Insecticides, preservatives, and other toxins can build up in and impair the liver. Even though a particular toxin may not accumulate in the liver, liver function may suffer if the toxin adversely affects the functioning of other organs, especially the pancreas and/or kidneys.

2. *An improper diet.* A diet that is low in protein and high in carbohydrates and fats, especially saturated fats, fried foods, and hydrogenated fats, is hard on the liver and may not provide sufficient protein building blocks necessary for repair. Poor food choices include processed foods, junk foods, refined white flour products, white sugar products, and imitation foods that are designed to appear and taste like an original product but that have been robbed of natural vitamins, minerals, and enzymes.

3. *Overeating.* Overeating is probably the most common cause of liver malfunction. Overeating creates excess work for the liver, resulting in liver fatigue. In addition, the liver must detoxify all of the various chemicals present in our food supply today. When the liver is overworked, it may not detoxify harmful substances properly. New studies show that the liver actually becomes fatty from overeating, just as it does from overdrinking. The syndrome is called non-alcoholic fatty liver disease.

4. *Drugs.* Drugs put a great strain on the liver. Drugs are substances that are foreign and unnatural to the body. These foreign substances cause the liver to work overtime in excreting these toxins. The liver neutralizes the effects of drugs on the body. Alcohol is particularly toxic to the liver. When excessive amounts of alcohol enter the liver, the liver begins to lose its functioning capacity. Other substances that can contribute to liver malfunction include oral contraceptives and caffeine.

❑ *See also* ALCOHOLISM and HEPATITIS, both in Part Two.

COLD

See COMMON COLD.

COLD SORES (FEVER BLISTERS)

Cold sores, or fever blisters, are caused by herpes simplex virus 1 (HSV-1), which is related to, but different from, the virus that causes genital herpes. Cold sores first appear three to ten days after exposure to the virus and may last up to three weeks. The virus then remains permanently in the body, and moves into the nervous system close to the lips.

It will lie dormant there until triggered by fever, a cold or other viral infection, exposure to sun and wind, stress, menstruation, high levels of the amino acid arginine, or depression of the immune system. These sores are very contagious and very common. By adulthood, 30 to 90 percent of people carry the virus.

There are said to be six stages of the development of the average cold sore. First comes stage one. In this first stage, no sore is visible but there is a feeling of prickling or itchiness around the affected area. In stage two, swelling may start and the area may be slightly red. Stage three brings with it the first signs of a blister or blisters. Stage four is the most painful, and generally comes on the fourth day. A soft crust or ulcer forms, and from this the cold sore moves into stage five, when a hard crust forms on the ulcer. This stage usually lasts for four days. The sixth and last stage, coming on or around the tenth day, leaves the sore red and slightly swollen, but without the hard scab.

An outbreak of cold sores may last more or less than ten days, depending on its severity.

Unless otherwise specified, the dosages recommended here are for adults. For a child between the ages of twelve and seventeen, reduce the dose to three-quarters the recommended amount. For a child between six and twelve, use one-half the recommended dose, and for a child under the age of six, use one-quarter the recommended amount.

NUTRIENTS

SUPPLEMENT	SUGGESTED DOSAGE	COMMENTS
Essential		
Herpanacine from Diamond-Herpancine Associates	As directed on label.	Proven effective in treating and stopping the outbreak of herpes. It contains many of the nutrients listed in this table.
L-lysine	500 mg twice daily.	Fights the virus that causes cold sores. *Caution:* Do not take lysine for longer than 6 months at a time. Do not take lysine pills if you are pregnant or nursing.
L-lysine cream	Apply topically as directed on label.	This amino acid fights herpes-viruses. (*See* AMINO ACIDS in Part One.)
Vitamin B complex	100–150 mg of each major B vitamin twice daily (amounts of individual vitamins in a complex will vary).	Important for healing and immune function. Use a high-stress formula.
Zinc lozenges	1 15-mg lozenge every 3 waking hours for 2 days, then 2 lozenges daily until healed. Do not exceed a total of 100 mg daily from all supplements.	Stimulates immune function to fight the virus. Zinc is absorbed quickly in lozenge form.
Very Important		
Acidophilus or Kyo-Dophilus from Wakunaga	As directed on label. Take on an empty stomach.	Inhibits pathogenic organisms.
Colloidal silver	Apply topically as directed on label.	An antiseptic and antibiotic that destroys bacteria, viruses, and fungi, and promotes healing.
Garlic (Kyolic from Wakunaga)	2 capsules 3 times daily.	Acts as a natural antibiotic and immunity enhancer.
Vitamin C	3,000–6,000 mg daily, in divided doses.	Fights the virus and boosts immune function. Use a buffered form.
Important		
Calcium and	1,500 mg daily.	To help relieve stress.
magnesium	750–1,000 mg daily.	
Essential fatty acids	As directed on label.	Aids skin in healing.
Helpful		
Herp-Eeze from Olympian Labs	As directed on label.	Contains lignans, nordihydro-gualaretic acid (NDGA), and other phytonutrients. Has antioxidant, anti-inflammatory, antiviral, and antimicrobal properties.
Maitake extract or	As directed on label.	To fight viruses and build resistance to disease.
shiitake extract or	As directed on label.	
reishi extract	As directed on label.	
Multivitamin and mineral complex	As directed on label.	All nutrients are necessary in balance.
Vitamin A plus carotenoid complex and	25,000 IU daily. If you are pregnant, do not exceed 10,000 IU daily.	Needed for healing of tissue in mouth and lip area. Use emulsion forms for easier assimilation and greater safety at higher doses.
vitamin E	200 IU daily.	Use d-alpha-tocopherol form.

Herbs

❏ For cold sores, use echinacea, goldenseal, pau d'arco, and red clover. Echinacea stimulates the immune system and may also aid in preventing an outbreak.

Cautions: Do not take echinacea for longer than three months. It should not be used by people who are allergic to ragweed. Do not take goldenseal internally on a daily basis for more than one week at a time. Do not use it during pregnancy or if you are breast-feeding, and use with caution if you are allergic to ragweed. If you have a history of cardiovascular disease, diabetes, or glaucoma, use it only under a doctor's supervision.

❏ Lemon balm contains a high concentration of polyphenols and appears to minimize herpes outbreaks. It can be applied topically in cream form. Or brew lemon balm tea and apply it directly to the sore. Taken internally, lemon balm tea has antiviral qualities.

❏ Olive leaf extract is good as a natural antibiotic for viral infections.

Recommendations

❏ Eat plenty of raw vegetables, as well as yogurt and other soured products.

❏ If cold sore outbreaks occur often, check for low thyroid function. (*See* HYPOTHYROIDISM in Part Two.)

Considerations

❏ The drug acyclovir (Zovirax), in capsule, liquid, or ointment form, is sometimes prescribed for cold sores.

❏ In studies, penciclovir (Denavir) cream has been shown to reduce the duration of the infection by one day, on average.

❏ An over-the-counter drug called docosanol (Abreva) has been approved by the FDA to reduce healing time and duration of symptoms of cold sores. The medication contains 10 percent docosanol, an antiviral agent. This is a topical medication that is rubbed into the sore five times a day for adults and children over age twelve. Children younger than twelve should use this medication under a doctor's supervision.

❏ Relaxation and visualization techniques (imagining the virus being destroyed by healing white blood cells, for example) may reduce the seriousness of cold sore outbreaks.

❏ If you are prone to allergies, you most likely have a malfunctioning immune system and may be susceptible to cold sores. (*See* ALLERGIES in Part Two.)

❏ Avoid touching others with the affected area until the sore is completely healed; the virus can be transmitted to others quite easily.

❏ *See also* HERPES INFECTION in Part Two.

COLITIS

See ULCERATIVE COLITIS.

COLORBLINDNESS

See under EYE PROBLEMS.

COMMON COLD

The common cold is an infection of the upper respiratory tract caused by a virus. Cold weather does not cause colds, although most colds are caught in the fall and winter. This is because most cold viruses thrive better in colder temperatures, when there is less humidity in the atmosphere.

There are more than two hundred viruses that can cause the common cold, but the most common ones are rhinoviruses. The well-known symptoms include head congestion, nasal congestion, sore throat, coughing, headache, sneezing, and watery eyes. Children may develop a low-grade fever, but this is rare in adults.

Colds usually strike eighteen to twenty-four hours after the virus enters the body. Most colds clear up on their own in a week to ten days, but occasionally a cold can lead to a more serious illness, such as bronchitis, a middle ear infection, or sinus infection. There is often confusion between the symptoms of the common cold, influenza, and allergies. Influenza, also a viral respiratory infection but caused by different types of virus, is by far the most serious complaint of the three and can lead to life-threatening complications, particularly in older or frail people. (*See* INFLUENZA in Part Two.) For an outline of the symptoms of colds as opposed to those of influenza and allergies, see COLD, FLU OR ALLERGY? on page 343.

It is estimated that healthy adults get an average of two colds per year. Children generally get many more because their immune systems are immature, and they have not yet developed immunity to many of the viruses that cause colds.

Unless otherwise stated, the dosages here are for adults. For a child between the ages of twelve and seventeen, reduce the dose to three-quarters of the recommended amount. For a child between six and twelve, use one-half of the recommended dose, and for a child under the age of six, use one-quarter of the recommended amount.

NUTRIENTS

SUPPLEMENT	SUGGESTED DOSAGE	COMMENTS
Essential		
ACES + Zn from Carlson Labs	As directed on label.	Contains vitamins A, C, and E, plus the minerals selenium and zinc.
Vitamin A plus carotenoid complex (Betatene)	15,000 IU daily. If you are pregnant, do not exceed 10,000 IU daily. As directed on label.	Helps heal inflamed mucous membranes and strengthens the immune system. Antioxidants and precursors of vitamin A.
Vitamin C with bioflavonoids	5,000–20,000 mg daily, in divided doses. (*See* ASCORBIC ACID FLUSH in Part Three.)	Fights cold viruses. For children, use buffered vitamin C or calcium ascorbate.
Zinc lozenges	For adults and children, 1 15-mg lozenge every 3 waking hours for 3 days, then 1 lozenge every 4 hours for 1 week. Do not exceed a total of 100 mg daily from all supplements.	Boosts the immune system. Keep these on hand and use them at the first sign of a cold. Note: Avoid lozenges containing citric acid, sorbitol, or mannitol. These ingredients inhibit absorption.
Important		
Free form amino acid plus N-acetylcysteine	As directed on label. As directed on label.	To supply needed protein for healing. A powerful antioxidant.
Garlic (Kyolic from Wakunaga)	2 capsules 3 times daily.	A natural antibiotic and immune system enhancer.
L-lysine	500 mg daily, on an empty stomach. Take with water or juice. Do not take with milk. Take with 50 mg vitamin B$_6$ and 100 mg vitamin C for better absorption.	Aids in destroying viruses and preventing cold sores in and around the mouth. (*See* AMINO ACIDS in Part One.) *Caution:* Do not take lysine for longer than six months at a time.
Helpful		
Acidophilus (Kyo-Dophilus from Wakunaga)	As directed on label. Take on an empty stomach. As directed on label.	To replace "friendly" bacteria. For adults.
Cold-X10 from Olympian Labs	As directed on label.	A combination of nutrients, herbal extracts, and enzymes that boost the immune system and fight viral and bacterial infection.
Maitake extract or shiitake extract or reishi extract	As directed on label. As directed on label. As directed on label.	Mushrooms with immune-boosting and antiviral properties.
Multimineral complex or kelp	As directed on label. 1,800–3,600 mg daily.	Minerals are needed for healing and for immune response. A rich source of necessary minerals.
Multivitamin complex with vitamin B complex	50–100 mg of each major B vitamin 3 times daily (amounts of individual vitamins in a complex will vary).	For healing and to reduce stress.
Olive leaf extract	As directed on label.	Supplements with antibiotic and antiviral properties.

Cold, Flu, or Allergy?

Since the common cold, influenza, and seasonal allergies all cause upper respiratory tract symptoms, it can sometimes be difficult to distinguish among them. There are certain notable differences, however. The following is a summary of the characteristic signs and symptoms of each.

Characteristic	Cold	Influenza	Seasonal Allergies
Chest infection or cough	Common. Mild to moderate.	Common. Can become severe. Pneumonia is a common complication.	Rare.
Fever	Rare (except in young children).	Usually high (102°–104°F). May last for 3–4 days.	Not present.
General aches and pains	Mild.	Usual. Can be severe.	Rare.
Headache	Rare.	Common.	Rare.
Sneezing/red, watery, itchy eyes	Usual, but more prevalent in allergies.	Rare.	Usual, especially sneezing. These symptoms come on quickly, without the warning signs of a cold, and can last longer.
Sore throat	Usual.	Occasional.	Occasional.
Stuffy nose	Usual.	Occasional.	Occasional.
Tiredness	Mild.	Severe.	Rare.
Primary season	Late August–April.	Winter.	March–September.
Duration	7–10 days.	Up to a month.	As long as the allergen is present.

Herbs

❑ Astragalus, native to Mongolia and China, helps promote the multiplication of the white blood cells that are vital for fighting infection.

Caution: Do not use astragalus in the presence of a fever.

❑ Wild pansy (*Viola tricolor*) grows wild in Europe, North Africa, the Near East, and parts of North America. When prepared as a tea or cough syrup, it is a good remedy for the common cold accompanied by fever, and for upper respiratory tract congestion. This is especially true if you have a dry cough along with the congestion. It has a high concentration of rutin, which strengthens capillary walls, and may have some beneficial effect in reducing arteriosclerosis. To make tea, pour 2 cups of hot water over 2 teaspoons of wild pansy, steep for ten minutes, and strain. Drink a cup of the tea two or three times a day after meals for a period of eight weeks. As a cough syrup, make an infusion by adding 1½ tablespoons of tea to ¾ cup of water and 1½ tablespoons of syrup. Take 1 tablespoon of this mixture three times daily.

❑ Boneset, a Native American herb, may be used to treat a fever.

Caution: Do not use boneset on a daily basis for more than one week, as long-term use can lead to toxicity.

❑ For fever, take catnip tea enemas and ¼ to ½ teaspoon of lobelia tincture every three to four hours until the fever drops. This dosage can be used for children also.

Caution: Lobelia is only to be taken under supervision of a health care professional as it is potentially toxic. People with high blood pressure, heart disease, liver disease, kidney disease, seizure disorders, or shortness of breath should not take lobelia. Pregnant and lactating women should avoid lobelia as well.

❑ Cat's claw is useful for easing the symptoms of a cold.

Caution: Do not use cat's claw during pregnancy.

❑ Chuan xin lian, a Chinese herbal remedy also known as Andrographis Anti-Inflammatory Tablets, clears the mucus from the respiratory tract.

❑ At the first sign of a cold, use an alcohol-free echinacea and goldenseal combination extract to boost your immune system and keep the virus from multiplying. For adults, place one dropperful in the mouth, hold it for five minutes, then swallow. Do this every three hours for three days. For

343

Common Cold Remedies

Americans spend billions of dollars every year on nonprescription treatments for coughs and colds. At best, these products can offer only temporary relief. The following is a list of some of the most common types of cold remedies, and what they can and cannot do:

- Analgesics, such as acetaminophen, aspirin, and ibuprofen, help to relieve aches and pains and reduce fever. By themselves, colds do not usually cause significant fever. Allowing a low-grade fever to run its course may actually be beneficial; an elevated temperature is one of the body's ways of fighting infection. If you have a fever that reaches 102°F or higher, chances are something other than the cold is causing it. It may be a sign of a developing bacterial infection somewhere in the body that requires treatment. By reducing fever, analgesics may mask this sign.

- Antihistamines decrease nasal secretions by blocking the action of histamine, a body chemical that causes swelling of small blood vessels, which results in sneezing and runny nose. These products may make you drowsy. In addition, it is better to allow the secretions that contain the virus to flow out of the body rather than trying to block them.

- Cough medicines come in two basic types: expectorants and antitussives. Expectorants make coughs more productive by increasing the amount of phlegm and decreasing its thickness. This helps remove irritants from respiratory airways. Guaifenesin, an expectorant found in many popular over-the-counter cough medicines, can be effective. The effectiveness of other over-the-counter expectorants is questionable. Antitussives reduce the frequency of coughing. An antitussive called dextromethorphan is generally considered reasonably safe and effective. It is often denoted by the initials "DM" on product labels. However, because coughing is the body's mechanism for clearing secretions from the lungs, it is probably best not to suppress it unless coughing is unusually severe or persistent, or it is interfering with sleep.

- Decongestants shrink nasal blood vessels to relieve swelling and congestion. These medications can cause side effects including jitteriness, insomnia, and fatigue.

Most over-the-counter cold remedies contain some combination of acetaminophen and various decongestants, antihistamines, and cough suppressants. Some experts believe that these ingredients may work against one another. For example, acetaminophen may increase nasal congestion, while the decongestant decreases it. If a cold is making you extremely uncomfortable and you feel you must take something for it, it is better to take a single-ingredient product appropriate for the particular symptom you are treating. Most are not tested in children so check with your pediatrician before using any over-the-counter cold remedy.

---

children, place 8 to 10 drops in the mouth; hold it for a few minutes (or as long as the child can manage), and then swallow. Do this every two hours for three days. Then take 8 to 10 drops of the liquid daily until symptoms are gone. Besides beating colds, flu, bronchitis, and other upper respiratory tract infections, echinacea is good for clearing up strep throat.

Cautions: Do not take echinacea for longer than three months. It should not be used by people who are allergic to ragweed. Do not take goldenseal internally on a daily basis for more than one week at a time. Do not use it during pregnancy or if you are breast-feeding, and use with caution if you are allergic to ragweed. If you have a history of cardiovascular disease, diabetes, or glaucoma, use it only under a doctor's supervision.

❏ Elderberry is recommended for upper respiratory tract infections and headaches associated with colds. It promotes sweating and can help to break a fever. Research has found that elderberry is effective against colds because it contains antioxidant flavonoids that protect cell walls against foreign substances.

❏ Eucalyptus oil is helpful for relieving congestion. Put 5 drops in a hot bath, or put 6 drops in 2 cups of boiling water and inhale the steam. It is best to remove the boiling water from the stove, then place a towel over your head and inhale deeply through your nose for three to five minutes (be careful not to get too close to the source of the hot steam—it can cause burns). Rosemary and sage oils can be added to the eucalyptus oil to aid in breaking up decongestion.

Caution: Do not use sage if you suffer from any type of seizure disorder, or are pregnant or nursing.

❏ Ginger, pau d'arco, slippery elm, and yarrow tea can help the common cold.

❏ Hyssop, an evergreen that can be taken as a tea, acts as an expectorant and has antiviral properties.

❏ Mullein is useful for coughs and congestion.

❏ Red clover helps clear accumulated toxins in the lymphatic system that may cause congestion and inflammation.

❏ For a sore throat, add 3 to 6 drops of pure tea tree oil to warm water and gargle. Repeat this up to three times daily. Take up to 2 tea tree oil lozenges and allow them to dissolve slowly in your mouth. Repeat this treatment as often as required, alternating it with goldenseal extract. These products can be found in most health food stores.

Caution: Do not take goldenseal internally on a daily basis for more than one week at a time. Do not use it during pregnancy or if you are breast-feeding, and use with caution if you are allergic to ragweed. If you have a history of cardiovascular disease, diabetes, or glaucoma, use it only under a doctor's supervision.

❑ Wild cherry bark soothes a cough.

Recommendations

❑ Take vitamin C and zinc lozenges at the first sign of a sore throat or stuffiness in the head or nose. This can shorten the duration of a cold, and may even stop it altogether. Take the lozenges every three hours for the first day of cold symptoms.

❑ Sip hot liquids such as turkey or chicken broth. Drink Potato Peeling Broth twice a day—make it fresh daily. You can add a carrot, a stalk of celery, garlic, and/or onions to your drink. Chicken soup is very effective in relieving the worst of the symptoms and in shortening the duration of a cold. (*See* THERAPEUTIC LIQUIDS in Part Three for both recipes.)

❑ Remain as active as possible. Not only is staying in bed for ordinary sniffles unnecessary, but it will probably make you feel worse. Moving around helps to loosen built-up mucus and fluids. Unless you have a fever, a brisk walk or any other type of moderate exercise should make you feel better.

❑ A study done between 1999 and 2000 in Florida has shown that taking antioxidants such as vitamins C and E, beta-carotene, selenium, zinc, fructooligosaccharides, and protein can significantly reduce the chance of getting an upper respiratory tract infection. This is particularly important for older adults due to the reduced efficiency of their immune systems. It has also proven to be useful in increasing the effectiveness of flu vaccines. This was originally published in the *Journal of the American Geriatrics Society*.

❑ Consider using homeopathic remedies for cold symptoms. *Calcarea carbonica* is excellent for sore throats, colds, or bronchitis. *Anas barbariae* (also available as Oscillococcinum from Boiron) and *Ferrum phosphoricum* (if there is a fever) are also good for treating the common cold.

❑ Flush facial tissues after they have been used. Because they harbor the virus, tissues can pass on the virus or cause you to reinfect yourself.

❑ Wash your hands often. Cold viruses can survive for several hours on hands, tissues, or hard surfaces. A healthy person can contract the virus by touching a contaminated surface, then touching his or her own mouth or nose. Using an antibiotic soap may prevent you from reinfecting yourself, but these soaps can also contribute to the development of antibiotic-resistant bacteria, so it is best to use them only when necessary.

❑ Try not to spread the cold to your family or colleagues. Refrain from close contact with loved ones. Even shaking hands is out; hand contact can spread the virus.

❑ Do not give aspirin, or any product containing aspirin, to a child with symptoms of any viral infection, including a cold. (*See* REYE'S SYNDROME in Part Two.) Taking large doses of aspirin also depletes the body of vitamin C.

Considerations

❑ Since there is no cure for the common cold, the best approach is prevention. Once a cold has a firm grip on you, it is hard to stop it.

❑ Bovine colostrum, taken in the cold and flu season, may help to ward off infection.

❑ There are many over-the-counter cold medications available. None of them can actually cure a cold, although they can be helpful for alleviating symptoms.

❑ It is unlikely that a vaccine will ever be developed to prevent the common cold because the viruses responsible have the ability to change in size and shape, and have hundreds of different forms. However, research being conducted in Britain may provide hope for cold sufferers. An experimental drug, tremacamra, appears to block cold viruses from finding a docking site in the nasal passages. So far, the drug's success rate has been impressive, cutting the risk of infection by 34 percent and symptoms by 45 percent. There have been no new developments with this drug since 1999 when the study was published.

❑ The possibility for real cold relief may lie in substances such as interferons, natural proteins that the body produces in response to viral infection. Interferons seem to improve the respiratory tract's ability to ward off viruses. Vitamin C promotes interferon production.

❑ Antibiotics are ineffective against viral infections, but many people still ask their doctors to prescribe them. It is important to understand that penicillin and most other antibiotics work only against bacterial infections—such as strep throat—not viral infections. Viruses and bacteria may produce similar symptoms, but they are very different kinds of microbes and do not respond to the same treatment. In fact, because antibiotics kill off "good" bacteria together with the bad, antibiotics actually inhibit the body's efforts to defend itself against viral invasion.

❑ You can, in a sense, catch a cold from yourself. When your immune system weakens from factors such as stress and/or a poor diet, viruses can take hold. These viruses are opportunistic and lie dormant in the body, taking hold when the immune system is at its weakest. Stress is often a factor.

❑ One study of young adults deliberately infected with a cold virus revealed that those given the drug naproxen or ibuprofen, which are commonly prescribed for arthritis, suffered fewer cold symptoms, such as sneezing, than those given a placebo. Coughing was not affected.

❑ Medical researchers at Dartmouth College gave a group of thirty-five cold sufferers zinc lozenges, and told these individuals to take a lozenge as often as every two hours. Another thirty-five cold sufferers were given placebos. The zinc takers' colds subsided in an average of four days, while the control group struggled with their colds for another nine days.

❑ Under experimental conditions, polysaccharides found in the herb echinacea have been shown to enhance the immune response.

Caution: Do not take echinacea for longer than three months. It should not be used by people who are allergic to ragweed.

❑ Allergies can cause symptoms that mimic those of colds and flu. Allergy testing is recommended. (*See* ALLERGIES in Part Two.)

❑ Anyone who has frequent colds or bouts with the flu should be checked for thyroid malfunction. When you are well, perform the thyroid function self-test. (*See under* HYPOTHYROIDISM in Part Two.) If your temperature is low, consult your health care provider.

❑ Congestion, cough, and/or sore throat are signs of a cold, but if these symptoms occur together with fever or fatigue, you may have the flu. (*See* INFLUENZA in Part Two.) If congestion develops in the chest, it is best to consult a physician, as chest (lung) infections can be serious. Also contact your health care provider if your fever goes above 102°F for more than three days, if yellow or white spots appear in the throat, if the lymph nodes under the jaw and in the neck become enlarged, and/or if chills and shortness of breath occur.

COMPLEXION PROBLEMS

See ACNE; DRY SKIN; OILY SKIN; PSORIASIS; ROSACEA; and WRINKLES.

CONJUNCTIVITIS

See under EYE PROBLEMS.

CONSTIPATION

Constipation is difficulty in passing stools or the infrequent passage of hard, dry stools as a result of food moving slowly through the large intestine. Most people experience constipation from time to time, but usually lifestyle changes and better eating habits help relieve the symptoms and prevent recurrences.

In most cases, constipation arises from insufficient amounts of fiber and fluids in the diet. Fiber is found in plant foods, such as whole grains, fruits, and vegetables. Fiber that is soluble in water takes on a soft texture and helps soften the stools. Insoluble fiber passes through the intestine largely unchanged and adds bulk to stools, which in turn helps to stimulate bowel contractions. Other factors that can cause constipation include inadequate exercise, advanced age, muscle disorders, structural abnormalities, bowel diseases, neurogenic disorders, and a poor diet, especially heavy consumption of junk food. Constipation may be a side effect of iron supplements and some drugs, such as painkillers and antidepressants. It is also common during pregnancy. High levels of calcium and low levels of thyroid hormone are two metabolic disturbances that can lead to constipation.

People with kidney failure or diabetes also tend to have problems with constipation. In older individuals, constipation is often caused by dehydration; in people of any age, depression can be a factor. Some medications can cause constipation, including cough syrups, pain medications that contain codeine, some antidepressants, iron supplements, blood pressure and heart medicines, calcium supplements, and some antihistamines.

A small percentage of people, such as persons with spinal injuries, have problems with constipation because the nerves that usually regulate bowel movement have been damaged or destroyed. In a condition called Hirschsprung's disease, normal excretion of feces is impossible because the nerves inside the bowel are missing. The nerve cells in the wall of the colon can also be damaged by long-term, habitual use of laxatives. When this happens, constipation is inevitable. A thrombosed hemorrhoid, an anal fissure, or a pocket of infection at the anus can create a spasm of pain strong enough to contract the muscles and hinder the evacuation of stools.

Constipation can give rise to many different ailments, including appendicitis, bad breath, body odor, coated tongue, depression, diverticulitis, fatigue, gas, headaches, hemorrhoids (piles), hernia, indigestion, insomnia, malabsorption syndrome, obesity, and varicose veins. It may even be involved in the development of serious diseases such as bowel cancer.

Regular bowel movements are an important mechanism for removing toxins from the body. The colon serves as a holding tank for waste matter. Antigens and toxins from bowel bacteria and undigested food particles may play a role in the development of diabetes mellitus, meningitis, myasthenia gravis, thyroid disease, candidiasis, chronic gas and bloating, migraines, fatigue, and ulcerative colitis. People can have bowel movements as infrequently as three times a week and still not be constipated, although there are some health practitioners who maintain that it is important to have a bowel movement every day.

Unless otherwise specified, the dosages recommended here are for adults. For a child between the ages of twelve and seventeen, reduce the dose to three-quarters the recommended amount. For a child between six and twelve, use one-half the recommended dose, and for a child under the age of six, it is suggested that one-quarter the recommended amount be used.

NUTRIENTS

SUPPLEMENT	SUGGESTED DOSAGE	COMMENTS
Important		
Garlic (Kyolic from Wakunaga)	2 capsules twice daily, with meals. (*See* ASCORBIC ACID FLUSH in Part Three.)	Destroys harmful bacteria in the colon.
Vitamin C with bioflavonoids	5,000–20,000 mg daily.	Has a cleansing and healing effect. Use a buffered form.
Helpful		
Apple pectin	500 mg daily. Take separately from other supplements and medications.	For fast results, use it in an enema. A source of fiber that aids in correcting . constipation.
Bio-Bifidus from American Biologics	As directed on label.	For bowel flora replacement to improve assimilation of nutrients from foods.
Chlorophyll liquid or alfalfa	1 tbsp daily, before meals.	Eliminates toxins and bad breath. *See* under Herbs, below.
Essential fatty acids (Kyolic-EPA from Wakunaga, flaxseed oil, and primrose oil)	As directed on label.	Restores proper fatty acid balance to aid in proper bowel movements.
Kyo-Dophilus from Wakunaga	As directed on label.	Aids in normal bowel function. Allows survival and rapid passage of "friendly" bacteria through the stomach into the small intestine.
Multienzyme complex	As directed on label. Take after meals.	To aid digestion.
Multivitamin and mineral complex with vitamin A and mixed carotenoids	As directed on label. If you are pregnant, do not exceed 10,000 IU daily.	Constipation blocks proper absorption of nutrients, resulting in vitamin and mineral deficiencies. Use a formula *without* iron.
Oxy-Cleanse from Earth's Bounty	As directed on label.	Removes harmful anaerobic pathogens from digestive tract.
Vitamin B complex plus extra vitamin B$_{12}$ and folic acid	50 mg of each major B vitamin 3 times daily, before meals (amounts of individual vitamins in a complex will vary). 1,000–2,000 mcg daily. 200 mcg daily.	Aids in proper digestion of fats, carbohydrates, and protein. Use a high-potency formula. A sublingual form is best. To aid in digestion and prevent anemia. Deficiency may result in constipation.
Vitamin D plus calcium and magnesium	400 mg daily. 1,500 mg daily. 750 mg daily.	Aids in preventing colon cancer. Needed for proper muscular contraction. May also help prevent colon cancer. Works with calcium to regulate muscle tone.
Vitamin E	200 IU daily. Take before meals.	Aids in healing of the colon. Use d-alpha-tocopherol form.

Herbs

❑ Alfalfa extract contains chlorophyll, which aids in detoxifying the body and cleansing the breath. Fennel seed tea also is good for freshening the breath.

❑ Aloe vera has a healing and cleansing effect on the digestive tract and aids in forming soft stools. Drink ½ cup of aloe vera juice in the morning and at night. It can be mixed with a cup of herbal tea if you wish. Warren Laboratories has a product called George's Aloe Vera Juice that is good.

❑ Ginger stimulates the digestive system and eases passage of food through the intestines. Try Ginger Dry Extract and Ginger Soft Extract from Sabinsa Corporation.

❑ Use milk thistle to aid liver function and to enhance bile output to soften stools.

❑ Naturalax 2 from Nature's Way is an herbal formula that is good for constipation.

❑ Triphala from Planetary Formulas is an herbal product that aids in the formation of odor-free, firm, and healthy stools.

❑ Other herbs that are helpful for constipation include cascara sagrada, goldenseal, rhubarb root, senna leaves, and yerba maté. If you take yerba maté, take 2 to 3 teaspoons in 16 ounces of hot water on an empty stomach.

Caution: Do not take goldenseal internally on a daily basis for more than one week at a time. Do not use it during pregnancy or if you are breast-feeding, and use with caution if you are allergic to ragweed. If you have a history of cardiovascular disease, diabetes, or glaucoma, use it only under a doctor's supervision.

Recommendations

❑ Eat high-fiber foods such as fresh fruits, raw green leafy vegetables, whole-grain oatmeal, and brown rice daily. Also eat asparagus, beans, Brussels sprouts, cabbage, carrots, garlic, kale, okra, peas, sweet potatoes, and whole grains. Foods that contain high levels of soluble fiber are adzuki beans, barley, dried beans, oats, and some fruits, especially apples, apricots, bananas, blackberries, blueberries, cranberries, figs, grapes, peaches, and prunes. Foods high in insoluble fiber are cereals, seeds, wheat bran, whole grains, and the skins of many fruits and vegetables. Eating in this way is a good idea for adults and children.

❑ Drink more water. This is important when adding fiber to the diet. Drink at least ten 8-ounce glasses of water every day, whether you are thirsty or not. As you age, you become less able to detect true thirst.

❑ Consume plenty of foods that are high in pectin, such as apples, carrots, beets, bananas, cabbage, citrus fruits, dried peas, and okra. Pectin is also available in supplement form.

❑ Follow a low-fat diet. Eat no fried foods.

❑ Avoid foods that stimulate secretions by the mucous membranes, such as dairy products, fats, and spicy foods.

Types of Laxatives

Laxatives are substances that are used to promote bowel movement. There are four basic types of laxatives: bulk-forming agents, stool softeners, osmotic agents, and stimulants. The following are basic descriptions of the way the different laxatives work to achieve their effects:

- Bulk-forming agents increase the bulk and water content of the stools. They are the only type of laxatives that can be safe to take on a daily basis. Examples include bran (both in foods and in supplement form), psyllium, and methylcellulose.

- Stool softeners, such as mineral oil and docusate sodium, soften fecal matter so that it passes through the intestines more easily. They should not be used on a regular basis because they can have other effects on the body. Mineral oil can damage the lungs if inhaled, and it reduces the absorption of fat-soluble vitamins. Docusate sodium (found in Colace and Dialose) may in-

crease the toxicity of other drugs taken at the same time, and may cause liver damage to occur.

- Osmotic agents contain salts or carbohydrates that promote secretion of water into the colon, initiating bowel movement. They are among the safest laxatives for occasional use, but if they are used more than occasionally, dependency can result. Examples include lactulose (a prescription medication sold under the brand names Cephulac and Chronulac), sorbitol (which is cheaper than lactulose but just as effective), milk of magnesia, citrate of magnesia, and Epsom salts.

- Stimulant laxatives irritate the intestinal wall, stimulating peristalsis. They can damage the bowels with habitual use, and can lead to dependency. Examples include bisacodyl (found in Dulcolax), casanthranol (Peri-Colace), cascara sagrada, castor oil, and senna (Perdiem, Senokot).

❑ Do not consume dairy products, soft drinks, meat, white flour, highly processed foods, salt, coffee, alcohol, or sugar. These foods are difficult to digest and have little or no fiber. For children, try a milk substitute such as soymilk.

❑ For quick relief of constipation, drink a large glass of quality water every ten minutes for half an hour. This can work wonders to flush out toxins and relieve constipation.

❑ Eat prunes or figs. These are the best natural laxatives.

❑ Eat smaller portions—no large, heavy meals or high-fat foods.

❑ Consume barley juice, Green Magma from Green Foods Corporation, Kyo-Green from Wakunaga, or wheatgrass for chlorophyll.

❑ Get some exercise. Physical activity speeds the movement of waste through the intestines. A twenty-minute walk can often relieve constipation. Regular exercise is also important for preventing constipation in the first place.

❑ Go to the toilet at the same time each day, even if the urge does not exist, and relax. Stress tightens the muscles and can cause constipation. Many people find reading helpful as a way to relax. Never repress the urge to defecate.

❑ Keep the bowel clean. (*See* COLON CLEANSING in Part Three.)

❑ If constipation is persistent, take cleansing enemas. (*See* ENEMAS in Part Three.)

❑ Do not consume products containing mineral oil, which can interfere with the absorption of fat-soluble vitamins. Also avoid taking Epsom salts, milk of magnesia, and citrate of magnesia, which draw volumes of fluid into the intestines and wash out minerals from the body.

❑ If you use laxatives, take acidophilus to replace the "friendly" bacteria. The continued use of laxatives cleans out the intestinal bacteria and leads to chronic constipation.

Considerations

❑ Psyllium seed is helpful for constipation. If you take psyllium seed, be sure to take it with a full glass of water.

❑ Some yogurts contain active cultures that help with constipation. Activia has bifidobacteria and fiber (fructo-oligosaccharide). In one study, women who consumed the yogurt twice a day experienced significant improvement.

❑ Flaxseed oil or freshly ground flaxseeds help to soften stools. Freshly ground flaxseeds have a pleasant, nutty taste and can be sprinkled over cereals, salads, and other foods.

❑ Fast periodically (adults only). (*See* FASTING in Part Three.)

❑ Laxatives can be used occasionally to relieve constipation, but if used regularly they can cause serious problems, including diarrhea, abdominal cramping, bloating, dehydration, and, ultimately, damage to the colon. Using laxatives too often also promotes dependence. Lifestyle changes, including getting regular exercise and eating a high-fiber diet, are better ways to avoid constipation.

❑ If added natural fiber and herbal laxatives do not improve constipation, you may have a problem with muscle coordination. Normally, the upper muscles in the bowel contract as the lower ones relax. Problems occur if the lower muscle tightens and goes into a spasm instead of relaxing.

❑ If constipation is more than an occasional problem, the possibility of a cancer or another obstruction in the lower bowel should not be dismissed unless a proctoscopic examination or a barium enema has shown that there is no blockage. Other symptoms of colon cancer include the presence of blood in the feces; severe cramping; a tender, distended abdomen; and markedly narrowed stools. However, cancer may be present even without these symptoms.

❑ Foul-smelling stools and a burning feeling in the anus may be signs of acidosis. (*See* ACIDOSIS *under* ACID/ALKALI IMBALANCE in Part Two.) Also, you could be malabsorbing fat and you may need medical attention to sort these issues out.

❑ Alternating constipation and diarrhea may be a sign of irritable bowel syndrome. While this disorder is chronic and unpleasant, it is not dangerous. Other common symptoms are cramps, gassiness, and variation in the consistency of the stool. The cause of irritable bowel syndrome is not known, but many experts believe it is stress related. (*See* IRRITABLE BOWEL SYNDROME in Part Two.)

❑ *See* DIVERTICULITIS and ULCERATIVE COLITIS, both in Part Two.

❑ *See also under* PREGNANCY-RELATED PROBLEMS in Part Two.

CHRONIC OBSTRUCTIVE PULMONARY DISEASE (COPD)

See ASTHMA; BRONCHITIS; and EMPHYSEMA.

COPPER DEFICIENCY

Copper is an essential trace mineral. Even a mild copper deficiency impairs the ability of white blood cells to fight infection. Copper is necessary for proper absorption of iron in the body, and it is found primarily in foods containing iron. If the body does not get a sufficient amount of copper, hemoglobin production decreases and copper-deficiency anemia can result.

Various enzyme reactions require copper as well. Copper is needed as a cross-linking agent for elastin and collagen, as a catalyst for protein reactions, and for oxygen transport. It is also used for the metabolism of essential fatty acids. Copper deficiency can produce various symptoms, including diarrhea, inefficient utilization of iron and protein, and stunted growth. In babies, the development of nerve, bone, and lung tissue can be impaired, and the structure of these body parts may be altered.

Since the body does not manufacture copper, it must be taken in through the diet. Too much copper produces a condition called copper toxicity or copper overload. (*See* COPPER TOXICITY in Part Two.) For the body to work properly, it must have a proper balance of copper and zinc; an imbalance can lead to thyroid problems. In addition, low (or high) copper levels may contribute to mental and emotional problems. Copper deficiency may be a factor in anorexia nervosa, for example.

The DRI for copper is 900 micrograms per day for adults nineteen to seventy years of age. For children, the DRI ranges from 200 micrograms for infants under six months to 890 for children fourteen to eighteen years of age. The DRI represents the recommended dietary allowance for copper. A normal healthy diet will provide the correct amount of copper for most people.

Copper deficiency is most likely to occur in babies who are fed only cow's milk (infant formulas are supplemented), persons suffering from sprue (a malabsorption syndrome) or kidney disease, and those who chronically take megadoses of zinc. Long-term use of oral contraceptives can upset the balance of copper in the body, causing either excessively high or excessively low copper levels. Copper levels can be determined through a blood test, urine samples, and hair analysis. Determining mineral levels and ratios is the basis for a nutritional program to balance body chemistry.

Unless otherwise specified, the dosages recommended here are for adults. For a child between the ages of twelve and seventeen, reduce the dose to three-quarters the recommended amount. For a child between six and twelve, use one-half the recommended dose, and for a child under the age of six, use one-quarter the recommended amount.

NUTRIENTS

SUPPLEMENT	SUGGESTED DOSAGE	COMMENTS
Important		
Copper	5 mg daily for 1 month, then reduce to 3 mg daily.	To restore copper in the body. Use copper amino acid chelate.
Zinc	30 mg daily. Do not exceed this amount.	Needed to balance with copper. Use zinc chelate form.
Helpful		
Iron	As directed by physician. Take with 100 mg vitamin C for better absorption.	Copper deficiency may cause anemia. Use a chelate form. *Caution:* Do not take iron unless anemia is diagnosed.
Multivitamin and mineral complex	As directed on label.	All nutrients are necessary in balance.

Recommendations

❑ If you suspect that you may have a copper deficiency, increase your intake of foods rich in copper, such as legumes (especially soybeans), nuts, cocoa, black pepper, seafood, egg yolks, raisins, molasses, avocados, whole grains, oats, and cauliflower. Pregnant women in particular should be sure to eat a well-balanced diet that includes these foods.

❑ Copper deficiency can be confirmed through hair analysis. (*See* HAIR ANALYSIS in Part Three.) If deficiency is confirmed, follow the supplementation plan above to restore proper mineral balance.

Considerations

❑ Copper deficiencies that have health consequences are thought to be linked to living in, and eating foods grown in, areas where the soil has been depleted of this mineral. However, deficiency is very rare in the United States.

❑ Patent ductus arteriosus is a congenital defect in which the ductus arteriosus, or fetal blood vessel, fails to close properly shortly after birth. It results in blood flow between the pulmonary artery, which goes to the lungs, and the aorta, which brings oxygenated blood to the rest of the heart. In a laboratory experiment reported in *Developmental Pharmacology and Therapy* the ductus arteriosus remained open in 100 percent of offspring of a copper-deficient group of rats, but in only 20 percent of the offspring of a control group not suffering from copper deficiency. This study underscores the importance of taking a multivitamin when you are pregnant.

COPPER TOXICITY

Trace amounts of copper are essential for the human body. Since copper is not manufactured by the body, it must be taken in through the diet. A number of biochemical processes depend on copper to function normally, plus copper is involved in the function of the nervous system. (*See* COPPER DEFICIENCY above.) However, as with all trace minerals, excess amounts of copper in the body can be toxic.

Too much copper in the system can cause a variety of ailments, including diarrhea, eczema, hemolytic anemia, high blood pressure, kidney disease, nausea, premenstrual syndrome, sickle cell anemia, stomach pain, and severe damage to the central nervous system. As with mercury and lead, high levels of copper are also associated with mental and emotional disorders, including autism, behavioral problems, childhood hyperactivity, clinical depression, anxiety, postpartum psychological problems, hallucinatory and paranoid schizophrenia, insomnia, mood swings, stuttering, and senile dementia (senility).

Sources of copper include beer, copper cookware, copper plumbing, industrial wastes, insecticides, pasteurized milk, tap water, and various foods, as well as swimming pool chemicals and permanent-wave solutions.

The DRI for copper is 900 micrograms per day for adults nineteen to seventy years of age. For children, the DRI ranges from 200 micrograms for infants under six months to 890 for children fourteen to eighteen years of age. The DRI represents the recommended dietary allowance for copper.

Copper levels can be determined through blood tests, urine samples, and hair analysis. Normal urine samples collected over a twenty-four-hour period contain 15 to 40 micrograms of copper. In people with diseases such as arthritis, heart disease, hypertension, schizophrenia, or cancer, serum copper levels tend to be high. During illness, copper is released from the tissues into the blood to promote tissue repair. High serum copper readings during illness should not be taken to mean that the copper is a cause of the illness; rather, it is an indication that the body's natural repair processes have been activated.

The use of oral contraceptives and/or tobacco can cause a rise in the amount of copper in the body. Excess serum copper is also characteristic of anemia, cirrhosis of the liver, leukemia, hypoproteinemia, and vitamin B_3 (niacin) deficiency.

Serum copper levels also tend to be higher than normal during pregnancy. Wilson's disease is a rare hereditary disorder in which the body is unable to properly metabolize copper, and the metal accumulates in the body. Treatment for Wilson's disease is high doses of zinc throughout childhood. Patients can grow and develop normally with this treatment. People with diminished adrenal gland function or abnormally slow metabolism can develop high copper levels. Zinc, another mineral, plays an important role in how much copper is stored in the tissues. A deficiency of zinc, especially when combined with a high copper intake, can cause too much copper to build up in the tissues. In addition, stress can cause a decrease in the amount of zinc available to the body, which can lead to copper overload.

With knowledge of how minerals interact in the body, it is possible to lower the amount of copper in the body and maintain a proper mineral balance. Unless otherwise specified, the dosages recommended here are for adults. For a child between the ages of twelve and seventeen, reduce the dose to three-quarters the recommended amount. For a child between six and twelve, use one-half the recommended dose, and for a child under the age of six, use one-quarter the recommended amount.

NUTRIENTS

SUPPLEMENT	SUGGESTED DOSAGE	COMMENTS
Important		
Vitamin C with bioflavonoids plus extra	1,000 mg 4 times daily.	Copper chelators. Use ascorbic acid form.
rutin	60 mg daily.	A bioflavonoid that is a by-product of buckwheat and lowers serum copper.
Zinc	50–80 mg daily. Do not exceed a total of 100 mg daily from all supplements.	Zinc deficiency predisposes one to excessive copper levels. Use zinc chelate form.
Helpful		
Calcium chelate or	1,500 mg daily.	Binds with metallic ions in the body.
calcium disodium edetate plus	As prescribed by physician.	Used by doctors to treat heavy metal poisoning. Available by prescription only.
magnesium	750 mg daily, at bedtime.	Works with calcium.
L-cysteine and L-cystine and L-methionine	As directed on label, on an empty stomach. Take with water or juice. Do not take with milk. Take with 50 mg vitamin B_6 and 100 mg vitamin C for better absorption.	Aids in elimination of copper from the body and protects the liver. (*See* AMINO ACIDS in Part One.)

Manganese	2–4 mg daily. Take separately from calcium.	Aids in excretion of excess copper.
Molybdenum	30 mcg daily.	Prevents accumulation of excess copper in the body.

Herbs

❏ Grape seed extract serves as a free radical scavenger and aids in protecting cells from damage.

Recommendations

❏ Have your drinking water tested. Drinking water can be a source of copper. The level of copper and other minerals in household drinking water can be tested by special labs. If there is more than 1 part per million of copper in your drinking water, an alternate source of water, such as bottled steam-distilled water, is advisable. If this is not feasible, always run the water for at least two minutes before using it to clear out some of the impurities.

❏ Increase your intake of sulfur, found in such foods as eggs, onions, and garlic. These help to rid the body of copper. In addition, supplement your diet with pectin, which can be found in apples.

❏ Do not take a multivitamin and/or mineral supplement that contains copper.

❏ Do not use copper pots or other cooking utensils.

Considerations

❏ Hair analysis has been shown to be a reliable test of the copper level in body tissues. (See HAIR ANALYSIS in Part Three.)

❏ If you have an extremely high level of copper, you may require medical treatment with chelation to remove the excess copper. Chelation therapy removes toxic metals from the body. (See CHELATION THERAPY in Part Three.) If the copper levels are higher than normal, but not extreme, this can often be managed with supplements.

❏ The trace minerals manganese, molybdenum, and zinc can prevent excess copper from accumulating in the body.

❏ Many people with schizophrenia have been found to have high levels of copper and iron, combined with deficiencies of zinc and manganese, probably as a result of lower than normal excretion of copper. Increasing the intake of zinc and manganese, whether through the diet or supplementation, increases elimination of copper and helps to return copper levels to normal.

❏ See also ENVIRONMENTAL TOXICITY and WILSON'S DISEASE, both in Part Two.

CORNEAL ULCER

See under EYE PROBLEMS.

CORNS AND CALLUSES

Corns and calluses are areas of hyperkeratosis, or overgrowth of skin tissue. The skin thickens and hardens. Calluses most commonly form on the soles of the feet and sometimes on the hands or knees. Corns are small cone-shaped areas of skin overgrowth that most often form on or between the toes. They can be either soft or hard. If they form between the toes, the moisture of the area keeps them soft; corns that form on top of the toes are typically hard.

Having a hammertoe or mallet toe may lead to a more severe form of callus called intractable plantar keratosis (IPK). This callus forms as a result of a serious imbalance in weight-bearing, with considerably more pressure being placed on one area of the foot than on others.

These growths can cause inflammation and pain. Corns especially may ache and be tender to the touch. Both corns and calluses usually form in response to repeated friction or pressure, such as from wearing ill-fitting shoes or performing certain tasks repeatedly. Other factors that may be involved include staphylococcus- or streptococcus-type infection, and an acid/alkaline imbalance in the body.

Herbs

❏ Use alternate applications of alcohol-free goldenseal extract and tea tree oil to keep down infection and speed healing.

Recommendations

❏ Consume raw vegetables and juices for three days to aid in balancing the acidity/alkalinity of your system. Umeboshi (Japanese salt plum) can quickly balance the body's pH. These are available in health food stores and Asian markets. Take one every three hours for two days.

❏ Avoid fried foods, meats, caffeine, sugar, and highly processed foods.

❏ To treat corns and calluses, soften the thickened skin by adding 2 tablespoons of Dr. Bronner's liquid soap (available in health food stores) or a mild dish soap to ½ gallon of warm water. Soak your feet in this mixture for fifteen minutes. Afterward, dry your feet with a soft towel and rub a couple of drops of vitamin E oil into the affected area. Then, using a pumice stone or a special callus file, gently file down the top layer of the corn or callus. Clean the area with mild soap and water, using a gauze pad or cotton ball, and apply a moisturizer to the area. Do this twice a day. Wear clean white cotton socks after treatment. This is effective only if the callus is not too thick.

❏ Apply a nonmedicated corn pad (a small round or oval-shaped foam pad with a hole in the center) around a corn to help to relieve the pressure. Stretch the pad so that it clears the corn by at least one-eighth inch on all sides. Then apply vitamin E oil to the corn, cover with a gauze square, and wrap the toe with adhesive tape. Alternate between using vitamin E oil and tea tree oil.

❏ For corns between the toes, dab on vitamin E oil and place a clean piece of cotton or a cotton ball over it. Make sure to use 100 percent cotton, not synthetic cosmetic puffs. Put on clean white cotton socks and leave them on overnight after treatment. Vitamin E oil mixed with a crushed garlic clove is good for softening corns and calluses.

❏ Never use a knife or any sharp instrument to cut the hardened area away, as infection can result.

❏ Always wear properly fitting shoes.

Considerations

❏ Compresses made from hot Epsom salts or Footherapy solution from Queen Helene/Hain Celestial Group are good.

❏ Medicated pads are available that are supposed to treat corns and calluses. Most of these products are fairly aggressive, however, and may attack good tissue as well, provoking an allergic reaction.

❏ If you suffer from diabetes, you may need to consult a doctor or podiatrist. In people with diabetes, poor circulation can lead to problems with the feet. You should also consult a professional if the area becomes infected.

❏ If the problem is persistent, a physician may suggest an X-ray to rule out an underlying bone spur.

❏ *See also* ACID/ALKALI IMBALANCE in Part Two.

CRAMPS

See MUSCLE CRAMPS; PREMENSTRUAL SYNDROME.

CROHN'S DISEASE

Crohn's disease is an inflammatory bowel disorder of unknown origin. Also called *ileitis* or *enteritis*, it usually affects the lowest portion of the small intestine, but it can occur in other parts of the digestive tract, from the mouth to the anus. Crohn's disease causes inflammation that extends deep into the lining of the intestinal wall, frequently causing crampy abdominal pain, diarrhea, rectal bleeding, loss of appetite, and weight loss.

A common complication of the disease is blockage of the intestine caused by scar tissue that narrows the passageway. The disease may also cause sores, or ulcers, that break through to the surrounding tissues. These tunnels are called *fistulas*, and while they can be treated using medication, surgery is sometimes required. People with Crohn's disease also suffer from nutritional deficiencies.

Crohn's disease affects men and women equally and tends to run in families. According to the Crohn's and Colitis Foundation of America (CCFA), people who have a relative with the disease have at least ten times the risk of

developing Crohn's disease compared with the general population. This disorder affects people in all age groups, but the onset usually occurs either between ages fifteen and thirty or between ages sixty and eighty. Children with Crohn's disease may suffer delayed development and stunted growth due to nutritional deficiencies.

Crohn's disease can be difficult to diagnose because its symptoms are similar to those of other intestinal disorders, particularly ulcerative colitis—another inflammatory bowel disease which affects only the colon. Crohn's symptoms can also appear intermittently, occurring every few months to every few years for some people. In rare cases, the symptoms may appear once or twice and not return. If the disease continues for many years, bowel function gradually deteriorates. Left untreated, it can become extremely serious, even life-threatening, and it may increase the risk of cancer by as much as twenty times.

Doctors believe that Crohn's disease has a genetic basis, but that it does not appear until triggered by the presence of bacteria or virus that provokes an abnormal activation of the immune system. The onset of Crohn's disease can be dramatic, with alarming symptoms such as sudden high fever, sudden weight loss of more than five pounds in a few days, significant rectal bleeding, severe abdominal pain that persists for more than an hour at a time, and persistent vomiting accompanied by a cessation of bowel movements.

A series of tests may be required to confirm Crohn's disease. Blood tests may be done to check for anemia and/or a high white blood cell count. A doctor may do an upper gastrointestinal X-ray series to look at the small intestine, or a colonoscopy, in which the doctor inspects the interior of the large intestine using a long, flexible lighted tube linked to a computer and monitor. If the tests show the presence of Crohn's disease, the doctor may do more X-rays of both the upper and lower digestive tract to find out how much is affected by the disease.

Since there is no cure for Crohn's disease, the goals of treatment are to control inflammation, relieve symptoms, and correct nutritional deficiencies—all of which can help keep Crohn's disease in remission. Two-thirds to three-quarters of patients with Crohn's disease will require surgery at some point in their lives. Surgery becomes necessary when medications can no longer control symptoms. Surgery is used either to relieve symptoms that do not respond to medical therapy or to correct complications such as blockage, perforation, abscess, or bleeding in the intestine. Surgery to remove part of the intestine can help people with Crohn's disease, but it is not a cure. It is not uncommon for people with Crohn's disease to have more than one operation, as inflammation tends to return to the area next to where the diseased intestine was removed.

Unless otherwise specified, the dosages recommended here are for adults. For a child between the ages of twelve and seventeen, reduce the dose to three-quarters of the recommended amount. For a child between six and twelve, use one-half of the recommended dose, and for a child under the age of six, use one-quarter of the recommended amount.

NUTRIENTS

SUPPLEMENT	SUGGESTED DOSAGE	COMMENTS
Essential		
Duodenal glandular	As directed on label.	Aids in healing gastrointestinal ulcers.
L-glutamine	500 mg twice daily, on an empty stomach. Take with water or juice. Do not take with milk. Take with 50 mg vitamin B_6 and 100 mg vitamin C for better absorption.	A major metabolic fuel for the intestinal cells; maintains the *villi*, the absorption surfaces of the gut. (*See* AMINO ACIDS in Part One.)
Liver extract injections plus	2 cc once weekly or as prescribed by physician.	Needed for proper digestion.
vitamin B complex and	1 cc once weekly or as prescribed by physician.	Helps to prevent anemia.
vitamin B_{12} and	1 cc twice weekly or as prescribed by physician.	Important for proper digestion and to prevent anemia. Deficiency aggravates malabsorption.
folic acid or	1/4 cc twice weekly or as prescribed by physician.	Needed for constant supply of new cells. Injections (under a doctor's supervision) are best.
vitamin B complex plus extra	100 mg 3 times daily.	If injections are not available, use a lozenge or sublingual form.
vitamin B_{12} and	1,000–2,000 mcg daily.	
folic acid	200 mcg daily.	
N-Acetylglucosamine (N-A-G from Source Naturals)	As directed on label.	A major constituent of the barrier layer that protects the intestinal lining from digestive enzymes and other potentially damaging intestinal contents.
Omega-3 essential fatty acids (Kyolic-EPA from Wakunaga, flaxseed oil, primrose oil, and salmon oil)	As directed on label.	Needed for repair of the digestive tract; reduces inflammatory processes. Studies show essential fatty acids may reduce Crohn's symptoms and aid in maintaining remission.
Pancreatin plus bromelain	As directed on label. Take with meals. As directed on label.	To break down protein and assist digestion.
Taurine Plus from American Biologics	500 mg daily, on an empty stomach. Take with 50 mg vitamin B_6 and 100 mg vitamin C for better absorption.	An important antioxidant and immune regulator. Use the sublingual form.
Vitamin C with bioflavonoids	1,000 mg 3 times daily	Prevents inflammation and improves immunity. Use a buffered type.
Vitamin D	800 IU.	68 percent of people with Crohn's disease have a vitamin D deficiency. Have your blood levels measured to see if this dose is right for you and correct it if not.
Vitamin K	As directed on label.	Vital to colon health. Deficiency is common in people with this disorder due to malabsorption and diarrhea.
Zinc	50 mg daily. Do not exceed a total of 100 mg daily from all supplements.	Needed for the immune system and for healing. Use zinc gluconate lozenges or OptiZinc for best absorption.
Important		
Free form amino acid (Amino Balance from Anabol Naturals)	1/4 tsp twice daily.	Protein is essential in the healing of the intestine. Use a sublingual form.
Garlic (Kyolic)	2 capsules 3 times daily, with meals.	Combats free radicals in Crohn's disease. Aids healing.
Lactobacilli (Kyo-Dophilus from Wakunaga) or Capricin from Probiologic	As directed on label. As directed on label.	Aids in digestion. Use a nondairy formula. A product containing both *L. acidophilus* and *L. bifidus* is best. Works in conjunction with butyric acid to reduce inflammation and seepage of undigested food particles.
Spiru-tein from Nature's Plus	2 capsules 3 times daily, between meals.	Supplies necessary protein. Helps stabilize blood sugar.
Helpful		
Calcium and magnesium	2,000 mg daily. 1,500 mg daily.	Aids in preventing colon cancer.
Floradix Iron + Herbs from Salus Haus	2 tsp daily.	To prevent anemia, if your physician agrees. Floradix is a readily absorbable form of iron that is nontoxic and derived from food sources.
Gastro-Calm from Olympian Labs	As directed on label.	A combination of herbs and digestive enzymes to help relieve indigestion and reduce gastrointestinal inflammation.
Multivitamin and mineral complex with copper and manganese and selenium plus extra potassium	As directed on label. 99 mg daily.	Malabsorption is often a result of this disorder. Copper, selenium, and manganese are important for treating this disorder and are often deficient because of absorption problems. Use a liquid, powder, or capsule formula. May reduce surgical complications and also the need for surgery.
Oxy-Caps from Earth's Bounty	As directed on label.	An oxygen supplement to counter nutritional deficiencies caused by Crohn's disease.
Quercetin plus bromelain or Activated Quercetin from Source Naturals	500 mg twice daily, before meals. 100 mg twice daily, before meals. As directed on label.	Slows histamine release; helps control food allergies. Needed for a variety of enzyme functions. Improves absorption of quercetin. Contains quercetin plus bromelain and vitamin C.

Vitamin A	25,000 IU daily. If you are pregnant, do not exceed 10,000 IU daily.	Antioxidants that aid in controlling infection and in repair of the intestinal tract. Use emulsion forms for easier assimilation.
and		
vitamin E	Up to 200 IU daily.	Use d-alpha-tocopherol form of vitamin E.

Herbs

❏ Aloe vera is beneficial for Crohn's disease because it softens stools and has a healing effect on the digestive tract. Drink ½ cup of aloe vera juice three times daily.

❏ There are many combination herbal products designed to offer gastrointestinal relief. Enzymatic Therapy, Olympian Labs, and Solaray are recommended sources.

❏ Other herbs that are good for this disorder include burdock root, echinacea, fenugreek, goldenseal, licorice, marshmallow root, pau d'arco, enteric-coated peppermint (do not use any other form), red clover, rose hips, silymarin (milk thistle extract), and yerba maté. These herbs support digestion, cleanse the bloodstream, and reduce inflammation and infection. For best results, use them on an alternating basis.

Cautions: Do not take echinacea for longer than three months. It should not be used by people who are allergic to ragweed. Do not take goldenseal internally on a daily basis for more than one week at a time. Do not use it during pregnancy or if you are breast-feeding, and use with caution if you are allergic to ragweed. If you have a history of cardiovascular disease, diabetes, or glaucoma, use it only under a doctor's supervision. Licorice root should not be used during pregnancy or nursing. It should not be used by persons with diabetes, glaucoma, heart disease, high blood pressure, or a history of stroke.

Recommendations

❏ Eat a diet consisting mainly of nonacidic fresh or cooked vegetables such as broccoli, Brussels sprouts, cabbage, carrots, celery, garlic, kale, spinach, and turnips. Steam, broil, boil, or bake your food.

❏ Drink plenty of liquids, such as steam-distilled water, herbal teas, and fresh juices. Fresh cabbage juice is very beneficial.

❏ Add papaya to your diet. Chew a couple of the seeds to aid digestion.

❏ During an acute attack, eat organic baby foods, steamed vegetables, and well-cooked brown rice, millet, and oatmeal.

❏ Try eliminating all dairy foods (including cheese), fish, hard sausage, pickled cabbage, and yeast products from your diet, and see if symptoms improve. These foods are high in histamine. Many people with Crohn's disease are histamine-intolerant. Milk and other dairy products also contain carrageenan, a compound extracted from red seaweed. Carrageenan, which is widely used in the food industry for its ability to stabilize milk proteins, has been shown to induce ulcerative colitis in laboratory animals.

❏ Avoid alcohol, caffeine, carbonated beverages, chocolate, corn, nuts, popcorn, eggs, foods with artificial additives or preservatives, fried and greasy foods, margarine, meat, dairy products such as milk and cheese, pepper, spicy foods, tobacco, white flour, and all animal products, with the exception of white fish from clear waters. These foods are irritating to the digestive tract. Mucus-forming foods such as processed, refined foods and dairy products should also be avoided. Limit your intake of barley, rye, and wheat.

❏ Avoid refined carbohydrates. Do not consume such foods as boxed dry cereals or anything containing any form of sugar. Diets high in refined carbohydrates have been associated with Crohn's disease. These foods must be eliminated from the diet.

❏ Check stools daily for bleeding.

❏ As much as possible, avoid stress. Our thoughts, nervous systems, and bodily functions are deeply interconnected. Our thoughts and moods affect our bodies. During an attack, rest is important.

❏ Make sure the bowels move daily, but do not use harsh laxatives. (*See* CONSTIPATION and/or DIARRHEA in Part Two.) Gentle enemas made by adding a dropperful of alcohol-free herbal extract and 1 teaspoon of nondairy acidophilus powder to 2 quarts of lukewarm water are good. Accumulations of toxic body wastes often become breeding grounds for parasitic infestation. Toxins can also be absorbed into the bloodstream through the colon wall. Psyllium husks should be used daily to add fiber to the diet; this aids in removing toxins before they are absorbed.

Note: Always take supplemental fiber separately from other supplements and medications.

❏ Do not use rectal suppositories that contain hydrogenated chemically prepared fats.

❏ If you are constipated, use a cleansing enema. (*See* ENEMAS in Part Three.)

❏ Use a heating pad to reduce abdominal pain.

Considerations

❏ There are no consistent dietary rules that apply to everyone, but people with Crohn's disease are generally encouraged to eat a healthy diet to help the body replace lost nutrients. Moreover, some nutrients, such as essential fatty acids and the amino acid glutamine, have been shown to help maintain a state of remission. However, one study using 4 grams of fish oil (up to 80 percent omega-3s) per day had no effect over one year's time on whether people who were in remission from Crohn's disease relapsed. It is possible that the dose was not large enough to see an effect, but the study was well done and included nearly 400 patients from around the world.

❏ It is important that nutritional deficiencies be corrected for healing. Persons with inflammatory bowel disorders require as much as 30 percent more protein than normal. If chronic diarrhea is present, electrolyte and trace mineral deficiencies should be considered. Chronic steatorrhea (fatty stools resulting from improper digestion of fats) may result in deficiencies of calcium and magnesium.

❏ Drugs such as corticosteroids and sulfasalazine (Azulfidine), which are prescribed for inflammatory bowel diseases, and cholestyramine (Questran), which is prescribed to bind bile in the gastrointestinal tract to prevent its reabsorption in people who had part of their intestine removed, increase the need for nutritional supplements. Corticosteroids depress protein synthesis and inhibit normal calcium absorption by increasing excretion of vitamin C in the urine. Deficiencies of other nutrients, such as zinc, potassium, vitamin B_6 (pyridoxine), folic acid, and vitamin D, decrease bone formation and slow healing. Sulfasalazine inhibits the transport of folic acid and iron, causing anemia.

❏ Antioxidants decrease a person's risk of developing Crohn's disease. The intestinal walls normally contain small amounts of the antioxidant enzymes superoxide dismutase (SOD), catalase, and glutathione peroxidase, but their ability to fight free radicals may be overwhelmed during periods of active inflammation that results in tissue damage.

❏ To reestablish a proper healing environment, it is necessary to maintain a generally alkaline (greater than 7.0) bodily pH.

❏ Adhering to an allergen-free diet, replacing lost nutrients, and using selected herbs can speed healing and may prevent future disturbances. Studies have proven that when a person who has achieved remission goes back to his or her former diet, Crohn's disease returns. Other things that have been implicated in this disorder include prolonged stress, trauma, and psychosomatic and vascular factors.

❏ Nutritional deficiencies resulting from malabsorption may weaken the immune system, in turn prolonging the time required for the inflammation and ulcers to heal.

❏ Many microorganisms have been considered as possible causes of Crohn's disease, including fungi, bacteria, viruses, mycobacteria, pseudomonas-like organisms, and chlamydia. However, the cause of Crohn's disease has not yet been established. It is likely that multiple factors are involved.

❏ Antigenic reactions may result from "leaky gut syndrome," in which minute particles of undigested or partially digested food pass through the swollen and inflamed mucosal wall into the bloodstream, where they cause reactions. The mucosal wall must be repaired to avoid this. Avoiding foods that cause a reaction is important. (*See* ALLERGIES in Part Two.) Treatment with butyric acid, a monounsaturated fatty acid, reduces inflammatory conditions, reduces seepage of undigested food particles, and aids in repair of the mucosal wall. N-acetylglucosamine (NAG) prevents leaky gut syndrome.

❏ Some foods—such as fruits and vegetables—are protective against getting Crohn's disease and some—such as fatty foods—increase the risk. Children are especially vulnerable to the effects of certain foods. In one study, four food patterns were identified and each had a different impact on the risk for Crohn's disease. Foods that seemed to prevent it were vegetables, fruits, olive oil, fish, grains, and nuts. Foods that were thought to cause it—only in girls—were meats, desserts, and fatty foods in general.

❏ If Crohn's disease continues for many years, bowel function gradually deteriorates. Surgery may be required to remove the diseased portion of the intestine. While this surgery doesn't cure the disease, it can relieve symptoms, and five years later at least 50 percent of people who undergo it are in good health, can work full-time, and enjoy life without being restricted by diarrhea or pain.

❏ People with Crohn's disease have a significantly higher than normal risk of developing colon cancer. If you have this disorder, you should undergo a colonoscopy at least once every two years, starting eight to ten years after diagnosis.

❏ Most people with Crohn's disease are initially treated with drugs, particularly corticosteroids, such as Budesonide, to help control inflammation. This newer drug has fewer side effects than the older corticosteroids. Drugs that suppress the immune system are also used, but they can increase susceptibility to infection. Currently, the drugs methotrexate (Trexall, Rheumatrex) and cyclosporine (Neoral, Sandimmune, SangCya) are being tried along with the traditional immunosuppressive drugs. Some of these drugs may be enhanced with 3 grams of fish oil containing 400 milligrams of EPA and 200 milligrams of DHA.

❏ The Food and Drug Administration (FDA) approved under an accelerated program a genetically engineered product called infliximab (Remicade). Remicade is an intravenously administered drug for people with moderate-to-severe Crohn's disease who have not responded to traditional treatments. Remicade works specifically against a protein that promotes inflammation, and it has been shown to reduce intestinal inflammation. In drug trials, one dose relieved many of the symptoms for two to four weeks, after which the benefits waned. Because the long-term toxic effects of the drug are unknown, scientists are still trying to better define risks and benefits. A new study showed that infliximab helped to improve symptoms over a five-year period and changed disease outcome by decreasing the rate of hospital admissions and surgery. A second drug, adalimumab (Humira), was also approved.

❑ Natalizumab (Tysabri) is another drug, approved in 2008, that appears to reduce symptoms and improve quality of life. This drug decreases inflammation by binding to immune cells and preventing them from getting to the intestines to cause inflammation. Antibiotics are used to treat the bacterial infections that often accompany Crohn's disease.

❑ Interleukin-10 is a cytokine that suppresses inflammation. It has shown some promise in treating Crohn's disease.

❑ Growth hormone seems to help adult patients with Crohn's disease to increase their activity levels. This must be done under a doctor's supervision. In one study, side effects were headaches and swelling (edema), but these resolved within the first month of treatment.

CROUP

Croup, or laryngotracheobronchitis, is a viral infection that causes the larynx or trachea (the upper part of the windpipe, near the vocal cords) to narrow due to swelling. The larynx goes into spasms, and the sufferer experiences difficulty breathing; a harsh, barking cough; hoarseness; tightness in the lungs; and feelings of suffocation. Mucus production may also increase, further clogging the airway.

At the beginning, croup has all the hallmarks of the common cold. It starts off with congestion, a runny nose, and a cough that develops into the distinctive barking cough associated with croup. Another trademark of croup is a harsh, wheezing noise that is made when air is breathed in through the constricted windpipe and over the inflamed vocal cords.

Croup accounts for approximately 15 percent of clinic and emergency room visits for pediatric respiratory infections. In North America, incidence peaks in the second year of life at 5 to 6 cases per 100 children. Approximately 5 percent of children experience more than one episode. Croup is most common in late fall and early winter but may be seen at any time of year. Attacks frequently occur at night. In the past, this illness was often caused by the measles virus, but now that children are immunized against measles, croup has become much less common than it once was. The virus usually runs its course in five to six days.

NUTRIENTS

SUPPLEMENT	SUGGESTED DOSAGE	COMMENTS
Essential		
Vitamin C with bioflavonoids	Children 6–12 months old: 60 mg 4 times daily. Children 1–4 years old: 100 mg 4 times daily. Children over 4 years: 500 mg 4 times daily.	Helps control infection and fever by boosting the immune system.
Zinc	Children 6–12 months old: 5 mg once daily for 3 days. Children 1–3 years old: 5 mg twice daily for 3 days. Children over 3 years: 5 mg 3 times daily.	Promotes immune function and is necessary in healing. Use lozenges for faster absorption.
Very Important		
Vitamin A with mixed carotenoids	2,000 IU daily.	Needed for healing of the mucous membranes. Use an emulsion form.
Vitamin E	Children 4–8 years old: 50 IU daily. Children 9–13 years old: 100 IU daily.	Destroys free radicals and carries oxygen to all cells. Use an emulsion form for best absorption. Use d-alpha-tocopherol form.

Herbs

The following herbs are recommended for croup: echinacea, fenugreek, goldenseal, and thyme. Echinacea tincture should be taken if a fever is present. Take 15 drops in liquid every three to four hours.

Cautions: Do not take echinacea for longer than three months. It should not be used by people who are allergic to ragweed. Do not take goldenseal internally on a daily basis for more than one week at a time. Do not use it during pregnancy or if you are breast-feeding, and use with caution if you are allergic to ragweed. If you have a history of cardiovascular disease, diabetes, or glaucoma, use it only under a doctor's supervision.

❑ Put a few drops of eucalyptus oil in a vaporizer and inhale the steam. It makes it easier for a child to breathe if the air is kept humidified.

❑ Give a child with croup very warm ginger herb baths; then immediately wrap the child in a heavy towel or blanket, and put him or her to bed to perspire. This helps loosen mucus and rid the body of toxins. You can also let your child stay in a steam-filled bathroom for ten or fifteen minutes. The moisture makes it easier to breathe.

Recommendations

❑ Give a child with croup plenty of fluids to help to thin mucus. Steam-distilled water, herbal teas, and homemade soups are good choices.

❑ Apply hot onion packs over the chest and back three times a day. Slice onions and place them between cloths, and then apply the pack and cover it with a heating pad. Onion packs open the pores and relieve congestion.

❑ If a child with croup is having difficulty breathing, take him or her to the emergency room of the nearest hospital for treatment and for X-rays of the larynx. Oxygen may be needed. Milder cases of croup can be treated at home, but parents should be alert for signs of increasing breathing difficulty.

Considerations

❏ Croup is a viral infection, so antibiotics will not help. In most cases, self-care measures at home—such as breathing moist air and drinking fluids—can speed your child's recovery. More aggressive treatment is rarely needed.

❏ If your child's symptoms persist or worsen, his or her doctor may prescribe corticosteroids, epinephrine, or another medication to open the airways. For severe croup, your child may need to spend time in a hospital receiving humidified oxygen. Rarely, a temporary breathing tube may need to be placed in a child's windpipe.

❏ Fresh cold air may also help a child with croup to breathe by reducing the swelling of the trachea and larynx.

CUSHING'S SYNDROME

See under ADRENAL DISORDERS.

CYSTIC FIBROSIS

Cystic fibrosis (CF) is the most common inherited illness among Americans of northern and western European ancestry. It occurs in people of all ethnic backgrounds and is most common in Caucasians. It occurs with approximately equal frequency in men and women. About 30,000 people in the United States (70,000 worldwide) have been diagnosed with CF and 1,000 new cases are diagnosed each year.

It is estimated that about 12 million Americans—adults and children—are silent carriers of the defective gene that leads to this disease. Many of them don't know that they are CF carriers. The gene responsible for CF was identified in 1989 on human chromosome 7, and it encodes instructions for a protein that regulates the passage of salt in and out of the cells of the body's exocrine glands. This defective gene transforms the protein called the cystic fibrosis transmembrane conductance regulator (CFTR) and causes it to produce a mucus too thick and too abundant for the body to excrete.

In most people with CF, the genetic instructions omit just one of the protein's 1,480 constituent amino acids—a tiny glitch, but a devastating one that affects many different glands in the body, including the pancreas, sweat glands, and glands of the digestive and respiratory systems.

All human cells (except red blood cells, eggs, and sperm) contain two copies of this gene, one inherited from each parent. CF results when both copies of the "CF gene" are abnormal. If one copy is abnormal and the other is normal, an individual is said to be a carrier. He or she will show no signs of CF, but can pass on a defective gene to offspring. Statistically, a child of two carrier parents has a 1-in-4 chance of inheriting CF; a 1-in-4 chance of being completely free of the mutant gene; and a 1-in-2 chance of being a carrier, like the parents.

The airway, gastrointestinal tract, bile ducts of the liver, ducts of the pancreas, and the male genitourinary tract all produce mucus. Cystic fibrosis alters this normally protective mucus and transforms it into a thick, abnormal excretion that obstructs airways and damages tissue. Symptoms of CF begin early in life. Glands in the lungs and bronchial tubes secrete large quantities of thick, sticky mucus that blocks lung passages and provides the perfect place for harmful bacteria to thrive. *Pseudomonas aeruginosa* (also seen in cancer and burn patients) is the bacteria that most commonly colonizes the lungs, resulting in chronic coughing and wheezing, difficulty breathing, and recurrent lung infections. Once established, the bacteria remain in the lungs and are responsible for repeated outbreaks of infection.

The bacteria form their own dense structure, called a biofilm, and are immune to most current treatments. They also produce toxic proteins that can cause tissue damage and weaken the immune system. The lungs of many children with CF are inhabited or colonized by the *Pseudomonas aeruginosa* bacteria before they are ten years of age.

Thick secretions also often obstruct the release of pancreatic enzymes, resulting in digestive difficulties and malabsorption problems, particularly problems with the metabolism of fats. Malnutrition may result because a lack of necessary digestive enzymes means that nutrients from foods are not properly absorbed. This in turn can cause pain after eating and, especially in young children, a failure to gain weight normally. Pancreatic enzymes need to be replaced to counter this.

Persons with this disease also lose excessive amounts of salt through their sweat glands. Sweating may be profuse, and the sweat itself contains abnormally high concentrations of sodium, potassium, and chloride salts. Other signs suggestive of CF include clubbing of the fingers and toes (a result of poor oxygenation due to weak lung function); greasy, bulky, foul-smelling stools; and salty-tasting skin. The reproductive organs may be affected, causing infertility in almost all men and some women.

The identification of the CF gene has enabled researchers to begin developing new approaches to diagnosis and treatment of the disease. A test is now available in which cells are swabbed from the inside of the cheek and then examined for the presence of defective genes. The presence of both normal and mutant CF genes indicates that the individual is a carrier. If only mutant genes are there, CF is indicated.

The most widely used test for CF is the electrolyte sweat test. Developed over forty years ago, the sweat test detects the excessive amounts of electrolytes (charged mineral salts) found on the skin of many people with CF. A physician would likely recommend that a sweat test be performed on a child who failed to gain weight despite adequate feeding, or who suffered from very frequent respiratory infections. CF testing is currently recommended only for those individuals with symptoms highly suggestive of the disease, or with a family history of the disorder. However, if there is doubt about the diagnosis, the sweat test can be confirmed by performing a genetic test.

Unless otherwise specified, the dosages recommended here are for adults. For children between the ages of twelve and seventeen, reduce the dose to three-quarters the recommended amount. For children between six and twelve, use one-half the recommended dose, and for children under the age of six, use one-quarter the recommended amount.

NUTRIENTS

SUPPLEMENT	SUGGESTED DOSAGE	COMMENTS
Very Important		
Complete Enzyme Blend	As directed on label, on an empty stomach. Take between meals.	Aids in controlling infection, helps digestion, and thins the mucous secretions of the lungs. Contact your physician to find a high-quality enzyme blend. Some of the food-based enzymes do not have the same potency as non-food-based enzymes.
Vitamin A plus carotenoid complex with beta-carotene	As directed on label. As directed on label.	Aids in the maintenance and repair of epithelial tissue, which makes up the mucous membranes. Use emulsion form for better absorption and greater safety at higher doses.
Vitamin B complex plus extra vitamin B$_2$ (riboflavin)	100 mg of each major B vitamin 3 times daily, with meals (amounts of individual vitamins in a complex will vary). 50 mg 3 times daily.	Aids in digestion, healing, and tissue repair.
Vitamin B$_{12}$	1,000–2,000 mcg daily, on an empty stomach.	Needed for proper digestion and assimilation of nutrients, including iron. Use a lozenge, sublingual, or spray form.
Vitamin C with bioflavonoids	3,000–6,000 mg daily, in divided doses.	For tissue repair and immune function.
Vitamin E	As directed on label. Do not to exceed 200 IU daily from all supplements.	Repairs tissue and prevents cell damage. Also helps in the utilization of vitamin A. Use d-alpha-tocopherol form.
Vitamin K or alfalfa	100 mcg twice daily.	Deficiency is common in those with this disorder. Needed for proper digestion. *See* under Herbs, below.
Important		
Essential fatty acids (fish oil, primrose oil)	As directed on label.	Relieves inflammation. *Caution:* DHA omega-3 oil had no effect on breathing in children with Delta 508 homozygous cystic fibrosis. So don't use DHA alone; use a blend of DHA and EPA.
Protein supplement or free form amino acid (Amino Balance from Anabol Naturals)	As directed on label. As directed on label.	Needed for healing. Use protein from a vegetable source or a free form amino acid. Speak to your doctor before using a protein supplement.
Zinc	50 mg daily. Do not exceed a total of 100 mg daily from all supplements.	Important in immune function and healing of tissue. Use zinc gluconate lozenges or OptiZinc for best absorption. Taking 30 mg a day may allow children to take less antibiotics to treat upper respiratory infections.
Helpful		
Coenzyme Q$_{10}$ plus	100 mg daily.	Acts as an immunostimulant.
Coenzyme A from Coenzyme-A Technologies	As directed on label.	Supports the immune system's detoxification of many dangerous substances.
Copper and selenium	3 mg daily. 200 mcg daily. If you are pregnant, do not exceed 40 mcg daily.	Low levels of copper and selenium have been linked to cystic fibrosis.
Kyo-Green from Wakunaga or chlorophyll	As directed on label. As directed on label.	To supply minerals and chlorophyll needed to control infection.
L-cysteine and L-methionine	500 mg each twice daily, on an empty stomach. Take with water or juice. Do not take with milk. Take with 50 mg vitamin B$_6$ and 100 mg vitamin C for better absorption.	Needed for repair of lung tissue and to protect the liver. (*See* AMINO ACIDS in Part One.)
Lipoic acid	As directed on label.	Helps the pancreas to function properly and controls the metabolism of sugar.
Methylsulfonyl-methane (MSM)	As directed on label.	Clinical tests have proven that this supplement combats lung damage.
Pycnogenol	As directed on label.	A powerful antioxidant that also protects the lungs.
Raw pancreas glandular and raw spleen glandular and raw thymus glandular	As directed on label. As directed on label. As directed on label.	To relieve inflammation. (*See* GLANDULAR THERAPY in Part Three.)
Vitamin D	400 IU daily.	Aids in protecting the lungs.

Herbs

❑ Alfalfa extract supplies vitamin K and necessary minerals, which are often deficient in those with cystic fibrosis due to absorption problems. It is also a good source of chlorophyll.

❑ Boswellia, bromelain, cayenne, ginger, and peppermint can aid in reducing inflammation.

❑ Expectorant herbs such as cayenne, elecampane, garlic, horehound, hyssop, and mullein may be effective in helping to clear some of the congestion.

❑ ClearLungs from RidgeCrest Herbals is a Chinese herbal formula that is highly recommended for this condition.

❑ Eucalyptus, garlic, onion, tea tree oil, and thyme have natural antiseptic properties and fight infection.

❑ Echinacea, licorice, and Siberian ginseng are good for building up the immune system.

Cautions: Do not take echinacea for longer than three months. It should not be used by people who are allergic to ragweed. Licorice root should not be used during pregnancy or nursing. It should not be used by persons with diabetes, glaucoma, heart disease, high blood pressure, or a history of stroke. Do not use Siberian ginseng if you have hypoglycemia, high blood pressure, or a heart disorder.

❑ Lung Tonic from Herbs, Etc., is a combination of many organic herbs designed to support the lungs.

❑ Other herbs beneficial for cystic fibrosis include ginger, goldenseal, and yarrow tea.

Caution: Do not take goldenseal internally on a daily basis for more than one week at a time. Do not use it during pregnancy or if you are breast-feeding, and use with caution if you are allergic to ragweed. If you have a history of cardiovascular disease, diabetes, or glaucoma, use it only under a doctor's supervision.

Recommendations

❑ Eat a diet consisting of 75 percent raw fruits and vegetables, and raw nuts and seeds.

❑ Make sure your intake of calories, protein, and other nutrients is adequate. People with CF require as much as 50 percent more of many nutrients than normal. Take supplements to provide required enzymes, vitamins, and minerals. Antioxidant supplements (vitamins A, E, and Coenzyme Q_{10}) have been shown to increase blood levels of these nutrients and reduce airway inflammation. The supplements were given in a novel micellar formulation to allow for better absorption.

❑ Include in the diet foods that are high in germanium, such as garlic, shiitake mushrooms, and onions. Germanium helps to improve tissue oxygenation at the cellular level.

❑ During hot weather, drink plenty of fluids and increase your salt intake.

❑ Do not eat foods that stimulate secretions by the mucous membranes. Cooked and processed foods cause excess mucus buildup and drain the body of energy. These foods are harder to digest. Do not eat animal products, dairy products, processed foods, sugar, or white flour products.

❑ When you must take antibiotics, take acidophilus to replace "friendly" bacteria.

Considerations

❑ Recent media reports on the beneficial effects of the spice turmeric (actually, its pigment, curcumin) in treating CF should not be taken to indicate that this is a cure. It is true that in animal tests conducted by Yale University, curcumin achieved beneficial results. Curcumin is a weak calcium-pump inhibitor and this enhances the energy transport mechanism of the cell, which appears to be defective in patients with CF. At this point, researchers caution that taking curcumin pills as a supplement, along with the existing CF drug therapies, has not been tested and could pose hazards. A phase I safety trial is being conducted. Research is still in the preliminary stages.

❑ The symptoms of cystic fibrosis are normally controlled with a number of different drugs. Antibiotics are used to combat the infections to which people with CF are prone, especially infection with *Pseudomonas aeruginosa,* a type of microbe that is attracted to the sticky mucus in the lungs.

❑ Pancrelipase (also sold under a variety of brand names, including Viokase) is a prescription product containing a combination of digestive enzymes that is often prescribed for people with CF and other pancreatic insufficiencies.

❑ Many people also take anti-inflammatory drugs such as ibuprofen (Advil, Nuprin, and others), naproxen (Naprosyn, Aleve), or prednisone (Deltasone and others).

❑ A small handheld device called the Flutter helps people with CF to dislodge mucus from the airways. It can replace conventional physiotherapy.

❑ The future of CF treatment may lie in gene therapy. In the laboratory, normal CF genes have been successfully introduced into cells from people with CF. Experiments in rats have indicated that replacing the defective CF genes with normal ones in just 10 percent of the lung-lining cells improves lung function. However, because the genes in the cells of the reproductive system are unaffected by this procedure, the defect can still be passed on to offspring. As part of this gene therapy, work is proceeding with vector aerosols. A vector is like a shuttle that can deliver a good copy of the defective gene to the appropriate place in the body.

❑ Dornase (Pulmozyme) is a naturally occurring enzyme that breaks down DNA molecules. Part of the reason the mucus that clogs the airways of people with CF is so thick and sticky is that it contains large molecules of DNA released by white blood cells as they die fighting chronic bacterial infection. This makes the mucus even denser and more difficult to expel. Breaking down the DNA molecules helps to thin the mucus. Other drugs that are used to increase sputum volume and decrease its thickness include N-acetylcysteine (Mucomyst) and guaifenesin (Humibid LA, Entex). Still others such as albuterol (Ventolin) and theophylline (Theo-Dur) open airways.

❑ Levels of two fatty acids—arachidonic acid (AA) and docosahexaenoic acid (DHA)—have been found to be out of balance in people with CF. This lipid imbalance is most noticeable in the lungs, pancreas, and intestine—all of the areas most affected by cystic fibrosis. Research in this area seems promising.

❑ When the antibiotic tobramycin (Nebcin) is administered by aerosol spray, it has proved to be more effective in reaching infected lung tissue than when administered through the traditional intravenous route.

❑ Low levels of selenium and vitamin E have been linked to cystic fibrosis and cancer.

❑ Further information about cystic fibrosis is available from the Cystic Fibrosis Foundation. (*See* Health and Medical Organizations in the Appendix.)

CYSTITIS

See BLADDER INFECTION.

DANDRUFF

Dandruff is a common scalp condition that occurs when dead skin is shed, producing irritating white flakes. It is usually a condition of oily, rather than dry, skin, and occurs as skin cells renew themselves and the old cells are shed.

Some people tend to generate and discard skin cells at a faster rate than others. Recent research shows that severe cases of flaking scalp, usually associated with seborrhea (a type of dermatitis), may be caused by an overgrowth of the yeast *Pityrosporum ovale,* which lives naturally on the skin.

Dandruff can be triggered by trauma, illness, hormonal imbalances, improper carbohydrate consumption, and the consumption of sugar. Deficiencies of nutrients such as the B-complex vitamins, essential fatty acids, and selenium have been linked to dandruff as well. Dandruff is normally worse in the winter months.

Dandruff is an annoying and embarrassing problem, but is rarely serious. There is no cure for dandruff, but the condition can be minimized.

NUTRIENTS

SUPPLEMENT	SUGGESTED DOSAGE	COMMENTS
Very Important		
Essential fatty acids (flaxseed oil, primrose oil, or salmon oil)	As directed on label.	Helps to relieve itching and inflammation; essential for healthy skin and scalp.
Kelp	1,000–1,500 mg daily.	Supplies needed minerals, especially iodine, for better hair growth and healing of the scalp.
Selenium	200 mcg daily. If you are pregnant, do not exceed 40 mcg daily.	An important antioxidant to aid in controlling dry scalp.
Vitamin B complex

plus extra | 100 mg of each major B vitamin twice daily, with meals (amounts of individual vitamins in a complex will vary). | B vitamins are needed for healthy skin and hair. Use a high-stress formula. Sublingual forms are best for absorption. |
vitamin B6 (pyridoxine) and	50 mg twice daily.	
vitamin B12	1,000–2,000 mcg daily.	
Vitamin E	200 IU daily.	For improved circulation. Use d-alpha-tocopherol form.
Zinc lozenges	One 15-mg lozenge 5 times daily for 1 week. Do not exceed a total of 100 mg daily from all supplements.	Protein metabolism depends on zinc. The skin is composed primarily of protein.
Important		
Free form amino acid (Amino Balance from Anabol Naturals)	As directed on label.	Needed for repair of all tissues and for proper hair growth. Use a formula containing both essential and nonessential amino acids.
L-cystine	500 mg daily, on an empty stomach. Take with water or juice. Do not take with milk. Take with 50 mg vitamin B6 and 100 mg vitamin C for better absorption.	Needed for flexibility of the skin and for hair texture. (*See* AMINO ACIDS in Part One.)
Vitamin A

plus mixed carotenoids | Up to 20,000 IU daily. If you are pregnant, do not exceed 10,000 IU daily. 15,000 IU daily. | Helps prevent dry skin. Aids in healing of tissue.

Antioxidants and precursors of vitamin A. |
Vitamin C with bioflavonoids	3,000–6,000 mg daily, in divided doses.	An important antioxidant to prevent tissue damage to the scalp and to aid in healing.
Helpful		
Lecithin granules or capsules	1 tbsp 3 times daily, before meals. 1,200 mg 3 times daily, before meals.	Protects the scalp and strengthens cell membranes of the scalp and hair.

Herbs

❑ An infusion of thyme may be used as a hair rinse.

❑ Aloe vera cream or gel is a powerful antiseptic and anti-inflammatory. Twice a day applications of the pure gel, or a shampoo containing aloe vera, should be beneficial.

❑ Those with dandruff can benefit from taking dandelion, goldenseal, and red clover.

Caution: Do not take goldenseal internally on a daily basis for more than one week at a time. Do not use it during pregnancy or if you are breast-feeding, and use with caution if you are allergic to ragweed. If you have a history of cardiovascular disease, diabetes, or glaucoma, use it only under a doctor's supervision.

Recommendations

❑ Eat a diet consisting of 50 to 75 percent raw foods. Eat soured products such as yogurt.

❑ Avoid fried foods, dairy products, sugar, flour, chocolate, nuts, and seafood.

❑ *See* FASTING in Part Three and follow the program once a month.

❑ Before washing your hair, add about 8 tablespoons of pure organic peanut oil to the juice of half a lemon and rub the mixture into your scalp. Leave it on for five to ten minutes, then shampoo.

❑ Try rinsing your hair with vinegar and water instead of plain water after shampooing. Use ¼ cup vinegar to 1 quart of water.

❑ If antibiotics are prescribed, take extra B-complex vitamins. Also take an acidophilus supplement to replace the "friendly" bacteria that are destroyed by antibiotics.

❑ Do not pick or scratch the scalp. Make sure to wash your hair frequently, and use a non-oily shampoo. Use natural hair products that do not contain chemicals. Avoid using irritating soaps and greasy ointments and creams. Massage your scalp first before washing your hair.

❑ Do not use a shampoo containing selenium on a daily basis, even if it aids in controlling dandruff.

❑ If dandruff is persistent or symptoms seem to be getting worse, or if it appears in areas other than the scalp, consult your health care provider.

Considerations

❑ Some people have found that sun exposure helps clear up dandruff, but others find that it seems to make the problem worse.

❑ It is best not to use over-the-counter ointments for dandruff. They can often do more harm than good.

❑ Nizoral A-D is an antifungal dandruff shampoo.

❑ *See also* SEBORRHEA in Part Two.

DEAFNESS

See HEARING LOSS.

DEPRESSION

Depression—including anxiety—affects one in five Americans aged eighteen and older every year, making it one of the most common medical problems in the United States. It affects young and old, and is twice as common in women as in men.

Depression is a whole-body illness, one that affects the body, nervous system, moods, thoughts, and behavior. It affects the way you eat and sleep, the way you feel about yourself, and the way you react to and think about the people and things around you. Symptoms can last for weeks, months, or years. There are many types of depression, with variations in the number of symptoms, their severity, and their persistence.

People with depression typically withdraw and hide from society. They lose interest in things around them and become incapable of experiencing pleasure. Symptoms of depression include chronic fatigue, sleep disturbances (either insomnia or excessive sleeping), changes in appetite, headaches, backaches, digestive disorders, restlessness, irritability, quickness to anger, loss of interest or pleasure in hobbies, and feelings of worthlessness and inadequacy.

Many think of death and consider suicide. Things appear bleak and time seems to pass slowly. A person with depression may be chronically angry and irritable, sad and despairing, or display little or no emotion at all. Some try to "sleep off" depression, or do nothing but sit or lie around.

Older adults with hardening of the arteries (atherosclerosis) are more likely to have depression than older adults without the coronary disorder, according to a study by Dutch researchers. This study, reported in the journal *Archives of General Psychiatry,* suggested a relationship between vascular factors, such as hardening of the arteries or calcium deposits in the blood vessels, and late-life depression. A theory has been put forward that atherosclerosis may have an effect on the brain that leads to depression. Depression is *not* a normal part of growing older, but rather a treatable condition that affects more than 5 million Americans over the age of sixty-five, according to the American Association for Geriatric Psychiatry.

There are three main types of clinical depression: major depressive disorder, dysthymic disorder, and bipolar depression (the depressed phase of bipolar disorder). Within these types are variations in the number of associated mental symptoms, their severity, and their persistence. Unlike major depressive disorder, dysthymic disorder—a chronic but less severe type of depression—does not strike in discrete episodes, but is instead characterized by milder, persistent symptoms that may last for years. Although it usually doesn't interfere with everyday tasks, people with this milder form of depression rarely feel like they are functioning at their full capacities. Bipolar disorders usually begin as depression, but as they progress, they involve alternating episodes of depression and mania, which is characterized by abnormally and persistently elevated mood, energy, restlessness, or irritability. As a result, bipolar depression is commonly known as manic depression. Other symptoms of mania include overly inflated self-esteem, a decreased need for sleep, and increased talkativeness, racing thoughts, distractibility, physical agitation, and excessive risk-taking. Because bipolar disorder requires different treatment than major depression or dysthymia, obtaining an accurate diagnosis is extremely important. (*See* BIPOLAR MOOD DISORDER in Part Two.)

This section focuses primarily on various types of unipolar depression.

The causes of depression are not fully understood, but they are probably many and varied. Depression may be triggered by tension, stress, a traumatic life event, a hyperstimulated immune system, chemical imbalances in the brain, thyroid disorders, nutritional deficiencies, poor diet, the consumption of sugar, mononucleosis, lack of exercise, endometriosis, any serious physical disorder, or even allergies. One of the most common causes of depression is food allergies. Hypoglycemia (low blood sugar) is another common cause of depression. Heredity is a significant factor in this disorder. In up to 50 percent of people suffering from recurrent episodes of depression, one or both of the parents also experienced depression. Death rates can be higher for depressed people, too. A recent study based on the Women's Health Initiative, the largest study of U.S. women's health ever undertaken, shows that depressed women had a 50 percent greater chance of dying of heart attack, and 30 percent higher chance of dying from other causes, than nondepressed women. This was in spite of the fact that the depression was only mild or moderate, and was under treatment. Why this should be is still unknown.

Whatever the factors that trigger it, depression begins with a disturbance in the part of the brain that governs moods. Most people can handle everyday stresses; their bodies readjust to these pressures. When stress is too great for a person and his or her adjustment mechanism is unresponsive, depression may be triggered.

Perhaps the most common type of depression is a chronic low-grade depression called *dysthymia*. This condition involves long-term and/or recurring depressive symptoms that are not necessarily disabling but keep a person from functioning normally and interfere with social interactions and enjoyment of life. Research has found that this type of depression often results from (unconscious) negative thinking habits. Double depression is a variation of dysthymia in which a person with chronic, low-grade depression periodically experiences major depressive episodes, then returns to his or her "normal," mildly depressed state.

Some people become more depressed in the winter months, when the days are shorter and darker. This type of disorder is known as seasonal affective disorder (SAD). Women are more likely to suffer from SAD than are men. People who suffer this type of depression in the winter months lose their energy, suffer anxiety attacks, gain weight as a result of craving the wrong foods, sleep too much, and have a reduced sex drive. Many people get depressed around the December holidays. While most of them probably just have the "holiday blues," some of them may be suffering from SAD. Suicides also seem to be highest during this time of year.

Foods greatly influence the brain's behavior. A poor diet, especially one with a lot of junk foods, is a common cause of depression. The levels of brain chemicals called neurotransmitters, which regulate our behavior, are controlled by what we eat, and neurotransmitters are closely linked to mood. The neurotransmitters most commonly associated with mood are dopamine, serotonin, and norepinephrine. When the brain produces serotonin, tension is eased. When it produces dopamine or norepinephrine, we tend to think and act more quickly and are generally more alert.

At the neurochemical and physiological levels, neurotransmitters are extremely important. These substances carry impulses between nerve cells. Serotonin, for example, plays a role in mood, sleep, and appetite. Low levels of serotonin can lead to depression, anxiety, and sleep disorders.

The substance that processes serotonin is the amino acid tryptophan. The consumption of tryptophan increases the amount of serotonin made by the brain. Thus, eating complex carbohydrates (not simple carbohydrates such as fructose, sucrose, and lactose), which raise the level of tryptophan in the brain (thereby increasing serotonin production), has a calming effect. High-protein foods, on the other hand, promote the production of dopamine and norepinephrine, which promote alertness.

The American Psychiatric Society estimates that most cases of depression can be treated effectively, but that 80 percent of people who suffer from depression do not get the help they need. Many people do not seek treatment because they are ashamed, or they feel lethargic and despondent. In many cases, people with major depression only seek help when they are at the point of breakdown, or when they are hospitalized following a suicide attempt (an estimated 15 percent of chronic depression cases result in suicide). A good support system from friends and family members is often crucial in getting a depressed person to seek help for his or her illness.

According to the National Institute of Mental Health (NIMH), most people with a depressive illness do not get the help they need, although the great majority—even those whose depression is severe—can be helped. Without treatment (nutrition is very important), the symptoms of depression can last for weeks, months, or even years. With treatment, many people can find relief from their symptoms and lead a normal, healthy life.

The following nutrients are helpful for those suffering from depression. Unless otherwise specified, the dosages recommended here are for adults. For children between the ages of twelve and seventeen, reduce the dose to three-quarters of the recommended amount. For children between six and twelve, use one-half of the recommended dose, and for children under the age of six, use one-quarter of the recommended amount.

NUTRIENTS

SUPPLEMENT	SUGGESTED DOSAGE	COMMENTS
Essential		
Essential fatty acids (Kyolic-EPA from Wakunaga, salmon oil, flaxseed oil, or primrose oil)	As directed on label. Take with meals.	Aid in the transmission of nerve impulses; needed for normal brain function.
5 Hydroxytryptophan (5-HTP)	As directed on label.	Increases the body's production of serotonin. It should not be used with other antidepressants.

362

L-tyrosine	Up to 50 mg per pound of body weight daily. Take on an empty stomach with 50 mg vitamin B$_6$ and 100–500 mg vitamin C for better absorption. Best taken at bedtime.	Alleviates stress by boosting production of adrenaline. It also raises dopamine levels, which influence moods. (*See* AMINO ACIDS in Part One.) *Caution:* Do not take tyrosine if you are taking an MAO inhibitor drug.
S-adenosylmethionine (SAMe) (SAMe Rx-Mood from Nature's Plus)	As directed on label.	Works as an antidepressant. *Caution:* Do not use if you have bipolar mood disorder or take prescription antidepressants. Do not give to a child under twelve.
Sub-Adrene from American Biologics	As directed on label.	A dietary supplement for adrenal support.
Taurine Plus from American Biologics	As directed on label.	An important antioxidant and immune regulator, necessary for white blood cell activation and neurological function. Use the sublingual form.
Vitamin B complex injections	2 cc once weekly or as prescribed by physician.	B vitamins are necessary for the normal functioning of the brain and nervous system. If depression is severe, injections (under a doctor's supervision) are recommended. All injectables can be combined in a single shot.
plus extra vitamin B$_6$ (pyridoxine) and	1/2 cc once weekly or as prescribed by physician.	Needed for normal brain function. May help lift depression.
vitamin B$_{12}$ or vitamin B complex	1 cc once weekly or as prescribed by physician. As directed on label.	Linked to the production of the neurotransmitter acetylcholine. If injections are not available, a sublingual form of B complex is recommended.
plus extra vitamin B$_5$ (pantothenic acid) and	500 mg daily.	The most potent anti-stress vitamin.
vitamin B$_6$ (pyridoxine) plus	50 mg 3 times daily.	
vitamin B$_3$ (niacin)	50 mg 3 times daily. Do not exceed this amount.	Improves cerebral circulation. *Caution:* Do not take niacin if you have a liver disorder, gout, or high blood pressure.
plus vitamin B$_{12}$ and	1,000–2,000 mcg daily.	
folic acid	400 mcg daily.	Found to be deficient in people with depression.
Zinc	50 mg daily. Do not exceed a total of 100 mg daily from all supplements.	Found to be deficient in people with depression. Use zinc gluconate lozenges or OptiZinc for best absorption.
Important		
Choline and inositol or lecithin	100 mg each twice daily. As directed on label.	Important in brain function and neurotransmission. *Caution:* Do not take these supplements if you suffer from bipolar mood disorder.
Helpful		
Calcium and magnesium	1,500–2,000 mg daily. 1,000 mg daily.	Has a calming effect. Needed for the nervous system. Works with calcium. Use magnesium asporotate or magnesium chelate form.
Chromium	300 mcg daily.	Aids in mobilizing fats for energy.

Gamma-aminobutyric acid (GABA)	750 mg daily. Take with 200 mg niacinamide for best results.	Has a tranquilizing effect, much as diazepam (Valium) and other tranquilizers do. (*See* AMINO ACIDS in Part One.)
Lithium	As prescribed by physician.	A trace mineral used to treat bipolar mood disorder. Available by prescription only.
Multivitamin and mineral complex	As directed on label.	To correct vitamin and mineral deficiencies, often associated with depression.
Nicotinamide adenine dinucleotide (NADH)	5–15 mg daily.	Enhances production of dopamine, serotonin, and noradrenaline, which are key neurotransmitters.
Vitamin C with bioflavonoids	2,000–5,000 mg daily, in divided doses.	Needed for immune function. Aids in preventing depression.
plus extra rutin	200–300 mg daily.	Buckwheat-derived bioflavonoid. Enhances vitamin C absorption.

Herbs

❑ Balm, also known as lemon balm, is good for the stomach and digestive organs during stressful situations.

❑ Ginger, ginkgo biloba, licorice root, oat straw, peppermint, and Siberian ginseng may be helpful.

Cautions: Do not take ginkgo biloba if you have a bleeding disorder, or are scheduled for surgery or a dental procedure. Licorice root should not be used during pregnancy or nursing. It should not be used by persons with diabetes, glaucoma, heart disease, high blood pressure, or a history of stroke. Do not use Siberian ginseng if you have hypoglycemia, high blood pressure, or a heart disorder.

❑ Kava kava helps to induce calm and relieve depression.

Caution: Kava kava can cause drowsiness. It is not recommended for pregnant women or nursing mothers, and it should not be taken together with other substances that act on the central nervous system, such as alcohol, barbiturates, antidepressants, and antipsychotic drugs.

❑ St. John's wort acts in the same way as monoamine oxidase (MAO) inhibitors do, but less harshly.

Caution: St. John's wort may cause increased sensitivity to sunlight. It may also produce anxiety, gastrointestinal symptoms, and headaches. It can interact with some drugs including antidepressants, birth control pills, and anticoagulants.

Recommendations

❑ Eat a diet that includes plenty of raw fruits and vegetables, with soybeans and soy products, whole grains, seeds, nuts, brown rice, millet, and legumes. A diet too low in complex carbohydrates can cause serotonin depletion and depression.

❑ If you are nervous and wish to become more relaxed, consume more complex carbohydrates. For increased alert-

Can Depression Be Caused by Testosterone Deficiency?

Testosterone deficiency is a factor in causing depression and a host of age-related ailments in men such as erectile dysfunction. Many people are leery of testosterone because of media hype concerning sports-related usage. But there is more than one type of testosterone, and one is beneficial. First of all, it is true that all the anabolic steroids are "bad" over the long term. Their molecules resemble those of natural testosterone but are chemically different and do not react the same way in the body. The notorious methyltestosterone may be the worst of these steroids.

In the body, natural testosterone is either free (unattached to anything else) or bound to a molecule known as sex hormone binding globulin (SHBG). While the total amount of testosterone in the body, as measured by a blood test, might be the same as a man ages, more and more of the testosterone is bound to SHBG. Bound testosterone cannot interact with testosterone receptors and thus is, in effect, biologically inert. The amount of free, or active, testosterone available declines as men age. As it turns out, this free testosterone is important to health in many ways. Men with low free testosterone levels are more prone to high blood sugar, high blood cholesterol and triglycerides, high blood pressure, obesity in general and abdominal obesity in particular, high levels of clotting factors, and low levels of clotting inhibitors. There is data suggesting that osteoporosis, which affects millions of men, and depression also are linked to low testosterone levels. Aside from testosterone therapy under a physician's care, there is an herbal product, the bioflavonoid chrysin, extracted from the plant *Passiflora coerula* (a type of passionflower), which can help the body produce testosterone naturally. Another useful herbal is an extract made from nettle root (*Urtica dioica*). This binds to SHBG better than testosterone does, thus helping to increase the body's level of free testosterone. If you choose to try this remedy, make sure you use a product made from the root, not the stems and leaves.

A word of caution here: Men with prostate cancer, or possible prostate cancer, should not take any herbal that increases the supply of free testosterone because it may enhance the cancer.

---

ness, eat protein meals containing essential fatty acids. The omega-3 fatty acids in particular are very necessary for healthy bodies and minds, and studies have shown that a deficiency can lead to mood disorders. Salmon and whitefish are good choices. In a study published in the *American Journal of Clinical Nutrition*, those who ate fish of any type had fewer depressive symptoms than those who didn't eat fish. Of the two major omega-3 fatty acids obtained from fish, EPA and DHA, only EPA seems to be protective against depression. Fish usually have a 50:50 mixture of the two fatty acids, which is a good ratio. If you are using dietary supplements, make sure they have the same ratio, or slightly more EPA than DHA.

❑ If you need your spirits lifted, you will benefit from eating foods like turkey and salmon, which are high in tryptophan and protein.

❑ The omega-3 fat DHA, docosahexaenoic acid, which is found in many cold-water fish such as salmon, tuna, and mackerel, is known to have cardioprotective effects. Researchers at the University of California–Los Angeles School of Medicine found that genetically engineered mice fed a diet rich in DHA also were found to have less brain cell damage than those fed a diet that substituted safflower oil, which is low in omega-3 fatty acids. We recommend at least two meals a week of fish (not fried) rich in omega-3 fatty acids. While this is for good cardiovascular health, it is possible that this diet can also favorably affect people with Alzheimer's disease or depression. Low levels of DHA have also been associated with postpartum depression. However, newer data from Holland showed that DHA when combined with another fatty acid did not prevent depressive symptoms associated with childbirth.

❑ Omit wheat products from the diet. Wheat gluten has been linked to depressive disorders in those who do not tolerate gluten protein.

❑ Avoid diet sodas and other products containing the artificial sweetener aspartame (in NutraSweet, Equal, and other products). This additive can possibly block the formation of serotonin and cause headaches, insomnia, and depression in individuals who are already serotonin-deprived.

❑ Limit your intake of supplements that contain the amino acid phenylalanine. It contains the chemical phenol, which is highly allergenic. Most depressed people are allergic to certain substances. If you take a combination free form amino acid supplement, look for a product that does not contain phenylalanine. Phenylalanine is one of the major components of aspartame.

❑ Avoid foods high in saturated fats; the consumption of meat or fried foods, such as hamburgers and French fries, leads to sluggishness, slow thinking, and fatigue. They interfere with blood flow by causing the arteries and small blood vessels to become blocked and the blood cells to become sticky and tend to clump together, resulting in poor circulation, especially to the brain.

❑ Avoid all forms of sugar, including normally "good" sweeteners such as honey, molasses, and fruit juice. The body reacts more quickly to the presence of sugar than it does to the presence of complex carbohydrates. The increase in energy supplied by the simple carbohydrates (sugars) is quickly followed by fatigue and depression. Stevia, a concentrated natural sweetener derived from a South American shrub, does not have the same effect on the body as sugar, and does not have the side effects of artificial sugar substitutes.

❑ Avoid alcohol, caffeine, and processed foods.

❑ Investigate the possibility that food allergies are causing or contributing to depression. (*See* ALLERGIES in Part Two.)

❑ Have a hair analysis to rule out heavy metal intoxication as the cause of depression. (*See* HAIR ANALYSIS in Part Three.)

❑ Keep your mind active, and get plenty of rest and regular exercise. Studies have shown that exercise—walking, swimming, or any activity that you enjoy—is most important for all types of depression. Avoid stressful situations.

❑ Learn to recognize, and then to "reroute," negative thinking patterns. Working with a qualified professional to change ingrained habits can be rewarding (cognitive behavioral therapists specialize in this type of work). Keeping a daily log also can help you to recognize distorted thoughts and develop a more positive way of thinking.

❑ If you are suffering from situational depression—depression that occurs in response to an event such as in the death of a loved one or the breakup of a relationship—try using *Ignatia amara*. This is a homeopathic remedy derived from a plant, the Saint Ignatius bean, that helps control emotions during periods of extreme grief and hysteria.

❑ If depression is seasonal (SAD), light therapy may help. For information about devices for this type of light treatment, contact either The SunBox Company or Apollo Health. (*See* Manufacturer and Distributor Information in the Appendix.)

❑ *See* HYPOTHYROIDISM in Part Two and take the underarm test to detect an underactive thyroid. If your temperature is low, consult your physician. Thyroid dysfunction is behind many depressive disorders.

❑ Try using color to alleviate depression. (*See* COLOR THERAPY in Part Three.)

Considerations

❑ Finding the right treatment for depression can be as difficult as convincing someone that he or she needs help. Even so, according to the National Institute of Mental Health, clinical depression is one of the most treatable of all medical illnesses. Today, most people with depression can be treated with antidepressant medications, "talk" therapy (psychotherapy), or a combination of the two. Experts agree that successful treatment also hinges on early intervention. Early treatment increases the likelihood of preventing serious recurrences. Medications, such as the selective serotonin reuptake inhibitors, or SSRIs, are help-

ful. (*See* CATEGORIES OF ANTIDEPRESSANT DRUGS on page 366.) SSRIs generally produce fewer side effects than the older drugs (tricyclics), making it easier for people, including older adults, to adhere to treatment. Both generations of medication are effective in relieving depression, although any given individual may respond to one type of drug and not another. It is difficult to predict which people will respond to which drug, or who will experience what side effects.

❑ Despite the relative safety and popularity of SSRIs and other antidepressants, some studies have suggested that they may have unintended effects on some people, especially adolescents and young adults. In 2004, the Food and Drug Administration (FDA) conducted a thorough review of published and unpublished controlled clinical trials of antidepressants that involved nearly 4,400 children and adolescents. The review revealed that 4 percent of those taking antidepressants thought about or attempted suicide (although no suicides occurred), compared to 2 percent of those receiving placebos. This information prompted the FDA, in 2005, to adopt a "black box" warning label on all antidepressant medications to alert the public about the potential increased risk of suicidal thinking or attempts in children and adolescents taking antidepressants. In 2007, the FDA proposed that makers of all antidepressant medications extend the warning to include young adults up through age twenty-four. A "black box" warning is the most serious type of warning on prescription drug labeling. Results of a comprehensive review of pediatric trials conducted between 1988 and 2006 suggested that the benefits of antidepressant medications likely outweigh their risks to children and adolescents with major depression and anxiety disorders. The study was funded in part by the National Institute of Mental Health.

❑ The FDA issued a warning that combining an SSRI or SNRI antidepressant with one of the commonly used triptan medications for migraine headache could cause a life-threatening serotonin syndrome, marked by agitation, hallucinations, elevated body temperature, and rapid changes in blood pressure. Although most dramatic in the case of the MAOIs, newer antidepressants may also be associated with potentially dangerous interactions with other medications.

❑ Seasonal affective disorder can be treated using light therapy, which involves exposing yourself to light of a certain frequency from a special light box for fifteen minutes to two hours per day. The reason this therapy works is that more melatonin, a hormone produced by the pineal gland in the brain, is produced in the dark, or on dark days, than in the light or on longer, brighter summer days. At certain levels, melatonin appears to trigger the onset of depression in some people. Most insurance companies now honor claims for these special light boxes.

❑ Atypical depression is a common but often undiagnosed disorder. Nearly fifty years ago, two English psychiatrists first described atypical depression as a type of depression that seemed to differ from classic forms of depression in both its symptoms and treatment. Experts in the field of psychiatric research continue to debate the finer points of this diagnosis. However, atypical depression is usually characterized by onset of symptoms at an early age, overeating, oversleeping, and mood reactivity. Mood reactivity refers to the observation that although people with atypical depression experience pervasive sadness, mood may improve or worsen in direct response to specific events. This is different from classically depressed individuals who experience persistent sadness. In addition, some research suggests that an older class of drugs, monoamine oxidase inhibitors (MAOIs), may be more effective in treating atypical depression than are newer drugs, including tricyclic antidepressants and selective serotonin reuptake inhibitors (SSRIs). However, research continues to try to define this more clearly. Atypical depression is more common in women than in men. Its exact cause isn't clear, but genetics and environmental factors play roles. If you're concerned that you or someone you know has atypical depression, seek help from a mental health professional.

❑ Pregnenolone is a naturally occurring hormone that may improve brain function, enhancing mood, memory, and thinking ability. (*See under* NATURAL FOOD SUPPLEMENTS in Part One.)

❑ Depression is not a natural part of aging, but it is frequently linked to age-related nutritional problems, such as B-vitamin deficiencies and poor eating habits. Older people who suffer from depression are as likely to benefit from treatment as a person in any other age bracket.

❑ Tyrosine is needed for brain function. This amino acid is directly involved in the production of norepinephrine and dopamine, two vital neurotransmitters that are synthesized in the brain and the adrenal medulla. A lack of tyrosine can result in a deficiency of norepinephrine in certain sites in the brain, resulting in mood disorders such as depression. The effects of stress may be prevented or reversed if this essential amino acid is obtained in the diet or by means of supplements. Mustard greens, beans, and spinach are good sources of tyrosine.

Caution: If you are taking an MAO inhibitor drug for depression, do not take tyrosine supplements, and avoid foods containing tyrosine, as drug and dietary interactions can cause a sudden, dangerous rise in blood pressure. Discuss food and medicine limitations thoroughly with your health care provider or a qualified dietitian.

❑ Some preliminary studies show promise in using dehydroepiandrosterone (DHEA)—a hormone naturally produced by the body—in the treatment of depression. In one study, nearly all patients taking DHEA for six weeks significantly improved, and about half of those were no longer considered clinically depressed.

Categories of Antidepressant Drugs

Following is a quick reference guide to the major categories of antidepressant medications currently in use, according to their mode of action and including both generic and brand names.

CATEGORY OF ANTIDEPRESSANT	GENERIC NAME	BRAND NAME(S)
Serotonin transport blocker (selective serotonin reuptake inhibitor or SSRI)	citalopram escitalopram fluoxetine paroxetine sertraline	Celexa Lexapro Prozac Paxil Zoloft
Tricyclic	amitriptyline amoxapine clomipramine desipramine doxepin imipramine nortriptyline trimipramine	Elavil Asendin Anafranil Norpramin Sinequan Tofranil Aventyl Pamelor Surmontil
Serotonin and norepinephrine reuptake inhibitor (SNRI)	venlafaxine duloxetine	Effexor Cymbalta
Monoamine oxidase inhibitor (MAOI)	isocarboxazid phenelzine tranylcypromine	Marplan Nardil Parnate
Tetracyclic	mirtazapine maprotiline	Remeron Ludiomil
Aminoketone	bupropion	Wellbutrin
Other	trazodone	Desyrel

❑ Selenium has been shown to elevate mood and decrease anxiety. These effects were more noticeable in people who had lower levels of selenium in their diets to begin with.

❑ Vigorous exercise can be an effective antidote to bouts of depression. During exercise, the brain produces pain-killing chemicals called endorphins and enkephalins. Certain endorphins and other brain chemicals released in response to exercise also produce a natural "high." Most of those who exercise regularly say that they feel really good afterward. This may explain why exercise is the best way to get rid of depression.

❑ Music can have powerful effects on mood and may be useful in alleviating depression. (*See* MUSIC AND SOUND THERAPY in Part Three.)

❑ In one study, people suffering from depression were found to have lower than normal levels of folic acid in their blood than nondepressed individuals. Other studies have shown that zinc levels tend to be significantly lower than normal when people suffer from depression.

❏ It may be possible to diagnose depression by using a computerized tomography (CAT) scan to measure a person's adrenal glands. Researchers at Duke University found that people suffering from clinical depression have larger adrenal glands than non-depressed people.

❏ A variety of different drugs are commonly prescribed to treat depression (see chart above). Antidepressant drugs fight depression by changing the balance of neurotransmitters in the body. These medications include the following:

- *Selective serotonin reuptake inhibitors (SSRIs).* A popular class of drugs known as "second-generation" antidepressants that have become available in recent years. These new drugs have not been shown to be more effective than the others, but they tend to have fewer serious side effects. They include fluoxetine (Prozac), paroxetine (Paxil), and sertraline (Zoloft), which specifically block the uptake of the neurotransmitter serotonin.

- *Tricyclics.* These drugs work by inhibiting the uptake of the neurotransmitters serotonin, norepinephrine, and dopamine, making more of the mood-enhancing chemical messengers available to nerve cells. Examples include amitriptyline (Elavil), desipramine (Norpramin), imipramine (Tofranil), amoxapine (Asendin), and nortriptyline (Aventyl, Pamelor). Possible side effects include blurred vision, constipation, dry mouth, irregular heartbeat, urine retention, and orthostatic hypotension, a severe drop in blood pressure upon sitting up or standing, which can lead to dizziness, falls, and fractures.

- *Serotonin and norepinephrine reuptake inhibitors (SNRIs).* These drugs increase the levels of both serotonin and norepinephrine by inhibiting their reabsorption (reuptake) into cells in the brain. Although the precise mechanism of action isn't clear, it's thought that these higher levels enhance neurotransmission—the sending of nerve impulses—and so improve and elevate mood. Medications in this group of antidepressants are sometimes called dual reuptake inhibitors. Examples include venlafaxine (Effexor) and duloxetine (Cymbalta).

- *Monoamine oxidase (MAO) inhibitors.* These drugs increase the amounts of mood-enhancing neurotransmitters in the brain by blocking the action of the enzyme monoamine oxidase, which normally breaks them down. Examples of MAO inhibitors include isocarboxazid (Marplan), phenelzine (Nardil), and tranylcypromine (Parnate). Possible side effects include agitation, elevated blood pressure, overstimulation, and changes in heart rate and rhythm. MAO inhibitors also have a high potential for dangerous interactions with other substances, including drugs and foods. Persons taking these drugs must adhere strictly to a diet that includes no foods containing the amino acid tyrosine. Refer to the detailed insert given out with the drug for details of the possible interactions. Over-the-counter cold and allergy remedies must also be avoided.

- *Tetracyclics.* These drugs have an action similar to that of the tricyclics, but have a slightly different chemical structure and appear to cause fewer side effects. Maprotiline (Ludiomil) and mirtazapine (Remeron) are in this category.

- Another drug, buproprion (Wellbutrin), is believed to act by inhibiting the uptake of dopamine but not serotonin or norepinephrine.

❏ Paxil (paroxetine) has been approved by the FDA for treatment of generalized anxiety disorders (GAD). The drug is already approved for treating social anxiety disorder, depression, panic disorder, and obsessive-compulsive disorder. GAD affects about 6.8 million adult Americans, and about twice as many women as men, according to the National Institute of Mental Health. People with GAD experience exaggerated, worrisome thoughts and tension about routine life events, lasting a minimum of six months. GAD is often accompanied by physical symptoms such as fatigue, trembling, muscle tension, headache, and nausea. The effectiveness of Paxil in long-term treatment of GAD (greater than eight weeks) was not evaluated, nor was Paxil studied in children and adolescents with GAD.

Caution: Paxil should not be used in children and adolescents for the treatment of major depressive disorder. Antidepressants in adults and children should be used with caution. Never discontinue use of antidepressants without first consulting a physician.

❏ Steroid drugs and oral contraceptives may cause serotonin levels in the brain to drop.

❏ Prozac and other "selective serotonin reuptake inhibitors" work to increase the activity of serotonin, while 5-hydroxy L-tryptophan (5-HTP) works to boost the body's production of serotonin.

❏ A study published in the *British Medical Journal* indicates that extracts of St. John's wort may be as effective as prescription antidepressants for mild and moderate depression. St. John's wort is the most-prescribed antidepressant in Germany, but is treated as a dietary supplement in the United States (it is not approved as a safe and effective drug by the FDA). Many studies are under way to determine the effectiveness and safety of long-term use of St. John's wort. Research published recently in the *British Medical Journal* indicates that, in a German study where St. John's wort was matched against Paxil, the supplement proved to be just as effective and subjects had fewer side effects.

In some patients with HIV, using St. John's wort and SSRIs may not be a good idea. It is expected that St John's wort may significantly decrease blood concentrations of all of the currently marketed HIV protease inhibitors (PIs) and possibly other drugs (to varying degrees) that are similarly metabolized, including the nonnucleoside reverse transcriptase inhibitors (NNRTIs).

Caution: St. John's wort may cause increased sensitivity to sunlight. It may also produce anxiety, gastrointestinal symptoms, and headaches. It can interact with some drugs including antidepressants, birth control pills, and anticoagulants.

❏ People who smoke are more likely than nonsmokers to be depressed. Smokers and nonsmokers alike may benefit from Zyban (a sustained-release preparation of buproprion, also sold as Wellbutrin SR), an antidepressant also approved to help people quit smoking. Buproprion elevates levels of dopamine and norepinephrine, substances that are also elevated by nicotine in tobacco products. It allows patients to obtain the same feeling while weaning themselves off nicotine.

❏ Allergies, hypoglycemia, hypothyroidism, and/or malabsorption problems can cause or contribute to depression. In people with these conditions, vitamin B_{12} and folic acid are blocked from entering the system, which can lead to depression.

❏ Individuals with depression are more likely than other people to have various disturbances in calcium metabolism.

❏ There is no doubt that attitude affects health. Study after study has shown that optimistic people are not only happier but also healthier. They suffer less illness, recover better from illness and surgery, and have stronger immune defenses.

❏ Many groups and organizations offer more information on depression. (*See* Health and Medical Organizations in the Appendix.)

DERMATITIS

Dermatitis is a general term for any type of inflammation of the skin. Types of dermatitis include atopic dermatitis, nummular dermatitis, seborrheic dermatitis, irritant contact dermatitis, and allergic contact dermatitis. The distinction between the use of dermatitis and eczema to describe skin disorders can be confusing. Often, the terms are used interchangeably, although many people use the term eczema to refer specifically to atopic dermatitis. The inflammation of the skin that accompanies dermatitis (or eczema) produces scaling, flaking, thickening, weeping, crusting, color changes, and, often, itching.

Several underlying problems can lead to eczema. Hypochlorhydria (low levels of hydrochloric acid in the stomach) has been cited, as has a condition known as "leaky gut syndrome," in which the intestines become porous and allow tiny particles of undigested food to enter the bloodstream, provoking allergic reactions. Candidiasis (an overgrowth of yeast in the system), food allergies, and a genetically based weakness in the enzyme delta-6-desaturase (which converts essential fatty acids into anti-inflammatory prostaglandins) are other possible causes of this condition.

Many cases of dermatitis are simply the result of allergies. This type of condition is called allergic contact dermatitis. Skin inflammation may be linked to contact with perfumes, cosmetics, rubber, medicated creams and ointments, latex, plants such as poison ivy, and/or metals or metal alloys such as gold, silver, and nickel found in jewelry or zippers. Some people with dermatitis are sensitive to sunlight. Whatever the irritant, if the skin remains in constant contact with it, the dermatitis is likely to spread and become more severe. Stress, especially chronic tension, can cause or exacerbate dermatitis.

Atopic dermatitis (AD; also known as atopic eczema or, in children, infantile eczema) is a condition known to affect allergy-prone individuals. It typically appears on the face, in the bends of the elbows, and behind the knees, and is very itchy. In children, it usually appears in the first year of life, and almost always in the first five years. Over half of the infants who have this condition get better by the age of eighteen months. Triggers vary from person to person, but tend to include cold or hot weather, a dry atmosphere, and exposure to allergens, stress, and infections such as colds. If other family members have histories of hay fever, asthma, or atopic dermatitis, it is more likely that a child will be diagnosed with AD. Women who take probiotics during pregnancy have had some success at reducing AD in their infants.

Nummular ("coin-shaped") dermatitis is a chronic condition in which round, scaling lesions appear on the limbs. It may be caused by an allergy to nickel and is often associated with dry skin. Dermatitis herpetiformis is a very itchy type of dermatitis associated with intestinal and immune disorders. This form of dermatitis may be triggered by the consumption of dairy products and/or gluten. Seborrhea is a form of dermatitis that most commonly affects the scalp and/or face.

Unless otherwise specified, the dosages recommended here are for adults. For a child between the ages of twelve and seventeen, reduce the dose to three-quarters of the recommended amount. For a child between six and twelve, use one-half of the recommended dose, and for a child under the age of six, use one-quarter of the recommended amount.

NUTRIENTS

SUPPLEMENT	SUGGESTED DOSAGE	COMMENTS
Essential		
Betaine HCl	As directed on label.	A form of hydrochloric acid. People with dermatitis often have low levels of hydrochloric acid. *Caution:* Do not take this supplement if you suffer from stomach acidity.
OptiMSM	As directed on label.	A patented form of methylsulfonylmethane. Reduces inflammation and contains a natural analgesic.

Vitamin B complex	50–100 mg of each major B vitamin 3 times daily, with meals (amounts of individual vitamins in a complex will vary).	Needed for healthy skin and proper circulation. Aids in reproduction of all cells. Use a high-stress, yeast-free formula. A sublingual form is recommended.
plus extra vitamin B$_3$ (niacin)	100 mg 3 times daily. Do not exceed this amount.	Important for proper circulation and healthy skin. Caution: Do not take niacin if you have a liver disorder, gout, or high blood pressure.
and vitamin B$_6$ (pyridoxine)	50 mg 3 times daily.	Deficiency has been linked to skin disorders.
and vitamin B$_{12}$	1,000–2,000 mcg daily.	Aids in cell formation and cellular longevity. Use a lozenge or sublingual form.
and biotin	300 mg daily.	Deficiency has been linked to dermatitis.

Important

Essential fatty acids (black currant seed oil, flaxseed oil, primrose oil, or salmon oil)	As directed on label.	Promotes lubrication of the skin.
Kelp	1,000 mg daily or as directed on label.	Contains iodine and other minerals needed for healing of tissues.
Vitamin C with bioflavonoids	As directed on label.	Inhibits inflammation and stabilizes cell membranes.
Vitamin E	200 IU daily.	Relieves itching and dryness. Use d-alpha-tocopherol form.
Zinc	100 mg daily. Do not exceed this amount.	Aids healing and enhances immune function. Use zinc gluconate lozenges or OptiZinc for best absorption.

Helpful

Aller Bee-Gone from CC Pollen	As directed on label.	For allergic dermatitis. A combination of herbs, enzymes, and nutrients designed to fight allergic flare-ups.
Borage oil and flaxseed oil	As directed on label.	Contain omega-6 and omega-3 essential fatty acids.
Coenzyme Q$_{10}$ plus Coenzyme A from Coenzyme-A Technologies	As directed on label. As directed on label.	Removes toxins from the body, boosts the immune system, improves overall physical and mental processes.
Free form amino acid (Amino Balance from Anabol Naturals)	As directed on label, on an empty stomach.	To supply protein, important for construction and repair of all tissues. Use a formula containing both essential and nonessential amino acids.
Herpanacine from Diamond-Herpanacine Associates	As directed on label.	Contains antioxidants, amino acids, and herbs that promote overall skin health.
Kyo-Dophilus from Wakunaga	As directed on label.	A nondairy probiotic formula. Prevents the overgrowth of yeasts in the body.

Kyolic-EPA from Wakunaga	As directed on label.	Restores fatty acid balance. Repairs tissue and aids in healing.
Shark cartilage	1 gram per 15 lbs of body weight daily, divided into 3 doses.	Reduces inflammation in eczema.
Vitamin A emulsion or capsules	100,000 IU daily for 1 month, then 50,000 IU daily for 2 weeks, then reduce to 25,000 IU daily. If you are pregnant, do not exceed 10,000 IU daily. 5,000 IU daily.	Needed for smooth skin. Aids in preventing dryness. Use emulsion form for easier assimilation and greater safety at high doses.
plus carotenoid complex	25,000 IU daily.	Antioxidants and precursors of vitamin A.
Vitamin D	400–1,000 IU daily.	Aids in healing of tissues.

Herbs

❑ Blackthorn, blueberry leaf, hawthorn berry, and rue contain flavonoids that are excellent for reducing inflammation.

❑ Chamomile can be taken internally or used to soothe the skin. It reduces inflammation.

Caution: Do not use chamomile if you are allergic to ragweed. Do not use during pregnancy or nursing. It may interact with warfarin or cyclosporine, so patients using these drugs should avoid it.

❑ Poultices combining dandelion and yellow dock root can be helpful. (*See* USING A POULTICE in Part Three.)

❑ The following herbs can be used in tea or capsule form: dandelion, goldenseal, myrrh, pau d'arco, and red clover. Alternate them for best results.

Caution: Do not take goldenseal internally on a daily basis for more than one week at a time. Do not use it during pregnancy or if you are breast-feeding, and use with caution if you are allergic to ragweed. If you have a history of cardiovascular disease, diabetes, or glaucoma, use it only under a doctor's supervision.

❑ To relieve itching and promote healing, mix goldenseal root powder with vitamin E oil, then add a little honey until it is the consistency of a loose paste. Apply this mixture to the affected area.

❑ Gotu kola contains powerful antioxidants and promotes the formation of lipids and proteins that are essential for healthy skin.

❑ Grape seed extract contains oligomeric proanthocyanadins (OPCs), which reduce inflammation and rid the body of toxins.

❑ Oregon grape root detoxifies the body and reduces inflammation.

❑ Wild pansy (*Viola tricolor*) can be used externally to treat bruises and various skin ailments. It is especially good against psoriasis and acne and can be used on eczema and cradle cap in infants.

Recommendations

❑ Add brown rice and millet to your diet.

❑ Avoid eggs, peanuts, soy foods, wheat, and dairy products.

❑ Avoid sugar, strawberries, chocolate, white flour, fats, fried foods, and processed foods.

❑ Try a gluten-free diet for six weeks, then add gluten-containing foods back to the diet one at a time, and see if the condition changes. A gluten-free diet is often of therapeutic benefit in controlling dermatitis. (See CELIAC DISEASE in Part Two for the recommended diet.)

❑ Do not eat foods containing raw eggs, which contain avidin, a protein that binds to biotin and prevents it from being absorbed. Biotin is needed for skin and scalp disorders.

❑ Try keeping your house humidified and take fewer showers and baths. Showers and baths deplete the skin of its natural oils.

❑ Use a perfume-free moisturizing lotion daily.

❑ For dermatitis of the scalp, make a strong, concentrated tea of rosemary, comfrey, tea tree oil (add the tea tree oil after the tea is made), dried nettles, and witch hazel, and apply it to the scalp after shampooing with a fragrance-free shampoo. Leave it on the scalp for ten or fifteen minutes.

❑ Massage tea tree oil antiseptic cream into the skin after contact with water or irritants.

❑ Keep the colon clean. Use a fiber supplement such as flaxseed, psyllium husk, or ABC Aerobic Bulk Cleanse from Aerobic Life Industries daily. Use occasional cleansing enemas for removing toxins for quicker healing. (See COLON CLEANSING and/or ENEMAS in Part Three.)

Note: Always take supplemental fiber separately from other supplements and medications.

Considerations

❑ Chemicals used in bubble bath products may cause dermatitis and may even irritate the tissues of the lower urinary tract sufficiently to cause bloody urine. This is most likely to occur if you soak in treated bathwater for too long.

❑ Primrose oil and vitamin B₆ (pyridoxine) have helped infants with dermatitis.

❑ Food allergies can cause dermatitis. (See ALLERGIES in Part Two.)

❑ See also FUNGAL INFECTION; HIVES; POISON IVY/POISON OAK/POISON SUMAC; PSORIASIS; ROSACEA; SCABIES; and/or SEBORRHEA, all in Part Two.

DETACHED RETINA

See DIMNESS OR LOSS OF VISION under EYE PROBLEMS.

DIABETES

Diabetes is a disease in which the body either does not produce or cannot properly use the pancreatic hormone insulin. Insulin controls the amount of glucose (sugar) in the blood and the rate at which glucose is absorbed into the cells. The cells need glucose to produce energy. Furthermore, the brain's only food is glucose; therefore the level of glucose must be maintained at a certain minimum for the brain to function normally. After eating a meal that contains carbohydrate or protein, the blood sugar normally rises, often to between 120 and 130 milligrams per decaliter (mg/dL), but generally not above 140 mg/dL. This increase triggers a release of insulin from cells in the pancreas called beta-cells. The insulin "opens the doors" of cells throughout the body, allowing glucose to enter them. As glucose enters the cells, the blood sugar level falls back toward normal and the release of insulin tapers off until the next time protein or carbohydrates are eaten. Every day, every hour, blood sugar levels vary, even in people who do not have diabetes. If blood sugar falls too low (hypoglycemia), a person's ability to reason can become impaired. If blood sugar is too high (hyperglycemia), the person has diabetes.

In people with diabetes, glucose builds up in the bloodstream instead of being taken into and used by the cells, leading to hyperglycemia. If it is not properly controlled, diabetes can lead to heart disease, kidney disease, edema, nerve damage, and infections of the mouth, gums, lungs, skin, feet, bladder, and genital areas. Skin sores may develop and fail to heal properly.

According to figures published by the American Diabetes Association (ADA), there are 23.6 million people in the United States with diabetes. The total prevalence of diabetes increased 13.5 percent from 2005 to 2007. Twenty-four percent of diabetes is undiagnosed, down from 30 percent in 2005 and from 50 percent ten years ago. About 57 million people have impaired fasting glucose (IFG) levels or pre-diabetes. More people are developing diabetes or IFG because of an increase in obesity and longer life spans. This disease is the seventh leading cause of death in the United States and the primary cause of new cases of blindness in people between the ages of twenty and seventy-four. The death rate for African-Americans with diabetes is 50 percent higher than the death rate for Caucasians who have the disease. Unfortunately, two-thirds of the people diagnosed with diabetes do not associate the disease with an increased risk of cardiovascular problems, such as heart disease and stroke. To someone with diabetes, controlling blood sugar must be done in conjunction with controlling cholesterol and blood pressure.

There are two major types of diabetes: type 1 (or insulin-dependent diabetes mellitus [IDDM]) and type 2 (non-insulin-dependent diabetes mellitus [NIDDM]).

Type 1 diabetes affects 5 to 10 percent of people with diabetes and usually starts at an early age. It is an autoimmune disease in which the body's immune system attacks and destroys the insulin-producing beta-cells in the pancreas. Experts believe this may result from an immune response after a viral infection or something related to nutrition.

Type 2 diabetes, by far the most common form of diabetes, affects 90 to 95 percent of diabetes sufferers. In type 2 diabetes, the pancreas does produce insulin in small quantities, but not enough to fuel the cells. The cells may also become resistant to the effects of what little insulin there is in the bloodstream. Many people have type 2 diabetes and are completely unaware of it. This type of diabetes usually begins in later years, although, unfortunately, it is now becoming more common in young people. The first clinical study sponsored by the National Institute of Diabetes and Digestive and Kidney Diseases (NIDDK) has begun in twelve medical centers around the country. The five-year study, called Treatment Options for type 2 Diabetes in Adolescents and Youth (TODAY), will compare three treatments of type 2 diabetes in children and teens to determine how well and how long each treatment approach controls blood glucose levels. The treatments will involve FDA-approved drugs and lifestyle changes. TODAY is the first clinical study aimed at showing the effects of lowering weight by cutting calories and increasing physical activity in youths with type 2 diabetes. It is now recognized that obesity and type 2 diabetes are among the most serious health challenges facing America's youth. During the last forty years, the percentage of overweight children (ages six to nineteen) in the United States has gone from 4 percent to 16 percent.

Known risk factors for type 2 diabetes include being overweight or obese; having a parent or sibling with diabetes; being Alaskan Native, American Indian, African American, Hispanic/Latino, Asian American, or Pacific Islander; having had gestational diabetes or having given birth to a baby over nine pounds; blood pressure of 140/90 mm/Hg or higher; abnormal cholesterol, including levels of HDL ("good") cholesterol less than 35 mg/dL and triglycerides of 250 mg/dL or higher; inactivity, defined as exercising fewer than three times per week; having polycystic ovary disease; having had a previous test showing impaired fasting glucose (IFG) or impaired glucose tolerance (IGT); clinical signs of insulin resistance like acanthosis nigricans (dark rash around the neck); and a history of heart disease. Epidemiological data from around the world show that the United States is not the only area that has this problem. Within the next thirty years, diabetes is projected to increase the most in the Middle East Crescent (163 percent); Sub-Saharan Africa (161 percent); Latin America, the Caribbean, and Asia (not including China and India) (148 percent); India (151 percent); China (104 percent); and overall around the world (114 percent).

Gestational diabetes is a form of the condition that develops during pregnancy, affecting about 5 percent of pregnant women. Hormonal changes during pregnancy can affect the body's resistance to insulin. Although this form of diabetes usually goes away after the baby is born, a woman who has had it is more likely to develop type 2 diabetes later in life.

Pre-diabetes is a condition in which blood glucose levels are higher than normal but not high enough for a diagnosis of diabetes. This condition is sometimes called impaired fasting glucose (IFG) or impaired glucose tolerance (IGT), depending on the test used to diagnose it. The U.S. Department of Health and Human Services estimates that about one in four U.S. adults aged twenty years or older—or 57 million people—had pre-diabetes in 2007. However, many people with IFG go on to develop type 2 diabetes. According to the American Diabetes Association, people with pre-diabetes can prevent or delay the development of type 2 diabetes by up to 58 percent through changes to their lifestyle that include modest weight loss and regular exercise. The expert panel recommends that people with pre-diabetes reduce their weight by 5 to 10 percent and participate in some type of modest physical activity for thirty minutes daily. For some people with pre-diabetes, intervening early can actually return elevated blood glucose levels to the normal range.

People with diabetes are subject to episodes of both high and low blood sugar. The symptoms of hyperglycemia (too much glucose in the blood) often include fatigue, a constant need to urinate, extreme thirst, constantly feeling hungry, loss of weight, and problems with eyesight. Episodes of hypoglycemia (less than normal amounts of glucose in the blood), which strike suddenly, can be caused by a missed meal, too much exercise, or a reaction to too much insulin.

The initial signs of hypoglycemia are hunger, dizziness, sweating, confusion, palpitations, and numbness or tingling of the lips. If not treated, the individual may go on to experience double vision, trembling, and disorientation, may act strangely, and may eventually lapse into a coma.

At present there is no cure for type 1 or type 2 diabetes. However, for people with type 2 diabetes, it is possible to reduce dependence on medications and diminish the effect of the disease on the body through weight loss and exercise. The major danger with diabetes is not the disease itself, but the complications that can arise if insulin levels are not maintained at a constant level. Consistently high blood sugar levels can, over time, lead to blindness, kidney failure, heart disease, limb amputations, and nerve damage. In fact, diabetes is the leading cause of blindness in adults between the ages of twenty and seventy-four, and it accounts for 44 percent of the people who have kidney failure. Cardiovascular disease is two to four times more common among people with diabetes, and is the leading cause of diabetes-related deaths. The risk of stroke is also two to four times higher in people with diabetes, and 73 percent have high blood pressure as well. Left untreated, diabetes can lead to diabetic ketoacidosis (DKA) or hyperosmolar syndrome. DKA occurs when the body is so low in insulin that it starts using stored fat as fuel. When this fat breaks down, substances known as ketones are produced as a by-product. In large quantities, ketones can cause the body to become excessively acidic. DKA is most often seen in people with type 1 diabetes. Symptoms include nausea, difficulty breathing, sweet breath, and confusion that can progress to coma. Hyperosmolar syndrome is a result of a combination of very high blood sugar levels (but without the presence of ketones) and dehydration. It is more common in older people with type 2 diabetes who are taking steroid medications. The condition may also be prompted by stress from a major illness. With hyperosmolar syndrome, blood sugar levels are so high that the blood thickens. Symptoms include confusion, tiredness, and coma. Hyperosmolar syndrome can sometimes be the first indication of diabetes in older adults. Both of these conditions require the immediate attention of a physician. Urinalysis can often detect unsuspected diabetes.

Monitoring blood sugar levels is a key component in treatment and management of the disease. Research has indicated that people who keep their blood sugar levels within individual target ranges set by their doctor stand a good chance of reducing the risk of associated complications. In many cases, intensive lifestyle changes in diet and exercise actually can prevent, reduce, or delay the risk of developing adult-onset diabetes.

Diabetes Self-Tests

There are several ways to test yourself for diabetes. The tests for type 1 diabetes are also used for self-monitoring by persons diagnosed with the condition. Home testing tends to be slightly less accurate than tests done in a doctor's office.

Type 1 Diabetes

To test for type 1 diabetes:

1. Purchase chemically treated plastic glucose testing strips at a drugstore.

2. Prick your finger and apply a drop of blood to the tip of the strip.

3. Wait one minute and compare the color on the strip to a color chart, which lists various glucose levels.

There are also electronic devices available that can analyze the test strip for you and give you a numerical readout of the glucose level. There are now more than a hundred different home-testing-type instruments available for testing blood glucose levels. Many of these devices are available free or have large rebates attached if you have a doctor's prescription. You simply prick your finger with the spring-loaded needle, apply a drop of your blood to the test strip, and place it in the machine for analysis. This test gives you an immediate blood sugar result and stores the result in memory for future reference. It is a device that all people with diabetes should own.

The following is an approximate guideline for fasting blood sugar levels for people who have not been diagnosed with diabetes. Fasting blood sugar levels should be measured from six to eight hours after eating. The measurement is milligrams of glucose per one-tenth liter (mg/dL) of blood:

- Less than 109 mg/dL: Normal

- 110–125 mg/dL: Fasting blood glucose/borderline, pre-diabetes

- 126 mg/dL and over: Diabetes

If you test at random, a number of 200 mg/dL or higher is considered diabetes when coupled with other signs of diabetes such as excessive thirst, unplanned weight loss, or fatigue. (*See* QUICK REFERENCE GUIDE—GOALS FOR PEOPLE WITH DIABETES, on page 375.)

There is another test that is used normally as a diabetes management tool rather than a screening test. This is the hemoglobin A1c lab test. It is based on the notion that sugar is sticky, and the longer it is around the harder it is to get off. The red blood cells in the bloodstream usually live for about three months, circulating around the body all that time. As they circulate, blood sugar sticks to them, and if it can be measured, it will tell how much sugar has been in the blood over the life of these cells, or about three months. The normal range for this test is 4 to 5.9 percent, but people can have 8 percent or above if they have poorly controlled diabetes. Those whose diabetes is under control usually have about a 7 percent or lower reading. There is a correlation between average blood sugar levels in mg/dL and A1c, as follows:

- A1c of 6: 135 mg/dL

- A1c of 7: 170 mg/dL

- A1c of 8: 205 mg/dL

- A1c of 9: 240 mg/dL

- A1c of 10: 275 mg/dL

- A1c of 11: 310 mg/dL

- A1c of 12: 345 mg/dL

Type 2 Diabetes

Testing for type 2 diabetes should begin at age forty-five. Younger people should get tested if they are overweight or have one of these risk factors:

- Physically inactive.

- Have a parent or sibling with diabetes.

- Are African American, Alaskan Native, American Indian, Asian American, Hispanic/Latino, or Pacific Islander.

- Have blood pressure of 140/90 or above.

- Have good cholesterol that is too low (less than 35 mg/dL).

- Have a history of heart disease.

People with type 2 diabetes often cannot perceive sweet tastes. This abnormality may play an important role in how individuals with diabetes perceive the taste of their food, and also in how well they comply with the dietary aspects of treatment. Because our society as a whole is addicted to sugar, this distorted taste perception is very common among the population in general.

The following test can detect an impaired ability to taste sweets:

1. Do not consume stimulants (coffee, tea, soda) or sweets for one hour before the test.

2. Fill seven identical glasses with 8 ounces of water each and label the glasses as having no sugar, ¼ teaspoon sugar, ½ teaspoon sugar, 1 teaspoon sugar, 1½ teaspoons sugar, 2 teaspoons sugar, and 3 teaspoons sugar. Add the appropriate amount of sugar to each glass, then ask someone else to rearrange the order of the glasses and hide the labels.

3. Take a straw and sip from each glass, then write down the amount of sugar you think it contains. Between sips, rinse your mouth with pure water. Healthy people generally notice a sweet taste when a teaspoon or less of sugar is added to 8 ounces of water. By contrast, people with adult-onset diabetes usually do not notice sweetness until 1½ to 2 teaspoons of sugar have been added to the water.

Unless otherwise specified, the dosages recommended here are for adults. For a child between the ages of twelve and seventeen, reduce the dose to three-quarters the recommended amount. For a child between six and twelve, use one-half the recommended dose, and for a child under the age of six, use one-quarter the recommended amount.

NUTRIENTS

SUPPLEMENT	SUGGESTED DOSAGE	COMMENTS
Essential		
Alpha-lipoic acid	As directed on label.	For treatment of peripheral nerve damage in diabetic patients. Helps control blood sugar levels.
Chromium picolinate or Diabetic Nutrition Rx from Progressive Research Labs or brewer's yeast	400–600 mcg daily. As directed on label. As directed on label.	Improves insulin's efficiency, which lowers blood sugar levels. A combination of chromium picolinate, vanadyl sulfate, and other vitamins and minerals that work synergistically to regulate blood sugar levels
with added chromium		and correct deficiencies. *Caution:* If you have diabetes, consult with your physician before taking any supplement containing chromium.
Garlic (Kyolic from Wakunaga)	As directed on label.	Decreases and stabilizes blood sugar levels. Enhances immunity and improves circulation.
L-carnitine plus L-glutamine plus taurine	500 mg twice daily, on an empty stomach. Take with water. Do not take with milk. Take with 50 mg vitamin B_6 and 100 mg vitamin C for better absorption. 500 mg twice daily, on an empty stomach. 500 mg twice daily, on an empty stomach.	Mobilizes fat. Reduces the craving for sugars. Aids in the release of insulin.
Quercetin (Activated Quercetin from Source Naturals)	100 mg 3 times daily.	Helps protect the membranes of the lens of the eyes from accumulations of polyols as a result of high glucose levels.
Raw adrenal glandular and raw pancreas glandular and thyroid glandular	As directed on label. As directed on label. As directed on label.	Aids in rebuilding and nourishing these organs. (*See* GLANDULAR THERAPY in Part Three.)
Vanadium	As directed on label.	Aids insulin's ability to move glucose into the cells. Use vanadyl sulfate form.
Vitamin B complex plus extra biotin and inositol	50 mg of each major B vitamin 3 times daily (amounts of individual vitamins in a complex will vary). Do not exceed 300 mg daily from all supplements. 50 mg daily. 50 mg daily.	The B vitamins work best when taken together. Improves the metabolism of glucose. Important for circulation and for prevention of atherosclerosis.
Vitamin B_{12} plus folic acid	As prescribed by physician or directed on label.	Needed to prevent diabetic neuropathy. Injections (under a doctor's supervision) are best. If injections are not available, use a lozenge or sublingual form.
Zinc	50–80 mg daily. Do not exceed a total of 100 mg daily from all supplements.	Deficiency has been associated with diabetes. Use zinc gluconate lozenges or OptiZinc for best absorption.
Very Important		
Coenzyme Q_{10} plus Coenzyme A from Coenzyme-A Technologies	80 mg daily. As directed on label.	Improves circulation and stabilizes blood sugar. Works well with coenzyme Q_{10} in protecting the cells and removing toxic substances from the body.

Magnesium	750 mg daily.	Important for enzyme systems and pH balance. Protects against coronary artery spasm in arteriosclerosis. Increases energy levels. Low readings of magnesium are often found in people with diabetes, and are associated with the complications of eye disease. Those who eat a healthy diet rich in foods with magnesium such as whole grains and nuts are less likely to develop diabetes.
Manganese	5–10 mg daily. Take separately from calcium.	Needed for repair of the pancreas. Also a cofactor in key enzymes of glucose metabolism. Deficiency is common in people with diabetes.
Psyllium husks or ABC Aerobic Bulk Cleanse from Aerobic Life Industries	As directed on label. Take with a large glass of water. Take separately from other supplements and medications.	Good fiber source and fat mobilizer.
Vitamin D	400–800 IU.	Helps maintain good blood flow in patients with diabetes who live in northern climates.
Important		
Vitamin A with carotenoids	15,000 IU daily. If you are pregnant, do not exceed 10,000 IU daily.	An important antioxidant needed to maintain the health of the eyes. Use emulsion form for best absorption.
Vitamin C with bioflavonoids	3,000–6,000 mg daily.	Deficiency may lead to vascular problems in people with diabetes. Vitamin C may slow or prevent complications that occur in diabetes.
Vitamin E	200 IU daily.	Improves circulation and prevents complications through its antioxidant properties. Use d-alpha-tocopherol form.
Helpful		
Calcium	1,500 mg daily.	Important for pH balance. Always take calcium with vitamin D. The combination at levels near or slightly above the DRI has been shown to prevent diabetes. Be sure to get calcium and vitamin D from foods (dairy products are the best sources of both) and supplements.
Copper complex	As directed on label.	Aids in protein metabolism and in many enzyme systems.
Maitake extract	1–4 gm (1,000–4,000 mg) daily.	May help to normalize blood sugar levels.
Multienzyme complex plus proteolytic enzymes	As directed on label. Take with meals. As directed on label. Take between meals.	To aid digestion. Proper digestion is essential in management of diabetes.
Pantethine	As directed on label.	A form of pantothenic acid that reduces LDL cholesterol and helps prevent buildup in the arteries.
Pycnogenol or grape seed extract	As directed on label. As directed on label.	Contains powerful antioxidants that also enhance the activity of vitamin C and strengthen connective tissue, including that of the cardiovascular system.

Herbs

❏ Beanpod tea, made up of kidney, white, navy, lima, and northern beans, detoxifies the pancreas.

❏ Bitter melon (*Momordica charantia*), gudmar (*Gymnema sylvestre*), and gulvel (*Tinospora cordifo*) are herbal remedies used in Ayurvedic medicine to regulate blood sugar levels.

❏ Cedar berries are excellent nourishment for the pancreas.

❏ Dandelion root protects the liver, which converts nutrients into glucose.

Note: If you suffer from gallbladder problems, avoid large quantities of dandelion.

❏ Fenugreek seeds have been shown to reduce cholesterol and blood sugar levels. They can be purchased under the brand name Sugar-Down.

❏ Ginseng tea is believed to lower blood sugar levels.

Caution: Do not use ginseng if you have high blood pressure, or are pregnant or nursing.

❏ Huckleberry helps to promote insulin production.

❏ Juniper berries have been found to lower blood glucose levels.

❏ In the premier diabetes medical journal, *Diabetes Care*, a review summary of 108 individual studies was published on herbal use in diabetic patients. The best herbs to control blood sugar according to the study were *Coccinia indica* and American ginseng. Other supplements included *Gymnema sylvestre*, aloe vera, vanadium, *Momordica charantia*, and nopal.

Caution: Do not use ginseng if you have high blood pressure, or are pregnant or nursing.

❏ Silymarin (200 mg per day) taken with a regular diabetes medication (glibenclamide) resulted in a reduction in fasting blood sugars as well as postprandial glucose levels. In addition, the patients lost weight and had improvements in the hemoglobin A1c.

❏ Other herbs that may be beneficial for diabetes include bilberry, buchu, goldenseal, and uva ursi.

Caution: Do not take goldenseal internally on a daily basis for more than one week at a time. Do not use it during pregnancy or if you are breast-feeding, and use with caution if you are allergic to ragweed. If you have a history of cardiovascular disease, diabetes, or glaucoma, use it only under a doctor's supervision.

Quick Reference Guide—Goals for People with Diabetes (Using a Finger Stick Blood Sample)

When Checked	Goal for People with Diabetes
Before breakfast (fasting)	80–120 mg/dL
Before lunch, dinner, and snack	80–120 mg/dL
Two hours after meals	Less than 170 mg/dL
Anytime (A1c hemoglobin)	Less than 7 percent

Recommendations

❏ Opinions may differ as to the optimal ratio of dietary carbohydrates, proteins, and fats for prevention and treatment of diabetes. However, it is safe to say that carbohydrates trigger the release of insulin. As more carbohydrates are consumed, more insulin is produced. The current epidemic of obesity and diabetes in the United States indicates that we are asking our bodies to burn the wrong fuel—refined carbohydrates in this case. It has been suggested by Dr. Gerald Reaven of Stanford University School of Medicine that a diet consisting of 45 percent carbohydrates, 40 percent "good" (polyunsaturated) fats, and 15 percent protein will benefit individuals with diabetes.

❏ In a study published in the *Journal of the American Medical Asssociation*, those with diabetes who adopted a healthy diet that included adequate protein (about 20 to 30 percent), fats—mainly from polyunsaturated fats (about 30 percent), and carbohydrates (40 to 50 percent) from fruits and non-starchy vegetables, and ate a limited amount of whole grains, starchy vegetables, and pasta had less ill effects from the disease as evidenced by a reduction in hemoglobin A1c. Those who followed a diet rich in high-glycemic-load foods such as white and brown rice, baked potatoes, and breads did not get this benefit.

❏ Eat a low-fat, high-fiber diet including plenty of raw fruits and vegetables as well as fresh vegetable juices. This reduces the need for insulin and also lowers the level of fats in the blood. Fiber helps to reduce blood sugar surges. For snacks, eat oat or rice bran crackers with nut butter or cheese. Legumes, root vegetables, and whole grains are also good. Remember to regulate your complex carbohydrate intake.

❏ The types of carbohydrates consumed are at least as important as the total carbohydrate loading. High-glycemic foods such as white rice, white flour products, starchy vegetables, and many processed foods are quickly converted into blood sugar during digestion, causing insulin levels to go up. Carbohydrates found in low-glycemic foods such as asparagus, broccoli, cabbage, green beans, and low-starch vegetables and fruits are converted into blood sugar more slowly, which only gradually raises insulin levels. Avoiding "white foods" might be best.

❏ For those who are trying to lose weight, following a low-carbohydrate diet appears to be safe and effective in patients with type 2 diabetes. In one study, those who followed a diet that contained 20 percent of the total calories from carbohydrates lost about 16 pounds and reduced their hemoglobin A1c levels to 6.6 percent from 8.0 percent over a twenty-two-month period.

❏ Supplement your diet with spirulina. Spirulina helps to stabilize blood sugar levels. Other foods that help normalize blood sugar include berries, brewer's yeast, dairy products (especially cheese), egg yolks, fish, garlic, kelp, sauerkraut, soybeans, and vegetables.

Caution: Brewer's yeast can cause an allergic reaction in some individuals. Start with a small amount at first, and discontinue use if any allergic symptoms occur.

❏ Get your protein from vegetable sources, such as grains and legumes. Fish and low-fat dairy products are also acceptable sources of protein. Kidney function in people with type 2 diabetes seems to benefit from dietary soy protein. This protein also raises the level of "good" cholesterol.

❏ Avoid saturated fats, trans fats, hydrogenated or partially hydrogenated oils, and simple sugars (except when necessary to balance an insulin reaction). While total fat intake doesn't seem to change the risk of getting diabetes, the trans saturated fats and hydrogenated oils found in most fast foods can greatly increase the risk. Beneficial fats and oils include extra virgin olive oil, fish oil, almond oil and butter, avocados, nuts, and seed oils such as sesame, flax, sunflower, and pumpkin. Substituting polyunsaturated fats such as these and other vegetable oils also reduces cognitive decline in people with diabetes. Getting saturated and trans fats out of your diet is key to maintaining good brain function. Trans fats now are out of most of the American food supply—except for at some restaurants. To reduce your saturated fat intake, read labels and limit the amount of animal fat you consume.

❑ Eat more complex carbohydrates or reduce your insulin dosage before exercise. Exercise produces an insulinlike effect in the body. Talk to your doctor about the right approach for you.

❑ Do not take supplements containing large amounts of para-aminobenzoic acid (PABA), and avoid salt and white flour products. Consumption of these products results in an elevation of blood sugar.

❑ Do not take supplements containing the amino acid cysteine. It has the ability to break down the bonds of the hormone insulin and interferes with absorption of insulin by the cells.

❑ Do not take extremely large doses of vitamins B_1 (thiamine) and C. Excessive amounts may inactivate insulin. These vitamins may, however, be taken in normal amounts.

Note: Consult the Nutrients table in this section for recommendations.

❑ If symptoms of hyperglycemia develop, go to the emergency room of the nearest hospital. This is a potentially dangerous situation. Intravenous administration of proper fluids, electrolytes, and insulin may be required.

❑ Avoid taking large amounts of vitamin B_3 (niacin). However, small amounts (50 to 100 milligrams daily), taken by mouth, may be beneficial.

❑ Chromium deficiency may be a key player in the type 2 diabetes problem. In addition, chromium may help improve body composition—that is, the ratio of fat to muscle. Chromium is not generally available in plant foods, as plants have no requirement for it and thus do not concentrate it. Brewer's yeast, beer, whole grains, cheese, broccoli, and meat are good dietary sources, but not all are good choices for people with diabetes. Inorganic forms of chromium are poorly absorbed. Chromium picolinate is an effective organic form that is readily available as a supplement. (*See* the Nutrients table in this section for dosage and details.)

Caution: Brewer's yeast can cause an allergic reaction in some individuals. Start with a small amount at first, and discontinue use if any allergic symptoms occur.

❑ If you have a child with diabetes, be sure his or her teacher knows how to respond to the warning signs of hypoglycemia and hyperglycemia.

❑ If symptoms of hypoglycemia develop, immediately consume fruit juice, soda pop, or anything else that contains sugar. If that fails to help within twenty minutes, repeat this regimen. If the second treatment fails, or if you cannot ingest food, seek immediate medical attention and/or administer a glucagon injection. Anyone who has insulin-dependent diabetes should always carry a glucagon kit and know how to use it.

❑ Avoid tobacco in any form; it constricts the blood vessels and inhibits circulation. Keep your feet clean, dry, and warm, and wear only white cotton socks and well-fitting shoes. Lack of oxygen (because of poor circulation) and peripheral nerve damage (with loss of pain sensation) are major factors in the development of diabetic foot ulcers. Try to avoid injury, and take measures to improve the circulation in the feet and legs. (*See* CIRCULATORY PROBLEMS in Part Two.)

❑ Exercise regularly. Women who exercised at least once a week had a reduced risk of developing type 2 diabetes.

❑ Moderate coffee consumption (up to 4 cups a day) of either caffeinated or decaffeinated coffee reduces the risk of getting type 2 diabetes. These surprising results were obtained from over 88,000 women and published in the prestigious diabetes journal *Diabetes Care*. Coffee contains natural compounds besides caffeine that have been shown to improve glucose control in laboratory animals.

Considerations

❑ To compensate for the lack of insulin production, a person with type 1 diabetes must inject insulin on a daily basis. Injections are necessary because insulin cannot be absorbed from the gastrointestinal tract into the bloodstream if taken orally. Insulin pumps and pens (individual, disposable prefilled insulin syringes in the form of a pen) are also available for the delivery of insulin. Because the management of type 1 diabetes is such a complex challenge, it is imperative that a person with this condition have a good relationship with the physician prescribing the insulin. There are many insulin formulations on the U.S. market. A table in this section shows what is available today.

❑ Since 1982, most of the newly approved insulin preparations have been produced by inserting portions of DNA (recombinant DNA) into special lab-cultivated bacteria or yeast. This process allows the bacteria or yeast cells to produce complete human insulin. Recombinant human insulin has all but completely replaced animal-derived insulin, such as pork or beef insulin. Recently, insulin analogs have been produced that have a structure differing slightly from human insulin (usually by one or two amino acids). This changes the onset and peak of action times. Refer to the table on page 381 for information about some of the more common insulin preparations.

❑ Strict glucose control in type 1 diabetes also reduces the risk of atherosclerosis, according to a study reported in *The New England Journal of Medicine*. Intensive glucose control was found to greatly reduce damage to the eyes, nerves, and kidneys. Researchers also concluded that the tight control benefited the heart. Strict glucose control involves at least three insulin injections per day, or the use of an insulin pump, plus frequent self-monitoring. However, some newer studies have refuted these results. Ask a trained diabetologist or endocrinologist what the latest thinking is on the subject.

❏ The FDA has approved pramlintide (Symlin), a new drug for people with diabetes who cannot adequately control their blood glucose levels with insulin. It is intended to be used along with insulin to help lower blood glucose levels during the three hours after meals. Pramlintide must be kept separately from insulin and never mixed, nor should the same syringe be used to administer both, to prevent alteration of the activity of the insulin.

❏ Gastroparesis, which affects up to 75 percent of people with diabetes, causes bloating, loss of appetite, vomiting, and dehydration. With this condition, the flow of food from the stomach to the intestine is blocked or slowed. Because the timing of the digestive process is disrupted, this can complicate efforts to control blood sugar levels with medication. Researchers at Johns Hopkins University School of Medicine have found that sildenafil (Viagra) could be an effective remedy for the condition. Sildenafil appears to cause muscles in the digestive tract to relax.

❏ Caiapo, an extract of white sweet potatoes that is taken as a supplement in Japan, has been studied for its efficacy and tolerability. Dr. Bernard Ludvik of the University of Vienna Medical School found that subjects with type 2 diabetes experienced improvement in both blood sugar and cholesterol levels when taking caiapo. Subjects who took a placebo experienced no significant change. The research was published in the journal *Diabetes Care*.

❏ Cinnamon, a spice third only to pepper and mustard in popularity, may be a possible and pleasant treatment for diabetes. In a small study, taking 1 or 2 teaspoonfuls a day in capsule form was shown to lower blood sugar, triglycerides, and cholesterol. Some investigators have shown that people with diabetes who took 1, 3, or 6 grams a day of cinnamon reduced serum glucose, triglycerides, and the bad cholesterol (LDL). Mostly associated with pastry products, cinnamon is also an excellent spice for teas, meats, and vegetables, as well as fruits such as apples, bananas, and peaches. The continuous ingestion of table cinnamon is, however, probably not advisable due to the potential toxic buildup of certain cinnamon compounds.

❏ Do not take too much selenium. One study showed that taking 200 micrograms a day for 7.7 years resulted in a nearly threefold increase in the risk of type 2 diabetes.

❏ Taking 600 milligrams of chromium picolinate and 2 milligrams of biotin each day helped patients with poorly controlled diabetes improve glucose management and blood lipid measurements. Larger amounts of chromium picolinate (1,000 micrograms) helped attenuate weight gain and abdominal fat accumulation, while at the same time improving blood sugar control.

❏ In the Nurses' Health Study, a study of over 80,000 women, higher zinc intake was associated with a slightly lower risk of developing type 2 diabetes. The lowest risk was associated with taking at least 18 milligrams a day of zinc.

❏ Cut back on soft drinks that contain sugar. That is the conclusion drawn by a study that appeared in the *Journal of the American Medical Association.* Women who drank more than one sugar-sweetened soft drink a day were found to be twice as likely to develop diabetes than those who did not. Even when other factors, such as weight, diet, and lifestyle differences, were factored in, researchers still found that the soft-drink group was 1.3 times more likely to develop the disease. It was hypothesized that in addition to the extra calories, the increase in risk might be attributable to the high amount of rapidly absorbed sugars that cause a dramatic rise in glucose and insulin. Neither diet soda nor fruit juice indicated a problem in the study, but sugared fruit punch showed results similar to the sugared soda.

❏ Cut back on soft drinks that contain artificial sweeteners. In a study of over 5,000 participants, those who drank one or more diet sodas a day had a 62 percent greater chance of developing diabetes. It is possible that the artificial sweetener increases the hedonistic desire for more sweet foods, or that incorporating diet sodas into one's life is just an indication that the rest of the diet is unhealthy.

❏ Some newly diagnosed patients with diabetes benefited from a whole-system Ayurvedic protocol that included an herbal blend of neem, bitter gourd, blackberry, and Bael fruit coupled with an Ayurvedic diet and meditation. These patients experienced higher hemoglobin A1c levels, which showed better control of blood sugar levels over the six-month study.

❏ People with type 2 diabetes are less able than most people to perceive sweet tastes, and this may make it more difficult for them to lose weight. Because they do not recognize the sweet taste of substances, they often consume sugary products that they do not appreciate as sweet. If a person with type 2 diabetes attains a better understanding of food, exercises greater care in choosing foods, and reads food product labels carefully, he or she should be able to control the problem and avoid the need for treatment with drugs or insulin. Adhering to a low-glycemic-load diet may help control cravings, as it reduces hunger.

❏ A higher magnesium intake lowers the risk of getting type 2 diabetes. The journal *Diabetes Care* published a study in which overweight women who consumed large amounts of magnesium were 22 percent less likely to develop type 2 diabetes than women who consumed lower amounts. A diet rich in nuts, whole grains, and vegetables that are high in magnesium may be beneficial.

❏ Type 2 diabetes can be controlled by diet and exercise alone, but oral medications or injections of insulin can be added if regulating the diet does not work. Obesity is a major factor in type 2 diabetes, and a weight reduction program is often all that is required to control it.

Oral Medications for Type 2 Diabetes

Type 2 diabetes may be managed with any number of different drugs. Following is a quick reference guide to the major medications currently used for this purpose, together with how they act in the body, generic and brand names, and general comments.

Action in the Body	Generic Name	Brand Name(s)	Comments
Sulfonylureas			
Stimulates beta cells to release more insulin	chlorpropamide	Diabinese	Taken one or two times daily before meals. First-generation drug.
	glipizide	Glucotrol	Second-generation drug. Used in smaller doses than first-generation agents.
	glyburide	DiaBeta Micronase Glynase	Second-generation drug. Smaller doses.
	glimepiride	Amaryl	Second-generation drug. Smaller doses.
Meglitinides			
Stimulates the pancreas to release more insulin.	repaglinide	Prandin	Taken before each of three meals.
Works similarly to sulfonylureas.	nateglinide	Starlix	Taken before each of three meals.
Biguanides			
Sensitizes the body insulin already present.	metformin metformin Extended Release metformin with glyburide	Glucophage Glucophage XR Glucovance	Taken two times daily with food for best results.
Thiazolidinediones (Glitazones)			
Helps insulin work better in muscle and fat and lowers insulin resistance.	rosiglitazone pioglitazone	Avandia ACTOS	Taken once or twice daily with food. Very rare but serious side effects on the liver are possible.
Alpha-Glucose Inhibitors			
Slows or blocks breakdown of starches and sugars; action slows rise in blood sugar after eating.	acarbose miglitol	Precose Glyset	Should be taken with first bite of meals
DPP-4 Inhibitors			
Increases the insulin made in the pancreas and decreases the sugar made in the liver.	sitagliptin	Januvia	Taken once daily with food.

❏ It was once thought that people with diabetes should avoid all sweetened foods. For weight control, this is still the case. However, research has shown that sugar—a simple carbohydrate—does not cause the greatest increase in blood glucose. Eating baked potatoes or some breakfast cereals causes a greater rise in blood sugar. Indeed, carrots raise blood sugar more than ice cream does. However, it is important to note that the extra vitamins and fiber in carrots probably make carrots a better choice for a diabetic than ice cream. Also, the amount of carrots consumed is usually not enough to cause concern. Carbohydrates are converted quickly into glucose in the body. It is on this principle that many high-protein, low-carbohydrate diets are based. It is essential, therefore, that people with diabetes measure their intake of both simple and complex carbohydrates—not simply those coming from sugar.

❑ Insulin inhalers are now in development. The dose is inhaled through the mouth into the lungs, and from there, the dry or dissolved insulin can easily be absorbed into the bloodstream. The benefits to this method of ingestion, as compared with injection, are obvious. The drawbacks, however, are in accurately administering the correct dose in the correct form. The inhalers deliver only up to 10 percent of the drug into the lungs, making it more expensive because more insulin is needed. The size of the drug particles is also critical—if they are too small, the drug will bind together; if too large, the insulin will not be able to reach the lungs.

❑ A continuous glucose monitoring system, the CGMS® System Gold™, is available from Medtronic, Inc. It records blood glucose levels at five-minute intervals for periods up to three days. Data can be downloaded into a computer for review by a doctor. This device should be used along with traditional finger stick tests for calibration purposes.

❑ A needle management system, called the Q-103 Needle Management System, is available to remove certain hypodermic needles from insulin syringes and to store them safely for later disposal. The device holds as many as 5,000 needles, and is produced by QCare International LLC.

❑ The FDA recently approved a wristwatch-like glucose-monitoring device for use by children and adolescents. The device, called the GlucoWatch G2 Biographer, manufactured by Cygnus, Inc., was previously approved for use by adults. Fluid is extracted through the skin as the device is worn and the glucose level is measured and displayed. Up to six painless measurements per hour for a thirteen-hour period are possible. The device must be warmed up and calibrated using a finger stick.

❑ A wound dressing, called Apligraf, is available that helps heal diabetic foot ulcers, open foot sores that can lead to amputation. It is manufactured by Organogenesis, Inc.

❑ Research indicates that supplementation with the hormone dehydroepiandrosterone in the form of 7-keto DHEA may help prevent diabetes. (See DHEA THERAPY in Part Three.)

❑ Hypothyroidism may be a leading cause of diabetes. Well-known researcher and author Stephen Langer, M.D., has noticed that neuropathies, together with other diabetic complications, disappear when thyroid hormone is administered. Many complications of diabetes and hypothyroidism are a result of clogged arteries, which prevent the blood from delivering nutrients and oxygen and carrying off waste and debris.

❑ Glycosylation—the binding of glucose and other sugars onto proteins in the blood, nerve cells, and lenses of the eyes—may be responsible for many of the long-term effects of diabetes. Researchers at the University of Surrey's School of Biological Sciences and the Academic Unit of Diabetes and Endocrinology of London's Whittington Hospital have shown that vitamin C may inhibit this destructive process. They say that if glycosylation is part of the normal aging process, taking vitamin C supplements may slow it.

❑ Magnet therapy helps some people with diabetes in coping with foot pain associated with the disorder. (See MAGNET THERAPY under PAIN CONTROL in Part Three.)

❑ A woman with diabetes who wants to become pregnant should watch her blood sugar levels long before she plans to conceive. The fetus has the greatest chance of developing birth defects during the first five to eight weeks of pregnancy, before most women know they are pregnant. It usually takes a few months to get the blood sugar under proper control; if a woman begins to monitor her blood sugar level the day she conceives, damage may already be done by the time it is under control. Pregnant women are routinely checked during pregnancy for gestational diabetes. This disorder usually resolves after giving birth. However, many women who have gestational diabetes will develop type 2 diabetes later in life.

❑ Retinopathy (damage to the retina) from diabetes is the leading cause of blindness in the United States. The incidence of blindness from diabetic retinopathy has dropped with the use of laser surgery. However, persons with untreated diabetes are said to be twenty-five times more at risk for blindness than the general population. The Diabetes Control and Complications Trial (DCCT), a ten-year study which ended in June 1993, showed that improved blood glucose control among type 1 patients prevents or delays diabetic retinopathy. Therapy that keeps blood sugar levels as close to normal as possible reduced damage to the eyes by 76 percent. Persons with diabetes should get annual retinal examinations to check on their condition.

❑ Diabetic nephropathy (damage to the kidneys caused by diabetes) is quite common, but is becoming less so as people recognize the necessity of maintaining a stable blood sugar level. It is important to monitor kidney function periodically. Treating high blood pressure is important. Diabetic neuropathy (damage to the nerves caused by diabetes) usually affects the peripheral nerves, such as those in the feet, hands, and legs. Symptoms include numbness, tingling, and pain. Amitriptyline and desipramine, common antidepressant drugs, have proved to be successful in the treatment of this condition. They work by increasing levels of the neurochemical that carries messages between cells, thus increasing sensation. Autonomic neuropathy may lead, among other complaints, to a buildup of gastric juices in the stomach. Too much stomach acid can cause nausea and diarrhea, but the condition can be relieved by either antibiotic treatment or by eating smaller, low-fat meals. For men, neuropathy or circulatory problems can lead to erectile dysfunction (ED). Sildenafil (Viagra) and tadalafil (Cialis) may be able to alleviate this problem. Your physician will probably want to do a stress test before prescribing this drug.

❑ In one study, large amounts of niacin raised blood sugar levels in people with non-insulin-dependent diabetes by as much as 16 percent. Over time, this could cause dependence on insulin or medication. Niacin can also cause the level of uric acid in the blood to rise, indicating probable kidney dysfunction and an increased risk of gout. However, niacinamide, a form of niacin, slows down the destruction and enhances the regeneration of the insulin-producing beta cells in the pancreas, and therefore may be helpful for those with type 1 diabetes.

❑ Elevated glucose levels in the lens of the eye can result in the accumulation of substances called polyols, whose presence can ultimately cause damage to the lens. High polyol concentrations resulting from high glucose levels can persist even if glucose levels subsequently return to normal. Flavonoids, such as quercetin, help to inhibit the accumulation of polyols.

❑ Diabetes and high blood pressure often go hand in hand, and both can lead to kidney disease. In one recent study, hypertensive diabetics who took drugs called angiotensin converting enzyme (ACE) inhibitors cut their risk of developing serious kidney disease in half.

❑ Coronary artery disease is common in people with diabetes. Women with diabetes are particularly at risk. A sixteen-year study published in *Circulation: Journal of the American Heart Association* by Frank B. Hu, M.D., lead author and associate professor of nutrition and epidemiology at the Harvard School of Public Health, indicates that women with type 2 diabetes who consumed fish five or more times a week had a 64 percent reduction in coronary heart disease and a 52 percent reduction in total mortality compared with women who ate fish less than once a month. This was attributed to the higher consumption of omega-3 fatty acids associated with this diet. Concerns with environmental toxins found in fresh fish point to fish oil supplements as an acceptable substitute for the actual consumption of fish. Dr. Hu did not study supplements specifically, but did not rule out their theoretical use as substitutes. It is probable that the consumption of omega-3 fatty acids would have the same effect on men.

❑ Researchers at the University of Colorado Health Sciences Center found that smokers who have diabetes are two to three times more likely than their nonsmoking counterparts to develop kidney damage, often leading to the need for dialysis or a transplant. Smoking constricts blood vessels. In people with diabetes, this helps to push large protein molecules out of the vessels and into the kidneys. That can eventually lead to kidney failure.

❑ Rosiglitazone (Avandia) is a drug sometimes prescribed for type 2 diabetes. This drug controls blood sugar by adjusting the sensitivity of fat and muscle tissue to the insulin in the body. Rosiglitazone may cause fluid retention (a condition where the body keeps excess fluid), which may lead to or worsen congestive heart failure.

❑ People with diabetes who experience the pain associated with nerve damage (diabetic peripheral neuropathy) have a new treatment option—the first FDA-approved drug for managing the burning, tingling, and numbing sensations in the extremities that mark this condition. The drug, duloxetine (Cymbalta), was approved in September 2004 for treating the condition, the most common complication of diabetes. In clinical trials, people treated with Cymbalta reported less pain than those given a placebo. Treated with Cymbalta, 58 percent of the people reported at least a 30 percent sustained reduction in pain. Only 34 percent of the people treated with a placebo reported sustained pain reduction. Most commonly reported side effects included nausea, dry mouth, constipation, and diarrhea. In a few cases, patients experienced dizziness and hot flashes.

❑ On days having high levels of airborne particulates, such as dust and soot, people with diabetes are twice as likely to be hospitalized for cardiovascular problems. Exposure to these particles may affect heart rate and increase inflammation in the heart. This places diabetics with cardiovascular problems at a greater risk. If you have diabetes, check air quality levels and stay indoors during periods of risk.

❑ Many nutrients recommended for people with diabetes are available in combination supplements. One company that produces a line of specialty supplements for people with diabetes is Progressive Research Labs of Austin, Texas.

❑ It is vital for people who have diabetes to take care of their feet. Nerve damage can lead to lack of sensation in the feet, and once the skin is broken, sores there may not heal. Treatments for diabetic foot problems include becaplermin (Regranex), a topical gel that encourages tissue growth in the wound, and Dermagraft. Dermagraft is a skin substitute used to help wound closure associated with diabetic foot ulcers. It helps replace and rebuild damaged tissue.

❑ People with diabetes should be vigilant about blood fat and cholesterol levels. Optimum cholesterol levels are LDL ("bad cholesterol"), less than 130; HDL ("good cholesterol"), 60 or above; triglycerides, 150 or under. Your doctor may set different levels for you if you are diagnosed with diabetes.

❑ For more information on diabetes and its potential complications, contact any of the organizations listed under Health and Medical Organizations in the Appendix.

Insulin Preparations for Type 1 Diabetes

Type 1 diabetes is managed with injections of the hormone insulin, as well as with close attention to diet and other lifestyle factors. Not all insulins are the same, however, and it may take some trial and error to find the one or ones that are right for any given individual. The principal differences are related to the speed with which they take effect, and the period of time they remain active in the body. Following is a quick reference guide to the major types of insulin available.

Examples	Onset of Action	Peak of Action	Duration of Action
Rapid-Acting Insulin			
Humalog (Lispro)	15 minutes	30–90 minutes	3–5 hours
Apidra (Glulisine)	15 minutes	30–90 minutes	3–5 hours
NovoLog (Aspart)	15 minutes	30–90 minutes	3–5 hours
Short-Acting Insulin (Regular)			
Humulin R	30–60 minutes	2–4 hours	5–8 hours
Novolin R	30–60 minutes	2–4 hours	5–8 hours
Intermediate-Acting Insulin (NPH)			
Humulin N	1–3 hours	8 hours	12–16 hours
Novolin N	1–3 hours	8 hours	12–16 hours
Intermediate- and Short-Acting Insulin Mixtures			
Humulin 70/30	30–60 minutes	Varies	10–16 hours
Novolin 70/30	30–60 minutes	Varies	10–16 hours
Humalog Mix 75/25	10–15 minutes	Varies	10–16 hours
Humalog Mix 50/50	10–15 minutes	Varies	10–16 hours
Novolog Mix 70/30	5–15 minutes	Varies	10–16 hours
Long-Acting Insulin			
Ultralente	4–8 hours	10–30 hours	36 hours
Levemir (Detemir)	1 hour	None	20–26 hours
Lantus (Glargine)	1 hour	None	20–26 hours

DIABETIC RETINOPATHY

See under EYE PROBLEMS.

DIARRHEA

Diarrhea is characterized by frequent and loose, watery stools. Symptoms that may accompany diarrhea include vomiting, cramping, thirst, and abdominal pain. Some people run a fever as well. It is rarely a serious condition, except in young children and older adults. Diarrhea causes the loss of both fluids and electrolytes (minerals), which can lead to troublesome problems. Diarrhea can exist alone or as a symptom of other problems.

Among the many possible causes of diarrhea are incomplete digestion of food; food poisoning; food allergies; excess alcohol consumption; bacterial, viral, or other infection; and consumption of contaminated water. Caffeine, magnesium, laxatives, and sorbitol and all sugar alcohols (especially for young children) are all known to cause diarrhea in some people. The use of certain drugs, including antibiotics such as tetracycline, clindamycin (Cleocin), or ampicillin can also contribute to diarrhea. Inflammatory bowel disease, such as ulcerative colitis, diverticulitis, or Crohn's disease; pancreatic disease; and cancer may all lead to severe intestinal upsets. Emotional stress also can cause diarrhea. Acute diarrhea accompanied by fever and mucus or blood in the stool can be a sign of infection or the presence of parasites.

Unless otherwise noted, the dosages recommended here are for adults. In any case, don't take too many supplements at once until your gastrointestinal tract has become quiescent. For a child between the ages of twelve and seventeen, reduce the dose to three-quarters of the recommended amount. For a child between the ages of six and twelve, use one-half the recommended dose, and for a child under six, use one-quarter of the recommended amount. If diarrhea is severe, seek medical attention.

NUTRIENTS

SUPPLEMENT	SUGGESTED DOSAGE	COMMENTS
Very Important		
ABC Aerobic Bulk Cleanse from Aerobic Life Industries or	As directed on label.	To provide bulk that aids in forming stools.
psyllium seeds	4 capsules daily, at bedtime. Take with a large glass of water.	
Charcoal tablets	4 tablets every hour with water until the diarrhea subsides. Take separately from other supplements and medications.	Absorbs toxins from the colon and bloodstream and aids in firming stools. *Note:* Do not take for more than 3 days at a time.
Essential fatty acid complex	As directed on label.	Aids in forming stools.
Kelp	1,000 mg daily.	To replace minerals lost through diarrhea.
L-glutamine	As directed on label.	Helps the gut to produce healthy new cells and boosts the immune system.
Potassium	99 mg daily.	To replace potassium lost in watery stools.
Important		
Acidophilus (Kyo-Dophilus or Probiata from Wakunaga)	1 tsp in distilled water, twice daily, on an empty stomach.	Replaces lost "friendly" bacteria. Use a nondairy powder form.
Garlic (Kyolic from Wakunaga)	2 capsules 3 times daily.	Kills bacteria and parasites. Enhances immunity.
Helpful		
Calcium and	1,500 mg daily.	To replace calcium depleted from the body. Also aids in forming stools.
magnesium and	1,000 mg daily.	Needed for calcium uptake. Promotes pH balance.
vitamin D	400 IU daily.	Needed for calcium uptake.
Multienzyme complex with pancreatin	Take with meals. As directed on label.	Needed for normal digestion.
Vitamin B complex	100 mg of each major B vitamin 3 times daily (amounts of individual vitamins in a complex will vary).	All B vitamins are necessary for digestion and absorption of nutrients. Sublingual forms are recommended for better absorption. Injections (under a doctor's supervision) may be necessary.
plus extra vitamin B₁ (thiamine) and	200 mg daily for 2 weeks.	
vitamin B₃ (niacin) and	50 mg daily.	
folic acid	50 mg daily.	
Vitamin C with bioflavonoids	500 mg 3 times daily.	Needed for healing and immunity. Use a buffered form.
Vitamin E	200 IU daily.	Protects the cell membranes that line the colon wall. Use d-alpha-tocopherol form.
Zinc	50 mg daily. Do not exceed a total of 100 mg daily from all supplements.	Aids in repair of damaged tissue of the digestive tract and enhances immune response. Use zinc gluconate lozenges or OptiZinc for best absorption.

Herbs

❏ If you suffer from occasional bouts of diarrhea, use blackberry root bark, chamomile, pau d'arco, and/or raspberry leaves. Herbs can be taken in tea form or added to applesauce, bananas, pineapple, or papaya juice.

Caution: Do not use chamomile if you are allergic to ragweed. Do not use during pregnancy or nursing. It may interact with warfarin or cyclosporine, so patients using these drugs should avoid it.

❏ Cayenne (capsicum) capsules, taken two to three times daily, may be beneficial.

❏ Fenugreek, taken as a tea, lubricates the intestines and reduces fever.

❏ Ginger tea is good for cramps and abdominal pain.

❏ Grapefruit seed extract has antiparasitic properties.

❏ Marshmallow root tea (also known as malva tea) helps calm the stomach and soothe intestinal problems.

❏ Slippery elm bark, taken in tea or extract form, is soothing to the digestive tract.

❏ Wild oregano oil contains antibacterial, antifungal, antiparasitic, and antiviral agents.

Recommendations

❏ Drink plenty of liquids, such as hot carob drink, "green drinks," and plenty of quality water. Do not drink very hot or cold liquids. The prolonged loss of fluids as a result of diarrhea can lead to dehydration and loss of necessary minerals, such as sodium, potassium, and magnesium. Liquid gelatin, clear broth, sodas such as ginger ale or flat cola, and weak tea with honey can be substituted for water if necessary. Carrot juice is also good, and makes the stools less watery. Do not drink apple juice, as this can make diarrhea worse. Most fruit juices are good sources of potassium, except cranberry juice. Include the potassium-rich juices, but try diluting them with half water until you can tolerate a stronger amount.

❏ Avoid high-fiber foods, which may stress the digestive system. Instead, stick to foods that are easy to digest, such as cooked potatoes, rice, bananas, applesauce, or toast.

❏ Drink 3 cups of rice water daily. To make rice water, boil ½ cup of brown rice in 3 cups of water for forty-five minutes. Strain out the rice and drink the water. Eat the rice as well. Rice helps to form stools and supplies needed B vitamins.

❏ Do not consume any dairy products (except for low-fat soured products). They are highly allergenic. Moreover, diarrhea causes a temporary loss of the enzyme needed to digest lactose (milk sugar). Limit your intake of fats and foods containing gluten, including barley, oats, rye, and wheat. Avoid alcohol, caffeine, and spicy foods.

❏ Let a mild case of diarrhea run its course. It is the body's way of cleaning out toxins, bacteria, and other foreign invaders. Do not take any medication to stop diarrhea for at least two days. Stick to a liquid diet for twenty-four hours to give the bowel a rest.

❏ Consider using homeopathic remedies. *Arsenicum album* is a homeopathic remedy for burning diarrhea that is troublesome at night. *Podophyllum* can be used for watery stools. *Sulfur* is excellent for diarrhea that comes on suddenly. *Pectin* is known to counteract diarrhea.

❏ Consult your health care provider if any of the following conditions occur: the diarrhea lasts for more than two days, there is blood in the stool, the stool looks like black tar, you have a fever above 101°F, you have severe abdominal or rectal pain or bleeding, you suffer from dehydration as evidenced by dry mouth or wrinkled skin, or urination is reduced or stops in any eight-hour period. If an infant has a dry diaper for more than four hours accompanied by a fever, it is wise to seek the advice of your physician.

Considerations

❏ Carob powder is high in protein and helps halt diarrhea.

❏ When traveling abroad, do not drink the water unless you know it is safe. Avoid ice cubes, raw vegetables, dairy products, and unpeeled fruit. Use bottled water when you brush your teeth. Diarrhea is common when traveling in other countries, so it may be advisable to take certain preparations with you. Lactobacillus GG, a type of probiotic, is a natural alternative to both antibiotics or bismuth subsalicylate (Pepto-Bismol).

❏ Chronic diarrhea in very young children is evident if the child has five or more watery stools a day. A baby with diarrhea can become dehydrated very quickly and should be evaluated by a health care provider.

❏ If diarrhea is chronic or recurrent, an underlying problem such as a food allergy, infection, or intestinal parasites may be the cause. Allergy testing can determine whether you have any food allergies. A stool culture can be done to check for infection or the presence of parasites.

DIVERTICULITIS

Diverticulitis is a condition in which diverticula are perforated and become infected and inflamed. Diverticula are saclike, pea- or grape-sized protrusions in the intestinal wall. They typically form if an individual suffers from frequent constipation. Eating a low-fiber diet, as is typical in industrialized countries such as the United States, may contribute to the development of diverticulitis. Without sufficient fiber to soften and add bulk, stools are harder to pass. Greatly increased pressure is required to force small portions of hard, dry stool through the bowel. This rise in pressure can cause pouches to form at weak points in the wall of the colon. Once diverticula develop, they do not go away. The diverticula themselves cause no symptoms.

Many people have diverticulosis (the pouchlike protrusions) and never develop diverticulitis (the inflamed pouches). However, if tiny cuts in the pouches become infected or inflamed, the result can be severe, causing fever, chills, nausea, and pain. Fifty percent of people over age sixty will develop diverticulosis. Complications including bleeding occur in 10 to 25 percent of this group. As many as 3,300 people die from it each year.

Diverticulitis can be either acute or chronic. Symptoms include cramping, bloating, tenderness on the left side of the abdomen that is relieved by passing gas or a bowel movement, constipation or diarrhea, nausea, and an almost continual need to eliminate. There may be blood in the stool. Peritonitis, an inflammation of the lining of the abdominal cavity, can develop if a diverticulum ruptures and intestinal contents flow into the abdomen.

Because the walls of the large intestine often weaken as a person ages, this is a condition affecting older rather than younger people. It usually strikes people between the ages of fifty and ninety. It affects millions of Americans, but many people do not even know they have the condition because they either experience no symptoms or accept their symptoms as simple indigestion.

Exactly why is not known, but it is known that smoking and stress make symptoms worse. In fact, this is a classic example of a stress-related disorder. Poor eating habits compound the problem. A poor diet, a family history of the disease, gallbladder disease, obesity, and coronary artery disease all increase the chances of developing diverticulitis.

There are several diagnostic tests available to help diagnose diverticulitis. A barium enema is a procedure in which the colon is filled with liquid barium and X-rays are taken to reveal pouches in the colon wall, narrowing of the colon, or other abnormalities. With sigmoidoscopy, a thin, flexible lighted tube is inserted into the rectum to give the physician a closer look at the lower colon. If necessary, tissue samples can be removed for examination. To see into other parts of the colon, a colonoscopy must be performed. This is similar to a sigmoidoscopy, but allows a view of the entire colon.

Unless otherwise noted, the dosages recommended here are for adults. For children between the ages of twelve and seventeen, reduce the dose to three-quarters of the recommended amount. For children between the ages of six and twelve, use one-half the recommended dose, and for children under six, use one-quarter of the recommended amount. Do not take too many different supplements at once if you are in pain. Go slowly and add one at a time.

NUTRIENTS

SUPPLEMENT	SUGGESTED DOSAGE	COMMENTS
Essential		
Bio-Bifidus from American Biologics and	As directed on label.	To replace flora in the small intestine, primarily to improve assimilation.
Kyo-Dophilus from Wakunaga	As directed on label. Take on an empty stomach.	For bowel flora replacement to improve elimination and assimilation.
Fiber (oat bran, psyllium, ground flaxseeds, and ABC Aerobic Bulk Cleanse from Aerobic Life Industries)	As directed on label. Take 1 hour before meals with a large glass of liquid. Take separately from other supplements and medications.	Helps prevent constipation. Prevents infection by preventing accumulation of wastes in pouches in the colon walls.
Vitamin B complex	100 mg of each major B vitamin 3 times daily (amounts of individual vitamins in a complex will vary).	Needed for all enzyme systems in the body and for proper digestion. Use a hypoallergenic formula.
Very Important		
Multienzyme complex with pancreatin	As directed on label. Take with meals.	Needed to break down proteins. Use a formula high in pancreatin.
Proteolytic enzymes	As directed on label. Take between meals.	Aids in digestion and reduces inflammation of the colon.
Important		
Essential fatty acids (flaxseed oil, primrose oil, salmon oil, or Kyolic-EPA from Wakunaga)	As directed on label 3 times daily, before meals.	Improves lymphatic function and aids in protecting the cells lining the wall of the colon.
Garlic (Kyolic from Wakunaga)	2 capsules 3 times daily, with meals.	Aids in digestion and destroys unwanted bacteria and parasites. Use a yeast-free formula.
Kyo-Green from Wakunaga	As directed on label.	Aids in normal bowel function.
L-glutamine	500 mg twice daily, on an empty stomach. Take with water or juice. Do not take with milk. Take with 50 mg vitamin B_6 and 100 mg vitamin C for better absorption.	A major metabolic fuel for the intestinal cells; maintains the villi, the absorption surfaces of the gut. (*See* AMINO ACIDS in Part One.)
Vitamin K or alfalfa	100 mcg daily.	Deficiency has been linked to intestinal disorders. *See* under Herbs, below.
Helpful		
Free form amino acid (Amino Balance from Anabol Naturals)	As directed on label, on an empty stomach, 1/2 hour before meals.	To supply protein, needed for healing and repair of tissue.
Raw thymus glandular	As directed on label.	*See* GLANDULAR THERAPY in Part Three for its benefits. *Caution:* Do not give this supplement to a child.
Vitamin A with mixed carotenoids	25,000 IU daily. If you are pregnant, do not exceed 10,000 IU daily.	Protects and heals the lining of the colon.
Vitamin C with bioflavonoids	3,000–8,000 mg daily, in divided doses.	Reduces inflammation and boosts immune response. Use a buffered form.
Vitamin E	Up to 200 IU daily.	A powerful antioxidant that protects the mucous membranes. Use d-alpha-tocopherol form.

Herbs

❑ Alfalfa is a good natural source of vitamin K and valuable minerals, which are often deficient in people with intestinal disorders. It also contains chlorophyll, which aids healing. Take 2,000 milligrams daily in capsule or extract form.

❑ Aloe vera promotes the healing of inflamed areas. It also helps to prevent constipation. Drink ½ cup of aloe vera juice three times daily. It can be mixed with a cup of herbal tea if you wish.

❑ Pau d'arco has antibacterial, cleansing, and healing effects. Drink two cups of pau d'arco tea daily.

❑ Other herbs beneficial for diverticulitis include cayenne (capsicum), chamomile, goldenseal, papaya, red clover, slippery elm bark, and yarrow extract or tea. The fibrous inner bark of slippery elm contains large quantities of a gentle laxative that soothes the digestive tract while keeping things moving. The U.S. Food and Drug Administration has declared slippery elm to be a safe and effective digestive soother. Prepare it like oatmeal, adding hot milk or water to the powdered bark to make a cereal. Capsules also are available.

Cautions: Do not use chamomile if you are allergic to ragweed. Do not use during pregnancy or nursing. It may interact with warfarin or cyclosporine, so patients using these drugs should avoid it. Do not take goldenseal internally on a daily basis for more than one week at a time. Do not use it during pregnancy or if you are breast-feeding, and use with caution if you are allergic to ragweed. If you have a history of cardiovascular disease, diabetes, or glaucoma, use it only under a doctor's supervision.

Recommendations

❑ The key to controlling this disorder is to consume an adequate amount of fiber and lots of quality water. You need at least 30 grams of fiber each day. You may prefer to supplement your diet with a bulk product and/or a stool softener that contains methylcellulose or psyllium, since these do not promote as much gas formation in the colon as other sources of fiber, especially wheat bran. Drink at least ten 8-ounce glasses of water daily. Herbal teas, broth, and live juices can account for some of the liquid needed. Liquid aids in keeping the pouchlike areas clean of toxic wastes, preventing inflammation.

❑ Eat a low-carbohydrate diet with high levels of protein from vegetable sources and fish. Do not eat grains, seeds, or nuts, except for well-cooked brown rice. These foods are hard to digest, resulting in bloating and gas. Also eliminate dairy products, red meat, sugar products, fried foods, spices, and processed foods. Make sure to get adequate calcium and vitamin D if you are eliminating dairy.

❑ Eat plenty of green leafy vegetables. These are good sources of vitamin K. Obtaining this vitamin through diet is especially important for people with intestinal disorders.

❑ Eat garlic for its healing and detoxifying properties.

❑ During an acute attack of diverticulitis, your health care provider may recommend a temporary low-fiber diet. Once the inflammation clears, you may slowly switch back to a high-fiber diet.

❑ When an attack or pain begins, give yourself a cleansing enema using 2 quarts of lukewarm water and the juice of a fresh lemon. (*See* ENEMAS in Part Three.) This helps to rid the colon of undigested and entrapped foods and to relieve pain. Make sure to first get the approval of your health care professional or your child's pediatrician.

❑ On the day of an acute attack, take 4 charcoal tablets or capsules with a large glass of water to absorb trapped gas. Charcoal tablets are available at health food stores. Always take charcoal separately from medications and other supplements, and do not take it for prolonged periods, as it absorbs beneficial nutrients as well as gas.

❑ During severe attacks, use liquid vitamin supplements for better assimilation and put all vegetables and fruits through a blender. Eat steamed vegetables only. Baby foods are good until healing is complete. Earth's Best produces organically grown baby foods that are available in health food stores and some supermarkets. Add supplemental fiber to the baby food. As healing progresses, gradually add raw fruits and vegetables to the diet. Drink carrot juice, cabbage juice, and "green drinks." Or take chlorophyll liquid or liquid alfalfa in juice.

❑ To relieve pain, massage the left side of the abdomen. Stand up and do stretching exercises.

❑ Clay tablets are beneficial. Take them as directed on the product label, on an empty stomach, when you get up in the morning.

❑ Check stools daily for blood. If the stool is black, take a portion of it to your physician for an analysis.

❑ Try to have a bowel movement at the same time each day. Take fiber first thing in the morning, before breakfast, to help the bowels move at this time.

Note: Always take supplemental fiber separately from other supplements and medications.

❑ Do not overuse laxatives; they can irritate the colon wall.

Considerations

❑ Food allergies are often a cause of intestinal disorders. Allergy testing is advised. (*See* ALLERGIES in Part Two.)

❑ One study of 47,000 males on high-fiber diets including hard, fibrous foods such as nuts, popcorn, and corn, did not show an increase in the risk of developing diverticulosis or diverticular complications.

❑ If the diverticula are infected, your doctor may prescribe antibiotics. Be sure to consume plenty of soured products and some form of nondairy acidophilus if you are taking antibiotics.

❑ Fasting is beneficial. (*See* FASTING in Part Three.)

❑ *See also* CROHN'S DISEASE; IRRITABLE BOWEL SYNDROME; and ULCERATIVE COLITIS, all in Part Two.

DIZZINESS

See MÉNIÈRE'S DISEASE; VERTIGO. *See also under* PREGNANCY-RELATED PROBLEMS.

DOG BITE

A bite or scratch from a dog (or cat) that breaks the skin poses the danger of infection, especially if the wound is deep. Bites also carry the risk of rabies. Most household pets are immunized against rabies, but the possibility of infection still exists. Rabies is always fatal if you don't get treated, so seek medical attention immediately. It is also possible to contract a tetanus infection from an animal bite. The microbe that causes tetanus, *Clostridium tetani*, lives in the top layers of soil, and in the intestinal tracts of cows and horses. It easily infects wounds that result in reduced oxygen flow in the tissue, particularly crushing and puncture wounds.

A dog bite can be nothing more than a minor graze, or it can be so severe as to be life-threatening. Children are at most risk from dog bites, and children under five years of age are victims of the most severe attacks—many of them requiring hospitalization.

Unless otherwise stated, the dosages recommended here are for adults. For a child between the ages of twelve and seventeen, reduce the dose to three-quarters of the recommended amount. For a child between the ages of six and twelve, use one-half the recommended dose, and for a child under six, use one-quarter of the recommended amount.

NUTRIENTS

SUPPLEMENT	SUGGESTED DOSAGE	COMMENTS
Very Important		
Vitamin C with bioflavonoids	4,000–10,000 mg daily for 1 week, then reduce to 3,000 mg daily.	Fights infection. Important for repair of collagen and connective tissue.
Important		
Proteolytic enzymes or Inf-zyme Forte from American Biologics	As directed on label. Take between meals. As directed on label.	Act as anti-inflammatories.
Helpful		
Colloidal silver	As directed on label.	To reduce the danger of infection. Can be placed on a sterile bandage covering the wound.
Garlic (Kyolic from Wakunaga)	2 capsules 3 times daily.	Acts as a natural antibiotic.
L-cysteine and L-methionine	500 mg each daily for 2 weeks. Take with water or juice on an empty stomach. Do not take with milk. Take with 50 mg vitamin B_6 and 100 mg vitamin C for better absorption.	Powerful detoxifying agents. (*See* AMINO ACIDS in Part One.)
ViraPlex from Enzymatic Therapy	As directed on label.	Aids in healing and fights infection.
Vitamin A plus mixed carotenoids plus vitamin E	25,000 IU daily. If you are pregnant, do not exceed 10,000 IU daily. 25,000 IU daily. 200 IU daily.	Powerful antioxidants that aid the immune system and assist healing of the skin. Use d-alpha-tocopherol form.
Vitamin B complex	50 mg of each major B vitamin 3 times daily (amounts of individual vitamins in a complex will vary).	Aids in tissue oxidation and antibody production.

Herbs

❏ Echinacea, goldenseal, pau d'arco, and red clover, taken in tea form, are good for dog bites. Goldenseal extract can also be applied directly on the affected area. This is a natural antibiotic that helps to fight infection.

Cautions: Do not take echinacea for longer than three months. It should not be used by people who are allergic to ragweed. Do not take goldenseal internally on a daily basis for more than one week at a time. Do not use it during pregnancy or if you are breast-feeding, and use with caution if you are allergic to ragweed. If you have a history of cardiovascular disease, diabetes, or glaucoma, use it only under a doctor's supervision.

Recommendations

❏ If you are bitten by a dog, the first thing you should do is seek medical attention. Rabies treatment needs to begin at once.

❏ If you know who the dog's owner is, inquire as to the animal's vaccination status. If the dog is unfamiliar, try to have someone confine it if possible so that its health can be checked and it can be placed under observation. But time is of the essence, so it is always better to be treated against rabies when you are not sure about the dog's vaccination status.

❏ Teach children how to behave around animals, and teach them not to approach strange animals. Never leave a young child alone with an animal—even the family pet.

Considerations

❏ Your physician may prescribe an oral antibiotic to prevent infection. If so, make sure that you take acidophilus to replace the "friendly" bacteria that antibiotics destroy. Your doctor will also likely recommend that you have a tetanus booster shot if you haven't had one in six years or more.

❏ In most states, dog bite incidents must be reported to the local health department, and the dog must then be kept under observation for any signs of rabies—viciousness, paralysis, growling, foaming at the mouth, or agitation. Rabies is an RNA-type virus that, once established in the human central nervous system, is invariably fatal. If the animal cannot be located so that rabies can be ruled out, a series of rabies injections will be necessary. The series of injections given today is no longer so painful, nor are injections given in the stomach, as in the past.

DOWN SYNDROME

Down syndrome is a condition caused by the presence of extra genetic material in the cells of a developing embryo. The disorder—named for English physician John Langdon Down—occurs in approximately 1 in every 733 births, and usually results in mental retardation with distinctive physical abnormalities.

The incidence of Down syndrome increases with the age of the parents, especially if the mothers are thirty-four or older. The risk is also higher for children of parents who have already given birth to a Down syndrome child. Life expectancy for people with Down syndrome has increased dramatically in recent decades—from twenty-five years in 1983 to sixty years today.

Down syndrome is usually caused by a phenomenon geneticists call nondisjunction, in which an error in cell division produces three copies of a chromosome—in this case, chromosome 21—instead of the normal two. In trisomy 21, which accounts for 95 percent of Down syndrome cases, the extra chromosome is due to an error in chromosome separation in the ovum before conception, although nondisjunction can also take place in the sperm. A small percentage of Down syndrome cases are linked to other kinds of chromosomal abnormalities, but all result in extra genetic material in some or all of the cells.

An infant born with Down syndrome typically—but not always—has characteristic physical traits such as a small head, poor muscle tone, a flat facial profile, slanted eyes, a depressed nose bridge, low-set ears, furrowed tongue, and a single deep crease across the center of the palm (known as a simian crease). People with Down syndrome are especially prone to having congenital heart disease and are more susceptible than most people to developing acute leukemia, thyroid disorders, and respiratory and digestive problems. While females with Down syndrome may menstruate and be fertile, males are almost always infertile.

Although the degree of mental retardation varies greatly among different individuals with Down syndrome, the average IQ falls within the range of 50 to 60. Generally, children with Down syndrome are able to learn everyday life skills and can be raised at home. Special education and training allow many individuals with Down syndrome to lead happy, useful, and love-filled lives. People with Down syndrome can live to middle or old age; however, as adults, they may be prone to developing Alzheimer's disease plus pneumonia and other lung diseases.

It is clear that the metabolism of people with Down syndrome differs considerably from those who have a normal complement of chromosomes. Immunological dysfunction, growth retardation, lipoprotein metabolism (cholesterol) problems, and an increased risk for Alzheimer's disease are among the issues raised by these metabolic differences.

It can be said that people with Down syndrome have a different genotype, and because of this their nutritional needs are very different from those of the general population. With proper, specialized nutrition, it is possible to improve metabolic and immune functions, as well as overall health, even though a definitive cure is probably not possible.

Unless otherwise specified, the dosages recommended here are for adults. For a child between the ages of twelve and seventeen, reduce the dose to three-quarters the recommended amount. For children between six and twelve, use one-half the recommended dose, and for children under the age of six, use one-quarter the recommended amount. Persons with malabsorption problems should consult a health care provider before starting any nutritional program.

NUTRIENTS

SUPPLEMENT	SUGGESTED DOSAGE	COMMENTS
Aangamik DMG from FoodScience of Vermont	50 mg 4 times daily.	Promotes the utilization of oxygen.
Acetyl-L-carnitine (ALC)	100–500 mg daily.	A carnitine derivative produced naturally in the body, involved in carbohydrate and protein metabolism and the transport of fats into the mitochondria. Increases carnitine in tissues, surpassing the metabolic potency of carnitine.
Coenzyme Q$_{10}$	10 mg daily.	Prevents heart damage by improving oxygenation of cells.
Essential fatty acids (Kyolic-EPA from Wakunaga, salmon oil, flaxseed oil, or primrose oil)	As directed on label. Take with meals.	Needed for proper brain and cardiovascular function.
Free form amino acid	As directed on label.	To provide needed protein and bolster the immune system.
Garlic (Kyolic from Wakunaga)	As directed on label.	Natural antibiotic that helps the body to eliminate toxins and strengthens the cardiovascular system.
Kelp	As directed on label.	To supply minerals helpful in establishing thyroid balance.
Lecithin granules or capsules	1 tsp 3 times daily. 2,400 mg 3 times daily.	Aids brain function.
Multivitamin and mineral complex with vitamin A and mixed carotenoids and selenium	As directed on label. 10,000 IU daily. 15,000 IU daily. 200 mcg daily.	All nutrients are needed for proper immune function.
Potassium	200 mg daily.	Helps transmit nerve impulses.
Taurine Plus from American Biologics	500 mg daily, on an empty stomach. Take with water or juice. Do not take with milk. Take with 50 mg vitamin B$_6$ and 100 mg vitamin C for better absorption.	Reduces stress and regulates nervous system.
Vitamin B complex with choline	As directed on label. 100 mg daily.	Prevents and/or treats memory loss and increases learning capacity. Also protects against cardiovascular disease.
Vitamin C with bioflavonoids	3,000 mg daily.	Enhances immune function and reduces cholesterol levels.
Vitamin E	200 IU daily.	Boosts immune system; facilitates absorption of lecithin. Use d-alpha-tocopherol form.
Zinc plus copper	50 mg daily. 2–3 mg daily.	Needed for proper brain function and a healthy immune system. Needed to balance with zinc.

Recommendations

❑ Be patient when feeding a child with Down syndrome, and be sure to provide a balanced diet. Include fresh and whole foods that are rich in vegetable proteins, as well as foods that are high in magnesium, such as fresh green vegetables, figs, meat, fish and seafood, nuts and seeds, tofu, blackstrap molasses, apples, kelp, soybeans, cornmeal, rice, apricots, and brewer's yeast. Reduce consumption of foods high in gluten, such as wheat, rye, barley, and oats. Avoid refined foods, sugars, dairy products, and alcohol.

Caution: Brewer's yeast can cause an allergic reaction in some individuals. Start with a small amount at first, and discontinue use if any allergic symptoms occur.

Considerations

❑ Vitamin/mineral supplements and extra nutrients can be nutritionally beneficial for people with Down syndrome. However, any kind of nutritional program should be designed with the help of a qualified physician or health care provider, who should take into account the individual makeup of any person with Down syndrome. However, in a review on the effect of vitamin supplementation on persons with Down syndrome, 337 studies showed no cognitive improvement. These authors cautioned parents about using mega-dosing vitamins for their children.

❑ One of the most common side effects seen in children with Down syndrome is hypothyroidism. One way to correct it in those whose zinc levels are too low is to supplement the diet with zinc. It is important to determine your child's zinc level before giving him or her zinc supplements.

❑ Care for the child with Down syndrome depends on the degree of mental and physical impairment. Carefully planned programs to promote development of motor and mental skills are important. Since learning potential is greatest during infancy, an early stimulation program of exercises based on the child's ability is necessary for teaching gross motor skills.

❑ The risk of giving birth to a child with Down syndrome increases markedly after the age of thirty-five. Amniocentesis is recommended if you become pregnant past this age. (For additional information on amniocentesis and other types of prenatal testing, *see under* PREGNANCY-RELATED PROBLEMS in Part Two.)

❑ Additional information on Down syndrome, parent support groups, and early intervention programs for children with Down syndrome is available from The National Down Syndrome Society. (*See* Health and Medical Organizations in the Appendix.)

DRUG ADDICTION (SUBSTANCE ABUSE)

Addiction is said to exist when the body becomes so accustomed to the presence of a foreign substance that it can no longer function properly if the substance is withdrawn.

Not everyone who uses drugs, legal or illegal, becomes addicted to them. The three most commonly used drugs—alcohol, tobacco, and caffeine—are legal and freely available, but they do not pose an addiction problem for all those who take them. Not everyone who drinks becomes an alcoholic; some people smoke only on weekends or special occasions. Many people who drink coffee don't crave it all the time.

Much research is focusing on the question of why some people become addicted while others do not, and scientists and nutritionists are providing some answers to the complex question of chemical dependency.

The reasons for addiction, according to most research, lie in the brain. A group of chemicals called neurotransmitters carry the signals between neurons in the brain. One of these neurotransmitters, dopamine, plays a pivotal role in transmitting feelings of satisfaction, arousal, and reward, so that every time we experience these feelings, we have the desire to replicate them by doing whatever it was that caused them before. This may account for the repetition inherent in addictive behavior.

Alcohol, nicotine, marijuana, cocaine, and amphetamines are a few of the substances that increase dopamine levels in the brain, and the more they are used, the more deeply these substances are associated with pleasure and reward, and the more profound the dependency. It is also thought that people who become addicted to a substance eventually take less pleasure in things they used to enjoy.

Positron-emission tomography (PET) brain scans of addicted people have shown that their brains show less response to other pleasurable pursuits, such as listening to their favorite music, than do the brain scans of people not involved in substance abuse.

The pleasure elicited by whatever substance the individual is addicted to is so strong that it is difficult to eradicate, and even after years of abstinence, there are triggers that may cause the person to relapse. Research has shown that long-term drug abuse results in significant changes in brain function that persist long after an individual stops using drugs.

Signs of drug addiction can include a decreased desire to work and/or socialize, extreme drowsiness, inattentiveness, frequent mood swings, restlessness, personality changes, and a loss of appetite. Persons addicted to drugs may want to be alone, and lose their tempers easily. Drug withdrawal symptoms may include headache, insomnia, sensitivity to light and noise, diarrhea, hot and cold flashes, sweating, deep depression, irritability, irrational thinking, and disorientation. Not surprisingly, individuals who are addicted to drugs can end up centering their lives on avoiding the excruciating pain of withdrawal—that is, on assuring a continuing supply of the drug. This need to obtain the drug at all costs leads ultimately to a disintegration of normal life, including broken personal relationships, loss of employment, and even criminal behavior.

People who become chemically dependent do so at different rates, and research is showing that susceptibility to addiction may be, in part, hereditary. Complicating the phenomenon of addiction is the problem of drug tolerance. Researchers have found that children who were diagnosed with ADHD (attention deficit hyperactivity disorder) are more likely than their peers to report alcohol-related problems, as well as drug and tobacco addictions, later in life. This study appeared in the *Journal of Abnormal Psychology*. Youngsters with severe inattention problems were five times more likely than others to use an illegal drug other than alcohol or marijuana at an early age. This turned out to be a uniquely important variable even when the presence of oppositional defiant disorder (ODD) and conduct disorder (CD) were considered. The risk factor for inattention paralleled the importance of family history as a predictor.

With prolonged drug use, the body often ends up needing more and more of the substance to produce the desired effect and to prevent withdrawal symptoms. Some users end up increasing the dosage to the point that they die, or come close to dying, from overdose. In addition, addiction almost always has a powerful psychological as well as a physical component.

The nutrient program outlined below is designed to help those recovering from drug addiction. Unless otherwise specified, the dosages recommended here are for adults. For a child under the age of seventeen, use one-half to three-quarters of the recommended amount.

NUTRIENTS

SUPPLEMENT	SUGGESTED DOSAGE	COMMENTS
Very Important		
Essential fatty acids complex	As directed on label.	Good for reversing the effects of malnourishment common in those with substance abuse problems.
Liquid Kyolic with B_1 and B_{12} from Wakunaga	As directed on label.	Fights stress and protects the liver.
Kyolic Neuro Logic from Wakunaga	As directed on label.	Nourishes the central nervous system. Detoxifies the body. Encourages normal brain function.
Vitamin B complex injections	2 cc daily or as prescribed by physician.	Needed when under stress to rebuild the liver. Injections (under a doctor's supervision) are most effective. If injections are not available, use a sublingual form.
plus extra vitamin B_{12} or vitamin B complex	1 cc daily or as prescribed by physician. 100 mg of each major B vitamin daily (amounts of individual vitamins in a complex will vary).	Can give the same energy boost as a cup of coffee.
plus extra vitamin B_5 (pantothenic acid)	500 mg 3 times daily.	Essential for the adrenal glands and for reducing stress.
and vitamin B_3 (niacinamide)	500 mg 3 times daily.	Important for brain function. *Caution:* Do not substitute niacin for niacinamide. Niacin should not be taken in such high doses.
Important		
Calcium and magnesium	1,500 mg at bedtime. 1,000 mg at bedtime.	Nourishes the central nervous system and helps control tremors by calming the body. Use chelate forms.
Free form amino acid plus extra L-glutamine	As directed on label, on an empty stomach. 500 mg 3 times daily, on an empty stomach.	To supply needed protein in a readily assimilable form. Passes the blood-brain barrier to promote healthy mental functioning. Increases levels of gamma-aminobutyric acid (GABA), which has a calming effect.
and L-tyrosine	500 mg twice daily, on an empty stomach. Take these supplements with water or juice, not milk. Take with 50 mg vitamin B_6 and 100 mg vitamin C for better absorption.	Tyrosine and valerian root taken every 4 hours have given good results for cocaine withdrawal. (See AMINO ACIDS in Part One.) *Caution:* Do not take this supplement if you are taking an MAO inhibitor drug.
Gamma-aminobutyric acid (GABA)	As directed on label, on an empty stomach.	Acts as a relaxant and lessens cravings. (See AMINO ACIDS in Part One.)
Glutathione	As directed on label.	Aids in detoxifying drugs to reduce their harmful effects. Also reduces the desire for drugs or alcohol.
Lithium	As prescribed by physician.	A trace mineral that aids in relieving depression. Available by prescription only.
L-phenylalanine	1,500 mg daily, taken upon arising.	Necessary as a brain fuel. Use for withdrawal symptoms. *Caution:* Do not take this supplement if you are pregnant or nursing, or suffer from panic attacks, diabetes, high blood pressure, or PKU.
S-Adenosylmethionine (SAMe)	As directed on label.	Aids in stress relief, depression, eases pain, and produces antioxidant effects that can improve the health of the liver. *Caution:* Do not use if you have bipolar mood disorder or take prescription antidepressants. Do not give to a child under twelve.
Vitamin C with bioflavonoids	2,000 mg every 3 hours.	Detoxifies the system and lessens the craving for drugs. Use a buffered form such as sodium ascorbate. Intravenous administration (under a doctor's supervision) may be necessary.
Zinc	As directed on label. Do not exceed a total of 100 mg daily from all supplements.	Promotes a healthy immune system and protects the liver from damage.

Helpful		
5-Hydroxytryptophan (5-HTP)	As directed on label.	Aids with both stress and withdrawal symptoms.
Multivitamin and mineral complex	As directed on label.	All nutrients are needed in high amounts. Use a high-potency formula.

Herbs

❏ Burdock root and red clover aid in cleansing toxins from the bloodstream.

❏ Siberian ginseng helps those experiencing cocaine withdrawal.

Caution: Do not use this herb if you have hypoglycemia, high blood pressure, or a heart disorder.

❏ Milk thistle helps to detoxify the liver.

❏ Pueraria, a Chinese herb, has been used for centuries as a cure for alcoholism.

❏ St. John's wort is a good antidepressant, and can help with withdrawal symptoms.

Caution: St. John's wort may cause increased sensitivity to sunlight. It may also produce anxiety, gastrointestinal symptoms, and headaches. It can interact with some drugs, including antidepressants, birth control pills, and antico-agulants.

❏ Valerian root has a calming effect. Used with the amino acid tyrosine, it has been found to be helpful for those undergoing withdrawal from cocaine.

Recommendations

❏ Eat a well-balanced, nutrient-dense diet that emphasizes fresh, raw foods.

❏ Add high-protein drinks to the diet.

❏ Avoid heavily processed foods, all forms of sugar, and junk food. These foods are a quick source of energy, but are followed by a low feeling that may increase cravings for drugs.

❏ *See* FASTING in Part Three, and follow the instructions.

❏ Consider consulting a qualified acupuncturist. Acupuncture has been known to help addicts by decreasing stress, anxiety, and the craving for drugs.

Considerations

❏ There is no single treatment that will help all addicted people. Treatment needs to be tailored to fit the different needs and problems facing the individual.

❏ To minimize withdrawal symptoms, withdrawal from any drug should be done slowly. The dosage should be decreased gradually over a period of four weeks or longer.

This task cannot be accomplished alone; most often hospitalization and/or professional help is required.

❏ Most people are aware that a drug overdose can kill, but many do not realize that these poisons kill in other ways as well. Angina, heart attack, coronary artery spasms, and life-threatening damage to the heart muscle may occur with the use of cocaine and heroin. All drugs weaken the immune system in one way or another. Chronic marijuana use can reduce the immune response by as much as 40 percent by damaging and destroying white blood cells. Without a strong immune system, the body is vulnerable to all kinds of infectious and degenerative diseases.

❏ Methadone may be prescribed as a substitute for illegal opiates.

❏ Many drug users suffer from malnutrition because they eat poorly. In addition, drugs rob the body of necessary nutrients, those addicted to drugs need to take high doses of supplemental nutrients.

❏ Research has found that children of alcoholics are more inclined than others to use drugs, including cocaine. These individuals are four hundred times more likely to use drugs than those who do not have a family history of alcohol addiction.

❏ An individual can be addicted to substances other than illegal drugs. Many are addicted to nicotine, caffeine, colas, alcohol, sugar, and even certain foods. Although these addictions may not pose as great a health risk, withdrawal still may be painful and difficult. Those who use these substances may also be more susceptible to illness and disease because these addictive substances deplete the body of needed nutrients. (*See* SUBSTANCES THAT ROB THE BODY OF NUTRIENTS on page 391.)

❏ A growing problem for substance abusers in these times, especially for those who use drugs intravenously and share needles, is the threat of AIDS (*see* AIDS in Part Two) and hepatitis. Unfortunately, for long-term drug users, even this is not enough to deter them from continuing the habitual use of drugs.

❏ *See also* ALCOHOLISM and SMOKING DEPENDENCY in Part Two.

DRY SKIN

A balance of oil and moisture is crucial for healthy, attractive skin. Oil is secreted by the sebaceous glands and lubricates the surface of the skin. Moisture is the water present inside the skin cells, and comes to the cells through the bloodstream. It is the water in the skin cells that keeps them plumped-up, healthy, and youthful-looking. Oil and moisture work together; there must be enough moisture in the skin cells, but there must also be enough oil to act as a shield, preventing excessive evaporation of moisture from the skin's top layers. Ichthyosis is one of several inherited skin conditions that cause the skin to lose moisture.

Substances That Rob the Body of Nutrients

Different substances deplete the body of different nutrients. Use the table below to determine which supplements you may need as a result of the use of prescription or over-the-counter drugs, including alcohol and caffeine.

Substance	Depleted Nutrients
Allopurinol (Zyloprim)	Iron.
Antacids B	B-complex vitamins; calcium; phosphate; vitamins A and D.
Antibiotics, general (*See also* isoniazid, penicillin, sulfa drugs, and trimethoprim)	B-complex vitamins; vitamin K; "friendly" bacteria
Antihistamines	Vitamin C.
Barbiturates	Vitamin C.
Beta-blockers (Corgard, Inderal, Lopressor, and others)	Choline; chromium; vitamin B_5 (pantothenic acid).
Caffeine	Biotin; inositol; potassium; vitamin B_1 (thiamine); zinc.
Carbamazepine (Atretol, Tegretol)	Dilutes blood sodium.
Chlorthiazide (Aldoclor, Diuril, and others)	Magnesium; potassium.
Cimetidine (Tagamet)	Iron.
Clonidine (Catapres, Combipres)	B-complex vitamins; calcium.
Corticosteroids, general (*See also* prednisone)	Calcium; potassium; vitamins A, B_6, C, and D; zinc.
Digitalis preparations (Crystodigin, Digoxin, and others)	Vitamins B_1 (thiamine) and B_6 (pyridoxine); zinc.
Diuretics, general (*See also* chlorthiazide, spironolactone, thiazide diuretics, and triamterene)	Calcium; iodine; magnesium; potassium; vitamins B_2 (riboflavin) and C; zinc.
Estrogen preparations	Folic acid; vitamin B_6 (pyridoxine).
Ethanol (alcohol) B	B-complex vitamins; magnesium; vitamins C, D, E, and K.
Fluoride	Vitamin C.
Glutethimide (Doriden)	Folic acid; vitamin B_6 (pyridoxine).
Guanethidine (Esimil, Ismelin)	Magnesium; potassium; vitamins B_2 (riboflavin) and B_6 (pyridoxine).
Hydralazine (Apresazide, Apresoline, and others)	Vitamin B_6 (pyridoxine).
Indomethacin (INH and others)	Vitamins B_3 (niacin) and B_6 (pyridoxine).
Laxatives (excluding herbs)	Potassium; vitamins A and K.
Lidocaine (Xylocaine)	Calcium; potassium.
Nitrate/nitrite coronary vasodilators	Niacin; pangamic acid; selenium; vitamins C and E.
Oral contraceptives	B-complex vitamins; vitamins C, D, and E.
Penicillin preparations	Vitamin B_3 (niacin); niacinamide; vitamin B_6 (pyridoxine).
Phenobarbital preparations	Folic acid; vitamin B_6 (pyridoxine); vitamin B_{12}; vitamins D and K.
Phenylbutazone (Cotylbutazone)	Folic acid; iodine.
Phenytoin (Dilantin)	Calcium; folic acid; vitamins B_{12}, C, D, and K.
Prednisone (Deltasone and others)	Potassium; vitamins B_6 (pyridoxine) and C; zinc.
Quinidine preparations	Choline; vitamin B_5 (pantothenic acid); potassium; vitamin K.
Reserpine preparations	Phenylalanine; potassium; vitamins B_2 (riboflavin) and B_6 (pyridoxine).
Spironolactone (Aldactone and others)	Calcium; folic acid.
Statins	Coenzyme Q_{10}
Sulfa drugs	Para-aminobenzoic acid (PABA); "friendly" bacteria.
Synthetic neurotransmitters	Magnesium; potassium; vitamins B_2 (riboflavin) and B_6 (pyridoxine).
Thiazide diuretics	Magnesium; potassium; vitamin B_2 (riboflavin); zinc.
Tobacco	Vitamins A, C, and E.
Triamterene (Dyrenium)	Calcium; folic acid.
Trimethoprim (Bactrim, Septra, and others)	Folic acid.

There are actually two types of dry skin—simple dry skin and complex dry skin. Simple dry skin results from a lack of natural oils. This condition most often affects women under the age of thirty-five. Complex dry skin lacks both oil and moisture, and is characterized by fine lines, brown spots, discolorations, enlarged pores, and sagging skin. It is usually associated with aging. The proteins that make up the skin—elastin, collagen, and keratin—may also be damaged by prolonged exposure to sunlight.

Dry skin tends to be dull-looking, even scaly and flaky, and readily develops wrinkles and fine lines. It usually feels "tight" and uncomfortable after washing unless some type of moisturizer or skin cream is applied. Chapping and cracking are signs of extremely dry, dehydrated skin.

Dry skin is most common on areas of the body that are exposed to the elements, such as the face and hands, but it also can be a whole-body problem, especially in winter. Dry skin can be caused (or aggravated) by a poor diet and by environmental factors such as exposure to sun, wind, cold, chemicals, or cosmetics, or excessive bathing with harsh soaps. Nutritional deficiencies, especially deficiencies of vitamin A and the B vitamins, can also contribute to the problem.

Fair-skinned people seem to be more likely than others to have dry skin, especially as they age. Most skin tends to become thinner and drier as people get older. If all other causes for dry skin, such as dermatitis, eczema, psoriasis, or seborrhea have been excluded, then it is most likely that the reason for dry skin lies in a combination of heredity, vitamin deficiencies, and poor nutrition. Many people have skin that is dry in some areas and oily in others. In the classic case of "combination skin," the skin on the forehead, nose, and chin tends to be oily, while the skin on the rest of the face is dry.

Unless otherwise specified, the dosages recommended here are for adults. For children between the ages of twelve and seventeen, reduce the dose to three-quarters the recommended amount. For children between six and twelve, use one-half the recommended dose, and for children under the age of six, use one-quarter the recommended amount. Persons with malabsorption problems should consult a health care provider before starting any nutritional program.

NUTRIENTS

SUPPLEMENT	SUGGESTED DOSAGE	COMMENTS
Very Important		
Primrose oil or Kyolic-EPA from Wakunaga	Up to 500 mg daily. As directed on label.	Contains linoleic acid, an essential fatty acid needed by the skin.
Vitamin A with mixed carotenoids or	25,000 IU daily for 3 months, then reduce to 15,000 IU daily. If you are pregnant, do not exceed 10,000 IU daily.	Strengthens and protects the skin tissue.
ACES + Zn from Carlson Labs	As directed on label.	Contains antioxidants that protect the skin by neutralizing free radicals.
Vitamin B complex plus extra vitamin B_{12}	As directed on label. 1,000–2,000 mcg daily.	Antistress and antiaging vitamins. Use a sublingual form.
Important		
Kelp	1,000–1,500 mg daily.	Supplies balanced minerals. Needed for good skin tone.
Vitamin E	200 IU daily.	Protects against free radicals. Used topically, it can minimize wrinkling. Use d-alpha-tocopherol form.
Zinc	50 mg daily. Do not exceed a total of 100 mg daily from all supplements.	Necessary for proper functioning of the oil-producing glands of the skin. Use zinc gluconate lozenges or OptiZinc for best absorption.
Helpful		
Ageless Beauty from Biotec Foods	As directed on label.	Protects the skin from free radical damage.
Collagen cream	Apply topically as directed on label.	Good for very dry skin. A nourishing cream that can restore a healthy tone to damaged skin.
Elastin	Apply topically as directed on label.	Helps prevent and smooth wrinkles.
Glucosamine sulfate or N-Acetylglucosamine (N-A-G from Source Naturals)	As directed on label. As directed on label.	Important for healthy skin and connective tissue.
Herpanacine from Diamond-Herpanacine Associates	As directed on label.	Contains antioxidants, amino acids, and herbs that promote skin health.
L-cysteine	500 mg daily, on an empty stomach. Take with water or juice. Do not take with milk. Take with 50 mg vitamin B_6 and 100 mg vitamin C for better absorption.	Contains sulfur, needed for healthy skin. (*See* AMINO ACIDS in Part One.)
Lecithin granules or capsules	1 tbsp 3 times daily, before meals. 1,200 mg 3 times daily, before meals.	Needed for better absorption of the essential fatty acids.
Pycnogenol or grape seed extract	As directed on label. As directed on label.	Contains a free radical scavenger that also strengthens collagen.
Selenium	200 mcg daily. If you are pregnant, do not exceed 40 mcg daily.	Encourages tissue elasticity and is a powerful antioxidant. Protects against ultraviolet-induced damage.
Superoxide dismutase (SOD)	As directed on label.	A free radical destroyer. Also good for brown age spots.
Vitamin C with bioflavonoids	3,000–5,000 mg daily, in divided doses.	Necessary for collagen production; strengthens the capillaries that feed the skin.

Herbs

❑ Used topically, aloe vera has excellent soothing, healing, and moisturizing properties. It also helps to slough off dead skin cells. Apply aloe vera gel topically on affected areas as directed on the product label.

❑ Calendula and comfrey have skin-softening properties. They can be used in a facial sauna or to make herbal or floral waters (see below). Comfrey also reduces redness and soothes irritated skin. Allantoin, an ingredient in many skin care products, is derived from comfrey.

Note: Comfrey is recommended for external use only.

❑ Spray an herbal or floral water mist on your skin throughout the day to replenish lost moisture. Almost all skin types, but particularly dry skin, benefit from lavender. You can purchase lavender water already made, or you can make your own by adding a few drops of essential oil to 4 ounces of distilled water, or by making an infusion of fresh lavender leaves and flowers.

❑ A weekly facial sauna using the herbs chamomile, lavender, and peppermint is good for dry skin. Using a glass or enameled pot, simmer a total of 2 to 4 tablespoons of dried or fresh herbs in 2 quarts of water. When the pot is steaming, place it on top of a trivet or thick potholder on a table, and sit with your face at a comfortable distance over the steam for fifteen minutes. You can use a towel to trap the steam if you wish. After fifteen minutes, splash your face with cold water and allow your skin to air-dry or pat it dry with a towel. Then either apply a good natural moisturizer or facial oil, or apply a clay mask (*see under* Recommendations, below). After the sauna, you can allow the herbal water to cool and save it for use as a toning lotion to be dabbed on your face with a cotton ball after cleansing.

Caution: Do not use chamomile if you are allergic to ragweed. Do not use during pregnancy or nursing. It may interact with warfarin or cyclosporine, so patients using these drugs should avoid it.

Recommendations

❑ Eat a balanced diet that includes vegetables, fruits, grains, seeds, and nuts. Eat quality protein from vegetable sources. Increase your intake of raw foods.

❑ Eat foods high in sulfur, which helps to keep the skin smooth and youthful. Good sources include garlic, onions, eggs, and asparagus. Sulfur is also present in the amino acid L-cysteine, which can be purchased in pill form.

❑ Consume plenty of yellow and orange vegetables. These are high in beta-carotene, a precursor of vitamin A.

❑ Drink at least 2 quarts of quality water every day to keep the skin well hydrated.

❑ Avoid fried foods, animal fats, and heat-processed vegetable oils such as those sold in supermarkets. Use cold-pressed oils only. Beware of any oils that have been subjected to heat, whether in processing or cooking. Heating oils leads to the production of free radicals, which have a destructive effect on the skin. Do take supplemental essential fatty acids (*see under* Nutrients, above). This may be the best supplement available for dry skin, but be patient; it may take a month or more to see results.

❑ Do not drink soft drinks or eat sugar, chocolate, potato chips, or other junk foods.

❑ Avoid alcohol and caffeine. These substances have a diuretic effect, causing the body—including the skin cells—to lose fluids and essential minerals.

❑ Twice weekly, use a loofah sponge and warm water for the face to boost circulation and remove dead skin cells. Avoid using the loofah around your eyes, however.

❑ Always moisturize your skin after cleansing, and at other times throughout the day, if necessary, to keep it from drying out. Use a liquid moisturizer or facial oil that contains nutrients and other natural ingredients. Do not use solid, waxy moisturizing creams. Vitamin A and E Wrinkle Treatment Oil and Vitamin A Retinyl Palmitate Wrinkle Treatment Gel are both good for dry age lines caused by the sun and the skin's natural aging. The Wrinkle Treatment Oil is also good for cleansing the skin. The moisturizing gel is non-oily and fast absorbing.

❑ Look for skin care products that contain humectants. Humectants are substances that attract water to the skin to hold in moisture. Natural humectants include vegetable glycerine, vitamin E, and panthenol, a form of pantothenic acid (vitamin B_5).

❑ Use a humidifier (or even a pan of water placed near a radiator) to humidify your environment, especially in winter. This helps to reduce the amount of moisture lost from the skin through evaporation.

❑ Once a week, use a facial mask to clarify the skin and remove dull, dry surface skin cells. (This can be done immediately after the facial sauna described under Herbs in this section.) Blend together well 1 teaspoon green clay powder (available in health food stores) and 1 teaspoon raw honey. Apply the mixture to your face, avoiding the eye area. Leave it on for fifteen minutes, then rinse well with lukewarm water. While your skin is still slightly damp, apply a natural skin oil or liquid moisturizer.

❑ If your skin is chapped or cracked, increase your consumption of water and essential fatty acids. Keep any chapped areas well lubricated and protected from the elements.

❑ For cracked, dry skin on the fingers, use calendula cream or oil with comfrey, vitamin E oil, and aloe vera. Apply the mixture to hands at bedtime, then wear plastic gloves overnight. Pure vitamin E oil can be found in health food stores.

❑ Do not smoke, and avoid secondhand smoke. Smoking has a harmful effect on the skin for several reasons. First, nicotine constricts the blood vessels, including the tiny capillaries that serve the skin. This deprives the skin of the oxygen and nutrients it needs for good health. Second, smoking involves the frequent repetition of certain facial postures, which eventually become etched in the skin in the form of wrinkles. The characteristic "smoker's face" has wrinkles radiating in a circle outward from the mouth. Smoking also can make the skin dry and leathery.

❑ Do not use harsh soaps, cold cream, or cleansing creams on your skin. Cleansing creams are made from hydrogenated oils, which can cause free radical damage to the skin, resulting in dryness and wrinkles. Instead, use pure olive, avocado, or almond oil to cleanse the skin. Pat the oil on, then wash it off with warm water and a soft cloth.

❑ Do not use very hot water when bathing or showering.

❑ As much as possible, stay out of the sun. The sun is responsible for most of the damage done to the skin. It causes dryness, wrinkles, and even rashes and blisters. Always apply a good sunscreen to all exposed areas of skin if you must be in the sun.

❑ To care for combination skin, simply treat the dry areas as dry skin and the oily areas as oily skin. (See OILY SKIN in Part Two.)

Considerations

❑ Dry skin can be a sign of an underactive thyroid. (See HYPOTHYROIDISM in Part Two.)

❑ Serious skin complications can arise for people with diabetes. (See DIABETES in Part Two.)

❑ Skin care for people of color used to be a hit-or-miss proposition. There is now more of an awareness that some of these problems are ethnic-specific. A clinic specifically to address this issue is the Multicultural Dermatology Clinic at Henry Ford Hospital in Detroit. There is also the book by Dr. Fran Cook-Bolden, director of the Ethnic Skin Specialty Group in New York—*Beautiful Skin of Color: A Comprehensive Guide to Asian, Olive and Dark Skin* (HarperCollins, 2005).

❑ Certain drugs, including diuretics, antispasmodics, and antihistamines, can contribute to dry skin.

❑ Balanced skin depends upon the production of natural moisturizing factors that help the skin attract and retain moisture. A group of acids known as alpha-hydroxy acids, applied topically, helps to stimulate production of these naturally occurring substances. Alpha-hydroxy acids also encourage the formation of new skin cells. These acids occur naturally in apples, milk, sugar cane, citrus fruits, tomatoes, grapes, and blackberries. Of the alpha-hydroxy acids, lactic acid appears to be the best for improving moisturization, while glycolic acid is more effective at sloughing off dead skin cells and promoting cell renewal.

❑ Cocoa butter is a good skin cream and is not expensive. It also helps reduce skin wrinkling. Keep it in the refrigerator after opening.

❑ A deficiency of vitamin A can result in scaly skin, particularly on the hands and feet. Cod liver oil is a good source of vitamins A and D. Although vitamin A deficiency is rare, vitamin D deficiency is much more common.

❑ GH3 cream from Gero Vita International, applied topically, is good for the prevention of wrinkles and can help with discoloration of the skin.

❑ Kinetin, a manufactured version of a plant hormone that prevents plants from withering, is proving effective in the treatment of fine facial lines.

❑ Hyper-C Serum from Jason Natural Cosmetics/Hain Celestial Group boosts collagen production and moisturizes and protects the skin.

❑ Pycnogenol Crème (or Gel) with Vitamins E, C, & A from Derma-E Skin Care is good for moisturizing, softening, and protecting the skin. Derma E also makes Vitamin E Deep Moisturizing Crème, a refreshing skin treatment, and Vitamin A with E Wrinkle Treatment for dry and aging skin.

❑ Tretinoin (Retin-A), applied topically, removes fine wrinkles and is also excellent for age spots, precancerous lesions, and sun-damaged skin. It is available by prescription only, and takes around six months to show results. Don't use Retin-A around your mouth, eyes, or nose.

DYSPEPSIA

See INDIGESTION.

DYSTHYMIA

See under DEPRESSION.

DYSTONIA

See under RARE DISORDERS.

EAR INFECTION

It has been estimated that 90 percent of all children suffer from some type of ear infection, most often between the ages of six months and four years. External otitis, also known as swimmer's ear, affects the outer ear. It may be preceded by an upper respiratory tract infection or an allergic reaction to some foods, most commonly dairy products.

The ear canal, extending from the eardrum to the outside, becomes inflamed and swollen. Symptoms can include slight fever, discharge from the ear, and pain, often severe and throbbing, that worsens when the earlobe is touched or pulled.

Middle ear infections (*otitis media*) are very common in infants and children. The site of this infection is behind the eardrum, where the small bones of the ear are located. Air pressure is regulated in this area by the eustachian or auditory tube, which runs from the ear to the back of the nasal cavity. If bacteria or viruses get into this space, the area becomes inflamed and fluid starts to build up, causing the sensation of pressure. Unfortunately, in small children the eustachian tube runs almost horizontally rather than sloping downward. This allows fluids to build up and lie stagnant, giving bacteria an ideal place to grow, rather than draining out. Other symptoms include earache; sharp, dull, or throbbing pain; a feeling of fullness in the ear; and a fever as high as 103°F or higher. Children often pull at their ears in an attempt to relieve the pressure. High altitudes and cold temperatures increase discomfort and can worsen an infection.

A severe middle ear infection can cause perforation of the eardrum. If this happens, it can actually cause a sudden reduction in pain. This is because the pain of an ear infection results when pressure builds up in restricted spaces; this pressure on sensitive nerve endings causes pain. A perforated eardrum results in hearing loss and a discharge of bloody fluid from the ear.

Recurring ear infections are generally an indication that an original infection has been resistant to the prescribed treatment. In babies, earache is often associated with teething. Living in a household where someone smokes can be a contributing factor to ear problems in children.

Unless otherwise specified, the dosages recommended here are for adults. For children between the ages of twelve and seventeen, reduce the dose to three-quarters the recommended amount. For children between six and twelve, use one-half the recommended dose, and for children under the age of six, use one-quarter the recommended amount.

NUTRIENTS

SUPPLEMENT	SUGGESTED DOSAGE	COMMENTS
Very Important		
Manganese	10 mg daily. Take separately from calcium.	Deficiency has been linked to ear disorders.
Vitamin C with bioflavonoids	3,000–7,000 mg daily, in divided doses. Children: 200 mg 4 times daily.	Boosts immunity and fights infection. Use an esterified or buffered form such as Ester-C or calcium or zinc ascorbate.
Zinc	10 mg in lozenge form 3 times daily for 5 days, then 50 mg daily in pill form. Do not exceed this amount.	Quickens immune response. Aids in reducing infection.
Important		
Kyolic-EPA from Wakunaga	As directed on label.	To reduce infection and inflammation.
Vitamin B complex	50 mg of each major B vitamin 3 times daily (amounts of individual vitamins in a complex will vary).	Essential for healing and immune function. A sublingual form is recommended. Important for immune function.
plus extra vitamin B₆ (pyridoxine)	50 mg daily.	
Vitamin E	200 IU daily.	Enhances immune function. Use d-alpha-tocopherol form.

Herbs

❑ Take alcohol-free echinacea extract by mouth; this will generally end an ear infection if you catch it early.

Caution: Do not take echinacea for longer than three months. It should not be used by people who are allergic to ragweed.

❑ Eardrops containing garlic (*Allium sativum*), mullein (*Verbascum thapsus*), and St. John's wort are available at drug and health food stores. Check with your doctor before putting anything into your child's ear.

Caution: St. John's wort may cause increased sensitivity to sunlight. It may also produce anxiety, gastrointestinal symptoms, and headaches. It can interact with some drugs including antidepressants, birth control pills, and anticoagulants.

❑ Olive leaf extract helps the body fight infection.

❑ Place ½ dropperful of alcohol-free goldenseal (*Hydrastis canadensis*) extract in your mouth and swish it around for a few minutes before swallowing. Do this every three hours for three days. Alternating echinacea (*Echinacea purpurea*) with goldenseal works wonders. For an infant, put the extract in formula or expressed breast milk, or in fruit-flavored sugar-free yogurt.

Cautions: Do not take echinacea for longer than three months. It should not be used by people who are allergic to ragweed. Do not take goldenseal internally on a daily basis for more than one week at a time. Do not use it during pregnancy or if you are breast-feeding, and use with caution if you are allergic to ragweed. If you have a history of cardiovascular disease, diabetes, or glaucoma, use it only under a doctor's supervision.

❑ Astragalus (*Astragalus membranaceus*) is an old Chinese remedy. Used as a tonic, it strengthens the body's resistance to disease.

Caution: Do not use astragalus in the presence of a fever.

❑ Onion poultices are good for ear infections. (*See* USING A POULTICE in Part Three.)

Recommendations

❑ Avoid the most common allergenic foods: wheat, dairy products, corn, oranges, peanut butter, and all simple carbohydrates, including sugar, fruits, and fruit juices.

❑ To help reduce and prevent the development of food allergies, do not repeat foods frequently. A four-day rotation diet may be beneficial. (*See* ALLERGIES in Part Two.) With a young child, introduce new foods one at a time and watch carefully for any reaction.

❑ If a bottle-fed baby has an ear infection, try eliminating milk and dairy products from the child's diet for thirty days to see if any benefits result. Try giving your baby soymilk instead of cow's milk, but do not do this without speaking to your child's pediatrician.

❑ Take garlic enemas if toxins accumulate to dangerous levels and cause the body to react. Signs of dangerous toxin levels include fever, chills, and general aches and pains. (*See* ENEMAS in Part Three.) Do not do this to a child without checking with a pediatrician.

❑ Apply hot compresses to the scalp, just behind the ear.

❑ For ringing in the ears, mix 1 teaspoonful of salt and 1 teaspoonful of glycerine (sold in drugstores) in 1 pint of warm water. Use a nasal spray bottle to spray each nostril with the solution until it begins to drain into the back of the throat. Spray the throat with the mixture as well. Do this several times a day.

❑ If you suffer from a chronic cough that lasts more than three weeks, see your health care provider. A chronic cough can be caused by impacted earwax that exerts pressure on a nerve in the ear canal, stimulating the coughing reflex. A physician can easily see if you have excessive earwax buildup and can remove it using careful suction or warm water with a slender blunt curette, plus a special microscope to aid in guiding the removal.

❑ Otoscopes (for examining the inside of the ear) are available for home use. Your physician can show you how to use one.

❑ Earache Tablets from Hyland's Inc. is a homeopathic combination remedy containing *Belladonna, Calcarea carbonica, Chamomilla, Lycopodium, Pulsatilla,* and *Sulfur* that appears to work well in reducing pain and fever.

❑ Do not blow your nose if you have an ear infection.

❑ Keep the ear canal dry. Retained soap and water in the ear canal can be dangerous. Put cotton in the ear canal when showering or bathing. Do not go swimming until healing is complete.

❑ Avoid unsanitary conditions. An ear infection may result from lowered resistance due to a recent illness. Nonprescription eardrops may relieve the pain. A nasal spray may help open up the eustachian tube and relieve the pressure.

❑ If there are symptoms of dizziness, ringing in the ears, bleeding or a bloody discharge, sudden pain (or a sudden lessening of pain), and hearing loss in one or both ears, contact your health care provider immediately. These symptoms could indicate a ruptured eardrum.

Considerations

❑ For children younger than two years of age, doctors often prescribe antibiotics. Older children can frequently go without antibiotics, as 80 percent of earaches clear up on their own. Antibiotics have only minimal effect on reducing pain and fever. Other considerations include the cost

and the risk that overuse of antibiotics may produce bacteria that are resistant to treatment.

❑ Use pain relievers like Tylenol to make your child comfortable. Do not give aspirin to anyone under twenty years of age, as it has been linked to Reye's syndrome, a serious illness that requires emergency treatment. Use only eardrops prescribed by your health care professional. Decongestants, antihistamines, and other over-the-counter cold remedies do not work for earaches. Antihistamines can cause sleepiness and thicken fluids, which may make your child worse.

❑ In most cases, with proper treatment, a perforated eardrum heals naturally, with no permanent loss of hearing. An eardrum may rupture as a result of infection or due to sudden inward pressure to the ear from swimming, diving, a slap, a nearby explosion, or even a kiss over the ear. For ruptured eardrums, keep water from getting into the ear. Don't use earplugs unless your doctor says it is safe to do so.

❑ Breast-fed babies are much less likely than bottle-fed babies to suffer from ear infections.

❑ Ear problems are much more common in the homes of smokers.

❑ *Branhamella catarrahalis* (B-cat), a common cause of ear infections, has developed strains that resist standard antibiotics. Fortunately, the antibiotic Augmentin (a combination of amoxicillin and clavulanate) can still destroy the B-cat bacterium.

❑ Ear infection is not the only cause of ear pain. Rapid changes in air pressure, such as occur during air travel, often cause ear pain and can even result in damage to the eardrum. This is called aerotitis or barotitis media. If an infection is present, the effects of pressure changes are magnified.

❑ Children who have frequent ear infections should be tested for food allergies. The role of allergies as a major cause of chronic otitis media has been firmly established. (*See* ALLERGIES in Part Two.)

EATING DISORDERS

See ANOREXIA NERVOSA; APPETITE, POOR; BULIMIA; OBESITY; UNDERWEIGHT.

ECZEMA

See DERMATITIS.

EDEMA

Edema is the accumulation of fluid in spaces between the cells in the soft tissue of the body. Any part of the body may develop edema. The swelling can be localized in the face, arms, and neck, or may involve the legs and ankles—a condition known as dependent edema. Periorbital edema is swelling around the eyes. Corneal stroma is edema of the cornea. Generalized edema is known as anasarca. Pre-eclampsia is a condition that occurs in approximately 5 percent of pregnant women, causing high blood pressure, fluid accumulation in the tissues, and albuminuria (protein in the urine).

The underlying causes of edema may be serious. Edema can indicate a much more profound illness, such as cirrhosis of the liver, congestive heart failure, diabetes, or vena cava syndrome (narrowing of the vein that supplies blood from the upper body to the heart). More simply, edema can occur as the result of infection or prolonged bed rest. Fluid retention can also be caused by allergies.

Unless otherwise specified, the dosages recommended here are for adults. For children between the ages of twelve and seventeen, reduce the dose to three-quarters the recommended amount. For children between six and twelve, use one-half the recommended dose, and for children under the age of six, use one-quarter the recommended amount.

NUTRIENTS

SUPPLEMENT	SUGGESTED DOSAGE	COMMENTS
Very Important		
Free form amino acid (Amino Balance from Anabol Naturals)	As directed on label.	Sometimes edema is caused by inadequate protein assimilation. Protein deficiency has been linked to water retention.
Vitamin B complex	50–100 mg of each major B vitamin twice daily, with meals (amounts of individual vitamins in a complex will vary).	B vitamins work best when taken together.
plus extra vitamin B₆ (pyridoxine)	50 mg 3 times daily.	Reduces water retention.
Important		
Alfalfa		*See* under Herbs, below.
Calcium and magnesium	1,500 mg daily. 1,000 mg daily.	To replace minerals lost with correction of edema.
Silica	As directed on label.	A natural diuretic.
Helpful		
Bromelain	As directed on label 3 times daily.	An enzyme derived from pineapples that helps digestion and allergies.
Garlic (Kyolic from Wakunaga)	2 capsules 3 times daily, with meals.	A detoxifier.
Kelp	1,000–1,500 mg daily.	Supplies needed minerals.
Potassium	99 mg daily.	Very important if taking diuretics. Helps to keep fluids on the inside of the cells.
Pycnogenol	As directed on label.	A powerful antioxidant that also strengthens the tissues of the circulatory system.
Superoxide dismutase (SOD)	As directed on label.	Helpful in heart and liver disorders.
Taurine	As directed on label.	Aids heart function.

Vitamin C with bioflavonoids	3,000–5,000 mg daily, in divided doses.	Essential for adrenal function and production of adrenal hormones, which are vital for proper fluid balance and control of edema.
Vitamin E	200 IU daily.	Aids circulation. Use d-alpha-tocopherol form.

Herbs

❑ Alfalfa is a good source of important minerals. It also contains chlorophyll, a potent detoxifier. Take 2,000 to 3,000 milligrams daily, in divided doses.

❑ Hawthorn berries, juniper, and uva ursi are diuretics. By increasing the output of urine, they help to counteract edema.

❑ Horse chestnut has been shown to reduce postsurgical edema.

❑ Rose hips contain bioflavonoids helpful in the treatment of edema.

❑ Kidney Blend SP-6 from Solaray contains corn silk and other herbs that aid the body in expelling excess fluids. Take 2 capsules three times daily.

❑ Other herbs that can be beneficial if you are suffering from edema include butcher's broom, dandelion root, juniper berries, lobelia, marshmallow, parsley, and pau d'arco tea.

Caution: Lobelia is only to be taken under supervision of a health care professional as it is potentially toxic. People with high blood pressure, heart disease, liver disease, kidney disease, seizure disorders, or shortness of breath should not take lobelia. Pregnant and lactating women should avoid lobelia as well.

Recommendations

❑ Eat a diet that is high in fiber.

❑ For protein, eat eggs, broiled whitefish, and broiled skinless chicken or turkey. Consume small amounts of buttermilk, cottage cheese, kefir, and low-fat yogurt.

❑ Use kelp to supply needed minerals.

❑ Avoid alcohol, animal protein, beef, caffeine, chocolate, dairy products (except for those listed above), dried shellfish, fried foods, gravies, olives, pickles, salt, soy sauce, tobacco, white flour, and white sugar. Salt, in particular, may exacerbate fluid retention.

❑ If you have swelling of the legs and feet, sit with your feet up as often as you can. Wear support hose for swelling in the legs.

❑ Exercise daily and take hot baths or saunas twice a week.

❑ Avoid stress.

❑ *See* FASTING in Part Three and follow the program. Fasting flushes excess water from the tissues.

□ If pressing with the fingers on your feet and ankles results in the formation of small "pits," consult your physician. This can be a sign of a serious health problem.

Considerations

□ According to traditional Chinese medicine, avoiding raw foods, cold drinks, and fatty foods helps to prevent water retention.

□ Food allergy testing is recommended. (*See* ALLERGIES in Part Two.)

□ *See also under* PREGNANCY-RELATED PROBLEMS in Part Two.

EMPHYSEMA

Emphysema is a degenerative lung disease that usually develops after many years of exposure to cigarette smoke or other toxins that pollute the air. It is one of a group of lung diseases referred to as chronic obstructive pulmonary disease (COPD). COPD, which also includes asthma and chronic bronchitis, can interfere with normal breathing. The predominant symptom of emphysema is shortness of breath and the feeling of not being able to get enough air during any kind of physical exertion.

In people with emphysema, damage to the alveoli (small air sacs in the lungs) causes the lungs to lose their elasticity. As a result, exhaling becomes difficult, and stale air remains trapped in the lungs, preventing the needed exchange of oxygen and carbon dioxide. A person with advanced emphysema may experience a near-constant state of breathlessness, chronic coughing and wheezing, and frequent discharge of sputum from the respiratory passages. Emphysema can also contribute to other health problems, such as lung infections and a condition called erythrocytosis, in which the blood contains abnormally high levels of red blood cells. Erythrocytosis can cause such symptoms as weakness, dizziness, fatigue, light-headedness, headache, and vision problems.

Most people who are diagnosed with emphysema are long-term smokers. Symptoms may not occur until middle age, when the individual's ability to exercise or do heavy work begins to decline, and a productive cough begins. The symptoms may be subtle at first, but worsen with time.

In rare cases, emphysema is caused by a genetic condition that leads to a deficiency of a blood protein called alpha-1-antitrypsin. The overwhelming majority of cases, however, are related to smoking. Regular smoking, whether of tobacco or marijuana, causes chronic low-level inflammation of the lungs, which increases the chance of developing this progressive disease.

In the United States, more than 12 million adults have been diagnosed with COPD. An additional 12 million likely have the disease and don't know it. COPD is the fourth leading cause of death in the United States, behind heart ailments, cancers, and stroke. The COPD death rate for women grew much faster than the rate for men from 1980 to 2000. This increase suggests that smoking, which increased dramatically among women from about 1940 onward, is now taking its toll.

In third-world countries, poor indoor air quality appears to be a major factor in the development and progression of the disease.

Unless otherwise specified, the dosages recommended here are for adults.

NUTRIENTS

SUPPLEMENT	SUGGESTED DOSAGE	COMMENTS
Essential		
Chlorophyll (Kyo-Green from Wakunaga	As directed on label 3 times daily.	Aids in clear breathing.
Dimethylglycine (DMG) (Aangamik DMG from FoodScience of Vermont)	250 mg 3 times daily.	Increases endurance and provides oxygen to cells. Use a sublingual form.
Essential fatty acids (Kyolic-EPA from Wakunaga, salmon oil, flaxseed oil, or primrose oil)	As directed on label. Take with meals.	Essential for rebuilding and producing new cells.
Zinc plus copper	80 mg daily. Do not exceed a total of 100 mg daily from all supplements. 3 mg daily.	Works as an antioxidant with specific protective effects on lung proteins. Needed to balance with zinc.
Very Important		
Coenzyme Q_{10} plus Coenzyme A from Coenzyme-A Technologies	60 mg daily. As directed on label.	A powerful antioxidant; enhances oxygen in the lungs. Aids in removing toxins from the body.
Free form amino acid	As directed on label.	Important for repair of lung tissue.
Garlic (Kyolic from Wakunaga)	2 capsules 3 times daily, with meals.	An immunity enhancer for protection against pneumonia.
L-cysteine and L-glutathione and L-methionine	500 mg each twice daily, on an empty stomach. Take with water or juice. Do not take with milk. Take with 50 mg vitamin B_6 and 100 mg vitamin C for better absorption.	To aid in repairing damaged lung tissue and act as antioxidants protecting lung tissue. (*See* AMINO ACIDS in Part One.)
Lung Support Formula from Gero Vita	As directed on label.	Promotes healing and improved breathing.
Pycnogenol or grape seed extract	30 mg 3 times daily. As directed on label.	Powerful antioxidants that help protect the lungs.
Vitamin A plus carotenoid complex	25,000 IU daily. If you are pregnant, do not exceed 10,000 IU daily. As directed on label.	Needed for repair of lung tissues and for the immune system. Emulsion form is recommended for easier assimilation and greater safety at higher doses. Powerful antioxidants that

		protect against excess levels of free radicals.
Vitamin C with bioflavonoids	5,000–10,000 mg daily, in divided doses.	Strengthens immune response and aids healing of inflamed tissue.
Vitamin E emulsion or capsules	200 IU daily.	An oxygen carrier and potent antioxidant. A deficiency can lead to destruction of cell membranes. Emulsion form is recommended for easier assimilation and greater safety at higher doses.
Helpful		
Aerobic 07 from Aerobic Life Industries	9 drops in water once daily.	Supplies oxygen and kills bacteria.
Beta-1,3-D-glucan	As directed on label.	Promotes healing and works as a highly effective free radical scavenger.
Calcium and magnesium	2,000 mg daily, at bedtime. 500–1,000 mg daily, at bedtime.	Act as a nerve tonic, protect nerve endings, and promote sound sleep. Use chelate forms.
Kelp	1,000–1,5000 mg daily.	Contains minerals needed for improved breathing and healing.
Multienzyme complex with pancreatin plus	As directed on label. Take with meals.	To keep infection in check by cleansing the lungs.
proteolytic enzymes or	As directed on label. Take with meals.	
Inf-zyme Forte from American Biologics or	As directed on label.	A balance of potent enzymes and cofactors that acts as a powerful inflammatory inhibitor.
Oxy-5000 Forte from American Biologics	As directed on label.	A potent nutritional antioxidant for health and stress that destroys free radicals.

Herbs

❑ Astragalus, a Chinese herb also known as huang qi, accelerates healing in the bronchial tubes and promotes better breathing.

Caution: Do not use astragalus in the presence of a fever.

❑ ClearLungs from RidgeCrest Herbals is an herbal combination that helps provide relief from shortness of breath, tightness in the chest, and wheezing due to bronchial congestion.

❑ Cordyceps may slow the progress of lung degeneration. Chinese medicine teaches that there is a synergistic connection between the kidneys and the lungs. Cordyceps reinforces this connection, opens up the bronchioles, and better oxygenates the blood to the kidneys. Cordyceps from R-Garden, Inc. (www.rgarden.com) is a good source of this herb.

❑ Licorice extract increases energy levels and helps to improve organ function. Use an alcohol-free extract.

Caution: Licorice root should not be used during pregnancy or nursing. It should not be used by persons with diabetes, glaucoma, heart disease, high blood pressure, or a history of stroke.

❑ Thyme is also very helpful for respiratory disorders.

❑ Other beneficial herbs for emphysema include alfalfa, fenugreek, fresh horseradish, mullein tea, and rosemary.

Recommendations

❑ Avoid any and all contact with tobacco. Tobacco smoke is the single most dangerous thing anyone suffering from emphysema can encounter. If you have emphysema and smoke, you must quit. Avoid areas where people smoke. Do not allow smoking in your home, your car, or anywhere near you.

❑ Eat a diet consisting of 50 percent raw foods. The other 50 percent should consist of soups, skinless chicken or turkey, fish, brown rice, millet, and whole-grain cereals.

❑ Consume onions and garlic daily.

❑ Do not eat a typical American breakfast. Instead, sip hot, clear liquids (such as herbal teas) in the morning to help clear the mucus from the airways. Drink at least eight glasses of quality water daily. Using a psyllium-based fiber product or ABC Aerobic Bulk Cleanse from Aerobic Life Industries (a colon cleanser available in health food stores and online) is helpful after consuming the liquids. Mix ABC with a glass of juice and drink it quickly. This will help rid the colon of excess mucus and reduce gas and distention.

❑ Avoid fried and greasy foods, salt, and all foods that cause excess mucus to be formed in the gastrointestinal tract, lungs, sinuses, and nasal cavity. Foods that lead to the formation of mucus include meats, eggs, all dairy products and cheese, processed foods, junk foods, and white flour products, as well as tobacco. Read labels carefully; these are sometimes "hidden" ingredients in food products.

❑ Avoid gas-forming foods such as legumes and cabbage. These foods cause abdominal distention that can interfere with breathing. Try using a product called Beano, available in local supermarkets, when you do eat foods that can cause gas. Place a few drops of the liquid on the first bite of food for best results.

❑ Avoid foods that require a great deal of chewing, such as meats and nuts. Chronic lung disease can make it difficult to breathe while chewing. If necessary, vegetables can be steamed to make them easier to eat.

❑ Get regular exercise. Daily exercise, especially walking, can be extremely beneficial for people with emphysema. It increases endurance, improves circulation, and generally leads to a reduced level of breathlessness. Start out with what you are able to do, even if it is only a minute or two of exercise every hour, then gradually increase the amount as you are able. Any exercise program should be started at a very low intensity and be gradually increased over time. Yoga or martial arts exercise, such as tai chi, may also be helpful. Consult your health care provider before beginning any exercise program.

❑ Try to lose weight, especially if you have abdominal fat, which could further impair breathing.

❑ Humidify your home, especially if you experience a lot of congestion or have heavy discharges of sputum.

❑ Go on a cleansing fast periodically, using carrot, celery, spinach, kale, and all dark green fresh juices. (See FASTING in Part Three.)

❑ Use warm castor oil packs on the chest and back to help reduce mucus and enhance breathing. To make a castor oil pack, place a cup or so of castor oil in a pan and warm but do not boil it. Dip a piece of cheesecloth or other white cotton material into the oil until the cloth is saturated. Apply the cloth to the affected area and cover it with a piece of plastic that is larger in size than the cotton cloth, then place a warm cloth or a hot water bottle on top. Keep the pack in place for one-half to two hours, as needed.

❑ Rest and avoid stress. Get plenty of fresh air.

❑ Leave the house during major housecleaning and other major household projects, and remain away for at least two hours afterward. Housecleaning stirs up dust and mold.

❑ Do daily breathing exercises, which can improve lung function. A technique known as deep breathing involves inhaling through the nose while pulling the abdominal muscles inward in order to allow more air to be inhaled. Exhaling takes place steadily and slowly through the mouth while the tongue is pressed between the roof of the mouth and top of the teeth, so that slight pressure is felt through the windpipe and chest. A hissing sound is produced as the air is expelled through the lips. Exhaling should take at least twice as long as inhaling, so that all air is forced out. Do this for about ten minutes, two to three times daily. This will aid in an exchange of air in the lungs and improve breathing capacity.

❑ Because every extra chemical adds potential risk to the lungs, use only essential (and unscented) laundry products. Avoid perfume and anything containing fragrance. Avoid gas stoves as well; electric stoves are better for people with respiratory disorders. Choose flooring made from hardwood, ceramic tile, or stone rather than carpeting, which holds dust, mold, and many chemicals that get into the air and that can irritate the lungs. Avoid using window curtains and draperies, which also can harbor dust. Decorate with paint (new "odorless" formulas are now available) rather than wallpaper; the glues used to make the paper adhere to the wall can have volatile chemicals that may bother some people. Avoid plastic chairs, plastic dishes, and other plastic items in furnishing your home. Do not use aerosol products.

❑ Avoid air pollution. If your current working environment is dirty, dusty, or toxic to inhale, change jobs.

❑ Avoid hot, humid climates. If you must live in such a climate, continuous central air-conditioning is essential. An air-conditioned car is also essential. Do not allow anyone to smoke or wear perfume in your car.

❑ Avoid letting furry or feathered animals into your home or car, as their hair and dander can irritate the lungs.

Considerations

❑ There is no known cure for emphysema, but the measures outlined in this section should slow the progression of the disease, ease discomfort, and make breathing a bit easier.

❑ Lung reduction surgery can be very effective in enhancing breathing function. This procedure involves making cuts in the damaged portions of the lungs and using a special stapling device that gives the healthy lung tissue more room to expand. In a similar procedure, surgeons section off the damaged lung tissue and buttress the folds using bovine pericardium (cow muscle) to enhance the viability of the tissue. Candidates for either type of surgery are carefully screened before being considered for treatment.

❑ In some cases, a lung transplant may be considered. This is a highly invasive, complex procedure that carries substantial risk. It is a viable option for only a small proportion of people with emphysema.

❑ Supplemental oxygen can benefit anyone with impaired lung function. Long-term oxygen therapy combats erythrocytosis and lowers the risk of heart failure.

❑ Older adults are at risk for magnesium deficiency, which can further compromise the ability to breathe. Taking magnesium supplements (500 to 1,000 milligrams daily) can significantly strengthen the muscles that power breathing and promote better oxygenation of the body's cells.

❑ The Air Supply personal air purifier from Wein Products is a miniature unit that is worn around the neck. It sets up an invisible pure air shield against microorganisms (such as viruses, bacteria, and mold) and microparticles (including dust, pollen, and pollutants). It also eliminates vapors, smells, and harmful volatile compounds in the air.

❑ The University of Pennsylvania Hospital Department of Allergy reports that having an air conditioner and an electrostatic air-cleaning machine in the bedroom of persons with respiratory disease is a major factor in the health of individuals with breathing trouble.

❑ A routine lung function test can determine lung capacity and other characteristics that can help identify various stages of emphysema. Several kinds of test are available:

• *Arterial blood gas (ABG)*. An ABG is a blood test that measures amounts of carbon dioxide and oxygen in the blood. This test is used to assess more-advanced stages of emphysema.

- *Pulse oximetry.* This test measures the amount of oxygen in the blood using a special light that is clipped onto a finger or earlobe.

- *Spirometry.* In this test, you take a deep breath and blow it out as quickly as possible through a tube that is connected to a machine that records airflow and capacity.

- *X-ray.* A plain chest X-ray and computerized axial tomography (CAT) scan can help diagnose moderate to severe cases of emphysema.

❏ *See also* ASCORBIC ACID FLUSH in Part Three and ENVIRONMENTAL TOXICITY in Part Two.

ENDOMETRIOSIS

Endometriosis is the abnormal growth of cells that form in the lining of the uterus. Some of these cells may, instead of being expelled from the body during the menstrual process, actually end up continuing their cycle elsewhere in the body. They then have no way of leaving the body, so the material builds up and may attach itself to other organs in the lower abdomen, such as the ovaries or bowel.

This can produce a host of different symptoms, including incapacitating pain in the uterus, lower back, and organs in the pelvic cavity prior to and during the menses; intermittent pain throughout the menstrual cycle; painful intercourse; excessive bleeding, including the passing of large clots and shreds of tissue during the menses; nausea, vomiting, and constipation during the menses; dyschezia (difficulty in passing stools due to weak pelvic muscles and anal sphincter); dysuria (pain while urinating); and, sometimes, infertility. Because menstruation is typically heavy, iron-deficiency anemia is common. Women whose cycles are shorter than twenty-seven days and/or whose periods last longer than one week are at increased risk of anemia.

Growths of endometrial tissue outside of the uterine cavity occur most often in or on the ovaries, the fallopian tubes, the urinary bladder, the bowel, the pelvic floor, and/or the peritoneum (the membrane that lines the walls of the abdominal cavity), and within the uterine musculature.

The most common site of endometriosis is believed to be the deep pelvic peritoneal cavity, or the cul-de-sac. The presence of endometrial implants outside the pelvic area is uncommon.

During the normal menstrual cycle, a continually changing hormonal environment stimulates the endometrium to grow in preparation for a possible pregnancy. This same cycle causes a follicle within one of the ovaries to ripen, and an egg is released. Fingerlike tissues on the fallopian tube grasp the egg, and the tiny, hairlike cilia inside the tube transport it toward the uterus, the lining of which is now spongy and well supplied with blood. If the egg is not

fertilized within twenty-four hours or so of being released, the uterine lining proceeds to "die," to be sloughed off, and to pass through the vagina during the menses.

Though not inside the uterus, the abnormal implants of endometriosis also respond to the hormonal changes controlling menstruation. Like the uterine lining, these fragments build tissue each month, then break down and bleed.

Unlike blood from the uterine lining, however, blood from the implants has no way to leave the body. Instead, it must be absorbed by surrounding tissue, which is a comparatively slow process. In the meantime, the blood accumulates in body cavities. The entire sequence, from bleeding through absorption, can be painful.

As the menstrual cycle recurs month after month, the implants may get bigger. They may seed new implants and form localized scar tissue and adhesions—scar tissue that attaches to pelvic organs and binds them together. This contributes to the pain of endometriosis, and it can cause extreme pain in a subsequent pregnancy, as the uterus enlarges and the organs within the abdomen are pushed into different positions. Sometimes a collection of blood called a sac or cyst forms. Endometrial or "chocolate" cysts are common on the ovaries. These are usually found to contain moderate amounts of oxidized blood, which looks something like chocolate syrup. If a cyst ruptures, it can cause excruciating pain.

No one knows what causes endometriosis, but several theories have been proposed. The reflux menstruation theory was developed by John Sampson, M.D., in 1920. According to this theory, menstrual fluid backs up into the fallopian tubes and drops into the peritoneal cavity, where endometrial cells implant themselves and grow. While this theory offers a possible answer to the question of what causes endometriosis, it has never been proven. Another popular theory states that endometriosis is caused when endometrial cells spread to other parts of the body through blood and lymphatic channels. Still another theory postulates that endometriosis is in effect a congenital condition (*see* AN ALTERNATIVE THEORY AND TREATMENT FOR ENDOMETRIOSIS on page 403).

Despite disagreement over the cause, more is known today about this condition than ever before. For example, research has shown that exposure to environmental polychlorinated biphenyls (PCBs) and dioxin, two types of hazardous waste materials, can cause spontaneous endometriosis.

This may account for the rising incidence in the condition over the last few decades. Most women who suffer from endometriosis have never been pregnant, and as many as 30 to 40 percent of women who report infertility problems actually have endometriosis. According to the Endometriosis Association, women who develop this condition have a history of more vaginal yeast infections, hay fever, eczema, and food sensitivities than most women. In addition, vulnerability to endometriosis appears to run in families. An estimated 10 percent of women of reproductive age suffer from endometriosis. Unfortunately, many women fail to seek medical help because they mistake the symptoms of this disease for normal menstrual discomfort.

Laparoscopy is the procedure most commonly used to diagnose endometriosis. This involves the insertion of a tiny lighted optical tube (a laparoscope or a smaller version, the microlaparoscope) through a small incision in the navel. The surgeon can then see inside the abdominal cavity. Laparoscopic procedures are usually done on an outpatient basis.

The nutrient program and other recommendations outlined below may help to keep endometriosis under control if it is diagnosed in the early stages.

NUTRIENTS

SUPPLEMENT	SUGGESTED DOSAGE	COMMENTS
Very Important		
Vitamin E	200 IU daily	Aids hormonal balance. Use d-alpha-tocopherol form.
Vitamin K or alfalfa	200 mcg daily.	Needed for normal blood clotting. *See* under Herbs, below.
Important		
Essential fatty acids (primrose oil and Kyolic-EPA from Wakunaga)	1,500 mg daily.	Provides essential fatty acids such as gamma-linolenic acid (GLA) that aid in regulating hormonal and prostaglandin balance.
Iron or Floradix Iron + Herbs from Salus Haus	As directed by physician. As directed on label.	Iron-deficiency anemia is common in those with this disorder. Use ferrous fumarate form. *Caution:* Do not take iron unless anemia is diagnosed. An easily assimilated and nontoxic source of iron.
Vitamin B complex plus extra vitamin B$_5$ (pantothenic acid) and vitamin B$_6$ (pyridoxine)	As directed on label. 50 mg 3 times daily. 25 mg 3 times daily.	Promotes blood cell productivity and proper hormone balance. Relieves stress. Needed for proper adrenal function. Aids the body in removing excess fluids.
Vitamin C with bioflavonoids	2,000 mg 3 times daily.	Important in the healing process. Use a buffered form.
Zinc	50 mg daily. Do not exceed a total of 100 mg daily from all supplements.	For tissue repair and immune function. Use zinc gluconate lozenges or OptiZinc for best absorption.
Helpful		
Beta-1,3-D-glucan	As directed on label.	Stimulates the activity of macrophages, which can remove foreign cellular debris.
Calcium and magnesium	1,500 mg daily. 1,000 mg daily, at bedtime.	To supply needed minerals. Use chelate forms.
Kelp	1,000–1,500 mg daily.	To supply needed iron and other minerals.
Multivitamin and mineral complex	As directed on label.	All nutrients are required for repair and healing.

Herbs

❑ Alfalfa is a good source of vitamin K (necessary for blood clotting and healing) and minerals, including iron. Many women with endometriosis are iron-deficient.

❑ Astragalus, garlic, goldenseal, myrrh gum, pau d'arco, and red clover have antibiotic and antitumor properties.

Cautions: Do not use astragalus in the presence of a fever. Do not take goldenseal internally on a daily basis for more than one week at a time. Do not use it during pregnancy or if you are breast-feeding, and use with caution if you are allergic to ragweed. If you have a history of cardiovascular disease, diabetes, or glaucoma, use it only under a doctor's supervision.

❑ Burdock root, dong quai, and red raspberry leaf help to balance hormones.

❑ Nettle is rich in iron.

Recommendations

❑ Eat a diet consisting of 50 percent raw vegetables and fruits and including soy foods. In addition, eat only whole-grain products (no refined flour products) and raw nuts and seeds. A diet rich in legumes and other fiber-rich foods is very important in managing endometriosis.

❑ Include "green drinks" made from dark green leafy vegetables in your diet.

❑ Avoid alcohol, caffeine, animal fats, butter, dairy products, fried foods, foods that contain additives, all hardened fats, junk foods or fast foods, red meats, poultry (except organically raised and skinless), refined and processed foods, salt, shellfish, and sugar.

❑ Fast for three days each month before the anticipated beginning of the menstrual period. Use steam-distilled water and fresh live juices. (*See* PREMENSTRUAL SYNDROME in Part Two and FASTING in Part Three.)

❑ Use a heating pad, hot water bottle, or a hot bath to help relieve pain. The warmth relaxes the muscles that cramp and cause pain.

❑ If you are taking medication for endometriosis, report any new or worsened symptoms to your doctor immediately, especially problems such as difficulty breathing or chest or leg pain. These symptoms may indicate the presence of a blood clot. Frequent checkups are needed to monitor possible side effects such as thinning of the bones. Be aware, however, that it is normal for endometriosis symptoms to worsen temporarily when a woman begins taking medicine.

An Alternative Theory and Treatment for Endometriosis

David Redwine, M.D., of St. Charles Medical Center in Bend, Oregon, has developed an alternative theory of the origin of endometriosis. Dr. Redwine disagrees with those obstetrician/gynecologists who accept reflux menstruation as the cause of endometriosis. Instead, he proposes that endometriosis is actually a type of birth defect. During fetal development, cells that are destined to become part of the female reproductive organs differentiate and migrate toward the appropriate locations. But, if the mechanisms that control this process do not function properly, some endometrial cells may be "left behind" in places they do not belong, where they become embedded and grow.

Initially, these bits of misplaced tissue are colorless, but over time the tissue begins to change into the lesions known as endometriosis, probably at least in part in response to stimulation from sex hormones. The lesions begin to change color and gradually become darker until they appear as the classic dark-colored implants found primarily in women in their thirties. Before they reach that stage, however, they may appear white, yellow, red, or brown, and many colors in between. Thus, according to Dr. Redwine, endometrial growths only *appear* to spread progressively throughout the pelvis—that is, they are there all the time, even before birth, but they are not usually recognized for what they are until they take on a sufficiently dark color, a process that occurs over time.

Based on his understanding of the disease, Dr. Redwine developed a treatment for endometriosis in which the implants are physically removed through surgery. Using a laparoscope, the surgeon examines the entire pelvic cavity and the entire peritoneal surface at very close range to identify any possible endometrial lesions. Then, all suspected endometrial growths are removed. Each lesion is biopsied, and a tissue sample is analyzed in a laboratory to determine whether or not it is endometrial in origin. With this identification method, Dr. Redwine says that he has been able to demonstrate that lesions other than the black "powder-burn" lesions normally considered characteristic of the condition have been endometrial in origin.

Many women who undergo surgery for endometriosis often are diagnosed with recurrences. This would seem to support the idea that this is a progressive disease that tends to come back despite treatment. However, Dr. Redwine maintains that the reason so many women have recurring problems with endometriosis is that only a portion of their endometrial implants are removed in surgery. Most surgeons remove only the "typical" black powder-burn lesions and chocolate cysts. Dr. Redwine estimates that a surgeon who excises only the black lesions may leave from 50 to 60 percent of the actual disease behind. He has found that only 40 percent of his patients have the typical lesions, while 60 percent have the multicolored, "atypical" type. He believes that endometriosis is indeed curable, so long as all the lesions—both typical and atypical, and not only within the pelvic cavity, but on the peritoneum as well—are removed. His follow-up studies indicate that after surgery, approximately 75 percent of his patients experience complete relief of symptoms, and approximately 20 percent experience an improvement in symptoms so that what was disabling pain becomes only minimal pain.

Only about 5 percent report no relief. Several other gynecological surgeons in the United States now use Dr. Redwine's treatment.

The following table outlines some of the key differences between Dr. Redwine's theory and conventional medical theory.

Endometriosis Theories Contrasted

Conventional Theory	Dr. Redwine's Theory
Caused by retrograde menstruation.	Caused by a defect in embryonic cell differentiation.
A progressive disease primarily of women over thirty.	A static disease affecting women of all ages.
Associated with menstruation.	Independent of menstruation.
Causes infertility.	May be associated with infertility, but is not the actual cause of it.
Lesions bleed monthly.	Lesions do not bleed.
Most lesions are black.	Lesions may be clear, white, pink, red, brown, black, or multicolored. Most are not black.
Peritoneal implants are not considered endometrial in origin.	Peritoneal implants have been proved to be to be endometrial in origin.
Recurrence following removal of lesions is common.	Recurrence following removal of lesions is rare if both typical and atypical lesions are removed.
Hysterectomy is recommended for severe cases. Surgery provides undependable levels of relief.	Surgical removal of all typical and atypical lesions is the treatment of choice for this disorder, and can provide complete relief in up to 75 percent of cases.

Further information on Dr. Redwine and his approach to endometriosis treatment can be obtained by contacting the Endometriosis Treatment Program (www.endometriosistreatment.org).

Considerations

❏ Daily moderate exercise such as walking or stretching is beneficial.

❏ If you suspect you may have endometriosis, you should see a gynecologist promptly so that the condition can be controlled at the earliest possible stage of development.

❏ Medical treatment recommended for endometriosis depends on how far the condition has progressed. Doctors may prescribe a drug called danazol (Danocrine), which stops the normal hormonal cycles, in an attempt to control the blood flow and pain, and in hopes of keeping the abnormal tissue from spreading and inducing the growths to heal and shrink. Some doctors prescribe oral contraceptives (birth control pills) for essentially the same reason. Danazol has been shown to improve symptoms in up to 90 percent of women who take it and to reduce the size and number of implants. Weight gain and a deepened voice are possible side effects, but are usually reversible when the medication is stopped. However, symptoms may also reappear after medication is stopped.

❏ The synthetic versions of a reproductive hormone, gonadotropin-releasing hormone (GnRH), such as leuprolide (Lupron), nafarelin (Synarel), and goserelin (Zoladex), can be used. Taken for six months, these drugs may help to lessen the symptoms of endometriosis for a year or more. They work by stopping the production of estrogen. The side effects of GnRH are the same as the effects of menopause.

❏ If endometriosis is severe and disabling, or if drug therapy fails and you do not wish to have any children at that point, hysterectomy may be recommended. However, hysterectomy does not always relieve all the symptoms, especially if there are implants of endometrial tissue throughout the pelvic region.

❏ An excision option less traumatic than hysterectomy that is used to treat milder cases is laparoscopy with laser surgery to identify and vaporize adhesions, cysts, and endometrial implants. The procedure has yet to be perfected; repeated laparoscopy may be necessary. Advances in this technique are being made at a rapid rate, however, and the need for repeat procedures may soon be a thing of the past.

❏ In one study, women who had surgery experienced less pain postoperatively, and improved quality of life with a vitamin and supplement mixture (multivitamin/mineral, probiotic, and fish oil) compared to a placebo group. These results were comparable to women who received hormonal suppression therapy. The patients were classified as stage III–IV, the most advanced stages.

❏ According to a report in the *Journal of the American Medical Association*, strenuous exercise lowers the level of estrogen in the body, and this may help suppress the symptoms of endometriosis. The more aerobic exercise a woman engages in and the earlier she starts, the lower her risk of developing the disease in the first place, according to a study of endometriosis led by Daniel W. Cramer of Brigham and Women's Hospital and Harvard Medical School. This study found that women who exercised more than seven hours a week had one-fifth the average risk of developing endometriosis. Unfortunately, this beneficial effect was limited to those who began exercising before the age of twenty-six.

❏ Because endometriosis depends on hormonal cycles, and pregnancy temporarily interrupts those cycles, many women find that their symptoms improve during pregnancy. In some cases, the improvement may be permanent, presumably because the break from cycles of growth, bleeding, and scarring finally allows the implants to heal and be shed. In other cases, however, the relief is only temporary, and once the hormonal cycles return to normal, the symptoms of endometriosis recur.

❏ Some nutrition researchers have theorized that endometriosis is related to an inability to absorb calcium properly. Another theory cites food allergies as part of the cause of endometriosis, and recommends removing all allergenic foods from the diet plus administering treatment for candida, using nystatin.

❏ Dioxins may be linked to endometriosis. Dioxins are chlorinated hydrocarbons and can be found in feminine hygiene products as a by-product of the bleaching process. Dioxin can be absorbed into the body, where it collects in fatty tissue. Pesticides are another source of dioxins, as is the effluent from some types of waste incinerators.

❏ Endometriosis is a benign (noncancerous) condition, but research shows that women who have endometriosis are at greater risk of developing breast cancer, melanoma, lymphoma, and ovarian cancer than women who do not.

❏ Adenomyosis is a condition similar to endometriosis in some respects, but it is confined to the uterus. This condition is common in women who have had several children. The uterine wall does not contract as it should, and blood flow continues after menstruation. Endometrial ablation is a thirty-minute outpatient treatment for adenomyosis. In this procedure, a balloon is inserted into the uterus and filled with water. The water is heated, causing the blood vessels to seal, thus stopping the bleeding.

❏ For more information about endometriosis, you can contact the Endometriosis Association. (*See* Health and Medical Organizations in the Appendix.)

ENLARGED PROSTATE

See PROSTATITIS/ENLARGED PROSTATE.

ENURESIS

See BED-WETTING.

ENVIRONMENTAL TOXICITY

Environmental issues such as global warming, ozone layer depletion, and the overuse of pesticides and other chemicals are cause for concern—particularly as they affect the quality of our water and food supply and our level of exposure to radiation and toxic metals. The body's immune system can be the last line of defense against these environmental assaults. It is a complex network that protects us from infectious agents (viruses, bacteria, and other microorganisms), allergens (substances that induce allergic reactions), and other pathogens (substances that cause disease). When something foreign threatens the body, the body responds by forming antibodies and producing increased numbers of white blood cells to combat the intruder. The kidneys and liver work to rid the body of toxins. Thus, a properly functioning immune system is vital for good health, and proper nutrition is becoming increasingly important to help the body detoxify itself.

Certain minerals, such as calcium and zinc, are necessary to sustain life. Other minerals, like copper, are essential in small amounts but are toxic in greater amounts. Some minerals not only have no nutritional value but also are toxic in almost any amount. These toxic metals—lead, aluminum, cadmium, and mercury—pervade our environment and threaten our health, impairing the function of our organs.

Pesticides, herbicides, insecticides, fungicides, fumigants, and fertilizers containing these metals and other toxic substances seep into our soil and food. Food additives, preservatives, and artificial coloring pervade the products in our supermarkets. Fruits and vegetables are sprayed, treated with ripening agents, and waxed to make them appear more appetizing. Toxic chemicals and hazardous waste have contaminated our air and water.

Indoor pollution is an especially serious issue. Studies conducted by the U.S. Environmental Protection Agency (EPA) have shown that indoor air pollution levels—in homes, schools, and workplaces—are often two to five times greater than outdoor levels, and sometimes as much as a hundred times greater. People spend up to 90 percent of their time indoors, which increases their exposure to toxic elements.

Such exposure is believed to have increased in recent years due to the construction of tightly closed, energy-efficient buildings and an increase in the use of synthetic building materials and chemical products. Indoor pollutants are as varied as the health problems they can cause. These substances include animal hair, asbestos, bedding, carbon monoxide, disinfectants, dust, electromagnetic fields, formaldehyde, hair sprays, household cleaning products, lead, low-level radiation from television screens and computer monitors, mold, paint, pesticides, pollen, radon, solvents, and tobacco smoke. Some products used in the home emit volatile components into the air, among them certain plastics (which emit styrene), solvents (benzene), carpets (4-phenylcyclohexene [4-PC]), and manufactured wood products such as pressed-wood furniture and kitchen cabinets (formaldehyde). Permanent-press clothes and plastics emit traces of toxic vapors. Smoke from cigarettes, cigars, or pipes raises the level of toxic substances not only in the smoker, but also in those exposed to secondhand smoke. Exposure to any such substances can aggravate allergies and compromise the immune system, paving the way for the development of serious illness.

When pollutants in our environment invade our bodies, they can cause such reactions as watery eyes, diarrhea, nausea, upset stomach, and ringing in the ears. The symptoms of environmental toxicity are so varied that they also include asthma, bronchitis, stuffy nose, arthritis, fatigue, headache, eczema, and depression. If you suffer from chronic flulike symptoms, the culprit may not be a virus. You may be reacting to some material or item in your home or workplace. Exposure to environmental toxins has been linked to immune deficiency and cancer. In children, poor academic performance, and some behavioral, emotional, and learning disabilities have also been linked to indoor environmental pollution.

The symptoms of environmental toxicity and environmental allergies can be very similar, but the mechanisms that cause them are different. Allergies result from an overreaction by the immune system to some substance encountered in the environment. Environmental toxicity, on the other hand, is not a result of an immune system reaction, but a direct poisoning of tissues or cells, so that they can no longer function as they should. Allergic reactions usually begin to subside when contact with the offending allergen ceases, whereas toxicity-based problems can persist long afterward, depending on the type and extent of the damage the toxins have caused.

Unless otherwise specified, the dosages recommended here are for adults. For children between the ages of twelve and seventeen, reduce the dose to three-quarters the recommended amount. For children between six and twelve, use one-half the recommended dose, and for children under the age of six, use one-quarter the recommended amount.

NUTRIENTS

SUPPLEMENT	SUGGESTED DOSAGE	COMMENTS
Essential		
Coenzyme Q$_{10}$ plus	As directed on label.	Help the immune system detoxify many dangerous substances.
Coenzyme A from Coenzyme-A Technologies	As directed on label.	
S-Adenosylmethionine (SAMe)	As directed on label.	Has antioxidant effects that can improve the health of the liver. *Caution:* Do not use if you have bipolar mood disorder or take prescription antidepressants. Do not give to a child under twelve.
Vitamin C with bioflavonoids and quercetin	3,000–10,000 mg daily, in divided doses.	Aids in removing toxins and heavy metals from the body.

Very Important		
Garlic (Kyolic from Wakunaga)	2 capsules 3 times daily.	A potent immunostimulant.
L-cysteine and L-methionine plus L-carnitine and L-glutathione	500 mg each 3 times daily, on an empty stomach. Take with water or juice. Do not take with milk. Take with 50 mg vitamin B_6 and 100 mg vitamin C for better absorption.	To protect the lungs, heart, and liver by destroying free radicals and harmful substances.
Proteolytic enzymes plus pancreatic enzymes	As directed on label. Take between meals. As directed on label. Take with meals.	Important for proper digestion and detoxification.
Superoxide dismutase (SOD) (Cell Guard from Biotec Foods)	As directed on label.	A powerful antioxidant that protects against free radical formation and radiation.
Taurine Plus from American Biologics	As directed on label.	An important antioxidant and immune regulator, necessary for white blood cell activation and neurological function. Use the sublingual form.

Important		
Apple pectin	As directed on label.	Binds with toxins and heavy metals to remove them from the body.
Grape seed extract	As directed on label.	A powerful antioxidant.
Vitamin A plus carotenoid complex with beta-carotene plus vitamin E	25,000 IU daily for 1 month, then reduce to 15,000 IU daily. If you are pregnant, do not exceed 10,000 IU daily. As directed on label. 200 IU daily.	Vitamins A and E both act as powerful antioxidants and detoxifiers. Use emulsion forms for easier assimilation and greater safety at high doses. Antioxidants and precursors of vitamin A. Use d-alpha-tocopherol form.
Vitamin B complex plus extra vitamin B_5 (pantothenic acid) and vitamin B_6 (pyridoxine) and niacinamide	100 mg of each major B vitamin 3 times daily, with meals (amounts of individual vitamins in a complex will vary). 100 mg 3 times daily. 50 mg 3 times daily. Up to 500 mg daily.	All B vitamins are vital for cellular function and repair; needed for proper digestion and to protect the lining of the digestive tract. Use a high-stress formula. Sublingual forms are recommended for best absorption.

Helpful		
Calcium plus copper and zinc	50 mg daily. 3 mg daily. 80 mg daily. Do not exceed a total of 100 mg daily from all supplements.	Minerals that aid the immune system. Use calcium pantothenate form. Use zinc gluconate lozenges or OptiZinc for best absorption.
Manganese	50 mg daily. Take separately from calcium.	Works with other trace minerals to aid the immune system. Use a chelate form.
Raw thymus glandular	500 mg daily.	Improves T cell production. (See GLANDULAR THERAPY in Part Three for its benefits.)

Herbs

❑ Burdock root and red clover assist in cleansing the bloodstream and lymphatic system.

❑ Milk thistle helps to protect the cells of the liver and also promotes the regeneration of damaged liver cells.

❑ Turmeric contains curcumin, which inhibits tumor growth and boosts the liver's ability to eliminate environmental toxins from the body.

Recommendations

❑ Include in your diet good sources of fiber, such as ABC Aerobic Bulk Cleanse from Aerobic Life Industries, oat bran, and wheat bran. Apple pectin also can be beneficial.

Note: Always take supplemental fiber separately from other supplements and medications.

❑ Drink only steam-distilled water.

❑ Try using an air cleaner or ionizer for symptomatic relief. These devices remove animal odors, bacteria, dust, pollen, smog, and smoke from the air.

❑ Use nontoxic cleaning products whenever possible; these are available at Whole Foods Market and other stores. Many disinfectants, drain cleaners, and other household chemicals have toxic properties. Fortunately, there are environmentally friendly alternatives. For example, an effective, nontoxic disinfectant can be made at home by mixing ½ cup borax with 1 gallon hot water. Try clearing your drains by pouring ¼ cup baking soda down your drain and follow it with ½ cup vinegar. Close the drain until the fizzling stops and then flush with hot water.

❑ To reduce your exposure to natural gas, pesticides, radon, smoke, and other chemicals in the household, ventilate your home well. Replace particleboard subflooring with exterior-grade plywood that does not contain formaldehyde. The wood should then be sealed with a nontoxic sealant.

❑ Have your home and workplace tested for radon. Radon is a radioactive gas that occurs naturally and seeps from the ground. It is believed to be the second leading cause of lung cancer. Simple test kits are available at most hardware stores. If radon is found, measures such as sealing cracks and increasing ventilation in basement areas can often correct the problem.

❑ If you have any fuel-burning appliances, such as furnaces, hot water heaters, kerosene heaters, or gas space heaters, be on the alert for carbon monoxide exposure. Be sure that all appliances are properly vented and that your house is well ventilated. Never run your car engine in the garage. Carbon monoxide is a colorless, odorless gas. When inhaled in sufficient quantities, it enters the bloodstream and combines with the hemoglobin in red blood cells, crowding out needed oxygen. Early symptoms of carbon monoxide poisoning include headaches, dizziness, nausea, vomiting, fatigue, and confusion. Continued exposure can lead to coma and, ultimately, death. About five hundred Americans die each year from carbon monoxide poisoning, many due to motor vehicle exhaust. Portable carbon monoxide detectors can be purchased at hardware stores. Most building codes require the installation of carbon monoxide detectors in new homes, and if you are selling a home, even an older home, most states require that the home be equipped with a carbon monoxide detector before it can be sold.

❑ Scrape any peeling paint inside and outside your home, using appropriate protective gear. Older paints can contain toxic lead residue. Any paint from before 1978 (when lead-based paint was banned) is probably lead-based. (*See* LEAD POISONING in Part Two.)

Caution: Some states require that this job be done by certified companies that have the proper protective gear, the ability to protect the environment from the paint scrapings, and the means to properly dispose of the hazardous waste when they are done.

❑ Change vacuum cleaner bags frequently. Most vacuum cleaner bags do a poor job of filtering out dust, pollen, dust mites, and other potentially harmful particles. When shopping for a new vacuum, look for models that encase the bag in a hard, impermeable shell or that have a HEPA filter.

❑ Do not smoke, and do not let anyone else smoke in your home or car.

❑ Do not use insect sprays or bug bombs. If you need the services of an exterminator, make sure that anyone you hire is licensed and can offer nontoxic insect repellents (such as diatomaceous earth).

Considerations

❑ Most metal pots and pans used for cooking leave residues of metal in your food. Some of these metals—like the iron from cast-iron skillets—actually can be beneficial. But other metals can be harmful. Some aluminum and coated cookware can leach off small amounts of metals that can be harmful over time.

❑ It is advisable to see an allergy specialist to have a radioallergosorbent test (RAST) if you experience any of the symptoms described above to rule out allergies as a cause of the problem. You may also want to have a hair analysis to determine the level of toxic substances in your system.

❑ Liver extract injections have produced good results for some people.

❑ Asbestos, once widely used in a variety of products and building materials, may still be present in buildings and homes that were built or renovated between 1900 and 1970. Asbestos is not dangerous if it is still intact and in solid form. It becomes dangerous when it breaks down and fibers are released into the air. The asbestos fibers—which are so small that they can pass through vacuum cleaner bags—can enter the lungs and get lodged in the delicate lung tissue. Asbestos exposure can cause a variety of illnesses, including lung cancer, asbestosis, and mesothelioma, a type of tumor. Cancers of the larynx, oral cavity, kidney, and colon are sometimes attributed to asbestos as well. Only qualified contractors should do asbestos removal.

❑ One household item that can cause a lot of problems is carpeting. Some of the chemicals commonly used in carpeting have been shown to have an adverse effect on health. One suspect chemical is 4-phenylcyclohexene (4-PC), a by-product of the production of styrene-butadiene. This substance is used for the backing of many carpets. Breakdown products from styrene-butadiene are also potentially toxic. Shampooing carpeting can be particularly bad for your health. When you shampoo a carpet, the bottom stays damp well after the surface you walk on is dry. This dampness becomes a breeding ground for thousands of microorganisms that can wreak havoc on your system. The moisture can also seep into the floor beneath, which in many buildings consists of particleboard made from formaldehyde-based glue and processed wood. When the particleboard gets wet, the formaldehyde can be released into the air in the home.

❑ *See also* ALUMINUM TOXICITY; ARSENIC POISONING; CADMIUM TOXICITY; CHEMICAL POISONING; COPPER TOXICITY; FOODBORNE/WATERBORNE DISEASE; LEAD POISONING; MERCURY TOXICITY; and NICKEL TOXICITY, all in Part Two.

EPILEPSY

An estimated 3 million people in America have epilepsy, a disorder characterized by recurring seizures. Seizures are a symptom of epilepsy, but not all people who have seizures have epilepsy. Even those who do may also have seizures that are not epileptic in nature. An epileptic seizure is a temporary malfunction of the brain caused by uncontrolled electrical activity from the nerve cells in the cerebral cortex. The seizures rarely damage the brain, but they can make life difficult. Seventy percent of people with epilepsy can be expected to enter remission, defined as five or more years seizure free on medication.

The underlying cause or causes of epilepsy is unknown. It is not caused by, nor is it related to, mental illness, developmental delays, or mental health issues. In fact, many famous people have or have had epilepsy and have contributed much to our society. Seizures may occur for no apparent reason or may be triggered by a wide range of things, including exposure to an allergen; drug or alcohol withdrawal; fever; flashing lights; hunger; hypoglycemia; infection; lack of sleep; metabolic or nutritional imbalances; or trauma, especially head injury. Some people have abnormally low levels of inhibitory neurotransmitters, brain chemicals that decrease neuronal activity in the brain, while others have abnormally high levels of excitatory neurotransmitters, the exact opposite situation. There is evidence for a genetic or hereditary link as well. Unfortunately, research into the genetic component is in its infancy. There are more than five hundred genes that could play roles in epilepsy, and identifying which one does what is the trick.

There are more than thirty different kinds of seizures, divided into two basic groups: focal seizures and generalized seizures:

1. *Partial seizures.* These may be classified as either simple or complex. Focal seizures occur in just one part of the brain and affect about 60 percent of the people who have epilepsy. Because they have a focus, an area of the brain they are associated with, they are usually categorized by the area of the brain where they originate. In a simple focal seizure, the person remains conscious, but experiences odd sensations or feelings such as sudden anger, joy, nausea, or sadness, and may even experience strange sounds, smells, or tastes or see and feel things that are not real to the rest of us. In a complex focal seizure, the person usually has a loss of consciousness, or at least a change in the conscious state. This may resemble a dreamlike experience. Repetitive behaviors, such as twitching, mouth movements (chewing), blinking, walking in a circle, and other automatic movements may occur. A person may experience a distinctive warning sign called an *aura* before this type of seizure. The aura is itself a form of seizure, but one the person remembers. The aura may be experienced as a peculiar odor, butterflies in the stomach, or a distorted sound. One man with epilepsy, an ardent racetrack gambler, said he always heard the roar of a crowd, followed by the name of a favorite racehorse, just before he lost consciousness. Temporal lobe epilepsy (TLE) is the most common epilepsy syndrome with focal features. It is often associated with an aura, and has been implicated in brain damage (to the hippocampus, which shrinks over time).

2. *Generalized seizures.* These include absence seizures, atonic seizures, tonic seizures, clonic seizures, and tonic-clonic seizures. Generalized seizures are the result of abnormal neuronal activity on both sides of the brain. With this type of seizure, loss of consciousness, falling down, and/or muscle spasms are common. There are numerous kinds of generalized seizure. Absence seizures (previously known as petit mal) are most common in children and teenagers. They are characterized by a blank stare lasting about half a minute. The person appears to be daydreaming. During this type of seizure, the individual is unaware of his or her surroundings. Staring or daydreaming children do not all have epilepsy, though. A daydreaming child can be aroused by a simple touch or someone talking. A child having an absence seizure cannot be aroused. Atonic seizure (drop attack) is a childhood seizure in which the child loses consciousness for about ten seconds and usually falls to the ground because of a complete loss of muscle tone. Tonic seizures cause stiffening of the body muscles, usually those in the back, arms, and legs. Clonic seizures cause repeated jerking movements of the muscles in both

sides of the body. Tonic-clonic seizures (previously known as grand mal) are characterized by sudden cries, a fall, and rigidity and jerking of the muscles, shallow breathing, and bluish skin. Loss of bladder control is possible. The seizure usually lasts two to five minutes, and is followed by confusion, fatigue, and/or memory loss. It can be frightening to witness, especially for the first-time observer. In myoclonic seizures, brief, massive muscle jerks occur, usually in the upper body, arms, or legs.

Another epilepsy syndrome, neocortical epilepsy, can be either focal or generalized in nature. Symptoms include strange sensations, hallucinations, emotional changes, muscle spasms, and convulsions, all of which can vary depending on the location, or focus, of the seizure.

Seizures in children can be particularly disturbing. They are the most common neurological problem affecting children—indeed, one-third of people with seizure disorders are children. Idiopathic epilepsy (seizures of unknown cause) or febrile seizures (nonepileptic seizures induced by fever) affect about 3 percent of children. Angelman syndrome (a rare congenital disorder seen in children) is associated with seizures or tremors. Lennox-Gastaut syndrome is a severe seizure disorder that usually develops in children between the ages of one and eight. The old-fashioned treatment was to start a course of anticonvulsant drugs after any seizure, including febrile seizure. The hope was that this would prevent epilepsy from developing in the future. However, long-term use of such drugs in children has proven to be harmful, and certainly febrile seizures generally require a less drastic therapy.

Seizures in very young children often stem from brain injury before birth, damage to the central nervous system, or metabolic inconsistencies. In older children, epilepsy is more likely to result from genetic factors, infections of the central nervous system, or head injury.

Nutritional supplementation is important for people with epilepsy. Pregnant women with epilepsy should take prenatal vitamins and get plenty of sleep to avoid seizures. They also should take vitamin K after thirty-four weeks of pregnancy to reduce the risk of the blood-clotting disorder called *neonatal coagulopathy,* which can result from the fetal exposure to epilepsy medication.

Unless otherwise specified, the dosages recommended here are for adults. For a child between twelve and seventeen, reduce the dose to three-quarters the recommended amount. For a child between six and twelve, use one-half the recommended dose, and for a child under the age of six, use one-quarter the recommended amount.

NUTRIENTS

SUPPLEMENT	SUGGESTED DOSAGE	COMMENTS
Essential		
Dimethylglycine (DMG)	As directed on label.	A powerful antioxidant. Increases oxygenation of tissues.

Supplement	Suggested Dosage	Comments
L-carnitine	As directed on label.	An amino acid required to make protein and deliver essential fatty acids to the cells. Carnitine is depleted by anticonvulsant drugs.
L-tyrosine	500 mg each 3 times daily, on an empty stomach. Take with water or juice. Do not take with milk. Take with 50 mg vitamin B_6 and 100 mg vitamin C for better absorption.	Important for proper brain function. *Caution:* Do not take tyrosine if you are taking an MAO inhibitor drug.
Magnesium	700 mg daily, in divided doses. Take between meals, on an empty stomach, with apple cider vinegar or betaine HCl.	Needed to calm the nervous system and muscle spasms. Use magnesium chloride form.
Omega-3s (fish oil)	1,000 mg daily.	Reduces risk of sudden death from heart problems.
Selenium	As directed on label. If you are pregnant, do not exceed 40 mcg daily.	Low selenium levels result in a deficiency of glutathione peroxidase, an enzyme that detoxifies peroxides in the cells.
Taurine Plus from American Biologics	10–20 drops daily, in divided doses.	Taurine is an important antioxidant and immune regulator, necessary for white blood cell activation and neurological function. Use the sublingual form.
or taurine	As directed on label.	Levels of taurine are often low in people with seizure disorders. Taurine is an essential building block of all other amino acids.
Vitamin B complex	100 mg of each major B vitamin 3 times daily, with meals (amounts of individual vitamins in a complex will vary). Injections (under a doctor's supervision) may be necessary.	Extremely important in the functioning of the central nervous system. Injections (under a doctor's supervision) may be necessary.
plus extra vitamin B_3 (niacin)	50 mg daily.	Improves circulation and is helpful for many brain-related disorders.
and vitamin B_6 (pyridoxine)	100–600 mg 3 times daily, under the supervision of a health care professional.	Needed for normal brain function.
and vitamin B_{12}	1,000–2,000 mcg daily, on an empty stomach.	Involved in maintenance of the myelin sheaths that cover and protect nerve endings.
and folic acid	400 mcg daily. If you are taking anticonvulsants, do not exceed 400 mg daily from all sources.	A brain food vital for the health of the nervous system.
and vitamin B_5 (pantothenic acid)	500 mg daily.	The anti-stress vitamin.

Very Important

Supplement	Suggested Dosage	Comments
Calcium	1,500 mg daily.	Important in normal nerve impulse transmission.
Liquid Kyolic with B_1 and B_{12} from Wakunaga	As directed on label.	Increases energy and acts as an antioxidant.
Zinc	50–80 mg daily. Do not exceed a total of 100 mg daily from all supplements.	Protects the brain cells. Use zinc gluconate lozenges or OptiZinc for best absorption.

Important

Supplement	Suggested Dosage	Comments
Coenzyme Q_{10} plus	30 mg daily.	Improves brain oxygenation.
Coenzyme A from Coenzyme-A Technologies	As directed on label.	Works with coenzyme Q_{10} for best results.
Oxy-5000 Forte from American Biologics	As directed on label.	A potent nutritional antioxidant for health and stress. Destroys free radicals.
Quercetin	As directed on label.	A flavonoid with anti-inflammatory and antioxidant properties. More powerful than vitamin C.

Helpful

Supplement	Suggested Dosage	Comments
Chromium picolinate	200 mcg daily.	Important in maintaining stable cerebral glucose metabolism.
Kelp or alfalfa	1,000–1,500 mg daily.	For necessary mineral balance. *See* under Herbs, below.
Melatonin	Start with 2–3 mg daily, taken 2 hours or less before bedtime. If necessary, gradually increase the dosage until an effective level is reached.	Helpful if symptoms include insomnia.
Proteolytic enzymes plus multienzyme complex	As directed on label. Take between meals. As directed on label. Take with meals.	Aids in healing if inflammation is the cause of seizures. Aids digestion, helping to make needed nutrients available.
Raw thymus glandular and thyroid glandular	As directed on label. As directed on label.	Both the thymus and thyroid are important in proper brain function. (*See* GLANDULAR THERAPY in Part Three.)
Vitamin A with mixed carotenoids	25,000 IU daily. If you are pregnant, do not exceed 10,000 IU daily.	An important antioxidant that aids in protecting brain function.
Vitamin C with bioflavonoids	2,000–7,000 mg daily, in divided doses.	Vital to functioning of the adrenal glands, which are the anti-stress glands. A potent antioxidant.
Vitamin E	200 IU daily.	Aids circulation. Compensates for anticonvulsant-induced vitamin depletion. An emulsion form is recommended for easier assimilation and greater safety at high doses. Use d-alpha-tocopherol form.

Herbs

❑ Alfalfa is a good source of needed minerals. Take 2,000 milligrams daily in capsule or extract form.

❑ Black cohosh, hyssop, and lobelia are beneficial for people with epilepsy because they aid in controlling the central nervous system and have a calming effect. For best results, they should be used on an alternating basis.

Caution: Do not use black cohosh if you are pregnant or have any type of chronic disease. Black cohosh should not be used by those with liver problems.

❑ Avoid the herb sage. It contains the chemical compound thujone, which can be poisonous. Do not use sage if you suffer from any type of seizure disorder.

Recommendations

❑ Eat cultured milk products like yogurt and kefir.

❑ Include beet greens, chard, eggs, green leafy vegetables, raw cheese, raw milk, raw nuts, seeds, and soybeans in the diet.

❑ Eat fish regularly (at least twice a week) and take a fish oil supplement. Patients with refractory seizures from epilepsy taking 9,600 milligrams of fish oil per day (2,880 milligrams omega-3s) had less severe seizures and better blood lipids, indicating lower heart attack risk. Some patients with epilepsy had heart rates that were variable, and the fish oil lowered their risk of sudden death.

❑ Drink fresh "live" juices made from beets, carrots, green beans, green leafy vegetables, peas, red grapes, and seaweed for concentrated nutrients. (See JUICING in Part Three.)

❑ Eat small meals, do not drink large quantities of liquids at once, and take 2 tablespoons of olive oil daily.

❑ Avoid alcoholic beverages, animal protein, fried foods, artificial sweeteners such as aspartame (found in Equal, NutraSweet, and other products), caffeine, and nicotine. Avoid refined foods and sugar.

❑ If the bowels do not move each day, before going to bed, take a lemon enema using the juice of two lemons and 2 quarts of water. (See ENEMAS in Part Three.)

❑ Take an Epsom salts bath twice a week.

❑ Work toward self-care. Keep drug dosages as low as possible, and work toward becoming as free from drugs and seizures as possible. The correct diet and nutritional supplements are very important in the control of epilepsy.

❑ Get regular moderate exercise to improve circulation to the brain.

❑ As much as possible, avoid stress and tension. Learn stress management techniques. (See STRESS in Part Two.)

Considerations

❑ Most people who have epilepsy are aware of their condition and take medication to control the seizures. Possible side effects of antiseizure medications include blood disorders, fatigue, liver problems, and mental fatigue and/or fogginess.

❑ Other types of drugs can interact with antiseizure medications, lessening or intensifying the effects of one drug or the other. Alcohol, birth control pills, the antibiotic erythromycin, and some types of asthma, ulcer, and heart medicines are known to interact with certain epilepsy drugs.

What to Do When Someone Is Having a Seizure

Seeing someone having a seizure can be disturbing and frightening, and many if not most people do not know exactly what to do. Complicating that are the many myths that surround seizure treatment. If you witness someone having a seizure, do the following:

- *Do not* restrain the person.
- *Do not* try to put anything in the person's mouth. A person having a seizure may bite his or her tongue, but this is not life-threatening.
- Try to restrain a fall so that the person does not hit something as he or she collapses. Often, the person knows he or she is about to have a seizure, and you can ask him or her to sit on the floor, or help him or her to sit down, before a fall.
- Leave the person lying flat on a safe surface. Do not put anything under the person's head. If possible, turn the person onto his or her side, propping him or her in that position with cushions at the back during the seizure. This way, any saliva or blood from a bitten tongue will be able to flow freely out of the mouth.
- In case of loss of bladder or bowel control, if possible, loosely cover the person with a blanket to protect his or her privacy.
- *Do not panic.* Loosen any tight clothing to make the person more comfortable. Stay with the person until the seizure has stopped. He or she may be confused and tired immediately after the seizure.
- If the person has repeated seizures, one after the other, seek medical assistance. With a baby or young child, medical help should be sought immediately.

Caution: Anyone who takes medication for epilepsy should always check with his or her doctor or pharmacist before taking other drugs, whether prescription or over-the-counter.

❑ Epilepsy is not the only cause of seizures. They can also be brought on by other factors, including alkalosis; excessive consumption of alcohol; arteriosclerosis; brain disorders such as a brain tumor, encephalitis, meningitis, or stroke; high fever (especially in children); the use of drugs; the formation of scar tissue as a result of an eye injury or a stroke; a lack of oxygen; and spasms of the blood vessels.

❑ High levels of aluminum have been found in the brains of some people with epilepsy. Studies in animals have shown that trace amounts of aluminum in the brain may initiate the type of disordered electrical activity that causes seizures. (See ALUMINUM TOXICITY in Part Two.)

❑ According to research done by Arizona State University's Biochemical Department, the artificial sweetener aspartame has been associated (rarely) with seizures in some people. But other toxic agents such as aluminum and lead may contribute to the problem. According to the Epilepsy Foundation of America, aspartame is safe for use by people with epilepsy.

❑ Doses of folic acid in excess of 400 micrograms (mcg) per day may increase seizure activity in people with epilepsy, especially if they are taking the commonly prescribed anticonvulsant phenytoin (Dilantin).

❑ At least 90 percent of women who take epilepsy drugs during pregnancy give birth to normal, healthy infants. Because a seizure during pregnancy carries its own risks, most doctors advise pregnant women with epilepsy to continue taking their medication unless it is likely they will be seizure-free without it.

❑ Some good results have been reported using hyperbaric (high-pressure) oxygen therapy in treating people with epilepsy. (See HYPERBARIC OXYGEN THERAPY in Part Three.)

❑ If epilepsy is due to tiny tumors in the brain, a type of surgery known as lesionectomy may be recommended. Using a computer, a surgeon can view and vaporize the tiny tumors that cause some cases of epilepsy. This procedure can be performed with minimal damage to healthy tissue in the brain.

❑ Diastat, a gel form of diazepam (better known as Valium) designed for rectal administration, may be prescribed for people who suffer from multiple seizures on a regular basis. The gel takes only minutes to work and should be administered two to three minutes into a seizure.

❑ A specialized dietary program called the ketogenic diet has been used with considerable success to control seizures in children. This is a rigidly controlled diet that is high in fats and extremely low in carbohydrates and proteins, which forces the body to use fats rather than the usual carbohydrates to generate cellular energy. When fats are burned, by-products called ketones are formed. Normally, ketosis—the presence of high levels of ketones in the body—occurs only in cases of starvation or uncontrolled diabetes mellitus. Eating a diet containing virtually no carbohydrates, however, can produce essentially the same effect, and also causes biochemical changes that enable the body's tissues to burn these ketones for needed energy. It is very much like the Atkins diet, which also produces ketones. Although it is not known exactly how, this process appears to control seizure activity. The mechanism may be a ketosis by-product with a tongue-twisting name, beta-hydroxybutyrate (BHB), but no human studies have yet confirmed this link. You should discuss this in detail with a physician before attempting it, and some drug therapy still may be required. The majority of children who have been put on this diet benefit from it, and many have been able to stop taking, or reduce their dosage of, antiseizure medication. Using this dietary program can be challenging for

parents because the child's foods, liquids, medications, and even personal hygiene products such as toothpaste must be strictly controlled, and the program must be followed to the letter (even slight deviations can negate its effects). It should be undertaken only under the direct supervision of a physician who is experienced in its use. Information about the ketogenic diet is available from the Johns Hopkins Epilepsy Center. (See Health and Medical Organizations in the Appendix.) The diet has been in use since the 1920s. In a recent study, seventy-three children were assigned to a ketogenic diet and seventy-two ate a regular diet. After three months, those on the ketogenic diet had fewer seizures and some were even seizure-free. Side effects of the ketogenic diet were constipation, vomiting, lack of energy, and hunger. This is a new, important study that shows the merits of a ketogenic diet.

❑ In a survey of doctors and nurses, 58 percent believed that there was a relationship between consumption of specific foods and the occurrence of seizures. Foods that were most likely to trigger a seizure as witnessed by the group were dairy products, sour foods, food additives, meat and fish, and fruits and vegetables.

❑ Pseudoseizures, also known as psychogenic or nonepileptic attack disorder, are nonepileptic seizures and may be a symptom of a number of different psychological factors.

❑ Huntington's disease (HD), also sometimes called Huntington's chorea, is a disorder that can cause tremors, jerking movements that may resemble myoclonic seizures. This is, however, not a seizure disorder. Huntington's disease is a result of a genetically transmitted chromosome irregularity that usually manifests itself during the third decade of life. There is no known cure for Huntington's disease, but following the diet designed for epilepsy may help slow the progression and ease symptoms of the condition.

EPSTEIN-BARR VIRUS

See under CHRONIC FATIGUE SYNDROME; FIBROMYALGIA SYNDROME; MONONUCLEOSIS.

ERECTILE DYSFUNCTION

Erectile dysfunction (ED), or chronic erectile dysfunction, is no longer a taboo subject. It is estimated that 30 million American men suffer from ED. For a great majority of them, the problem is solvable. A man is considered to have erectile dysfunction if he does not have the ability to achieve or maintain an erection adequate for normal sexual intercourse. Erections result from a complex combination of brain stimuli, blood vessel and nerve function, and hormonal actions. Anything that interferes with any of these factors can lead to erectile dysfunction, and that can include arteriosclerosis, metabolic syndrome, and peripheral vascular disease; the use of certain medications listed later in this section; alcohol, or cigarettes; a history of sexually transmitted disease; and chronic illness such as diabetes and high blood pressure.

Erectile dysfunction is extremely common in men who have diabetes. Men who have diabetes are two to three times more likely to have erectile dysfunction than men who do not have diabetes. Hormonal imbalances such as low levels of thyroid hormone may also contribute to the problem. Low levels of the hormone testosterone are rarely the cause of ED. Lack of desire may be the problem. If desire is not there in the first place, it is difficult to either get or maintain an erection. Loss of libido (sexual desire) may be caused by depression, illness, or medications, and a waning attraction to one's partner.

ED may be chronic or recurring, or it may occur as a single isolated incident. One or two occurrences, however, are rarely thought of as erectile dysfunction, although they may be upsetting at the time. Most of the men who have this problem are age forty or over (one in three men over sixty is affected), but those under forty may also have the problem.

In the past, it was assumed that erectile dysfunction was primarily a psychological problem, but many therapists and physicians today believe that as many as 85 percent of all cases of ED have some physical basis. There are many drugs that may cause erectile dysfunction as a side effect. Some of the most common are alcohol, antidepressants, antihistamines, antihypertensives, blood pressure medication, cancer chemotherapy, diuretics, narcotics, nicotine, sedatives, steroids (if abused), stomach acid inhibitors, and ulcer medications. Atherosclerosis, or hardening of the arteries (one type of arteriosclerosis), poses a risk to the condition of both the heart and the penis (erectile dysfunction can, in fact, be a symptom of this disorder). Most people today know smoking and eating fatty foods lead to the production of plaques that clog arteries and block the flow of blood to the heart. These plaques also can block the arteries leading to the genitals, interfering with the ability to attain an erection.

The following nutrient dosages are for adult males.

NUTRIENTS

SUPPLEMENT	SUGGESTED DOSAGE	COMMENTS
Essential		
Essential fatty acid complex	As directed on label.	Aids in the formation of sperm and seminal fluid in the prostate gland.
Iodine	As directed on label (usually 150 mg daily).	Iodine is a component of the thyroid hormones and necessary for development of the reproductive organs. Toxicity results if it is taken in large quantities.
or kelp	2,000–3,000 mg daily.	A natural source of iodine.
Selenium	As directed on label.	Found in high concentration in the testicles. Caution: Do not take this supplement if you have heart, liver, or kidney disease.
Vitamin C with bioflavonoids	500 mg 3 times daily.	Helps boost testosterone levels.
Vitamin E	200 IU daily or 400 IU every other day.	Increases circulation. Use d-alpha-tocopherol form. Caution: Vitamin E is a blood-thinning agent. Do not use if you take prescription blood-thinners.
Zinc	80 mg daily. Do not exceed this amount.	Important in prostate gland function and reproductive organ growth. Also helps boost testosterone levels. Use zinc gluconate lozenges or OptiZinc for best absorption.
Important		
Dimethylglycine (DMG) (Aangamik DMG from FoodScience of Vermont)	As directed on label.	Increases oxygen supply in the blood to all tissues. Blood vessels must be dilated for an erection to occur. Use a sublingual form.
GH3 from Gero Vita	As directed on label.	Stimulates the activity of sex hormones. Caution: Do not use GH3 if you are allergic to sulfites.
Multi-Glandular from American Biologics	As directed on label.	A supplement for the endocrine, hormonal, and enzyme systems.
Octacosanol	1,000–2,000 mcg 3 times weekly.	Natural source of vitamin E. Good for hormone production.
Helpful		
L-tyrosine	500 mg twice daily, on an empty stomach. Take with water or juice. Do not take with milk. Take with 50 mg vitamin B6 and 100 mg vitamin C for better absorption.	Helps stabilize moods and alleviate stress. (See AMINO ACIDS in Part One.) Caution: Do not take tyrosine if you are taking an MAO inhibitor drug.
Raw orchic glandular	As directed on label.	Glandular extracts from the male reproductive organs that promote their function. (See GLANDULAR THERAPY in Part Three.)
Vitamin A plus	15,000 IU daily.	Antioxidants that enhance immunity.
mixed carotenoids or	15,000 IU daily.	Antioxidants and vitamin A precursors.
carotenoid complex (Betatene)	As directed on label.	
Vitamin B complex	50 mg of each major B vitamin 3 times daily (amounts of individual vitamins in a complex will vary).	Needed for a healthy nervous system. B vitamins are important in all cell activities.
plus extra vitamin B6 (pyridoxine)	50 mg 3 times daily.	Required for the synthesis of RNA and DNA, which govern cellular reproduction.

Herbs

❑ Ashwagandha and schizandra, both Ayurvedic herbs, are said to ensure potency and increase fertility.

❑ Damiana is good for improving blood flow to the genital area and increasing desire.

❑ Sarsaparilla contains a testosterone-like substance for men.

❑ Wild yam contains natural steroids that rejuvenate and give vigor to lovemaking. This hormone is found in the human body as dehydroepiandrosterone (DHEA). Take twice the amount recommended on the label for two weeks, then stop for two weeks. Continue this on-and-off cycle, taking the recommended amount.

❑ Yohimbe bark, which comes from west Africa, is said to expand the blood vessels in the penis and increase blood flow. It also claims to increase nitrous oxide (NO), which is important for producing an erection.

Caution: Yohimbe should not be used by women who are pregnant or nursing. Do not use yohimbe if you have high blood pressure, heart disease, stomach ulcers, depression, or other psychiatric conditions. There have been cases of people dying from taking too much yohimbe.

❑ Other herbs that may be beneficial include dong quai, gotu kola, hydrangea root, pygeum, saw palmetto, and/or Siberian ginseng.

Caution: Do not use Siberian ginseng if you have hypoglycemia, high blood pressure, or a heart disorder.

❑ There are herbal products on the market that claim to help sexual potency; they include:

- Prostata from Gero Vita International normalizes prostate function, increasing libido and erectile ability.

- Saw Palmetto Supercritical Extract from Gaia Herbs is an herbal tincture that helps to normalize prostate function.

Recommendations

❑ Eat a healthy, well-balanced diet. Include in the diet pumpkin seeds, bee pollen, or royal jelly.

Caution: Bee pollen may cause an allergic reaction in some individuals. Start with a small amount at first, and discontinue use if a rash, wheezing, discomfort, or other symptom occurs.

❑ Avoid alcohol, particularly before sexual encounters.

❑ Some men have found benefit from pomegranate juice, according to the International Index of Erectile Function (IIEF).

❑ In one study, men with erectile dysfunction and low levels of the hormone dehydroepiandrosterone (DHEA) derived benefit from taking supplemental doses of the hormone. Long-term studies are not available, however.

❑ Do not consume animal fats, sugar, or fried or junk foods.

❑ Do not smoke. Avoid being around cigarette smoke.

❑ Avoid stress.

❑ Consult a urologist for testing to determine whether ED is caused by an underlying illness that requires treatment.

❑ Consider possible psychological factors that may be contributing to ED, especially repressed anger or a fear of intimacy. Exploring psychological issues with a qualified therapist can help.

❑ If you suspect ED may be related to a drug you are taking, discuss this with your physician. There may be satisfactory alternatives that will not cause this problem. Certain blood pressure medications and tranquilizers often cause erectile difficulties. The drugs cimetidine (Tagamet) and ranitidine (Zantac), which are used to treat ulcers and heartburn, also have significant side effects in some men.

Caution: Do not stop taking a prescription drug or change the dosage without consulting your physician.

❑ Investigate the possibility of heavy metal intoxication. A hair analysis can reveal possible heavy metal poisoning. (*See* HAIR ANALYSIS in Part Three.)

❑ Keep in mind that sexual function changes with age. As you age, you may require more stimulation and a longer period of time to achieve an erection.

Considerations

❑ A study done at the Boston University School of Medicine linked overall health to erectile dysfunction. Researchers studied the medical histories of 1,300 men aged forty to seventy years. They found some ED in a total of 52 percent of those under study. Men who were being treated for heart disease, high blood pressure, or diabetes were one and a half to four times more likely than the overall group to be completely impotent later in life. The situation was even worse for men with heart disease or hypertension who also smoked.

❑ Men with metabolic syndrome (a combination of medical disorders such as high blood pressure and high cholesterol, sugar, and insulin levels that increase the risk of cardiovascular disease and diabetes) who followed a Mediterranean diet were able to regain their erectile function. In this study, the men followed the diet—which included more fruits, vegetables, nuts, whole grains, and olive oil—for two years and were compared to a group who ate their regular diet. Nearly half the men in the Mediterranean diet group improved their symptoms, while only 6 percent did in the regular diet group.

❑ In one study published in the *Journal of the American Medical Association (JAMA),* losing 10 percent of body weight coupled with an exercise program seemed to be enough to get rid of ED in 31 percent of men compared to a group who did not change their diet or who did not exercise.

❑ Alcohol intake decreases the body's ability to produce testosterone. Research at Chicago Medical School revealed that drinking alcohol may cause the hormonal equivalent of menopause in men. Alcohol not only affects sexual function, but also helps set the stage for a heart attack and other dangerous conditions.

❏ Arteriosclerosis, which restricts blood supply to the penis and to the nerves that govern sexual arousal, may result in a "failure to perform." If ED is related to clogged blood vessels, a diet low in fats can actually help reverse the problem. (*See* ARTERIOSCLEROSIS/ATHEROSCLEROSIS; CARDIOVASCULAR DISEASE; and/or CIRCULATORY PROBLEMS in Part Two.)

❏ A study done at Boston University showed that men who smoked one pack of cigarettes a day for five years were 15 percent more likely to develop clogging in the arteries that serve the penis, a situation that can cause ED. In addition, heavy smoking decreases sexual capability by damaging the tiny blood vessels in the penis. The use of marijuana and cocaine can also result in ED.

❏ Duplex ultrasonography, a noninvasive method of measuring penile blood flow, is a reliable method of determining whether arterial occlusion plays a role in ED. If your doctor believes atherosclerosis to be the underlying problem, he or she may advise vascular surgery to improve blood flow to the penis.

❏ Urologists differ in the types of treatment they recommend for ED, but many opt first for nonsurgical treatment. Sildenafil (Viagra) is probably the best-known drug for dealing with ED. It is not, however, a drug that will make you feel like having sex, but rather a drug that will help you to have an erection. In other words, if desire is not there, it will not help. Partners of men who take Viagra may have difficulty adjusting to the higher level of potency shown by their partners, so taking an enhancement drug such as sildenafil should always be discussed with your partner.

Caution: Sildenafil may not be suitable for men with certain cardiovascular or blood disorders, or for men with advanced kidney or liver disease. There are some concerns about sildenafil and high blood pressure.

❏ Tadalafil (Cialis) is another oral medication that relaxes muscles in the penis and increases blood flow, and it has been shown to stay in the body longer. However, like sildenafil, serious side effects can occur, and tadalafil should only be taken under the direction of a physician.

❏ Apomorphine (Uprima) is a newer prescription drug for ED that works through the brain to produce erections—unlike sildenafil, which works by increasing blood flow to the penis.

Caution: This drug can cause unpleasant side effects, most notably nausea, vomiting, dizziness, or sweating.

❏ Injections of the drugs papaverine (Pavabid) and phentolamine (Regitine) or prostaglandin E1 (PGE1) into the base of the penis before intercourse have proven effective in producing "satisfactory erection" in men with ED. The drug alprostadil also is available in an injection kit (Caverject). These drugs work by relaxing smooth muscle, which causes the blood vessels in the penis to dilate, promoting an erection that can last an hour or more. Possible side effects include priapism (prolonged, painful erections). Also, although the injections are done with a tiny needle, and are supposed to be painless when done properly (proper technique is crucial), this prospect is unappealing to many men. A less invasive technique involves instilling alprostadil into the urethra with a suppository applied with a tiny plunger.

❏ If ED is linked to high levels of the hormone prolactin, bromocriptine (Parlodel) may be prescribed to correct the problem.

❏ A number of vacuum devices are used to promote erection. With these devices, a cylinder is placed over the penis and a hand pump is used to create a vacuum in the cylinder. This in turn causes blood to flow into the penis, creating an erection. The user then puts a constriction band around the base of the penis, causing the erection to last up to thirty minutes.

❏ Some men turn to inflatable penile implants to mechanically create erections. Penile implants are surgically installed devices that are made of silicone or polyurethane. One type is made of two semirigid but bendable rods; another type consists of a pump, a fluid-filled reservoir, and two cylinders into which the fluid is pumped to create an erection. With the development of more effective agents, implants are now considered to be a last resort, to be tried only when all other methods have failed.

❏ Premature ejaculation (PE) is considered sexual dysfunction. It is not the same thing as ED, but it too can diminish the quality of one's sex life. Premature ejaculation—reaching orgasm too quickly to satisfy one's partner—is thought to be a learned trait, acquired through the habit of masturbation and immediate gratification, that can be unlearned through counseling. However, if PE begins suddenly, when there was no history of it before, it is probably due to problems with the arteries and veins that run to the penis. Venous leaks may be one of these problems because the extra blood that should be going to the penis and making it erect is draining away, so it is difficult to maintain a good erection for any length of time. This problem is common with older men.

❏ Peyronie's disease results in a twisting of the penis when it is erect. This is due to plaque or scars blocking the tunica albuginea, a membrane containing the corpora cavernosa, the two long, thin chambers in the penis that fill with blood and create the erection. This prevents the penis from retaining its overall elasticity. When erect, the penis may look deformed and contorted.

❏ *See also* HYPERTHYROIDISM and HYPOTHYROIDISM in Part Two.

EYE PROBLEMS

Two of the most complex organs of the body, the eyes provide us with instantaneous visual feedback of the world around us. We have all experienced eye trouble at one time or another—eyes that are tired, bloodshot, dry, irritated, itchy, sensitive to light, or watery, to name just a few. While some eye disorders—nearsightedness or cataracts, for example—are localized problems, eye disturbances can be a symptom of disease elsewhere in the body. Watery eyes, for example, can be a symptom of the common cold; protruding or bulging eyes and reading difficulties may indicate a thyroid problem; dark circles under the eyes and eyes that are red, swollen, and/or watery may indicate allergies; yellowing of the eyes from jaundice can be a sign of hepatitis, gallbladder disease, or gallstone blockage; droopy eyes are often an early sign of myasthenia gravis, a disorder in which the eye muscles weaken. A drastic difference in the sizes of the pupils can indicate a tumor somewhere in the body, whereas high blood pressure and diabetes may manifest themselves in periodic blurring of vision.

The eyeball is a sphere about an inch in diameter that is covered by a tough outer layer called the sclera, the "white of the eye." Underneath the sclera is the middle layer of the eye, the choroid, which contains the blood vessels that serve the eye. The front of the eye is covered by a transparent membrane called the cornea. Behind the cornea is a fluid-filled chamber called the anterior chamber; behind that—in the center of the sclera, on the front of the eyeball—is the highly pigmented iris, and in the center of the iris is the pupil. Behind the iris is the transparent lens. Inside, at the back of the eye, is the retina, a delicate light-sensitive membrane that is connected to the brain by the optic nerve.

The eye also contains two important fluids. The ciliary body, whose muscles are responsible for focusing the lens of the eye, also produces a waterlike substance called the aqueous humor, which fills the space between the cornea and the lens. The aqueous humor contains all of the constituents of blood except for red blood cells. The other fluid is the vitreous humor, a jellylike substance that fills the back of the eyeball, the space between the lens and the retina.

On the outside of the eyeball are six muscles that move the eyes. Under the upper eyelids are the lacrimal glands, which secrete tears. At the inner corners of the eyelids are the tear ducts, small openings through which the tears drain into the nose and the back of the throat. At the edges of the eyelids, where the eyelashes are, are glands that produce oils, sweat, and other secretions.

What we think of as the simple act of seeing is actually a complex, multistep process that goes on continuously and at breathtaking speed. Light enters the eye through the pupil, which changes size depending on the amount of light entering it. When there is very little light, the pupil dilates; in bright light, the pupil constricts. As light enters the eye, it is focused by the lens, which adjusts its shape by means of the action of the muscles and ligaments of the ciliary body.

The lens becomes fatter or flatter depending upon the distance to the object being focused on. The lens projects

Maintaining Healthy Eyes

Like all other parts of the body, the eyes need to be nourished properly. In addition to making sure that the eyes are not strained by too much intense close work or inadequate light, proper eye care includes a healthy diet containing sufficient amounts of vitamins and minerals.

In order to promote good eyesight, you must make sure your diet contains the proper amounts of the B vitamins; vitamins A, C, and E; and the minerals selenium and zinc. Fresh fruits and vegetables are good sources of these vitamins and minerals; include plenty of these in your diet, especially yellow and yellow-orange foods such as carrots, yams, and cantaloupes. A well-balanced diet with plenty of fresh fruits and vegetables can help keep your eyes healthy.

When you are outdoors, exposure to sunlight can be damaging. The recommendation is that people who must deal with prolonged exposure should wear ultraviolet (UV) protective sunglasses that block both types of UV rays, UV-A and UV-B. UV-A is ultraviolet radiation with a wavelength of 320–400 nanometers. It passes right through the earth's ozone layer. UV-B is ultraviolet radiation with a wavelength of 280–320 nanometers. The ozone layer absorbs most of this radiation, but a small amount gets through and can cause cataracts, pterygia (benign lesions that grow on either side of the cornea), and skin cancer. This especially is true for children, and their sunglasses should be as good or better than those of an adult. In other words, buy real sunglasses, not the kiddie models. Look for polycarbonate lenses, which are light, shatterproof, and optically sound.

light onto the retina, where special pigment absorbs the light and forms a corresponding image. Finally, this image is transmitted by means of the optic nerve to the brain, which interprets the image. Anything that interferes with any link in this chain of events can result in impaired vision.

Many cases of eye damage and vision loss are linked to underlying diseases of one type or another. Diabetes often leads to hemorrhages in the retina and the vitreous humor, eventually producing blindness. Early cataracts also may be related to diabetes. High blood pressure produces a gradual thickening of the blood vessels inside the eyes that can result in visual impairment and even blindness. Other factors linked to declining eyesight include too much sun exposure, poor nutrition, exposure to tobacco smoke or other pollutants, and dehydration.

One major contributor to eye trouble is poor diet, specifically the denatured, chemical- and preservative-laden foods that most Americans consume daily. A deficiency of just one vitamin can lead to various eye problems. Supplementation with the correct vitamins and minerals can help prevent or correct eye trouble. Some of these supplements also protect against the formation of free radicals, which can damage the eyes. Specific eye problems that can be helped by supplementing the diet with vitamins and other nutrients are discussed in this section.

Unless otherwise specified, the nutrient dosages given in the tables within this section are for adults. For a child between the ages of twelve and seventeen, reduce the dose to three-quarters of the recommended amount. For a child between six and twelve, use one-half of the recommended dose, and for a child under the age of six, use one-quarter of the recommended amount.

NUTRIENTS

SUPPLEMENT	SUGGESTED DOSAGE	COMMENTS
Desiccated liver	As directed on label.	A good source of many important vitamins and minerals. Use only liver derived from organically raised beef.
Free form amino acid plus	As directed on label.	For necessary protein. Free form amino acids are assimilated best.
glutathione	500 mg daily, on an empty stomach.	Powerful antioxidants that protect the lenses of the eyes.
or		
N-acetylcysteine	500 mg daily, on an empty stomach. Take with water or juice. Do not take with milk. Take with 50 mg vitamin B$_6$ and 100 mg vitamin C for better absorption.	
Multivitamin and mineral complex with	200 mcg daily.	All nutrients are needed in balance.
selenium	If you are pregnant, do not exceed 40 mcg daily.	Destroys free radicals that can damage the eyes.
Ocu-Care from Nature's Plus or	As directed on label.	These formulas provide many eye-strengthening nutrients, as well as protective and antioxidant substances, to support and nourish the eyes.
OcuGuard from Twinlab or	As directed on label.	
Visual Eyes from Source Naturals	As directed on label.	
Taurine Plus from American Biologics	As directed on label.	Taurine is associated with zinc in maintaining eye function. It is present in the retina of the eye in high concentrations. Use the sublingual form.
Vitamin A emulsion	25,000 IU daily. If you are pregnant, do not exceed 10,000 IU daily.	Absolutely necessary for proper eye function. Protects the eye from free radicals. Emulsion form is recommended for easier assimilation and greater safety at higher doses.
or		
capsules plus	15,000 IU daily.	
carotenoid complex with lutein and zeaxanthin	As directed on label.	Precursors of vitamin A.
Vitamin B complex	100 mg of each major B vitamin twice daily (amounts of individual	Needed for intracellular eye metabolism.
	vitamins in a complex will vary).	
Vitamin C with bioflavonoids	2,000 mg 3 times daily.	An antioxidant that reduces intraocular pressure.
Vitamin E	200 IU daily.	Important in healing and immunity. Use d-alpha-tocopherol form.
Zinc	50 mg daily. Do not exceed a total of 100 mg daily from all supplements.	Deficiency has been linked to retinal detachment. Use zinc gluconate lozenges or OptiZinc for best absorption.

Herbs

❑ Bayberry bark, cayenne (capsicum), and red raspberry leaves, taken by mouth, are beneficial.

❑ Bilberry extract has been shown to improve both normal and night vision.

Recommendations

❑ Include the following in your diet: broccoli, raw cabbage, carrots, cauliflower, green vegetables, squash, sunflower seeds, and watercress.

❑ Drink fresh carrot juice. This can help to prevent or alleviate some eye problems.

❑ Eliminate sugar and white flour from your diet.

❑ If you wear glasses, wear clear spectacles that have been treated to keep out ultraviolet rays. This will help protect against damage from ultraviolet exposure. Avoid wearing tinted eyeglasses for this purpose, especially on a regular basis; dark glasses prevent needed light from entering the eyes. The functioning of the pineal gland, which plays an important role in the regulation of metabolism, behavior, and physiological functions, is largely governed by sunlight.

❑ Never use hair dyes containing coal tar on the eyelashes or eyebrows; doing so can cause injury or blindness. Although coal tar dyes are legal, marketing them for the eyebrows and eyelashes is not.

❑ Be careful when using drugs, whether prescription or over-the-counter. Some may cause eye problems. Drugs that can cause light sensitivity, blurriness, dizziness, or damage to the optic nerve, retina, or other vital parts of the eye include:

• Adrenocorticotropic hormone, or ACTH (HP Acthar, Cortrosyn).

• Anticoagulants such as heparin and warfarin (Coumadin).

• Corticosteroids, such as hydrocortisone (Cortenema Enema, Hydrocortone, Solu-Cortef, VoSol HC), prednisolone (Blephamide, Hydeltra-T.B.A.), and prednisone (Deltasone).

• Chlorpropamide (Diabinese), which is used for non-insulin-dependent diabetes.

- Diuretics, antihistamines, and digitalis preparations.

❏ Consult your health care provider if you develop any of the following conditions: change in pupil size; eye pain or pain on eye movement; impaired vision; intolerance to light; known exposure to gonorrhea or chlamydia; seeing floating black bits that you hadn't seen before; or swelling, tenderness, or redness around the eyes.

❏ If you have a baby or young child who exhibits any signs of eye infection, have the child evaluated by a professional.

Considerations

❏ There are three types of specialists who deal with the eyes:

1. Ophthalmologists are medical doctors who are eye specialists. They diagnose and treat eye disease, perform eye surgery, give eye tests, and prescribe corrective lenses.

2. Optometrists are not medical doctors, but they are licensed by the states to give eye tests and treat nonsurgical eye problems. They can prescribe corrective lenses. In some states, they can prescribe medication.

3. Opticians fill prescriptions for glasses and contact lenses. Only twenty-two states require opticians to be licensed.

❏ Because the light-absorbing retinal pigment is composed of vitamin A and protein, which are continually being used up as images are formed, adequate supplies of these nutrients are vital for proper eye function.

❏ The combination of nicotine, sugar, and caffeine may temporarily affect vision.

❏ Sea mussel is a source of protein that aids in the functioning of eye tissues and the secretion of eye fluids.

❏ Zinc may help reduce vision loss because it is a factor in the metabolic functioning of several enzymes in the chorioretinal complex (the vascular coating of the eye). Never take more than 100 milligrams a day.

❏ People who work at computers every day are at risk for eyestrain, headaches, blurred vision, dry or irritated eyes, sensitivity to light, double vision, and afterimages.

❏ People who wear contact lenses need to take precautions against eye damage because of the increased risk of injury and infection associated with them.

❏ Two studies have shown that leaving contact lenses in place for more than twenty-four consecutive hours can result in ulcerative keratitis, a condition in which the cells of the cornea are rubbed away by the contact lens, leading to infection and scarring. If not properly treated, this condition can cause blindness. Users of extended-wear lenses are ten to fifteen times more likely than other people to develop ulcerative keratitis, according to *The New England Journal of Medicine*. If ordinary daily-wear lenses are left in place overnight, the risk rises to the same level.

❏ Abnormalities in one or more of the six muscles that move the eyes, or a lack of coordination among these muscles, can result in a cross-eyed or walleyed condition. These muscles can be exercised and relaxed to improve their function. The internal muscles likewise can be exercised to improve the focusing ability of the eyes, both near and far.

Astigmatism

See under BLURRED VISION in this section.

Bags Under the Eyes

Skin loses some of its elasticity with age, and muscles within the eyelids lose tone, causing what is known as bags under the eyes. In addition, fat can gather in the eyelid, and fluids can accumulate and cause swelling. Puffiness around the eyes can also be caused by allergies or excessive consumption of salt. Smoking can aggravate the problem.

Recommendations

❏ Avoid drinking fluids before bed.

❏ Avoid monosodium glutamate (MSG) and limit your salt intake.

❏ Do not smoke, and avoid secondhand smoke.

❏ Get plenty of sleep.

❏ Place a washcloth moistened in ice water, or a chilled gel-filled compress, over your eyes for fifteen minutes once or twice daily. You can also try using a lukewarm wet tea bag or cold cucumber slices. The cold shrinks the swollen blood vessels.

❏ *See* ALLERGIES in Part Two and take the self-test to determine allergens that may be causing the problem.

Bitot's Spots

Bitot's spots are distinct elevated white patches on the conjunctiva, the membrane that covers most of the visible part of the eye. They may signify a severe deficiency of vitamin A. Before taking large doses of vitamin A, establish that you have a deficiency. Large doses are usually given to children living in areas prone to vitamin A deficiency.

NUTRIENTS

SUPPLEMENT	SUGGESTED DOSAGE	COMMENTS
Vitamin A	25,000 IU daily for two weeks, then 15,000 IU daily for 1 month, then reduce to 10,000 IU daily. If you are pregnant, do not exceed 10,000 IU daily.	Aids in dissolution of Bitot's spots, which may be caused by vitamin A deficiency. Use emulsion form for easier assimilation and greater safety at higher doses.
plus carotenoid complex with lutein and zeaxanthin	As directed on label.	

Recommendations

❏ Avoid eyestrain and smoke-filled rooms.

Blepharitis

Blepharitis is an inflammation of the outer edges of the eyelids that causes redness, itching, burning, and, often, a sensation that something is in your eye. Other possible symptoms include swelling of the eyelids, loss of eyelashes, excessive tearing, and sensitivity to light. Secretions may form crusts that "glue" the eyes together during sleep.

This condition may be caused by an infection of the eyelash follicles or glands at the outer edges of the eyelids. Eyestrain, poor hygiene, poor living and sleeping habits, poor nutrition, and systemic disease with resulting immunodepression commonly contribute to the problem. Blepharitis may also be associated with seborrhea of the face or scalp. (*See* SEBORRHEA in Part Two.)

NUTRIENTS

SUPPLEMENT	SUGGESTED DOSAGE	COMMENTS
Inf-zyme Forte from American Biologics	As directed on label.	Aids in reducing inflammation.
Vitamin A plus carotenoid complex with lutein and zeaxanthin	25,000 IU daily. If you are pregnant, do not exceed 10,000 IU daily. As directed on label.	Important in all eye disorders. Important antioxidants and precursors of vitamin A.
Vitamin C with bioflavonoids	6,000 mg daily, in divided doses.	A powerful antioxidant that protects the eyes and reduces inflammation.
Zinc	50 mg daily. Do not exceed a total of 100 mg daily from all supplements.	Needed for proper immune function. Use zinc gluconate lozenges or OptiZinc for best absorption.

Herbs

❏ Warm eyebright, goldenseal, or mullein compresses are soothing and help reduce inflammation. Prepare a tea using one of these herbs, cool it to a comfortably warm temperature, and soak a clean cloth or a piece of sterile cotton in it to make the compress. Apply the compress and relax for ten to fifteen minutes. Then make a fresh compress and gently wipe the edge of the eyelid and the area around and between the eyelashes to remove any scaly matter or dandruff-like debris. Do this twice a day or as needed. Use each compress only once before laundering or discarding it.

Recommendations

❏ Eat a well-balanced diet that emphasizes fresh, raw vegetables, plus grains, legumes, and fresh fruits.

❏ Keep the eyelids clean, especially along the edges (see the procedure described under Herbs, above), but do not touch or rub your eyes except when necessary. Always wash your hands before touching your eyes.

❏ Get sufficient sleep, and avoid eyestrain. Anything that increases eye fatigue makes the discomfort worse.

Considerations

❏ *See also* SEBORRHEA in Part Two.

Bloodshot Eyes

Bloodshot eyes occur when the small blood vessels on the surface of the eye become inflamed and congested with blood, usually in response to an insufficient supply of oxygen in the cornea or tissues covering the eyes. They are usually a consequence of eyestrain, fatigue, and improper diet, especially the consumption of alcohol. But they can also indicate bodywide capillary fragility, the presence of a blood clot, or high blood pressure.

A bloodshot appearance can also result from deficiencies in vitamins B_2 (riboflavin) and B_6 (pyridoxine), and the amino acids histidine, lysine, or phenylalanine. Once the body receives the nutrients it needs, the congestion in the blood vessels should disappear.

NUTRIENTS

SUPPLEMENT	SUGGESTED DOSAGE	COMMENTS
Vitamin A plus carotenoid complex with lutein and zeaxanthin	25,000 IU daily. If you are pregnant, do not exceed 10,000 IU daily. As directed on label.	Needed for all eye disorders.
Vitamin B complex plus free form amino acid	100 mg of each major B vitamin 3 times daily (amounts of individual vitamins in a complex will vary). As directed on label.	Deficiencies have been linked to bloodshot eyes. Use a formula containing both essential and nonessential amino acids.
Vitamin C with bioflavonoids	1,000–2,500 mg 4 times daily.	Important antioxidants and necessary free radical destroyers. Required for tissue growth and repair.

Herbs

❏ Use raspberry leaf to alleviate redness and irritation. Prepare a raspberry leaf tea, allow it to cool, and soak a clean cloth or piece of sterile cotton in the tea to make a compress. Apply the compress to the eyes with the lids closed for ten minutes or as needed.

Blurred Vision

Vision may become blurred for any number of reasons. Refractive error (nearsightedness, farsightedness, and/or astigmatism) results in chronically blurry vision that can usually be overcome with corrective lenses. Eyestrain, fatigue, and excessive tearing can result in a temporary blurring of vision. A disturbance in the fluid balance in the body can also result in blurry vision.

A recurring tendency to periodic blurring can result from an inadequate supply of the light-sensitive pigment in the eye called rhodopsin, or visual purple, which is composed of vitamin A and protein. Any light that enters the eyes breaks down part of the visual purple, and the products of this purposeful breakdown set up nerve impulses that tell the brain what the eyes are seeing. If there is not enough pigment present, a time delay occurs between the time the eyes focus on an object and the time the brain forms an image of it. This is experienced as blurred vision.

NUTRIENTS

SUPPLEMENT	SUGGESTED DOSAGE	COMMENTS
Potassium	99 mg daily.	Needed to maintain proper fluid balance.
Vitamin A plus carotenoid complex with lutein and zeaxanthin	25,000 IU daily. If you are pregnant, do not exceed 10,000 IU daily. As directed on label.	Necessary for pigment formation and proper balance of intraocular fluid. Needed for all eye disorders.

Considerations

❑ Laser surgery is an increasingly popular method for correcting refractive errors that cause myopia (nearsightedness) and hyperopia (farsightedness). Three laser surgery procedures—photorefractive keratectomy (PRK), conductive keratoplasty, and laser in situ keratomileusis (LASIK)—may be used to correct mild to moderate nearsightedness. These are outpatient procedures with relatively short recovery times. They also have very high rates of success, but neither procedure is foolproof. Some people have improved vision as a result of the laser surgery, but still have to wear corrective lenses afterward. Others have to have follow-up surgery to improve results. In rare cases, people who have laser surgery end up with worse vision. People who tend to heal slowly or who have ongoing medical problems such as glaucoma or diabetes are not good candidates for laser surgery. The same is true of those with uncontrolled high blood pressure, autoimmune diseases, or certain eye diseases involving the cornea or retina. Pregnant women should not have refractive surgery of any kind because the refraction of the eye may change during pregnancy.

Cataracts

A cataract is a clouding of the eye's lens that can lead to vision problems. If the lens of the eye thickens and becomes clouded or opaque, it becomes unable to focus or admit light properly. Some causes of cataracts include aging, diabetes, heavy metal poisoning, exposure to radiation, injury to the eye, and the use of certain drugs, such as steroids. High blood sugar levels are a major risk factor for developing cataracts.

The main symptom of a developing cataract is a gradual, painless loss of vision. Cataracts are the number-one cause of blindness in the world, although the vast majority of cataract conditions can be successfully treated with surgery. Occasionally, a cataract may swell and cause secondary glaucoma.

The most common form of cataract is the senile cataract, which typically affects people over sixty-five. This type of cataract is often caused by free radical damage. Exposure to ultraviolet rays and low-level radiation from X-rays leads to the formation of reactive chemical fragments in the eye's lens. The resistance of the lens begins to decline in older people. Free radicals attack the structural proteins, enzymes, and cell membranes of the lens. The free radicals in our food, water, and environment are probably a major factor in the increasing number of cataracts in our population.

NUTRIENTS

SUPPLEMENT	SUGGESTED DOSAGE	COMMENTS
Copper and manganese	3 mg daily. 10 mg daily. Take separately from calcium.	These minerals are important for proper healing and for retarding the growth of cataracts.
Glutathione	As directed on label.	An amino acid that is a potent antioxidant and aids in maintaining a healthy lens and protects against toxins. Has been shown to slow the progression of cataracts.
Grape seed extract	As directed on label.	A powerful antioxidant.
L-lysine	As directed on label, on an empty stomach. Take with water or juice. Do not take with milk. Take with 50 mg vitamin B6 and 100 mg vitamin C for better absorption.	Important in collagen formation, which is necessary for lens repair. Also neutralizes viruses implicated in lens damage. Caution: Do not take lysine for longer than 6 months at a time.
Vitamin B5 (pantothenic acid)	500 mg daily.	An anti-stress vitamin.
Selenium	200 mcg daily. If you are pregnant, do not exceed 40 mcg daily.	An important free radical destroyer that works synergistically with vitamin E.
Vitamin A plus carotenoid complex with lutein and zeaxanthin	25,000 IU daily. If you are pregnant, do not exceed 10,000 IU daily. As directed on label.	Vital for normal visual function. Precursors of vitamin A. Needed for all eye disorders.

Vitamin B complex plus extra	As directed on label.	B vitamins work best when taken together.
vitamin B$_1$ (thiamine) and	50 mg daily.	Important for intracellular eye metabolism.
vitamin B$_2$ (riboflavin)	50 mg daily.	Deficiency has been linked to cataracts.
Vitamin C with bioflavonoids	3,000 mg 4 times daily.	A necessary free radical destroyer that also lowers intraocular pressure.
Vitamin E	200 IU daily.	An important free radical destroyer. Has been shown to arrest and reverse cataract formation in some cases. Use d-alpha-tocopherol form.
Zinc	50 mg daily. Do not exceed a total of 100 mg daily from all supplements.	Protects against light-induced damage. Use zinc gluconate lozenges or OptiZinc for best absorption.

Herbs

❑ Bilberry extract, taken orally, supplies bioflavonoids that aid in removing toxic chemicals from the retina of the eye.

❑ Ginkgo biloba improves microcapillary circulation.

Caution: Do not take ginkgo biloba if you have a bleeding disorder, or are scheduled for surgery or a dental procedure.

Recommendations

❑ Increase your consumption of green leafy vegetables—especially collard greens, kale, mustard greens, spinach, and turnip greens—legumes, and yellow vegetables. Also, flavonoid-rich berries—such as blueberries and blackberries—cherries, and foods rich in vitamins E and C, such as raw fruits and vegetables.

❑ Follow a low-glycemic-load diet. It can reduce the risk of cataracts by 77 percent. Such a diet is rich in fruits and vegetables, low-fat dairy products, and proteins (meat and vegetable sources). It has smaller amounts of whole grains, refined grains, and sugars.

❑ Avoid dairy products, saturated fats, and any fats or oils that have been subjected to heat, whether by cooking or processing. These foods promote formation of free radicals, which can damage the lens. Use cold-pressed vegetable oils only. Get calcium and vitamin D from other sources such as soymilk or supplements.

❑ Drink quality water, preferably steam-distilled water. This is absolutely necessary in cataract prevention. Avoid fluoridated and chlorinated water. Even water from deeply driven wells may not be safe, since many aquifers (underground water sources), especially those located near or under farmland, are contaminated with toxic residue from farm runoff.

❑ Avoid direct sunlight. Wear a wide-brimmed hat when outdoors, and protect your eyes by wearing sunglasses (polarized) that block ultraviolet rays. Make sure the sunglasses are large enough to adequately protect your eyes.

❑ If you have cataracts, avoid antihistamines.

Considerations

❑ Several studies have found that people who eat foods rich in lutein and zeaxanthin—broccoli, collard greens, kale, mustard greens, spinach, and turnip greens—are much less likely to develop age-related cataracts than those who do not include these foods in their diets. These foods also are effective in reducing risk of macular degeneration. Researchers believe lutein and zeaxanthin act as antioxidants, protecting the cells in the eyes from free radical damage.

❑ Selected vitamins have been shown to reduce the risk of cataracts. In one study of 35,000 women who did not yet have cataracts, those who consumed a diet highest in lutein/zeaxanthin (6,700 micrograms) had an 18 percent reduced risk for cataracts; those who consumed the most vitamin E (262 milligrams) had a 14 percent reduced risk. The lutein/zeaxanthin came from fruits and vegetables and the vitamin E from supplements and diet.

❑ Taking vitamin C supplements (400 milligrams a day) for at least a decade and eating a diet rich in antioxidants can lower the risk of cataracts, according to researchers at the Harvard Medical School.

❑ A study published by the *Journal of Pineal Research* showed that melatonin was very effective in preventing laboratory-induced cataracts in rats. A control group of rats not given melatonin developed cataracts in 89 percent of the cases, whereas only 7 percent of the rats that had received melatonin developed cataracts. It is known that melatonin production slows with age, and most cataract cases develop in people who are sixty or older. Melatonin is known to be a powerful antioxidant, with the ability to permeate every level of the cell. Its effectiveness against cataract formation in humans needs to be further studied.

❑ A number of heavy metals increase in concentration in the lenses of both aging people and people with cataracts. Cadmium, for instance, is found at levels two or three times higher than normal in lenses with cataracts. Concentrations of other metals, such as cobalt, nickel, iridium, and bromine, also are elevated.

❑ An article in *Science* magazine reported that the single greatest cause of cataracts is the body's inability to cope with food sugars. Lactose (milk sugar) was the worst offender, followed by refined white sugar. Many eye specialists note that most people with cataracts eat diets that include substantial amounts of dairy products and refined white sugar. Cataracts can also develop if the diet is inadequate and prolonged stress is endured.

❑ People who are deficient in the enzyme that converts galactose into glucose (ordinary blood sugar) develop cataracts much sooner than the rest of the population.

❑ Smoking is a risk factor for cataracts, probably because the free radicals it generates increase the oxidant stress on the body. A study of cigarette smoking and the risk of cataracts reported in the *Journal of the American Medical Association* found a significant association between smoking and the incidence of cataracts.

❑ The conventional treatment for cataracts is surgery. In cataract surgery, the eye's own dysfunctional lens is removed, and usually is replaced with a prosthetic intraocular lens implant made of plastic or silicone. The lens may be removed whole, or a surgical procedure called phacoemulsification (often called the "phaco" technique) may be used. In this operation, the surgeon makes one minuscule incision, inserts the tip of a vibrating instrument into the cataract, and beats it until it turns liquid. The liquid is then sucked out and a new lens is implanted. With this type of surgery, the incision is only one-tenth of an inch long, compared to conventional one-third inch or one-half inch incisions. Another method used is extracapsular surgery, in which a slightly longer incision is made on the side of the cornea. The surgeon then removes the hard center of the lens, and the remainder of the lens is removed by suction.

Colorblindness

Colorblindness is a general term for the inability to see colors as most people see them. Specialized cells in the retina known as cones, which are vital for translating light waves into a perception of color, may be completely or partially lacking, or may not function properly, resulting in colorblindness.

There are different types and varying severities of this condition. Most colorblind people confuse certain colors (they may not be able to tell red from green, for example); in rare cases, an individual may see no color at all. Some can distinguish colors only in certain lights.

There are also certain diseases, including pernicious anemia and sickle cell disease, as well as a number of different medications, that can cause disturbances in color vision.

Because few people are tested for color vision, colorblindness is probably an underdiagnosed condition, especially among women. In most cases, colorblindness is present from birth, although the dimming of vision caused by cataracts can diminish a person's ability to distinguish colors later in life. Colorblindness is passed along through the mother and is more common in males.

NUTRIENTS

SUPPLEMENT	SUGGESTED DOSAGE	COMMENTS
Vitamin A plus carotenoid complex with lutein	25,000 IU daily. If you are pregnant, do not exceed 10,000 IU daily. As directed on label.	May be helpful because it is essential for proper functioning of the cones in the retina. Also improves night blindness. Use emulsion form, which is safe at higher doses than capsules.
Vitamin B$_{12}$	1,000–2,000 mcg daily.	Deficiency can lead to yellow-blue colorblindness.

Conjunctivitis (Pinkeye)

Conjunctivitis is an inflammation of the conjunctiva—the membrane that lines the eyelid and wraps around to cover most of the white of the eye. The eyes may appear swollen and bloodshot; they are often itchy and irritated. Because the infected membrane is often filled with pus, the eyelids are apt to stick together after being closed for an extended period.

Factors that can contribute to conjunctivitis include bacterial infection, virus, injury to the eye, allergies, and exposure to substances that are irritating to the eye, such as fumes, smoke, contact lens solutions, chlorine from swimming pools, chemicals, makeup, or any other foreign substance that enters the eye. Conjunctivitis is highly contagious if it is caused by a viral infection.

NUTRIENTS

SUPPLEMENT	SUGGESTED DOSAGE	COMMENTS
Vitamin A plus carotenoid complex with lutein and zeaxanthin	25,000 IU daily for 1 month; then reduce to 15,000 IU daily. If you are pregnant, do not exceed 10,000 IU daily. As directed on label.	Vitamin A, vitamin C, and zinc all help to promote immunity, which is especially important in common viral conjunctivitis. Use an emulsion form for easier assimilation and greater safety at high doses.
Vitamin C with bioflavonoids	2,000–6,000 mg daily, in divided doses.	Protects the eye from further inflammation. Enhances healing.
Zinc	50 mg daily. Do not exceed a total of 100 mg daily from all supplements.	Enhances immune response. Use zinc gluconate lozenges or OptiZinc for best absorption.

Herbs

❑ Calendula, chamomile, fennel, and/or eyebright herbal teas can be used to make hot compresses. Eyebright can also be taken orally in capsule or tea form. It is good for any eye irritation or inflammation. The tea can also be used to rinse the eyes.

Caution: Do not use chamomile if you are allergic to ragweed. Do not use during pregnancy or nursing. It may interact with warfarin or cyclosporin, so patients using these drugs should avoid it.

❑ The homeopathic remedy Similasan can help with pinkeye.

❑ Goldenseal, used as an alternative or in addition to eyebright, is very useful if conjunctivitis is caused by infection.

Caution: Do not take goldenseal internally on a daily basis for more than one week at a time. Do not use it during pregnancy or if you are breast-feeding, and use with caution if you are allergic to ragweed. If you have a history of cardiovascular disease, diabetes, or glaucoma, use it only under a doctor's supervision.

Recommendations

❑ Increase your consumption of green leafy vegetables—especially collard greens, kale, mustard greens, spinach, and turnip greens—legumes, and yellow vegetables. Also, flavonoid-rich berries such as blueberries and blackberries, cherries, and foods rich in vitamins E and C, such as raw fruits and vegetables.

❑ Apply hot compresses several times a day. Many of the microorganisms that cause conjunctivitis cannot tolerate heat. For greater benefit, use one of the herbal teas recommended above to make the compresses.

❑ If pain or blurred vision occurs, seek medical attention immediately. These can be signs of a more serious problem.

❑ If your eyelids are swollen, try peeling and grating a fresh potato, wrapping it with gauze, and placing it over your eyes. This acts as an astringent and has a healing effect.

Considerations

❑ Pinkeye associated with hay fever can be treated with prescription drops containing steroids.

❑ A bacterial infection is typically treated with antibiotics if the eye does not improve within four days of using compresses and taking supplements.

Corneal Ulcer

If the cornea—the membrane covering the front of the eye—is damaged, the eye becomes inflamed and vulnerable to infection that can result in ulceration. Damage may occur as a result of injury, a foreign body in the eye, or excessive or inappropriate wearing of contact lenses. The infections that can result in ulceration of the cornea may be caused by viruses, bacteria, or fungi.

NUTRIENTS

SUPPLEMENT	SUGGESTED DOSAGE	COMMENTS
Vitamin A plus carotenoid complex with lutein and zeaxanthin	25,000 IU daily. If you are pregnant, do not exceed 10,000 IU daily. As directed on label.	Needed for all eye disorders.
Vitamin C with bioflavonoids	6,000 mg daily, in divided doses.	A healing and antiviral substance.

Recommendations

❑ If you suspect that a corneal ulcer may be developing, consult a physician immediately.

Diabetic Retinopathy

Diabetes can cause retinopathy, a disorder in which some of the tiny capillaries that nourish the retina leak fluid or blood that can damage the rod and cone cells. New capillaries then begin to form in the injured area, and these also interfere with vision. Problems with the blood vessels can cause retinal hemorrhage (leakage from the vessels that transmit the fluids of the eye), microaneurysms (abnormally enlarged blood vessels in the eye), retinal edema (the accumulation of fluid in the eye), and, perhaps, loss of vision.

Diabetic retinopathy affects nearly every patient with type 1 or type 2 diabetes, and causes blindness among about 12,00 to 14,000 persons each year.

Unfortunately, there are few warning signs; the condition usually causes no symptoms until it is relatively advanced.

NUTRIENTS

SUPPLEMENT	SUGGESTED DOSAGE	COMMENTS
Shark cartilage	1 gm per 15 lbs of body weight daily, divided into 3 doses. If you cannot tolerate taking it orally, it can be administered rectally in a retention enema.	To prevent or possibly halt the progression of the condition by inhibiting the growth of tiny blood vessels in the eye that contribute to vision loss.
Vitamin A plus carotenoid complex with lutein and zeaxanthin	25,000 IU daily. If you are pregnant, do not exceed 10,000 IU daily. As directed on label.	Needed for all eye disorders.

Recommendations

❑ See DIABETES in Part Two and follow the dietary recommendations.

❑ If you have diabetes, make sure to have an annual eye examination to detect the onset of retinopathy. If the disorder is detected in time, laser surgery to seal leaking blood vessels can help stem vision loss.

Considerations

❑ One study reported that people with insulin-dependent (type 1) diabetes who controlled their blood sugar levels tightly were able to slow the pace of retinopathy by about 60 percent.

❑ Researchers at the National Eye Institute induced a condition resembling diabetic retinopathy in dogs and then treated the animals with an experimental drug called sorbinil, which suppresses the action of an enzyme that converts excess sugar in the blood into an alcohol that seems to damage the retinal blood vessels. In this study, the sorbinil treatment totally blocked the progression of retinopathy.

Dimness or Loss of Vision

Many different conditions can lead to a dimming or loss of vision. Among the most common are cataracts, glaucoma, and diabetic retinopathy. Macular degeneration and retinitis pigmentosa are less common, but do occur with some frequency. There are others as well:

- *Retinal detachment.* This causes a loss of vision often compared to having a curtain drawn across one's field of vision. Loss of vision may be preceded by a shower of "sparks" or lightning-like flashes of light, or by a dramatic increase in the number of black floaters in the field of vision. (*See* FLOATERS in this section.)

- *Uveitis.* This is an inflammation in the middle layer of the eye, which consists of the iris, the ciliary body, and the choroid. In many cases it is caused by an underlying systemic disease such as rheumatoid arthritis or infection. Pain and redness may be present, but often symptoms consist primarily of diminished or hazy vision. Another condition that can lead to loss of vision is blockage of a blood vessel serving the retina, usually by a blood clot. Visual loss is generally sudden if the affected blood vessel is an artery, but it may be less rapid if the blocked vessel is a vein. Usually only one eye is affected.

- *Inflammation of the optic nerve.* This inflammation is another possible cause of vision loss. Such inflammation may occur as a result of a systemic illness or infection, but in many cases the cause cannot be determined. This condition usually affects only one eye but it may affect both, causing varying degrees of vision loss over the course of a few days.

- *Toxic amblyopia.* This is a condition in which a toxic reaction damages the optic nerve, creating a small "hole" in the field of vision that enlarges over a period of time and may even lead to blindness. In most cases, both eyes are affected. This disorder is most common in people who smoke—in fact, it is sometimes referred to as tobacco amblyopia—and is seen most often in pipe smokers. It may also occur in those who consume excessive amounts of alcohol or who come into contact with lead, methanol, chloramphenicol, digitalis, ethambutol, and other chemicals.

Recommendations

❑ If any of the above symptoms develop, consult a physician. For most of these conditions, prompt treatment may help to preserve sight or at least slow vision loss.

❑ Do not smoke, and avoid those who do. Even people who have already developed toxic amblyopia as a result of smoking can have their vision improve if they quit.

Considerations

❑ The syndromes discussed here are usually painless. Physical discomfort is not a reliable indicator of visual health. Regular ophthalmic examinations are recommended for everyone over thirty-five.

❑ *See also* CATARACTS; DIABETIC RETINOPATHY; GLAUCOMA; MACULAR DEGENERATION; and RETINITIS PIGMENTOSA in this section.

Dry Eyes

Dry eyes occur when the tear ducts do not produce enough fluid (tears) to keep the eyes moist, resulting in burning and irritation. This problem is more common in women than in men, and women's susceptibility increases after menopause.

Contact lens wearers are particularly prone to developing dry eye problems. Dry eyes generally stem from a lack of vitamin A, and are more likely to affect people over the age of sixty-five. Some drugs are known to inhibit tear production or change the composition of tears, including antihistamines, decongestants, and various drugs used to control Parkinson's disease and high blood pressure.

NUTRIENTS

SUPPLEMENT	SUGGESTED DOSAGE	COMMENTS
Primrose oil	1,000 mg 2–3 times daily.	A source of essential fatty acids.
Vitamin A ointment and/or	As directed on label.	Beneficial for eyes that seem dry and scratchy. Tears
vitamin A	25,000 IU daily. If you are pregnant, do not exceed 10,000 IU daily.	contain vitamin A.
plus carotenoid complex with lutein and zeaxanthin	As directed on label.	Needed for all eye disorders.

Recommendations

❑ Drink at least ten glasses (80 ounces) of water every day. Steam-distilled water is best.

❑ See your health care provider if you have dry eyes. It may be a symptom of a more serious condition, such as rheumatoid arthritis or lupus. Also, constant irritation to the eye as a result of dryness can result in injury and damage.

❑ If your tear ducts are swollen, add more calcium to your diet and avoid processed foods.

❑ Artificial tears are safe and effective for keeping the eyes moist. Choose a product that is preservative-free, such as Cellufresh from Allergan or Tears Naturale from Alcon.

❑ Similasan Dry Eye Relief is a soothing homeopathic eye-drop product containing *Belladonna*, *Euphrasia*, and *Mercurius sublamitus*.

❑ Use a humidifier to add moisture to the dry air.

❑ Wear wraparound glasses on windy days.

❑ Avoid cigarette smoke and other types of smoke.

❑ Avoid products that claim they can "get the red out." Some over-the-counter drops used to relieve red and sore eyes contain vasoconstrictors that can further dry your eyes, especially if used for an extended period of time.

❑ Limit your use of hair dryers. Allow your hair to dry naturally. Shield your eyes from direct heat blasts from hair dryers and other heat sources.

Considerations

❑ In some cases, an ophthalmologist may perform a procedure to close the internal tear ducts, through which some tears drain from the eyes into the nose, to conserve tears and keep the eyes moist.

❑ Contact lenses made of a material called sulfoxide hydrogel may hold promise for people who currently cannot wear contact lenses because they are prone to dry eyes or frequent eye infections. The new material holds more water than current lens materials. It is currently being tested in clinical trials.

❑ Sjögren's syndrome is a disorder that can cause dryness in the eyes.

Eyestrain

Eyestrain causes a dull, aching sensation around and behind the eyes that can expand into a generalized headache. It may feel painful or fatiguing to focus the eyes. Eyestrain is commonly a result of overuse of the eyes for activities requiring close, precise focus, such as reading or computer work. People in certain occupations, such as jewelers, are particularly prone to eyestrain. Wearing improper lenses (whether the wrong prescription or an incorrectly made pair of glasses) can also cause eyestrain.

Acute closed-angle glaucoma can cause pain around the eyes as well, but the sensation is usually sharp and throbbing and accompanied by other symptoms. Most other eye disorders, even serious ones, cause little or no discomfort.

NUTRIENTS

SUPPLEMENT	SUGGESTED DOSAGE	COMMENTS
Vitamin A plus carotenoid complex with lutein and zeaxanthin	25,000 IU daily. If you are pregnant, do not exceed 10,000 IU daily. As directed on label.	Needed for all eye disorders.
Vitamin B complex plus extra vitamin B₂ (riboflavin)	50–100 mg of each major B vitamin daily (amounts of individual vitamins in a complex will vary). 25 mg 3 times daily.	Improves intraocular cellular metabolism. Helps to alleviate eye fatigue.

Herbs

❑ Taking eyebright in capsule or tea form can be helpful. Eyebright tea can also be used to rinse the eyes.

❑ Goldenseal can be used as an alternative or in addition to eyebright.

Caution: Do not take goldenseal internally on a daily basis for more than one week at a time. Do not use it during pregnancy or if you are breast-feeding, and use with caution if you are allergic to ragweed. If you have a history of cardiovascular disease, diabetes, or glaucoma, use it only under a doctor's supervision.

Recommendations

❑ Lie down, close your eyes, and place a cold compress over your eyes. Relax for ten minutes or longer, replacing the compress with a fresh one as necessary. This often helps to alleviate discomfort. You can also try using a wet tea bag or cold cucumber slices. The cold shrinks the swollen blood vessels.

❑ Take measures to avoid eyestrain. Try to vary your tasks so that your eyes change focusing distance every so often. When doing close work for prolonged periods, take periodic "focus breaks." Every twenty minutes or so, look away from your work and focus your eyes on something in the distance for a minute or two.

❑ If you work with computers for long periods of time, take a five- or ten-minute break every hour. Focus on distant objects as often as possible. Position the computer monitor to reduce glare from all light sources. Try a glare-reduction filter that carries a seal of approval by the American Optometric Association. If possible, use an active-matrix LCD flat display, which is sharper and brighter than a typical CRT-based display.

❑ Get sufficient sleep. Fatigue promotes eyestrain.

❑ If pain is severe and comes on suddenly, and especially if vision is disturbed or the pain is accompanied by nausea and vomiting, seek professional help at once. This may be a sign of an acute glaucoma attack. (*See* GLAUCOMA in Part Two.)

Floaters

Bits of cellular debris floating within the eye are commonly referred to as floaters. Because these floaters cast shadows over the retina, the individual sees small specks that move slowly before the eyes, especially in certain lights and against certain backgrounds. Older adults and nearsighted people are most likely to complain of floaters. Most floaters are considered benign, but seek medical attention anyway if you get them.

Floaters that coalesce into long, stringy strands may be caused by a disorder called fibrillar degeneration of the vitreous. This condition is usually caused by excessive exposure to sunlight.

NUTRIENTS

SUPPLEMENT	SUGGESTED DOSAGE	COMMENTS
Apple pectin	As directed on label.	Chelates heavy metals that can circulate through the eyes.
L-methionine	As directed on label, on an empty stomach. Take with water or juice. Do not take with milk. Take with 50 mg vitamin B_6 and 100 mg vitamin C for better absorption.	Chelates heavy metals. (See AMINO ACIDS in Part One.)
Oxy-5000 Forte from American Biologics	As directed on label.	A potent nutritional antioxidant for health and stress that destroys free radicals.
Vitamin A plus carotenoid complex with lutein and zeaxanthin	25,000 IU daily. If you are pregnant, do not exceed 10,000 IU daily. As directed on label.	Needed for all eye disorders.

Recommendations

❑ It is normal to see a few floaters at times, but if you suddenly see a large number of them, consult an ophthalmologist. This may be a sign of developing retinal detachment. Delaying treatment can result in a detached retina requiring lengthy surgery.

Glaucoma

Glaucoma is a serious eye disease marked by an increase in the pressure that the fluids within the eyeball exert on other parts of the eye. If this pressure is unrelieved, it may harm the retina and ultimately damage the optic nerve, resulting in vision loss, even blindness. It is most common in people over thirty-five, in nearsighted people, and in people with high blood pressure. *See* GLAUCOMA in Part Two for a more complete discussion of this condition.

Hyperopia

See under BLURRED VISION in this section.

Itchy or Tired Eyes

Itchy or tired eyes can be the result of many different factors, including allergies, eyestrain, fatigue, infection (conjunctivitis), and an inadequate supply of oxygen to the cornea and outer eye tissues.

NUTRIENTS

SUPPLEMENT	SUGGESTED DOSAGE	COMMENTS
Vitamin A plus carotenoid complex with lutein and zeaxanthin	25,000 IU daily. If you are pregnant, do not exceed 10,000 IU daily. As directed on label.	Needed for all eye disorders.
Vitamin B complex plus extra vitamin B_2 (riboflavin)	50–100 mg daily. 50 mg daily.	Improves intraocular cellular metabolism. Helps improve oxygenation of eye tissues.

Recommendations

❑ For quick relief of occasional itchy or tired eyes, close your eyes and apply a cold compress. Leave the compress in place for ten minutes. Compresses can be used as often as necessary.

Considerations

❑ If the problem is a recurrent one, allergies are a likely culprit. (See ALLERGIES in Part Two.)

❑ If itching and aching are accompanied by a bright pink or red color and thick secretions, you may have conjunctivitis. (See CONJUNCTIVITIS in this section.)

❑ If itchy and tired eyes persist over a long period of time, there may be an underlying nutritional cause. Supplement your diet with the B vitamins as described under Nutrients, above.

Macular Degeneration

This disorder causes a progressive visual loss due to degeneration of the macula, the portion of the retina responsible for fine vision. It is basically caused by hardening of the arteries that nourish the retina, depriving the tissue of oxygen and nutrients. Macular degeneration is the leading cause of severe visual loss in the United States and Europe in people over fifty-five years old. This loss of vision may appear suddenly or it may progress slowly. Usually peripheral and color vision are unaffected.

There are two types of macular degeneration: atrophic (or "dry"), which is the more common (90 percent of cases); and exudative ("wet"). In the latter type, the degeneration of the macula is accompanied by hemorrhaging or leaking of fluid from a network of tiny blood vessels that develop under the center of the retina. This results in scarring and loss of vision. In both cases, because the macula alone is affected, central vision is lost but total blindness is avoided. Some side vision usually is retained.

Macular degeneration is probably the result of free radical damage similar to the type of damage that induces cataracts. Factors that predispose a person to developing macular degeneration include aging, atherosclerosis, hypertension, and environmental toxins. Heredity may play a role as well.

NUTRIENTS

SUPPLEMENT	SUGGESTED DOSAGE	COMMENTS
Coenzyme Q$_{10}$ plus	60 mg daily.	Powerful antioxidants protect against macular degeneration.
Coenzyme A from Coenzyme-A Technologies	As directed on label.	
Grape seed extract	As directed on label.	A powerful antioxidant that protects against free radical damage.
Selenium	400 mcg daily.	An important antioxidant.
Shark cartilage	1 gm per 15 lbs of body weight daily, divided into 3 doses. If you cannot tolerate taking it orally, it can be administered rectally in a retention enema.	To prevent and possibly halt the progression of exudative macular degeneration by inhibiting the growth of tiny blood vessels in the eye that contribute to vision loss.
Vitamin A plus	25,000 IU daily. If you are pregnant, do not exceed 10,000 IU daily.	Potent antioxidant and important in eye function.
carotenoid complex with lutein and zeaxanthin	As directed on label.	Use an emulsion form for easier assimilation and greater safety at high doses. The macula selectively concentrates zeaxanthin and lutein to levels over 1,000 times greater than those found in any other body tissues. The macula places zeaxanthin in its center, where the greatest protection is required and which is the last to degenerate.
Vitamin C plus bioflavonoids	1,000–2,500 mg 4 times daily.	An important antioxidant and a necessary free radical destroyer. Prevents eye damage; also relieves pressure from cataracts.
Vitamin E	200 IU daily.	An important antioxidant and free radical destroyer. Use d-alpha-tocopherol form.
Zinc plus copper	45–80 mg daily. Do not exceed a total of 100 mg daily from all supplements. 3 mg daily.	Deficiency has been linked to eye disorders. Use zinc picolinate form. Needed to balance with zinc.

Herbs

❑ Taking bilberry extract (160 milligrams and up daily) and eating fresh blueberries (8 to 10 ounces per day), plus taking ginkgo biloba extract and zinc, can help halt the loss of vision. Blueberries are rich in valuable bioflavonoids. Treatment at an early stage is most effective.

Caution: Do not take ginkgo biloba if you have a bleeding disorder, or are scheduled for surgery or a dental procedure.

Recommendations

❑ Increase your consumption of green, leafy vegetables—especially collard greens, kale, mustard greens, spinach, and turnip greens—legumes; yellow vegetables; flavonoid-rich berries—such as blueberries and blackberries—cherries; and foods rich in vitamins E and C, such as raw fruits and vegetables.

❑ Avoid alcohol, cigarette smoke, all sugars, saturated fats, and foods containing fats and oils that have been subjected to heat and/or exposed to the air, such as fried foods, hamburgers, luncheon meats, and roasted nuts.

❑ Broccoli contains sulforaphane, which may help prevent macular degeneration, according to Peter Gehlbach, assistant professor of ophthalmology at Johns Hopkins University School of Medicine. Some doctors recommend as many as five servings of broccoli a day, along with the green vegetables listed above.

❑ Reduce dietary fat to less than 24 grams per day and trans fats to less than ½ gram per day. Eat more nuts and fish (to increase omega-3s) and less animal fat in general. Eating fish one to three times a week supplied omega-3 fats and was associated with a 40 to 75 percent reduction in macular degeneration. No association was found for butter, margarine, or nuts. Another study showed that eating fish just once a week reduced the chance of getting macular degeneration by 50 percent.

Considerations

❑ In a study reported in the *Archives of Ophthalmology*, ophthalmologists at Louisiana State University Medical School tested the effects of supplemental zinc on people suffering from macular degeneration. Half the group received a 100-milligram tablet of zinc twice a day; the other half received a placebo. After twelve to twenty-four months, the zinc group showed significantly less deterioration than the placebo group.

❑ In general, eating a low-glycemic-load, healthy diet (fruit, vegetables, whole grains) was related to a 53 percent lower risk of macular degeneration. The risk was even lower—77 percent—when vitamin C supplements were used.

❑ Eating a diet rich in sugars and refined grains increases the risk of developing a worse form of macular degeneration. Specifically, retinal pigment abnormalities, characteristics of the condition, were associated with the high-glycemic-load diet but not the total carbohydrate dietary intake.

❑ Antioxidant nutrients are known to protect against macular degeneration, but two in particular—lutein and zeaxanthin—are believed to play critical roles in the prevention of the disease. A study by Johanna M. Seddon, M.D., of the Massachusetts Eye and Ear Infirmary in Boston, compared the diets of 356 patients with macular degeneration with 520 patients with other eye diseases. The data revealed that beta-carotene was not especially effective, but that lutein and zeaxanthin were. Some foods that contain lutein and zeaxanthin are collard greens, kale, mustard greens, and turnip greens. In a subsequent study, the risk of macular degeneration was reduced 65 percent with high amounts of lutein and zeaxanthin. Also, zinc was found to be important to lower risk, but at levels of about 13 milligrams per day. This was confirmed in the 2007 major eye and vitamin study in the United States, called AREDS (Age-Related Eye Disease Study). However, other studies have not shown any benefit from antioxidant supplementation to prevent macular degeneration. In a compilation of nine studies including nearly 150,000 people, no effect was seen for the following: vitamins A, C, and E, zinc, lutein, zeaxanthin, and alpha- and beta-carotene. Similarly, taking 6 milligrams of lutein with a vitamin and mineral supplement did not reduce the risk of getting macular degeneration.

❑ The FDA has approved the drug pegaptanib sodium (Macugen). This drug is particularly suited for treatment of wet age-related macular degeneration. The drug must be administered by injection. Macugen was co-developed by Eyetech Pharmaceuticals and Pfizer, Inc.

❑ Coenzyme Q₁₀ improves retinal function in patients with age-related macular degeneration, according to Dr. Janos Feher, a researcher at the University of Rome, Italy. A small study, reported in the journal *Ophthalmologica,* compared a group getting a Coenzyme Q₁₀ preparation to a control group getting vitamin E alone. The subjects who received the Coenzyme Q₁₀ mixture showed slight improvement or no degeneration over two years, while the control group continued to slowly decline.

Mucus in the Eyes

A number of different conditions can cause mucus to accumulate in the eyes, such as allergies, head colds, and infection (conjunctivitis).

Herbs

❑ Gently and very carefully wash each eye with diluted alcohol-free goldenseal extract or cool goldenseal tea.

Caution: Do not take goldenseal internally on a daily basis for more than one week at a time. Do not use it during pregnancy or if you are breast-feeding, and use with caution if you are allergic to ragweed. If you have a history of cardiovascular disease, diabetes, or glaucoma, use it only under a doctor's supervision.

Myopia

See under BLURRED VISION in this section.

Photophobia

Photophobia is an abnormal inability of the eyes to tolerate light; exposure to light hurts the eyes. It is more common in people with light-colored eyes, and usually is not a serious problem. In some cases, however, it may be associated with irritation or damage to the cornea, acute glaucoma, or uveitis. It can also be a symptom of developing measles.

NUTRIENTS

SUPPLEMENT	SUGGESTED DOSAGE	COMMENTS
Vitamin A plus carotenoid complex with lutein and zeaxanthin	25,000 IU daily. If you are pregnant, do not exceed 10,000 IU daily. As directed on label.	Needed for all eye disorders.

Considerations

❑ *See also* GLAUCOMA and/or MEASLES, both in Part Two.

❑ *See also* the discussion of uveitis *under* DIMNESS OR LOSS OF VISION in this section.

Pinkeye

See CONJUNCTIVITIS in this section.

Retinal Edema

See DIABETIC RETINOPATHY in this section.

Retinal Hemorrhage

See DIABETIC RETINOPATHY in this section.

Retinitis Pigmentosa

Retinitis pigmentosa is a group of inherited diseases that affects approximately 100,000 people in the United States. The retina is the innermost layer that lines the eyeball. It contains photoreceptor cells that are directly connected to the brain by the optic nerve. Retinitis pigmentosa causes these photoreceptor cells to degenerate over time. The first symptom usually is loss of night vision, beginning in adolescence or young adulthood. This is followed by loss of peripheral vision and, ultimately, blindness, which sets in anywhere between the ages of thirty and eighty. Usher syndrome is a variation of retinitis pigmentosa that also impairs hearing. (*See* HEARING LOSS in Part Two.)

NUTRIENTS

SUPPLEMENT	SUGGESTED DOSAGE	COMMENTS
Coenzyme Q₁₀	60 mg daily.	A powerful antioxidant that can improve retinitis pigmentosa symptoms.
Vitamin A plus carotenoid complex with lutein and zeaxanthin	15,000 IU daily. If you are pregnant, do not exceed 10,000 IU daily. As directed on label.	Helpful for all eye disorders. Use an emulsion form for easier assimilation and greater safety at higher doses.

Recommendations

❑ Get a thorough eye evaluation by an eye care professional who specializes in retinitis pigmentosa. An accurate diagnosis sometimes can be difficult to obtain, but it is getting better through increased awareness and more sophisticated technology.

Considerations

❑ High doses of vitamin A may be able to slow the loss of remaining eyesight by about 20 percent per year in some cases, according to a study led by Eliot Berson, M.D., professor of ophthalmology at Harvard Medical School. At the same time, the study found that high doses of supplemental vitamin E (400 international units or more daily) can be detrimental to people with retinitis pigmentosa.

Caution: Check with your eye doctor before exceeding the DRI for vitamin A.

❑ Retinal cell transplantation and gene therapy are still in the preliminary stages of research, but both may prove to be effective in treating retinitis pigmentosa. Photoreceptor cells have been transplanted successfully into the retinas of animals. The Foundation Fighting Blindness reports that it remains to be seen whether or not this procedure will be effective with retinitis pigmentosa–type disorders. Meanwhile, researchers have identified many of the mutated genes that contribute to the condition. It may become possible in the future to use gene therapy—to replace defective genes with normal ones—as a treatment for the disorder.

❑ More information on this disorder can be obtained by calling the Foundation Fighting Blindness. (*See* Health and Medical Organizations in the Appendix.)

Scotoma

A scotoma is a blind spot in the visual field. Unless a scotoma is large or is located in the center of the field of vision, it may not be noticed. However, a professional can detect scotomas with a type of examination called a visual field test.

Scotomas are considered a symptom of disease, not a disease in themselves. They may be a sign of a problem with the retina or damage to the optic nerve, such as that caused by glaucoma.

NUTRIENTS

SUPPLEMENT	SUGGESTED DOSAGE	COMMENTS
Very Important		
Vitamin A plus carotenoid complex with lutein and zeaxanthin	25,000 IU daily for 2 months. If you are pregnant, do not exceed 10,000 IU daily. As directed on label.	Essential for eye health. Use emulsion form for easier assimilation and greater safety at higher doses.

Shingles (Herpes Zoster)

Shingles is an infection caused by the varicella-zoster virus, a member of the herpes family and the same virus that causes chickenpox. The characteristic symptom is a rash of painful blisters. Shingles can appear anywhere on the body.

If shingles occurs on the forehead near the eyes or on the tip of the nose, the eyes are likely to become involved, and damage to the cornea can occur. Taking the proper supplements when blisters first appear can make the blisters dry up quickly, and the discomfort may be alleviated.

NUTRIENTS

SUPPLEMENT	SUGGESTED DOSAGE	COMMENTS
L-lysine	1,000 mg daily, on an empty stomach. Take with water or juice. Do not take with milk. Take with 50 mg vitamin B_6 and 100 mg vitamin C for better absorption.	Fights herpesviruses. (*See* AMINO ACIDS in Part One.) *Caution:* Do not take lysine longer than six months at a time.
Vitamin A plus carotenoid complex with lutein and zeaxanthin	25,000 IU daily. If you are pregnant, do not exceed 10,000 IU daily. As directed on label.	Needed for all eye disorders.
Vitamin B_{12}	1,000–2,000 mcg daily, on an empty stomach.	Prevents damage to the nerves in the eyes. Use a lozenge or sublingual form.
Vitamin C with bioflavonoids	2,000–6,000 mg daily and up.	An antiviral and immune system enhancer.
Vitamin E	200 IU daily.	Helps to prevent scarring and tissue damage. Use d-alpha-tocopherol form.

Recommendations

❑ If shingles appear on the forehead near the eyes or on the tip of the nose, seek treatment from an ophthalmologist.

❑ Apply zinc oxide cream to the blisters and the affected area. After the blisters have healed over, apply aloe vera gel and vitamin E to the area.

Considerations

❑ If zinc oxide, aloe vera gel, and/or vitamin E do not work to heal the blisters within three days, intravenous injections of large doses of vitamin C should provide relief almost immediately. Large intravenous doses of vitamin C can cause diarrhea. Let your doctor decide how much to give. The normal dose given is between 10 and 50 centigrams (a centigram is one-hundredth of a gram).

❑ *See also* SHINGLES in Part Two.

Stye

A stye is a bacterial infection within an oil gland on the edge of the eyelid. Because the tissues of the eye become inflamed from the infection, the stye takes on the appearance of a small pimple. This pimple gradually comes to a head, opens, and drains. Early treatment speeds the healing process and helps to avoid further complications.

Herbs

❏ Prepare raspberry leaf tea and use it as an eyewash to alleviate styes.

Recommendations

❏ Apply a hot compress to the affected area for ten minutes four to six times daily to help relieve discomfort and bring the stye to a head so that it can drain and healing can begin.

❏ If you frequently suffer from styes, supplement your diet with vitamin A. Recurring styes are often a sign of vitamin A deficiency.

Considerations

❏ If a stye does not heal promptly, it may need to be drained. This is a procedure that must be done by a health care professional. Do not squeeze the lump or attempt to drain it at home. This can cause the infection to spread into the bloodstream, leading to systemic illness.

❏ In severe and/or stubborn cases, treatment with antibiotics may be necessary.

Thinning Eyelashes

Many problems can lead to a thinning or even the total loss of the eyelashes. Among these are allergies, especially contact allergies to eye makeup; the use of certain drugs; exposure to environmental toxins; hypothyroidism; eye surgery; a poor diet and/or nutritional deficiencies; and trauma.

NUTRIENTS

SUPPLEMENT	SUGGESTED DOSAGE	COMMENTS
Vitamin A	25,000 IU daily. If you are pregnant, do not exceed 10,000 IU daily.	Promotes healthy skin and hair.
plus carotenoid complex with lutein and zeaxanthin	As directed on label.	Needed for all eye disorders.
Vitamin B complex plus extra	50–100 mg daily.	The B vitamins help prevent loss of eyelashes.
vitamin B$_2$ (riboflavin) and	As directed on label.	
vitamin B$_3$ (niacin) plus	As directed on label.	

brewer's yeast	2 tbsp daily	Can cause an allergic reaction in some individuals. Start with a small amount at first, and discontinue if any allergic symptoms occur.

Recommendations

❏ Gently rub vitamin E oil on your eyelashes and into your eyelids at bedtime. This helps to thicken the lashes and promote normal growth.

Ulcerated Eye

See CORNEAL ULCER in this section.

Ulcerated Eyelid

If an eyelid is scratched and the scratch becomes infected, an ulcerated area may develop. Ulcerated eyelids also can occur as a result of chronic blepharitis.

Xerophthalmia

Xerophthalmia is an inflammation of the cornea that is associated with nutritional deficiency, especially a deficiency of vitamin A. The cornea becomes dry, and infection and/or ulceration may set in. Bitot's spots may appear, and night blindness may occur.

NUTRIENTS

SUPPLEMENT	SUGGESTED DOSAGE	COMMENTS
Vitamin A	25,000 daily. If you are pregnant, do not exceed 10,000 IU daily.	Specifically for dry eyes.
plus carotenoid complex with lutein and zeaxanthin	As directed on label.	Needed for all eye disorders.
Vitamin B$_6$ (pyridoxine) and	50 mg daily.	Nutrients that work well together to heal dry eyes.
vitamin C with bioflavonoids and	2,000–14,000 mg daily, in divided doses.	
zinc	50 mg daily. Do not exceed a total of 100 mg daily from all supplements.	Use zinc gluconate lozenges or OptiZinc for best absorption.

Considerations

❏ See also BITOT'S SPOTS in this section.

FABRY'S DISEASE

See under RARE DISORDERS.

FATIGUE

See CHRONIC FATIGUE SYNDROME.

FEVER

A fever is an elevation in body temperature. Fever is not a disease, but a symptom that may indicate the presence of disease.

Normal body temperature ranges from 97°F to 99°F. It varies from individual to individual. Rectal temperature is usually about 1°F higher than oral temperature, and body temperature varies in the course of the day—it usually increases in the afternoon. Women have a higher temperature after ovulation than before ovulation.

One should not have undue concern unless body temperature rises above 102°F (103°F in children). Often, running a temperature is helpful to the body. This defense mechanism of the body acts to destroy harmful microbes. A part of the brain called the hypothalamus regulates body temperature by regulating heat loss, mainly from the skin.

When destructive microbes or tumor cells invade the body, the immune cells rushing to fight them release proteins that tell the hypothalamus to raise the temperature. Moderate temperatures (under 103°F for adults) encourage the body to manufacture more immune cells.

There are some situations, however, in which fever can cause problems. A high fever (104°F or higher) may pose a risk for people with cardiac problems, since it makes the heart beat faster and work harder, and can cause irregular heart rhythms, chest pain, or heart attack. Fever over 106°F, especially for prolonged periods, can cause dehydration and brain injury.

Unless otherwise specified, the dosages recommended here are for adults. For a child between the ages of twelve and seventeen, reduce the dose to three-quarters the recommended amount. For a child between six and twelve, use one-half the recommended dose, and for a child under the age of six, use one-quarter the recommended amount.

NUTRIENTS

SUPPLEMENT	SUGGESTED DOSAGE	COMMENTS
Very Important		
Inf-zyme Forte from American Biologics	As directed on label.	A balanced, potent enzyme complex that moderates the inflammatory response.
Vitamin A emulsion or capsules with carotenoids	As directed on label. Adults: 25,000 IU daily. If you are pregnant or nursing, do not exceed 10,000 IU daily. Children over 2 years: 1,000–10,000 IU daily.	Essential in immune system function. Needed to fight infection and to strengthen the immune system. Emulsion form is recommended because it enters the system more quickly.
Important		
Bio-Bifidus from American Biologics	As directed on label.	For bowel flora replacement to improve elimination and assimilation.
Free form amino acid (Amino Balance	As directed on label 3 times daily, on an empty stomach. Take	A readily absorbed form of protein that helps repair tissue damaged by fever.
from Anabol Naturals or Amino Blend from Carlson Labs)	with 50 mg each of vitamins B_6 and C for better absorption.	
Taurine Plus from American Biologics	As directed on label.	An important antioxidant and immune regulator, necessary for white blood cell activation and neurological function. Use the sublingual form.
Vitamin C with bioflavonoids	5,000–20,000 daily, in divided doses. (See ASCORBIC ACID FLUSH in Part Three.)	To flush out toxins and reduce fever. For a child, use calcium ascorbate form—it does not produce heavy diarrhea.
Helpful		
Garlic (Kyolic from Wakunaga)	2 capsules 3 times daily.	A natural antibiotic and powerful immunostimulant.
Royal jelly	As directed on label 3 times daily.	Has antifungal properties and improves adrenal function.
Spiru-tein from Nature's Plus	As directed on label, between meals.	A protein drink that contains all the amino acids, vitamins, and minerals needed for nourishment.

Herbs

❏ To bring a high fever down, use catnip tea enemas twice daily. These also relieve constipation and congestion, which keep fever up. (*See* ENEMAS in Part Three.)

❏ Catnip tea with dandelion and lobelia, taken in tea or extract form, is good for lowering fever. Lobelia can also be used on its own. Taking ½ teaspoon of lobelia extract or tincture every four hours helps to lower fever. If an upset stomach occurs, cut the dosage back to ¼ teaspoon.

Caution: Lobelia is only to be taken under supervision of a health care professional as it is potentially toxic. People with high blood pressure, heart disease, liver disease, kidney disease, seizure disorders, or shortness of breath should not take lobelia. Pregnant and lactating women should avoid lobelia as well.

❏ Elderberry tea and hot steam baths may help.

❏ You can make a poultice from echinacea root to lower fever. (*See* USING A POULTICE in Part Three.)

Caution: Do not take echinacea for longer than three months. It should not be used by people who are allergic to ragweed.

❏ A combination of hyssop, licorice root, thyme, and yarrow tea can help a fever.

Caution: Licorice root should not be used during pregnancy or nursing. It should not be used by persons with diabetes, glaucoma, heart disease, high blood pressure, or a history of stroke.

❏ Other beneficial herbs include blackthorn, echinacea, fenugreek seed, feverfew, ginger, and poke root.

Cautions: Do not take echinacea for longer than three months. It should not be used by people who are allergic to ragweed. Do not use feverfew when pregnant or nursing. People who take prescription blood-thinning medications should consult a health care provider before using feverfew, as the combination can result in internal bleeding. Do not use feverfew during pregnancy.

Recommendations

❑ Replace fluid loss by drinking as much quality water as you can. This will also help to bring down body temperature.

❑ Get plenty of rest.

❑ Avoid radical changes in atmospheric temperature.

❑ Drink plenty of distilled water, broths, and juices, but avoid solid food until the fever breaks.

❑ While feverish, avoid taking any supplements that contain iron or zinc. When an infection is present, the body attempts to "hide" iron in the tissues in an attempt to keep the infecting organism from using it for nourishment. Taking a supplement containing iron therefore causes undue strain on a body that is fighting an infection. Zinc is not properly absorbed while a fever is present.

❑ Take cool sponge baths. Do not use rubbing alcohol to cool off, however; it gives off noxious fumes.

❑ To induce sweating, which may shorten the length of the fever, wrap up in a warm blanket or robe for twenty minutes. Replace lost fluids as soon as you can.

❑ *Belladonna* and *Aconite* napellus are homeopathic remedies used to reduce fever. Use a 123 strength and dilute 5 drops of one or both of these remedies in a glass of water. Take this every half-hour or as needed.

❑ It should be noted that lowering a fever is not always the best thing to do for an otherwise healthy adult. As long as a fever does not get too high (above 102°F), let it run its course. It helps to fight infection and eliminate toxins.

❑ If body temperature rises above 102°F (103°F in a child), take measures to reduce the fever, and consult your health care provider. This can be a sign of a serious condition.

❑ If a baby of three months or under has a temperature of 103°F or higher, take the child to a doctor immediately.

❑ In a child of any age, fever accompanied by a stiff neck, swelling of the throat, or disorientation needs immediate attention from a physician, as these symptoms may indicate meningitis.

❑ See a health care professional immediately if you develop a fever associated with any of the following:

• Frequent urination, a burning sensation while urinating, or blood in the urine.

• Pain concentrated in one area of the abdomen.

• Shaking chills or alternating chills and sweats.

• Severe headache and vomiting.

• Profuse watery diarrhea lasting more than twenty-four hours.

• Swollen glands or rashes.

❑ Never give aspirin to a child with a fever. (*See* REYE'S SYNDROME in Part Two.)

Considerations

❑ Lingering or recurring flulike symptoms can be associated with chronic fatigue syndrome, diabetes (especially in children), hepatitis, Lyme disease, or mononucleosis (especially in adolescents). (*See* CHRONIC FATIGUE SYNDROME; DIABETES; HEPATITIS; LYME DISEASE; and/or MONONUCLEOSIS in Part Two.)

❑ Vigorous exercise, in which the muscles generate heat faster than the body can dissipate it, can cause a temporary rise in temperature.

FIBROCYSTIC BREASTS

Fibrocystic breast disease is a noncancerous condition characterized by the presence of cysts, or lumps, in the breasts. This condition is also known as fibrocystic changes, chronic cystic mastitis, mammary dysphasia, and—although it is not actually a disease—fibrocystic breast disease. It is caused by monthly changes in levels of estrogen and progesterone. It affects more than half of all women of childbearing age, most often those between the ages of thirty and fifty.

Fibrocystic breasts are characterized by the presence of round lumps, or cysts, that move freely and are either firm or soft. Symptoms include tenderness and lumpiness in the breasts. The discomfort is usually most pronounced before menstruation.

Normally, fluids from breast tissues are collected and transported out of the breasts by means of the lymphatic system. However, if there is more fluid than the system can cope with, small spaces in the breast may fill with fluid. Fibrous tissue surrounds them and thickens like a scar, forming cysts. Many breast cysts swell before and during menstruation, and the resulting pressure can cause a feeling of fullness, a dull ache, increased sensitivity, or a burning sensation. Some women also experience significant pain.

Breast cysts may change in size, but they are benign. A cyst is tender and moves freely—it feels like an eyeball behind the lid. In contrast, a cancerous growth usually does not move freely, is most often not tender, and does not go away.

Most cysts are harmless. In fact, the normal structure of the breasts has a lumpy texture. However, this does not mean that any lumps should be disregarded. Each woman should be familiar with the normal feel of and cyclical changes in her breasts so that she can easily detect any new lumps. Ideally, she should check her breasts weekly, and if any new lumps become apparent between menstrual cycles, she should consult her health care practitioner promptly.

A physician can diagnose fibrocystic breasts with a simple office procedure. Using a fine needle, he or she attempts to remove fluid from the lump. If fluid is present, the lump is a cyst. A biopsy may be recommended to determine the risk, if any, of developing cancer. Routine mammograms are recommended as well after the age of thirty-five if you have fibrocystic breasts.

NUTRIENTS

SUPPLEMENT	SUGGESTED DOSAGE	COMMENTS
Essential		
Coenzyme Q10 plus Coenzyme A from Coenzyme-A Technologies	As directed on label. As directed on label.	Powerful antioxidants that help to remove toxins from the body, boost the immune system, and improve overall physical and mental processes.
Kelp	1,500–2,000 mg daily, in divided doses.	A rich source of iodine. Iodine deficiency has been linked to fibrocystic breasts.
Primrose oil	1,500 mg daily.	May reduce the size of the lumps.
Vitamin E	200 IU daily.	Protects the breast tissue because of its antioxidant ability. Use d-alpha-tocopherol form.
Very Important		
Vitamin A plus carotenoid complex with beta-carotene	15,000 IU daily, with meals. If you are pregnant, do not exceed 10,000 IU daily. As directed on label.	Needed for the ductal system of the breast. Antioxidants and precursors of vitamin A.
Vitamin B complex plus extra vitamin B6 (pyridoxine)	50 mg of each major B vitamin 3 times daily, with meals (amounts of individual vitamins in a complex will vary). 50 mg 3 times daily.	B-complex vitamins are important for all enzyme systems in the body. Needed for proper fluid balance and hormone regulation.
Important		
Vitamin C with bioflavonoids	2,000–4,000 mg daily, in divided doses.	Needed for proper immune function, tissue repair, and adrenal hormone balance.
Zinc	50 mg daily. Do not exceed a total of 100 mg daily from all supplements.	For repair of tissues and immune function. Use zinc gluconate lozenges or OptiZinc for best absorption.
Helpful		
Multimineral complex	As directed on label.	Balanced body minerals are important. Take one with iron if you are still menstruating.
Proteolytic enzymes plus bromelain	As directed on label. Take with meals and between meals. As directed on label.	To reduce inflammation and soreness due to swelling.

Herbs

❏ The following herbs are good for fibrocystic breasts: echinacea, goldenseal, mullein, pau d'arco, red clover, squaw vine, and turmeric (curcumin).

Cautions: Do not take echinacea for longer than three months. It should not be used by people who are allergic to ragweed. Do not take goldenseal internally on a daily basis for more than one week at a time. Do not use it during pregnancy or if you are breast-feeding, and use with caution if you are allergic to ragweed. If you have a history of cardiovascular disease, diabetes, or glaucoma, use it only under a doctor's supervision.

❏ Use poke root or sage poultices to relieve breast inflammation and soreness. (*See* USING A POULTICE in Part Three.)

Cautions: Poke root is recommended for external use only. Do not use sage if you suffer from any type of seizure disorder, or are pregnant or nursing.

Recommendations

❏ Eat a low-fat, high-fiber diet. Eat more raw foods, including seeds, nuts, and grains. Be sure nuts have not been subjected to heat. Although some newer data does not confirm that a low-fat diet rich in fruits and vegetables is beneficial for someone with fibrocystic breast disease, such a diet is necessary for optimal health and maintaining a healthy body weight. The women in the study followed a diet where dietary fat was 20 percent of total calories; however, a diet with 25 to 35 percent fat is currently recommended. Include in your diet three or more servings daily of apples, bananas, grapes, grapefruit, raw nuts, seeds, fresh vegetables, and yogurt. Whole grains and beans should also be important parts of the diet.

❏ Include in your diet foods that are high in germanium, such as garlic, shiitake mushrooms, and onions. Germanium helps to improve tissue oxygenation at the cellular level.

❏ Do not consume any coffee, tea (except herbal teas), cola drinks, or chocolate. These foods contain caffeine, which has been implicated in fibrocystic breasts. However, newer data published in the *Archives of Internal Medicine* from a rigorous review of the published literature showed there was no association between caffeine consumption and fibrocystic breast disease. Talk to your doctor.

Considerations

❏ Good results have been achieved using primrose oil to reduce the size of cysts.

❏ In one study, a diet that included one soy food a day was shown to reduce the development of fibrocystic disease.

❏ The drug danazol (Danocrine), a hormone, acts through the pituitary gland, reducing the function of the ovaries. This in turn decreases the amount of estrogen in the breast, shrinking the lumps. Danocrine is not effective for all women, but many notice results within a few weeks. Many report less pain or tenderness. The drug may have some unpleasant side effects and it should be used only if the suggestions above fail to give the desired results.

❑ Thyroid function is important in fibrocystic breasts; iodine deficiency can cause an underactive thyroid and has also been linked to fibrocystic changes. (*See* HYPOTHYROIDISM in Part Two.) Other factors include hormonal imbalance and abnormal production of breast milk brought about by high levels of the hormone estrogen.

❑ The National Cancer Institute recommends that all women examine their own breasts once a month. Self-examination should be done five to ten days after menstruation, after all swelling has subsided. Postmenopausal women should conduct a self-examination on the same date every month.

FIBROIDS, UTERINE

Uterine fibroids (also called leiomyomas or myomas) are benign growths that can form on the interior muscular wall as well as the exterior of the uterus. These tumors can be microscopic to several pounds in size. The disorder involves not only the uterus but sometimes also the cervix. The term *fibroid* may be somewhat misleading because the tumor cells are not fibrous. They are abnormal muscle cells, and their position within the uterus determines what they are called—submucosal, intramural, or subserosal. Fibroids attached to the uterus by a stalk are referred to as pedunculated.

It is estimated that 20 to 50 percent of women of reproductive age have fibroids, although not all are diagnosed. In more than 99 percent of fibroid cases, the tumors are benign; they are not associated with cancer and do not increase a woman's risk for uterine cancer. For reasons not yet understood, they tend to form during a woman's late thirties and early forties, and then shrink after menopause. This would seem to suggest that estrogen is involved in the process. However, while all women produce estrogen, only some develop fibroid tumors. The presence of fibroid tumors does seem to be genetically linked (they are known to run in families). African-American women are over two to five times more likely to develop fibroids than women of other ethnic backgrounds.

Most women who have fibroid tumors never even know it, unless they are discovered during the course of a routine pelvic examination. In roughly half of all cases, fibroid tumors cause no symptoms at all. In other cases, however, these growths can cause abnormally heavy and frequent menstrual periods. Other possible signs and symptoms include anemia, bleeding between periods, fatigue and weakness as a result of blood loss, increased vaginal discharge, and painful sexual intercourse or bleeding after intercourse.

Depending upon their precise location, fibroids can cause pain in the legs, back, and/or pelvis, and exert pressure upon the bowels or the bladder, or even block the urethra and create a kidney obstruction.

NUTRIENTS

SUPPLEMENT	SUGGESTED DOSAGE	COMMENTS
Coenzyme Q$_{10}$	30 mg daily.	Promotes immune function and tissue oxygenation.
Floradix Iron + Herbs from Salus Haus	As directed on label. Do not take at the same time as vitamin E; iron depletes vitamin E in the body.	To supply iron in easily assimilable natural formula. Women with heavy menstrual flow as a result of fibroids are often anemic.
Garlic (Kyolic from Wakunaga)	As directed on label.	Powerful immune stimulant and antioxidant. Inhibits tumor growth.
L-arginine	500 mg daily, on an empty stomach. Take with water or juice. Do not take with milk. Take with 50 mg vitamin B$_6$ and 100 mg vitamin C for better absorption.	Enhances immune function and may retard tumor growth. (*See* AMINO ACIDS in Part One.)
and L-lysine	500 mg daily, on an empty stomach.	Needed to balance with arginine.
Maitake extract and/or shiitake extract	As directed on label. As directed on label.	To strengthen the body and improve overall health; have potent immunostimulant properties that inhibit tumor growth.
Multivitamin and mineral complex	As directed on label.	All nutrients are necessary in balance.
Vitamin A with mixed carotenoids	25,000 IU daily. If you are pregnant, do not exceed 10,000 IU daily.	Important in immune function and to promote tissue repair. Use emulsion form for easier assimilation and greater safety at higher doses.
Vitamin C with bioflavonoids	3,000–10,000 mg daily, in divided doses.	Promotes immune function and acts as an antioxidant.
Zinc plus copper	30–80 mg daily. Do not exceed a total of 100 mg daily from all supplements. 3 mg daily.	Needed for a healthy immune system. Needed to balance with zinc.

Herbs

❑ Dandelion root, milk thistle, scutellaria (also known as Chinese skullcap) root, and turmeric rhizome are all powerful antioxidants that support the liver while promoting the elimination of toxins.

❑ Green tea is a powerful antioxidant.

Caution: Green tea contains vitamin K, which can make anticoagulant medications less effective. Consult your health care professional if you are using them. The caffeine in green tea could cause insomnia, anxiety, upset stomach, nausea, or diarrhea.

❑ Red clover and burdock root both aid in cleansing the bloodstream.

Recommendations

❑ If you have unpleasant symptoms such as those outlined in this section, or if menstrual bleeding is so heavy that you saturate a sanitary pad or tampon more often than once an hour, consult your health care practitioner.

❏ If a fibroid is found, do not take oral contraceptives with a high estrogen content. High-estrogen birth control pills may stimulate the growth of fibroid tumors. Consider other forms of contraception, such as condoms and foam, a diaphragm, or a cervical cap.

Considerations

❏ Fibroids are almost never malignant, so treatment is not usually required as long as they remain relatively small and do not produce unpleasant symptoms.

❏ Women with fibroids may have higher levels of human growth hormone than other women.

❏ A woman's chance of developing fibroids may be decreased if she avoids the use of oral contraceptives.

❏ In the past, it was a matter of general practice to perform surgery to remove fibroids if they grew to a point that the uterus was enlarged to the same extent it would be in a twelfth-week pregnancy. Increasingly, however, physicians are becoming more reluctant to remove these tumors based solely upon the "twelve-week rule" unless they are causing medical problems for the patient. Since these tumors usually shrink with the onset of menopause, the problem may well take care of itself over time.

❏ In the past, the conventional treatment for uterine fibroids was removal of the uterus (hysterectomy). Today, an alternative to hysterectomy is a procedure known as myomectomy. This operation removes the fibroids, but leaves the uterus intact. This is an attractive alternative for a woman who wishes to bear children in the future, although it can be performed on any woman, regardless of age. Myomectomy is a more exacting surgery and places greater demands on the woman during recovery. There is also a slightly higher chance of complications with myomectomy than with hysterectomy, and the results are not always permanent. There is a good chance that new tumors will form later, although they probably will not grow as large as the original fibroid tumors. If fibroids recur and cause symptoms, a repeat myomectomy can be performed.

❏ Laparoscopic myolysis is a procedure that may be recommended for the treatment of larger fibroids. In this technique, the surgeon uses a laser or electric current, delivered by means of special needles, to burn the fibroid and shrink it. This can be done on an outpatient basis.

❏ Uterine fibroid embolization (UFE) is a technique that involves making a tiny incision in the groin and placing a catheter into the femoral artery. The catheter is then guided up into the blood vessels that supply the fibroid. The idea is to cut off the blood supply to the fibroid, thus making it shrink. This technique is relatively new. Certain risks and side effects should be discussed with your doctor if you are considering this path.

❏ Hysteroscopic resection can be used to remove uterine fibroids. In this procedure, a surgical instrument is inserted though the vagina into the uterus, the fibroids are removed vaginally, and the remaining area is cauterized. This can be performed on an outpatient basis.

❏ Any woman pondering a hysterectomy should give the matter close and careful consideration, and should ask her physician about less radical ways to treat fibroids. There are alternative procedures that may be suitable for some women. More than 600,000 hysterectomies are performed each year in the United States, many of them unnecessary. (See HYSTERECTOMY-RELATED PROBLEMS in Part Two.)

FIBROMYALGIA SYNDROME

Fibromyalgia syndrome (FMS) is a rheumatic disorder characterized by chronic achy muscular pain that has no obvious physical cause. It most commonly affects the lower back, the neck, the shoulders, the back of the head, the upper chest, and/or the thighs, although any area or areas of the body may be involved. The pain is usually described as burning, throbbing, shooting, and stabbing. The pain and stiffness are often greater in the morning than at other times of day, and may be accompanied by chronic headaches, strange sensations in the skin, insomnia, irritable bowel syndrome, and temporomandibular joint syndrome (TMJ). Other symptoms often experienced by people with fibromyalgia include premenstrual syndrome, painful periods, anxiety, palpitations, memory impairment, irritable bladder, skin sensitivities, dry eyes and mouth, a need for frequent changes in eyeglass prescription, dizziness, and impaired coordination. Such activities as lifting and climbing stairs are often very difficult and painful. Depression often accompanies this disorder, and stress may trigger the development of problems similar to those associated with cardiovascular disease and adrenal gland disorders.

Because the immune system is typically compromised in this disorder, opportunistic viral and bacterial infections are common as well.

The most distinctive feature of fibromyalgia, one that differentiates it from similar conditions, is the existence of certain "tender points"—eighteen specific spots where the muscles are abnormally tender to the touch. The eighteen points tend to cluster around the neck, shoulders, chest, knees, elbow region, and hips, and include the following:

• Around the lower vertebrae of the neck.

• At the insertion of the second rib.

• Around the upper part of the thigh bone.

• In the middle of the knee joint.

• In muscles connected to the base of the skull.

• In muscles of the neck and upper back.

• In muscles of the mid-back.

- On the side of the elbow.
- In the upper and outer muscles of the buttocks.

There are approximately 5 million people known to be suffering from FMS in the United States. However, the real number of cases is probably much higher, as this condition is often misdiagnosed. Fibromyalgia manifests itself in similar ways to chronic fatigue syndrome (CFS), chemical sensitivities, rheumatoid arthritis, and chronic myofascial pain (shortened muscle fiber syndrome). As a result, it often takes a long time for a proper diagnosis to be made. In the past, FMS was known as fibrositis or fibromyositis, but both of these terms are now considered inappropriate because they imply inflammation of some sort (the suffix -itis is medical terminology for "inflammation") and inflammation is not a major factor in fibromyalgia.

Most people with fibromyalgia also have an associated sleep disorder known as alpha-EEG anomaly. In this disorder, the individual's deep sleep periods are interrupted by bouts of waking-type brain activity, resulting in poor sleep. Some people with fibromyalgia are plagued by other sleep disorders, such as sleep apnea, restless leg syndrome, bruxism, and sleep myoclonus (a sudden rapid contraction of a muscle or a group of muscles during sleep or as one is falling asleep). Not surprisingly, given all these sleep difficulties, people with fibromyalgia often suffer from chronic fatigue that can range from mild to incapacitating.

Other disorders common in people with fibromyalgia include the following:

- Chemical and/or food allergies.
- Dizziness and loss of balance.
- Extreme fatigue.
- Headaches.
- Irritable bowel syndrome (diarrhea and/or constipation, often alternating).
- Jaw pain.
- Memory loss and difficulty in concentrating.
- Menstrual pain.
- Sensitivity to bright lights or loud noises.
- Sensitivity to dairy products.
- Skin sensitivities.
- Stiffness in the morning and, often, when walking.

Fibromyalgia is much more common in females than in males, and most often begins in young adulthood. For unknown reasons, between 80 and 90 percent of those diagnosed with fibromyalgia are women. In most cases, symptoms come on gradually and slowly increase in intensity. They can be triggered (or made worse) by a number of different factors, including overexertion, stress, lack of exercise, anxiety, depression, lack of sleep, grief, trauma, extremes of temperature and/or humidity, and infectious illness. In the majority of cases, symptoms are severe enough to interfere with normal daily activities; a significant number of people with fibromyalgia are actually disabled by the condition.

The course of the disorder is unpredictable. Some cases clear up on their own, some become chronic, and some go through cycles of flare-ups alternating with periods of apparent remission.

The cause or causes of fibromyalgia are not known, and there are no tests that can diagnose FMS with complete certainty. It is thought by some that the disorder, which was only recognized as such in 1990, is caused by a disruption in the brain's ability to process pain. Some evidence also points to a problem with the immune system. Certain immunologic abnormalities are common among people with fibromyalgia. Their significance and relationship to the syndrome are, however, not understood. A disturbance in brain chemistry may also be involved; many people who develop fibromyalgia have a history of clinical depression. Some research has found FMS is more likely to occur in people who have a history of sexual abuse, domestic violence, and even alcoholism. Other possible causes that have been proposed include infection with the Epstein-Barr virus (EBV), the virus that causes infectious mononucleosis, or with the fungus *Candida albicans;* chronic mercury poisoning from amalgam dental fillings; anemia; parasites; hypoglycemia; and hypothyroidism. Some experts believe that fibromyalgia may be related to chronic fatigue syndrome (CFS), which causes similar symptoms, except that in fibromyalgia, muscle pain predominates over fatigue, whereas in CFS, fatigue predominates over pain. FMS has even been misdiagnosed as multiple sclerosis or Parkinson's disease.

Because malabsorption problems are common in people with this disorder, it is best to use sublingual vitamins and other supplements because they are more easily absorbed than tablets or capsules.

NUTRIENTS

SUPPLEMENT	SUGGESTED DOSAGE	COMMENTS
Essential		
Acidophilus (Kyo-Dophilus from Wakunaga) or bifidis (Bifido Factor from Natren)	As directed on label. As directed on label.	Candida infection is common in people with fibromyalgia. Probiotics replace "friendly" bacteria destroyed by candida. Use a nondairy formula.
Coenzyme Q$_{10}$ plus Coenzyme A from Coenzyme-A Technologies	75 mg daily. As directed on label.	Improves oxygenation of tissues, enhances the effectiveness of the immune system, and protects the heart. Works with coenzyme Q$_{10}$ to increase energy supply to the cells.
Lecithin	As directed on label, with meals.	Promotes energy, enhances immunity, aids in brain function, and improves circulation.

Supplement	Suggested Dosage	Comments
Malic acid and magnesium	As directed on label.	Involved in energy production in many cells of the body, including the muscle cells. Needed for sugar metabolism.
Manganese	5 mg daily. Take separately from calcium.	Influences the metabolic rate by its involvement in the pituitary hypothalamic-thyroid axis.
Nicotinamide adenine dinucleotide (NADH) (Enada)	10–15 mg first thing in the morning, on an empty stomach.	Increases level of energy.
Proteolytic enzymes or Inf-zyme Forte from American Biologics	As directed on label, 6 times daily, with meals, between meals, and at bedtime.	Reduces inflammation and improves absorption of foods, especially protein, which is needed for tissue repair.
Vitamin A with mixed carotenoids plus vitamin E or ACES + Zn from Carlson Labs	25,000 IU daily for 1 month, then slowly reduce to 10,000 IU daily. If you are pregnant, do not exceed 10,000 IU daily. 200 IU daily. As directed on label.	Powerful free radical scavengers that protect the body's cells and enhance immune function. Use emulsion forms for easier assimilation. Use d-alpha-tocopherol form. Contains vitamins A, C, and E plus the minerals selenium and zinc, to protect immune function.
Vitamin C with bioflavonoids	5,000–10,000 mg daily.	Has a powerful antiviral effect and increases the body's energy level. Use a buffered form.

Very Important

Supplement	Suggested Dosage	Comments
Dimethylglycine (DMG) (Aangamik DMG from FoodScience of Vermont)	50 mg 3 times daily.	Enhances oxygen utilization by the muscles and destroys free radicals that can damage cells.
5-Hydroxy L-tryptophan (5-HTP)	50 mg daily for 1 week, then increase to 100 mg daily.	Enhances synthesis of serotonin in the brain. Excellent for pain relief. Caution: Do not use if you take an MAO inhibitor, commonly prescribed for depression.
Free form amino acid (Amino Balance from Anabol Naturals or Amino Blend from Carlson Labs)	As directed on label.	To supply protein essential for repair and rebuilding of muscle tissue and for proper brain function. Use a formula containing all the essential amino acids.
Garlic (Kyolic from Wakunaga) plus Kyo-Green from Wakunaga	2 capsules 3 times daily, with meals. As directed on label.	Promotes immune function and increases energy. Also destroys common parasites. To improve digestion and cleanse the bloodstream.
Grape seed extract or Pycnogenol	As directed on label. As directed on label.	Powerful antioxidants that protect the muscles from free radical damage and enhance immunity.
Methylsulfonyl-methane (MSM)	As directed on label.	Provides support for tendons, ligaments, and muscles. Note: Because this supplement contains sulfur, you may notice an odor to your urine.
Methylsulfonyl-methane (MSM) cream	As directed on label.	Relieves pain.

Supplement	Suggested Dosage	Comments
S-Adenosylmethio-nine (SAMe)	As directed on label.	Aids in relief of stress and depression, eases pain, and produces antioxidant effects that can improve the health of your liver. Caution: Do not use if you have bipolar mood disorder or take prescription antidepressants. Do not give to a child under twelve.
Vitamin B complex injections plus extra vitamin B$_6$ (pyridoxine) and vitamin B$_{12}$ plus raw liver extract or vitamin B complex	2 cc twice weekly for 1 month or as prescribed by physician. ¼ cc twice weekly for 1 month or as prescribed by physician. 1 cc twice weekly for 1 month or as prescribed by physician. 2 cc twice weekly for 1 month or as prescribed by physician. 100 mg of each major B vitamin 3 times daily, with meals (amounts of individual vitamins in a complex will vary).	Essential for increased energy and normal brain function. Injections (under doctor's supervision) are best. All injectables can be combined in a single syringe. A source of B vitamins and iron. Caution: Do not take a supplement containing iron unless prescribed by your physician. If injections are not available, or once the course of injections has been completed, use a sublingual form of all the B vitamins listed.

Important

Supplement	Suggested Dosage	Comments
Calcium and magnesium and vitamin D	2,000 mg daily. 1,000 mg daily. 400 IU daily.	Needed for proper functioning of all muscles, including the heart; relieves muscle spasms and pain. Deficiencies are common in people with this disorder.
Chromium	200–400 mcg daily.	To help balance blood sugar levels and aid in preventing night sweats.
Creatine	As directed on label. Do not take with fruit juices, as this combination produces creatinine, which is difficult for the kidneys to process.	To combat muscle depletion. Should be used in conjunction with a balanced, nutritious diet.
DL-phenylalanine (DLPA)	500 mg daily every other week.	Can be very effective for controlling pain. Also increases mental alertness. Caution: Do not take this supplement if you are pregnant or nursing, or suffer from panic attacks, diabetes, high blood pressure, or PKU.
Essential fatty acids (black currant seed oil, flaxseed oil, Kyolic-EPA from Wakunaga, or primrose oil)	As directed on label 3 times daily, with meals.	Protects against cell damage. Helps to reduce pain and fatigue.
Fibroplex from Metagenics	As directed on label.	A formula containing vitamins B$_1$ and B$_6$ plus magnesium, manganese, and malic acid.
Fibro-X from Olympian Labs	As directed on label.	To relieve pain. Contains many nutrients listed in this table, plus shark cartilage.

Gamma-amino-butyric acid (GABA)	As directed on label.	For proper control of brain function and to control anxiety.
Kelp	As directed on label.	Contains minerals that support the thyroid.
L-leucine plus L-isoleucine and L-valine	500 mg each daily, on an empty stomach. Take with water or juice. Do not take with milk. Take with 50 mg vitamin B₆ and 100 mg vitamin C for better absorption.	These amino acids are found primarily in muscle tissue. They are available in combination formulas. (*See* AMINO ACIDS in Part One.)
plus L-carnitine	As directed on label.	Increases energy.
L-tyrosine	500–1,000 mg daily, at bedtime.	Helps to relieve depression and aids in relaxing the muscles. *Caution:* Do not take this supplement if you are taking an MAO inhibitor drug.
Melatonin	As directed on label, 1–2 hours or less before bedtime.	Promotes sound sleep. A sustained-release formula is best. Take a sublingual form during the night if you wake up and cannot go back to sleep.
Multivitamin and mineral complex plus carotenoid complex (Advanced Carotenoid Complex from Solgar)	As directed on label. 15,000 IU daily.	All nutrients are necessary in balance. Use a high-potency hypoallergenic formula.
Ocu-Care from Nature's Plus	As directed on label.	Contains essential nutrients to protect and nourish the eyes.
Raw thymus glandular and raw spleen glandular plus multiglandular complex	As directed on label. As directed on label. As directed on label.	To boost the immune system. (*See* GLANDULAR THERAPY in Part Three.)
Reishi extract	As directed on label.	A mushroom extract that helps the body deal with stress and increases energy levels.
Taurine	500 mg daily, on an empty stomach.	An important antioxidant and immune system regulator necessary for white blood cell activation and neurological function.
Vanadyl sulfate	As directed on label.	Protects the muscles and reduces overall body fatigue.

Herbs

❑ Astragalus and echinacea enhance immune function.

Cautions: Do not take astragalus in the presence of a fever. Do not take echinacea for longer than three months. It should not be used by people who are allergic to ragweed.

❑ Black walnut and garlic aid in removing parasites.

❑ Boswellia is excellent for morning stiffness and joint pain.

❑ Teas brewed from burdock root, dandelion, and red clover promote healing by cleansing the bloodstream and enhancing immune function. Combine or alternate these herbal teas, and drink 4 to 6 cups daily.

❑ Calendula or rosemary oil (or a combination of the two), diluted with an equal amount of water or vegetable oil and massaged into the skin, helps to relieve pain.

❑ Topical applications of cayenne (capsicum) powder mixed with wintergreen oil can help relieve muscle pain. Cayenne contains capsaicin, a substance that appears to inhibit the release of neurotransmitters responsible for communicating pain sensations. Use 1 part cayenne powder to 3 parts wintergreen oil. Cayenne can also be taken orally, in capsule form.

❑ Put 4 to 6 ounces of ginger powder into a moderately hot bath. This will induce sweating and help remove toxins from the body. Drinking hot ginger tea will have the same effect.

❑ Ginkgo biloba improves circulation and brain function.

Caution: Do not take ginkgo biloba if you have a bleeding disorder, or are scheduled for surgery or a dental procedure.

❑ Kava kava decreases anxiety and elevates the mood.

Caution: Kava kava can cause drowsiness. It is not recommended for pregnant women or nursing mothers, and it should not be taken together with other substances that act on the central nervous system, such as alcohol, barbiturates, antidepressants, and antipsychotic drugs.

❑ Licorice root supports the glandular system, especially the adrenal glands.

Caution: Licorice root should not be used during pregnancy or nursing. It should not be used by persons with diabetes, glaucoma, heart disease, high blood pressure, or a history of stroke.

❑ Milk thistle protects the liver.

❑ Pau d'arco, taken in tea or tablet form, is good for treating candida infection.

❑ Skullcap and valerian root improve sleep.

Recommendations

❑ Eat a well-balanced diet of 50 percent raw foods and fresh "live" juices. The diet should consist mostly of vegetables, fruits, whole grains (primarily millet and brown rice), raw nuts and seeds, soy products, skinless turkey or chicken, and deepwater fish. These quality foods supply nutrients that renew energy and build immunity.

❑ Include pomegranates and pomegranate juice in your diet. They have anti-inflammatory and antioxidant properties.

❑ Eat four to five small meals daily to keep a steady supply of protein and carbohydrates available for proper muscle function. If the body does not have enough fuel for energy, it will rob the muscles of essential nutrients, causing muscle wasting and pain.

❏ Drink plenty of liquids to help flush out toxins. The best choices are steam-distilled water and herbal teas. Fresh vegetable juices supply necessary vitamins and minerals.

❏ Limit your consumption of green peppers, eggplant, tomatoes, and white potatoes. These foods contain solanine, which interferes with enzymes in the muscles, and may cause pain and discomfort.

❏ Do not eat meat, dairy products, or any other foods that are high in saturated fats. Saturated fats raise cholesterol levels and interfere with circulation. Also avoid fried foods, processed foods, shellfish, and white flour products such as bread and pasta. Make up your calcium, magnesium, and vitamin D needs from supplements.

❏ In one study there seemed to be no benefit from eating a vegetarian diet for those with fibromyalgia. Still, another study showed that a raw, pure vegetarian diet—consisting mainly of raw fruits, salads, carrot juice, tubers, grain products, nuts, seeds, and a dehydrated barley grass juice product—improved quality of life, reduced pain, and improved range of motion and flexibility in people with the disease.

❏ Do not consume any caffeine, alcohol, or sugar. Eating sugar in any form—including fructose and honey—promotes fatigue, increases pain, and disturbs sleep. If these substances have been a regular part of your diet, your symptoms may actually get worse for a short period as a result of the "withdrawal" effect, but after that, you should experience a noticeable improvement in your condition.

❏ Avoid wheat and brewer's yeast until your symptoms improve.

Caution: Brewer's yeast can cause an allergic reaction in some individuals. Start with a small amount at first, and discontinue use if any allergic symptoms occur.

❏ Use wheatgrass retention enemas to detoxify the system. To make the enema, add 1 ounce of wheatgrass juice to 1 cup of warm water. If fresh wheatgrass is not available, powdered Sweet Wheat from Sweet Wheat, Inc., is a good substitute. Use this treatment every other day for two weeks. (*See* ENEMAS in Part Three.)

❏ Maintain a regular program of moderate exercise. A daily walk followed by some gentle stretching exercises is good. If you have been sedentary before, start slowly and be careful not to overexert yourself; this can aggravate symptoms. Keep in mind that what you need is some amount of daily exercise, not a strenuous workout two or three times a week. Once your body is accustomed to regular exercise, symptoms are likely to improve. Moderate exercise and stretching help to keep muscles flexible and prevent joints from stiffening up.

Caution: If you are thirty-five or older and/or have been sedentary for some time, consult with your health care provider before beginning an exercise program.

❏ Be sure to give your body sufficient rest. Set aside at least eight hours for sleep each night.

❏ Take a hot shower or a bath upon arising to stimulate circulation and help relieve morning stiffness. Or alternate between hot water and cold water while showering. Recent studies have shown cold showers to be beneficial for relieving the pain of fibromyalgia. Hot baths help to relax the muscles.

❏ Consider trying massage therapy, which can help to relax muscles and reduce stiffness of the joints.

❏ Take chlorophyll in tablet form or in "green drinks" such as Kyo-Green from Wakunaga of America. Spiru-tein from Nature's Plus is a good protein drink to use between meals to aid in maintaining energy levels and to reduce muscle pain. Chlorella pyrenoidosa, a unicellular freshwater green algae rich in protein, vitamins, and minerals, was shown to help with the management of symptoms for patients with fibromyalgia.

❏ Have your doctor check your thyroid function. Symptoms of hypothyroidism can mimic those of FMS.

Considerations

❏ Chronic pain sufferers, especially those with fibromyalgia and chronic fatigue syndrome, tend to be deficient in magnesium.

❏ Common painkillers such as aspirin, acetaminophen, and ibuprofen are not usually effective at relieving the pain of fibromyalgia. Other approaches, including attention to diet, exercise, and nutritional supplementation, are more likely to be of benefit.

Caution: If you are thirty-five or older and/or have been sedentary for some time, consult with your health care provider before beginning an exercise program.

❏ There are two FDA-approved treatments for fibromyalgia—Lyrica and Savella. Sevella is a selective serotonin and norepinephrine reuptake inhibitor (SNRI). It was shown to reduce pain, fatigue, and improve cognition. In addition, two studies indicate that a majority of people who suffer from the disorder can find relief by taking duloxetine (Cymbalta), an antidepressant drug. A report on the latest study of the drug was reported in the medical journal *Arthritis and Rheumatism.* Duloxetine may be effective because it works by boosting levels of two neurotransmitters that play a role in pain processing. New drugs such as sodium oxybate are under study.

❏ Many different disorders can cause symptoms similar to those of fibromyalgia, including anemia, depression, hepatitis, and Lyme disease, among others. Anyone who experiences muscular pain and/or fatigue that persists for longer than a week or two should consult a health care professional. There may be an underlying medical disorder that requires treatment.

❏ Recent research points to the possible involvement of chemical and/or food sensitivities in fibromyalgia, chronic fatigue syndrome, and the pain associated with these disorders. This would hardly be surprising, as humans have been exposed to more chemicals in the last fifty years than in all the rest of our history combined.

❑ Studies are being conducted on the possible role of a genetic defect that interferes with the formation of adenosine triphosphate (ATP, the source of cellular energy) in this disorder.

❑ Some experts suggest that people with fibromyalgia should avoid salt-free diets.

❑ Plant sterols and sterolins (plant fats that are present in fruits, vegetables, seeds, and nuts) stimulate the immune system, thus helping the body fight off infection.

❑ Because malabsorption problems are common in this disorder, all nutrients are needed in greater than normal amounts, and a proper diet is essential. Colon cleansing is recommended to rid the gastrointestinal tract of mucus and debris, and to improve nutrient absorption. (*See* COLON CLEANSING in Part Three.)

❑ A vegetarian, Mediterranean-type diet and intermittent fasting were tested for their effect on changing bowel bacteria and immune function; neither therapy affected the flora or serum IgA levels.

❑ Many doctors prescribe low-dose antidepressants for fibromyalgia. These drugs can be beneficial in some cases, but can also cause a number of side effects, such as drowsiness. Other medical treatments that may or may not be of help to any given individual include muscle relaxants and/or local anesthetic sprays or injections for relief of pain. Antianxiety drugs are sometimes prescribed as well. These drugs can cause a loss of equilibrium.

❑ Physical therapy, relaxation techniques, exercise therapy, massage therapy, deep heat therapy, and biofeedback are all helpful in some cases. Massage therapy is particularly beneficial for improved muscle function and pain relief. Acupuncture has also been shown to be effective at reducing pain and improving quality of life. Neither Reiki nor touch therapy, frequently used by patients with fibromyalgia, were shown to improve symptoms of the condition. If you are diagnosed with fibromyalgia, it is wise to seek out a health care practitioner who has specific experience in the management and treatment of this condition.

Caution: If you are thirty-five or older and/or have been sedentary for some time, consult with your health care provider before beginning an exercise program.

❑ In one study, children (aged eight to eighteen years) who underwent an aerobic exercise program experienced improved physical function, fewer fibromyalgia symptoms, better quality of life, and less pain. Another group participated in qi gong, which did not show these improvements.

❑ An eight-month supervised program led to both physical and mental improvements. Women who exercised in warm water experienced significant improvements in physical function, and had less pain, stiffness, and anxiety. In another study, older women who were postmenopausal

had reduced fatigue and increased strength by undergoing an exercise program that incorporated weights, strength-training equipment, and speed walking.

Caution: If you are thirty-five or older and/or have been sedentary for some time, consult with your health care provider before beginning an exercise program.

❑ Food allergies can exacerbate the discomfort of many disorders. (*See* ALLERGIES in Part Two.)

❑ *See* CHRONIC FATIGUE SYNDROME and DEPRESSION in Part Two. *See also* PAIN CONTROL in Part Three.

❑ For names and addresses of organizations that can provide further information about fibromyalgia, *see* Health and Medical Organizations in the Appendix.

FLU

See influenza.

FOODBORNE/WATERBORNE ILLNESS

Food- or waterborne illness occurs when a person consumes substances containing harmful toxins, chemicals, parasites, or microorganisms (usually bacteria). Foodborne illness, commonly referred to as food poisoning, causes some 76 million cases of illness and 5,000 deaths every year in the United States according to the U.S. Centers for Disease Control and Prevention (CDC). The actual number of cases is almost certainly well above any reported number, because people often mistake the symptoms of food poisoning for a simple upset stomach.

There are different types of food poisoning, depending on the agent that causes it. (For a quick summary of some of these, *see* Types of Food Poisoning on page 443.)

One type is salmonellosis, or *Salmonella* infection. *Salmonella* bacteria are part of the natural intestinal flora of many animals. They are easily transmitted through the food supply, the hands of food preparers, and the surfaces of objects such as knives and tabletops. Salmonellosis is typically associated with eggs.

External contamination from fecal matter, once a common source of salmonellosis, has almost been eliminated as a cause due to more stringent testing and inspection regimens implemented in the 1970s. The principal danger now comes from eggs because *Salmonella enteritidis*, the organism responsible for the majority of *Salmonella* infections, is now present in the ovaries of a significant percentage of egg-producing hens in the United States, and it contaminates the eggs before the shells form. Thus, eggs do not need to be cracked or unclean on the outside to be contaminated.

Foods made from raw eggs, including Caesar salad dressing, eggnog, hollandaise sauce, and ice cream, have also been found to contain these bacteria. Salmonellosis as a result of the consumption of raw clams, oysters, and sushi made from raw fish has also been reported. Although this does not occur as often as *Salmonella* infection from fresh produce, eggs, meat, and poultry, it does happen.

Symptoms of *Salmonella* infection can range from mild abdominal pain to severe diarrhea and dehydration to typhoid-like fever. Symptoms usually develop within eight to thirty-six hours of eating contaminated foods. Diarrhea is often the first sign. *Salmonella* can also weaken the immune system and cause kidney and cardiovascular damage as well as arthritis.

Outbreaks of salmonellosis occur primarily in the warmer months. Most cases are the result of the consumption of contaminated foods, primarily chicken, eggs, beef, and pork products. People who eat raw or incompletely cooked meats are at greater risk of developing the disorder.

Cooks who first handle raw meat or poultry and then handle other foods, without washing their hands in between, endanger others; cooks who lick their hands or fingers after handling raw meat or poultry put themselves at risk of *Salmonella* infection. People taking antibiotics are also at greater risk.

Salmonella infections usually resolve in five to seven days and often do not require treatment other than oral fluids. Persons with severe diarrhea may require rehydration with intravenous fluids. Antibiotics, such as ampicillin, trimethoprim-sulfamethoxazole, or ciprofloxacin, are not usually necessary unless the infection spreads from the intestines. Some *Salmonella* bacteria have become resistant to antibiotics, largely as a result of the use of antibiotics to promote the growth of food animals. Antibiotics can also promote infection by destroying good, competing bacteria and permitting the growth of bacteria that are antibiotic-resistant. A Taiwanese strain of *Salmonella,* called the "super *Salmonella*" by some, is completely resistant to all known antimicrobials.

Staphylococcus aureus is another cause of foodborne illness. *Staphylococcus* (staph) infection can manifest itself in a variety of ways, from food poisoning to skin infections to septicemia (blood infection). In severe cases, it can be life-threatening. This microorganism is commonly found in the nose and throat, but if a food product becomes contaminated with the bacteria (by being sneezed or coughed on, for example), the bacteria can grow and produce an enterotoxin, a toxin that specifically targets the cells of the intestines.

It is this toxin, rather than the bacteria itself, that causes the food poisoning. Symptoms include diarrhea, nausea, vomiting, abdominal cramps, and prostration, usually beginning from two to eight hours after consumption of the contaminated food. Staphylococcal toxin is found most often in meat, poultry, egg products, tuna, potato and macaroni salads, and cream-filled pastries.

The bacterium *Clostridium botulinum,* which commonly inhabits the soil in the form of harmless spores, can cause a particularly dangerous type of food poisoning. Of the various types of food poisoning, botulism is among the most severe. It affects the central nervous system. As with *Staph-*

ylococcus, it is not the bacteria but rather nerve toxins produced by the bacteria that cause the poisoning—and like staph, the bacteria can infect surface wounds. Woundborne botulism is not common, but it can occur if an open sore becomes infected with the botulism bacteria. People who use intravenous drugs can also be infected by using dirty or shared needles. Infant botulism is a type of the disorder that usually affects children under twelve months of age. It can occur if a young child ingests anything contaminated by botulism spores. This can include soil, cistern water, dust, and even some foods, such as honey.

The toxins produced by *C. botulinum* block the transmission of impulses from nerves to muscles, thus paralyzing the muscles. The paralysis often begins with the muscles that are responsible for eye movement, swallowing, and speech, and progresses to those in the torso and the extremities. Early symptoms of botulism include extreme weakness, double vision, droopy eyelids, and trouble swallowing. These symptoms typically appear twelve to forty-eight hours after ingestion of the contaminated food. Eventually, muscle weakness affecting the entire body, including the muscles required for breathing, can result. Paralysis and death may occur in severe cases.

There are seven recognized types of botulin bacteria, designated A, B, C, D, E, F, and G. The A, B, E, and F varieties cause human botulism. Types C and D are isolated to animals. Type G has been found in soil samples in Argentina, but no cases of illness involving type G have yet been reported. A total of about 145 cases of botulism are reported each year. Of these, 65 percent are infant botulism, 15 percent are foodborne botulism, and 20 percent are woundborne botulism.

Botulin toxin has been found in home-canned foods with a low acidity level, such as asparagus, beets, corn, and green beans. Less common sources include chopped garlic in oil, tomatoes, baked potatoes that have been improperly handled and then kept in aluminum foil, and home-canned or fermented fish. A bulging lid or cracked jar can be a sign that the food within is contaminated, but botulism can occur even if a food container shows no signs of damage. Keeping certain foods at room temperature for prolonged periods also can be a problem. In one reported case, a restaurant allowed a large batch of sautéed onions to be kept out throughout the day, instead of keeping them refrigerated, and small amounts were used as needed. Several people became very ill from botulin toxin in the onions.

Freezing, drying, and treatment with chemicals such as sodium nitrite prevent *C. botulinum* spores from growing and producing toxins. Although it does not kill the spores themselves, heating food to a temperature of at least 176°F for thirty minutes prevents food poisoning by destroying the lethal toxins.

Another microorganism that can cause food poisoning is *Campylobacter jejuni.* With this type of food poisoning, people tend not to associate the illness with food because it takes three to five days for the bacteria to produce symptoms, which include abdominal cramps, diarrhea, fever, and possibly blood in the stool. *C. jejuni* can be present in the intestinal tracts of apparently healthy cattle, sheep, chickens, turkeys, dogs, and cats, and can be contracted by eating or drinking food or water that has somehow become contaminated by the feces of an infected person or animal.

Chickens, turkeys, and waterfowl are the most common carriers. Fortunately, heat destroys these bacteria, so it is possible to avoid this type of food poisoning by eating meat only if has been cooked thoroughly.

Another type of bacteria that can cause food poisoning is *Clostridium perfringens,* sometimes called the "food service germ." It is one of the most common causes of foodborne illness. This microorganism thrives in previously cooked food that is kept for a long time at room temperature. Meat products and gravy are the most likely sources of the toxin. As foods cool, the bacteria multiply, forming spores and generating toxins. The toxins are often heat resistant. The symptoms of *C. perfringens* poisoning usually are limited to mild nausea and vomiting that last a day or less, but that can be a very serious problem for older adults or people with Crohn's disease or HIV.

Not all foodborne illness is the result of bacterial contamination. *Giardia lamblia* is a protozoan (single-celled parasitic microorganism) that infects the small intestine. Giardiasis is associated with the consumption of contaminated water. It can also be transmitted to raw foods that have grown in contaminated water. Cool, moist environments are conducive to the growth of this microorganism. Symptoms generally occur within one to three weeks of infection and include diarrhea, constipation, abdominal pain, flatulence, loss of appetite, nausea, and vomiting.

Norwalk virus is a very common virus that can be transmitted in food and water, and causes many cases of nausea, fever, headache, stomachache, vomiting, and diarrhea in both children and adults. The Norwalk virus is getting a reputation as the "cruise ship virus" because of the great number of recent shipboard outbreaks. The symptoms usually start one or two days after infection and last from one to ten days.

Hepatitis A and E viruses can be transmitted by direct contact with fecal matter or with foods contaminated by fecal matter. They can also be transmitted by contaminated water.

Trichinella spiralis is a parasitic roundworm that causes the infection known as trichinosis. It is most often the result of eating raw or improperly cooked or processed pork or pork products (ham and sausage) and wild game.

Escherichia coli (*E. coli*) is a type of bacteria naturally found in the intestines of humans and some animals, where it actually serves a useful function—it helps to suppress harmful bacteria and aid in the absorption of vitamins. But sometimes, under the right circumstances, *E. coli* can cause serious illness. The reason for the change from benign or friendly to pathogenic is not known. But this can be a very

serious illness, particularly for the very young, the elderly, and those with compromised immune systems. This bacteria has been found in meat, vegetables, and some unpasteurized juices and fruits. In 2006, a specific strain, 0157:H7, was found in spinach.

Scombroid poisoning (also called histamine poisoning) is a relatively rare type of food poisoning that can occur after the consumption of fish such as tuna, mackerel, mahi mahi, sardines, bluefish, and abalone. After a fish is caught, decomposition carried on by bacteria in the fish can trigger the production of high levels of a chemical called histamine. When the fish is eaten, in a matter of minutes the histamine can cause symptoms including facial flushing, nausea, vomiting, abdominal pain, and/or hives. Fortunately, symptoms usually subside in twenty-four hours. Vibriobacteria, which comprise a group of different species of bacteria that can cause food poisoning, are mostly found in raw or improperly cooked fish and shellfish.

Thanks to our food safety, labeling, and inspection laws, our supermarket shelves are stocked with a nearly endless variety of foods that must meet strict government standards. Yet the truth is that food poisoning remains a major problem in this country, and it strikes with a frequency that is both surprising and alarming. The CDC offers several reasons for this. First, food animals are now raised in very close, confined quarters, a situation that is conducive to the spread of bacteria such as *Salmonella.* At the same time, food processing is becoming more and more centralized, so a single ingredient that is tainted with a contaminant can eventually show up in a multitude of different products. The United States now also imports record amounts of food from overseas, often from developing countries where proper hygiene in food production may not be as reliable as it is in this country.

Then there is the matter of food preparation. An increasing number of Americans are simply unaware of the prevalence of potentially dangerous microorganisms in the food supply, and lack knowledge of basic techniques for handling, preparing, and storing food safely. Most cases of food poisoning are easily preventable, provided you know how (*see* Tips for Preventing Food Poisoning on page 444). Also, more and more Americans, rather than eating meals prepared at home, purchase ready-made food at restaurants and from takeout establishments. Younger workers, who have no experience with or education in the consequences of improper food handling and the diseases that can be transmitted, staff many of these establishments.

If you contract food- or waterborne illness, the following supplements should be helpful. Unless otherwise specified, the dosages recommended here are for adults. For children between the ages of twelve and seventeen, reduce the dose to three-quarters the recommended amount. For children between six and twelve, use one-half the recommended dose, and for children under the age of six, use one-quarter the recommended amount.

NUTRIENTS

SUPPLEMENT	SUGGESTED DOSAGE	COMMENTS
Very Important		
Charcoal tablets	5 tablets at first signs of illness and again 6 hours later. Take separately from other medications and supplements.	Removes toxic substances from the colon and bloodstream.
Garlic (Kyolic from Wakunaga)	2 capsules 3 times daily, with meals.	A powerful detoxifier that also destroys bacteria in the colon.
Potassium	99 mg daily.	To restore proper electrolyte balance.
Vitamin C with bioflavonoids	8,000 mg daily, in divided doses.	Detoxifies the body and aids in removing bacteria and toxins.
plus vitamin E	200 IU daily.	Reduces symptoms by enhancing immune function. Use d-alpha-tocopherol form.
Important		
Acidophilus (Kyo-Dophilus from Wakunaga)	As directed on label, twice daily, on an empty stomach.	Replaces essential intestinal bacteria. Use a nondairy source.
Aerobic 07 from Aerobic Life Industries	20 drops in a glass of water every 3 hours.	Destroys harmful bacteria such as *Salmonella*.
Fiber (ABC Aerobic Bulk Cleanse from Aerobic Life Industries or oat bran)	As directed on label 6 hours after second dose of charcoal tablets and twice daily thereafter. Take separately from other supplements and medications.	Removes bacteria that have attached themselves to the colon walls, preventing them from entering the bloodstream; this reduces symptoms and speeds recovery.
Kelp	1,000–1,500 mg daily.	Contains needed minerals to restore electrolytes.
L-cysteine and L-methionine and selenium and superoxide-dismutase (SOD)	500 mg each daily, on an empty stomach. Take with 50 mg each of vitamins B6 and C for better absorption. 200 mcg daily. If you are pregnant, do not exceed 40 mcg daily. 5,000 mg daily.	All of these nutrients are essential in immune function.
plus glutathione	500 mg daily.	A powerful antioxidant.

Herbs

❏ At the first sign of food poisoning, take a dropperful of alcohol-free goldenseal extract. Repeat this every four hours for one day. Goldenseal is a natural antibiotic that aids in destroying bacteria in the colon.

Caution: Do not take goldenseal internally on a daily basis for more than one week at a time. Do not use it during pregnancy or if you are breast-feeding, and use with caution if you are allergic to ragweed. If you have a history of cardiovascular disease, diabetes, or glaucoma, use it only under a doctor's supervision.

❏ Milk thistle and red clover aid in liver and blood cleansing.

❏ Use lobelia tea enemas to rid the body of the poison. (*See* ENEMAS in Part Three.) Adding a dropperful of alcohol-free goldenseal extract to the enema is beneficial as well.

Cautions: Lobelia is only to be taken under supervision of a health care professional as it is potentially toxic. People with high blood pressure, heart disease, liver disease, kidney disease, seizure disorders, or shortness of breath should not take lobelia. Pregnant and lactating women should avoid lobelia as well. Do not take goldenseal internally on a daily basis for more than one week at a time. Do not use it during pregnancy or if you are breast-feeding, and use with caution if you are allergic to ragweed. If you have a history of cardiovascular disease, diabetes, or glaucoma, use it only under a doctor's supervision.

Recommendations

❏ If you suspect food poisoning, call your regional poison control center immediately. Poison control centers can be reached twenty-four hours a day, and can provide you with up-to-date information regarding treatment. It is a good idea to keep the number of your local center posted by your telephone and/or entered into your telephone's automatic dialing program.

❏ At the first suspicion of food poisoning, protect your immune system by taking 6 charcoal tablets. These are available at most health food stores and should be kept on hand for emergencies. The agents in these tablets circulate through the bloodstream and help to neutralize and eliminate poisons. After six hours, take 6 more tablets. Consume a lot of quality water to aid in flushing toxins from the system.

❏ Use cleansing enemas to remove toxins from the colon and bloodstream. (*See* ENEMAS in Part Three.)

❏ If vomiting occurs, make sure that the individual does not choke. If vomiting does not subside in twenty-four hours, collect a sample of the vomit for analysis to aid in pinpointing the cause of the illness.

❏ If you have been vomiting and have diarrhea, you may become seriously dehydrated. Replace lost fluids and electrolytes with clean water or other liquids designed specifically for rehydration. If you become lethargic or dizzy, have diarrhea for more than three days, or a fever over 101.5°F, seek medical attention right away. You may require intravenous fluids and electrolytes.

❏ If you suspect that you have been poisoned by food from a public restaurant or other eating place, contact your local health department right away. It may be possible to save others from food poisoning.

❏ For some cases of poisoning, it may be desirable to induce vomiting to help expel the toxin that is the cause of the problem. Keep syrup of ipecac (available in drugstores) on hand for this purpose.

Types of Food Poisoning

There are many different types of food poisoning, some more common than others. The following is a summary of some of these, together with the relative incidence and typical symptoms of each.

Type	Relative Incidence	Symptoms	Time Between Exposure and Onset of Symptoms
Bacterial Origin			
Botulism	Rare.	Double vision; difficulty speaking, breathing, and swallowing; nausea, vomiting, and abdominal pain; diarrhea; muscular weakness.	12–48 hours, but may be as long as 8 days.
Campylobacter infection	Common.	Muscular pain, nausea, vomiting, fever, abdominal cramps.	2–10 days.
Clostridium perfringens poisoning	Common.	Diarrhea, abdominal cramps.	9–15 hours.
Escherichia coli (*E. coli*) poisoning	Common.	Diarrhea, abdominal cramps, vomiting.	1–7 days.
Listeriosis	Rare.	Flulike symptoms, including fever, chills; can cause spontaneous abortion or stillbirth; can cause severe illness in newborns and immune-depressed people. Spreads to the nervous system; stiff neck, confusion, and loss of balance can occur.	2–4 weeks.
Salmonellosis	Common.	Nausea, vomiting, diarrhea, abdominal cramps, fever, headache.	6–48 hours.
Staphylococcal food poisoning	Common.	Vomiting, diarrhea; occasionally weakness, dizziness.	30 minutes–8 hours.
Vibriobacteria	Not common, but occurs in occasional outbreaks during warmer months.	Diarrhea, fever, chills, cramps, headache, vomiting.	4–96 hours.
Parasitic Origin			
Giardiasis	Common.	Nausea, gas, abdominal pain and/or cramping, diarrhea; in severe cases, malabsorption problems and weight loss.	1–3 weeks.
Trichinosis	Rare.	Fever, edema of eyelids, muscle pain.	1–2 days.
Viral Origin			
Hepatitis A/ hepatitis E	Sporadic outbreaks.	Fever, nausea, lethargy, and pain in abdominal area. Hepatitis A infection may cause jaundice.	Hepatitis A: 10–50 days. Hepatitis E: 2–9 weeks.
Norwalk virus infection	Common.	Nausea, vomiting, diarrhea, headache.	1–2 days.
Rotavirus infection	Common.	Vomiting, diarrhea, possible temporary lactose intolerance.	1–3 days.
Toxin-caused scombroid poisoning	Uncommon.	Headache, dizziness, burning throat, hives, nausea, vomiting, abdominal pain.	5 minutes–1 hour.

Tips for Preventing Food Poisoning

Here are some fast, easy rules to help prevent food poisoning at home and while eating out:

• Keep food either hot or cold. Leaving food at room temperature encourages the growth of bacteria.

• Keep perishable products refrigerated. Oils containing herbs or garlic should also be refrigerated.

• Refrigerate leftovers as soon as possible. Do not refrigerate foods in the same containers they were cooked or served in; transfer leftovers into clean containers so that they will cool more quickly. Most foods should be discarded after twenty-four to thirty-six hours.

• Organize your refrigerator so that raw meats are kept away from, or do not drip blood onto, other foods. Do not leave raw meats in the refrigerator for more than forty-eight hours. If you are not using it right away, freeze it.

• Cook meat, poultry, and seafood thoroughly. Meats should be cooked to an internal temperature of at least 165°F.

• If you bake potatoes in aluminum, keep them either hot or refrigerated.

• Never use raw eggs that are cracked.

• Wash your hands before handling food, and after handling raw meat or poultry. Harmful bacteria can be transmitted if you handle food after diapering a baby or blowing your nose.

• Keep two cutting boards, one for meat and the other for vegetables. This will prevent the transfer of bacteria from meat to vegetables. At least three times a week, wash your cutting boards with a solution of ¼ cup of 3 percent hydrogen peroxide and 2 gallons of water. As an alternative, you can use a mixture of ½ cup of chlorine bleach and 1 quart of water, then rinse the board thoroughly with clean water.

• Go home directly after grocery shopping, especially in warm weather. Store foods immediately according to the instructions on the labels.

• Clean any utensil that has come in contact with raw hamburger, poultry, eggs, or seafood. Such utensils should not be allowed to come into contact with other foods until they have been disinfected.

• Wash out lunch boxes and Thermos bottles after every use.

• Beware of bulging cans, cracked jars, or loose lids on products. These can indicate botulism. Throw away cans that are bulging, rusted, bent, or sticky. Beware of cracks in jars and leaks in paper packaging, and exercise caution when consuming home-canned foods.

• When reheating food, bring it to a rapid boil, if possible, and cook it at that temperature for at least four minutes.

• Set your refrigerator temperature at 40°F or below. Freezers should be set at 0°F or below.

• Wash kitchen towels and sponges with a bleach-and-water solution (1 part bleach to 20 parts water) daily.

• Do not leave foods such as mayonnaise, salad dressing, and milk products at room temperature or, worse, out in the sun. Be especially careful at picnics and cookouts.

• Do not give honey to a young baby. This can lead to infant botulism, in which botulinal spores colonize the digestive tract and produce botulin toxin there. Honey is safe for babies after age one.

• Mold commonly grows on spoiled food products. The following foods should be avoided if mold is growing on them: bacon, bread, cured luncheon meats, soft dairy products, flour, canned ham, hot dogs, dried nuts, peanut butter, roast poultry, soft vegetables, and whole grains. Throw away any cooked or raw foods that are covered with mold.

• Thaw all frozen foods, especially meats and poultry, in the refrigerator, not at room temperature.

• Eat hamburger and other meats only if they have been cooked at least until they turn brown. Meat or poultry that is even a little pink in color may still harbor bacteria. To ensure that all bacteria have been destroyed, it is best to cook meat until it is well done.

• When preparing a chicken or turkey with dressing, do not stuff the bird until you are ready to put it in the oven. Either cook the stuffing separately or place it in the poultry immediately before putting it in the oven and then remove it as soon as the bird is done.

• Exercise caution when eating at restaurants and salad bars. Do not eat at salad bars that do not look fresh and clean or that do not have protective glass over them. Avoid the following foods when eating at salad bars: chicken, fish, creamed foods, foods containing mayonnaise, undercooked foods, and soups that are not kept at near-boiling temperatures.

• Before eating out, take 2 garlic tablets to help prevent food poisoning, as well as a product called ACES + Zn from Carlson Labs to destroy any free radicals created by unknown toxins and oxidized fats in the food.

Caution: Syrup of ipecac should be used only at the direction of a physician or poison control center.

❑ If symptoms of food poisoning are severe or prolonged, consult your health care provider.

Considerations

❑ David Hill, a microbiologist at Musgrove Park Hospital in Somerset, England, monitored all the bacteria present in the intestines and found that in the presence of garlic, disease-causing microbes were eliminated. According to Hill, the sulfur compounds in garlic are the secret weapon that knocks out dangerous bacteria.

❏ It was once believed that nylon or plastic cutting boards were preferable to the wooden variety. Since then, research has indicated that wood is probably better after all. Researchers have discovered that when cutting boards are contaminated with organisms that can cause food poisoning, almost all the bacteria on the wooden boards die off within three minutes, while almost none die on the plastic ones. For added security, you can wash your wooden cutting board periodically with hydrogen peroxide and water or a bleach-and-water solution. The ideal solution is to use one cutting board exclusively for vegetables and one for meat (*see* Tips for Preventing Food Poisoning on page 444). Glass or polished ceramic cutting boards are probably safest of all.

❏ Certain strains of bacteria found in eggs are not destroyed if the eggs are poached or prepared over-easy or sunny-side up.

❏ Food allergies are a common cause of illness and stomach upsets. For instance, a person who experiences severe headache and vomiting soon after eating may be suffering from food allergies. If this is the case, you should be able to develop a pattern associated with certain foods. (*See* ALLERGIES in Part Two.) In the meantime, charcoal tablets and a coffee retention enema can help rid the body of substances that cause allergic reactions. (*See* ENEMAS in Part Three.)

FOOD POISONING

See FOODBORNE/WATERBORNE illness.

FRACTURE

A fracture is a break or a crack in a bone. If the skin over the bone remains intact, a fracture is referred to as a closed or simple fracture; if the bone breaks the skin, it is termed an open or compound fracture. A fracture may cause extreme pain and tenderness in the injured area; swelling; a protruding bone or blood under the skin; and numbness, tingling, or paralysis below the fracture. A major fracture, such as of an arm or leg, may also cause a loss of the pulse below the fracture, as well as weakness and an inability to bear weight. Broken arms, fingers, or legs may be bent out of alignment.

Fractures occur most often in the very young and in older adults. Indeed, fractures pose an increasing problem as we grow older and our bones become more brittle. Falls account for more than 90 percent of all fractures in people aged sixty-five or older. An estimated 300,000 hip fractures occur in people over fifty years of age each year. People aged eighty-five or older are ten to fifteen times more likely to suffer from a fracture if they fall than people between sixty and sixty-five. Osteoporosis is a factor in many of

these cases. Hip fractures are by far the most troublesome fractures for older adults, and, unfortunately, many cannot live an independent life after a hip fracture. In fact, about one out of every five hip fracture patients dies within a year of their injury.

A broken bone calls for prompt professional help. After a bone has been set, the following supplements and other recommendations will aid in healing. Unless otherwise specified, the dosages recommended here are for adults. For a child between the ages of twelve and seventeen, reduce the dose to three-quarters the recommended amount. For a child between six and twelve, use one-half the recommended dose, and for a child under the age of six, use one-quarter the recommended amount.

NUTRIENTS

SUPPLEMENT	SUGGESTED DOSAGE	COMMENTS
Very Important		
Bone Builder with Boron from Ethical Nutrients	As directed on label.	A microcrystalline hydroxyapatite concentrate (MCHC) that contains the organic protein-calcium matrix of raw bone. Available only through health care professionals.
Bone Defense from KAL	As directed on label.	To supply essential nutrients for bone health.
Boron	3 mg daily. Do not exceed this amount.	Important in bone health and healing. Studies show boron can increase calcium uptake by as much as 30 percent.
Calcium	1,000–2,000 mg daily, in divided doses, after meals and at bedtime.	Vital for proper bone repair.
and magnesium	1,000 mg daily.	Needed to balance with calcium.
and potassium	99 mg daily.	Useful for maintaining good muscle and heart function.
Glucosamine and chondroitin	As directed on label.	Helps the body maintain joint flexibility by building cartilage.
plus methylsulfonyl-methane (MSM)	As directed on label.	Makes cell walls permeable, allowing water and nutrients to freely flow into cells and allowing wastes and toxins to properly flow out.
Kelp	1,000–1,500 mg daily.	Rich in calcium and minerals in a natural balance.
Neonatal Multi-Gland from Biotics Research	As directed on label.	Promotes healing. *See* GLANDULAR THERAPY in Part Three for its benefits.
Proteolytic enzymes	As directed on label. Take between meals and with meals.	Taken between meals, reduces inflammation. Taken with meals, aids digestion of proteins. *Caution:* Do not give this supplement to a child under sixteen years of age.
S-Adenosylmethio-nine (SAMe)	As directed on label.	A natural alternative to prescribed antidepressants. Can also be used in a lower dose as an anti-inflammatory agent for joint stiffness.

		Caution: Do not use if you have bipolar mood disorder or take prescription antidepressants. Do not give to a child under twelve.
Silica	As directed on label.	Supplies silicon, needed for calcium uptake and connective tissue repair.
Vitamin C with bioflavonoids	3,000–6,000 mg daily, in divided doses.	Important in repair of bones, connective tissue, and muscles.
Vitamin D	400–1,000 IU daily.	Needed for calcium absorption and bone repair. May help to prevent fractures.
Zinc	80 mg daily. Do not exceed a total of 100 mg daily from all supplements.	Important in tissue repair. Use zinc gluconate lozenges or zinc methionate (OptiZinc) for best absorption.
Helpful		
Free form amino acid (Amino Balance from Anabol Naturals or Amino Blend from Carlson Labs)	As directed on label.	Speeds healing.
Octacosanol	3,000 mg daily.	Improves tissue oxygenation.
Raw liver extract	As directed on label.	Supplies balanced B vitamins and other needed vitamins and minerals. (*See* GLANDULAR THERAPY in Part Three.)
Vitamin B complex	As directed on label.	Helps maintain healthy muscle tone and proper brain function. Important for older adults because these nutrients are less well absorbed as we age.
plus extra vitamin B_5 (pantothenic acid) and	100 mg 3 times daily.	Antistress vitamin. Aids in vitamin utilization.
folic acid	400–600 mcg per day from all sources.	Reduces homocysteine, high levels of which raise the risk of osteoporosis-related fractures.

Herbs

❑ Boswellia, an herb used commonly in Ayurvedic medicine, aids in the process of recovery from a fracture, easing pain and acting as an excellent anti-inflammatory.

❑ Turmeric paste makes a good poultice. Combine turmeric with a little hot water and apply it to the site of the injury on a gauze dressing. This is also good for bruises and helps to reduce swelling. A poultice of fresh mullein leaves is also good. (*See* USING A POULTICE in Part Three.)

Recommendations

❑ Eat half of a fresh pineapple every day until the fracture is healed. Pineapple contains bromelain, an enzyme that acts to reduce swelling and inflammation. Use only fresh pineapple, not canned or processed. If you don't like pineapple, the food supplement bromelain will provide the same benefits. Bromelain should be taken on an empty stomach.

❑ Avoid red meat, as well as colas and any other products containing caffeine. Foods with preservatives should also be avoided due to their phosphorus content. Phosphorus can lead to bone loss.

❑ Use clay poultices for bruises and swelling.

❑ Make your home safer by taking measures such as the following:

- Use nonslippery floor coverings. If you have carpets that are not fitted, make sure the edges are taped down.

- Make sure you have enough light so that you can see properly.

- Keep your path clear. If you have pets, they should be trained to keep out of your way. Do not leave things on the floor.

- Wipe up any spilled liquids immediately.

- Wear shoes or slippers with rubber soles.

- Take extra precautions when using stairs. Install handrails if necessary.

- Keep the telephone in a readily accessible place. Do not rush to answer it. Portable phones are available with a simple large red button that will connect you directly with the 911 emergency number.

- Medical alert devices that are worn around the neck are also available for people living alone.

- Talk to your physician about the medications you are taking and discuss whether they might impair your balance or orientation.

❑ If you are in any discomfort after a fall, have an X-ray taken of the painful area. If there is a fracture, you need to have it attended to immediately.

❑ If you suffer a hip fracture, ask your physician about nerve blocks before you have an operation to fix it. A nerve block can lessen the amount of oral analgesic administered during surgery.

Considerations

❑ Ultrasound therapy after a fracture may speed healing. If you want to try this at home, there is an FDA-approved device called Sonic Relief. Check with your doctor first.

❑ *See also* OSTEOPOROSIS and SPRAINS, STRAINS, AND OTHER INJURIES OF THE MUSCLES AND JOINTS in Part Two.

FRIEDREICH'S ATAXIA

See ATAXIA *under* RARE DISORDERS.

FUNGAL INFECTION

Certain types of fungi (most commonly *Candida* and *Tinea*) can infect the skin and/or mucous membranes; they can also grow under the nails, between the toes, or on internal surfaces of the colon and other organs. Fungal infection of the skin is most common in places where skin tends to be moist and one skin surface is in contact with another, such as the groin area ("jock itch") and between the toes ("athlete's foot"). A type of scalp infection known as tinea capitis is found mainly in schoolchildren, although adults also may be affected. Moist, possibly itchy, red patches anywhere on the body can indicate fungal infection. In babies, a fungal infection can manifest itself as diaper rash that makes the skin bright red in light-skinned babies and darker brown in dark-skinned babies.

Fungal infection of the mouth is referred to as oral thrush, a condition in which creamy-looking white patches form on the tongue and the mucous membranes of the mouth. If the patches are scraped off, bleeding may result. This condition is most common in infants and in those with compromised immune systems.

Nursing mothers sometimes develop a candida infection of the nipples that causes severe pain while feeding. This can be further complicated if the baby develops oral thrush; it can lead to a "ping-pong" effect in which mother and baby continually reinfect each other.

Fungal infection under the nails (paronychia) or between the toes may cause discoloration and swelling, and the nails may become raised above the surface of the nail bed. In fungal infection of the vagina (yeast infection), a cheesy discharge is present, usually accompanied by intense itching.

Ringworm, also known as tinea infection, is a fungal infection of the skin or scalp. Caused by various species of fungi—mainly microspora, trichophyta, and epidermophyta—it is characterized by the development of small red spots that grow to a size of about one-quarter inch in diameter.

As the spots expand, the centers tend to heal and clear while the borders are raised, red, and scaly, giving them a ringlike appearance. Like other fungal infections, ringworm can be very itchy.

Recurrent fungal infections are a common sign of depressed immune function. The people most likely to be affected are those who have diseases such as diabetes or cancer, or who are infected with human immunodeficiency virus (HIV). Women who use oral contraceptives and people taking antibiotics are at higher risk as well, as are people who are obese and/or who perspire heavily.

Unless otherwise specified, the dosages recommended here are for adults. For children between the ages of twelve and seventeen, reduce the dose to three-quarters the recommended amount. For children between six and twelve, use one-half the recommended dose, and for children under the age of six, use one-quarter the recommended amount.

NUTRIENTS

SUPPLEMENT	SUGGESTED DOSAGE	COMMENTS
Essential		
Acidophilus (Kyo-Dophilus from Wakunaga)	As directed on label.	To supply the "friendly" bacteria that are usually deficient in people with fungal infections.
Garlic (Kyolic from Wakunaga)	2 capsules 3 times daily, with meals.	Neutralizes most fungi.
Kyolic-EPA from Wakunga	As directed on label.	For relief of pain and inflammation.
Important		
Colostrum (Colostrum Plus from Symbiotics or Colostrum Prime Life from Jarrow Formulas)	As directed on label.	Possesses healing properties, boosts the immune system, and fights fungal infection.
Vitamin B complex plus extra vitamin B$_5$ (pantothenic acid)	50 mg 3 times daily, with meals. 50 mg 3 times daily.	Needed for correctly balanced "friendly" bacteria in the body. Plays a role in the formation of antibodies and aids in the utilization of nutrients.
Vitamin C with bioflavonoids	5,000–20,000 mg daily, in divided doses. (*See* ASCORBIC ACID FLUSH in Part Three.)	Needed for proper immune function.
Vitamin E	200 IU daily.	Needed for proper immune function. Use emulsion form for easier assimilation. Use d-alpha-tocopherol form.
Zinc	50 mg daily. Do not exceed a total of 100 mg daily from all supplements.	Needed for proper immune function. Use zinc gluconate lozenges or OptiZinc for best absorption.
Helpful		
Essential fatty acids (black currant seed oil, primrose oil, or salmon oil)	As directed on label.	For relief of pain and inflammation.
Vitamin A with mixed carotenoids	25,000 IU daily. If you are pregnant, do not exceed 10,000 IU daily.	Aids healing of skin and mucous membranes. Needed for proper immune function.

Herbs

☐ Berberine is a phytochemical that has antifungal action. Goldenseal, a berberine-containing herb, works against a variety of fungi, including candida. Bloodroot, another herb that contains berberine, has shown action against skin fungi and is also an anti-inflammatory. Other herbs that contain berberine and are recommended for fungal infections include barberry, Oregon grape, and yellowroot.

Caution: Do not take goldenseal internally on a daily basis for more than one week at a time. Do not use it during pregnancy or if you are breast-feeding, and use with caution if you are allergic to ragweed. If you have a history of cardiovascular disease, diabetes, or glaucoma, use it only under a doctor's supervision.

❑ Horopito, or pepper tree (*Pseudowintera colorata*), a shrub native to New Zealand, contains polygodial, an antifungal agent that has been shown to act against bacteria as well. The leaves can be bruised, steamed, and applied topically to treat skin diseases such as ringworm. *Licaria puchuri-major,* a medicinal plant found in the Brazilian rain forest, has been found to augment the antifungal activity of polygodial and increase its effectiveness against fungal infection.

❑ Kolorex from Nature's Sources is an herbal product that has been shown to be effective in treating ringworm and tinea fungi infections. It is available in both capsule and cream form.

❑ Pau d'arco has strong antifungal properties. Drink 3 cups of pau d'arco tea daily.

❑ For toenail or fingernail fungus, soak nails in a mixture of pau d'arco and goldenseal. In a wide pan, make pau d'arco tea using 6 tea bags and a gallon of water. Bring to a boil, then allow to cool to a very warm but tolerable temperature. Add the contents of 4 capsules of goldenseal. Soak your feet or hands in this mixture for fifteen minutes twice a day.

Caution: Do not take goldenseal internally on a daily basis for more than one week at a time. Do not use it during pregnancy or if you are breast-feeding, and use with caution if you are allergic to ragweed. If you have a history of cardiovascular disease, diabetes, or glaucoma, use it only under a doctor's supervision.

❑ Tea tree oil is a natural antifungal for external use. It can be applied to the affected area several times a day, either full strength or diluted with distilled water or cold-pressed vegetable oil. For trichomonal vaginitis or vaginal candidiasis, apply a few drops of the oil on a tampon, or mix it with water and use it as a douche. You can also use black walnut extract.

❑ Wild oregano oil is a powerful antifungal agent that has the ability to destroy even resistant forms of fungi.

Recommendations

❑ Eat a diet of 60 to 70 percent raw foods. Eat plenty of fresh vegetables and moderate amounts of broiled fish and broiled skinless chicken.

❑ Do not eat any foods containing sugar or refined carbohydrates. Fungi thrive on sugar.

❑ Eliminate those foods from the diet that tend to promote secretion of mucus, especially meat and dairy products.

❑ Avoid cola drinks, grains, processed foods, and fried, greasy foods.

❑ *See* FASTING in Part Three and follow the program.

❑ Keep the skin clean and dry. Expose the affected area to the air as much as possible.

❑ Wear clean cotton clothing and underwear. Do not wear clothing or use towels more than once without washing them, preferably in hot water with chlorine bleach added.

❑ To replace necessary "friendly" bacteria in the colon, use a *B. bifidus* retention enema. (*See* ENEMAS in Part Three.)

❑ Try not to allow an infected area of the body to come in contact with healthy skin. People who have fungal infections in one area often also have infections in other areas.

❑ If you are nursing a baby and your baby has thrush, or you develop sharp, shooting pains during feedings, or both, consult both your child's and your own health care provider. You may have a fungal infection. Both you and your baby should be treated to ensure a cure.

❑ To treat ringworm, use a sterile pad and apply colloidal silver to the affected area. Hands and feet can also be soaked in this solution, a natural antibiotic that destroys some 650 different microorganisms.

❑ For ringworm, mix ½ clove crushed garlic with ¼ cup vegetable oil. Coat the affected area with honey, then apply the garlic mixture (avoid healthy skin). Cover loosely with sterile gauze that allows air to penetrate. Leave in place for four hours.

❑ If you have been treating a fungal infection on your own and you develop symptoms of a worsening infection, such as increased redness and swelling or fever, consult your physician. You may have developed a bacterial infection on top of the fungal infection.

❑ For fungal infections underneath the fingernails, soak your nails in a mixture of 50 percent white distilled vinegar and 50 percent pure water for ten to twenty minutes daily.

Considerations

❑ There are numerous topical antifungal preparations available in drugstores.

❑ *See also* ATHLETE'S FOOT; CANDIDIASIS; and/or YEAST INFECTION in Part Two.

GALLBLADDER DISORDERS

The gallbladder is a three- to four-inch-long pear-shaped organ located on the right side of the body, directly under the liver. One of the functions of the liver is to remove poisonous substances from the blood so that they can be expelled from the body. The liver excretes all these gathered toxins mixed with a digestive agent called bile. Bile also contains cholesterol, bile salts, lecithin, and other substances. The bile—about one pint of it every day—goes first to the gallbladder, which holds it until food arrives in the small intestine. The gallbladder then releases the bile, which passes through the cystic and bile ducts into the small intestine. Ultimately, the toxins are passed out of the body through the feces.

Abnormal concentration of bile acids, cholesterol, and phospholipids in the bile can cause the formation of gallstones. The presence of gallstones is known to doctors as cholelithiasis. It has been estimated that over 25 million Americans have gallstones and almost 1 million new cases are diagnosed each year. As many as one in ten people might have gallstones without knowing it. However, if a stone is pushed out of the gallbladder and lodges in the bile duct, this can cause nausea, vomiting, and pain in the upper right abdominal region. These symptoms often arise after the individual has eaten fried or fatty foods.

Gallstones can range from the size of a tiny grain of sand to larger than a pea-sized mass. More than 75 percent of gallstones are cholesterol stones, with the remaining being pigment stones. Pigment stones are composed of calcium salts. Although the cause of pigment stones is unknown, factors such as intestinal surgery, cirrhosis of the liver, and blood disorders can increase the rate risk.

The presence of gallstones creates a possibility that cholecystitis, or inflammation of the gallbladder, may develop. This can cause severe pain in the upper right abdomen and/or across the chest, possibly accompanied by fever, nausea, and vomiting. Other symptoms of gallbladder disease include constant pain below the breastbone that shoots into the right or left shoulder area and radiates into the back.

The pain can last from thirty minutes to several hours. The urine may be tea- or coffee-colored, and there may be shaking, chills, and jaundice (a yellowish discoloration of the skin and eyes). Gallbladder attacks often occur in the evening and can take place sporadically. Abdominal pain that occurs on a daily basis might be a problem unrelated to the gallbladder. A gallbladder attack may mimic a heart attack, with severe pain in the chest area. Biliary dyskinesia is a condition in which all the symptoms of gallbladder disease are present, but there are no stones.

Inflammation of the gallbladder requires immediate treatment. If left untreated, it can be life-threatening. If you experience pain in your upper abdomen that lasts for more than an hour, your doctor may recommend an ultrasound to confirm signs of gallbladder disease.

NUTRIENTS

SUPPLEMENT	SUGGESTED DOSAGE	COMMENTS
Alfalfa		See under Herbs, below.
Esential fatty acid complex or Kyolic-EPA from Wakunaga	As directed on label.	Important constituents of every living cell. Needed for repair and prevention of gallstones.
Lecithin granules or capsules	1 tbsp 3 times daily, before meals. 1,200 mg 3 times daily, before meals.	A fat emulsifier; aids digestion of fats.
L-glycine	500 mg daily, on an empty stomach. Take with water or juice. Do not take with milk. Take with 50 mg vitamin B6 and 100 mg	Essential for the biosynthesis of nucleic and bile acids. (See AMINO ACIDS in Part One.)
	vitamin C for better absorption.	
Magnesium	400 mg daily.	Magnesium may reduce insulin levels that are associated with gallbladder disease.
Multienzyme complex with ox bile (D.A, #34 from Carlson Labs)	As directed on label. Take before meals.	Aids in digestion if too little bile is secreted from the gallbladder. Ox bile is needed especially if you have had gallbladder removal surgery. Caution: Do not give this supplement to a child. If you have a history of ulcers, do not use a formula containing HCl.
Taurine Plus from American Biologics	As directed on label.	Necessary for the formation of an important bile acid and may prevent the formation of gallstones. Use the liquid form.
Vitamin A with carotenoids	25,000 IU daily. If you are pregnant, do not exceed 10,000 IU daily.	Needed for repair of tissues. Use emulsion form for easier assimilation.
Vitamin B complex plus extra vitamin B12 and choline and inositol	50 mg 3 times daily, with meals. 2,000 mcg daily. 500 mg daily. 500 mg daily.	All B vitamins are necessary for proper digestion. Use a high-potency formula. Important in cholesterol metabolism and liver and gallbladder function.
Vitamin C with bioflavonoids	3,000 mg daily.	Deficiency can lead to gallstones.
Vitamin D	400 IU daily.	Gallbladder malfunction interferes with vitamin D absorption.
Vitamin E	200 IU daily.	Prevents fats from becoming rancid. Use d-alpha-tocopherol form.

Herbs

❑ Alfalfa cleanses the liver and supplies necessary vitamins and minerals. Twice a day for two days, take 1,000 milligrams in tablet or capsule form with a glass of warm water.

❑ Fumitory (Fumaria officinalis) has long been used in traditional medicine to treat liver disorders. Research has shown that it does stimulate the flow of bile. However, this antispasmodic contains many alkaloids and is toxic in large doses. Dry extracts found as capsules, tablets, or drops are available, especially in Europe. It is recommended that these be taken before meals. If the dried leaves are available, a tea can be made by pouring ½ cup of boiling water over 1 to 2 teaspoons of fumitory. Steep for ten minutes, strain, and drink at least one-half hour before meals.

Caution: Consult with your physician before using fumitory.

❑ Peppermint oil capsules are used in Europe to cleanse the gallbladder.

❑ If you have gallstones, or are prone to developing them, turmeric can reduce your risk of further problems.

❏ Other beneficial herbs include barberry root bark, catnip, cramp bark, dandelion, fennel, ginger root, parsley, and wild yam.

Recommendations

❏ If you have an attack, drink 1 tablespoon of apple cider vinegar in a glass of apple juice. This should relieve the pain quickly. If the pain does not subside, go to the emergency room to rule out other disorders such as gastroesophogeal reflux disease (GERD) or heart problems.

❏ For inflammation of the gallbladder, eat no solid food for a few days. Consume only distilled or spring water. Then drink juices such as pear, beet, and apple for three days. Then add solid foods: shredded raw beets with 2 tablespoons of olive oil, fresh lemon juice, and freshly made uncooked applesauce made in a blender or food processor. Apple juice aids in softening gallstones.

❏ For gallstones, take 3 tablespoons of olive oil with the juice of a lemon before bed and upon awakening. Stones are often passed and eliminated in the stool with this technique—look for them. You can substitute grapefruit juice if desired.

❏ To relieve acute pain, call your doctor. You can ask him or her about using hot castor oil packs on the gallbladder area. Place castor oil in a pan and heat but do not boil it. Dip a piece of cheesecloth or other white cotton material into the oil until the cloth is saturated. Apply the cloth to the affected area and cover it with a piece of plastic that is larger in size than the cotton cloth. Place a heating pad over the plastic and use it to keep the pack warm. Keep the pack in place for one-half to two hours, as needed.

❏ Eat a diet consisting of 75 percent raw foods. Include in the diet applesauce, eggs, yogurt, cottage cheese, broiled fish, fresh apples, and beets.

❏ Eat protein from vegetable sources. This is particularly important for men. The iron (called heme) in meats (fish, poultry, and beef) accumulates in men and is associated with a 20 percent increased risk of gallbladder disease. Postmenopausal women would also likely benefit from eating a diet low in animal products.

❏ The kind of dietary fat consumed also is important. In one study, those who ate polyunsaturated and monounsaturated fats, while maintaining a healthy weight, had an 18 percent reduction in risk of developing gallstones.

❏ To cleanse the system, consume as much pure apple juice as possible for five days. Add pear juice occasionally. Beet juice also cleanses the liver.

❏ Avoid sugar and products containing sugar. People who consume an excessive amount of sugar are much more likely to form gallstones. Avoid all animal fat and meat, saturated fats (found primarily in meat), full-fat dairy products, fried foods, spicy foods, margarine, soft drinks, commercial oils, chocolate, and refined carbohydrates.

❏ While you have pain, nausea and/or vomiting, and fever, follow a fasting program and use coffee enemas for a few days. The coffee enema is important. You can also use garlic in the enema. (See ENEMAS and FASTING in Part Three.)

❏ A detoxification program for the liver and colon is important for improved gallbladder function. Use cleansing enemas if you have chronic problems.

❏ Do not overeat. Obesity and gallbladder disease are related. Females age forty and over who are overweight and who have had children are more likely than most people to suffer from disorders of the gallbladder.

Considerations

❏ Rapid weight changes can cause gallbladder problems. A study published in the *Annals of Internal Medicine* revealed that "yo-yo" dieting—repeatedly losing and gaining weight due to dieting—increases the risk of gallstones and the necessity for surgery by as much as 70 percent.

❏ The recommended treatment for gallstones used to be surgical removal of the gallbladder. However, if gallstones show up on an X-ray but do not cause symptoms, there may be no need for surgery.

❏ A gallstone may slip into a bile duct, one of the structures that drain the gallbladder and the liver. If this occurs, extraction or surgical removal by a technique called laparoscopic cholecystectomy may be necessary. Also known as keyhole surgery, this is now the most common method of removing the gallbladder. The surgeon uses a trocar (a hollow tube) and enters the abdomen through the navel. Three more of these tubes are inserted into the abdomen so that instruments can be inserted through them. The surgeon inserts a laparoscope (a small camera) through one of these tubes, so that he or she can see inside the patient without the large incision normally required to remove a gallbladder. The procedure requires four small incisions in total, instead of a single six- to nine-inch incision, and recovery time is greatly reduced. However, research from Washington University suggests that people with a history of gallbladder inflammation or ten or more gallbladder attacks, or who are over sixty-five years of age, may be more likely to have complications with this type of surgery. The risk is mitigated if your surgeon is adept at the procedure. If complications do arise after surgery, this may be because the gallbladder was not in fact the source of the initial problem, or because of a bile leak.

❏ Sometimes stones in the gallbladder can be fragmented or dissolved without surgery, using the drug deoxycholic acid or lithotripsy (the use of sound waves to break up stones). Bile acid preparations used to dissolve stones work very slowly and can be used only on small stones.

❏ Eighty percent of gallstones produce no symptoms and require no treatment. Discuss any recommended treatment with your doctor and surgeon and make sure an operation is absolutely necessary before proceeding.

❏ Physical activity may reduce the risk of gallstones.

❏ A study reported in the *Journal of the American Medical Association* found that drinking three cups of coffee a day might lower men's (and possibly women's) risk of developing gallstones. However, it is not recommended that you start drinking more coffee due to the results of one study.

❏ People with pigment stones, which consist of calcium salts, should probably avoid using calcium supplements, although some researchers believe it is all right for them to continue taking calcium supplements.

❏ In one study, men who took 400 milligrams per day of magnesium had 33 percent less chance of developing gallbladder disease compared to men who took less than 288 milligrams a day. The magnesium can come from food or supplements.

❏ Gallstones run in families, and women are twice as likely to form gallstones as men.

GANGRENE

Gangrene is a condition in which body tissues die, and ultimately decay, as a result of an inadequate oxygen supply. It can affect any body part, but most frequently affects extremities—the toes, feet, fingers, hands, and arms. Gangrene of the internal organs is especially dangerous.

There are two types of gangrene: wet gangrene and dry gangrene. Wet gangrene is the result of a wound or injury that becomes infected with bacteria. The infection prevents adequate venous drainage, depriving the area of needed blood supply and oxygen. The disruption in oxygen supply in turn promotes the infection. Symptoms of wet gangrene include severe and rapidly worsening pain, swelling, and tenderness in the area. As the infection progresses, the affected tissue changes color, usually from pink to deep red to gray-green or purple. Left untreated, wet gangrene can lead to shock and death in a matter of days. Fortunately, careful hygiene can usually prevent this type of gangrene.

Dry gangrene does not involve bacterial infection. It is caused by stopped or reduced blood flow, which results in oxygen-deprived tissue. Reduced blood flow may be caused by injury, hardening of the arteries, poor circulation, diabetes, or blockage in a blood vessel. The condition most often occurs in the feet and toes. Symptoms of the most common type of dry gangrene are a dull, aching pain and coldness in the area. Pain and pallor of the affected area are early signs.

Sometimes gangrene is caused by frostbite. In frostbite, the oxygen-deprived area dies, but the gangrene does not spread to any other area. As the flesh dies, it may be painful, but once the skin is dead, it becomes numb and slowly darkens.

The risk of developing gangrene is higher than normal for people with diabetes, who smoke or drink excessively, or who have poor circulation in general. Proper nutrition and a healthy lifestyle decrease the likelihood of developing gangrene and also aid in recovery should you require surgery for this condition.

Unless otherwise specified, the dosages recommended here are for adults. For children between the ages of twelve and seventeen, reduce the dose to three-quarters of the recommended amount. For children between six and twelve, use one-half of the recommended dose, and for children under the age of six, use one-quarter of the recommended amount.

NUTRIENTS

SUPPLEMENT	SUGGESTED DOSAGE	COMMENTS
Essential		
Dimethylglycine (DMG) (Aangamik DMG from FoodScience of Vermont)	100 mg 3 times daily.	Enhances oxygen utilization by affected tissue.
Dioxychlor	As directed on label.	Antiviral, antifungal, and antibacterial. Assists the immune system in defending against invading microorganisms, with little or no toxicity to normal tissues.
Garlic (Kyolic from Wakunaga)	As directed on label.	Speeds healing and increases circulation. Cleanses the blood. Use the liquid form.
Methylsulfonyl-methane (MSM)	As directed on label.	Aids in the healing of injuries and can help to detoxify the body on a cellular level. It has also been found to be an aid to the organs, connective tissue, and immune functions.
plus vitamin C with bioflavonoids	5,000–20,000 mg daily. (*See* ASCORBIC ACID FLUSH in Part Three.)	For tissue repair and improved circulation. Improves the. benefits of MSM.
Silicon (JarroSil from Jarrow Technologies)	As directed on label.	Needed for skin and tissue repair.
Very Important		
Liquid chlorophyll	As directed on label.	A source of minerals, enzymes, and vitamins. Also used as a blood detoxifier and nutrient.
Coenzyme Q10 plus Coenzyme A from Coenzyme-A Technologies	As directed on label. As directed on label.	Powerful antioxidants that help to improve circulation and boost the immune system.
Essential fatty acids (flaxseed oil, primrose oil, or salmon oil)	As directed on label.	Protects and aids in the repair of new tissues and cells.
Free form essential amino acid plus extra	As directed on label.	For repair of tissues.
L-arginine	As directed on label.	Facilitates natural synthesis of nitric oxide, which promotes healthy blood vessels.

451

Note: Do not use if you are pregnant or have cataracts, colitis, or a viral infection such as herpes.

Kyo-Green from Wakunaga	As directed on label.	Acts as a blood cleanser and builds up the blood supply.
Micellized Vitamin A and E from American Biologics	As directed on label.	Vitamin A is essential for tissue repair; vitamin E (see below) improves circulation. Both enhance immune function. Use emulsion form for easier assimilation and safety at higher doses.
Proteolytic enzymes	As directed on label. Take with meals and between meals.	Aids in damaged tissue "cleanup" and repair. *Caution:* Do not give this supplement to a child under sixteen years of age.
Vitamin E	200 IU daily.	Improves circulation. Use d-alpha-tocopherol form.
Important		
Kelp	1,000–1,500 mg daily.	A rich source of chlorophyll and minerals good for circulation. A blood cleanser.
Helpful		
Aerobic 07 from Aerobic Life Industries	As directed on label. Also apply a few drops directly on the affected area.	A stabilized oxygen product. Kills infecting bacteria.
Beta-1,3-D-glucan	As directed on label.	Helps to recruit immune T cells to the site of infection and aids in the growth of new blood vessels.
Calcium and magnesium	2,000 mg daily. 1,000 mg daily.	For connective tissue repair. Dilates blood vessels, improving blood flow. Needed to balance with calcium.
Multivitamin and mineral complex with potassium	As directed on label.	All nutrients are necessary for healing. Helps reduce tissue swelling.
Zinc	50–80 mg daily. Do not exceed a total of 100 mg daily from all supplements.	Speeds healing. Necessary for tissue repair and immune function. Use zinc gluconate lozenges or zinc methionate (OptiZinc) for best absorption.

Herbs

❏ Butcher's broom is important for circulation.

❏ Bromelain and turmeric (curcumin) are good for reducing swelling and inflammation.

❏ Olive leaf is good for fighting infections.

❏ Other beneficial herbs include bayberry, cayenne (capsicum), echinacea, ginkgo biloba, goldenseal, and red seal.

Cautions: Do not take echinacea for longer than three months. It should not be used by people who are allergic to ragweed. Do not take ginkgo biloba if you have a bleeding disorder, or are scheduled for surgery or a dental proce-

dure. Do not take goldenseal internally on a daily basis for more than one week at a time. Do not use it during pregnancy or if you are breast-feeding, and use with caution if you are allergic to ragweed. If you have a history of cardiovascular disease, diabetes, or glaucoma, use it only under a doctor's supervision.

Recommendations

❏ Eat a high-protein, high-calorie diet to promote fast tissue repair.

❏ Include in the diet foods that are high in germanium, such as garlic, shiitake mushrooms, and onions. Germanium helps to improve tissue oxygenation.

❏ Drink six to eight 8-ounce glasses of quality water (preferably steam-distilled) every day.

❏ Add "green drinks" made from vegetables to your diet. (*See* JUICING in Part Three.)

❏ If you smoke, stop. Avoid all contact with tobacco.

❏ If you have diabetes, be vigilant in your treatment.

❏ If an injured area becomes red, swollen, and painful, or develops an odor, see your health care practitioner without delay.

Considerations

❏ The only treatment for established gangrene is surgical removal of the affected area.

❏ For wet gangrene, treatment with antibiotics and surgical removal of the dead tissue are usually necessary. Hyperbaric oxygen therapy may be employed as well. (*See* HYPERBARIC OXYGEN THERAPY in Part Three.)

❏ Slowly developing dry gangrene may be reversed by arterial surgery. Chelation is an alternative. (*See* CHELATION THERAPY in Part Three.) If an acute arterial obstruction is involved, emergency surgery must be performed.

❏ *See also* ARTERIOSCLEROSIS and CIRCULATORY PROBLEMS in Part Two.

❏ Raynaud's syndrome, a condition that affects the small arteries of the fingers and toes, can lead to gangrene if not treated. *See* RAYNAUD'S DISEASE/RAYNAUD'S PHENOMENON in Part Two for a more complete discussion of this condition.

GAS

See HEARTBURN/GASTROESOPHAGEAL REFLUX DISEASE (GERD); INDIGESTION (DYSPEPSIA). *See also under* PREGNANCY-RELATED PROBLEMS.

GASTROENTERITIS

See FOODBORNE/WATERBORNE ILLNESS. *See also under* INFLUENZA.

GASTROESOPHAGEAL REFLUX DISEASE (GERD)

See HEARTBURN/GASTROESOPHAGEAL REFLUX DISEASE (GERD).

GERMAN MEASLES (RUBELLA)

German measles, or rubella, is a contagious viral disease that generally produces mild symptoms but is potentially dangerous to a fetus if a pregnant woman contracts the disease during the first trimester. Before a rubella vaccine was developed in the late 1960s, thousands of babies in the United States were born with severe birth defects because their mothers were exposed to the virus. Today, most children receive a vaccine (the MMR vaccine) that protects against measles, mumps, and rubella, but the virus exists worldwide and outbreaks still occur sporadically, usually in large population areas.

German measles mostly affects children, adolescents, and young adults. It initially causes swelling of the lymph glands in the neck and behind the ears. Other symptoms include coughing, fatigue, headache, mild fever, muscle aches, and stiffness, mainly in the neck. A pink rash often develops, usually starting on the face and neck and then spreading to the rest of the body. The rash typically lasts for about three days, thus the old name *three-day measles*. The virus usually runs its course in five to seven days, and is generally not treated since the patient gradually gets well. A person who has had German measles has a lifetime immunity against the virus. This disease is *not* related to regular measles and is caused by a different virus.

The communicable period probably begins two to four days before the rash appears, and the virus most often disappears from the nose and throat by the time the rash on the body disappears, one to three days after the onset of symptoms. However, because of the danger it poses to pregnant women, German measles should be considered contagious from one week before the rash appears until one week after the rash fades.

Unless otherwise specified, the dosages recommended here are for adults. For children between the ages of twelve and seventeen, reduce the dose to three-quarters the recommended amount. For children between six and twelve, use one-half the recommended dose, and for children under the age of six, use one-quarter the recommended amount.

NUTRIENTS

SUPPLEMENT	SUGGESTED DOSAGE	COMMENTS
Helpful		
Bio-Strath from Nature's Answer	As directed on label.	Acts as a tonic. Contains the vitamin B complex. Use the liquid form.
Calcium and magnesium	As directed on label. As directed on label.	Needed for tissue repair.
Essential fatty acids (flaxseed oil, Kyolic-EPA from Wakunaga, primrose oil, or salmon oil)	As directed on label.	Helps prevent scarring and promotes healing of tissue cells.
Garlic (Kyolic from Wakunaga)	2 capsules 3 times daily, with meals.	Improves immune function.
Kyo-Dophilus from Wakunaga	As directed on label.	Aids in normal bowel function. Allows survival and rapid passage of "friendly" bacteria through the stomach into the small intestine. Use a dairy-free, yeast-free formula.
Micellized Vitamin A and E from American Biologics	As directed on label.	Supplies vitamins A and E, needed to reduce infection and repair tissues. For a child under ten, substitute cod liver oil.
Proteolytic enzymes	As directed on label. Take on an empty stomach. Also take between meals.	Reduces infection and aids digestion. *Caution:* Do not give this supplement to a child.
Raw thymus glandular plus adrenal glandular	500 mg twice daily. As directed on label.	To stimulate the immune system. *Caution:* Do not give these supplements to a child.
Vitamin C with bioflavonoids	5,000–20,000 mg daily, in divided doses. (*See* ASCORBIC ACID FLUSH in Part Three.)	Very important for immune function. Controls fever and infection. Has antiviral properties. Use ascorbate or esterified form.
Zinc lozenges	1 15-mg lozenge 3 times daily for 4 days. Then reduce to 1 lozenge daily. Use this dosage for adults and for children over five.	For immune response and tissue repair.

Herbs

❑ If necessary, catnip tea or garlic enemas can be used to lower fever. (*See* ENEMAS in Part Three.)

❑ Clove and peppermint tea are useful in relieving symptoms.

❑ Alcohol-free goldenseal extract, placed directly under the tongue, aids in destroying bacteria and viruses and also relieves coughing. Use 3 drops for a child from three to ten years of age; for an adult or a child over ten, use one dropperful. Hold the extract under the tongue for a few minutes, then swallow. Repeat this three times daily for three days. As an alternative, use an echinacea and goldenseal combination extract, available in health food stores. Echinacea is good for the immune response.

Cautions: Do not take echinacea for longer than three months. It should not be used by people who are allergic to ragweed. Do not take goldenseal internally on a daily basis for more than one week at a time. Do not use it during pregnancy or if you are breast-feeding, and use with caution if you are allergic to ragweed. If you have a history of cardiovascular disease, diabetes, or glaucoma, use it only under a doctor's supervision.

❑ Take ½ teaspoon of lobelia extract every four to five hours for pain.

Caution: Lobelia is only to be taken under supervision of a health care professional as it is potentially toxic. People with high blood pressure, heart disease, liver disease, kidney disease, seizure disorders, or shortness of breath should not take lobelia. Pregnant and lactating women should avoid lobelia as well.

❑ Maitake, reishi, and shiitake mushrooms are all effective in boosting the body's immune system.

❑ Olive leaf extract is good for reducing symptoms and controlling the virus.

Recommendations

❑ Drink plenty of fluids such as water, juices, and vegetable broths.

❑ Avoid processed foods.

❑ Rest until the rash and fever have disappeared.

❑ Avoid contact with healthy individuals, especially women of childbearing age and their children, until one week after the rash disappears.

❑ Do not give aspirin to a child with German measles. *See* REYE'S SYNDROME in Part Two.

Considerations

❑ Antibiotics are useless against viruses, so they are not called for in the treatment of German measles.

❑ A person infected with German measles should be kept isolated in a dimly lit room. Extra care should be taken if a rash breaks out close to the eyes. Be sure your child does not go to school.

❑ A woman who has had German measles will pass immunity to any child she has for the first year of his or her life.

❑ Immunity to German measles can be determined by a blood test. Any woman who wishes to become pregnant and who is not sure whether she has achieved immunity to German measles should be tested and vaccinated, if necessary. Pregnancy must then be avoided for at least three months following immunization.

❑ It is a good idea for any woman who is (or who may be) pregnant to take precautions to avoid exposure to anyone who has, or has recently been exposed to, German measles. A pregnant woman who suspects she may have been exposed to German measles and who knows she has not achieved immunity (either through vaccination or from having the disease) should consult her doctor immediately concerning a gamma-globulin injection. If given soon after exposure, gamma-globulin may reduce the severity of the

illness or even prevent it from developing, although it is not known how effective this approach is.

❑ Many doctors believe that children should be immunized against German measles at about fifteen months of age and again a few years later. Non-pregnant women of childbearing age also should be immunized. People who should not be immunized include women who may be pregnant and individuals with impaired immune function, such as those with AIDS or cancer, or those currently taking cortisone or anticancer drugs or undergoing radiation therapy. Those with an illness that causes a fever should defer vaccination until healthy.

GIGANTISM

See under GROWTH PROBLEMS.

GINGIVITIS

See under PERIODONTAL DISEASE.

GLAUCOMA

Glaucoma is a group of diseases that affect the optic nerve and can lead to irreversible vision loss. It is usually, but not always, associated with elevated fluid pressure within the eye. All forms of glaucoma can cause damage to the optic nerve and lead to vision loss, even blindness, if left untreated.

More than 2 million Americans have been diagnosed with glaucoma and as many as 2 million more could have it and not yet know. It is the second leading cause of blindness, and is expected to become more prevalent in years to come due to the growing population of older adults. Those at greatest risk are people over the age of sixty; people of African ancestry; and people with diabetes, high blood pressure, severe myopia (nearsightedness), or a family history of glaucoma. Smokers also have an elevated risk, as do those who have sustained eye injuries or who have used steroids for an extended period of time.

Open-angle glaucoma is the most common form of the disease; it is estimated that 1 million people have it. Yet because this disorder causes no symptoms until it is quite advanced, only about half of those who have it are aware of it. In open-angle glaucoma, there is no physical blockage and the structures of the eye appear normal, but the drainage of fluid nevertheless is inadequate to keep the intraocular pressure at a normal level. The most pronounced symptoms of open-angle glaucoma are the gradual loss or "darkening" of peripheral vision and a marked decrease in night vision or the ability of the eye to adjust to darkness. Peripheral vision is the ability to see "out of the corner of the eye." The loss of this ability leaves a person with "tunnel vision." Other possible symptoms include chronic low-grade headaches (often mistaken for tension headaches), the need for frequent changes in eyeglass prescription, and/or seeing halos around electric lights.

A far less common, yet more serious, form of glaucoma is closed-angle glaucoma. Closed-angle glaucoma is much more insidious than open-angle forms because it almost never manifests any symptoms until very late in the condition. By that time, vision may be irreversibly damaged.

Attacks of this type of glaucoma occur when the channels through which the eye's fluids drain suddenly become constricted or obstructed. This is usually due to narrowing or hardening of the exit channels from the eyes, and it results in extreme pain, poor vision, and even blindness. It is considered a medical emergency. Early warning signs that a problem may be developing include eye pain or discomfort mainly in the morning, blurred vision, seeing halos around lights, and inability of the pupils to adjust to a dark room. Symptoms of the acute attack itself include throbbing eye pain and loss of sight, especially peripheral vision; pupils that are fixed in a mildly dilated condition and do not respond to light properly; and a sharp increase in the pressure in the inner eye, especially on one side. These symptoms come on very rapidly and may be accompanied by nausea and even vomiting. Permanent vision damage can occur in as little as three to five days, making treatment within the first twenty-four to forty-eight hours imperative.

In some cases, glaucoma manifests itself even though there is normal fluid pressure within the eye. This form of glaucoma is called normotensive (normal-tension) glaucoma, or NTG. With this condition, the optic nerve is damaged and vision is impaired much the same way as in open-angle glaucoma, but without the increased fluid pressure. This has led many researchers to shift their focus in recent years to the optic nerve itself. Mechanisms other than pressure may cause changes in the eye that can cause damage to the optic nerve.

Glaucoma probably has many causes. Many scientists believe it may be closely linked to stress and nutritional problems, or disorders such as diabetes and high blood pressure. Some suspect that excessive amounts of glutamic acid, a nonessential amino acid also known as glutamate, may be involved. Glaucoma has also been linked with a deficiency in nitric oxide, a molecule that is critical for healthy blood vessels. Problems with collagen, the most abundant protein in the human body, have been linked to glaucoma.

Collagen acts to increase the strength and elasticity of tissues in the body, especially those of the eye. Collagen and tissue abnormalities at the back of the eye contribute to the "clogging" of the tissues through which intraocular fluid normally drains. The result is elevated inner eye pressure that leads to glaucoma and related vision loss. Conditions characterized by errors of collagen metabolism are frequently associated with eye disorders.

Experts now believe that a simple pressure test is inadequate for diagnosis of glaucoma. An eye exam should also include a close examination of the optic nerve itself while the pupil is dilated, plus a test of the peripheral vision to see if any vision loss has occurred. People who are at risk for glaucoma should be tested frequently so that any loss of peripheral vision can be documented early.

NUTRIENTS

SUPPLEMENT	SUGGESTED DOSAGE	COMMENTS
Very Important		
Choline and inositol	1,000–2,000 mg daily.	Important B vitamins for the eyes and brain.
or lecithin	As directed on label.	A good source of choline and inositol.
Essential fatty acids (flaxseed oil, Kyolic-EPA from Wakunaga, primrose oil, or salmon oil)	As directed on label. Take with meals.	Protects and aids repair of new tissues and cells.
Glutathione	500 mg twice daily, on an empty stomach. Take with 50 mg vitamin B$_6$ and 100 mg vitamin C for better absorption.	A powerful antioxidant that protects the lens and maintains the molecular integrity of the lens fiber membranes.
Rutin	50 mg 3 times daily.	An important bioflavonoid that works with vitamin C and aids in reducing pain and intraocular pressure.
Vitamin A	50,000 IU daily. If you are pregnant, do not exceed 10,000 IU daily.	Needed for good eyesight. Essential in formation of visual purple, the substance necessary for night vision.
plus carotenoid complex with lutein and zeaxanthin	As directed on label.	
Vitamin B complex	100 mg of each major B vitamin 3 times daily (amounts of individual vitamins in a complex will vary).	B vitamins work best when taken together. Use a sublingual form or injections (under a doctor's supervision). Whenever stress is a factor, B-complex injections are a good idea.
plus extra vitamin B$_5$ (pantothenic acid)	100 mg 3 times daily.	Antistress vitamin needed for the adrenal glands, and an essential constituent of coenzyme A, needed for many vital metabolic processes.
Vitamin C with bioflavonoids	10,000–15,000 mg daily, in divided doses. Under a doctor's supervision, you can increase the dose to 30,000 mg daily.	Reduces intraocular pressure.
Vitamin E plus	200 IU daily.	Helpful in removing particles from the lens of the eye. Has antioxidant properties to protect the lens and other eye tissues. Use d-alpha-tocopherol form.
L-arginine	As directed on label.	Facilitates natural synthesis of nitric oxide, which promotes healthy blood vessels.

Note: Avoid arginine if you are pregnant or have cataracts, colitis, or a viral infection such as herpes.

Helpful		
Alpha-lipoic acid	150 mg daily.	An important antioxidant. Improves visual functions.
Magnesium	500–1,000 mg daily.	Dilates blood vessels, enhancing flow to the eyes.
Multivitamin and mineral complex with	As directed on label.	All nutrients are needed to aid in healing and to reduce intraocular pressure.
selenium	200 mcg daily.	A potent antioxidant that works with vitamin E.
Taurine Plus from American Biologics	As directed on label.	An antioxidant that protects the lens of the eye.
Zinc	50 mg daily. Do not exceed a total of 100 mg daily from all supplements.	Essential in activating vitamin A from the liver. Very beneficial in glaucoma therapy. Use zinc sulfate form.

Herbs

❑ Bilberry contains flavonoids and nutrients needed to protect the eyes from further damage. Fresh blueberries and red raspberry leaf can be used also.

❑ Chickweed and eyebright are good for all eye disorders.

❑ *Coleus forskohli,* an Ayurvedic herb, has been shown to reduce eye pressure.

❑ Eye baths using warm fennel tea, alternating with chamomile and eyebright, are helpful. Or use an eye dropper and apply three drops to each eye three times a day. Always dilute any herbal preparations used in the eyes with high-quality water.

Caution: Do not use chamomile if you are allergic to ragweed. Do not use during pregnancy or nursing. It may interact with warfarin or cyclosporine, so patients using these drugs should avoid it.

❑ A combination of ginkgo biloba extract and zinc sulfate may slow progressive vision loss.

Caution: Do not take ginkgo biloba if you have a bleeding disorder, or are scheduled for surgery or a dental procedure.

❑ Jaborandi is a rain-forest herb that contains pilocarpine, used for more than 120 years to relieve intraocular pressure in glaucoma.

Caution: Do not use this herb if you have pleurisy, are nursing, or have excess fatty tissue around the heart.

❑ Rose hips supply valuable flavonoids and vitamin C.

❑ Completely avoid the herb ephedra (ma huang), no longer legally sold in the United States, and licorice.

Caution: Licorice root should not be used during pregnancy or nursing. It should not be used by persons with diabetes, glaucoma, heart disease, high blood pressure, or a history of stroke.

Recommendations

❑ Follow the supplementation program outlined above.

❑ Exercise regularly. Research has shown that people with open-angle glaucoma who exercise at least three times a week may reduce intraocular pressure. If they stop exercising, the pressure again begins to build up. Exercise does not appear to have the same benefits for people with closed-angle glaucoma.

Caution: If you are thirty-five or older and/or have been sedentary for some time, consult with your health care provider before beginning an exercise program.

❑ Control blood pressure and blood sugar levels through diet and exercise, if they are elevated.

Caution: If you are thirty-five or older and/or have been sedentary for some time, consult with your health care provider before beginning an exercise program.

❑ If your ophthalmologist recommends medication to control glaucoma and it is working to your satisfaction, continue to use it faithfully. Also take vitamin C in high doses, but only under supervision.

❑ If you are using eye drops to reduce intraocular pressure, make sure you know how to administer the eye drops properly to ensure that your eyes receive a sufficient amount of the medication. If improperly administered, eye drops can roll off the eye, spill down your cheek, or even get absorbed into your own tear duct. It can be difficult to gauge how effective you are at administering your own eye drops. Ask your ophthalmologist for help in finding the best method. It also helps to occasionally have someone watch you administer the drops to make sure they are getting into the eye. It is also a good idea to close your eye gently for a minute or two after administering eye drops to give time for the medication to be absorbed.

❑ Avoid prolonged eye stress such as watching television, reading, and using a computer for long periods. If you must engage in close work for any length of time, take periodic "focus breaks." Every twenty minutes or so, raise your eyes and focus on something in the distance for a minute or so.

❑ Avoid tobacco smoke, coffee, alcohol, nicotine, and all caffeine.

❑ Drink only small amounts of liquid at any given time.

❑ Avoid taking high doses of niacin (over a total of 200 milligrams daily).

Considerations

❑ There is no cure for glaucoma, and any damage to vision is irreversible. Chronic open-angle glaucoma can often be controlled through the use of medication, usually in the form of eye drops. Several types of these medications are available. Often an ophthalmologist has to experiment a little to find the specific one that works most effectively for a particular individual. However, many people with glaucoma find that the eye drops cause severe headaches and other side effects. This problem can often be alleviated by changing the prescription. If headaches persist, it may help to adjust the schedule for taking the medication so that it interferes with normal activities as little as possible.

❑ Several studies have shown that smoking marijuana can help reduce intraocular pressure. However, marijuana is not recommended in the treatment of glaucoma for a variety of reasons, not least of which is its illegal status. Marijuana tends to increase the heart rate and lower blood pressure, which could compromise blood flow to the optic nerve. Also, the mechanisms by which marijuana lowers intraocular pressure are not fully understood, nor has it been shown that marijuana can work as safely and effectively as many FDA-approved drugs currently on the market.

❑ If eye drops fail to control intraocular pressure, a doctor may use a procedure called argon laser trabeculoplasty, or ALT. With this technique, a laser beam makes tiny holes in the meshwork through which the aqueous fluid normally drains, opening up blocked drainage channels.

❑ A technique called selective laser trabeculoplasty, or SLT, is used to lower pressure inside the eye. The outpatient procedure works by activating only pigment-containing cells, which through a series of events causes the release of cytokines that lead to microphage recruitment, along with other changes, to lower the pressure within the eye. SLT can zero in on specific cells without causing thermal damage to surrounding tissue; thus it can be repeated if necessary. The older argon laser therapy can be used only twice in a lifetime due to collateral damage.

❑ Surgery has certain advantages over medication, such as reduced out-of-pocket costs. However, it has disadvantages as well. An estimated 60 to 80 percent of people who undergo surgery for glaucoma experience improvement, although the procedure may have to be repeated.

❑ For acute closed-angle glaucoma attacks, surgery is usually necessary. Even though only one eye may be affected initially, the ophthalmologist performing the surgery will likely recommend that you have the surgical procedure on both eyes to prevent a second attack.

❑ The conventional treatment for acute closed-angle glaucoma is to immediately reduce eye pressure by employing an osmotic diuretic agent, followed by surgery. These osmotic agents (applied as eye drops) almost always act immediately to alleviate symptoms. However, surgery is still recommended because without it, the attacks are likely to recur, and each attack can cause additional irreversible vision damage. Using only osmotic agents can lull a person into thinking that his or her condition is improving while in fact it is worsening rapidly.

❑ Agents that act to dilate the pupils, such as belladonna, should be avoided at all costs.

❑ Vitamin C supplementation has been demonstrated to lower intraocular pressure in several clinical studies. Nearly normal tension levels have been achieved in some people who were unresponsive to conventional therapies. Intravenous administration of vitamin C has yielded even greater initial pressure reduction, but close monitoring by a physician is necessary to determine the required dosage. The role vitamin C plays in collagen formation may be the key to its action.

❑ Bioflavonoid supplementation prevents the breakdown of vitamin C in the body before it is metabolized. It also improves capillary integrity and stabilizes the collagen matrix by preventing free radical damage. The bioflavonoid rutin is known to help in lowering ocular pressure when used in conjunction with conventional drugs. Bilberry extract is particularly rich in this beneficial flavonoid compound. It is also good for diabetic retinopathy.

❑ Corticosteroids can induce glaucoma by destroying collagen structures in the eye. If you must take corticosteroids, you should take the smallest amount possible and for the shortest possible time. If you have glaucoma, you should avoid these medications entirely.

❑ There are many types of glaucoma medications available. Most are in eye drop form and are administered several times a day. Types of medications your doctor may prescribe include:

- Miotics, which increase the outflow of aqueous (liquid) from the eye. Examples include pilocarpine (Isopto Carpine, Pilopine, and others) and carbachol (Carboptic or Isopto Carbachol).

- Beta-blockers, which can reduce the amount of aqueous humor produced in the eye. Examples include betaxolol (Betoptic) and timolol (Timoptic-XE).

- Carbonic anhydrase inhibitors and alpha-adrenergic agonists, which also work to reduce the amount of aqueous humor. Examples include acetazolamide (Sequels, Diamox, and others) and dorzolamide (Trusopt).

- Prostaglandin analogs, which work near the drainage area of the eye to increase the secondary route of aqueous outflow to lower pressure. Travoprost (Travatan) is one such drug.

❑ Many of the same medications used to treat open-angle glaucoma are also used to treat closed-angle glaucoma. Several medications that help to reduce intraocular pressure can have potentially serious side effects, such as headaches or respiratory problems.

❑ Beta-blocking eye drops, which are often prescribed for people with glaucoma, have some undesirable side effects. Talk to your doctor if you experience any ill effects.

❑ Some laser surgery treatments are being used to improve fluid drainage in the eyes, frequently in conjunction with other medications. Other surgical procedures have a fairly high success rate, but are usually used only when traditional medications fail.

❑ The best way to prevent vision loss due to glaucoma is to receive regular eye exams from a qualified ophthalmologist—especially if you fall into one of the risk categories mentioned earlier in this section.

❑ For names and addresses of organizations that can provide additional information about glaucoma, *see* Health and Medical Organizations in the Appendix.

GLOMERULONEPHRITIS

See under KIDNEY DISEASE (RENAL FAILURE).

GOUT

Gout is a common type of arthritis that occurs when there is too much uric acid (sodium urate) in the blood, tissues, and urine. Uric acid is the end product of the metabolism of a class of chemicals known as purines. In people with gout, the body does not produce enough of the digestive enzyme uricase, which oxidizes relatively insoluble uric acid into a highly soluble compound. As a result, uric acid accumulates in the blood and tissues and, ultimately, crystallizes. When it crystallizes, uric acid takes on a shape like that of a needle and, like a needle, it jabs its way into the joints.

Uric acid seems to prefer the joint of the big toe, but other joints can be vulnerable as well, including the midfoot, ankle, knee, wrist, and even the fingers. Uric acid is more likely to crystallize at lower temperatures, which may explain why roughly 90 percent of gout attacks affect cooler extremities like the big toe.

Acute pain is usually the first symptom. Then the affected joints become inflamed, almost infected-looking—red, swollen, hot, and extremely sensitive to the touch. Repeated attacks of gout over a long period of time can lead to joint damage.

It should be noted that uric acid is not a fundamentally harmful substance, but a powerful antioxidant, almost as effective as vitamin C, that helps to protect cells from oxidative damage. It is only when levels become abnormally elevated that it becomes a problem. Elevated levels of uric acid in the blood can also be an indicator of poor kidney function.

Uric acid is a by-product of certain foods, so gout is closely related to diet. Obesity and an improper diet increase the risk of developing gout. Gout has been called the rich man's disease, since it is associated with too much rich food and alcohol. But in fact it affects people from all walks of life, most commonly men between the ages of forty and fifty. It may be inherited or brought on by crash dieting, drinking, certain medications, overeating, stress, surgery, or injury to a joint. Approximately 90 percent of the people who suffer from gout are male. Uric acid kidney stones may be a related problem.

Diagnosing gout can be difficult when the symptoms appear in the joints—several other diseases can mimic gout, including rheumatoid arthritis and infections. Pseudogout (false gout), another form of arthritis, produces joint inflammation, redness, and swelling in the larger joints (usually the knees, wrists, or ankles) caused by the development of calcium pyrophosphate dihydrate crystals in one or more joints. The best way to get a definitive diagnosis of gout is for a physician to insert a needle into the affected joint, remove some fluid, and examine the fluid under a microscope for the characteristic uric acid crystals.

NUTRIENTS

SUPPLEMENT	SUGGESTED DOSAGE	COMMENTS
Very Important		
Essential fatty acids (Kyolic-EPA from Wakunaga)	As directed on label. Take with meals.	Needed to repair tissues, aid in healing, and restore proper fatty acid balance. An excess of saturated fats is often behind this disorder.
Liquid Kyolic with B$_1$ and B$_{12}$ from Wakunaga	As directed on label.	Stress reducer. Antioxidant free radical quencher. Excellent for joint problems.
Proteolytic enzymes (Inf-zyme Forte from American Biologics)	2 capsules with meals and 2 capsules between meals.	Taking with meals improves digestion of protein; taking between meals reduces inflammation.
Vitamin B complex	100 mg of each major B vitamin twice daily (amounts of individual vitamins in a complex will vary).	Needed for proper digestion and all bodily enzyme systems.
plus extra vitamin B$_5$ (pantothenic acid) and	500 mg daily, in divided doses.	The antistress vitamin.
folic acid	400–800 mcg daily.	An important aid in nucleoprotein metabolism.
Vitamin C with bioflavonoids	3,000–5,000 mg daily, in divided doses.	Lowers serum uric acid levels.
Vitamin E	200 IU daily.	Improves circulation. Use d-alpha-tocopherol form.
Important		
Free form amino acid	As directed on label.	Uric acid production increases if essential amino acids are lacking. Use a supplement containing all the essential amino acids.
Kelp or alfalfa	1,000–1,500 mg daily.	Contains complete protein and vital minerals to reduce serum uric acid. *See* under Herbs, below.
Micellized Vitamin A and E from American Biologics	As directed on label.	Aids in reducing uric acid in the blood and is a potent antioxidant.
Potassium	99 mg daily.	Needed for proper mineral balance.
Pycnogenol or grape seed extract	As directed on label. As directed on label.	Powerful antioxidants.

Superoxide dismutase (SOD)	As directed on label, on an empty stomach (first thing in the morning is best). Take with a full glass of water.	An antioxidant and potent free radical destroyer.
Zinc	50–80 mg daily. Do not exceed a total of 100 mg daily from all supplements.	Important in protein metabolism and tissue repair. Use zinc gluconate lozenges or OptiZinc for best absorption.
Helpful		
Calcium and magnesium	1,500 mg daily. 750 mg daily.	To reduce stress caused by this disorder. Works well during sleep. Use chelate forms.
Glucosamine and chondroitin plus methylsulfonyl- methane (MSM)	As directed on label. As directed on label.	Important for joint tissue. Has anti-inflammatory and pain-relieving properties.
Sea cucumber (bêche-de-mer)	As directed on label.	Marine animals that have been used as an arthritis treatment in China for thousands of years.

Herbs

❑ Alfalfa is a good source of minerals and other nutrients that help to reduce serum uric acid. Take 2,000 to 3,000 milligrams daily in tablet or capsule form.

❑ Bilberry extract is a good source of anthocyanidins and proanthocyanidins—powerful antioxidant compounds.

❑ Boswellia and turmeric (curcumin) have powerful anti-inflammatory properties.

❑ Apply cayenne (capsicum) powder, mixed with enough wintergreen oil to make a paste, to affected areas to relieve inflammation and pain. This may cause a stinging sensation at first, but with repeated use, pain should diminish markedly. Cayenne can also be taken in capsule or liquid form.

❑ Celery seed extract contains numerous anti-inflammatory compounds.

❑ Try using chamomile, lady's mantle (yarrow), peppermint, or skullcap, in either capsule or tea form.

Caution: Do not use chamomile if you are allergic to ragweed. Do not use during pregnancy or nursing. It may interact with warfarin or cyclosporine, so patients using these drugs should avoid it.

❑ Devil's claw and yucca can aid in relieving pain.

❑ Other beneficial herbs include birch, burdock, colchicum tincture, hyssop, and juniper.

Recommendations

❑ When an attack of gout strikes, eat only raw fruits and vegetables—especially those rich in vitamin C—for two weeks. Juices are best. Frozen or fresh cherry juice is excellent. Also drink celery juice diluted with distilled water—use distilled water only, not tap water. Blueberries, cherries, and strawberries neutralize uric acid and have antioxidant properties, so eat lots of them. Also include grains, seeds, and nuts in your diet.

❑ Maintain a diet low in purines at all times. Purines are organic compounds that contribute to uric acid formation. Purine-rich foods to avoid include anchovies, mackerel, shellfish, asparagus, consommé, herring, meat gravies and broths, mushrooms, mussels, sardines, peanuts, baker's and brewer's yeast, mincemeat, and sweetbreads. Thyme and thyroid extracts can also pose a problem if taken for long periods of time.

❑ Enjoy foods like rice, millet, starchy vegetables, green vegetables, corn, cornbread, fruit, cheese, eggs, nuts, and milk.

❑ Consume plenty of quality water. Fluid intake promotes the excretion of uric acid.

❑ Eat no meat of any kind, including organ meats. Meat contains extremely high amounts of uric acid. Increase your intake of vegetarian protein sources.

❑ Consume no alcohol. Alcohol both increases the production of uric acid and reduces uric acid elimination. Beer and wine also contain yeast.

❑ Do not eat any fried foods, roasted nuts, or any other foods containing (or cooked with) oil that has been subjected to heat. When heated, oils become rancid. Rancid fats quickly destroy vitamin E, resulting in the release of increased amounts of uric acid.

❑ Avoid rich foods such as cakes and pies. Leave white flour and sugar products out of your diet.

❑ Avoid the amino acid glycine. Glycine can be converted into uric acid more rapidly in people who suffer from gout.

❑ Limit your intake of caffeine, cauliflower, dried beans, lentils, fish, eggs, oatmeal, peas, poultry, spinach, and yeast products.

❑ If you are overweight, lose the excess pounds and lower your serum uric acid levels. Avoid very restricted weight-loss diets (crash diets), however. Abruptly cutting back on foods or fasting for longer than three days may result in increased uric acid levels.

❑ Consider using homeopathic remedies. One helpful homeopathic regimen for gout involves using a combination of *Belladonna* for severe pain, *Arnica* for less intense pain, and *Rhus toxicodendron* for joint pain and itching. Use 33 to 123 strength and take one dose of each three times each day.

❑ Avoid taking high doses of niacin (over 50 milligrams daily).

Considerations

❑ Very few women develop gout. Most of those who do are in their seventies, when estrogen levels are low.

❑ Some people can have high levels of uric acid with no gout symptoms.

❑ Dimethylsulfoxide (DMSO) is helpful for flare-ups of gout. This oily liquid is applied topically and is reportedly very effective at relieving pain and reducing swelling.

❑ Treatment with honeybee venom has provided relief for some gout sufferers. In this practice, called apitherapy, honeybee venom is administered by injection, either with a hypodermic needle or by the bees themselves. The venom appears to act as both an anti-inflammatory and immune system stimulant.

❑ Deficiencies of certain nutrients can provoke an attack. A deficiency of pantothenic acid (vitamin B_5) produces excessive amounts of uric acid. A study in animals found that a diet deficient in vitamin A could produce gout. Vitamin E deficiency causes damage to the nuclei of cells that produce uric acid, causing more uric acid to form.

❑ New research from the *Archives of Internal Medicine* shows that getting 1,500 to 2,000 milligrams of vitamin C a day from food and supplements reduces the risk of gout by 45 percent.

❑ People who have candida infections, or who have taken antibiotics on and off for long periods, often have increased levels of uric acid in their blood.

❑ Because of the cellular destruction associated with chemotherapy in cancer treatment, uric acid is often released in extreme amounts, resulting in gouty arthritis.

❑ In rare cases, a secondary type of gout called saturnine gout can result from a toxic overload in the body.

❑ Allopurinol (Zyloprim), which inhibits uric acid synthesis, is often prescribed for gout. This drug has been linked directly to skin eruptions, inflammation of the blood vessels, and liver toxicity. If you have kidney problems, treatment with this drug should be carefully monitored.

❑ Colchicine, a drug derived from the autumn crocus (*Colchicum autumnale*), is used to both alleviate acute attacks and prevent further attacks from occurring. While often dramatically effective, this drug can cause serious side effects such as nausea and vomiting and toxicity, especially when taken in high doses and/or for prolonged periods.

❑ Other medications sometimes prescribed for gout are nonsteroidal anti-inflammatory drugs (NSAIDs) such as ibuprofen (Advil) and naproxen (Aleve).

❑ Cortisone is commonly prescribed for relief of acute attacks. However, this may put added strain on the adrenal glands, which are already under stress as a result of this painful disorder.

❑ For pseudogout, injections of NSAIDs and steroids directly into the joint may provide relief. Unfortunately, there is no thorough procedure to extract the calcium crystals that cause this condition.

❑ *See also* ARTHRITIS in Part Two and PAIN CONTROL in Part Three.

GRAVES' DISEASE

See under HYPERTHYROIDISM.

GROWTH PROBLEMS

Growth problems usually occur when the pituitary gland fails to function as it should. The pituitary gland distributes hormones, including the growth hormone somatotropin, to various parts of the body. Somatotropin stimulates the growth of muscle and bone in growing children.

Either overproduction or underproduction of this hormone can cause growth abnormalities. The secretion of too little growth hormone by the pituitary causes dwarfism; too much causes the body to grow in an exaggerated fashion, resulting in abnormally large hands, feet, and jaw. Some cases of malfunction of the pituitary are caused by the growth of a tumor on the gland.

In some cases, growth problems are caused by the failure of the thyroid gland to function properly. The thymus gland may also be involved. If the thymus gland of an infant is damaged, development can be retarded. The child can then develop a greater than normal susceptibility to infection. Nutrition can also play a significant role in the growth and development of a child.

Dwarfism is a condition characterized by abnormally short stature. In some cases, individuals are very small, but normally proportioned; in others, the limbs are short as compared to the size of the rest of the body. Causes of dwarfism include unrecognized or untreated congenital hypothyroidism (once known as cretinism), Down syndrome, achondroplasia, hypochondroplasia, and spinal tuberculosis.

Achondroplasia is a primary bone disorder caused by chemical changes within a single gene. People with achondroplasia have large heads and arms and legs that are short in comparison with the length of the trunk. They usually also have a large forehead, a flat area between the eyes, and a protruding jaw. Often, the teeth are crowded together. In most cases, intelligence is normal, although motor development may occur a bit more slowly than normal. Both children and adults with achondroplasia must be particularly attentive to diet and nutrition, as obesity can be a problem. People with achondroplasia are at greater than normal risk for a number of other health problems, including certain neurolgic and respiratory problems, orthopedic problems, fatigue, and numbness or pain in the lower back and thighs.

Congenital hypothyroidism is a condition characterized by the absence of sufficient quantities of thyroxine, a hormone secreted by the thyroid gland. In most cases, this is a result of the absence of a thyroid gland, an inborn defect. If congenital hypothyroidism is not detected and treated within a very short time, a number of developmental abnormalities may result, including short stature, disproportionately short arms and legs, coarse hair, and mental retardation.

Gigantism is a growth disorder characterized by an abnormally great height, usually due to excessive cartilage and bone formation at the ends of the long bones. Pituitary gigantism is the most common form of this condition. It is a result of the pituitary gland secreting excessive amounts of growth hormone. (For further information, *see* GIGANTISM *under* RARE DISORDERS in Part Two.)

Nutritional imbalances, delayed puberty, obesity, and certain diseases (including congenital heart disorders and chronic kidney failure) can be other factors involved in growth problems. If you are concerned about your child's growth rate, you should have him or her examined by an endocrinologist to determine if there is a problem and, if so, what the exact nature of the problem is. It is important to remember that some people are just naturally shorter or taller than average.

Unless otherwise specified, the dosages recommended here are for adults and teenagers over age seventeen. For children between ages twelve and seventeen, use three-quarters of the recommended amount. For children between six and twelve, use half the recommended dose. For children under six, use a quarter of the recommended dose.

NUTRIENTS

SUPPLEMENT	SUGGESTED DOSAGE	COMMENTS
Very Important		
Alfalfa		*See* under Herbs, below.
Cod liver oil	As directed on label.	Contains vitamins A and D, needed for proper growth and for strong tissues and bones.
Essential fatty acid complex or primrose oil	As directed on label. As directed on label.	For normal growth.
Kelp	As directed on label.	Contains natural iodine. An iodine deficiency can cause growth problems.
L-lysine	As directed on label, on an empty stomach. Take with water or juice. Do not take with milk. Take with 50 mg vitamin B$_6$ and 100 mg vitamin C for better absorption.	Needed for normal growth and bone development. (*See* AMINO ACIDS in Part One.) *Caution:* Do not take this supplement for longer than six months at a time.
Zinc	As directed on label. Do not exceed a total of 100 mg daily from all supplements.	Deficiency has been linked to growth problems. Use zinc gluconate lozenges or OptiZinc for best absorption.
Important		
Calcium and magnesium	As directed on label. As directed on label.	Needed for normal bone growth.
Free form amino acid	As directed on label.	Deficiency has been linked to growth disorders.
Raw pituitary glandular	As directed on label.	For children. Stimulates growth.
Helpful		
Bio-Bifidus from American Biologics	As directed on label.	For bowel flora replacement to improve assimilation and elimination.
L-ornithine	As directed by physician.	Helps to promote release of growth hormone. Use only under a physician's supervision.
Multiglandular complex	As directed on label.	For the endocrine, hormonal, and enzyme systems.
Vitamin B complex	50 mg of each major B vitamin daily (amounts of individual vitamins in a complex will vary).	B vitamins work best when taken together.
plus extra vitamin B$_6$ (pyridoxine)	50 mg 3 times daily, with meals.	Needed for uptake of the amino acids and for proper growth.

Herbs

❑ Alfalfa is a valuable source of vitamins, minerals, and other nutrients that promote the proper functioning of the pituitary gland. It can be taken in tablet or capsule form, as well as eaten in a natural form such as alfalfa sprouts.

Recommendations

❑ Eat a well-balanced diet high in healthful sources of protein. Protein is necessary for growth.

❑ Include in the diet foods high in the amino acid arginine. Arginine is used by the body to synthesize another amino acid, ornithine, which promotes the release of growth hormone. Good food sources of arginine include carob, coconut, dairy products, gelatin, oats, peanuts, soybeans, walnuts, wheat, and wheat germ.

Considerations

❑ When evaluating a child's growth, it is the overall growth pattern, rather than size, that is important. If a child seems to "fall off" a previously steady growth curve, he or she should be evaluated for possible nutritional deficiencies and other underlying health problems.

❑ There is currently no treatment to promote growth in people with achondroplasia. Therapy is directed toward prevention and treatment of complications.

❑ Surgery is now being performed on an experimental basis to lengthen the arms and legs of those with achondroplasia. It is an arduous procedure, often involving many complications.

❑ The addition of iodine to public drinking water supplies has shown a decrease in the occurrence of neonatal and congenital hypothyroidism in some areas of the United States.

❏ If growth is slowed because of insufficient growth hormone production, a doctor may prescribe growth hormone therapy.

❏ If growth problems are the result of a tumor of the pituitary gland, surgical removal or treatment of the tumor with drugs or by other means may be recommended.

❏ Kwashiorkor is a protein deficiency disorder that causes children to grow slowly and have very little resistance to disease. It is most common among very poor people in developing countries. However, it can occur anywhere if a child's protein requirements are not met over a period of time. If detected early, it can be treated. Malabsorption syndromes, such as that associated with celiac disease, can cause similar problems even though nutritional intake appears to be adequate.

❏ High levels of lead, a toxic metal, may cause growth problems. A hair analysis can be done to rule out this metal toxicity. (*See* LEAD POISONING in Part Two and HAIR ANALYSIS in Part Three.)

❏ A large amount of research is being done on growth problems. Interestingly, some studies have indicated that shorter people may live longer than people of average height.

❏ *See also* HYPERTHYROIDISM and HYPOTHYROIDISM in Part Two.

GUM DISEASE

See under PERIODONTAL DISEASE. *See also* BLEEDING GUMS under PREGNANCY-RELATED PROBLEMS.

HAIR LOSS

Baldness or loss of hair is referred to as *alopecia*. *Alopecia totalis* means loss of all the scalp hair. *Alopecia universalis* means loss of all body hair, including eyebrows and eyelashes. If hair falls out in patches, it is termed *alopecia areata*. This condition is usually temporary and rarely leads to baldness. Factors that are involved in hair loss include heredity, hormones, and aging. Researchers have yet to determine the exact cause of hair loss, but some scientists believe the body's immune system mistakes hair follicles for foreign tissue and attacks them. Many suspect a genetic component.

A less dramatic, but more prevalent, type of hair loss is *androgenetic alopecia* (AGA), or male pattern baldness. AGA is common in men. As the name implies, a genetic or hereditary predisposition to the disorder and the presence of androgens—male sex hormones—are involved in this condition. Research indicates that the hair follicles of individuals susceptible to AGA may have receptors programmed to slow down or shut off hair production under the influence of androgens.

Women sometimes have the same type of hair loss, but it is not usually as extensive and most often does not occur until after menopause. All women experience some hair thinning as they grow older, especially after menopause, but in some it begins as early as puberty. In addition, most women lose some hair two or three months after having a baby because hormonal changes prevent normal hair loss during pregnancy.

A species of tiny mite, *Demodex follicularum*, may be the cause of, or a contributing factor to, balding. These mites are present in virtually all hair follicles by the time a person reaches middle age, and in most cases cause no harm. Researchers believe that the difference between people who lose their hair and those who do not may lie in how the scalp reacts to the presence of these mites. If the body initiates the inflammatory response as it tries to reject the mites, this may close down the hair follicles, thus killing the mites but also killing the hair.

In addition to heredity, factors that promote hair loss include poor circulation, acute illness, surgery, radiation exposure, skin disease, sudden weight loss, high fever, iron deficiency, diabetes, thyroid disease, drugs such as those used in chemotherapy, stress, poor diet, ringworm and other fungal infections, chemicals such as hair dyes, and vitamin deficiencies.

NUTRIENTS

SUPPLEMENT	SUGGESTED DOSAGE	COMMENTS
Very Important		
Essential fatty acids (flaxseed oil, Kyolic-EPA from Wakunaga, primrose oil, or salmon oil)	As directed on label.	Improves hair texture. Prevents dry, brittle hair.
Raw thymus glandular	500 mg daily.	Stimulates immune function and improves functioning capacity of glands. *Caution:* Do not give this supplement to a child.
Ultra Hair from Nature's Plus	As directed on label.	Contains nutrients necessary to stimulate hair growth. If the condition is not severe, you can use this complex alone.
Vitamin B complex with		B vitamins are important for the health and growth of the hair.
vitamin B₃ (niacin) and	50 mg 3 times daily.	
vitamin B₅ (pantothenic acid) and	50 mg 3 times daily.	
vitamin B₆ (pyridoxine) plus extra	50 mg 3 times daily.	
biotin and	300 mcg daily. Also use hair care products containing biotin.	Deficiencies have been linked to skin disorders and hair loss.
inositol and	100 mg twice daily.	Vital for hair growth.
methylsulfonyl-methane (MSM)	As directed on label.	Aids with the manufacture of keratin, a protein that is the major component of hair.

Vitamin C with bioflavonoids	3,000–10,000 mg daily.	Aids in improving scalp circulation. Helps with the antioxidant action in hair follicles.
Vitamin E	200 IU daily, or 400 IU every other day.	Increases oxygen uptake, which improves circulation to the scalp. Improves health and growth of hair. Use d-alpha-tocopherol form.
Zinc	50–100 mg daily. Do not exceed this amount.	Stimulates hair growth by enhancing immune function. Use zinc gluconate lozenges or OptiZinc for best absorption.
Important		
Coenzyme Q10 plus Coenzyme A from Coenzyme-A Technologies	60 mg daily. As directed on label.	Improves scalp circulation. Increases tissue oxygenation.
Dimethylglycine (DMG) (Aangamik DMG from FoodScience of Vermont)	100 mg daily.	Good for circulation to the scalp.
Kelp	500 mg daily.	Supplies needed minerals for proper hair growth.
Helpful		
Copper	3 mg daily.	Works with zinc to aid in hair growth. Use a chelate form.
Dioxychlor	5 drops in water twice daily.	Destroys harmful bacteria and supplies oxygen to the tissues.
Grape seed extract	As directed on label.	A powerful antioxidant to protect hair follicles from free radical damage.
L-cysteine and L-methionine plus glutathione	500 mg each twice daily, on an empty stomach. Take with water or juice. Do not take with milk. Take with 50 mg vitamin B6 and 100 mg vitamin C for better absorption.	Improves quality, texture, and growth of hair. Helps prevent hair from falling out, and also promotes blood supply to the scalp. (*See* AMINO ACIDS in Part One.)
Methylsulfonyl-methane (MSM)	As directed on label.	Required for the building blocks of protein, which provides stronger hair.
Silica (Body Essential Silica gel from NatureWorks or JarroSil from Jarrow Formulas).	As directed on label.	Aids in hair growth and also makes the hair stronger.

Herbs

❑ Use apple cider vinegar and sage tea as a rinse to help hair grow.

❑ Ginkgo biloba improves circulation to the scalp.

❑ Green tea, pygeum, and saw palmetto may aid in reducing hair loss in men.

❑ Tea tree oil combats bacteria and mites that may cause hair loss. Massage 10 drops into the scalp, then shampoo your hair in the usual fashion.

Recommendations

❑ Eat a diet high in fruits and vegetables and low in starch. This may help to slow down the process of hair loss. Fruits and vegetables contain flavonoids, many of which are antioxidants that may provide protection for the hair follicles and encourage hair growth.

❑ Eat plenty of foods high in biotin and/or take supplemental biotin as recommended under Nutrients in this entry. Biotin is needed for healthy hair and skin, and may even prevent hair loss in some men. Good food sources of biotin include brewer's yeast, brown rice, bulgur, green peas, lentils, oats, soybeans, sunflower seeds, and walnuts.

Caution: Brewer's yeast can cause an allergic reaction in some individuals. Start with a small amount at first, and discontinue use if any allergic symptoms occur.

❑ Include soy foods such as soybeans, tempeh, and tofu in your diet. Soy foods appear to inhibit the formation of dihydrotestosterone, a hormone implicated in the process of hair loss.

❑ Do not eat foods containing raw eggs. Raw eggs not only pose a risk of *Salmonella* infection (*see* FOODBORNE/ WATERBORNE DISEASE in Part Two), but are high in avidin, a protein that binds to biotin and prevents it from being absorbed. Cooked eggs are acceptable.

❑ Lie head down on a slant board fifteen minutes a day to allow the blood to reach your scalp. Massage your scalp daily.

❑ Use shampoos and conditioners that contain biotin and silica. Aloe vera gel, vitamins C and E, and jojoba oils also are very good for the hair. Conditioners containing chamomile, marigold, ginseng, and/or passionflower help to keep hair healthy as well.

❑ Be careful of using products that are not natural on the hair. Allergic reactions to chemicals in these products occur frequently. Alternate among several different hair care products, using only all-natural and pH-balanced formulas. Most health food stores carry a variety of natural hair care products.

❑ Hair is fragile when it is wet. Gently pat your hair dry and squeeze out remaining moisture with a towel.

❑ Cover your hair when it is exposed to sunlight. Long exposure to sunlight and seawater can damage the hair.

❑ Avoid rough treatment. Do not use a brush or fine-toothed comb, or towel-dry your hair. Also, do not use a blow-dryer or other heated appliances on your hair; let it dry naturally. Do not comb your hair until it is dry, as wet hair tends to break off. Use a pick to put wet hair in place. Do not wear tight ponytails, cornrows, or other styles that pull on the hair.

❑ Avoid crash diets and diets that neglect any of the food groups. These can cause deficiencies in nutrients that are detrimental to the hair.

❑ If you are losing large amounts of hair, see a physician.

Considerations

❑ It is normal to lose 50 to 100 hairs a day.

❑ Taking large doses of vitamin A (100,000 IU or more daily) for a long period can trigger hair loss, but stopping the vitamin A will reverse the problem. Often the hair grows back when the cause is corrected.

❑ Pregnancy, a high concentration of metals in the body, and autoimmune diseases can sometimes cause hair loss.

❑ Hypothyroidism can cause hair loss. (*See* HYPOTHYROIDISM in Part Two.)

❑ Hair transplantation can be a very successful treatment for hair loss if you have enough of your own hair to graft onto the bald area. Make sure to find a physician skilled in the technique if you decide to pursue a hair transplant.

❑ Rogaine, a topical solution containing 5 percent minoxidil, has been approved by the FDA for the treatment of male pattern baldness. Five percent minoxidil topical solution is not intended for frontal baldness or receding hairline. This product is available over the counter in drugstores. There is also a 2 percent minoxidil solution available for women. Rogaine may cause heart changes if used for long periods of time. Read the warning label on the box carefully and tell your doctor if you have heart disease. Also, although using minoxidil does result in hair growth, the quality of the hair is usually poor and hair growth ceases when use is discontinued.

❑ Finasteride (Propecia), a prescription medication, is said to be effective for younger men with male pattern baldness who have at least half of their hair remaining. It usually takes at least three months to be effective, and results last only as long as the medication is continued.

❑ In some people with alopecia areata, cortisone injections into the hairless patches of the head can trigger hair growth. Anthralin (Dritho-Scalp) cream, applied to the scalp and washed off after an hour, can sometimes stimulate hair growth after a few months of use. For extensive alopecia areata, a treatment called psoralen plus ultraviolet A radiation therapy, abbreviated PUVA, may be recommended. It involves the administration of light-sensitizing medication followed by exposure to ultraviolet-A light rays. In clinical trials, approximately 55 percent of people achieve cosmetically acceptable hair growth using this method. However, the relapse rate is high, and patients must go to a treatment center where the equipment is available at least two to three times per week. Furthermore, the treatment carries the risk of developing skin cancer.

❑ Research conducted at Cornell University suggests that gene therapy may someday be used to stimulate hair growth. Researchers discovered that hair follicles that have genetically been "turned off" can, in effect, be "turned on" again.

❑ For names and addresses of organizations that can provide more information on treatments for alopecia areata, *see* Health and Medical Organizations in the Appendix.

HALITOSIS (BAD BREATH)

Halitosis is typically caused by poor dental hygiene. However, other factors may be involved, including gum disease, tooth decay, heavy metal buildup, infection of the respiratory tract (throat, lungs, nose, and windpipe), improper diet, constipation, smoking, fever, diabetes, foreign bacteria in the mouth, indigestion, inadequate protein digestion, liver or kidney malfunction, postnasal drip, stress, and too much unfriendly bacteria in the colon. Halitosis can also be caused by a buildup of toxins in the gastrointestinal tract, salivary gland disorders, chronic bronchitis, sinusitis, or diabetes. Dieting, alcohol abuse, or fasting can cause bad breath as well. "Morning breath" results from dehydration and a reduction in the amount of saliva, which is needed to wash away bacteria in the mouth. Dieters and people who are fasting may experience bad breath because the lack of food causes the body to break down stored fat called ketones and protein for fuel; metabolic wastes resulting from that process have an unpleasant odor as they are exhaled from the lungs.

NUTRIENTS

SUPPLEMENT	SUGGESTED DOSAGE	COMMENTS
Very Important		
ABC Aerobic Bulk Cleanse from Aerobic Life Industries or oat bran or psyllium husks or rice bran	1 tbsp in juice or water twice daily, on an empty stomach. Take separately from other supplements and medications.	For needed fiber. Fiber removes toxins from the colon that can result in bad breath.
Chlorophyll (alfalfa liquid, wheatgrass, or barley juice are good sources) or	1 tbsp in juice twice daily. Chlorophyll can also be used as a mouth rinse— add 1 tbsp to ½ glass of water.	"Green drinks" are one of the best ways to combat bad breath.
Kyo-Green from Wakunaga	As directed on label.	Contains chlorophyll to cleanse the body of toxins.
Vitamin C with bioflavonoids	2,000–6,000 mg daily.	Important in healing mouth and gum disease and in preventing bleeding gums. Also rids the body of excess mucus and toxins that can cause bad breath.
Important		
Acidophilus (Kyo-Dophilus from Wakunaga)	As directed on label. Take on an empty stomach.	Needed to replenish "friendly" bacteria in the colon. Insufficient "friendly" bacteria and an overabundance of harmful bacteria can cause bad breath.
Garlic (Kyolic from Wakunaga)	2 capsules 4 times daily, with meals and at bedtime.	Acts as a natural antibiotic, destroying foreign bacteria in both the mouth and colon. Use an odorless form.

Zinc	30 mg 3 times daily. Do not exceed 100 mg daily.	Has an antibacterial effect and neutralizes sulfur compounds, a common cause of mouth odor.
Helpful		
Bee propolis	As directed on label.	Aids in healing the gums, aids control of infection in the body, and has an antibacterial effect.
Vitamin A plus carotenoid complex	15,000 IU daily. If you are pregnant, do not exceed 10,000 IU daily.	Needed for control of infection and in healing of the mouth.
Vitamin B complex	100 mg of each major B vitamin daily (amounts of individual vitamins in a complex will vary).	Needed for proper digestion.
plus extra vitamin B$_3$ (niacin)	50 mg 3 times daily. Do not exceed this amount.	Dilates tiny capillaries to help blood flow to infection sites. *Caution:* Do not take niacin if you have a liver disorder, gout, or high blood pressure.
and vitamin B$_6$ (pyridoxine)	50 mg daily.	Needed for all enzyme systems in the body.

Herbs

❑ Alfalfa supplies chlorophyll, which cleanses the bloodstream and colon, where bad breath often begins. Take 500 to 1,000 mg in tablet form or 1 tablespoon of liquid in juice or water three times daily.

❑ Gum disease is a major factor in bad breath. If infection is present, place alcohol-free goldenseal extract on a small piece of cotton and place the cotton over infected gums or mouth sores. Do this for two hours per day for three days. It should quickly heal the infected parts.

Caution: Do not take goldenseal internally on a daily basis for more than one week at a time. Do not use during pregnancy or if you are breast-feeding, and use with caution if you are allergic to ragweed. If you have a history of cardiovascular disease, diabetes, or glaucoma, use it only under a doctor's supervision.

❑ Use myrrh (to brush your teeth and rinse your mouth), peppermint, rosemary, and sage.

Caution: Do not use sage if you suffer from any type of seizure disorder, or are pregnant or nursing.

❑ Chewing a sprig of parsley after meals is an excellent treatment for bad breath. Parsley is rich in chlorophyll, the active ingredient in many popular breath mints.

❑ Other herbs that may be helpful for bad breath include anise, cloves, and fennel.

Recommendations

❑ Go on a five-day raw foods diet. After the fast, eat at least 50 percent of your food raw every day. This is a good routine diet to adhere to on an ongoing basis.

❑ Drink generous amounts of quality water.

❑ Avoid spicy foods, whose odors can linger for hours. Foods like anchovies, blue cheese, Camembert, garlic, onions, pastrami, pepperoni, Roquefort cheese, salami, and tuna leave oils in the mouth that can release odor for up to twenty-four hours, no matter how much you brush or gargle. Beer, coffee, whiskey, and wine leave residues that stick to the soft, sticky plaque on teeth and get into the digestive system. Each exhalation releases their odor back into the air.

❑ Avoid foods that get stuck between the teeth easily or that cause tooth decay, such as meat, stringy vegetables, and sweets, especially sticky sweets.

❑ Go on a cleansing fast with fresh lemon juice and water to detoxify the system. (*See* FASTING in Part Three.)

❑ Brush your teeth *and tongue* after every meal.

❑ Use a tongue scraper to help remove bacterial plaque and shed dead cells and food debris from the surface of the tongue.

❑ Replace your toothbrush every month, as well as after any infectious illness, to prevent bacteria buildup.

❑ Use dental floss and a chlorophyll mouthwash daily. Use a small brush or rubber-tipped dental tool in between teeth to remove any remaining food after you have flossed.

❑ Use Stim-U-Dent wooden toothpicks, available in most drugstores, after every meal to massage between the teeth and remove plaque. This is important for the prevention of gum disease.

❑ Keep your toothbrush clean. Between uses, store it in hydrogen peroxide or grapefruit seed extract to kill germs (if using hydrogen peroxide, rinse it well before brushing). There are bacteria-destroying toothbrush sanitizers available that turn on automatically at intervals throughout the day.

❑ Do not use commercial mouthwashes. Most contain nothing more than flavoring, dye, and alcohol. While they may kill the bacteria that cause bad breath, the bacteria soon return in greater force. Mouthwashes can also irritate the gums, tongue, and mucous membranes in the mouth.

❑ Have your teeth professionally cleaned every six months.

❑ Bad breath may be a sign of an underlying health problem. Consult your health care provider for a thorough checkup if the suggestions in this section do not improve the condition.

Considerations

❑ *See also* PERIODONTAL DISEASE; SINUSITIS; and/or SORE THROAT in Part Two.

HAMBURGER DISEASE

See HEMORRHAGIC COLITIS *under* RARE DISORDERS.

HAY FEVER

Hay fever (allergic rhinitis) is an allergy to proteins in the pollen of trees, grasses, some plants, or mold that affects the mucous membranes of the nose, eyes, and air passages. Symptoms include itchy, red eyes; watery discharge from the nose and eyes; sneezing; fatigue; and nervous irritability. Many of the symptoms of hay fever are similar to those of the common cold. However, allergies cause a distinctive clear, thin nasal discharge, whereas secretions caused by colds usually become thick and yellow-greenish as the illness progresses. Also, colds are often associated with mild fever and are usually gone within a week, while allergy sufferers often have a feeling of being "wiped out" for weeks on end.

At least 50 million Americans suffer from the seasonal sneezes, runny nose, and itchy eyes that come with hay fever. There are actually three hay fever seasons, distinguished by the different types of pollen present at different times. Tree pollens appear first, usually between February and May, depending on the local climate. The biggest problems come later in spring and in summer, when trees, weeds, and grass pollens—and people—are out at the same time. The fall is ragweed pollen season. Depending on which pollen or pollens an individual is allergic to, hay fever may be present at any or all of these times. Following is a more detailed summary of the types of plants according to the times of year they are most likely to cause problems (again, blooming times are somewhat approximate, as they depend on the climate where you live):

- February through May: Alder, hazelnut, and elm trees.
- March through June: Birch, maple, and oak trees.
- April through June: Beech and spruce trees.
- April through August: Horse chestnut trees.
- April through September: Asters, pine trees, plantain, sorrel, stinging nettle, and various grasses.
- May through July: Buttercups.
- June through September: Goosefoot.
- July through September: Mugwort.

People who suffer from hay fever often also suffer from other so-called *atopic disorders,* such as asthma and dermatitis. Those who suffer from hay fever symptoms throughout the year are said to have *perennial rhinitis.* Animal hair, dust, feathers, fungus spores, molds, and/or some other environmental agent may trigger the symptoms. A susceptibility to hay fever tends to be inherited.

People who are prone to allergies are most often aware of the time of year and conditions under which they are most sensitive. For a definitive diagnosis, the radioallergosorbent (RAST) test is easily done and gives reliable results.

The nutrient program outlined below is beneficial for hay fever. Hay fever sufferers should always choose hy-poallergenic supplements. Unless otherwise specified, the dosages recommended here are for adults. For children between the ages of twelve and seventeen, reduce the dose to three-quarters the recommended amount. For children between six and twelve, use one-half the recommended dose, and for children under the age of six, use one-quarter the recommended amount.

NUTRIENTS

SUPPLEMENT	SUGGESTED DOSAGE	COMMENTS
Very Important		
Bromelain (Ultra Bromelain from Nature's Plus)	1,000 mg 3 times daily, between meals.	Reduces inflammation associated with hay fever symptoms.
Coenzyme Q$_{10}$	30 mg twice daily.	Improves oxygenation and immunity.
Quercetin	400 mg twice daily, before meals.	A bioflavonoid that stabilizes the membranes of the cells that release histamine, which triggers allergic symptoms.
or Activated Quercetin from Source Naturals	As directed on label.	Contains quercetin plus bromelain and vitamin C for better absorption.
or Anti-Allergy formula from Freeda Vitamins	As directed on label.	A combination of quercetin, calcium pantothenate, and calcium ascorbate.
Raw thymus glandular plus adrenal glandular	500 mg twice daily. As directed on label.	To promote immune function. *Caution:* Do not give these supplements to a child under sixteen years of age.
Vitamin A with mixed carotenoids	25,000 IU daily. If you are pregnant, do not exceed 10,000 IU daily.	Powerful immunostimulants. An emulsion form is recommended for easier assimilation and greater safety at high doses.
Vitamin B complex plus extra vitamin B$_5$ (pantothenic acid) and vitamin B$_6$ (pyridoxine)	As directed on label. 100 mg 3 times daily. 50 mg twice daily.	All B vitamins are necessary for proper functioning of the immune system. Use hypoallergenic formulas.
Vitamin C with bioflavonoids	3,000–10,000 mg 3 times daily.	A potent immunostimulant and anti-inflammatory. Use an esterified or buffered form.
Important		
Proteolytic enzymes	As directed on label. Take with meals and between meals.	Necessary for digestion of essential nutrients that boost immune function. *Caution:* Do not give this supplement to a child.
Zinc	50–80 mg daily. Do not exceed a total of 100 mg daily from all supplements.	Boosts immune function. Use zinc gluconate lozenges or OptiZinc for best absorption.
Helpful		
Aller Bee-Gone from CC Pollen	As directed on label.	A combination of herbs, enzymes, and nutrients to fight acute symptoms.

Calcium and magnesium	1,500 mg daily. 1,000 mg daily.	Minerals that have a calming effect on the system.
Dioxychlor or Aerobic 07	5 drops in water twice daily. Also use topically: Mix 30 drops in 2 oz water and instill 1 dropperful in each nostril. As directed on label.	To supply stabilized oxygen and fight bacteria, fungi, and viruses.
Garlic (Kyolic from Wakunaga)	As directed on label.	Helpful for sinus inflammation. Use a liquid formula.
Kelp	As directed on label twice daily.	A rich source of minerals.
Manganese	10–30 mg daily. Take separately from calcium.	Aids in metabolism of vitamins, minerals, enzymes, and carbohydrates.
Pycnogenol or grape seed extract	As directed on label. As directed on label.	Powerful free radical scavengers that also act as anti-inflammatories and enhance the activity of vitamin C.
Superoxide dismutase (SOD) (Cell Guard from Biotec Foods)	As directed on label.	A powerful antioxidant.
Vitamin E	200 IU daily or 400 IU every other day.	Boosts the immune system. Use d-alpha-tocopherol form.

Herbs

❑ Alfalfa supplies chlorophyll and vitamin K. Use a liquid form. Take 1 tablespoon in juice or water twice daily.

❑ For red, itchy eyes, place slices of cool cucumber over the eyes. Rotate this treatment with steeped, cooled black tea bags placed directly on the eyelids.

❑ Eucalyptus oil can relieve congestion if used in a steam inhalation (see STEAM INHALATION in Part Three) or added to bathwater.

❑ Alcohol-free eyebright and lady's mantle (yarrow) liquid extracts are good for relieving hay fever symptoms. Use 20 to 30 drops two times daily to make a tea or place the extract under your tongue and hold it there for a few minutes before swallowing. Drink a glass of water after you take the extract.

❑ If your throat is itchy or you feel a need to cough, use alcohol-free goldenseal extract. Hold a dropperful in your mouth for a few minutes, then swallow. This will halt a sore throat.

Caution: Do not take goldenseal internally on a daily basis for more than one week at a time. Do not use it during pregnancy or if you are breast-feeding, and use with caution if you are allergic to ragweed. If you have a history of cardiovascular disease, diabetes, or glaucoma, use it only under a doctor's supervision.

❑ Horehound, mullein leaf, stinging nettle, and/or wild cherry bark help to ward off severe allergic reactions.

❑ Use turmeric to reduce inflammation.

❑ Nettle leaf is very good for all types of allergies.

❑ Noni juice aids in relieving symptoms of hay fever.

Recommendations

❑ The best defense against hay fever is to try to avoid the substance that is causing your allergies. Following are some tips to help you avoid contact with pollen:

• When allergy season arrives, spend as little time as possible outdoors, particularly after 10:00 A.M. Grasses generally pollinate in midday, and the wind keeps the pollen floating until it drops to the ground at night.

• Try to avoid working in the yard. If you must do so, wear a mask and goggles to keep the pollen from getting into your eyes.

• Keep windows and doors shut during your local blossoming season. Use air conditioning if possible.

• Keep all car windows closed while driving. Use your car air conditioner instead.

• Shower thoroughly, wash your hair, and change your clothes when you come indoors after spending time outside to remove pollen collected during the day. Pollen can stick to your hair, skin, and clothing, especially on a windy day. A shower before bedtime is also a good idea.

• Have your lawn mown regularly—before the grass flowers.

• Avoid placing laundry outdoors to dry, as the pollen collects on the surface of fabrics.

• Keep pets either inside or outside. Dogs and cats can pick up pollen on their fur and bring it indoors with them.

❑ Eat more fruits (especially bananas), vegetables, grains, and raw nuts and seeds. Stay on a high-fiber diet.

❑ If you enjoy the flavor of horseradish, use it liberally. Horseradish is good for a runny nose and congestion.

❑ Eat yogurt or any soured products three times a week. Homemade yogurt is best. However, beware of the possibility that you may be allergic to casein, the principal protein found in milk.

❑ Consume no cakes, chocolate, coffee, dairy products (except yogurt), packaged or canned foods, pies, soft drinks, sugar, tobacco, white flour products, or any junk food.

❑ Avoid tobacco smoke, which irritates the lungs and eyes, and alcohol, which increases the production of mucus.

❑ Consider using homeopathic remedies. *Sabadilla* is good for watery eyes, runny nose, and a dry throat. Another good choice for these symptoms is *Wyethia*.

❑ Perform a cleansing fast. (See FASTING in Part Three.)

❏ Try using a good-quality air purifier and filter in your home. The Air Supply personal air purifier from Wein Products is a miniature unit that is worn around the neck. It sets up an invisible pure air shield against microorganisms (such as viruses, bacteria, and mold) and microparticles (including dust, pollen, and pollutants) in the air. It also eliminates vapors, smells, and harmful volatile compounds in the air.

Considerations

❏ The best and safest way to control allergies is the natural way—by avoiding allergens and taking steps to normalize immune function and prevent or lessen the symptoms. Allergies can usually be controlled if you are willing to make changes in your lifestyle, diet, and mental state.

❏ A study conducted at the University of California–Davis found that eating yogurt every day significantly reduced the incidence of hay fever attacks, especially those triggered by grass pollens.

❏ If you are a man with facial hair, cleaning your mustache and/or beard with soap and water or shampoo twice a day will cut down on the symptoms associated with hay fever.

❏ Researchers at Giessen University in Germany found that three bananas contain enough magnesium—180 milligrams—to quell a hay fever attack. Other foods rich in magnesium are kidney beans, soybeans, almonds, lima beans, whole wheat flour, brown rice, molasses, and peas. Magnesium can also be taken in supplement form.

❏ Antihistamines are the most commonly recommended conventional treatment for hay fever. They can reduce itching in the eyes, ears, and throat; dry up a runny nose; and reduce sneezing attacks. However, they can also cause drowsiness, depression, and other side effects. Antihistamines such as fexofenadine (Allegra) and loratidine (Claritin) do not cause drowsiness and depression. But they are expensive and they might not work for everyone. Do not take these with grapefruit juice.

❏ Some physicians recommend desensitization shots for people with hay fever. These are expensive, painful, and not risk-free. And a disappointingly low percentage of people experience satisfactory relief, even after years of injections. The typical person requires weekly shots for up to a year and monthly shots for up to five years, at a total cost that can run into thousands of dollars.

❏ The following types of treatments are available for hay fever sufferers: antihistamines, decongestants, topical corticosteroids, leukotriene antagonists, immunotherapy, and surgery (for those with structural problems in which airways are open, making medications ineffective). Unfortunately, most of these treatments have drawbacks. You should consider them only if your symptoms substantially interfere with the quality of your daily life.

❏ *See also* ALLERGIES in Part Two and ASCORBIC ACID FLUSH in Part Three.

HEADACHE

Virtually everyone gets a headache at one time or another. Headaches are as common—and as difficult to cure—as the common cold and flu. Common causes of headache include stress; tension; anxiety; allergies; constipation; coffee consumption; eyestrain; hunger; sinus pressure; muscle tension; hormonal imbalances; temporomandibular joint (TMJ) syndrome; trauma to the head; nutritional deficiencies; the use of alcohol, drugs, or tobacco; fever; and exposure to irritants such as pollution, perfume, or aftershave lotions. (*See* Types of Headaches on page 470.) Migraines result from a disturbance in the blood circulation in the head. (*See* MIGRAINE in Part Two.)

Headache experts estimate that about 90 percent of all headaches are tension headaches and 6 percent are migraines. Tension headaches, as the name implies, are caused by muscular tension. Another type of headache is the cluster headache. These are severe, recurring headaches that strike about 1 million Americans, and are widely considered to be the most painful type of headache.

Headaches can also be a sign of an underlying health problem. People who suffer from frequent headaches may be reacting to certain foods and food additives, such as wheat, chocolate, monosodium glutamate (MSG), sulfites (used in restaurants on salad bars), sugar, hot dogs, luncheon meats, dairy products, nuts, citric acid, fermented foods (cheeses, sour cream, yogurt), alcohol such as spirits and red wine, vinegar, and/or marinated foods. Other possibilities to consider are anemia, bowel problems, brain disorders such as tumors, bruxism (tooth-grinding), hypertension (high blood pressure), hypoglycemia (low blood sugar), sinusitis, spinal misalignment, toxic overdoses of vitamin A, vitamin B deficiency, and diseases of the eye, nose, and throat. Dehydration also can cause headaches—often accompanied by a feeling of being flushed, a warm face, and a sense of heaviness in the head.

Unless otherwise specified, the dosages recommended here are for adults. For children between the ages of twelve and seventeen, reduce the dose to three-quarters the recommended amount. For children between six and twelve, use one-half the recommended dose, and for children under the age of six, use one-quarter the recommended amount.

NUTRIENTS

SUPPLEMENT	SUGGESTED DOSAGE	COMMENTS
Helpful		
Bromelain	500 mg as needed.	An enzyme that helps to regulate the inflammatory response.
Calcium and	1,500 mg daily.	Minerals that help to alleviate muscular tension. Use chelated forms.

magnesium	1,000 mg daily.	Deficiency may be a cause of migraines. Relaxes muscles and blood vessels.
Coenzyme Q₁₀ plus	30 mg twice daily.	Improves tissue oxygenation.
Coenzyme A from Coenzyme-A Technologies	As directed on label.	Supports the immune detoxification of many dangerous substances, increases energy, and facilitates the manufacture of connective tissue.
Dimethylglycine (DMG) (Aangamik FoodScience of Vermont)	125 mg twice daily.	Improves tissue oxygenation. Use a sublingual form.
DL-Phenylalanine (DLPA)	750 mg daily.	For pain relief. *Caution:* Do not take this supplement if you are pregnant or nursing a baby, or if you suffer from panic attacks, diabetes, high blood pressure, or PKU.
5-Hydroxy L-tryptophan (5-HTP)	As directed on label.	Many clinical studies have shown excellent results with both tension headaches and migraines.
Glucosamine sulfate	As directed on label.	A natural alternative to aspirin and other nonsteroidal anti-inflammatory drugs (NSAIDs).
L-tyrosine plus L-glutamine plus quercetin	As directed on label. 500 mg twice daily. 500 mg twice daily.	For relief of cluster headaches. *Caution:* Do not take tyrosine if you are taking an MAO inhibitor drug, commonly prescribed for depression.
Methylsulfonyl-methane (MSM)	As directed on label.	Relieves pain.
Potassium	99 mg daily.	For the proper sodium and potassium balance, which is needed to avoid water retention. Water retention may put undue pressure on the brain.
Primrose oil	500 mg 3–4 times daily.	Supplies essential fatty acids, which promote healthy circulation, help regulate the inflammatory response, and relieve pain.
Vitamin B₃ (niacin) and niacinamide	Up to 300 mg combined daily. Do not exceed this amount. Stop and maintain the dosage that provides relief.	Improves circulation and aids in the functioning of the nervous system. Professional supervision is advised. *Caution:* Do not take niacin if you have a liver disorder, gout, or high blood pressure.
Vitamin B complex plus extra vitamin B₆ (pyridoxine)	50 mg of each major B vitamin 3 times daily (amounts of individual vitamins in a complex will vary). 50 mg 3 times daily.	B vitamins work best when taken together. Use a yeast-free formula. In severe cases, injections (under a doctor's supervision) may be advisable. Removes excess water from tissues.
Vitamin C with bioflavonoids	2,000–8,000 mg daily, in divided doses.	Protects against harmful effects of pollution and aids production of antistress hormones. Use an esterified or buffered form.
Vitamin E	200 IU daily or 400 IU every other day.	Improves circulation. Use d-alpha-tocopherol form.

Herbs

❑ Cayenne thins the blood, which reduces pain and allows beneficial blood flow.

❑ Chamomile relaxes muscles and soothes tension.

Caution: Do not use chamomile if you are allergic to ragweed. Do not use during pregnancy or nursing. It may interact with warfarin or cyclosporine, so patients using these drugs should avoid it.

❑ A salve made from ginger, peppermint oil, and wintergreen oil rubbed on the nape of the neck and temples can help to relieve tension headaches. For sinus headaches, rub the salve across the sinus area.

❑ Ginkgo biloba extract improves circulation to the brain, and may be helpful for certain types of headache.

Caution: Do not take ginkgo biloba if you have a bleeding disorder, or are scheduled for surgery or a dental procedure.

❑ Guarana can alleviate cluster headaches. It has caffeine in it, so don't use this herb if you are sensitive to caffeine.

❑ Several clinical studies have shown ginger to be helpful for pain relief.

❑ Jamaica dogweed is good for sinus headaches.

❑ Kava kava is helpful for tension headaches.

Caution: Kava kava can cause drowsiness. It is not recommended for pregnant women or nursing mothers, and it should not be taken together with other substances that act on the central nervous system, such as alcohol, barbiturates, antidepressants, and antipsychotic drugs.

❑ Meadowsweet is an anti-inflammatory agent.

❑ Periwinkle flower has been found to increase the cerebral flow of oxygen, which helps to alleviate headache pain.

❑ Skullcap acts as an antispasmodic agent and has a sedative effect. It is good for headaches related to muscular tension and spasms.

❑ Valerian root is a good sedative to take during a headache.

❑ Other herbs that may help relieve headache pain include brigham, burdock root, fenugreek, feverfew, goldenseal, lavender, lobelia, marshmallow, mint, rosemary, skullcap, and thyme.

Cautions: Do not use feverfew when pregnant or nursing. People who take prescription blood-thinning medications should consult a health care provider before using feverfew, as the combination can result in internal bleeding. Do not take goldenseal internally on a daily basis for more than one week at a time. Do not use it during pregnancy or if you are breast-feeding, and use with caution if you are allergic to ragweed. If you have a history of cardiovascular disease, diabetes, or glaucoma, use it only under a doctor's supervision. Lobelia is only to be taken under supervision of a health care professional as it is potentially toxic. People with high blood pressure, heart disease, liver

Types of Headaches

Headaches come in a number of forms, differentiated by their causes and specific symptoms. The appropriate treatment depends on the type of headache. The table below lists some of the more common types of headaches and possible treatments for them.

Type of Headache	Symptoms	Causes/Triggers	Treatment
Aneurysm-associated headache	Early symptoms mimic those of cluster headaches and migraines. If an aneurysm ruptures, it can cause sudden extreme pain, double vision, rigid neck, and stroke leading to unconsciousness.	A balloonlike bulge or weak spot on a blood vessel wall; high blood pressure.	Keep blood pressure low. If found early, surgery may be necessary.
Arthritis headache	Pain at the back of the head or neck, made worse by movement; inflammation of joints and shoulder and/or neck muscles.	Unknown.	Take feverfew supplements. *Caution:* Do not use feverfew during pregnancy.
Bilious headache	Dull pain in forehead and throbbing temples.	Indigestion; overeating; lack of exercise.	Colon cleansing may be helpful. (*See* COLON CLEANSING in Part Three.)
Caffeine headache	Throbbing pain caused by blood vessels that have dilated.	Caffeine withdrawal.	Ingest a small amount of caffeine, then taper off.
Cluster headache	Severe, throbbing pain on one side of the head around the eye area, flushing of the face, tearing of eyes, nasal congestion, occurring 1–3 times a day over a period of weeks or months and lasting from a few minutes to several hours each time. One of the most painful headaches.	Stress, alcohol, smoking.	Take supplemental L-tyrosine, DL-phenylalanine, ginkgo biloba extract, L-glutamine, quercetin. *Caution:* Do not take L-tyrosine if you are taking an MAO inhibitor drug. Do not take phenylalanine if you are pregnant or suffer from panic attacks, diabetes, high blood pressure, or phenylketonuria (PKU).
Exertion headache	Generalized headache during or after physical exertion such as running or sexual intercourse, or passive exertion such as sneezing or coughing.	Usually related to migraine or cluster headaches. About 10 percent are related to organic diseases such as tumors or blood vessel malformation.	Take nutritional supplements; apply ice packs at the site of pain. If the pain worsens in intensity and duration after exercising and exertion, see your physician.
Eyestrain headache	Usually frontal pain on both sides.	Overuse of the eyes; eye muscle imbalance; uncorrected vision; astigmatism.	Correct vision.
Fever headache	Headache develops with fever due to inflammation of blood vessels of the head.	Infection.	Reduce fever, apply ice packs.
Hangover headache	Migraine-like, with throbbing pain and nausea.	Alcohol causes dehydration and dilation of blood vessels in the brain.	Drink plenty of quality water. Take a B-complex supplement. Apply ice to neck.
Hunger headache	Strikes just before mealtime due to low blood sugar, muscle tension, and rebound dilation of blood vessels.	Skipping meals; too-stringent dieting.	Eat regular meals with adequate amounts of complex carbohydrates and protein.

Hypertension headache	Dull, generalized pain affecting a large area of the head and aggravated by movement or exertion.	Severe high blood pressure.	Get blood pressure under control.
Menstrual headache	Migraine-type pain shortly before, during, or after menstruation, or at midcycle, at time of ovulation.	Variation in estrogen levels.	Take supplements of vitamin B_6, potassium, and extra magnesium.
Migraine, classic	Similar to common migraine, but preceded by auras such as visual disturbances, numbness in arms or legs, smelling of strange odors, hallucinations.	Excessive dilation or contraction of blood vessels of the brain.	See MIGRAINE in Part Two.
Migraine, common	Severe throbbing pain, often on one side of the head; nausea; vomiting; cold hands; dizziness; sensitivity to light and sounds.	Excessive dilation or contraction of blood vessels of the brain.	See MIGRAINE in Part Two.
Sinus headache	Gnawing, nagging pain over nasal/sinus area, often increasing in severity as the day goes by. Fever and discolored mucus may be present.	Allergies, infection, nasal polyps, food allergies. Often caused by blocked sinus ducts or acute sinus infection.	Increase intake of vitamins A and C; use moist heat to help get sinuses to drain.
Temporal headache	Jabbing, burning, boring pain; pain in temple or around ear on chewing; weight loss; flulike symptoms; problems with eyesight. Usually seen in people over fifty-five. Untreated, can lead to blindness, stroke, heart attack, or a tear in the aorta.	Inflammation of temporal arteries.	Consult physician for steroid therapy.
Temporo-mandibular joint (TMJ) headache	Temporal, above-ear, or facial pain; muscle temple pain upon awakening.	Stress, contraction of one side of face; clicking or malocclusion (poor bite); jaw clenching, gum chewing; jaw, neck or upper back popping.	Reduce stress; use relaxation techniques, biofeedback, nutritional supplements, ice packs.
Tension headache	Constant pain, in one area or all over the head; sore muscles with trigger points in neck and upper back; light-headedness; dizziness. The most common type of headache.	Emotional stress, anxiety, worry, depression, anger, food allergies, poor posture, too-shallow breathing.	Apply ice packs on neck and upper back; take supplements of vitamin C with bioflavonoids, DLPA, bromelain, magnesium, primrose oil, and ginger for relief of muscle spasms.
Tic douloureux	Short, jabbing pains around the mouth, jaw, or forehead. More common in women over fifty-five years old.	Unknown.	Take nutritional supplements. In some cases, surgery may be necessary.
Tumor headaches	Progressively worsening pain; projectile problems with vision, speech, and equilibrium; personality changes.	Usually unknown.	Surgery and/or radiation.
Vascular headaches	Throbbing on one side of the head, sensitivity to light, and often nausea. Related to cluster headaches and migraines.	Disturbances in the blood vessels.	Lie down and keep your blood pressure under control.

disease, kidney disease, seizure disorders, or shortness of breath should not take lobelia. Pregnant and lactating women should avoid lobelia as well.

Recommendations

❑ Eat a well-balanced diet, including protein with every meal. Avoid chewing gum; do not consume ice cream, iced beverages, or salt (unless you suspect that your headache is caused by dehydration); and guard against excessive sun exposure.

❑ Try eliminating foods containing tyramine and the amino acid phenylalanine. Then reintroduce one food at a time and see which ones produce headaches. Phenylalanine is found in aspartame (sold in the form of Equal, NutraSweet, and other products), monosodium glutamate (MSG), and nitrites (preservatives found in hot dogs and luncheon meats). Foods that contain tyramine include alcoholic beverages, bananas, cheese, chicken, chocolate, citrus fruits, cold cuts, herring, onions, peanut butter, pork, smoked fish, sour cream, vinegar, wine, and fresh-baked yeast products. Tyramine causes the blood pressure to rise, resulting in a dull headache.

❑ Practice deep-breathing exercises. A lack of oxygen can cause headaches. (*See* BREATHING EXERCISES *under* PAIN CONTROL in Part Three.)

❑ Maintain good posture habits.

❑ Use fiber daily and a cleansing enema weekly. (*See* COLON CLEANSING and ENEMAS in Part Three.)

Note: Always take supplemental fiber separately from other supplements and medications.

❑ If you feel a headache coming on, drink a large glass of water every three hours until symptoms subside. If you tend to get headaches after travel by plane, it is probably due to dehydration. Try to drink at least a cup of water or other non-caffeine-containing beverage each hour of the flight.

❑ When a headache strikes, take a cleansing enema. This removes the toxins that cause many headaches. If not eliminated, toxins can be absorbed into the bloodstream and circulated throughout the body. For a headache brought on by fasting, use a coffee retention enema. (*See* ENEMAS in Part Three.)

❑ Apply cold compresses to the spot from which the pain is radiating. This helps to relieve headaches by constricting blood vessels and easing muscle spasms. To make a cold compress, place a damp washcloth in the freezer for ten minutes or use a cold gel-pack.

❑ Use a heating pad, hot water bottle, or hot towel to relax neck and shoulder muscles, which can cause tension headaches when they are too tight.

❑ Use a homeopathic remedy suitable for the particular headache symptoms you are experiencing. *Belladonna* helps with sudden, severe pain that is worse on the right side of the body. *Natrum muriaticum* is recommended for tension headaches and periodic headaches. *Sanguinaria* is good for pain that is sharp and splitting. *Arsenicum album, kali bichromium, Mecurius solubilis,* and *Pulsatilla* all encourage drainage of the sinuses.

❑ Acupressure is helpful for tension headaches and pain. Take your thumb and press up firmly underneath your skull, at the back of your neck, for one to two minutes.

❑ For headaches caused by sinus congestion, try self-massage. By applying pressure to specific areas of the head, you can open up the sinuses and ease tension. Rub the area surrounding the bones just above and below the eyes, and massage the cheeks directly in line with these points. Lean your head forward slightly to facilitate sinus drainage. Applying heat to the sinuses, either with compresses or with steam inhalation, can also be beneficial.

❑ Always seek and treat the cause of the headache, not the symptom. Long-term overreliance on aspirin, acetaminophen, and other nonprescription painkillers can make chronic headaches worse by interfering with the brain's natural ability to fight headaches. If you are using nonprescription painkillers more than four times a week, talk to your health care provider about other ways to control the pain.

❑ If you experience a headache that does not subside, but instead progressively worsens over the course of a week, consult your physician. This can be a sign of an underlying organic problem such as a tumor.

❑ To help prevent headaches, eat small meals and eat between meals to help stabilize wide swings in blood sugar. Include almonds, almond milk, watercress, parsley, fennel, garlic, cherries, and pineapple in your diet.

❑ Be sure to get sufficient sleep. Inositol and/or calcium, if taken before bedtime, aid sleeping. A grapefruit half also helps. Do not eat sweet fruit or anything else sweet after 5:00 P.M.

❑ If you suffer from headaches while taking birth control pills, talk to your doctor about switching to a low-estrogen formulation or going off the pills for a while. Oral contraceptives can cause a vitamin B_6 deficiency that results in headaches and migraines.

❑ If you must eat a food to which you suspect you may be sensitive, use charcoal tablets (available in health food stores). Take five tablets within an hour before eating and three tablets after eating. As soon as possible, take a cleansing enema and a coffee retention enema. If you have severe headaches after consuming a food, this will relieve it quickly by eliminating the allergenic substances. Do not take charcoal tablets daily, however, as they also absorb the good nutrients.

❑ If any of the following symptoms accompany the headache, consult your health care provider: blurred vision, confusion or loss of speech, fever and stiffness in the neck, sensitivity to light, pressure behind the eyes that is relieved by vomiting, pressure in the facial sinus area, throbbing of the head and temples, a pounding heartbeat, visual color changes, and feeling as though your head will explode. Seek immediate medical attention if you experience a sudden, severe headache like a "thunderclap," or if you experience a headache after a head injury, even a minor fall or bump. Chronic headache pain that worsens after coughing, exertion, straining, or sudden movement is also reason to seek professional attention.

❑ If you suffer from more than the occasional tension headache, keep a headache log to help your health care provider diagnose your condition. Keep the log for at least two months, noting the time of each headache and describing the pain (throbbing or dull), its severity, location, and duration.

❑ If you get a headache every time you exercise, see your health care provider to rule out heart problems. A headache that begins with exercise and then subsides after rest can be a cardiac headache.

Considerations

❑ Headaches are often caused by allergies. A food allergy diary can help identify offending foods. (*See* ALLERGIES in Part Two.)

❑ Poor vertebral alignment may cause reduced blood flow to the brain. This is often caused by flat feet or by wearing high heels. Chiropractic adjustment can help.

❑ Routine chiropractic spinal manipulation and deep neck muscle massage can reduce the frequency of headaches and the need for pain-relieving medications.

❑ Regular exercise can help prevent headaches caused by tension and may also reduce the frequency and severity of migraines. But headaches with organic causes can be made worse by exercise. Talk to your health care provider about your headaches before using exercise to control the pain.

❑ Cluster headaches occur when a nerve pathway in the base of the brain (the trigeminal nerve pathway) is activated. The trigeminal nerve is the main nerve of the face responsible for sensations such as pain. When activated, the trigeminal nerve causes eye pain associated with cluster headaches. It becomes activated by a part of the brain called the hypothalamus. Serotonin causes the blood vessels in the head to contract, and this lowers the pain threshold. Before a migraine, serotonin levels are high, but during the attack, they drop. The low serotonin levels cause the blood vessels to be unusually large. The expansion of the blood vessels is thought to cause the throbbing pain in the temple or behind the eye. The area around the expanded blood vessels becomes inflamed and irritates the nerve endings. These dramatic changes in serotonin levels and reduced blood flow may cause headaches, but also nausea and distorted speech and vision.

❑ The FDA has approved three over-the-counter medications to treat migraines: Excedrin Migraine (a combination aspirin, acetaminophen, and caffeine), Advil Migraine (ibuprofen), and Motrin Migraine Pain (ibuprofen).

❑ Prescription medications for treating the pain of a migraine include: Dihydroergotamine (DHE) injection and as a nasal spray (Migranal); a combination product containing DHE plus isometheptene (Midrin) is not very effective. Triptans (5-hydroxytryptamine [5-HT], serotonin, agonists) are a class of medications used to treat migraines that are categorized as acute. They include: Sumatriptan (Imitrex), an injection, nasal spray, and rapid-dissolving tablet; almotriptan (Axert); naratriptan (Amerge); rizatriptan (Maxalt); zolmitriptan (Zomig); frovatriptan (Frova); and eletriptan (Relpax). These migraine-specific therapies are most effective when taken early in an attack. The goal is to relieve the pain and associated symptoms. Triptans should not be used by those who have a past history of, or risk factors for, heart disease, high blood pressure, high cholesterol, angina, peripheral vascular disease, impaired liver function, stroke, or diabetes.

❑ The FDA has approved four drugs for migraine prevention: propranolol (Inderal), timolol (Blocadren), topiramate (Topamax), and divalproex sodium (Depakote). Amitriptyline is also sometimes used. If patients have frequent migraine attacks, attacks that do not respond consistently to the treatments above, or if the migraine-specific medications are ineffective or contraindicated because of other medical problems, then these preventive medications should be given to reduce the migraine frequency and improve the response to the acute migraine medicines.

❑ Some doctors prescribe the drug lidocaine (Anestacon, Xylocaine) for cluster headaches and migraines. Used in nose drop form, it gives relief in minutes.

❑ In one study, twenty adults suffering from long-term cluster headaches squirted a capsaicin solution in their noses daily for five days. Within ten days of the last dose, there was a 67 percent drop in the number of attacks.

❑ Research shows that sleeping in a bedroom kept at a cooler temperature can help to prevent cluster headaches. Headaches are more frequent when environmental heat increases body temperature, which causes blood vessels to dilate.

❑ One study reported that taking 10 milligrams of melatonin near bedtime was effective in reducing the frequency of episodic cluster headaches. Chronic cluster headaches did not show improvement with this treatment, however.

❑ Women who suffer from migraines may benefit from using progesterone cream topically. Check with your health care provider first, as this cream may also affect hormones in your body unrelated to headaches.

❑ There are a number of common misdiagnoses of headache, including sinus pain, allergies, and temporomandibular joint syndrome (TMJ). What many people think are sinus headaches are really migraines. Sinus infections can cause brief, intense bouts of head pain, but recurring headaches are more likely to be tension headaches, migraines, or cluster headaches. Facial pain, pain in the temples, or pain above the ear is sometimes diagnosed as TMJ headache, caused by the joint of the jawbone being out of alignment. But this too may actually be one of the common types of headache, which may be triggered or aggravated by the joint.

❑ Carbon monoxide poisoning can cause headache, in addition to nausea, vomiting, and neurological problems. Some 400 Americans die each year, and another 20,000 are treated in emergency rooms, for carbon monoxide exposure from leaking furnaces, gas ranges, and water heaters. Early signs of carbon monoxide poisoning are sometimes misdiagnosed. One way to protect yourself is to invest in a carbon monoxide detector. These can be purchased at hardware stores.

❑ *See* HYPOGLYCEMIA; MIGRAINE; and TMJ SYNDROME, all in Part Two. *See also* PAIN CONTROL in Part Three.

❑ For the names and addresses of organizations that can provide additional information and other services for people with headaches, see Health and Medical Organizations in the Appendix.

HEARING LOSS

Loss of hearing occurs when the passage of sound waves to the brain is impaired. Hearing loss may be partial or complete, temporary or permanent, depending on the cause. Hearing loss is not technically the same thing as deafness, or hearing deficit. While hearing loss can lead to hearing deficit, deafness is an inability to hear that most often occurs at, or before, birth or as a result of a major illness or infection.

An estimated 50 to 60 percent of hearing loss has a genetic component. Hearing loss can occur at any age, but it is most commonly diagnosed in the very young or very old.

Hearing loss is divided into three categories: conductive hearing loss, sensorineural hearing loss, and central hearing loss. Conductive hearing loss occurs when the passage of sound waves is impeded in the external or middle ear. It may result from factors such as earwax buildup, middle ear infection and inflammation, Paget's disease, arthritis, or trauma to the eardrum. Sensorineural hearing loss is a consequence of damage to the structures or pathways of the inner ear. It may result from damage to the acoustic nerve (the eighth cranial nerve, also known as the auditory nerve), which carries information from the inner ear to the brain, or from damage to tiny cells called hair cells in the inner ear. The hair cells are responsible for translating sound waves into nerve impulses for transmission to the brain. If the hair cells die, they are unable to repair themselves and the resulting hearing loss is permanent. Sensorineural hearing loss can be present from birth, or it can be caused by certain prescription medications, including certain antibiotics, nonsteroidal anti-inflammatory drugs (NSAIDs), aspirin taken over a long period of time in high doses, quinine, viral infection of the inner ear, and Ménière's disease. This type of hearing loss affects both the acuity and clarity of hearing. Initially, it is noticed at higher pitches, and then, as it progresses, it is noticed at lower pitches, where speech is

heard. It is also possible to have mixed hearing loss, in which both conductive and sensorineural loss are present. Neural hearing loss usually occurs as a result of a brain tumor or stroke. Central hearing loss is very rare and is usually due to severe brain damage.

Hearing loss can be sudden or gradual, occurring over a period of days, weeks, or years. Infection, trauma, changes in atmospheric pressure, and earwax buildup or impaction can cause a sudden loss of hearing. Infection and inflammation often follow an upper respiratory tract infection or trauma to the ear, such as from the overuse or improper use of cotton swabs. Bathing or swimming in water that is overly chlorinated or contains high levels of bacteria and/ or fungi can also lead to ear infections. Persistent and recurrent ear infections are often linked to fungal infection (candidiasis) and are frequently seen in people with allergies, cancer, diabetes, or other chronic diseases.

If hearing loss develops gradually, the individual experiencing it may be unaware of it until it reaches a fairly advanced stage. In fact, it is not uncommon for friends and family members to notice signs of hearing loss before the person experiencing it does. Some signs that may point to a hearing problem include perceived inattentiveness, unusually loud speech, irrelevant comments, inappropriate responses to questions or environmental sounds, requests for statements to be repeated, a tendency to turn one ear toward sound, and unusual voice quality.

Aging is the major factor in loss of the ability to hear the full range of frequencies in everyday communication. Eighteen percent of American adults forty-five to sixty-four years old, 30 percent of adults sixty-five to seventy-four years old, and 47 percent of adults seventy-five years old or older have a hearing impairment. Loss of the ability to hear high-frequency noises usually comes first. This type of age-related hearing impairment is called *presbycusis*. Presbycusis can be caused by a change in the blood supply to the ear due to heart disease, some diabetic conditions, or circulatory problems.

Suspected hearing deficits in infants deserve close and immediate attention, as an undiagnosed hearing impairment can lead to delayed and/or diminished acquisition of language skills and, possibly, learning disabilities. Risk factors for hearing loss in infancy include a family history of hearing loss; known hereditary disorders; congenital abnormalities of the ears, nose, or throat; maternal exposure to rubella or syphilis, or to the 130 or so ototoxic drugs such as tobramycin (Nebcin), streptomycin, gentamicin (Garamycin), quinine (Quinamm), furosemide (Lasix), or ethacrynic acid (Edecrin); chemotherapy agents such as cisplatin and carboplatin; glucocorticosteroids (cortisone, steroids); and birth-related problems such as prematurity, trauma and/or lack of oxygen during delivery, low birth weight, Usher syndrome, or jaundice. Otitis media (middle ear infection) is the most common cause of hearing loss in children. For the most part, this is temporary, but chronic or recurrent ear infections can cause permanent hearing loss due to inflammation and infection of the middle ear. (*See* EAR INFECTION in Part Two.)

Sensorineural hearing loss in children can also be caused by childhood diseases such as meningitis, mumps, and rubella. Signs of hearing problems in infancy include failure to blink or startle at loud noises; failure to turn the head toward familiar sounds; a consistent ability to sleep through loud noises; greater responsiveness to loud noises than to voices; a failure to babble, coo, or squeal; and monotonal babbling. In toddlers, warning signs include failure to speak clearly by age two, showing no interest in being read to or in playing word games, habitual yelling or shrieking when communicating or playing, greater responsiveness to facial expressions than to speech, shyness or withdrawal (often misinterpreted as inattentiveness, dreaminess, and/or stubbornness), and frequent confusion and puzzlement. In older children, signs of hearing loss are similar to those in adulthood—a failure to respond to verbal requests, inappropriate responses to questions or other sound stimuli, and a seeming inattentiveness.

Many children suffer from auditory processing disorders (APD), which are disruptions, or dysfunctions, in the neural pathways that transmit hearing information from the ear to the brain. A child with APD might have excellent hearing but cannot effectively process what is heard. Despite having normal hearing, they often miss what people are saying. Signs of APD are:

- Frequent response is "What?" or "Huh?"

- Trouble following or inability to follow multistage directions.

- Considerable difficulty understanding speech in the presence of background noise.

Hearing loss caused by exposure to loud noises (noise pollution) is an increasing problem in our society today. When the delicate mechanisms of the inner ear are assaulted by loud noises, a phenomenon called *temporary threshold shift* (TTS) occurs. If you have ever walked away from a concert or a construction site with a buzzing or hissing in your ears, or with everything sounding as if you are underwater, you have experienced temporary threshold shift. When this condition occurs, you hear only noises above a certain level. While overnight rest usually restores normal hearing, this is a sign that damage has occurred to the hair cells in your inner ear. If this type of damage is lengthy and/or repeated, permanent threshold shift (PTS), with permanent damage and hearing loss, is the result. There are a number of terms—some clinical, some informal—used to distinguish among the sources of noise-related hearing loss. Boilermaker's ear is a condition caused by heavy exposure to broad-band noise. The affected individual loses the ability to hear high-frequency sounds and has difficulty understanding spoken words. Diplacusis is a form of hearing loss experienced as sound distortion—the pitch of a given tone is heard differently by each ear. Hy-peracusis is an extreme sensitivity to loud noises that can be caused by damage to the eardrum. Sociocusis is a term used to denote hearing loss from non-work-related exposure to noise. Most people who develop noise-related hearing loss say they were unaware that anything was wrong until they developed tinnitus or speech became inaudible, but in fact, the damage begins long before that and temporary threshold shift is a clear sign of it.

Noise-related hearing loss is common in train engineers, military personnel, and workers subjected to constant industrial noise, as well as in hunters and musicians, especially rock musicians. National Institutes of Health (NIH) statistics indicate that 15 percent of Americans between the ages of twenty and sixty-nine have high-frequency hearing loss due to exposure to loud sounds or noise. Be sure your child does not blast the music in headphones. If you can hear the radio or CD player when he or she is wearing headphones, the volume is too loud.

Tinnitus is a condition that occurs in about 25 million people with hearing loss. Tinnitus is experienced as constant or recurring ringing, buzzing, or hissing noises not caused by anything in the external environment. It is now thought that the noise originates in the brain and not in the ear, as was previously believed. If the ear is damaged by exposure to loud noises or certain medications (including aspirin), the brain may try to compensate and end up producing electrical signals that a person hears as a ringing noise in the ears. Experts at the University of Iowa claim that listening strategies could break the pattern responsible for the problem in the brain.

Unless otherwise specified, the dosages recommended here are for adults. For a child between the ages of twelve and seventeen, reduce the dose to three-quarters the recommended amount. For a child between six and twelve, use one-half the recommended dose, and for a child under the age of six, use one-quarter the recommended amount.

Hearing Loss Self-Test

The following is a quick test for hearing loss that you can do easily on your own: Rub your thumb and index finger together a few inches from your ear. If you can hear a scratching sound, your hearing is probably intact. If not, you may be experiencing hearing loss. Consult a doctor or audiologist for further evaluation.

NUTRIENTS

SUPPLEMENT	SUGGESTED DOSAGE	COMMENTS
Important		
Coenzyme Q$_{10}$	30 mg daily.	Powerful antioxidant. Crucial in the effectiveness of the immune system and circulation to the ears.
plus		
Coenzyme A from Coenzyme-A Technologies	As directed on label.	Works well with coenzyme Q$_{10}$ in supporting the immune system.

Magnesium	1,500 mg daily.	Prevents damage to the hair cells in the inner ear.
Manganese	10 mg daily.	Deficiency has been linked to ear disorders.
Multivitamin and mineral complex	As directed on label.	To provide a balance of all nutrients.
Potassium	99 mg daily.	Important for a healthy nervous system and transmission of nerve impulses.
Ultimate Oil from Nature's Secret	As directed on label.	A blend of essential fatty acids. Helps to reduce the tendency to produce excessive amounts of earwax.
Vitamin A plus carotenoid complex	15,000 IU daily. If you are pregnant, do not exceed 10,000 IU daily. 15,000 IU daily.	To boost immunity, increase resistance to infection, and strengthen mucous membranes. Studies haveshown benefits to hearing-impaired people from taking vitamin A. Antioxidants and precursors of vitamin A.
Vitamin B-complex injections or vitamin B complex plus extra folic acid and vitamin B$_{12}$	As prescribed by physician. 50 mg of each major B vitamin 3 times daily (amounts of individual vitamins in a complex will vary). 400 mcg daily. 1,000–2,000 mcg daily.	Essential for healing; reduces ear pressure. Injections (under a doctor's supervision) are best. If injections are not available, use a sublingual form. Often depleted in people with hearing loss.
Vitamin C with bioflavonoids plus N-acetylcysteine	3,000–6,000 mg daily. As directed on label.	Needed for proper immune function and to aid in preventing ear infections. To remove excess fluids from the ear canal.
Vitamin E	200 IU daily, or 400 IU every other day.	Powerful antioxidant that increases circulation. Use d-alpha-tocopherol form.
Zinc lozenges	50 mg daily. Do not exceed a total of 100 mg daily from all supplements.	Quickens immune response; aids in reducing infection.

Herbs

❑ Bayberry bark, burdock root, goldenseal, hawthorn leaf and flower, and myrrh gum purify the blood and counteract infection.

Caution: Do not take goldenseal internally on a daily basis for more than one week at a time. Do not use it during pregnancy or if you are breast-feeding, and use with caution if you are allergic to ragweed. If you have a history of cardiovascular disease, diabetes, or glaucoma, use it only under a doctor's supervision.

❑ Echinacea aids equilibrium and reduces dizziness. It also fights infection and helps reduce congestion. It can be taken in tea or capsule form.

Caution: Do not take echinacea for longer than three months. It should not be used by people who are allergic to ragweed.

❑ Eucalyptus, hyssop, mullein, and thyme have decongestant properties, which may help to alleviate ringing in the ears.

❑ Ginkgo biloba helps to reduce dizziness and improve hearing loss related to reduced blood flow. Other herbs that may help to improve circulation and blood flow to the ear area include butcher's broom, cayenne, chamomile, ginger root, turmeric, and yarrow.

Cautions: Do not use chamomile if you are allergic to ragweed. Do not use during pregnancy or nursing. It may interact with warfarin or cyclosporine, so patients using these drugs should avoid it. Do not take ginkgo biloba if you have a bleeding disorder, or are scheduled for surgery or a dental procedure.

❑ To soothe inflammation and fight infection, mullein oil can be used as ear drops. If mullein is not available, garlic oil or liquid extract (Kyolic) may be substituted.

❑ Take supplemental antioxidants. According to research published in the medical journal *Laryngoscope*, supplemental antioxidants may protect the inner ear from traumatic and age-related hearing loss.

Recommendations

❑ Eat fresh pineapple frequently to reduce inflammation. Also include plenty of garlic, kelp, and sea vegetables in your diet.

❑ Limit your consumption of alcohol and sugars, which encourage the growth of yeast. This is particularly important if you have recurrent ear infections and have been treated with antibiotics. Also eliminate or keep to a minimum your intake of caffeine, chocolate, and sodium.

❑ For earwax buildup, clean or irrigate your ears using either a solution of 1 part vinegar to 1 part warm water, or a few drops of hydrogen peroxide. Using an eyedropper, place a few drops in your ear, allow them to settle for a minute, then drain. Repeat the process with the other ear. Do this two or three times a day. Do not use cotton swabs to clean inside the ear canal, as this can push wax farther into the ear canal and exacerbate the problem. If the wax is hard and dry, apply garlic oil for a day or two to soften it. Then wash out the ear with a steady stream of warm water. Be patient, continue to irrigate the ear canal, and flush with warm water. Most cases of earwax buildup can be treated by this method. Another method of removing excess earwax, called ear candling, uses special candles available at health food stores. Instructions for the procedure are included with the candles. The candling procedure requires assistance, so do not attempt this by yourself.

❑ For an ear infection, put 2 to 4 drops of warm (not hot) liquid garlic extract in the affected ear. (If both ears are infected, do not use the same dropper for both ears, as it may spread the infection.) This treatment is very helpful for children.

❑ If you are experiencing ear pain, tug on your earlobe. If this tug makes the ear hurt, you probably have an ear infection and should seek medical treatment. If the tug on the lobe does not hurt, the pain may be due to a dental problem.

❑ When flying, chew gum during the plane's descent to prevent the discomfort and hearing loss associated with changes in atmospheric pressure. Or pop your ears by holding your nose and *gently* blowing air through your closed mouth. This clears the eustachian tubes. A decongestant such as pseudoephedrine (found in Sudafed and other products) may also be helpful, but remember, these medications are dehydrating (and so is the lack of humidity in an airplane cabin). If you use them, be sure to drink plenty of water and juice during the flight, and skip the cocktail and coffee, as alcohol and caffeine also are dehydrating.

❑ Always wear ear protection (disposable plugs or an earphone-style headset) when using loud appliances such as power tools or lawn mowers and when you know you will be exposed to sudden loud noises, such as when shooting a gun.

❑ Protect your hearing when listening to music. A general guideline is to keep the volume low enough that you can easily hear the telephone and other sounds over the music. If you are using a personal stereo unit with headphones, you should be the only one able to hear your music. If someone standing next to you can hear it, it's too loud.

❑ Take measures to reduce your cholesterol level. Studies suggest that people with high cholesterol levels have greater hearing loss as they age than people with normal cholesterol levels. (*See* HIGH CHOLESTEROL in Part Two.)

❑ If you are prone to ear infections, wear earplugs while swimming.

❑ If you are planning to become pregnant, make sure you have achieved immunity to German measles, either through having had the disease or through vaccination. A doctor can perform a blood test to determine immunity. If vaccination is necessary, you must guard against becoming pregnant for at least three months to avoid the risk of serious birth defects, such as hearing loss.

❑ If you become ill during pregnancy and medication is required, question your doctor or pharmacist thoroughly about possible effects on the developing fetus and do some research on your own. This will reduce the risk of giving birth to a child with impaired hearing.

❑ If you have an infant, pay very close attention to his or her reactions to noises. If you have any doubt about your child's hearing, consult your physician. Be aware, however, that many physicians fail to pick up on hearing loss. If your doctor seems too quick to dismiss your concerns, talk to another doctor. Keep in mind that early detection is vitally important; detection of hearing loss before a child's first birthday greatly reduces the chances that he or she will be disadvantaged by hearing problems in the years to come.

❑ If you have experienced permanent hearing loss, advise family members, friends, and coworkers to speak slowly and distinctly, and avoid shouting. Depending on the nature of the hearing loss, a hearing aid may be helpful. There are now several different types of hearing aids on the market, including the following:

• Behind-the-ear (BTE) devices. These hook behind the ear and a tube carries the sound to a microphone fitted in the ear. The earpiece can also be attached to a pair of glasses. BTE devices work well, but some people find them aesthetically unappealing.

• In-the-ear (ITE) devices. These are placed partly in the outer portion of the ear and partly in the ear canal. They are less obvious than BTE hearing aids. They can cause problems with feedback, however, because the microphone part is so close to the receiver and the controls are rather small.

• In-the-canal (ITC) devices. As the name suggests, these are placed in the ear canal so they are difficult to see. This makes them very popular, but they too have problems with feedback due to the close proximity of the microphone and the receiver.

• Digital devices. These represent the most exciting potential advance in hearing aid technology. They are able to suppress background noise, which is something other hearing aids cannot do. Unfortunately, the price of these devices, at least at present, is prohibitively high, and more work is needed before they exceed the efficacy of the older analogue hearing aids. For information on affordable, digital hearing aids, see www.project-impact.net.

❑ Hearing loss due to infection that has destroyed or damaged the sound-conducting mechanism of the inner ear can now be corrected with surgery. Surgeons can rebuild the damaged section with artificial bone and restore the eardrum to its original state.

Considerations

❑ Appropriate treatment for hearing loss depends on the underlying cause. Sometimes a high dose of steroids is given to see if sudden hearing loss can be rectified.

❑ Food allergies, especially allergies to wheat and dairy products, can be the culprit in recurrent middle ear infections. (*See* ALLERGIES in Part Two.)

❑ In one study, women aged sixty-one to seventy who had low B_{12} and folic acid levels were found to be more likely to have impaired hearing. Those who took supplements of these vitamins were less likely to experience hearing loss.

❑ If your infant is suffering from atopic dermatitis, eczema of the external ear, resulting in red, itchy, and scaling skin of the pinna, then avoid common food triggers such as eggs, peanuts, soy, wheat, and milk. Speak to your child's pediatrician before removing any foods from your child's diet.

❑ You can minimize the level of hearing loss you will experience as you grow older if you reduce your exposure to loud noises in the earlier years of your life. Hearing can also be improved with proper diet and supplements.

❑ If you have to raise your voice to be heard over your surroundings, your environment is too noisy. You should try to limit your exposure to such places. If such exposure cannot be avoided, you should wear ear protection.

❑ Most cases of early childhood hearing deficit are first detected by the parents, not health care providers.

❑ The Occupational Safety and Health Administration (OSHA) has established guidelines for workplace noise levels. For any eight-hour day, the noise level should not be above 90 decibels (dBA). Protective headphones should be provided if noise levels exceed 85 dBA for any period of time.

❑ The average rock concert or stereo headset set at full blast (about 100 decibels) can damage your hearing in as little as half an hour. Similar damage can occur after about two hours spent in a video game arcade.

❑ Some researchers say that in addition to causing hearing loss, constant exposure to noise may lead to (or exacerbate) impaired vision, heart disease, psychological disorders, and other health problems.

❑ Any hearing loss that does not resolve on its own within two weeks should be evaluated by a health care professional. Some of the symptoms associated with hearing loss can be a sign of a serious health problem that requires treatment.

❑ If you are concerned about your hearing, you can arrange to take a free hearing test over the telephone. The Dial-a-Hearing Screening Test is provided as a public service by Occupational Hearing Services (800-222-3277). It is not a definitive test, but can give some indication as to whether you have a hearing problem you may need to talk to a hearing specialist about.

❑ Researchers at the Massachusetts Institute of Technology (MIT) have developed a cochlear implant, which is an electronic device containing electrodes that are surgically inserted into one of the structures of the inner ear to activate nerve fibers and allow sound signals to be transmitted to the brain. Hearing-impaired individuals who are candidates for this device are able to hear normal, everyday sounds.

See also EAR INFECTION and MÉNIÈRE'S DISEASE in Part Two.

HEART ATTACK

The heart is a muscle that pumps blood around the body. It is made up of four separate chambers, two *atria* and two *ventricles*. Between the four chambers are valves that allow the blood to flow in one direction only—forward. With each beat of the heart, the right ventricle pumps deoxygenated blood to the lungs while the left ventricle pumps oxygenated blood into the arteries for circulation around the body. The heart in turn depends on oxygenated blood coming to it through the coronary arteries (the arteries around the heart) for necessary oxygen and nutrients. If the coronary arteries are constricted due to atherosclerosis (the deposit of fatty plaques in the arteries), an embolus (a piece of tissue or air lodged in the artery), or a thrombus (a blood clot in the artery), the heart may be deprived of sufficient oxygen, causing a heart attack. The medical term for a heart attack is *myocardial infarction* (death of cardiac tissue). When the supply of blood to the heart is sharply reduced or cut off, the heart is deprived of needed oxygen. If blood flow is not restored within minutes, portions of the heart muscle begin to die, permanently damaging the heart muscle. Because this happens when the coronary arteries cannot provide the heart with sufficient oxygen, physicians also commonly refer to a heart attack as a "coronary."

With the onset of a heart attack, the primary symptom is usually a consistent deep, often severe, discomfort or pain in the chest (often described as a heavy substernal pressure that makes it feel as if the chest is being squeezed). Also common are discomfort in the arm(s), back, neck, jaw, or stomach, plus shortness of breath, breaking out in a cold sweat, nausea, vomiting, and light-headedness. It is important to know, however, that heart attack symptoms for men can be different than symptoms for women, the latter manifesting themselves as back pain, flulike symptoms, or a sense of impending doom. Heart attack symptoms may be present for up to twelve hours. In addition, a heart attack can cause abnormal heartbeat rhythms called *arrhythmias.* But the symptoms often are not at all as clear as this. They may also vary from person to person, and from heart attack to heart attack. This cannot be emphasized enough—especially for women, who are more likely to have "atypical" symptoms such as pain between the shoulder blades rather than crushing chest pain, and who therefore tend to delay seeking treatment or help.

There are three basic scenarios that can produce a heart attack. The first, and by far the most common, is partial or complete blockage of one of the arteries that supply the heart with oxygen, most often by a blood clot. Usually the arteries have been narrowed by years of coronary artery disease in which plaque, which is composed of cholesterol-rich fatty deposits, proteins, calcium, and excess smooth muscle cells, builds up on the arterial walls. The arterial walls thicken, inhibiting the flow of blood to the heart muscle. The roughening of arterial walls by deposits of plaque not only narrows the arteries, but also makes it easier for blood clots to form along their inner surfaces. When a clot grows, or detaches from its place of origin and travels through the blood vessels, it may block a coronary artery completely, resulting in a heart attack.

In the second heart attack scenario, an arrhythmia may set in, so that the heart is no longer pumping enough blood to ensure its own supply.

In the third, a weak spot in a blood vessel, called an aneurysm, may rupture, causing internal bleeding and disrupting normal blood flow.

No one knows exactly why some people develop heart disease and others do not, but a number of significant clues and risk factors have been identified. One risk factor that has been receiving a great deal of attention is homocysteine, an amino acid formed as a result of the metabolism of another amino acid, methionine, which is essential for normal growth and normal metabolism. Homocysteine in turn is converted back into methionine in a constant recycling process. The proper balance between homocysteine and methionine is essential. Too much homocysteine is toxic to the vascular system, and is very strongly associated with atherosclerosis. High homocysteine levels can be detected in over 20 percent of people with heart disease.

High levels of blood fats—specifically, certain lipoproteins and triglycerides—are also associated with an increased risk of heart disease. Lipoproteins are molecules that transport cholesterol in the bloodstream. There are two principal types: low-density lipoprotein (LDL) and high-density lipoprotein (HDL). High levels of LDL can lead to the formation of fatty plaques that can narrow the arteries and cause reduced blood flow. Lipoprotein(a) is a cholesterol-carrying protein closely related to LDL. It appears to be an important contributing factor in atherosclerosis, although the reason for this is not clear. High levels of HDL, on the other hand, appear to carry cholesterol away from the arteries and back to the liver for processing. Triglycerides are lipids (fats) that bind to proteins to form the high- and low-density lipoproteins. As with LDL, high triglyceride levels are associated with atherosclerosis and heart attack. Eating too many fatty foods, drinking too much alcohol, or having high insulin levels can result in elevated triglyceride levels.

Another possible factor in heart disease is an insufficient supply of antioxidants. Antioxidants render free radicals harmless and help the body dispose of toxic substances that may cause cellular damage. High levels of fibrinogen, a blood-clotting protein, may also be involved. If fibrinogen levels are high, the blood is more likely to form clots that obstruct blood flow, resulting in heart attack or stroke.

Still other research into the origins of heart disease focuses on the possible role of infectious bacteria. The presence of the bacteria *Helicobacter pylori* (*H. pylori*), normally associated with ulcers, has been found to be present in a significant number of people who have suffered heart attack. *Chlamydia pneumoniae,* a type of bacteria responsible for nearly 10 percent of cases of pneumonia, may also be associated with an increased likelihood of developing heart disease. Researchers believe that the chronic presence of low levels of these bacteria may result in chronic low-level inflammation in the blood vessels, which in turn makes them more vulnerable to developing deposits of fatty plaques. In support of this hypothesis, high levels of a substance called C-reactive protein (CRP) have been found helpful in predicting an individual's potential for developing heart disease. CRP is released into the bloodstream when the blood vessels serving the heart have been damaged due to inflammation. Another sign of inflammation is a substance known as intracellular adhesion molecule (ICAM-1) or CD54. A type of molecule found on the surface of certain cells, ICAM-1 interacts with other body chemicals to trigger the inflammatory process. The more prevalent ICAM-1 is, the more likely you are to develop atherosclerosis, although CRP levels are still considered a better indicator of inflammation than ICAM-1 levels.

In general, people who are considered to be at greater than normal risk of heart attack are those with a family history of heart disease; those who smoke and/or abuse drugs; people with diabetes, high blood pressure, high blood cholesterol and/or triglyceride levels, or high homocysteine levels; sedentary people; and those who are under stress and/or who have "type A" personalities.

Some heart attacks occur without warning. The remainder are preceded by months or even years of symptoms, most commonly angina pectoris—chest pain that is typically aggravated by stress or physical exertion and relieved by rest. Like a heart attack, angina is caused by a lack of oxygen in the heart muscle, but the extent of oxygen deprivation is not sufficient to actually damage heart tissue. Many people complain of intermittent angina, shortness of breath, and/or unusual fatigue in the days or weeks leading up to a heart attack. A constant sensation of heartburn that persists for days and from which antacids provide no relief can be a sign of an impending heart attack.

The dietary, nutritional, and lifestyle recommendations in this section are designed to help prevent, or to support recovery from, a heart attack. They are not meant as a substitute for proper emergency treatment. If you think you may be having a heart attack, do not waste any time in seeking medical assistance. Any delay in obtaining help can result in greater damage to the heart.

Unless otherwise specified, the dosages recommended here are for adults. For children between the ages of twelve and seventeen, reduce the dose to three-quarters the recommended amount. For children between six and twelve, use one-half the recommended dose, and for children under the age of six, use one-quarter the recommended amount.

NUTRIENTS

SUPPLEMENT	SUGGESTED DOSAGE	COMMENTS
Essential		
Alpha-linolenic acid (ALA)	As directed on label.	An omega-3 fatty acid found in a long-term French study to lower the risk of a fatal heart attack by over one-third.

Alpha-lipoic acid	As directed on label.	An antioxidant; lowers LDL levels.
Chinese red yeast rice extract	As directed on label.	Promotes blood circulation and regulates cholesterol levels.
Coenzyme Q_{10}	100 mg daily.	Improves heart muscle oxygenation and may help to prevent second heart attacks. A patented form of coenzyme Q_{10} that is more easily absorbed than standard forms, so you can take less with the same effect. Works well with coenzyme Q_{10} to streamline metabolism, ease depression and fatigue, increase energy, support adrenal glands, process fats, remove toxins from the body, and boost the immune system.
or Q-Gel	As directed on label.	
plus Coenzyme A from Coenzyme-A Technologies	As directed on label.	
Grape seed extract or Pycnogenol	150–300 mg daily. As directed on label.	Powerful antioxidants. Reduce the clotting tendency of the blood. Best used in combination with phosphatidylcholine, a natural component of lecithin.
Inositol hexaphosphate (IP_6)	As directed on label.	Protects the heart by preventing blood clots and reducing cholesterol and triglyceride levels.
L-arginine	As directed on label.	An amino acid that boosts production of nitric oxide, which dilates the arteries to allow better blood flow. *Note:* If you are prone to herpes outbreaks, do not take L-arginine without L-lysine.
Lecithin	As directed on label.	Contains choline and inositol, important parts of the vitamin B complex. Aids in lowering cholesterol levels.
Potassium	99 mg twice a day.	Needed to maintain regular heart rhythm. Lowers cholesterol.
S-Adenosylmethio-nine (SAMe)	As directed on label.	A natural antidepressant (depression has been linked to heart disease). Lowers homocysteine levels. *Note:* If you take SAMe, be careful to maintain a correct balance of vitamins B_6 and B_{12} and folic acid.
or Trimethylglycine (TMG)	As directed on label.	Is converted into SAMe in the body. Lowers homocysteine levels. *Caution:* Do not use if you have bipolar mood disorder or take prescription antidepressants. Do not give to a child under twelve.
Selenium	300 mcg daily. If you are pregnant, do not exceed 40 mcg daily.	Deficiency has been implicated in heart disease.
Vitamin B complex	50 mg of each major B vitamin 3 times daily (amounts of individual vitamins in a complex will vary).	B vitamins work best when taken together.
plus extra vitamin B_3 (niacin) and	50 mg daily.	B vitamins that lower homocysteine levels. Sublingual forms are best.

vitamin B_6 (pyridoxine) and	50 mg daily.	
vitamin B_{12} and	1,000–2,000 mcg daily.	
folic acid	400 mcg daily. If you take anticonvulsant medication for epilepsy, do not exceed 400 mcg of folic acid per day from all sources, as it may induce seizures.	Deficiency of folic acid in the heart muscle leads to heart disease. Low folate levels may be more dangerous than high cholesterol for people with heart disease.
or No Shot B-6/B-12/ Folic from Superior Source	As directed on label.	A combination of these three important B vitamins.
Vitamin E capsules or liquid vitamin E with tocotrienols	200 IU daily, or 400 IU every other day. As directed on label.	A powerful antioxidant that improves circulation and thins the blood, reducing the risk of clots. Use d-alpha-tocopherol form. *Note:* If you take prescription blood-thinners, consult your doctor before taking supplemental vitamin E.

Very Important

Acetyl-L-carnitine or L-carnitine plus L-cysteine and L-methionine	500 mg each daily, on an empty stomach. Take with water or juice. Do not take with milk. Take with 50 mg vitamin B_6 and 100 mg vitamin C for better absorption.	To reduce blood lipid levels, increase cellular glutathione and coenzyme Q_{10}, protect against lipid peroxidation, and assist in the breakdown of fats, preventing fatty buildup in the arteries, which helps restore blood flow to the heart.
Calcium and magnesium	1,500 mg daily. 1,000 mg daily, in divided doses, between meals and at bedtime.	Important for maintaining proper heart rhythm and blood pressure. Use chelate or citrate forms.
Cardio Logic from Wakunaga	As directed on label.	Increases oxygenation of heart tissue.
Chromium	100 mcg daily.	Helps raise levels of HDL ("good") cholesterol.
Essential fatty acids (Kyolic-EPA from Wakanuga, primrose oil, or salmon oil)	As directed on label.	Protect heart muscle cells. Reduce triglyceride levels in the blood.
Garlic (Kyolic from Wakunaga)	2 capsules 3 times daily.	Beneficial for the heart, promotes circulation, and aids in reducing high blood pressure.
Glucosamine Plus from FoodScience of Vermont	As directed on label.	Plays an important role in the formation of heart valves.
Heart Science from Source Naturals	As directed on label.	Contains antioxidants, cholesterol-fighters, herbs, and vitamins that work together to promote cardiovascular function.
Multienzyme complex	As directed on label. Take with meals.	For proper digestion and to prevent heartburn.
Proteolytic enzymes	As directed on label 3 times daily. Take between meals for better protein absorption.	Anti-inflammatory agents that prevent free radical damage to the arteries.

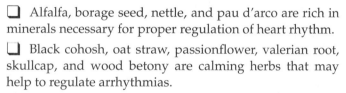

Sea mussel	As directed on label.	Aids in the functioning of the cardiovascular system, the lymphatic system, and the endocrine system.
7-Keto DHEA	As directed on label.	Has been found to reduce depression.
Vitamin A with mixed carotenoids	As directed on label. If you are pregnant, do not exceed 10,000 IU daily.	Helps to prevent free radical damage to the arteries. Use emulsion form for easier assimilation.
Zinc plus copper	50 mg daily. Do not exceed a total of 100 mg daily from all supplements. 3 mg daily.	Necessary for proper balance with copper and for thiamine utilization. Use a chelate form. Deficiency has been linked to heart disease.
Important		
Dimethylglycine (DMG) (Aangamik DMG from FoodScience of Vermont)	As directed on label.	Improves oxygenation of heart tissue.
Vitamin C with bioflavonoids	3,000–6,000 mg daily.	Aids in thinning the blood. Prevents blood clots and free radical damage.

Herbs

❑ Alfalfa, borage seed, nettle, and pau d'arco are rich in minerals necessary for proper regulation of heart rhythm.

❑ Black cohosh, oat straw, passionflower, valerian root, skullcap, and wood betony are calming herbs that may help to regulate arrhythmias.

Caution: Do not use black cohosh if you are pregnant or have any type of chronic disease. Black cohosh should not be used by those with liver problems.

❑ Butcher's broom, hawthorn berries and leaf, motherwort, and red sage strengthen the heart muscle.

Caution: If you are taking a blood-thinning medicine, consult you health care professional first before using red sage.

❑ Cayenne (capsicum), ginger root, and ginkgo biloba strengthen the heart and are helpful for chest pain.

Caution: Do not take ginkgo biloba if you have a bleeding disorder, or are scheduled for surgery or a dental procedure.

❑ Cordyceps is a Chinese herb that lowers both blood pressure and LDL ("bad") cholesterol levels.

❑ Gotu kola, primrose, and rosemary are helpful in managing angina.

❑ Green tea has superb antioxidant properties and may provide protection against heart disease and many other illnesses.

Note: If you take prescription blood-thinners, consult your doctor before taking green tea in capsule form. Green tea capsules—not the tea itself—contain fairly large quantities of vitamin K, which promotes blood clotting.

❑ Turmeric contains curcumin, an anti-inflammatory that also lowers blood cholesterol.

Recommendations

❑ If you experience any of the following warning signs of heart attack, seek emergency medical care *immediately*:

- Chest discomfort in the center of the chest that lasts more than a few minutes or that goes away and then comes back. Discomfort can be defined as pressure, squeezing, fullness, or pain.

- Pain or discomfort in one or both arms, the back, neck, jaw, or stomach.

- Shortness of breath.

- Sweating (possibly profuse).

- Nausea and/or vomiting.

- Light-headedness.

If you think you may be having a heart attack, follow the steps outlined below:

- Stop what you are doing and sit down.

- Assess the situation. Try to remain calm. If there is someone else around you, let him or her know what is happening. If there is no one else there and you are still feeling pain or discomfort after a few minutes, or if you are sweating and weak without any other obvious symptoms, call for emergency help and tell the person on the other end of the line that you may be having a heart attack. *Do not* drive yourself to the hospital. *Do not* delay getting treatment.

- After calling for medical help, if you are unable to leave your telephone number and address, you may want to leave the telephone off the hook so that your number and address can be traced. If you have given your address and telephone number successfully, hang up and call a friend or relative who may be of assistance.

- If you have nitroglycerin tablets, take one every five minutes, up to three tablets in total. If you have aspirin in the house, take one and chew it. This may prevent a blood clot.

- Perform a technique called *cough CPR,* which involves vigorous coughing. This may help you to remain conscious long enough to call for help. Obviously, it is something that must be learned before it is needed; if you are considered at increased risk of a heart attack, discuss this with your health care professional.

- If a friend or relative is with you, have him or her check your pulse and respiration (breathing) at regular intervals. If your pulse or breathing stops, this person should start cardiopulmonary resuscitation (CPR) immediately. He or she should then call the emergency number again, so that when the ambulance arrives, emergency personnel know that this is indeed a heart attack.

- If it is later established that the episode was *not* a heart attack, consider having your potential for a heart attack assessed by a doctor to relieve any doubts and concerns you may have.

❑ If you have suffered a heart attack, or if you are considered at risk for a heart attack, modify your diet. Important dietary measures include the following:

- Make sure your diet is high in fiber. Not all types of fiber decrease the risk of heart attack, however. The most beneficial fiber appears to come from whole grains, fruits, and vegetables.

- Eat lots of foods that are rich in vitamins B_6 and B_{12} and folic acid, which are needed to keep homocysteine levels in check. Vitamins B_6 and B_{12} come naturally from leafy green vegetables and fruits. Folic acid can be found in some breakfast cereals, asparagus, spinach, chickpeas, and beans.

- Include almonds, brewer's yeast, grains, and sesame seeds in your diet.

  Caution: Brewer's yeast can cause an allergic reaction in some individuals. Start with a small amount at first, and discontinue use if any allergic symptoms occur.

- Enjoy onions frequently. Onions—especially red onions—contain valuable antioxidants. Chop them and allow them to stand for ten minutes before cooking for optimal benefit.

- Add kelp and sea vegetables to your diet for necessary minerals.

- Drink fresh vegetable juices.

- Drink steam-distilled water only.

- Do not eat red meat, salt, sugars, or white flour. A diet high in red meat can elevate homocysteine levels. Eat soy-based protein foods instead. Soy protein can effectively lower high LDL cholesterol levels.

- Avoid salt, sugars, and white flour. Refined sugars produce adverse reactions in all cells by causing wide variations in blood sugar. The high surges are followed by hypoglycemic drops, causing dangerous instability in vital intracellular sugar levels.

- Eliminate fried foods, coffee, black tea, colas, and other stimulants from the diet.

- Refrain from excessive alcohol use, as it has an adverse effect on the heart. Drinking alcohol in moderation may actually be heart-healthy, but do not start to drink if you have not done so before—the potential benefit simply does not justify it.

- Sip barley water throughout the day for its healing and fortifying properties. (*See* THERAPEUTIC LIQUIDS in Part Three.)

❑ Learn to make heart-smart food substitutions, such as the following:

- Instead of whole or 2 percent milk and cream, use 1 percent or skim milk.

- Instead of fried foods, eat baked, steamed, boiled, or broiled foods.

- Instead of lard, butter, palm oil, or coconut oils, cook with unsaturated vegetable oils such as corn, olive, canola, safflower, sesame, soybean, sunflower, or peanut.

- Instead of eating fatty cuts of meat, choose extra-lean cuts or cut off the fatty parts. Or substitute skinless chicken or fish.

- Instead of one whole egg in recipes, use two egg whites.

- Instead of sauces, butter, and salt, season vegetables with herbs and spices.

- Instead of regular hard and processed cheeses, eat low-fat, low-sodium cheeses.

- Instead of salted potato chips, eat low-fat, unsalted tortilla and potato chips and unsalted pretzels and popcorn.

- Instead of sour cream and mayonnaise, use plain low-fat yogurt, low-fat cottage cheese, or low-fat, light sour cream.

❑ Fast three days a month to cleanse and detoxify the body. (*See* FASTING in Part Three and follow the program.)

❑ To relieve stress and promote relaxation, add a few drops of lavender, sandalwood, or ylang ylang essential oil to a bath, or simply place a few drops on a tissue and inhale the aroma from time to time throughout the day.

❑ *Arnica* is a homeopathic remedy used to support recovery from a heart attack.

❑ Do not smoke. Avoid secondhand smoke.

❑ The tests you'll need to diagnose your heart disease depend on what condition your doctor thinks you might have. No matter what type of heart disease you have, your doctor will likely perform a physical exam and ask about your personal and family medical history before doing any other tests. If you think you may be at risk for cardiovascular disease, you should discuss the following tests with your doctor: blood tests, chest X-ray, electrocardiogram (ECG), Holter monitoring, echocardiogram, catheterization, cardiac computerized tomography (CT) scan, and cardiac magnetic resonance imaging (MRI). (*See* box "Common Heart Problems and Procedures" under CARDIOVASCULAR DISEASE in Part Two.)

Considerations

❏ Research has shown that people typically wait two hours or more before seeking emergency care after the onset of heart attack symptoms. It could be because they are uncertain about their symptoms or are concerned that it might be a false alarm. However, clot-busting medications and other effective treatments that restore blood flow and save heart muscle are most effective in the first hour following a heart attack.

❏ Heart attacks are directly related to a number of other conditions, such as arteriosclerosis, circulatory problems, hypertension (high blood pressure), high cholesterol, and cardiovascular disorders (including aneurysms, angina pectoris, and arrhythmias). These conditions are discussed separately in Part Two. It is advisable to refer to all of the sections on these interrelated diseases to learn about all aspects of, and contributing causes to, heart attacks.

❏ The severity of first heart attacks has dropped significantly in the United States—propelling a decline in coronary heart disease deaths, researchers reported in *Circulation: Journal of the American Heart Association*. This study suggests that better prevention and better management in the hospital have contributed to the reduction in deaths.

❏ Similarly, a study published in *The Journal of the American Medical Association (JAMA)* found that the chance of dying thirty days after a heart attack dropped from 18.8 percent in 1995 to 15.8 percent in 2006. The drop can be attributed in part to the fact that treatment in hospitals across the United States has become more consistent.

❏ Heart attacks are not, as many think, a male disorder. In fact, women account for nearly half of all heart attack deaths. Forty-four percent of women die within a year, whereas only 27 percent of men do. Heart attacks, not cancer, are the leading cause of death for American women. Twice as many women die of heart attacks each year as die from all forms of cancer combined.

❏ New guidelines call for women to maintain HDL levels above 50 mg/dL, a 25 percent increase over the previous recommendation, 40 mg/dL. Women are also advised to keep triglycerides below 150 mg/dL, rather than the previously recommended 200 mg/dL.

❏ Women experience a heart attack on average nine years later than men. However, many of the risk factors for having one are the same in men and women. These include high cholesterol, smoking, abdominal obesity, poor diet, and stress. These factors explain more than 90 percent of the risk for heart attack, and all are controllable.

❏ A guide to some of the language doctors use in talking about cardiovascular disease and heart attacks appears on page 311. This is not a definitive list, but it may provide a handy reference guide for major terms and tests for heart attacks.

❏ It is highly recommended that at least one person in every household receive thorough training in CPR.

Stress Testing

Many physicians recommend that certain individuals undergo stress testing to determine the fitness and health of their hearts and cardiovascular systems. There are actually a number of different variations on stress testing. Following are some points you should know about them.

The most common stress test is an exercise test, which involves walking on a treadmill that increases in speed and grade (steepness) every three minutes. This test normally is stopped when the person undergoing it becomes fatigued or is short of breath, or experiences chest pressure. Heart rhythm and blood pressure are continuously monitored during the test.

Traditional stress testing sometimes can be combined with other techniques to take images of the heart before and after exercise. An exercise (treadmill or bicycle) echocardiogram, informally known as an echo, can be made that takes ultrasound pictures of the heart to see how it responds.

A nuclear thallium or sestamibi test is another type of imaging stress test. In this procedure, an intravenous (IV) line is placed in the arm and a small amount of radioactive material is injected before and after exercise. Images of the heart's blood supply then can be made.

For those who are unable to exercise, a medicine such as dobutamine or dipyridamole is given via an IV to gradually increase the workload of the heart, just as if it were exercising. Echo or nuclear images of the heart are then made to determine how well the heart's overall pumping action increases and whether or not there are any problems with blood supply to one of the walls of the heart.

An angiogram looks at the blood vessels around the heart and can also give information concerning the heart muscle and heart valves. A special catheter is threaded into the body through a blood vessel in the groin or arm. This catheter reaches the arteries around the heart. Dye is injected via the catheter into the blood vessels while pictures are being shot with an X-ray machine. These X-rays will show blockages in the arteries and their severity.

Your doctor will choose the best stress test for you, if needed, based on your symptoms, risk factors, and a physical exam. Regular checkups by a health care professional, regular exercise, eating lots of fruits and vegetables, and quitting smoking are key to a healthy heart.

❏ A technique known as thermography can be used to test for the presence of atherosclerosis by detecting fluctuations in the temperature of the arteries. In healthy arteries, the temperature remains constant, while in arteries that contain plaque, the temperature is different in diseased areas and the healthy areas. Another test for detecting harmful levels of calcium or plaque buildup in the arteries is gated helical computerized tomography (GHCT) scanning. Ask your doctor if he or she thinks either of these is a test you should have.

❏ Tirofiban (Aggrastat) is an injectable drug that may help people recover from acute cardiac episodes, including severe angina or severe chest pain. It is a type of agent called a glycoprotein blocker that stops blood from clotting. Trials conducted in New Zealand found that tirofiban was more effective at preventing a second heart attack than aspirin or heparin. Tirofiban was recommended by the American Heart Association in 2007 for patients who have had a type of heart attack called non-ST-segment elevation myocardial infarction (NSTEMI).

❏ Some compounds known as plant sterols and stanols have been shown to lower LDL cholesterol levels and can be found in some types of margarine and salad dressing. They are also available in tablet form.

❏ Carnitine, coenzyme Q_{10}, fish oil, magnesium, and antioxidants are recommended for the prevention of cardiac arrhythmia, heart attack, and angina. Carnitine protects the heart muscle from damage due to poor circulation or partial arterial blockage.

❏ An Austrian study found that coughing vigorously ("cough CPR") until help arrives can help to save the lives of people experiencing heart attack or cardiac arrest.

❏ The omega-3 fatty acids docosahexaenoic acid (DHA) and eicosapentaenoic acid (EPA) help to reduce the risk of heart attack. Taking both DHA and EPA supplements was shown to reduce the chances of dying from all causes, including heart disease. These data were based on twelve studies including more than 32,000 individuals. Although the best dose is not yet known, the FDA is getting closer to making a DRI for omega-3s. The recommendation will likely be between 250 milligrams and 500 milligrams a day.

❏ Diet is important after a heart attack. Both a low-fat diet and a Mediterranean diet, which is also low in fat but has more omega-3s, were shown to reduce the chance of having a second heart attack or dying from a heart attack.

❏ Very large doses of vitamin D—over 1,000 international units daily—can be dangerous for people with heart disease. In large quantities, vitamin D is toxic and can cause hypercalcemia (excessively high levels of calcium in the blood), which in turn may lead to deposits of calcium in the arteries.

❏ Among the more recently identified risk factors that may be linked to cardiovascular disease is C-reactive protein (CRP). This is a compound produced by the liver in response to injury or infection, and is a sign of inflammation in the body. Research correlates high levels of CRP with an increased risk of heart attack and stroke. Although the evidence is conflicting, some researchers believe that CRP itself is not a risk factor, but elevated levels of CRP could mean that some part of the cardiovascular system is inflamed, which can lead to stroke or heart attack. Information about CRP and other new risk factors is still emerging.

❏ There is ongoing debate about whether or not taking synthetic estrogen protects the heart after menopause. Some studies have suggested that it may, but there have also been studies showing it may actually increase the risk of a heart attack.

❏ There are many different medications that may be prescribed for people with heart disease. These include the following:

- Angiotensin-converting enzyme (ACE) inhibitors inhibit the formation of the hormone angiotensin, which narrows the blood vessels. Angiotensin II receptor blockers interfere with the action, rather than the formation, of the same hormone.

- Anticoagulants (blood-thinners) are commonly prescribed for people in particular danger of developing blood clots, such as people who are bedridden, cancer patients, people with certain types of arrhythmias, and those who have had heart valve replacement surgery. There are also newer drugs known as platelet-aggregation inhibitors that may be prescribed for the same purposes. Sometimes just an aspirin is recommended when a patient is at risk for heart disease, but does not need anticoagulation drugs. The dose is small (81 milligrams per day) and less likely to cause stomach erosion, but effective enough to slightly thin the blood.

- Beta-blockers induce the heart to beat more slowly and with less force.

- Calcium channel blockers relax blood vessel muscle.

- Central adrenergic inhibitors (central-acting agents) prevent the nervous system from increasing heart rate and narrowing blood vessels.

- Diuretics (water pills) help the kidneys get rid of sodium and water, reducing the volume of blood in the body and, therefore, the strain on the heart.

❏ Most people who have heart attacks experience the characteristic chest pain. However, not all do. Some people have a sensation that feels like indigestion; others have no noticeable symptoms at all. This phenomenon is often referred to as a "silent" heart attack. Older adults and people with diabetes are probably more likely than others to have this type of heart attack.

❏ Many illnesses can mimic heart attacks, such as a gallbladder attack, fibromyalgia that causes pain in the chest wall, or gastroesophageal reflux disease (GERD), but if you have chest pain, you must see a physician. Chest pain or even ill-defined symptoms that you cannot explain just may be a heart attack—these are not conditions you can afford to ignore.

❏ People with high blood pressure should avoid cold weather, which might trigger heart attacks because the lower temperatures increase blood pressure, putting more strain on the heart.

❏ In some cases, heart attacks are caused by spasms of the arteries that suddenly shut off the flow of blood to the heart.

❑ Sensible, moderate exercise and a proper diet with nutritional supplements can prevent arteriosclerosis of the coronary arteries and myocardial infarction.

Caution: If you are over thirty-five and/or have been sedentary for some time, consult with your health care provider before beginning an exercise program.

❑ Studies have shown that people who take supplemental coenzyme Q_{10} following a heart attack are less likely to have a second attack within five years than those who do not.

❑ Researchers have found that eating just an ounce of walnuts a day (about seven nuts) may reduce the risk of a heart attack by 8 to 10 percent.

❑ A heart attack is not the same thing as heart failure. In heart failure, the heart does not supply enough blood to the body; in a heart attack, the heart does not receive enough blood to meet its needs. However, the damage produced by a heart attack can lead to heart failure.

❑ An underactive thyroid may increase the risk of heart attacks. An article in the *Annals of Internal Medicine* reported that women who had a condition termed *subclinical hypothyroidism* were about two times more likely to suffer from blockage in the aorta that could lead to a heart attack than women who had normally functioning thyroids.

❑ Depression and heart attacks often go hand in hand. It is therefore wise to actively treat depression.

❑ *See* ARTERIOSCLEROSIS/ATHEROSCLEROSIS; CARDIOVASCULAR DISEASE; CIRCULATORY PROBLEMS; HIGH BLOOD PRESSURE (HYPERTENSION); HIGH CHOLESTEROL; and RHEUMATIC FEVER, all in Part Two.

❑ *See also* CHELATION THERAPY in Part Three.

HEART DISEASE

See CARDIOVASCULAR DISEASE; HEART ATTACK.

HEARTBURN/GASTROESOPHAGEAL REFLUX DISEASE (GERD)

Heartburn is a burning sensation and pain in the stomach and/or chest, behind the breastbone. It may be accompanied by bloating, gas, nausea, shortness of breath, and/or an acidic or sour taste in the throat. Most people suffer from heartburn at some time in their life. It often occurs when hydrochloric acid, which is used by the stomach to digest food, backs up into the esophagus (the tube between the throat and stomach), causing sensitive tissues to become irritated.

Normally, the esophageal sphincter muscle pinches itself shut and prevents stomach acid from surging upward. However, if the sphincter is not functioning properly, the acid can slip past it and into the esophagus. This is gastroesophageal reflux. Conditions that affect the esophagus and cause a reflux of stomach acids into the esophagus are now referred to as *gastroesophageal reflux disease* (GERD) rather than dyspepsia, chronic heartburn, or acid indigestion.

GERD can strike anyone, at any age. GERD can scar the esophagus, and if stomach acids make their way into the lungs, it can cause asthma-like symptoms. GERD can also lead to a condition called *Barrett's esophagus,* which is characterized by changes in the cells lining the esophagus that can induce cancer.

People with hiatal hernia often experience heartburn. It can also be triggered by certain foods. Common trigger foods include alcohol, caffeine, chocolate, citrus fruits and products, fats and fatty or fried foods, peppermint, spicy foods, and tomatoes and tomato-based foods. Gallbladder problems, stress, allergies, and enzyme deficiencies are other possible contributing factors.

Unless otherwise specified, the dosages recommended here are for adults. For children between the ages of twelve and seventeen, reduce the dose to three-quarters the recommended amount. For children between six and twelve, use one-half the recommended dose, and for children under the age of six, use one-quarter the recommended amount.

NUTRIENTS

SUPPLEMENT	SUGGESTED DOSAGE	COMMENTS
Very Important		
Pancreatin plus bromelain	As directed on label. Take with meals. 80 mg daily, in divided doses. Do not exceed a total of 100 mg daily from all supplements.	Enzymes necessary for proper digestion.
Papaya tablets	As directed on label.	To relieve symptoms. Use chewable tablets from a health food store.
Vitamin B complex plus extra vitamin B_{12}	50 mg of each major B vitamin 3 times daily, with meals (amounts of individual vitamins in a complex will vary). 1,000–2,000 mcg daily.	Needed for proper digestion. Use lozenge or sublingual forms.
Helpful		
Acid-Ease from Enzymatic Therapy	As directed on label.	A soothing plant enzyme and herb formula that aids in the breakdown and assimilation of foods.
Acidophilus	As directed on label.	Replaces "friendly" bacteria in the stomach.
Calcium and magnesium and potassium	300 mg twice daily. 150–200 mg twice daily. 100 mg twice daily.	These minerals have an alkalizing effect that binds up stomach acid. Take these together between meals. Use calcium carbonate or calcium chelate form.
Methylsulfonyl-methane (MSM)	As directed on label.	Relieves hyperacidity without disturbing the normal acid-alkaline balance.

485

Herbs

❏ Aloe vera juice aids healing of the intestinal tract.

❏ Catnip, fennel, ginger, marshmallow root, and papaya tea all aid in proper digestion and act as buffers to stop heartburn.

❏ Drinking chamomile tea can relieve esophageal irritation.

Caution: Do not use chamomile if you are allergic to ragweed. Do not use during pregnancy or nursing. It may interact with warfarin or cyclosporine, so patients using these drugs should avoid it.

❏ Deglycyrrhizinated licorice (DGL) has effectively treated both heartburn and ulcers of the stomach and esophagus.

Caution: Licorice root should not be used during pregnancy or nursing. It should not be used by persons with diabetes, glaucoma, heart disease, high blood pressure, or a history of stroke.

Recommendations

❏ At the first sign of heartburn, drink a large glass of water. This often helps.

❏ Try raw potato juice. Do not peel the potato—just wash it and put it in a juicer. (*See* JUICING in Part Three.) Mix the juice with an equal amount of water. Drink it immediately after preparation, three times a day.

❏ Try drinking a glass of fresh cabbage or celery juice every day.

❏ Change your eating habits. Eat more raw vegetables. Eat smaller, more frequent meals. Chew your food well. Eat slowly and enjoy your food. Following a disciplined diet is an important aspect of managing GERD.

❏ Sip 1 tablespoon of raw apple cider vinegar, mixed with a glass of water, while eating a meal. Do not drink any other liquids with meals.

❏ Eat fresh papaya and/or pineapple to aid digestion. Chew a few of the papaya seeds as well.

❏ Do not eat for three hours before bedtime. Wait at least three hours after eating before lying down.

❏ Avoid acidic foods such as citrus fruits and juices (*see* ACID/ALKALI IMBALANCE in Part Two).

❏ Do not consume caffeine-containing products, carbonated beverages, creamy cheeses, desserts, eggnog, fats, fried foods, gravies, rich sauces, marbled meats, onions (especially raw), peppermint, poultry skin, processed foods, spearmint, spicy or highly seasoned foods, sugar, tobacco, or tomatoes. These seem to be the main cause of heartburn.

❏ Avoid overeating at a meal.

❏ If you are overweight, weight loss may help reduce symptoms.

❏ *See* FASTING in Part Three and follow the instructions.

Also see the self-tests *under* ACID/ALKALI IMBALANCE and CARDIOVASCULAR DISEASE in Part Two.

❏ Do not take a multienzyme complex containing hydrochloric acid (HCl).

❏ Maintain an exercise program that includes walking, biking, or low-impact aerobics. Avoid running and weight lifting, as these activities put pressure on the stomach. Do not exercise after eating, however.

Caution: If you are thirty-five or older and/or have been sedentary for some time, consult with your health care provider before beginning an exercise program.

❏ Elevate the head of your bed.

❏ As much as possible, avoid stress and anger.

❏ If you are taking any medications, ask your doctor if heartburn may be a side effect.

❏ Do not wear clothes that fit tightly around the waist. Do not wear tight clothing to bed.

❏ Do not ignore symptoms of GERD. This condition can cause serious health problems. If heartburn lasts longer than two weeks, you should seek medical attention.

❏ The early symptoms of angina and heart attack sometimes mimic those of "acid stomach." If symptoms persist, if the pain begins to travel down into your left arm, or if the sensation is accompanied by a feeling of weakness, dizziness, or shortness of breath, seek emergency medical help at once. (*See* HEART ATTACK in Part Two.)

Considerations

❏ Estrogens can weaken the esophageal hiatus muscle, which keeps stomach acids in the stomach. Women who are pregnant and women who take birth control pills that contain estrogen and progesterone are therefore more likely to suffer from heartburn.

❏ Some nutrients such as melatonin, L-tryptophan, vitamins B_6 and B_{12}, folic acid, methionine, and betaine were shown to be just as effective as drug therapy in reducing symptoms.

❏ People with certain illnesses, such as cancer, often have excessive amounts of acid in their systems. The consumption of too much processed and cooked food can also create an acidic environment in the body.

❏ Aspirin and ibuprofen can cause heartburn.

❏ Lying on your left side can help relieve heartburn. This keeps the stomach below the esophagus, helping to keep it acid-free.

❏ Antacids often provide relief of symptoms. However, in so doing, they may mask an underlying problem. In addition, many over-the-counter antacids contain excessive amounts of sodium, aluminum, calcium, and magnesium. With prolonged use of these products, dangerous mineral imbalances can occur. Excess sodium can aggravate hypertension, and excess aluminum has been implicated in Alzheimer's disease. Reading the label of the antacids you intend to use will provide you with information concerning possible harmful ingredients contained in the product. Some types of antacids and the products they are found in are:

- Aluminum salts or gels: AlternaGEL, Amphojel.

- Aluminum-magnesium mixtures: Aludrox, Di-Gel, Gaviscon, Gelusil, Maalox, Mylanta, Riopan.

- Calcium carbonate: Alka-Mints, Chooz, Titralac, Tums.

- Calcium-magnesium mixtures: Rolaids.

- Magnesium salts or gels: Phillips' Milk of Magnesia.

- Sodium bicarbonate: Alka-Seltzer, Bromo Seltzer, Citrocarbonate.

❑ Calcium carbonate works as an antacid and contains no aluminum.

❑ A product called Acid-Ease, from Enzymatic Therapy, has shown promising results. It can be purchased at health food stores. Acid-Ease is aluminum-free.

❑ Drugs that suppress the production of stomach acid are sometimes recommended for people who suffer from frequent heartburn. These include cimetidine (Tagamet), famotidine (Pepcid), nizatidine (Axid), omeprazole (Prilosec), and ranitidine (Zantac). It has been suggested that long-term use of these medications may lead to damage to the stomach lining, thus increasing the risk of benign or malignant tumors. According to an item in the *Johns Hopkins Medical Letter,* excessive (more than 3 grams a day) and prolonged use of the heartburn medication cimetidine may lower the libido or cause breast enlargement. These conditions usually go away when the medication is discontinued.

❑ The prescription drug famotidine (Pepcid) is now available in generic form. The over-the-counter Pepcid-AC is also now available as a generic.

❑ One study showed that 57 percent of heartburn sufferers had hiatal hernias, almost half had damage to the esophageal lining, and 6 percent had developed *Barrett's esophagus.*

❑ If you are taking antacids more than three times a week, you should consult your physician.

❑ Free information about GERD is available from the International Foundation for Functional Gastrointestinal Disorders. (*See* Health and Medical Organizations in the Appendix.)

❑ *See* PEPTIC ULCER in Part Two. *Also see under* PREGNANCY-RELATED PROBLEMS in Part Two.

HEEL OR BONE SPUR

A bone spur is a pointed growth on a bone, most commonly in the heel. Extreme stress and strain on the heel bone and soft tissues are the main causes of heel spurs. The stress results in inflammation of the plantar fascia, a ligament on the bottom of the foot that attaches the ball of the foot to the heel bone. This condition is known as plantar fasciitis. If it is not relieved, the repeated pulling of the ligament aggravates the heel bone and eventually the body, in an attempt to protect itself, forms a bone spur. The most common sign of a bone spur is severe pain with the first step in the morning and after periods of inactivity.

Bone spurs can be caused by, or be associated with, physical injury, obesity, gout, lupus, muscle inflammation, nerve problems (such as tarsal tunnel syndrome), strain of the plantar arch, or excessive exercise, standing, or walking. Heel spurs are also common in people who have alkalosis, arthritis, neuritis, or tendinitis. A bone spur may be caused by calcium deposits in unwanted areas of the body. Most people who have heel disorders are middle-aged or overweight. Shoes that are uncomfortable, fit poorly, or lack cushioning for the heel may contribute to the pain.

X-rays may reveal a bony spur within the heel. The presence of this may lead to the formation of tiny tumors at the end of several nerves, and these may be very painful.

Unless otherwise specified, the dosages recommended here are for adults. For children between the ages of twelve and seventeen, reduce the dose to three-quarters the recommended amount. For children between six and twelve, use one-half the recommended dose, and for children under the age of six, use one-quarter the recommended amount.

NUTRIENTS

SUPPLEMENT	SUGGESTED DOSAGE	COMMENTS
Very Important		
Betaine hydrochloride (HCl)	As directed on label.	Needed for proper calcium uptake. A deficiency of HCl is more common in older people. *Caution:* Do not use HCl if you have a history of ulcers.
Calcium and magnesium	1,500 mg daily. 750 mg daily.	A proper balance of calcium and magnesium helps prevent abnormal calcium deposition. Use chelate or aspartate forms.
Important		
Proteolytic enzymes or Inf-zyme Forte from American Biologics or Intenzyme Forte from Biotics Research	As directed on label. As directed on label. As directed on label.	To aid in absorption of nutrients and in control of inflammation and irritation. *Caution:* Do not give these supplements to a child.
Vitamin C with bioflavonoids	2,000–4,000 mg daily.	Acts as an anti-inflammatory; important for collagen and connective tissue.
Helpful		
Bioflavonoids	100 mg daily.	Vitamin C activators that also help relieve pain.
Methylsulfonyl-methane (MSM)	As directed on label. It can be applied as a	Very effective for pain relief.

	cream or taken by mouth in the pill form.	
Vitamin B complex	50–100 mg of each major B vitamin daily (amounts of individual vitamins in a complex will vary).	B vitamins work best when taken together.
plus extra vitamin B$_6$ (pyridoxine)	50 mg daily.	Necessary for production of hydrochloric acid, which helps prevent bone spurs by aiding proper calcium absorption.

Herbs

❑ Use arnica and chamomile to bathe the foot. You can also wrap the herbs in a cloth and apply it to the affected area as a poultice. (*See* USING A POULTICE in Part Three.)

❑ Bromelain, derived from pineapple, and curcumin, from turmeric, reduce pain and inflammation.

Recommendations

❑ Drink steam-distilled water only.

❑ Do not eat any citrus fruits, especially oranges. Eliminate alcohol, coffee, and sugar from your diet. These inhibit the healing process and upset the body's mineral balance.

❑ To alleviate pain, try stretching exercises; deep, localized massage; physical therapy; and anti-inflammatory herbs. You can also use hot linseed oil packs. Place linseed oil in a pan and heat but do not boil it. Dip a piece of cheesecloth or other white cotton material into the oil until the cloth is saturated. Apply the cloth to the affected area and cover it with a piece of plastic that is larger in size than the cotton cloth. Place a heating pad over the plastic and use it to keep the pack warm. Keep the pack in place for one-half to two hours, as needed.

❑ Ice massages on the bottoms of the feet can be helpful. Alternate between hot and cold foot baths.

❑ Select well-made, rubber-heeled shoes; these are better for the feet than leather. Choose footwear for comfort—not for looks. Some jogging shoes can be very comfortable. Adding heel cushions to footwear helps to relieve pain.

❑ Use night splints to provide a mild, constant stretching function across the sole of the foot at night while sleeping.

❑ If you normally walk or jog for exercise, try bicycling or swimming instead.

❑ Avoid walking on hard surfaces such as concrete, wood, or hard floors without carpeting.

Considerations

❑ A two-week raw food fast or a cleansing fast can be beneficial. (*See* FASTING in Part Three.)

❑ It is best not to have a heel spur surgically removed unless it is extremely irritating or painful.

❑ Steroid injections have been used to treat this condition. They are not without potential complications, however. They may cause loss of the fatty tissue pad at the bottom of the heel and bring about a condition that is painful and irreversible.

❑ Foot surgery is a last-resort option that is usually reserved for extremely rare, severe cases. An incision is made over the heel to release the attached fascia from the heel bone. Recovery time is approximately six to ten weeks before walking can be resumed comfortably. However, if you find that you are unable to exercise or engage in normal activities because of a heel or bone spur, you should consider surgery. Lack of exercise could lead to weight gain and other problems such as diabetes and heart disease.

❑ *See also* ARTHRITIS in Part Two.

HEMOPHILIA

In a healthy individual, a minor bump can damage a blood vessel, causing blood to leak into the surrounding tissue, producing a bruise. A process called hemostasis (coagulation) plugs the hole in the damaged vessel and forms a clot that stops the blood loss and limits the size of the bruise.

In people with hemophilia and related problems, bleeding can take a very different course. The blood does not clot normally because one or another of the blood proteins that collaborate to repair damaged vessels and form clots is defective, deficient, or totally absent. Approximately 20,000 people in the United States suffer from hemophilia.

There are two main types of hemophilia. They are classified according to the particular protein, or clotting factor, that is deficient. Hemophilia A, caused by a deficiency of factor VIII, accounts for almost 80 percent of people with this disorder. It is usually inherited by male children of mothers who are carriers. Hemophilia B, sometimes called *Christmas disease,* is caused by a problem with clotting factor IX. It too is passed on by carrier mothers to male children. It is also possible to have a bleeding disorder due to factor XI deficiency. Unlike hemophilia A and B, this problem can be carried by either the male or female parent, and can be passed on to both male and female offspring.

The idea that people with hemophilia can bleed to death from a minor cut or injury is a misconception. In fact, external bleeding is seldom a serious problem. People with hemophilia may bleed somewhat longer than other people, but minor bleeding episodes can generally be controlled by ordinary first aid measures.

Injuries also commonly cause bleeding inside the body— bleeding we may neither see nor feel. Unchecked internal bleeding can be serious—even life-threatening—for a person with hemophilia. Blood that leaks into the knee joint, a common site of internal bleeding, can cause painful swelling. Repeated bleeding eventually destroys the cartilage that enables the knee to work smoothly and easily. The joint becomes permanently stiff and painful, the result of hemophilic arthritis. Other joints—the ankle, wrist, or elbow—can be similarly affected by internal bleeding. People with hemophilia can also bleed into muscle and other soft tissue. Internal bleeding can ultimately obstruct air passages or damage the brain or other vital organs.

Hemophilia can be mild, moderate, or severe, depending on how impaired an individual's production of clotting factors is. In severe hemophilia, clotting factor activity is less than 1 percent of normal. Injury, surgery, or dental care can present significant problems for such people. Spontaneous bleeding can require infusion of clotting factor concentrate as often as several times a week. People with moderate hemophilia (factor levels between 1 and 5 percent of normal) do not usually experience spontaneous bleeding, but even a minor injury, if untreated, can cause prolonged bleeding. In mild hemophilia, factor activity ranges between 5 and 50 percent of normal. Bleeding can be expected from surgery, major dental care, or trauma. These individuals rarely bleed into joints, and their disease usually does not interfere with normal living.

The National Hemophilia Foundation estimates that nearly 450 American boys with hemophilia are born each year. The number of females with hemophilia is not known. Hemophilia primarily affects males and is passed down through females because the two primary genes involved in the production of clotting factors are located on the X chromosome. And while females have two X chromosomes, males have only one. For a female to develop the disease, both of her X chromosomes would have to carry the defective gene (which is unlikely), whereas a male has only a single X chromosome, so if one of its clotting factor genes is defective, he will be affected.

A woman who has one defective gene will not develop hemophilia herself, but is a carrier of the condition. All children of (female) carriers have a 50 percent chance of inheriting the defective gene. For sons, this means a 50 percent chance of developing the disease; for daughters, it means a 50 percent chance of being carriers, like their mothers. For the children of (male) hemophiliacs, the story is somewhat different. Sons are not affected (unless the mother is a carrier), but daughters always become carriers. For hemophilia to occur in a female, she would have to have both a father with the condition and a mother who either has hemophilia or is a carrier.

People with hemophilia are commonly treated with plasma concentrates prepared from pooled blood plasma. As a result, as many as two-thirds of all Americans with hemophilia became infected with HIV before the virus was identified and a screening test developed. Blood donors are now screened for HIV, and clotting factor products are routinely subjected to heat to minimize, if not eliminate, the risk of transmission of the virus, but the chance of con-

tracting HIV understandably remains a source of concern for people with hemophilia. Hepatitis viruses had also been a problem for people using blood products.

Unless otherwise specified, the dosages recommended here are for adults. For children between the ages of twelve and seventeen, reduce the dose to three-quarters the recommended amount. For children between six and twelve, use one-half the recommended dose, and for children under the age of six, use one-quarter the recommended amount.

NUTRIENTS

SUPPLEMENT	SUGGESTED DOSAGE	COMMENTS
Helpful		
Calcium and	1,500 mg daily.	Essential for blood clotting.
magnesium	1,000 mg daily.	Needed to balance with calcium.
Liver extract injections or raw liver extract	1 cc once weekly or as prescribed by physician. As directed on label.	Contains vital nutrients for blood clotting.
Multivitamin and mineral complex	As directed on label.	Provides necessary vitamins and minerals.
Vitamin B complex plus extra vitamin B$_3$ (niacin) and niacinamide	As directed on label. As directed on label. As directed on label.	All B vitamins are essential in blood formation and clotting. *Caution:* Do not take niacin if you have a liver disorder, gout, or high blood pressure.
Vitamin C with bioflavonoids	3,000 mg daily.	Important in normal blood coagulation.
Vitamin K or alfalfa	300 mcg daily.	Essential in blood-clotting mechanism. *See* under Herbs, below.

Herbs

❑ Alfalfa is a good source of vitamin K, which is vital in the process of blood clotting. It can be taken in tablet form or eaten in a natural form, such as alfalfa sprouts.

Recommendations

❑ Eat a diet high in vitamin K. Foods that contain a measurable amount of this vitamin are alfalfa, broccoli, cauliflower, egg yolks, kale, liver, spinach, and all green leafy vegetables.

❑ "Green drinks" made from the vegetables listed above are very healthful. Drink one of these each day for vitamin K and other essential clotting factors.

❑ Be alert for early warning signs of internal bleeding, including a bubbling or tingling sensation or a feeling of warmth, tightness, or stiffness in the affected area. A blow to the head, headache, confusion, drowsiness, or other evidence of neurological impairment may signal intracranial bleeding.

❑ Wear an identity bracelet so that, in an emergency, people will know that you have hemophilia.

❑ *Do not* take aspirin. Aspirin is an anticlotting agent.

❑ If you care for an infant or toddler with hemophilia, be alert for signs of joint or muscle pain caused by internal bleeding. The child may cry for no apparent reason, refuse to use an arm or leg, refuse to walk, or have swelling or excessive bruising. If you suspect internal bleeding, seek treatment immediately.

Considerations

❑ Treatment of hemophilia consists of intravenous infusions of the missing clotting factor. This is now usually done at home. How much antihemophilic factor an individual needs and when depends on the severity of his or her disease.

❑ Gene therapy may hold the key to curing hemophilia, although the factor VIII gene is extremely complex, and it may be some time before scientists are able to replace these defective genes in people with hemophilia.

❑ For names and addresses of organizations that may be of assistance in obtaining information and/or treatment options, *see* Health and Medical Organizations in the Appendix.

HEMORRHOIDS

Hemorrhoids are swollen veins around the anus and in the rectum (the very lowest portion of the colon) that may protrude from the anus. The word *hemorrhoid* comes from *hemo* (Greek for "blood") and *rrhoos* ("discharging"). They are also known as piles, from the Latin word *pila,* meaning "ball." Hemorrhoids are very much like varicose veins; they enlarge and lose their elasticity, resulting in saclike protrusions into the anal canal. They are not tumors or growths. They can be caused, and aggravated, by sitting or standing for prolonged periods, violent coughing, lifting heavy objects (or lifting even relatively light objects improperly), and straining at bowel movements (especially when constipated, although bouts of diarrhea accompanied by involuntary spasms can exacerbate the problem). Other factors that can cause or contribute to the formation of hemorrhoids include obesity, lack of exercise, liver damage, food allergies, and insufficient consumption of dietary fiber. Hemorrhoids are common during pregnancy and after childbirth. Hormonal changes and pressure exerted by the growing fetus may be the reasons. Approximately half of all Americans have had hemorrhoids by the age of fifty. The incidence increases with age until age seventy, then begins to decrease again.

The most common symptoms of hemorrhoids include itching, burning, pain, inflammation, swelling, irritation,

seepage, and bleeding. The bleeding, which is usually bright red during bowel movements, can be startling, even frightening. Although it does signal that something is amiss in the digestive system, rectal bleeding is not necessarily an indication of serious disease.

There are different types of hemorrhoids, depending on their location, severity, and the amount of pain, discomfort, or aggravation they cause. These are:

- *External.* These develop under the skin at the opening of the anal cavity. They may form a hard lump and cause painful swelling if a blood clot forms. When an external hemorrhoid swells, the tissue in the area becomes firm but sensitive and turns blue or purple in color. This type of hemorrhoid most often affects younger people and can be extremely painful.

- *Internal.* Internal hemorrhoids are located inside the rectum. They are usually painless, especially if located above the anorectal line, because rectal tissues lack nerve fibers. Internal hemorrhoids do, however, tend to bleed. When they do, the blood appears bright red.

- *Prolapsed.* A prolapsed hemorrhoid is an internal hemorrhoid that collapses and protrudes outside the anus, often accompanied by a mucous discharge and heavy bleeding. Prolapsed hemorrhoids can become *thrombosed*— that is, they can form clots within that prevent their receding. Thrombosed hemorrhoids can also be excruciatingly painful.

As far as we know, hemorrhoids are unique to human beings. No other creature develops this problem. This can be taken as an indication that our dietary and nutritional habits probably play a greater role in this disorder than anything else. Hemorrhoids can occur at any age, but they tend to become more common as people age. Among younger people, pregnant women and women who have had children seem to be the most susceptible. The tendency to develop hemorrhoids also appears to be hereditary. Although hemorrhoids can be quite painful, they do not usually pose a serious threat to health.

Unless otherwise specified, the dosages recommended here are for adults. For children between the ages of twelve and seventeen, reduce the dose to three-quarters the recommended amount. For children between six and twelve, use one-half the recommended dose, and for children under the age of six, use one-quarter the recommended amount.

NUTRIENTS

SUPPLEMENT	SUGGESTED DOSAGE	COMMENTS
Very Important		
ABC Aerobic Bulk Cleanse from Aerobic Life Industries	As directed on label. Mix with ½ glass fruit juice and ½ glass aloe vera juice, and drink it down quickly before the fiber thickens. Take separately from other supplements and medications.	Keeps the colon clean, relieving pressure on the rectum.

Calcium	1,500 mg daily.	Essential for blood clotting. Helps prevent cancer of the colon. Use calcium chelate or aspartate form.
and magnesium	750 mg daily.	Needed to balance with calcium.
Vitamin C plus mixed bioflavonoids with hesperidin and rutin	3,000–5,000 mg daily. 100 mg 3 times daily.	Aid in healing and normal blood clotting.
Vitamin E	200 IU daily or 400 IU every other day.	Promotes normal blood clotting and healing. Use d-alpha-tocopherol form.

Important

Vitamin B complex plus extra vitamin B$_6$ (pyridoxine) and vitamin B$_{12}$ plus choline and inositol	50–100 mg of each major B vitamin 3 times daily, with meals (amounts of individual vitamins in a complex will vary). 50 mg 3 times daily, with meals. 1,000 mcg twice daily. 50 mg each twice daily.	All B vitamins are vital for digestion. Improved digestion results in reduced stress on the rectum. Use lozenge or sublingual forms.

Helpful

Coenzyme Q$_{10}$	100 mg daily.	Increases cellular oxygenation and assists in healing.
Dimethylglycine (DMG) (Aangamik DMG from FoodScience of Vermont)	125 mg twice daily.	Improves cellular oxygenation.
Garlic (Kyolic from Wakunaga)	As directed on label.	A natural antibiotic and immune system stimulant. Use the liquid form.
Key-E Suppositories from Carlson Labs	As directed on label.	Shrinks inflamed hemorrhoidal tissue. Check with your doctor before placing anything transrectally.
Potassium	99 mg daily.	Constipation, which can cause hemorrhoids, is common in those with potassium deficiencies.
Shark cartilage	1 gram per 15 lbs of body weight daily, divided into 3 doses. Can be taken either orally or rectally, in a retention enema.	Treats pain and inflammation.
Vitamin A with mixed carotenoids	15,000 IU daily. If you are pregnant, do not exceed 10,000 IU daily.	Aids in healing of mucous membranes and tissues.
Vitamin D	600 IU daily.	Aids in healing of mucous membranes and tissues. Also needed for calcium absorption.

Herbs

☐ Aloe vera gel, applied directly on the anus, has properties similar to aspirin. It can relieve pain and soothe the burning sensation. The fresh pulp is best.

☐ Bayberry, goldenseal root, myrrh, and white oak, used in a salve form, work like conventional hemorrhoid preparations—possibly better.

Caution: Do not take goldenseal internally on a daily basis for more than one week at a time. Do not use it during pregnancy or if you are breast-feeding, and use with caution if you are allergic to ragweed. If you have a history of cardiovascular disease, diabetes, or glaucoma, use it only under a doctor's supervision.

☐ A paste made from powdered comfrey root can be used in a poultice to heal bleeding hemorrhoids.

Caution: Comfrey is recommended for external use only.

☐ An elderberry poultice can relieve the pain associated with hemorrhoids. A mullein poultice can be used as well. (*See* USING A POULTICE in Part Three.)

☐ Brew a strong, warm tea using the herb lady's mantle (yarrow), and apply with a cotton ball several times a day.

☐ Witch hazel is helpful because of its astringent properties. Apply it three times daily with a sterile cotton pad to shrink the swollen vein.

☐ Other beneficial herbs include buckthorn bark, collinsonia root, parsley, red grapevine leaves, and stone root. These can be taken in capsule or tea form.

Recommendations

☐ Eat foods that are high in dietary fiber, such as wheat bran, fresh fruits, and nearly all vegetables. Apples, beets, Brazil nuts, broccoli, foods in the cabbage family, carrots, green beans, guar gum, oat bran, lima beans, pears, peas, psyllium seed, and whole grains are recommended. A high-fiber diet is probably the most important consideration in the treatment and prevention of hemorrhoids. Psyllium has been shown to be particularly effective in patients with internal bleeding hemorrhoids. It may take one month to take effect, but its continued use is advised.

☐ To help bleeding hemorrhoids, eat foods such as alfalfa, blackstrap molasses, and dark green leafy vegetables, which are high in vitamin K.

☐ Drink plenty of liquids, especially water (preferably steam-distilled). Water is the best, most natural stool softener in existence. It also helps prevent constipation.

☐ Avoid animal products, coffee, alcohol, and hot spices. Red meat and high-protein diets are especially hard on the lower digestive tract.

☐ Eat a healthy low-fat diet that is rich in fruits and vegetables. Include protein at each meal, mostly from vegetable sources, fish, or lean poultry.

❑ Take 1 or 2 tablespoons of flaxseed oil daily. Flaxseed oil helps to soften stools.

❑ If you decide to use a fiber supplement, start with a moderate amount and increase your intake gradually. If you take too much at first, this will cause painful bloating, gas, and possibly diarrhea.

Note: Always take supplemental fiber separately from other supplements and medications.

❑ Use cayenne (capsicum) and garlic enemas to keep the bowels clean. A plain warm-water enema is fast-acting and relieves discomfort in most cases. (*See* ENEMAS in Part Three.) Check with your health care provider before using.

❑ Use a peeled clove of garlic as a suppository three times a week. Raw potato suppositories help heal hemorrhoids and relieve pain. Cut a peeled potato into small cone-shaped pieces.

❑ If you are bothered by persistent bleeding, take vitamin and mineral supplements to prevent anemia. An iron supplement together with a powerful vitamin B complex and vitamin C will keep the blood healthy. Coenzymate B Complex from Source Naturals is among the most efficiently absorbed forms of the B vitamins. Consult your physician before taking iron.

Caution: See your physician if bleeding persists.

❑ Learn not to strain when moving the bowels. Keep the bowels clean and avoid constipation. Don't sit on the commode for longer than ten minutes at a time, as this causes blood to pool in the hemorrhoidal veins.

❑ Cleanse the problem area frequently with warm water. A hot bath for fifteen minutes a day is quite helpful. Do not add bath beads, oils, or bubbles to the water, as this can irritate sensitive tissues. Many people add Epsom salts, but this has no proven clinical value. It is the warm water that reduces swelling and eases the pain. Avoid using soap products to cleanse the anus.

❑ Warm sitz baths are especially beneficial. Take a mineral sitz bath daily. (*See* SITZ BATH in Part Three.) I recommend Batherapy from Queen Helene, a powder that contains many valuable minerals and is added to bathwater. This can be found in many health food stores.

❑ Sit on a soft cushion, not on hard surfaces. Use an ordinary cushion, not a donut-shaped one. The old-fashioned inflated doughnut cushion actually increases pressure upon the hemorrhoidal blood vessels, aggravating the swelling and bleeding.

❑ Learn proper lifting techniques. Bend your knees, not your back. Do not hold your breath as you lift; this puts enormous strain and pressure upon the hemorrhoidal vessels. Instead, take a deep breath and exhale at the moment of lifting. Make your thighs do the work, not your back. Avoid heavy lifting as much as possible.

❑ Get regular moderate exercise.

Caution: If you are thirty-five or older and/or have been sedentary for some time, consult with your health care provider before beginning an exercise program.

❑ Avoid strong or harsh laxatives. Most of these products induce unnecessary straining at bowel movements and often "overdo" their jobs by creating a condition similar to diarrhea. Also, using chemical laxatives does not provide the healthful benefits that natural substances provide. Laxative products can also cause the bowels to become dependent upon them for normal functioning, much like an addiction. Instead of chemical preparations, use a stool softener such as aloe vera or prune juice if constipation or straining at defecation is a problem.

❑ Avoid using rough toilet paper. Use moistened toilet paper or baby wipes instead.

❑ Avoid sitting or standing for prolonged periods of time. If sitting for extended periods of time cannot be avoided, take frequent breaks to stretch and move around (this is also good for circulation, the back, and the legs).

❑ Do not use products containing ibuprofen or aspirin for hemorrhoid pain—they can encourage bleeding. Instead, choose pain medications such as acetaminophen (in Tylenol, Datril, Anacin, Valadol, and other products).

❑ If home treatments bring no relief, consult your health care provider, especially if the problem is recurrent and bleeding persists for more than three days. Although the amount of blood loss might seem insignificant, even a slow loss of blood will eventually result in anemia and its associated problems. (*See* ANEMIA in Part Two.) In addition, persistent rectal bleeding can lead to infections and even a compromised immune system. If the blood is dark red, it can indicate a more serious problem such as an abscess, an anal fissure, a fistula, or cancer. Anal fissures are common in people with Crohn's disease.

Considerations

❑ Depending upon the location and severity of the problem, physicians today use the following treatment approaches in dealing with hemorrhoids:

- *Bipolar electrocoagulation.* Also called BiCap coagulation, this procedure uses spurts of electrical current to shrink hemorrhoids. It is comparable to infrared photocoagulation in that it has the equivalent advantages and disadvantages.

- *Conservative measures.* A dietary regimen with fiber supplements and self-help treatments is helpful in most cases, except in instances where a hemorrhoid has thrombosed.

- *Infrared photocoagulation.* This involves the employment of infrared heat to treat minor internal hemorrhoids. It is less painful than ligation but is not always as effective.

- *Injection sclerotherapy.* In this procedure, used to shrink internal hemorrhoids and stop bleeding, a solution containing either quinine and urea or phenol is injected directly into the hemorrhoids.

- *Laser coagulation.* This approach has gained popularity over the last several years as the easiest and least painful method of dealing with internal hemorrhoids. There is controversy about its efficacy, however. Repeated treatments are frequently required. Most researchers believe that more study should be done to improve effectiveness before laser treatment is routinely recommended.

- *Ligation.* This is now the most common treatment approach for internal hemorrhoids. A small rubber band is used to tie off the base of the blood vessel. Once blood circulation is eliminated from the offending vessel, it soon detaches and the rubber band is eliminated with body waste. This approach often requires repeat treatments and is painful.

- *Surgery.* Some hemorrhoids are not helped very much by any of the above approaches and respond to nothing short of aggressive surgery. If you have very painful hemorrhoids or are losing significant amounts of blood, you should receive a thorough examination from a physician, preferably a proctologist, as soon as possible. Improved surgical techniques have resulted in less painful operations and quicker recovery periods than in the past. In most cases surgery is successful. However, additional surgery may be required if the hemorrhoids recur.

❑ Anurex is a chemical-free product that helps give prompt, soothing, and lasting relief from the burning, itching, and bleeding caused by hemorrhoids. It is a small plastic device that contains a permanently sealed cold-retaining gel. It works best if kept in the freezer. When placed at the site of pain, it imparts a controlled degree of cooling to the inflamed tissue. Each Anurex device is reusable for up to six months. This product can be found in many pharmacies and health food stores, or can be ordered directly from Anurex Labs. (*See* Manufacturer and Distributor Information in the Appendix.)

❑ Eating certain foods, especially beets, can cause the stool to become reddish and can be mistaken for blood.

❑ The most common cause of anal itching is tissue trauma resulting from the use of harsh toilet paper. *Candida albicans,* allergies, and parasitic infections can also cause anal itching.

❑ *See also under* PREGNANCY-RELATED PROBLEMS in Part Two.

HEPATITIS

Hepatitis is an inflammation of the liver, usually caused by a viral infection. The liver is responsible for filtering out from the bloodstream harmful substances such as dead cells, toxins, fats, an overabundance of hormones, and a yellowish substance called bilirubin that is a by-product of the breakdown of old red blood cells. If the liver is in-flamed, tender, and enlarged, it becomes unable to function normally. As a result, toxins that would normally be filtered out by the liver build up in the body, and certain nutrients are not processed and stored as they should be. The symptoms of hepatitis include fever, weakness, nausea, vomiting, headache, appetite loss, muscle aches, joint pains, drowsiness, dark urine, light-colored stools, abdominal discomfort, and often, jaundice (yellowing of the skin due to an accumulation of bilirubin) and elevated liver enzymes in the blood. Flulike symptoms may be mild or severe.

There are different types of hepatitis, classified according to the virus that causes the condition. Scientists have identified the viruses responsible for three leading types of the disease, called hepatitis A, hepatitis B, and hepatitis C. There are also other, less common types known as hepatitis D, hepatitis E, and hepatitis G. All are contagious to some extent.

Hepatitis A virus (HAV), also known as *infectious hepatitis,* can cause acute liver disease. In most cases, however, the liver heals within a few months. Hepatitis A can develop without sudden signs or symptoms. It is easily spread through person-to-person contact, fecal contamination of food or water, and raw shellfish taken from polluted water. It is contagious between two to three weeks before, and one week after, jaundice appears.

Hepatitis B virus (HBV), also referred to as serum hepatitis, is spread through contact with infected blood (for example, from mother to child at birth or through the use of contaminated syringes, needles, and transfused blood) from adults to children living together in close contact, through sexual activity, and through blood transfusions. Most people—85 percent—recover from hepatitis B, although 15 percent go on to develop cirrhosis or cancer of the liver.

Hepatitis C virus (HCV), the most serious form of hepatitis, accounts for approximately 10,000 deaths a year in America. It is estimated that 4 million Americans are infected with HCV, 3.2 million of them chronically. Hepatitis C is the primary reason for liver transplants in this country. Hepatitis C is four times more prevalent than AIDS and twenty times easier to contract. About 85 percent of infections lead to chronic liver disease. Currently, 1 to 5 out of 100 people with HCV die. The virus causes slowly progressing but ultimately devastating damage to the liver. In addition, people with hepatitis CV often have elevated levels of iron in the liver. This also can cause liver damage. Tests can detect HCV antibodies in donated blood, but an infected individual may take up to six months to develop the antibodies, so it is still impossible to identify all infected blood. The U.S. Food and Drug Administration (FDA) maintains that only 7 percent of current hepatitis C cases were acquired as a result of blood transfusions, and that the risk of contracting the virus from a unit of blood is near zero. The incidence of hepatitis C infection from blood transfusions or the use of blood products has dropped substantially since 1992, when screening was introduced, but there is always a minuscule risk—and the lack of testing before 1992 has left a huge legacy of HCV-infected people. You may be at risk for hepatitis C if you have:

- Had a blood transfusion prior to 1992, when screening for HCV antibodies started.

- Shared needles for intravenous (IV) drug use (even one incident, years ago).

- Shared straws for inhaling cocaine.

- Had body piercing or tattoos with nonsterile equipment.

- Had hemodialysis (used a kidney machine).

- Had frequent exposure to blood products (due to hemophilia, chronic renal failure, chemotherapy, organ transplantation, or any other reason).

- Had a needle-sticking incident (health care workers are at high risk).

- Used an infected person's toothbrush, razor, or other item that had blood on it.

- Engaged in high-risk sexual behavior, such as having multiple partners and using no protection.

Hepatitis D virus (HDV), or delta hepatitis, occurs in some people already infected with hepatitis B. It is the least common of all the hepatitis viruses, but the most serious because it means that there are two types of hepatitis working together. It can be transmitted through sexual contact or from mother to child at birth.

Hepatitis E virus (HEV) is rare in the United States, but more common in other parts of the world, notably Mexico, India, and Asian and African countries. It is usually spread through fecal contamination and appears to be dangerous for pregnant women, but generally does not lead to chronic hepatitis in others.

It is also possible to develop hepatitis as a result of exposure to certain toxins or alcohol or drug use, including the overuse of over-the-counter medications such as acetaminophen or ibuprofen. This is called *toxic hepatitis*. Environmental toxins absorbed through the skin can also damage the liver. Chlorinated hydrocarbons and arsenic are examples of toxic agents. In toxic hepatitis, the amount of exposure to the toxin determines the extent of liver damage.

Unless otherwise specified, the dosages recommended here are for adults. For children between the ages of twelve and seventeen, reduce the dose to three-quarters the recommended amount. For children between six and twelve, use one-half the recommended dose, and for children under the age of six, use one-quarter the recommended amount.

NUTRIENTS

SUPPLEMENT	SUGGESTED DOSAGE	COMMENTS
Essential		
Alpha-lipoic acid (ALA)	As directed on label.	Has antioxidant properties that protect the liver.
Beta-1,3-D-glucan	As directed on label.	An excellent antioxidant. Stimulates the activity of macrophages, which surround and digest cellular debris.
Free form amino acid (Amino Balance from Anabol Naturals)	As directed on label.	To supply necessary protein. The liver breaks down protein; taking free form amino acids takes strain off the liver.
Glutathione	500 mg twice daily, on an empty stomach.	Protects the liver.
plus L-arginine	As directed on label.	Detoxifies the liver.
and L-cysteine and L-methionine	500 mg each twice daily, on an empty stomach. Take with water or juice. Do not take with milk. Take with 50 mg vitamin B_6 and 100 mg vitamin C for better absorption.	Detoxifies harmful hepatotoxins and protects glutathione. (*See* AMINO ACIDS in Part One.)
Inositol hexaphosphate (IP_6)	As directed on label.	A powerful antioxidant that has many positive effects on the body, including protecting the liver. Also known as phytic acid.
Liquid Kyolic with B_1 and B_{12} from Wakunaga	As directed on label.	Powerful liver protectors and potent antioxidants.
Raw liver extract or desiccated liver	As directed on label. As directed on label.	Promotes liver function. (*See* GLANDULAR THERAPY in Part Three.) Consider injections (under a doctor's supervision).
S-Adenosylmethionine (SAMe)	As directed on label.	Promotes the health of the liver. *Caution:* Do not use if you have bipolar mood disorder or take prescription antidepressants. Do not give SAMe to a child under twelve.
or Trimethylglycine (TMG)	As directed on label.	Needed for conversion of harmful homocysteine into methionine, the basis for production of SAMe.
Selenium Forte from American Biologics	As directed on label.	Studies have shown selenium to protect against liver cancer.
Very Important		
Coenzyme Q_{10} plus Coenzyme A from Coenzyme-A Technologies	60 mg daily. As directed on label.	Counteracts immuno-suppression and enhances tissue oxygenation.
Dimethylglycine (DMG)(Aangamik DMG from FoodScience of Vermont)	As directed on label.	Improves cellular oxygen concentration.
Lecithin granules or capsules	1 tbsp 3 times daily, before meals. 1,200 mg 3 times daily, before meals.	Protects cells of the liver and is a fat mobilizer. Aids in preventing fatty liver.
Multivitamin complex with vitamin B complex	50–100 mg of each major B vitamin 3 times daily, with meals (amounts of individual vitamins in a complex will vary). Do not exceed a total of 100 mg vitamin B_3 (niacin) in any one day until healing is complete.	All nutrients are necessary in balance. All B vitamins are absolutely essential for normal liver function. Sublingual forms are recommended. Injections (under a doctor's supervision) may be necessary, especially of vitamin B_{12} and folic acid.

494

plus extra vitamin B$_{12}$	1,000 mcg twice daily.	
plus chloline	As directed on label.	
and inositol	As directed on label.	
Superoxide dismutase (SOD)	As directed on label.	Powerful antioxidants that neutralize damaging superoxide free radicals, improving liver function.
or Cell Guard from Biotec Foods	As directed on label.	
or Oxy-5000 Forte from American Biologics	As directed on label.	
Vitamin C with bioflavonoids	5,000–10,000 mg daily and up.	A powerful antiviral agent. Studies show improvement quickly with high doses.
Vitamin E	200 IU daily, or 400 IU every other day over the course of one month.	A potent antioxidant. Use d-alpha-tocopherol form.
Important		
Calcium and magnesium	1,500 mg daily. 1,000 mg daily.	Essential for blood clotting, which is a problem for people with liver disease. Use chelated forms. Do not use bone meal.
Essential fatty acids (primrose oil or salmon oil)	As directed on label.	Important sources of essential lipids. To combat inflammation of the liver and lower serum fats.
or shark liver oil	As directed on label.	
or squalene	As directed on label.	
or Kyolic-EPA from Wakunaga	As directed on label.	
Multienzyme complex with betaine hydrochloride (HCl)	As directed on label.	Important for proper digestion.
Helpful		
Maitake extract	As directed on label.	To boost the immune system and fight viral infection.
or reishi extract	As directed on label.	
or shiitake extract	As directed on label.	
Raw pancreas glandular	As directed on label.	Aids in digestion and pancreatic function.
7-Keto DHEA	50–75 mg daily.	Increases antibody and interleukin-2 formation.
Vitamin A (Micellized Vitamin A and E from American Biologics)	25,000 IU daily. If you are pregnant, do not exceed 10,000 IU daily.	Needed for healing. Use an emulsion form for easier assimilation and greater safety. Avoid using beta-carotene or capsule forms of vitamin A until healing is complete.

Herbs

❏ Artichoke increases the effectiveness of liver function.

❏ Ayurvedic medicine has used beets to promote the regeneration of liver cells.

❏ Burdock and dandelion are important for cleansing the liver and the bloodstream.

❏ Fumitory has been shown to stimulate bile flow and strengthen the liver.

Caution: Consult with your physician before using fumitory.

❏ Studies have shown licorice to be effective in treating viral hepatitis, particularly chronic active hepatitis, due to its well-documented antiviral activity.

Caution: Licorice root should not be used during pregnancy or nursing. It should not be used by persons with diabetes, glaucoma, heart disease, high blood pressure, or a history of stroke.

❏ Ligustrum is a good immune restorative and anti-inflammatory agent.

❏ Milk thistle extract contains silymarin, a flavonoid that has been shown to aid in healing and rebuilding the liver. It can be taken in capsule or alcohol-free extract form. Take 200 to 400 milligrams three times daily.

❏ Olive leaf extract is a potent antifungal agent.

❏ Phyllanthus, an Ayurvedic herb, is useful for hepatitis B. After an initial bout with the virus, you can become symptom-free but still remain a carrier of the disease. This herb is said to eradicate carrier-status hepatitis B in some cases.

❏ Schizandra is a Chinese herb used to protect the liver.

❏ Scutellaria, also known as Baikal skullcap or Chinese skullcap, is a Chinese herb that is a powerful antioxidant.

❏ Turmeric is a potent anti-inflammatory.

❏ Other herbs beneficial for hepatitis include black radish, green tea, red clover, and yellow dock.

Caution: Green tea contains vitamin K, which can make anticoagulant medications less effective. Consult your health care professional if you are using them. The caffeine in green tea could cause insomnia, anxiety, upset stomach, nausea, or diarrhea.

Recommendations

❏ Eat a raw vegetable and fruit diet for two to four weeks. Start this diet with a cleansing fast. (*See* FASTING in Part Three.)

❏ Include artichokes in the diet. Artichokes protect the liver. Globe artichoke extract also is available.

❏ Drink "green drinks," carrot juice, and beet juice. (*See* JUICING in Part Three.)

❏ Drink only steam-distilled water.

❏ Consume no alcohol in any form. Propylene glycol is a compound related to alcohol that is commonly used in medicines that are supposed to be alcohol-free. It too should be avoided.

❏ Avoid most fats, sugar, and highly processed foods.

❏ Avoid all raw fish and shellfish, and eat no animal protein. Also avoid chemicals and food additives.

❏ Get plenty of bed rest.

❏ Use chlorophyll-containing enemas such as fresh wheatgrass juice or Kyo-Green from Wakunaga, three times a week. Use one pint and retain it for fifteen minutes. (*See* ENEMAS in Part Three.)

❏ Keep a person with hepatitis A in isolation to avoid spreading the infection. Wash hands and all clothing often. The clothing and bed linens of a person with hepatitis A require special handling. Wash them separately from other laundry in hot water with chlorine bleach or a disinfectant added. Because the feces are infectious, bathrooms should be decontaminated frequently. Clean toilets and floors with a disinfectant.

❏ Especially when traveling, beware of contaminated water or foods from polluted waters.

❏ Do not take any drugs that have not been prescribed by your doctor. Read package inserts carefully for information regarding liver toxicity.

Considerations

❏ Taking excessive amounts of vitamin A over long periods may cause liver enzyme levels to become elevated. Anyone who has been taking over 50,000 international units of vitamin A daily for over a year should reduce his or her intake or switch to an emulsion form, which is less harmful to the liver.

❏ If you have hepatitis C, it is best to reduce the iron levels in the body before starting any treatment. High iron levels inhibit therapy for the liver.

❏ Catechin, a flavonoid found in green and black Indian teas, has been shown to decrease serum bilirubin levels in people with all types of acute viral hepatitis.

❏ Liver extract supplements contain nutritional substances that aid liver regeneration. Only products derived from organically raised beef should be used.

❏ In laboratory experiments, injections of whole liver cells have rapidly repaired liver tissue in experimental animals with lethal, acute liver failure.

❏ Silymarin, the active ingredient in milk thistle, has been known to lower liver enzymes and reverse the kind of liver damage common in people with hepatitis C. Some studies have found that milk thistle can cure liver cancer in rats.

❏ Ribavirin (Virazole) and interferon may be prescribed for hepatitis C and are proving to be effective in the treatment of this disease.

❏ Adefovir dipivoxil (Hepsera) tablets slow the progression of chronic hepatits B by blocking an enzyme needed for the virus to reproduce within the body.

Caution: Do not stop taking adefovir dipivoxil unless under guidance by a physician.

❏ Hepatitis is diagnosed by means of a blood test. In some cases, it may be necessary to double-check a test for the hepatitis C virus by means of a test called the RIBA HCV 3.0 Strip Immunoblot Assay (SIA).

❏ A home test called the Home Access Hepatitis C Check is available. It can be purchased in drugstores or ordered directly from the manufacturer, Home Access Health. (*See* Manufacturer and Distributor Information in the Appendix.)

❏ If you require surgery and may need a blood transfusion, discuss this with your doctor or surgeon. You may be able to bank your own blood or the blood of a relative or friend before the procedure.

❏ There is a vaccine available to protect against hepatitis A. It is recommended for members of high-risk groups such as those suffering from liver disease, those in contact with hepatitis A–infected people, those who engage in anal sex with multiple partners, and those traveling to areas where hepatitis A is common, including Africa, the Middle East, the Caribbean, and South and Central America. The U.S. Centers for Disease Control (CDC) now recommends that children living in high-risk states in this country be vaccinated against this disease as well. The high-risk states include Arizona, Alaska, California, Idaho, New Mexico, Oregon, South Dakota, and Washington. Some other states have *areas* where hepatitis A is common. Ask your health care provider about possible side effects from the vaccine.

❏ There is a vaccine available that gives protection against hepatitis B. Ask your health care provider about both the benefits and side effects. If you work in a hospital, you will likely need to get vaccinated.

❏ Because the hepatitis C virus has many genotypes, or forms, and can mutate rapidly, no vaccine has yet been developed to successfully protect against this virus. Likewise, there are no vaccines against hepatitis D or E.

HEREDITARY FRUCTOSE INTOLERANCE

See under RARE DISORDERS.

HERPES INFECTION

There are at least seven types of herpesviruses. Herpes simplex type 1 (HSV-1) and type 2 (HSV-2) cause cold sores and genital herpes. Many experts suspect HSV-1 may be involved in Bell's palsy and some other neurological disorders. Herpes zoster is responsible for chickenpox and shingles. Cytomegalovirus, another member of the herpes family, can cause some cardiovascular diseases and eye disorders, and is particularly dangerous to developing fetuses, newborns, and people with depressed immune systems. The Epstein-Barr virus (EBV) is the virus that causes infectious mononucleosis. Human herpesvirus type 6 (HHV-6) and 7 (HHV-7) are suspected of being capable of triggering autoimmune disorders, including multiple sclerosis, and roseola, a common illness of early childhood. Human herpesvirus type 8 (HHV-8) is very closely related to the Epstein-Barr virus, and may lead to cancer of the bone, chronic fatigue syndrome, Kaposi's sarcoma, and infection of the lymphatic system. This section primarily addresses genital herpes.

Genital herpes is the most prevalent sexually transmitted disease in the United States. More than 45 million Americans—one out of every five persons over the age of twelve—have it, though more than half never develop serious symptoms. This viral infection can range in severity from a silent infection to a serious inflammation of the liver with fever. It is more common among blacks than whites, and more likely to infect women than men. It is especially dangerous to infants. A baby whose mother is infected can pick up the virus in the birth canal, creating a risk of brain damage, blindness, and death.

For those whose symptoms do not remain dormant, genital herpes causes outbreaks of red, sensitive skin; itching; burning; and painful, fluid-filled blisters that are highly infectious until they are completely healed, which can take up to three weeks. It is, however, fairly common to have virtually no symptoms of the infection.

A mild tingling and burning in the vaginal area may be the first sign of genital herpes in women. Within a matter of a few hours, blisters develop around the rectum, clitoris, and cervix, and in the vagina. There is often a watery discharge from the urethra and pain when urinating. In men, blisters break out on the penis, groin, and scrotum, often with a urethral discharge and painful urination. Sometimes the penis and foreskin swell. A man may also have tender, swollen lymph nodes in the groin.

The first attack of genital herpes usually comes within twenty days after exposure to the virus. It may be so mild that it isn't noticed, or it may cause itching and burning at the site of viral entry as well as painful sores that can last a week or more, plus fever, headache, and other flulike symptoms. After a few days, pus erupts from the blisters and painful ulcers form. These sores crust over and dry while healing. Usually, they leave no scars.

It has traditionally been believed that HSV-1 causes cold sores and skin eruptions and HSV-2 is responsible for genital herpes. The difference between HSV-1 and HSV-2 is often debated, however. The current theory is that the two viruses are more alike than once was thought—the two viruses share about 50 percent of their DNA—but that they do have different characteristics. For example, when HSV-1 is in a dormant state, the virus usually establishes its home in the nerve cells near the ear, so it is more inclined to cause an outbreak around the mouth. HSV-2, on the other hand, prefers to live near the base of the spine, so when an outbreak occurs, it is more likely to occur in the genital area. The two viral agents can, however, live in either place, and it has been suggested that social pressures are the real reason we like to think of the two as being very different.

Many people have a tendency to associate genital herpes with a promiscuous lifestyle (which in fact is not justified), but the same stigma is not attached to cold sores.

If HSV-1 exchanges its usual site with HSV-2, or vice versa, outbreaks are normally less severe. If you have a sexual partner who has a genital HSV-1 infection and you have genital HSV-2, you can contract HSV-1, but it is extremely rare that HSV-1 is transmitted to a person who already has HSV-2. Oral sex with a person who has genital HSV-2 is unlikely to result in an HSV-2 infection affecting the mouth. HSV-2 is almost wholly transmitted through genital sex.

Experts now believe that HSV-2 can be transmitted even when an infected individual is experiencing no symptoms. In the first year after infection, people shed the virus between 6 and 10 percent of the time when there are no visible signs of the infection, a phenomenon called *asymptomatic viral shedding.*

There is growing evidence that people with genital herpes are at greater than normal risk of contracting human immunodeficiency virus (HIV) if they have unprotected sex with someone who is HIV-positive. HIV-infected people who are also infected with genital herpes are more likely to have more frequent and severe herpes outbreaks, which may result in episodes that are more difficult to treat.

It is now possible to diagnose herpes by means of a blood test, even if no symptoms are apparent or after sores have healed. While there is no cure for herpes, antiviral drugs have been approved that greatly reduce the frequency of outbreaks and shorten their duration and severity. Although it is a serious illness, herpes is not normally life-threatening. Having the virus means that you have to adjust your lifestyle to protect yourself and others, but there are few cases of herpes infecting other organs of the body. If you already have the infection, it is equally important to protect yourself as much as you can from repeated outbreaks and to avoid passing the infection on to others.

Unless otherwise specified, the dosages recommended here are for adults. For children between the ages of twelve and seventeen, reduce the dose to three-quarters the recommended amount. For children between six and twelve, use one-half the recommended dose, and for children under the age of six, use one-quarter the recommended amount.

NUTRIENTS

SUPPLEMENT	SUGGESTED DOSAGE	COMMENTS
Very Important		
Beta 1,3-D-glucan	As directed on label.	Useful for treating any bacterial, viral, or fungal disease. Stimulates the activity of macrophages, immune cells that surround and digest invading microorganisms and cellular debris.

Coenzyme A from Coenzyme-A Technologies	As directed on label.	Supports the immune system's detoxification of many dangerous substances.
Herp-Eeze from Olympian Labs	As directed on label.	Possesses antiviral, anti-inflammatory, and antioxidant properties for the treatment of herpes.
L-lysine	1,500 mg daily, on an empty stomach. Take with water or juice. Do not take with milk. Take with 50 mg vitamin B6 and 100 mg vitamin C for better absorption.	If the amount of lysine present in the body exceeds the amount of arginine, the growth of the herpesvirus is inhibited. (See AMINO ACIDS in Part One.) Caution: Do not take this supplement for longer than 6 months at a time without a break. Resume the therapy again if you have further outbreaks.
Vitamin A with mixed carotenoids	25,000 IU daily. If you are pregnant, do not exceed 10,000 IU daily.	Important for healing. Prevents spreading of infection. Use emulsion form for easier assimilation and greater safety at higher doses.
Vitamin B complex	50 mg and up of each major B vitamin, 3 times daily (amounts of individual vitamins in a complex will vary).	Combats the virus and helps to keep it from spreading. Also works with lysine to prevent outbreaks. Use hypoallergenic form.
Vitamin C plus bioflavonoids	5,000–10,000 mg daily. 30–60 mg daily, in divided doses.	Needed to prevent sores and inhibit the growth of the virus. Use esterified or buffered form. Work with vitamin C.
Zinc	50–100 mg daily, in divided doses. Do not exceed 100 mg daily from all supplements.	Boosts immune function. For genital herpes, use chelate form. For oral herpes, use zinc gluconate lozenges.
Important		
Acidophilus (Kyo-Dophilus from Wakunaga)	As directed on label, 3 times daily, on an empty stomach.	Needed for the production of the B vitamins. Prevents overgrowth of harmful micro-organisms in the intestines. Use nondairy formula.
Dioxychlor	As directed on label.	An important antiviral, anti-bacterial, and antifungal agent.
Egg lecithin	As directed on label.	Helps to control the virus.
Essential fatty acids (primrose oil, salmon oil, or Kyolic-EPA from Wakunaga)	As directed on label.	Needed for cell protection.
Garlic (Kyolic from Wakunaga)	3 tablets 3 times daily, with meals.	An immune system stimulant and a natural antibiotic.
Superoxide dismutase (SOD) or Cell Guard from Biotec Foods	As directed on label. As directed on label.	Reduces infection and speeds healing. A powerful free radical destroyer. An antioxidant complex that contains SOD.
Vitamin E	200 IU daily.	Important in healing. Prevents spread of the infection. Use emulsion form for easier assimilation. Use d-alpha-tocopherol form.

Helpful		
Calcium and magnesium	1,500 mg daily. 750 mg daily.	To relieve stress and anxiety. Use chelated forms.
Dimethylglycine (DMG) (Aangamik DMG from FoodScience of Vermont)	2 tablets dissolved in the mouth twice daily.	Enhances utilization of oxygen by tissue.
Maitake extract or shiitake extract or reishi extract	As directed on label. As directed on label. As directed on label.	Mushroom extracts that have immune-boosting and antiviral properties.
Multivitamin and mineral supplement	As directed on label.	Needed to enhance healing. Take hypoallergenic form.
Proteolytic enzymes	As directed on label 2–3 times daily. Take between meals.	Helps to protect against infection; works on undigested food remaining in the colon. Caution: Do not give this supplement to a child.
Raw thymus glandular	500 mg twice daily.	Enhances immune function. Caution: Do not give this supplement to a child.

Herbs

❑ Astragalus, or huang qi, enhances the immune system and acts as an antibiotic.

Caution: Do not use astragalus in the presence of a fever.

❑ Applying black walnut or goldenseal extract to the affected area may help.

❑ Cat's claw has immune-enhancing properties and acts against viral infection.

Caution: Do not use cat's claw during pregnancy.

❑ Goldenseal is a natural antibiotic. It can be taken in capsule or tea form.

Caution: Do not take goldenseal internally on a daily basis for more than one week at a time. Do not use it during pregnancy or if you are breast-feeding, and use with caution if you are allergic to ragweed. If you have a history of cardiovascular disease, diabetes, or glaucoma, use it only under a doctor's supervision.

❑ Licorice root inhibits both the growth and cell-damaging effects of herpes simplex. If you are using licorice, increase your potassium intake.

Caution: Licorice root should not be used during pregnancy or nursing. It should not be used by persons with diabetes, glaucoma, heart disease, high blood pressure, or a history of stroke.

❑ Olive leaf extract appears to help curb the growth of viral diseases such as herpes.

❏ Red marine algae contains antiviral carbohydrates that are effective, both topically and orally, for the treatment of herpes.

❏ Spirulina contains phytonutrients that appear to boost the immune system.

❏ Tea tree oil is a powerful natural antiseptic. During a herpes outbreak, dab it lightly on the affected area several times a day, either full strength or, if that is too strong, diluted with distilled water or cold-pressed vegetable oil. Do not get tea tree oil close to the eye area.

❏ Other herbs useful for herpes treatment include cayenne (capsicum), echinacea, myrrh, red clover, and St. John's wort.

Cautions: Do not take echinacea for longer than three months. It should not be used by people who are allergic to ragweed. St. John's wort may cause increased sensitivity to sunlight. It may also produce anxiety, gastrointestinal symptoms, and headaches. It can interact with some drugs, including antidepressants, birth control pills, and anticoagulants.

Recommendations

❏ Avoid alcohol, processed foods, colas, white flour products, sugar, refined carbohydrates, coffee, and drugs to lessen the chance of an outbreak. Herbal teas are beneficial (*see* Herbs, above), but all other teas should be avoided.

❏ Drink steam-distilled water.

❏ Eat the following in moderation during outbreaks: almonds, barley, cashews, cereals (grains), chicken, chocolate, corn, dairy products, meat, nuts and seeds, oats, and peanuts. These contain L-arginine, an amino acid that suppresses L-lysine, the amino acid that retards virus growth.

❏ Do not consume citrus fruits and juices while the virus is active.

❏ Get plenty of rest. Stress reduction is important.

❏ To ease swelling and pain in the genital area, use ice packs. Warm Epsom salts or baking soda baths help itching and pain. After the bath, pat dry gently and keep the lesions dry.

❏ Apply vitamin E and vitamin A, alternately, directly on the sores. Or try using L-lysine cream from a health food store.

❏ Wear cotton underwear. Practice good genital hygiene—keep clean and dry.

❏ If you have active lesions, refrain from sex until the sores have completely healed. Do not have intercourse with a person with visible genital lesions of any kind.

❏ If you are pregnant and know you have genital herpes, tell your health care provider. If an attack occurs late in the pregnancy, your baby may have to be delivered by cesarean section to protect against exposure during birth. If there are no lesions present, the risk to the baby is probably low.

Considerations

❏ Genital herpes infections in women increase the risk of cervical cancer. Women with herpes should be conscientious about having Pap smears done periodically, as recommended by a qualified health care provider.

❏ A virus identified by the National Cancer Institute as the human B cell lymphotropic virus (HBLV) is believed to be a member of the herpes family and may also be a factor in fatigue.

❏ L-lysine has been shown to be effective in treating symptoms. In one study, a dose of 1,248 milligrams a day decreased the recurrence rate of herpes and the severity of symptoms if an outbreak occurred.

❏ Research suggests that capsaicin may be able to prevent outbreaks of genital lesions.

❏ High levels of the amino acid arginine may cause outbreaks of herpes. Foods containing arginine include chocolate, peanuts, and soybeans.

❏ One study in the UK looked at differences in dietary intake of fruits, vegetables, and selected micronutrients. Those with the herpesvirus who ate fewer servings of fruits (one per week) had three times the risk of getting herpes. In individuals over sixty years of age, those who consumed five or more servings of vegetables a day and got adequate iron from food, antioxidants (zinc, vitamin A, and vitamin B$_6$), folic acid, vitamin C, and vitamin E had the lowest risk of developing herpes. The immune system weakens with age, so a healthy diet and supplementation are important.

❏ Dimethylsulfoxide (DMSO), a by-product of wood processing, is a liquid that can be applied topically to relieve pain and promote the healing of herpes outbreaks.

Caution: Only pure DMSO from a health food store should be used. Commercial-grade DMSO such as that found in hardware stores is not suitable for healing purposes. Any contaminants on the skin or in the product can be taken into the tissues by action of the DMSO.

Note: The use of DMSO may result in a garlicky body odor. This is temporary, and is not a cause for concern.

❏ There are a number of antiviral drugs that may be recommended to relieve symptoms and/or to reduce the severity and frequency of genital herpes outbreaks. All are available by prescription only. They include the following:

• Acyclovir (sold in generic form or under the brand name Zovirax or generic) may be prescribed for the initial infection at a dosage of 200 milligrams taken five times a day for ten days. Thereafter, for acute outbreaks, the usual dosage is 200 milligrams five times a day for five days; and to suppress future outbreaks, 400 milligrams twice a day for one year, after which your doctor should reassess your condition. Acyclovir comes in both capsule and lotion forms. Applying the lotion when an imminent outbreak is first sensed usually weakens the attack.

- Famcyclovir (Famvir) generally is not used for initial infection. To combat acute outbreaks, the usual prescription is for 125 milligrams taken twice a day for five days; to suppress future outbreaks, 250 milligrams a day for up to one year, after which your doctor should reassess your condition.

- Valcyclovir (Valtrex) may be prescribed for the initial infection at a dosage of 1,000 milligrams (1 gram) taken twice a day for ten days. Thereafter, for acute outbreaks, the usual prescription is for 500 milligrams taken twice a day for three days; to suppress future outbreaks, 1 gram once a day (for those who have a history of nine or fewer recurrences per year, an alternate dosage of 500 milligrams once a day may be used). As with the other antivirals, your doctor should reassess your condition after a year of suppressive therapy.

You should exercise caution if you use one of these drugs on a regular basis, however. When the drug is stopped, a "rebound" effect may result in a more serious outbreak than usual. Discuss with your doctor the correct method for discontinuing the medication—don't just stop taking it on your own.

❑ A vaccine for prevention of genital herpes in women called Herpevac is currently undergoing testing. As of July 2009, the study was fully enrolled, and results should be forthcoming within a couple of years. Approximately 7,550 women were enrolled from forty states and Canada.

❑ Some physicians have used butylated hydroxytoluene (BHT) to treat herpes. This can have dangerous consequences, however, especially if taken on an empty stomach. Irritation and even perforation of the stomach can result. We do not recommend this treatment for herpes.

❑ Choraphor is a trademarked topical antiseptic formula containing ammoniated acid sulfate and trace minerals that is said to promote an immune response to herpes and clear up outbreaks. It has not yet undergone clinical testing, however.

❑ *See also* COLD SORES; SEXUALLY TRANSMITTED DISEASE; and SHINGLES in Part Two.

HERPES ZOSTER

See SHINGLES. *See also under* EYE PROBLEMS.

HIATAL HERNIA

See under HEARTBURN/GASTROESOPHAGEAL REFLUX DISEASE (GERD).

HIGH BLOOD PRESSURE (HYPERTENSION)

When the heart pumps blood through the arteries, the blood presses against the walls of the blood vessels. In people who suffer from hypertension, this pressure is abnormally high. If blood pressure is elevated, the heart must work harder to pump an adequate amount of blood to all the tissues of the body.

Whether blood pressure is high, low, or normal depends on several factors: the output from the heart, the resistance to blood flow of the blood vessels, the volume of blood, and blood distribution to the various organs. All of these factors in turn can be affected by the activities of the nervous system and certain hormones.

Blood pressure is represented as a pair of numbers. The first is the *systolic* pressure, which is the pressure exerted by the blood when the heart beats, forcing blood into the blood vessels. This reading indicates blood pressure at its highest. The second reading is the *diastolic* pressure, which is recorded when the heart is at rest in between beats, when the blood pressure is at its lowest. Both figures represent the height (in millimeters, or mm) that a column of mercury (Hg) reaches under the pressure exerted by the blood. The combined blood pressure reading is then expressed as a ratio of systolic blood pressure to diastolic blood pressure, such as 120/80.

About 73.6 million people in the United States—or one in every three American adults age twenty and older—have hypertension. From 1995 to 2005, the death rate from high blood pressure increased 25.2 percent, and the actual number of deaths rose 56.4 percent.

While high blood pressure was once thought of as a "man's disease," in fact women are as likely to suffer from this condition as men are—30.3 percent of American women and 31.8 percent of American men have high blood pressure. Furthermore, more women than men die from complications of high blood pressure because women and, to some extent, their medical practitioners, often ignore or fail to detect their high blood pressure until it is too late.

Because high blood pressure usually causes no symptoms until complications develop, it is known as the "silent killer." According to a national survey, 78 percent of Americans with high blood pressure are aware of it, 69 percent are being treated, and 45 percent have it under control. Unfortunately, many people stop taking their medications because they don't feel sick and it takes effort and is expensive. Warning signs associated with advanced hypertension may include headaches, sweating, rapid pulse, shortness of breath, dizziness, and visual disturbances.

High blood pressure is usually divided into two categories, designated *primary* and *secondary*. Primary hypertension is high blood pressure that is not due to another underlying disease. The precise cause is unknown, but a number of definite risk factors have been identified. These include cigarette smoking, stress, obesity, excessive use of stimulants such as coffee or tea, drug abuse, and high sodium intake. The use of oral contraceptives used to be considered a contributing factor, but with the low-dose pills now available, this is not as much of a problem as it once was. Because too much water retention can exert pressure on the blood vessels, those who consume foods high in sodium may be at a greater risk for high blood pressure. Elevated blood pressure is also common in people who are overweight. Blood pressure can rise due to stress as well, because stress causes the walls of the arteries to constrict. Also, those with a family history of hypertension are more likely to suffer from high blood pressure.

When persistently elevated blood pressure arises as a result of another underlying health problem, such as a hormonal abnormality or an inherited narrowing of the aorta, it is called secondary hypertension. A person may also have secondary hypertension because the blood vessels are chronically constricted or have lost elasticity from a buildup of fatty plaque on the inside walls of the vessel, a condition known as atherosclerosis. Arteriosclerosis and atherosclerosis are common precursors of hypertension. In addition, high blood pressure is often associated with coronary heart disease, arteriosclerosis, kidney disorders, obesity, diabetes, hyperthyroidism, and adrenal tumors.

The narrowing and/or hardening of the arteries makes circulation of blood through the vessels difficult. As a result, blood pressure becomes elevated. Secondary hypertension can also be caused by poor kidney function, which results in the retention of excess sodium and fluid in the body. This increase in blood volume within the vessels causes elevated blood pressure levels. The kidneys may also elevate blood pressure by secreting substances that cause blood vessels to constrict.

To diagnose high blood pressure, a physician uses a device called a *sphygmomanometer*. It is impossible, however, for a health care provider to make a correct diagnosis of high blood pressure with a single reading. The test must be repeated throughout the day to be accurate. Home testing is best because it enables you to monitor your condition periodically. Measuring blood pressure at home on a regular schedule may:

- Help to determine whether your blood pressure is high only when taken during a medical visit.

- Enable you to collaborate with your health care provider in controlling your high blood pressure.

- Reduce the frequency with which you need to visit your health care provider for blood pressure evaluation.

Blood pressure monitoring devices fall into two basic categories: mechanical gauges and automated electronic gauges. The mechanical gauge is the type most often used in physicians' offices. It consists of an instrument to measure the pressure, an air bladder (inflatable cuff), and a pressure bulb with a release valve to pump up the cuff. The standard-size arm cuff on blood pressure monitors fits arms up to thirteen inches around (if your arm is larger than this, you will need to obtain a larger cuff). With most of these devices, the pressure is read on a gauge dial.

Mechanical gauges are much less expensive than electronic ones and many physicians feel they give more accurate readings, at least in the hands of an experienced user. However, if you use this type of device to take your own blood pressure, you must pump up the cuff with one hand, read a dial, and listen with a stethoscope more or less simultaneously. (*See* How to Measure Your Blood Pressure on page 505.) In other words, using these devices correctly requires dexterity, good eyesight, acute hearing, and some training and practice.

An alternative to the mechanical gauge is the digital sphygmomanometer. With this device, the machine automatically gauges your blood pressure when the cuff is inflated and presents the result in a digital format. These are more expensive than the mechanical types, but because they are much easier to use accurately, they are generally preferred for home use.

There are also other electronic devices available, including wrist and finger cuff monitors. Although they are easy to operate, most doctors do not recommend them because they tend to be less accurate and also more sensitive to the effects of temperature and poor blood circulation.

Basic guidelines for what the blood pressure numbers mean, as revised in 2004 by the National Heart, Lung, and Blood Institute (NHLBI) are as follows:

- Normal: Lower than 120 (systolic) over lower than 80 (diastolic)—lower than 120/80.

- Prehypertension: 120–139 (systolic) over 80–89 (diastolic)—120–139/80–89.

- Stage 1 hypertension: 140–159 (systolic) over 90–99 (diastolic)—140–159/90–99.

- Stage 2 hypertension: 160 or higher (systolic) over 100 or higher (diastolic)—higher than 160/100.

Treatment seeks to lower blood pressure to less than 140 systolic and less than 90 diastolic for most people. Treatment for those with diabetes and chronic kidney disease aims to lower blood pressure to less than 130 systolic and less than 80 diastolic. For people aged fifty and older, systolic blood pressure may be a more important cardiovascular risk factor than diastolic pressure.

Studies have found that an increased risk of death from cardiovascular causes (heart attack and stroke) can begin at pressures as low as 115/75, and that it doubles for each additional 20/10 increase. High blood pressure also can lead to kidney failure and heart failure.

Unless otherwise specified, the nutrient and other dosages recommended here are for adults. For children between the ages of twelve and seventeen, reduce the dose to three-quarters the recommended amount. For children between six and twelve, use one-half the recommended dose, and for children under the age of six, use one-quarter the recommended amount.

NUTRIENTS

SUPPLEMENT	SUGGESTED DOSAGE	COMMENTS
Essential		
Calcium	1,500–3,000 mg daily.	Deficiencies have been linked to high blood pressure.
and magnesium	750–1,000 mg daily.	
and potassium	As directed on label.	If you take cortisone or high blood pressure medication, take extra potassium to counteract depletion of this mineral.
Coenzyme Q_{10}	As directed on label.	Improves heart function.
plus Coenzyme A from Coenzyme-A Technologies	As directed on label.	Works effectively with coenzyme Q_{10} to support the immune system's detoxification of many dangerous substances.
Essential fatty acids (black currant seed oil, flaxseed oil, olive oil, primrose oil, or Kyolic-EPA from Wakunaga)	As directed on label.	Important for circulation and for lowering blood pressure.
Garlic (Kyolic from Wakunaga)	2 capsules 3 times daily.	Effective in lowering blood pressure.
L-arginine	As directed on label.	Shown to play an increasingly important role in heart health by lowering blood pressure and cholesterol levels.
L-carnitine	500 mg twice daily, on an empty stomach.	Transports long fatty acid chains. Together with L-glutamic acid and L-glutamine, aids in preventing heart disease.
plus L-glutamic acid and L-glutamine	500 mg each daily, on an empty stomach. Take with water or juice. Do not take with milk. Take with 50 mg vitamin B_6 and 100 mg vitamin C for better absorption.	To detoxify ammonia and aid in preventing heart disease. (See AMINO ACIDS in Part One.)
Selenium	200 mcg daily.	Deficiency has been linked to heart disease.
Vitamin E	100 IU daily for first month, then increase to 200 IU daily.	Improves heart function. Vitamin E also acts as a blood-thinning agent; use with caution if you are taking prescription blood-thinners. Use d-alpha-tocopherol form. Use emulsion form for easier assimilation and greater safety at high doses.
and/or octacosanol	As directed on label.	
Very Important		
Vitamin C with bioflavonoids	3,000–6,000 mg daily, in divided doses.	Improves adrenal function; reduces blood-clotting tendencies.
Important		
Lecithin granules	1 tbsp 3 times daily, before meals.	To emulsify fat, improve liver function, and lower blood pressure.
or capsules	1,200 mg 3 times daily, before meals.	
or lipotropic factors	As directed on label.	

Helpful		
Bromelain	As directed on label.	An enzyme that aids in the digestion of fats.
Chinese red yeast rice extract	As directed on label.	Has cholesterol-lowering properties.
Kelp	1,000–1,500 mg daily.	A good source of minerals and natural iodine.
Kyo-Green from Wakunaga	As directed on label twice daily.	This concentrated barley and wheatgrass juice contains important nutrients.
Maitake extract	As directed on label.	To help reduce high blood pressure and prevent heart disease.
or shiitake extract	As directed on label.	
or reishi extract	As directed on label.	
Multivitamin and mineral complex	As directed on label.	All nutrients are needed in balance.
with vitamin A	15,000 IU daily. If you are pregnant, do not exceed 10,000 IU daily.	
and zinc	50 mg daily.	
Proteolytic enzymes	As directed on label. Take with meals and between meals.	Aids in cleansing the circulatory system. Completes protein digestion.
Raw heart glandular	As directed on label.	Strengthens the heart.
plus Heart Science from Source Naturals	As directed on label.	Contains antioxidants, cholesterol-fighters, herbs, and vitamins that work together to promote cardiovascular function.
Vitamin B complex	100 mg of each major B vitamin twice daily, with meals (amounts of individual vitamins in a complex will vary).	Important for circulatory function and for lowering blood pressure. Take niacin only under the supervision of a physician.
plus extra vitamin B_3 (niacin)	50 mg twice daily.	
and choline	50 mg twice daily.	
and inositol	50 mg twice daily.	
Vitamin B_6 (pyridoxine)	50 mg 3 times daily.	Reduces water content in tissues to relieve pressure on the cardiovascular system.

Herbs

❑ Use cayenne (capsicum), chamomile, fennel, hawthorn berries, parsley, and rosemary for high blood pressure.

Caution: Do not use chamomile if you are allergic to ragweed. Do not use during pregnancy or nursing. It may interact with warfarin or cyclosporine, so patients using these drugs should avoid it.

❑ Hops and valerian root are good for calming the nerves.

❑ Studies show that mistletoe can reduce symptoms of high blood pressure, especially headaches and dizziness.

❑ Drink 3 cups of suma tea daily.

❑ *Avoid* licorice, as this herb can elevate blood pressure.

Recommendations

❑ Follow a strict salt-free diet. This is essential for lowering blood pressure. Lowering your salt intake is not enough; eliminate all added salt from your diet. Read labels carefully and avoid those food products that have "salt," "soda," "sodium," or the symbol "Na" on the label. Some foods and food additives that should be avoided on this diet include monosodium glutamate (Accent, MSG); baking soda; canned vegetables (unless marked sodium- or salt-free); commercially prepared foods; over-the-counter medications that contain ibuprofen (such as Advil or Nuprin); diet soft drinks; foods with mold inhibitors, preservatives, and/or sugar substitutes; meat tenderizers; softened water; and soy sauce.

❑ Eat a high-fiber diet and take supplemental fiber. Oat bran is a good source of fiber.

Note: Always take supplemental fiber separately from other supplements and medications.

❑ Eat plenty of fruits and vegetables, such as apples, asparagus, bananas, broccoli, cabbage, cantaloupe, eggplant, garlic, grapefruit, green leafy vegetables, melons, peas, prunes, raisins, squash, and sweet potatoes.

❑ Include fresh "live" juices in the diet. The following juices are healthful: beet, carrot, celery, currant, cranberry, citrus fruit, parsley, spinach, and watermelon.

❑ Eat grains like brown rice, buckwheat, millet, and oats.

❑ Drink steam-distilled water only.

❑ Take 2 tablespoons of flaxseed oil daily.

❑ Avoid all animal fats. Bacon, beef, bouillons, chicken liver, corned beef, dairy products, gravies, pork, sausage, and smoked or processed meats are prohibited. The only acceptable animal foods are broiled whitefish and skinless turkey or chicken, and these should be consumed in moderation only. Get protein from vegetable sources, grains, and legumes instead.

❑ Avoid foods such as aged cheeses, aged meats, anchovies, avocados, chocolate, fava beans, pickled herring, sherry, sour cream, wine, and yogurt.

❑ Avoid all alcohol, caffeine, and tobacco.

❑ If you are taking an MAO inhibitor (one of a class of drugs prescribed to counter depression, lower blood pressure, and treat infections and cancer), avoid the chemical tyramine and its precursor, tyrosine. Combining MAO inhibitors with tyramine causes the blood pressure to soar and could cause a stroke. Tyramine-containing foods include almonds, avocados, bananas, beef or chicken liver, beer, cheese (including cottage cheese), chocolate, coffee, fava beans, herring, meat tenderizer, peanuts, pickles, pineapples, pumpkin seeds, raisins, sausage, sesame seeds, sour cream, soy sauce, wine, yeast extracts (including brewer's yeast), yogurt, and other foods. In general, any high-protein food that has undergone aging, pickling, fermentation, or simi-

lar processes should be avoided. Over-the-counter cold and allergy remedies should also be avoided.

Caution: Brewer's yeast can cause an allergic reaction in some individuals. Start with a small amount at first, and discontinue use if any allergic symptoms occur.

❑ Keep your weight down. If you are overweight, take steps to lose the excess pounds. (*See* OBESITY in Part Two.) Losing 10 percent of your body weight will reduce blood pressure, and may even allow you to use less of your medications, if you are currently taking medications—or avoid them altogether, if you are not.

Caution: You should not stop taking your medication without consulting your physician.

❑ Fast for three to five days each month. Periodic cleansing fasts help to detoxify the body. (*See* FASTING in Part Three.)

❑ Get regular light to moderate exercise. Take care not to overexert yourself, especially in hot or humid weather.

Caution: If you are thirty-five or older and/or have been sedentary for some time, consult with your health care provider before beginning an exercise program.

❑ Be sure to get sufficient sleep.

❑ Have your blood pressure checked at least every four to six months. Because hypertension often shows no signs, regular blood pressure checks by a professional are important, especially if you are in a high-risk category.

❑ Take your blood pressure at home. This is a good way to track your blood pressure levels throughout the day. Any minute your blood pressure is elevated, there is stress on your blood vessels, which increases your chance of a stroke.

❑ If you are pregnant, have your blood pressure monitored frequently by your health care provider. Untreated hypertension in pregnancy can progress suddenly and pose a serious threat to both mother and child.

❑ Do not take antihistamines except under a physician's direction.

❑ Do not take supplements containing the amino acids phenylalanine or tyrosine. Also avoid the artificial sweetener aspartame (Equal, NutraSweet), which contains phenylalanine.

❑ As much as possible, avoid stress.

Considerations

❑ The most vital lifestyle changes you can make to reduce hypertension can be summarized as follows:

• Maintaining a normal weight.

• Eating plenty of fruits, vegetables, and low-fat dairy products.

• Eating less saturated fat and salt.

- Getting a minimum of thirty minutes of aerobic exercise per day. Walking is an excellent exercise.

Caution: If you are thirty-five or older and/or have been sedentary for some time, consult with your health care provider before beginning an exercise program.

- Limiting consumption of alcohol to a maximum of two drinks per day for men and one drink per day for women.

❑ The DASH diet (Dietary Approaches to Stop Hypertension) was developed by scientific experts in the field to help patients with high blood pressure lower it. The diet recommends:

- less than or equal to 27 percent of calories from fat,

- less than or equal to 6 percent saturated fat as a percentage of calories,

- more than or equal to 18 percent of calories as protein,

- less than or equal to 150 milligrams of cholesterol a day,

- more than or equal to 31 grams of fiber,

- at least 4,700 milligrams of potassium,

- 500 milligrams of magnesium, and

- 1,240 milligrams of calcium.

❑ If you have high blood pressure or wish to prevent it, it is important to follow the DASH diet guidelines and be aware of any personal food preferences you have that may keep you from meeting these guidelines. In another study (the PREMIER study), researchers looked at patients with high blood pressure and found that a 12 to 14 percent reduction in heart disease risk was possible by following the DASH diet or just a simpler version of a low-salt diet combined with regular exercise and weight loss.

Caution: If you are thirty-five or older and/or have been sedentary for some time, consult with your health care provider before beginning an exercise program.

❑ Fruits and vegetables cause the release of a hormone that opens up blood vessels. Eating up to six servings a day of both fruits and vegetables can reduce blood pressure.

❑ Hypertension is directly related to a number of other conditions, such as arteriosclerosis, cardiovascular disease, heart attack, and high cholesterol. These conditions are discussed separately in Part Two. It is advisable to refer to all of the sections on these interrelated conditions mentioned, even if you are concerned with only one of these illnesses.

❑ Because the use of diuretic drugs causes increased urinary excretion of magnesium, it can cause hypomagnesemia (magnesium depletion), particularly in older adults. Magnesium is needed in conjunction with calcium to prevent bone deterioration, as well as to maintain a normal heart rhythm and muscular contraction. Losses of potassium due to diuretics also are common and may be dangerous, causing

heart malfunction. Often potassium supplements are prescribed. Consult your physician before using diuretics.

❑ People with hypertension often suffer from sleep apnea, in which they stop breathing for ten seconds or more throughout the night. Apnea is associated with loud snoring and restless sleep, and can cause the individual to feel excessively sleepy during the day. Evaluation and treatment of apnea may help reduce high blood pressure.

❑ Some risks for hypertension cannot be changed—a family history of the disease, for instance. However, many risk factors can be avoided by making changes in diet and lifestyle.

❑ According to the National Stroke Association, hypertension is the most important controllable risk factor for stroke, increasing the risk of stroke by seven times.

❑ Approximately 26 percent of Americans with normal blood pressure and about 58 percent of those with hypertension are salt sensitive.

❑ Research has revealed that people with variations in two specific genes are twice as likely to develop high blood pressure from salt consumption. This discovery may make it possible to identify children prone to high blood pressure; if such people can be identified in early childhood, it may be possible to modify their diets so that they can avoid developing high blood pressure later in life.

❑ Heavy snorers are more likely to have high blood pressure or angina than silent sleepers. Research suggests that snorers may suffer from a malfunctioning of the part of the brain responsible for fluent breathing; this can put an unnatural strain on the heart and lungs due to oxygen shortage.

❑ Researchers at the State University of New York found that the lower the level of magnesium in the body, the higher the blood pressure. This double-blind, placebo-controlled trial showed that taking supplemental magnesium can result in a significant, dose-dependent reduction in both systolic and diastolic blood pressure.

❑ Apple pectin aids in reducing blood pressure.

❑ A synthetic heart hormone that appears to be very effective in lowering blood pressure is currently undergoing testing at some twenty-five medical centers.

❑ Certain colors have a beneficial effect on blood pressure. (*See* COLOR THERAPY in Part Three.) Music also can be used to reduce stress and thereby lower blood pressure. (*See* MUSIC AND SOUND THERAPY in Part Three.)

❑ Taking medication for high blood pressure may lead to low blood pressure (hypotension). Hypotension can cause fainting, fatigue, and weakness, possibly with nausea, sweating, and restlessness preceding a loss of consciousness. Postural hypotension, or orthostatic hypotension, a very temporary lowering of blood pressure, is usually caused by standing up too suddenly. This leads to dizziness and wears off quickly. (*See* Orthostatic Hypotension *under* RARE DISORDERS in Part Two for further information.) For older adults, low blood pressure can simply result from

How to Measure Your Blood Pressure

Your blood pressure measurement actually tells you how much pressure it takes to move the flow of blood through your arteries. This is assumed to be equivalent to the pressure at the pump end, the heart.

Blood pressure is measured at two points in the heart's pumping rhythm: *systolic pressure* is taken at the moment the heart beats; *diastolic pressure* is taken when the heart is at rest between beats. To measure blood pressure, the soft, inflatable cuff of the sphygmomanometer is wrapped around the upper arm and inflated. Slowly deflate the cuff. The systolic pressure is measured when the first pounding sound begins. Then the cuff is further deflated and the diastolic pressure is taken when the sound is no longer audible. The combined pressure is usually expressed as a fraction—120/80, for example.

Ideally, blood pressure should be taken with the arm bare. A tight sleeve may constrict the arm or make it impossible to apply the blood pressure cuff properly. The cuff should be placed around the arm about one inch above the bend in the elbow. Before beginning to work with the sphygmomanometer, check the following four items:

1. Be sure that the sphygmomanometer reads 0 when there is no pressure in the system.

2. Check to be sure that the needle stays in place when the valve is closed.

3. Check the valve screw to make sure that it operates smoothly.

4. Inspect your stethoscope for cracks or leaks in the tubing, earpieces, bell, or diaphragm.

Next, use the stethoscope to take the blood pressure. Follow this procedure:

1. Position the disc of the stethoscope snugly against the skin where the elbow bends—a little to the left of center on the right arm, and a little to the right of center on the left arm. There should be no gaps between the stethoscope and the skin, but you should not apply any undue pressure. Make sure that the stethoscope is not touching the cuff at any point.

2. Position the earpieces of the stethoscope in your ears (with the earpieces directed forward).

3. Hold the stethoscope disc snugly in position with one hand while you pump the cuff with the other hand.

4. Pump the cuff until the gauge registers about 180–200 mm Hg.

5. Loosen the valve slightly and permit the pressure to drop slowly. Listen carefully for the first sound of a beat—the number on the scale when you hear the first beat is the systolic pressure. (If you think that you missed the first beat or are unsure, tighten the valve again and pump the cuff up; repeat the process, listening carefully.)

6. Continue to deflate the cuff slowly until the last sound of blood pumping through the blood vessels is heard. When you hear no more blood flowing, the number on the scale is the diastolic pressure.

When taking your blood pressure, follow these general guidelines for best results:

• Avoid eating, smoking, or exercising for at least one-half hour before measuring your blood pressure.

• Test yourself at about the same times each day. Plan ahead to give yourself time to get over any feelings of anger or anxiety.

• Sit quietly and eliminate extraneous noise.

• Follow the manufacturer's instructions carefully.

• Position your arm at heart level, palm up. If you are using a cuff device, wrap the cuff just above the elbow—with your sleeve rolled up above the cuff—and be sure it is not too tight.

• Make sure the hoses from the cuff are not tangled or pinched.

• Take care not to move the hoses during the reading.

• Wait at least five minutes in between readings, with the cuff fully deflated.

• Take the device along on medical visits once a year or more to check its accuracy against your physician's measurements.

eating. This is called *postprandial hypotension.* It happens because blood is diverted to the gastrointestinal tract to help with digesting the food. In older people, the heart is not as efficient at increasing blood flow by pumping more quickly, so, with too much blood going to help with digesting a meal, there is too little traveling to the brain. Drinking lots of fluids increases blood volume, which may alleviate this condition. In some cases, low blood pressure can be a sign of heart disease or blood loss, especially a sudden loss of blood such as in an accident. In very many cases though, moderately low blood pressure is a sign of good health, especially in younger people.

❑ *See also* ARTERIOSCLEROSIS/ATHEROSCLEROSIS; CARDIOVASCULAR DISEASE; CIRCULATORY PROBLEMS; and HEART ATTACK in Part Two.

HIGH CHOLESTEROL

A high blood cholesterol level, especially elevated low-density lipoproteins (LDL), is considered to be a contributor to plaque building up in the arteries and impeded blood flow to the brain, kidneys, genitals, extremities, and heart. It is among the primary causes of heart disease, because cholesterol produces deposits in arteries. High cholesterol levels may also be implicated in gallstones, erectile dysfunction (although it is often the drugs prescribed to deal with high cholesterol that cause this), mental impairment, and high blood pressure.

Cholesterol is an essential part of every cell structure and is needed for proper brain and nerve function. It is also the basis for the manufacture of sex hormones. Cholesterol is manufactured in the liver and transported through the bloodstream to the sites where it is needed. It is a fatty substance and, because blood is mainly water, it has to latch on to molecules called lipoproteins to travel around successfully. Low-density lipoproteins (LDLs) are the major transporters of cholesterol in the bloodstream and, because LDLs seem to encourage the deposit of cholesterol in the arteries, it is known as bad cholesterol. High-density lipoproteins (HDLs), on the other hand, are considered good cholesterol because they carry unneeded cholesterol away from the cells and back to the liver, where it is broken down for removal from the body. If everything is functioning as it should, this system remains in balance.

However, if there is too much cholesterol for the HDLs to pick up promptly, or if there are not enough HDLs to do the job, cholesterol can form plaque that sticks to artery walls and may eventually cause heart disease.

It is important to distinguish between serum cholesterol and dietary cholesterol. Serum cholesterol is the cholesterol in the bloodstream. Dietary cholesterol is cholesterol that is present in food. While eating foods high in dietary cholesterol can raise serum cholesterol, it is not the only source of serum cholesterol. Indeed, you would have some amount of serum cholesterol even if you never ate any food containing dietary cholesterol because the body produces its own cholesterol.

Cholesterol levels are greatly influenced by diet, but they are also affected by your genetic makeup. The consumption of foods high in cholesterol and/or saturated fat increases cholesterol levels, while a vegetarian diet, regular exercise, and the nutrients niacin and vitamin C may lower cholesterol.

The National Heart, Lung and Blood Institute guidelines for cholesterol levels are:

LDL cholesterol

Less than 100 mg/dL	Optimal
100–129 mg/dL	Near optimal/less than optimal
130–159 mg/dL	Borderline high
160–189 mg/dL	High
Greater than or equal to 190 mg/dL	Very high

Total cholesterol

Less than 200 mg/dL	Desirable
200–239 mg/dL	Borderline high
Greater than or equal to 240 mg/dL	High

HDL cholesterol

Less than 40 mg/dL	Low; a major risk factor for heart disease
60 mg/dL and above	Considered protective against heart disease

If you have an abnormal reading on any of these, speak to your doctor about how to correct them. It will probably involve adjusting your diet, increasing your exercise, and possibly taking medication.

NUTRIENTS

SUPPLEMENT	SUGGESTED DOSAGE	COMMENTS
Very Important		
Apple pectin	As directed on label.	Lowers cholesterol levels by binding fats and heavy metals.
Calcium	As directed on label.	To prevent hypocalcemia, or low calcium levels. Use calcium aspartate form.
Chinese red yeast rice extract	2.4 g daily.	Has cholesterol-lowering properties.
Chromium picolinate	400–600 mcg daily.	Lowers total cholesterol levels and improves HDL-to-LDL ratio.
Coenzyme Q$_{10}$ plus	60 mg daily.	Improves circulation.
Coenzyme A from Coenzyme-A Technologies	As directed on label.	Works well with coenzyme Q$_{10}$ to streamline metabolism, process fats, remove toxins from the body, and boost the immune system.
Fiber (oat bran or guar gum)	As directed on label, ½ hour before the first meal of the day. Take separately from other supplements and medications.	Helps to lower cholesterol.
Garlic (Kyolic from Wakunaga)	2 capsules 3 times daily.	Lowers cholesterol levels and blood pressure.

L-carnitine	As directed on label.	Studies conducted using 4 grams of carnitine daily for 12 months showed lowered death rates and lowered cholesterol levels in people who had had heart attacks.
Lecithin granules or capsules	1 tbsp 3 times daily, before meals. 1,200 mg 3 times daily, before meals.	Lowers cholesterol. A fat emulsifier.
Lipotropic factors	As directed on label.	Substances that prevent fat deposits (as in atherosclerosis).
Vitamin A with mixed carotenoids	As directed on label.	If you are taking cholesterol-lowering drugs, your lycopene levels will be reduced. Lycopene is one of the carotenoids that boosts the immune system.
Vitamin B complex plus extra vitamin B$_1$ (thiamine) and vitamin B$_3$ (niacin)	As directed on label. 300 mg daily. Do not exceed this amount.	B vitamins work best when taken together. Important in controlling cholesterol levels. Lowers cholesterol. Do not use a sustained-release formula, and do not substitute niacinamide for niacin. Caution: Do not take niacin if you have a liver disorder, gout, or high blood pressure.
Vitamin C with bioflavonoids	3,000–8,000 mg daily, in divided doses.	Lowers cholesterol.
Vitamin E	200 IU daily or 400 IU every other day.	Improves circulation. Use an emulsion form for rapid assimilation. Use d-alpha-tocopherol form.
Helpful		
Essential fatty acids (black currant seed oil, borage oil, fish oil, primrose oil, or Kyolic-EPA from Wakunaga)	As directed on label. Take with vitamin E as recommended above.	Thins the blood.
Heart Science from Source Naturals	As directed on label.	Contains antioxidants to lower cholesterol, plus herbs, vitamins, and other nutrients that protect the heart and promote healthy cardiovascular function.
Proteolytic enzymes	As directed on label. Take with meals and between meals.	Aids digestion. Caution: Do not give this supplement to a child.
Selenium	200 mcg daily. If you are pregnant, do not exceed 40 mcg daily.	Deficiency has been linked to heart disease.
Shiitake extract or reishi extract	As directed on label. As directed on label.	Helps to control and lower cholesterol levels.

Herbs

❑ Cayenne (capsicum), goldenseal, and hawthorn berries help to lower cholesterol.

Caution: Do not take goldenseal internally on a daily basis for more than one week at a time. Do not use it during pregnancy or if you are breast-feeding, and use with caution if you are allergic to ragweed. If you have a history of cardiovascular disease, diabetes, or glaucoma, use it only under a doctor's supervision.

❑ Cinnamon has been shown to lower cholesterol. Use Cinnulin PF from Nutrivitals rather than the culinary spice.

Recommendations

❑ Include the following cholesterol-lowering foods in your diet: almonds, apples, bananas, carrots, cold-water fish, dried beans, garlic, grapefruit, oats, olive oil, salmon, strawberries, and walnuts. Strawberries in particular were shown to reduce damage from oxidation to the bad (LDL) cholesterol, thereby lowering the risk of heart disease.

❑ Make sure to take in plenty of fiber in the form of fruits, vegetables, and whole grains. Water-soluble dietary fiber is very important in reducing serum cholesterol. It is found in barley, beans, brown rice, fruits, glucomannan, guar gum, and oats. Oat bran and brown rice bran are the best foods for lowering cholesterol. Whole-grain cereals (in moderation) and brown rice are good as well. Since fiber absorbs the minerals from the food it is in, take extra minerals separately from the fiber.

❑ In 1999, the FDA granted a health claim for products that contain plant stanols and sterol esters from any plant, especially soybeans. Any product containing 0.65 gram of plant sterols or 1.7 grams of plant stanols per serving can claim to reduce the risk of heart disease. Foods such as Minute Maid's HeartWise orange juice or Rice Dream HeartWise rice drink, or supplements are good sources, but they must be consumed as part of a low-saturated-fat and low-cholesterol diet. The sterols and stanols were shown to lower total cholesterol by 9 percent and bad cholesterol by 12 percent. Adding fish oil to the diet along with sterols or stanols had an added benefit of lowering triglycerides.

❑ Drink fresh juices, especially carrot, celery, and beet juices. Carrot juice helps to flush out fat from the bile in the liver and this helps lower cholesterol.

❑ Go on a monthly spirulina fast, with carrot and celery juice or lemon and steam-distilled water. (*See* FASTING in Part Three.)

❑ Use only unrefined cold- or expeller-pressed oils. Cold-pressed oils are those that have never been heated above 110°F during processing—at this temperature, enzyme destruction begins. Use vegetable oils that are liquid at room temperature, such as olive, soybean, flaxseed, primrose, and black currant seed oil. Olive oil is recommended.

❑ Do not eat any nuts except raw, unsalted pecans, walnuts, and almonds. Almonds are rich in the amino acid arginine, and were found in one study to cut cholesterol levels by sixteen points over a four-week period.

❑ Reduce the amount of saturated fat and cholesterol in your diet. Saturated fats include all fats of animal origin as well as coconut and palm oils. Eliminate from the diet all hydrogenated fats and hardened fats and oils such as margarine, lard, and butter. Margarine that contains plant sterols, however, is a relatively healthy option. Consume no heated fats or processed oils, and avoid animal products (especially pork and pork products) and fried or fatty foods. Always read food product labels carefully. You may consume nonfat milk, low-fat cottage cheese, and skinless white poultry meat (preferably turkey), but only in moderation.

❑ Do not consume alcohol, cakes, candy, carbonated drinks, coffee, gravies, nondairy creamers, pies, processed or refined foods, refined carbohydrates, tea, tobacco, or white bread.

❑ Get regular moderate exercise. Always consult with your health care provider before beginning any new exercise program.

❑ Try to avoid stress and sustained tension. Learn stress management techniques. (See STRESS in Part Two.)

Considerations

❑ High cholesterol is directly related to conditions such as Alzheimer's disease, arteriosclerosis, cardiovascular disease, circulatory problems, heart attack, hypertension, and osteoporosis. These conditions are discussed separately in Part Two. It is advisable to refer to all of the sections on these interrelated diseases to learn about all aspects of, and contributing causes to, high cholesterol.

❑ Meat and dairy products are primary sources of dietary cholesterol. Grains, vegetables, and fruits are free of cholesterol.

❑ Many people use margarine or vegetable shortening as substitutes for butter because they contain no cholesterol. Now most products are free of harmful trans fatty acids. These are good alternatives to butter.

❑ In large amounts, coffee can elevate blood cholesterol levels, more than doubling the risk of heart disease. According to a report published in *The New England Journal of Medicine,* observation of 15,000 coffee drinkers revealed that as the intake of coffee rises, the amount of cholesterol in the blood goes up.

❑ Cream substitutes (nondairy coffee creamers) are actually poor alternatives to cholesterol-heavy dairy products. Many contain coconut oil, which is a highly saturated fat. Soymilk or almond milk is preferable.

❑ The body does need some fats, but they must be the right kind. Good fats supply essential fatty acids, which are a very important link in our health chain. Fats supply energy, and they stay in the digestive tract for longer periods than proteins or carbohydrates, giving a feeling of fullness. They act as an intestinal lubricant, generate body heat, and carry the fat-soluble vitamins A, D, E, and K in the body. The protective myelin sheaths that protect nerve fibers are composed of fats. All cell membranes are composed of fats as well. Unfortunately, most Americans consume much too much of the wrong fats—that is, saturated, hydrogenated, and heated fats—which are linked to obesity, cardiovascular disease, and certain types of cancer.

❑ Human growth hormone therapy has been found to decrease cholesterol levels. (See GROWTH HORMONE THERAPY in Part Three.)

❑ Some fast-food restaurants use beef tallow (fat) to make their hamburgers, fish, chicken, and French-fried potatoes. Not only do these fried foods contain high amounts of cholesterol, but this fat is subjected to high temperatures in the deep-frying process, resulting in oxidation and the formation of free radicals. Heating fat, especially frying food in fat, also produces toxic trans-fatty acids, which seem to behave much like saturated fats in clogging the arteries and raising blood cholesterol levels.

❑ Certain drugs can worsen cholesterol levels. Beta-blockers, often prescribed to control high blood pressure, can cause unfavorable changes in the ratio of LDL to HDL in the blood, by lowering HDL. Check with your physician if you are taking any medications that you suspect might be affecting your cholesterol levels.

❑ Some people claim that taking charcoal tablets lowers blood cholesterol. However, charcoal also absorbs good nutrients along with the cholesterol. Activated charcoal should not be consumed daily, and it should not be taken at the same time as other supplements or medications. Other experts recommend taking fish oil capsules to lower cholesterol, but fish oil is 100 percent fat, and the evidence is lacking that the ingestion of fish oil reduces serum fats. Although fish oil does not lower cholesterol levels, it can reduce the risk of illness and death from heart disease by other mechanisms related to inflammation and heart rhythm.

❑ Pure virgin olive oil appears to help reduce serum cholesterol. A monounsaturated-fatty-acid-rich diet that includes olive oil may be the reason for the low serum cholesterol levels found in people living in Italy and Greece.

❑ Studies have shown that diets consisting of grains, fruits, and vegetables result in lower blood cholesterol levels. In the United States and northern Europe, where people consume large amounts of meat and dairy products, extremely high rates of heart and circulatory disease are present. Even children in these nations show signs of progressive vascular disease due to hypercholesterolemia (an excess of cholesterol in the blood).

❑ There are a number of cholesterol-lowering drugs on the market. Available by prescription only, these tend to be costly, and they can have serious side effects. We believe that these drugs should be used only as a last resort. The sensible way to keep the serum fats within a safe range is to follow a diet that excludes animal fats (including meat, milk, and all dairy products) and includes ample amounts of fiber and bulk (whole grains, fruits, and vegetables).

❑ Sunlight, or rather the lack of it, has been shown to have adverse effects of cholesterol levels.

❑ Lowering your blood cholesterol level may help to stop clogging of the arteries.

❑ Some people have hereditary disorders that prevent even the healthiest diet from lowering LDL levels. For these people, researchers are working on a device that uses an enzyme to break down LDL and accelerate its removal before it can fasten onto artery walls to form plaque. The device would be implanted under the skin to control the LDL levels in the blood.

❑ There are opposing theories about high cholesterol levels. Some medical practitioners believe that it has little to do with heart disease and that a direct correlation has never been fully established. Studies in India, Guatemala, Poland, and the United States claim to have proved that there is no relationship between atherosclerosis and cholesterol levels. However, it is probably best to take cholesterol levels seriously, and also to consider other tests that may help to assess your likelihood of developing heart disease as outlined in HEART ATTACK in Part Two.

❑ *See* ARTERIOSCLEROSIS/ATHEROSCLEROSIS; CARDIOVASCULAR DISEASE; CIRCULATORY PROBLEMS; HEART ATTACK; and HYPERTENSION, all in Part Two. *Also see* CHELATION THERAPY in Part Three.

HIV/HUMAN IMMUNODEFICIENCY VIRUS

See AIDS.

HIVES

Hives, called *urticaria* by the medical profession, is a skin condition that is characterized by sudden outbreaks of red, itchy welts on the skin. Any area of the body may be affected. The welts may vary in appearance, from tiny, goose-bump-like spots to rashes that cover significant areas of the body. Hives usually go away within a few hours to two days, but in rare cases they become chronic and may last for six weeks or more.

Many cases of hives are brought on as allergic reactions and coincide with the release of histamine in the body. The release of histamine into the skin produces an inflammatory reaction, with itching, swelling, and redness. Hives can cause significant discomfort, but it does not cause injury or damage to any vital organs.

The skin is the largest organ of the body. It is an important part of the excretory system. The skin acts in conjunction with other systems in the body to remove toxins and waste. Hives can be a natural reaction to the presence of a foreign substance in the body. However, an offending substance need not enter the body to trigger an outbreak of hives. Merely coming into contact with various substances, such as pesticides, soaps, shampoos, hair sprays, residues from laundry products or dry cleaning chemicals on cloth-

ing, or any other of a vast array of other seemingly innocuous household items can unleash a maddening attack of hives.

The severity of a hives outbreak can vary from case to case as well as from person to person. Some people can break out in hives if they merely touch a certain type of plant or bush; others may develop hives only with considerable exposure, such as overconsumption of a certain food. Chemicals are a major cause of hives for many people; anything from perfumes to household cleaners can trigger a reaction, as can nervous conditions, stress, certain foods, and alcohol.

Viruses also can cause hives. Hepatitis B and Epstein-Barr virus, the virus that causes infectious mononucleosis, are the two most common culprits. Some bacterial infections likewise can cause outbreaks of hives, both chronic and acute. An association between *Candida albicans* and chronic hives has been established in several clinical studies over the past twenty years.

Antibiotics such as penicillin and related compounds are the most common cause of drug-induced hives. Persons who are allergic to penicillin may have various reactions including hives, angioedema (a condition that is similar to hives but affects deeper layers of the skin and causes larger wheals), laryngeal angioedema (angioedema that affects the throat, and can have an adverse effect on breathing), or anaphylaxis (a systemic allergic reaction causing generalized itching and difficulty breathing) if they ingest penicillin. The symptoms get worse with increased use. If you are allergic to penicillin, make sure your health care provider does not give it to you. Also inform your dentist. If you are traveling, make sure someone else knows about your allergy in case you become ill and are unable to communicate the information yourself.

The following are some of the disorders, drugs, and other substances that most commonly cause outbreaks of hives in susceptible people. This list is not exhaustive, and we do not mean to imply that these items *will* cause a hives outbreak, only that they at least contribute to the condition in some people:

- *Allopurinol* (Zyloprim), a gout medication.

- *Animals,* especially animal dander and dog saliva.

- *Antimony,* a metallic element that is present in various metal alloys.

- *Antipyrine,* an agent used to relieve pain and inflammation.

- *Aspirin.*

- *Barbiturates.*

- *BHA and BHT,* preservatives used in many food products.

- *Bismuth,* another metallic element present in certain metal alloys.

- *Cancer,* especially leukemia.

- *Chloral hydrate,* a sedative used in the treatment of tetany.

- *Chlorpromazine* (Thorazine), a tranquilizer and antiemetic.

- *Cologne or perfume.*

- *Corticotropin* (also known as adrenocorticotropic hormone, or ACTH, and sold for medicinal purposes under the brand names Acthar and Cortrosyn).

- *Environmental factors,* especially heat, cold, water, and sunlight.

- *Eucalyptus,* a tree whose leaves yield an aromatic oil that is used in cough remedies and other medicines.

- *Exercise.*

- *Fluorides,* which are found in certain dental care products and in fluoridated drinking water.

- *Food allergies,* especially allergies to shellfish, eggs, fruits, and various nuts.

- *Food colorings and preservatives.*

- *Gold.*

- *Griseofulvin* (Fulvicin, Grisactin, and others), an antifungal medication.

- *Hyperthyroidism.*

- *Infections,* especially strep infections, hepatitis, and parasites.

- *Insect bites.*

- *Insulin.*

- *Iodines,* used in certain antiseptics and dyes.

- *Liver extract.*

- *Makeup.*

- *Menthol,* an extract of peppermint oil used in perfumes, as a mild anesthetic, and as a mint flavoring in candy and cigarettes.

- *Meprobamate* (Miltown, Equanil, Meprospan), a tranquilizer.

- *Mercury,* a toxic metallic element found in dental fillings, certain antacids, and some first-aid preparations, among other things.

- *Morphine.*

- *Opium.*

- *Para-aminosalicylic acid,* an anti-inflammatory drug.

- *Penicillin.*

- *Phenacetin,* an ingredient in some pain medications.

- *Phenobarbital,* a sedative and anticonvulsant.

- *Pilocarpine,* a glaucoma medication.

- *Plants.*

- *Poliomyelitis vaccine.*

- *Potassium sulfocyanate,* a preservative.

- *Preservatives.*

- *Procaine* (Novocain), an anesthetic.

- *Promethazine* (Phenergan), an antihistamine, sedative, and antiemetic.

- *Quinine,* used in quinine water and antimalaria medications.

- *Reserpine,* a heart medication.

- *Saccharin,* an artificial sweetener found in Sweet'N Low, many toothpastes, and many dietetic and sugarless products.

- *Salicylates,* chemicals used as food flavorings and preservatives.

- *Shampoo.*

- *Soaps,* including laundry soap.

- *Sulfites,* chemicals used as food preservatives and in the production of dried fruits such as raisins.

- *Tartrazine,* a food dye and an ingredient in Alka-Seltzer.

- *Thiamine hydrochloride,* an ingredient in some cough medicines.

Other hives-provoking substances are being identified with increasing frequency. Meat, dairy, and poultry products, especially in frozen or fast foods, are increasingly being associated with hives, probably because many farmers and ranchers routinely give their livestock antibiotics in an effort to prevent disease or infection. These antibiotics are not affected by subsequent freezing, processing, or cooking. Allergic reactions have been traced to antibiotics in milk, soft drinks, and even frozen dinners.

Unless otherwise specified, the dosages recommended here are for adults. For children between the ages of twelve and seventeen, reduce the dose to three-quarters the recommended amount. For children between six and twelve, use one-half the recommended dose, and for children under the age of six, use one-quarter the recommended amount.

NUTRIENTS

SUPPLEMENT	SUGGESTED DOSAGE	COMMENTS
Helpful		
Acidophilus	As directed on label.	Reduces allergic reactions and helps replenish "friendly" bacteria. Use a nondairy formula.
Flaxseed oil or primrose oil	1,000 mg twice daily. 1,000 mg twice daily.	Has anti-inflammatory effects.
Garlic (Kyolic from Wakunaga)	As directed on label.	Aids in destroying bacteria.

Herpanacine from Diamond-Herpanacine Associates	As directed on label.	A nutrient and herb combination that supports overall skin health.
Multivitamin and mineral complex	As directed on label.	To correct any nutrient or mineral deficiencies that may be contributing to outbreaks. Use a hypoallergenic formula.
Quercetin	As directed on label.	Reduces inflammation and reactions to substances that may cause hives.
or		
Anti-Allergy formula from Freeda Vitamins	As directed on label.	A combination of quercetin, calcium pantothenate, and calcium ascorbate.
Vitamin B complex	As directed on label, with meals (amounts of individual vitamins in a complex will vary).	Needed for the functioning of the nervous system and for healthy skin. Aids with the body's immune response.
plus extra vitamin B5 (pantothenic acid)	250 mg 3–4 times daily at first outbreak. Reduce to 1–2 times daily when hives subside.	
and vitamin B12	1,000–2,000 mcg daily.	Prevents nerve damage and promotes normal growth of the skin. Use a lozenge or sublingual form.
Vitamin C with bioflavonoids	1,000 mg 3 times daily.	Enhances immune response; acts as an anti-inflammatory.
Vitamin D	400 IU daily.	To reduce outbreaks.
Vitamin E	200 IU daily or 400 IU every other day.	A powerful antioxidant that improves circulation to the skin tissues. Use d-alpha-tocopherol form.
and zinc	50 mg daily. Do not exceed a total of 100 mg daily from all supplements.	Promotes a healthy immune system and healing of skin tissues. Needed for proper concentrations of vitamin E in the blood. Use zinc gluconate lozenges or OptiZinc for best absorption.

Herbs

❑ Alfalfa, bilberry extract, cat's claw, chamomile, echinacea, ginseng, licorice, nettle, sarsaparilla, and yellow dock are all beneficial to the hives sufferer. Alfalfa can also be used as a preventive blood tonic. It cleanses the blood and helps keep the body free of toxins.

Cautions: Do not use cat's claw during pregnancy. Do not use chamomile if you are allergic to ragweed. Do not use during pregnancy or nursing. It may interact with warfarin or cyclosporine, so patients using these drugs should avoid it. Do not take echinacea for longer than three months. It should not be used by people who are allergic to ragweed. Do not use ginseng if you have high blood pressure, or are pregnant or nursing. Licorice root should not be used during pregnancy or nursing. It should not be used by persons with diabetes, glaucoma, heart disease, high blood pressure, or a history of stroke.

❑ Applying aloe vera gel to the affected area can be helpful.

❑ Black nightshade leaves may help. Wash and boil the leaves in water, put them on a cloth, and apply as a poultice to the affected area. (*See* USING A POULTICE in Part Three.)

Caution: Do not take this herb internally, and avoid getting it in your eyes.

❑ The leaves and the bark of the red alder tree, when brewed into a strong tea, can help hives. Apply it locally to the affected area, and take a couple of tablespoons internally as well. Reapply several times daily until the hives abate. Red alder contains the astringent tannin.

Recommendations

❑ Avoid alcohol and all processed foods, which put added stress on the body by depleting nutrients. Also avoid dairy products, eggs, chicken, and nuts. Especially avoid foods high in saturated fats, cholesterol, and sugar.

❑ Do not take any medications (including aspirin, pain killers, sedatives, laxatives, cough syrups, and antacids) that are not prescribed for you.

❑ Use only hypoallergenic skin care products.

❑ For the typical case of hives, avoid using prednisone or other steroids. Instead, use the nutrients and herbs listed above. Try nettle first.

❑ For topical treatment, use cornstarch or colloidal oatmeal added to bathwater. A good oatmeal product for this purpose is Aveeno Bath Treatment, available at drugstores. Bathing in cool water with baking soda added also may relieve symptoms.

❑ Take a cool shower when you see the first signs of hives appearing. Make sure that it is cool, not hot. This may slow the spreading of hives.

❑ Wear loose-fitting clothing.

❑ Try using homeopathic remedies. *Bovista, Cantharis,* and *Rhus toxicodendron* are homeopathic remedies that may alleviate symptoms of hives.

❑ If you have had hives and they are bothering you or if you are developing an acute case of hives, consult your health care provider.

❑ If sun exposure is the cause of your hives, apply a strong sunscreen—this will usually alleviate the problem.

❑ If hives develop in your mouth or throat, and especially if they cause swelling around the throat or interferes with swallowing or breathing *to any extent at all,* seek medical help immediately. Go to the emergency room of the nearest hospital or call for emergency assistance. Hives can signal or accompany the onset of anaphylaxis, a dangerous allergic reaction that can block the breathing passages. The possibility of anaphylaxis is what makes allergies to insect stings, such as those from bees, a potentially serious concern. If you have ever had this type of reaction, you should be under a physician's care and have an epinephrine injection kit on hand. Make sure you know how to use it, and keep the kit with you at all times.

Considerations

❏ Many people who suffer acute attacks find at least temporary relief from the symptoms of hives by taking antihistamines such as hydroxyzine (Atarax, Vistaril), chlorpheniramine (Chlor-Trimeton, Teldrin, and others), or diphenhydramine (Benadryl and others). Chronic sufferers have less success with this approach, as antihistamines are suppressive agents and may actually contribute to the persistence of hives. Antihistamines in gel or spray form can be applied topically for immediate but temporary relief of itchiness or burning.

❏ Depending on the nature and severity of the symptoms, health care providers may prescribe antihistamines, cortisone, or a bronchodilator such as terbutaline or ephedrine for people with hives. They may also prescribe sedatives for anxiety in severe cases.

❏ If a hives outbreak is the result of a food or drug that you have ingested, you obviously do not want that substance in your body again. If you cannot isolate whatever food or drug it might be that causes hives, having a physician do some blood work to find the allergen may be your only solution, even though this approach can be relatively expensive.

❏ Occasionally, hives can persist for weeks or even months, resisting all attempts at treatment. For this reason alone, it is best to learn what the cause of the outbreak is in order to avoid it. If you suffer from chronic hives and cannot isolate the cause, eliminating all the possible allergens from your home may be your only resort. This can be a long, drawn-out, and painstaking process. (*See* ALLERGIES in Part Two.)

❏ Chronic hives may be linked to *Candida albicans*. If you suspect this may be the cause of hives, adopting a yeast-free diet can be of some benefit. (*See* CANDIDIASIS in Part Two.)

❏ An elimination diet is important. (*See* ALLERGIES in Part Two.)

HOT FLASHES

See under MENOPAUSAL AND PERIMENOPAUSAL PROBLEMS.

HYPERTENSION

See HIGH BLOOD PRESSURE.

HYPERTHYROIDISM

This disorder occurs when the thyroid gland produces too much thyroid hormone, resulting in an overactive metabolic state. All of the body's processes speed up with this disorder. Symptoms of hyperthyroidism include nervousness, irritability, a constant feeling of being hot, increased perspiration, insomnia and fatigue, increased frequency of bowel movements, less frequent menstruation and decreased menstrual flow, weakness, hair and weight loss, change in skin thickness, separation of the nails from the nail bed, hand tremors, intolerance of heat, rapid heartbeat, goiter, and, sometimes, protruding eyeballs. Hyperthyroidism is sometimes also called *thyrotoxicosis*. The most common type of this disorder is Graves' disease.

The thyroid gland is the body's internal thermostat. It regulates the temperature by secreting two hormones that control how quickly the body burns calories and uses energy. If the thyroid secretes too much hormone, hyperthyroidism results; too little hormone results in hypothyroidism. Many cases of hypothyroidism and hyperthyroidism are believed to result from an abnormal immune response. The exact cause is not understood, but the immune system can produce antibodies that invade and attack the thyroid, disrupting hormone production. Hyperthyroidism can also be caused by lumps or tumors that form on the thyroid and disrupt hormone production. Infection or inflammation of the thyroid can cause temporary hyperthyroidism, as can certain prescription drugs.

Hyperthyroidism is not as common as hypothyroidism. Both of these thyroid disorders affect women more often than men. A malfunctioning thyroid can be the underlying cause of many recurring illnesses.

Unless otherwise specified, the dosages recommended here are for adults. For a child between the ages of twelve and seventeen, reduce the dose to three-quarters of the recommended amount. For a child between six and twelve, use one-half of the recommended dose, and for a child under the age of six, use one-quarter of the recommended amount.

NUTRIENTS

SUPPLEMENT	SUGGESTED DOSAGE	COMMENTS
Very Important		
Multivitamin and mineral complex	As directed on label.	Increased amounts of vitamins and minerals are needed for this "hyper" metabolic condition. Use a super-high-potency formula.
Vitamin B complex plus extra	50 mg of each major B vitamin 3 times daily, with meals (amounts of individual vitamins in a complex will vary).	Needed for thyroid function. Injections (under a doctor's supervision) may be necessary.
vitamin B₁ (thiamine) and	50 mg twice daily.	Needed for blood formation and energy levels.
vitamin B₂ (riboflavin) and	50 mg twice daily.	Required for normal functioning of all cells, glands, and organs in the body.
vitamin B₆ (pyridoxine)	50 mg twice daily.	Activates many enzymes and is needed for immune function and antibody production.
Helpful		
Brewer's yeast	1–3 tbsp and up daily.	Rich in many basic nutrients, especially the B vitamins.

Essential fatty acids (Kyolic-EPA from Wakunaga)	As directed on label.	Needed for correct glandular function.
Lecithin granules or capsules	1 tbsp 3 times daily, before meals. 1,200 mg 3 times daily, before meals.	Aids in digestion of fats and protects the lining of all cells and organs.
Vitamin C with bioflavonoids	3,000–5,000 mg and up daily.	Especially important in this stressful condition.
Vitamin E	200 IU daily or 400 IU every other day.	An antioxidant and necessary nutrient. However, excessive amounts may stimulate the thyroid gland. Use d-alpha-tocopherol form.

Recommendations

❑ Eat plenty of the following foods: broccoli, Brussels sprouts, cabbage, cauliflower, kale, mustard greens, peaches, pears, rutabagas, soybeans, spinach, and turnips. These help to suppress thyroid hormone production.

❑ Avoid dairy products for at least three months. Also avoid stimulants, coffee, tea, nicotine, and soft drinks.

Considerations

❑ Along with other bodily processes, digestion speeds up with this disorder. Malabsorption occurs, so a proper diet is important.

❑ Radioactive sodium iodine (iodine 131, or I-131) is often recommended for treatment of hyperthyroidism. Many people are concerned because the treatment uses radioactive substances. There is no proof that radioactive iodine increases the incidence of tumors, leukemia, thyroid cancer, or birth defects in children born to women who became pregnant later in life and used this therapy. However, this treatment is not for use during pregnancy.

❑ Researchers in England studied ten people who were being treated for Parkinson's disease and found that all of them also had hyperthyroidism. Once the thyroid condition was treated, the Parkinson's disease improved dramatically.

❑ If a goiter affects breathing or swallowing, surgery may be needed to remove part or all of the thyroid. It may be necessary to take thyroid hormone pills after surgery.

❑ The pituitary gland, parathyroid glands, and sex glands all work together and are influenced by thyroid function. If there is a problem in one place, they all may be affected.

❑ The parathyroid glands, small endocrine glands that are positioned near or within the rear surface of the thyroid, secrete parathyroid hormone (PTH), which aids in controlling calcium levels. Hyperparathyroidism is a rare disorder in which these apple-seed-sized organs become enlarged and overactive. When too much PTH is released,

excess calcium leaches out of the bones and into the blood. Routine blood tests may reveal excess calcium in the blood. If left untreated, it can lead to other problems such as bone pain and kidney stones. The standard treatment for this disorder is surgery. Permanent hoarseness is a possible side effect, if the nerves supplying the voice box are injured.

❑ An undiagnosed thyroid condition can be mistaken for menopausal symptoms. Symptoms such as fatigue, mood swings, and depression are often present in both circumstances. If you are experiencing menopausal symptoms, you should have your thyroid function tested.

❑ For names and addresses of organizations that can provide additional information about thyroid disorders, see Health and Medical Organizations in the Appendix.

HYPOGLYCEMIA (LOW BLOOD SUGAR)

Hypoglycemia, or low blood sugar, is a condition in which there is an abnormally low level of glucose (sugar) in the blood. Reactive hypoglycemia occurs when blood sugar drops to abnormally low levels two to five hours after eating a meal. Symptoms of reactive hypoglycemia include sweating, tremors, rapid heartbeat, anxiety, and hunger. Most often, this results from the oversecretion of insulin by the pancreas. Insulin facilitates the transport of glucose from the bloodstream into the cells, especially those of muscle and fatty tissue, and causes glucose to be synthesized in the liver. If the pancreas is not functioning properly, normal carbohydrate metabolism is impossible. As the blood sugar drops, stress hormones such as adrenaline and cortisol kick in at high levels to prevent the blood sugar level from dropping dramatically. Another type of hypoglycemia is known as *fasting hypoglycemia*. This occurs as a result of abstaining from food for eight or more hours. The symptoms are often more severe than those of reactive hypoglycemia and can include seizures, loss of consciousness, and a loss of mental acuity. Liver disease or a tumor of the pancreas is generally the underlying cause of this type of hypoglycemia.

A person with hypoglycemia may display any or all of the following symptoms: fatigue, dizziness, heart palpitations, nausea, blurred vision, an inability to concentrate, light-headedness, headache, irritability, fainting spells, depression, nervousness, anxiety, cravings for sweets, confusion, night sweats, weakness in the legs, swollen feet, a feeling of tightness in the chest, constant hunger, pain in various parts of the body (especially the eyes), nervous habits, mental disturbances, and insomnia. If blood sugar levels drop below 40 milligrams (mg) of glucose per 100 cubic centimeter (cc) of blood (80 to 100 is normal), an individual may become unconscious. People with hypoglycemia can become very aggressive and lose their tempers easily. Any or all of these symptoms may occur a few hours after eating sweets or fats. The onset and severity of symptoms are directly related to the length of time since the last meal was eaten and the type of foods that meal contained.

More and more Americans today may have this condition, due to poor dietary habits that include eating large quantities of simple carbohydrates, sugars, alcohol, caffeine, and soft drinks, and insufficient amounts of complex carbohydrates. High stress levels are believed to be a contributing factor in the increasing incidence of hypoglycemia.

Hypoglycemia can be inherited, but most often it is precipitated by an inadequate diet. This is referred to as *functional hypoglycemia* (FH). Many other bodily disorders can cause hypoglycemic problems as well, among them adrenal insufficiency, stomach surgery, thyroid disorders, pituitary disorders, kidney disease, and pancreatitis and other pancreatic disorders such as pancreatic cancer. Immune deficiency and candidiasis are strongly linked to hypoglycemia. Glucose intolerance and hyperinsulinemia (high blood insulin levels), producing hypoglycemia, frequently occur in people with chronic liver failure. Other common causes are smoking and the consumption of large amounts of caffeine, found in colas, chocolate, and coffee. Though it may seem paradoxical, low blood sugar can also be an early sign of diabetes (high blood sugar).

Diagnosis of hypoglycemia can be difficult because the symptoms often mimic those of other disorders, including adrenal dysfunction, allergies, asthma, candidiasis, chronic fatigue syndrome, digestive or intestinal disorders, eating disorders, food allergies, hypothyroidism, kidney failure, malabsorption syndrome, menopause, mental disorders, neurological problems, nutritional deficiencies, sepsis (blood infection), stress, and weight problems.

To diagnose hypoglycemia, a health care provider may perform a glucose tolerance test (GTT). However, many people have symptoms of hypoglycemia even though the results of a five-hour GTT are within normal limits. A useful diagnostic test may be to follow the dietary and nutritional supplement regimen outlined in this section and see if symptoms improve.

Unless otherwise specified, the dosages recommended here are for adults. For children between the ages of twelve and seventeen, reduce the dose to three-quarters the recommended amount. For children between six and twelve, use one-half the recommended dose, and for children under the age of six, use one-quarter the recommended amount.

NUTRIENTS

SUPPLEMENT	SUGGESTED DOSAGE	COMMENTS
Very Important		
Brewer's yeast	As directed on label.	Aids in stabilizing blood sugar levels.
Chromium picolinate	300–600 mcg daily.	Vital in glucose metabolism. Essential for optimal insulin activity.
Garlic (Kyolic from Wakunaga)	As directed on label.	Very good for relieving low blood sugar when an attack occurs.
Glutathione	As directed on label.	A compound consisting of three amino acids that is associated with the breakdown of glucose into energy.
Kyo-Dophilus from Wakunaga	As directed on label.	To replace the "friendly" bacteria lacking in this disorder. Use the liquid form.
Pancreatin	As directed on label. Take with meals.	For proper protein digestion. Use a high-potency formula.
Proteolytic enzymes	As directed on label. Take between meals.	People with this disorder often fail to digest protein properly, resulting in "leaky gut syndrome" and allergies. *Caution:* Do not give this supplement to a child.
Quercetin	As directed on label.	Aids in stopping allergic reactions. Helpful if food allergies are a factor.
Vitamin B complex	50–100 mg and up of each major B vitamin daily (amounts of individual vitamins in a complex will vary).	Important in carbohydrate and protein metabolism, and proper digestion and absorption of foods; helps the body tolerate foods that produce low blood sugar reactions. Also helps counteract the effects of malabsorption disorders, common in people with hypoglycemia.
plus extra vitamin B_1 (thiamine)	100 mg daily.	Aids in the production of hydrochloric acid, needed for proper digestion.
and vitamin B_3 (niacin) and vitamin B_5 (pantothenic acid)	100 mg daily. Do not exceed this amount. 1,000 mg daily, in divided doses.	Aids in the functioning of the nervous system and in proper digestion. *Caution:* Do not take niacin if you have a liver disorder, gout, or high blood pressure.
and vitamin B_{12}	1,000–2,000 mcg daily, on an empty stomach.	Important in adrenal gland function and conversion of glucose to energy. Crucial for prevention of anemia, common because malabsorption disorders result in deficiency.
Zinc	50 mg daily. Do not exceed a total of 100 mg daily from all supplements.	Needed for proper release of insulin. People with hypoglycemia are often zinc deficient. Use zinc gluconate lozenges or OptiZinc for best absorption.
Important		
L-carnitine plus	As directed on label.	Converts stored body fat into energy.
L-cysteine and	As directed on label.	Blocks the action of insulin, which lowers blood sugar.
L-glutamine	1,000 mg daily, on an empty stomach. Take with water or juice. Do not take with milk. Take with 50 mg vitamin B_6 and 100 mg vitamin C for better absorption.	Reduces cravings for sugar.
Magnesium plus	750 mg daily, in divided doses, after meals and at bedtime.	Important in carbohydrate (sugar) metabolism.
calcium	1,500 mg daily, in divided doses, after meals and at bedtime.	Works with magnesium.

Manganese	As directed on label. Take separately from calcium.	Important for the maintenance of blood glucose levels. Most people with hypoglycemia have low levels of this trace mineral in their blood.
Vitamin C with bioflavonoids	3,000–8,000 mg daily, in divided doses.	For adrenal insufficiency, common in people with hypoglycemia.
Vitamin E	200 IU daily or 400 IU every other day.	Improves energy and circulation. Use d-alpha-tocopherol form.
Helpful		
ABC Aerobic Bulk Cleanse from Aerobic Life Industries or psyllium husks	As directed on label. Take with aloe vera juice on an empty stomach in the morning. Take separately from other supplements and medications.	Aids in slowing down blood sugar reactions and keeping the colon clean.
Liver extract injections or desiccated liver	1 cc twice weekly for 3 months, then once weekly for 2 months or more, or as prescribed by physician. As directed on label.	Liver glandulars supply B vitamins and other valuable nutrients.
Multivitamin and mineral complex	As directed on label.	All nutrients are required for healing.
Cravex from Natrol	As directed on label.	Controls sugar cravings and helps balance metabolism.

Herbs

❑ The following herbs help to normalize blood sugar: angostura bitters (or any combination of bitters), artichoke leaf, and gentian root.

❑ To help your body respond to stress, try astragalus or licorice root.

Cautions: Do not use astragalus in the presence of a fever. Licorice root should not be used during pregnancy or nursing. It should not be used by persons with diabetes, glaucoma, heart disease, high blood pressure, or a history of stroke.

❑ Dandelion root is an excellent source of calcium and supports the pancreas and liver.

❑ Gudmar (*Gymnema sylvestre*), an Ayurvedic herb, suppresses the intestinal absorption of saccharides, which prevents blood sugar fluctuations.

❑ Licorice nourishes the adrenal glands.

Caution: Licorice root should not be used during pregnancy or nursing. It should not be used by persons with diabetes, glaucoma, heart disease, high blood pressure, or a history of stroke.

❑ Milk thistle rejuvenates the liver.

❑ Other beneficial herbs include echinacea, parsley, pau d'arco, raspberry leaves, and uva ursi.

Caution: Do not take echinacea for longer than three months. It should not be used by people who are allergic to ragweed.

Recommendations

❑ Remove from the diet all alcohol, canned and packaged foods, refined and processed foods, dried fruits, salt, sugar, saturated fats, soft drinks, and white flour. Also avoid foods that contain artificial colors or preservatives.

❑ Avoid sweet fruits and juices such as grape and prune. If you drink these, mix the juice with an equal amount of water.

❑ Sweeten food with natural sweeteners such as stevia, a South American herb available in liquid form that is two hundred times sweeter than sugar. Other acceptable sweeteners include barley malt syrup, molasses, and brown rice syrup.

❑ Eat a diet high in fiber and include large amounts of vegetables, especially broccoli, carrots, Jerusalem artichokes, raw spinach, squash, and string beans. Vegetables should be eaten raw or steamed. Also eat beans, brown rice, lentils, oats, oat bran, potatoes, soy products (tofu), and fruits, especially apples, apricots, avocados, bananas, cantaloupes, grapefruits, lemons, and persimmons.

❑ For protein, eat low-fat cottage cheese, fish, grains, kefir, raw cheese, raw nuts, seeds, skinless white turkey or white chicken breast, and low-fat yogurt.

❑ Eat starchy foods such as corn, hominy, noodles, pasta, white rice, and yams in moderation only.

❑ Include maitake mushrooms in your diet. They are beneficial for helping the body adapt to stress.

❑ Do not eat fatty foods such as bacon, cold cuts, fried foods, gravies, ham, sausage, or dairy products (except for low-fat soured products).

❑ Do not go without food or consume large, heavy meals. Eat six to eight small meals throughout the day. Some people find that eating a small snack before bedtime helps. In addition, if the hypoglycemia is related to a previous stomach surgery, don't take fluids with the meals or snacks—wait thirty to sixty minutes.

❑ Use a rotation diet; food allergies are often linked to hypoglycemia and can make the symptoms more pronounced. (*See* ALLERGIES in Part Two.)

❑ Try taking 200 micrograms of chromium picolinate daily. This can alleviate many symptoms and raise blood glucose levels if symptoms occur after sugar or a heavy meal is consumed. Chromium, also known as glucose tolerance factor or GTF, has been known to alleviate sudden shock.

❑ During a low blood sugar reaction, eat something that combines fiber with a protein food, such as bran or rice crackers with raw cheese or almond butter.

❑ Instead of eating applesauce, have a whole apple, which has more fiber. The fiber in the apple will inhibit fluctuations in blood sugar. Fiber alone (found in popcorn, oat bran, rice bran, crackers, ground flaxseed, and psyllium husks) will slow down a hypoglycemic reaction. Take fiber half an hour before meals. Spirulina tablets taken between meals further help to stabilize blood sugar.

❑ Maintain a regular exercise regimen. This helps to maintain steady blood sugar levels. Eat one to three hours prior to exercise.

Caution: If you are over thirty-five and/or have been sedentary for some time, consult with your health care provider before beginning an exercise program.

❑ Stress is a major factor in hypoglycemia, as it affects adrenal function and blood sugar levels. Practice stress reduction by meditating, listening to soothing music, getting a massage, or using deep breathing techniques.

❑ Fast once a month with fresh vegetable juices and a series of lemon juice enemas. (*See* FASTING and ENEMAS in Part Three.) To prevent a low blood sugar reaction while fasting, use spirulina or a protein powder supplement. Many people find this makes them start to feel better very quickly.

Considerations

❑ Hypoglycemia is usually an indication of any number of health problems, all of which can be serious. If you suspect that you have it, see your physician so he or she can figure out why. The body is very sensitive to fluctuations in blood glucose levels. It metes out insulin based on how much sugar is in the blood. The brain in particular primarily uses glucose for energy, and it likes levels under a tight range. Deviations can usually be diagnosed and treated.

❑ Avocados contain a seven-carbon sugar that depresses insulin production, which make them an excellent choice for people with hypoglycemia.

❑ The production of insulin is affected by the functioning of the adrenal glands. The adrenal glands produce epinephrine, which acts to "turn off" insulin production, among other things. If the adrenal glands are overstressed and exhausted, they cannot function properly and an overabundance of insulin may result. This causes the blood sugar level to sink below normal, creating a low energy syndrome in the body.

❑ Injections of vitamin B complex plus extra vitamin B$_6$ (pyridoxine) and liver extract have produced good results for those with hypoglycemia. Liver extract supplements contain a nutritional substance that aids liver regeneration. Only liver from organically raised beef should be used.

❑ Hypoglycemia can mimic menopausal symptoms, especially since it often escalates during midlife.

❑ In rare cases, hypoglycemia can be triggered by large doses of aspirin or by sulfonamides (sulfa drugs), a class of antibiotics often prescribed for urinary tract infections.

❑ People who are most prone to hypoglycemia are those taking medications for high blood sugar or diabetes.

❑ Hypoglycemia is often the underlying cause of misdiagnosed cases of attention deficit disorder (ADD). (*See* ATTENTION DEFICIT DISORDER [ADD]/ATTENTION DEFICIT HYPERACTIVITY DISORDER [ADHD] in Part Two.)

❑ Caffeine, alcohol, and tobacco cause profound swings in blood sugar levels. Insomnia can result if any type of sugar is consumed after dinner. Consuming sugar at any time tends to cause drowsiness and fatigue.

❑ Some studies have shown that reducing the amount of meat protein in the diet and adding some starches, such as potatoes, may be beneficial.

❑ Milk allergy is common as this disorder progresses. Allergy testing is recommended. (*See* ALLERGIES in Part Two.)

HYPOTHYROIDISM

Hypothyroidism is caused by an underproduction of thyroid hormone. Symptoms include chronic fatigue, loss of appetite, inability to tolerate cold, low body temperature, a slow heart rate, easy weight gain, elevated cholesterol, painful premenstrual periods, heavy periods, a milky discharge from the breasts, fertility problems, muscle weakness, muscle cramps, dry and scaly skin, a yellow-orange coloration in the skin (particularly on the palms of the hands), yellow bumps on the eyelids, hair loss (including the eyebrows), recurrent infections, migraines, hoarseness, respiratory infections, constipation, depression, difficulty concentrating, slow speech, goiter, and drooping, swollen eyes. The most common symptoms are fatigue and intolerance to cold. If you consistently feel cold while others around you are hot, you may be suffering from reduced thyroid function.

The thyroid gland is the body's internal thermostat, regulating the temperature by secreting two hormones that control how quickly the body burns calories and uses energy. If the thyroid secretes too much hormone, hyperthyroidism results; too little hormone results in hypothyroidism. It affects an estimated 5 percent of the population in the United States, and women are much more likely than men to develop it. Women between the ages of thirty and fifty seem to be most prone to this condition. It is estimated that one in ten women will develop a thyroid condition at some point in her lifetime. Thyroid problems can cause many recurring illnesses and fatigue. The thyroid can be affected by poor diet, fluoride in the water, excessive consumption of unsaturated fats, endurance exercise, pesticide residues on fruits and vegetables, radiation from x-rays, alcohol, and drugs.

A condition called *Hashimoto's disease* is believed to be the most common cause of underactive thyroid. In this disorder, the body in effect becomes allergic to thyroid hormone. It then produces antibodies against its own thyroid tissue. Hashimoto's disease is a common cause of goiter, a swelling of the thyroid gland, among adults, and it can occur in association with other disorders, such as pernicious anemia, lupus, yeast infections, and rheumatoid arthritis. Congenital hypothyroidism in children, if left untreated, can lead to mental retardation and dwarfism. Generally, however, hypothyroidism is detected within a baby's first few months, when routine blood tests are performed.

A rare condition that can result from long-term undiagnosed hypothyroidism is called *myxedema coma*. The coma can occur during illness, after an accident, from exposure to cold, or as a result of the ingestion of narcotics and/or sedatives. This is a medical emergency that requires immediate treatment.

Measuring levels of different hormones in the blood can determine if the thyroid gland is working properly. A physician may order a blood test to measure levels of thyroid hormone or thyroid-stimulating hormone (TSH). This hormone is secreted by the pituitary gland and in turn helps regulate thyroid hormone production. Even a minuscule drop in thyroid function registers as a distinctly elevated TSH level. Most endocrinologists believe that TSH levels rise when a person is in the earliest stages of thyroid failure.

An iodine absorption test may also be performed. This test involves ingesting a small amount of radioactive iodine. An X-ray then shows how much of the iodine was absorbed by the thyroid. A low uptake of the iodine may indicate hypothyroidism.

Unless otherwise specified, the dosages recommended in this section are for adults. For children between the ages of twelve and seventeen, reduce the dose to three-quarters of the recommended amount. For children between six and twelve, use one-half of the recommended dose, and for children under the age of six, use one-quarter of the recommended amount.

Thyroid Self-Test

To test yourself for an underactive thyroid, keep a thermometer by your bed at night. When you awaken in the morning, place the thermometer under your arm and hold it there for fifteen minutes. Keep still and quiet. Any motion can upset your temperature reading. A temperature of 97.6°F or lower may indicate an underactive thyroid. Keep a temperature log for five days. If your readings are consistently low, consult your health care provider.

NUTRIENTS

SUPPLEMENT	SUGGESTED DOSAGE	COMMENTS
Essential		
Kelp	2,000–3,000 mg daily.	Contains iodine, the basic substance of thyroid hormone. *Caution:* Check with your health care professional before using this if you are diagnosed with thyroid problems.
L-tyrosine	500 mg twice daily, on an empty stomach. Take with water or juice, not with milk. Take with 50 mg vitamin B$_6$ and 100 mg vitamin C for better absorption.	Low plasma levels have been associated with hypothyroidism. (*See* AMINO ACIDS in Part One.)
Very Important		
Multi-Glandular from American Biologics	As directed on label.	A nutritional supplement for the endocrine, hormonal, and enzyme systems.
Raw thyroid glandular	As prescribed by physician.	To replace deficient thyroid hormone (see GLANDULAR THERAPY in Part Three). A natural thyroid extract such as Armour Desiccated Thyroid Tablets is best. Available by prescription only.
Important		
Vitamin B complex plus extra vitamin B$_2$ (riboflavin) and vitamin B$_{12}$	100 mg of each major B vitamin 3 times daily, with meals (amounts of individual vitamins in a complex will vary). 50 mg twice daily. 1,000–2,000 mcg 3 times daily, on an empty stomach.	B vitamins improve cellular oxygenation and energy and are needed for proper digestion, immune function, red blood cell formation, and thyroid function. Use a lozenge or sublingual form for best absorption.
Helpful		
Brewer's yeast	As directed on label.	Rich in basic nutrients, especially B vitamins.
Essential fatty acids (Kyolic-EPA from Wakunaga)	As directed on label.	Necessary for proper functioning of the thyroid gland.
Iron or Floradix Iron + Herbs from Salus Haus	As directed by physician. Take with 100 mg vitamin C for better absorption. As directed on label.	Essential for enzyme and hemoglobin production. Use ferrous chelate form. *Caution:* Do not take iron unless anemia has been diagnosed. A natural, nontoxic form of iron from food sources.
Selenium	As directed on label. If you are pregnant, do not exceed 40 mcg daily.	A vital antioxidant that protects the immune system.
Vitamin A with mixed carotenoids plus natural beta-carotene or carotenoid complex (Betatene)	15,000 IU daily. If you are pregnant, do not exceed 10,000 IU daily. 15,000 IU daily. As directed on label.	Needed for proper immune function and for healthy eyes, skin, and hair. May be taken in a multivitamin complex. Antioxidant and precursor of vitamin A. *Note:* If you have diabetes, omit the beta-carotene; people with diabetes cannot convert beta-carotene into vitamin A.
Vitamin C with bioflavonoids	500 mg 4 times daily. Do not exceed this amount.	Needed for immune function and stress hormone production. *Caution:* Do not take extremely high doses of vitamin C—this may affect the production of thyroid hormone.
Vitamin E	200 IU daily or 400 IU every other day.	An important antioxidant that improves circulation and immune response. Use d-alpha-tocopherol form.
Zinc	50 mg daily. Do not exceed a total of 100 mg daily from all supplements.	An immune system stimulant. Use zinc gluconate lozenges or OptiZinc for best absorption.

Herbs

❑ Bayberry, black cohosh, and goldenseal can help this thyroid condition.

Cautions: Do not use black cohosh if you are pregnant or have any type of chronic disease. Black cohosh should not be used by those with liver problems. Do not take goldenseal internally on a daily basis for more than one week at a time. Do not use it during pregnancy or if you are breastfeeding, and use with caution if you are allergic to ragweed. If you have a history of cardiovascular disease, diabetes, or glaucoma, use it only under a doctor's supervision.

❑ Gentian and mugwort extracts are helpful for hypothyroidism.

❑ Herbal bitters such as Swedish bitters may help alleviate the symptoms associated with thyroid malfunctions.

Recommendations

❑ Include in your diet apricots, dates, egg yolks, molasses, parsley, potatoes, prunes, raw seeds, and whole grains. Eat fish or chicken and raw milk and cheeses.

❑ Eat these foods in moderation: broccoli, Brussels sprouts, cabbage, kale, mustard greens, peaches, pears, radishes, spinach, and turnips. If you have severe symptoms, omit these foods entirely. They may further suppress thyroid function.

❑ Avoid processed and refined foods, including white flour and sugar.

❑ Drink steam-distilled water only.

❑ Begin a moderate exercise program such as yoga or walking.

Caution: If you are thirty-five or older and/or have been sedentary for some time, consult with your health care provider before beginning an exercise program.

❑ Do not take sulfa drugs or antihistamines unless specifically directed to do so by a physician.

❑ Avoid fluoride (including that found in toothpaste and tap water) and chlorine (also found in tap water). Chlorine, fluoride, and iodine are chemically related. Chlorine and fluoride block iodine receptors in the thyroid gland, resulting in reduced iodine-containing hormone production and finally in hypothyroidism.

❑ Taking the homeopathic remedy *Calcarea carbonica* may help. It can sometimes increase thyroid function.

❑ Because thyroid medication can interact with other medications, take them several hours apart. Ask your physician if any other medications will interfere with the effectiveness of your thyroid prescription. Aluminum hydroxide (an antacid found in Alu-Tab, Amphojel, and Nephrox) and a drug used to lower cholesterol, cholestyramine (Questran) are a couple of the drugs that affect thyroid medications. Do not take thyroid medication at the same time you take carbonate supplements or calcium as they can block the absorption of thyroxine (T_4).

Considerations

❑ Because sugar intolerance, menopause, and depression can cause many of the same symptoms as thyroid disorders, a simple thyroid test should be considered to rule out any errors in diagnosis.

❑ Treatment for a regular morning temperature of 96°F is 3 to 4 grains of Armour Desiccated Thyroid Tablets (available by prescription) daily. A person with a regular morning temperature of 97°F should take 1 to 2 grains. If you have side effects, speak to your physician about reducing the dosage.

❑ Synthroid and Levothroid are synthetic versions of T_4 that are most frequently prescribed by physicians for people with hypothyroidism. Some side effects of these medications include headache, irritability, nervousness, loss of sleep, diarrhea, weight loss, and changes in appetite. If a person shows no response to this medication, the physician may prescribe liothyronine (Cytomel). It contains T_3, which is needed to regulate metabolism. A study done at the University of Massachusetts found that thyroxine can cause a loss of bone mass.

❑ The conventional treatment for Hashimoto's disease is usually a prescription of a thyroid hormone that must be taken for the duration of one's lifetime.

❑ The presence of too much thyroid hormone in the system can cause a condition known as *thyroid storm.* The heart rate increases rapidly and, in exceptionally severe cases, a heart attack can occur.

❑ Recent evidence indicates that an underactive thyroid may put you at an increased risk of heart attack—even if your thyroid is only slightly underactive.

❑ Applying a natural progesterone cream, which is available at most health food stores, may increase thyroid activity.

❑ Lithium, a trace mineral used as a drug to treat bipolar mood disorders, can sometimes cause thyroid malfunction.

❑ Wilson's syndrome is a condition that results from a problem in the conversion of one thyroid hormone, T_4, to another thyroid hormone, T_3. This causes symptoms of decreased thyroid function, especially triggered by significant physical or emotional stress. These symptoms can be debilitating, and may persist even after the stress has passed. People with Wilson's syndrome have many of the symptoms of hypothyroidism, including low body temperature, fatigue, headaches, menstrual dysfunction, memory loss, loss of concentration, loss of sex drive, anxiety and panic attacks, depression, unhealthy nails, dry skin, frequent infections, allergies, insomnia, intolerance to cold, and lack of energy and motivation. Their blood test results are often normal, however. (*See* WILSON'S DISEASE in Rare Disorders in Part Two.)

❏ For names and addresses of organizations that can provide more information about thyroid disorders, *see* Health and Medical Organizations in the Appendix.

HYSTERECTOMY-RELATED PROBLEMS

Hysterectomy is the surgical removal of the uterus. This is done for many different reasons. A common reason is fibroid tumors, benign growths in the uterus that can cause problems. More than 30 percent of the hysterectomies performed in the United States are done to remove fibroids. (*See* FIBROIDS, UTERINE, in Part Two.) Other conditions for which hysterectomy is performed include endometriosis (20 percent) and prolapse of the uterus (16 to 18 percent).

Hysterectomy is the second most common surgery among reproductive-age women in the United States—more than 600,000 are performed each year. One in three women in the United States will have had one by age sixty. Very few of these operations are performed because of a life-threatening situation, and it is likely that many of them are actually unnecessary. Per capita, half as many hysterectomies are performed in Great Britain as in the United States, and, statistically, American women show no health benefits for their higher incidence of surgery. Outside the United States, very few hysterectomies are performed for what doctors often term "quality of life" reasons. Hysterectomy effectively and permanently causes sterility, and this may be a motive (conscious or unconscious) for some women and/or their doctors to make this choice. Financial motives may be another possibility. U.S. Department of Health and Human Services statistics show that far fewer hysterectomies are performed under managed care plans, in which doctors receive a set fee for their services each year, than in situations in which surgeons are compensated directly for each operation performed.

The symptoms that lead women to consider hysterectomy are varied but include the following: a constant heavy, bloated feeling; urinary tract problems or incontinence; unusually long and heavy menstrual periods; unusual swelling in the abdominal region (due to fibroid tumors); infertility (due to fibroid tumors or endometriosis); complications of childbirth; cancer; and intolerance to drug therapy usually prescribed for endometriosis.

The following are three different ways in which hysterectomy may be performed:

- *Total hysterectomy.* In this procedure, the cervix is removed along with the uterus.
- *Partial (also known as subtotal or supracervical) hysterectomy.* In partial hysterectomy, the uterus is removed but the cervix and other female reproductive organs remain intact.
- *Pan (or radical) hysterectomy.* In this, the most extensive form of hysterectomy, the ovaries, cervix, supporting ligaments, tissues, fallopian tubes, upper portion of the vagina, pelvic lymph nodes, and uterus are removed.

To remove the uterus surgically, doctors may choose one of the following three options:

- *Abdominal hysterectomy.* In some circumstances, the physician may choose to perform the hysterectomy by making an incision in the abdomen. This option is usually chosen if the woman undergoing the procedure has a large ovarian cyst or tumor. It is the most invasive type of hysterectomy, and the most traumatic due to the incision in the abdomen.
- *Total laparoscopic hysterectomy* (TLH). This involves performing the entire operation with a laparoscope (a tiny telescope), inserted through a very small incision in the navel and using small surgical instruments. This is used in situations in which the doctor needs an extensive picture of the pelvic region.
- *Vaginal hysterectomy.* In this type of procedure, the uterus is removed through the vagina. A doctor may choose to perform the procedure using a laparoscope. This method is called the *laparoscopically assisted vaginal hysterectomy* (LAH).

Many women who have hysterectomies experience significant problems as a result. The most obvious of these occurs when the ovaries are removed together with the uterus; menopause begins abruptly, with its attendant difficulties and discomforts, because the body is suddenly deprived of estrogen. This hormonal loss in turn can lead to a greatly increased risk of bone mass loss, which often precedes osteoporosis, and to an increased likelihood of heart disease, as well as depression, urinary tract problems, joint pain, headaches, dizziness, insomnia, and fatigue.

Even women who retain their ovaries often experience a drastic reduction in estrogen production, and menopause comes earlier—sometimes years earlier—than it would have naturally. This is believed to be because the supply of blood to the ovaries is disrupted and decreased by removal of the uterus. Over half of women who have ovary-sparing "partial" hysterectomies experience early menopause.

Another problem common among women who have undergone hysterectomy is diminished sexual interest and desire after surgery. Research indicates that one-third of all women who have hysterectomies find their sexual desire and enjoyment greatly diminished. Removal of the ovaries may result in loss of sexuality because they secrete about half of a woman's supply of androgens, hormones that are responsible for sex drive in both men and women. However, diminished sexuality may occur whether or not the ovaries are removed. In Finland, studies have shown that the removal of the cervix in hysterectomy also resulted in diminished capacity for orgasm. Hormone replacement therapy can alleviate this problem.

Not all of the problems that can follow hysterectomy are directly hormone related. Some women experience depression because of the knowledge that once the uterus is gone, it is too late to change one's mind about having children. Also, no surgical procedure is entirely 100 percent safe, foolproof, or guaranteed. There is a 50 percent chance of at least one minor postoperative complication (usually fever, bleeding, or wound trouble). It is estimated that 11 women in 10,000 who have a hysterectomy will die as a result of complications. If there is a possibility that you may require a transfusion as a result of this type of surgery, you should talk to your doctor about donating your own blood for use during the operation. (SEE HEPATITIS in Part Two for information about blood transfusions.)

The following supplements can help to counteract the unpleasant side effects of hysterectomy. The dosages given here are for adults.

NUTRIENTS

SUPPLEMENT	SUGGESTED DOSAGE	COMMENTS
Very Important		
Boron	3 mg daily. Do not exceed this amount.	Aids in calcium absorption and prevention of bone loss that can occur after hysterectomy.
Calcium and magnesium	2,000 mg daily, at bedtime. 1,000 mg daily, at bedtime.	Lack of estrogen hinders calcium uptake. Needed for the central nervous system. Enhances calcium absorption.
Essential fatty acids (primrose oil)	1,000 mg 3 times daily.	Helps the body manufacture estrogen.
Garlic (Kyolic from Wakunaga)	As directed on label.	May inhibit tumor growth.
Potassium	99 mg daily.	Needed if hot flashes occur to replace electrolytes lost through perspiration.
Raw thymus glandular	As directed on label.	Potentiates immune function.
Vitamin B complex	100 mg of each major B vitamin twice daily, with meals (amounts of individual vitamins in a complex will vary).	Needed for the nervous system and to reduce stress. Use a high-stress formula. Injections (under a doctor's supervision) may be necessary.
Vitamin C with bioflavonoids	3,000–6,000 mg and up daily, in divided doses.	An antistress vitamin also needed for tissue repair.
Vitamin E	200 IU daily, or 400 IU every other day.	Important in estrogen production. Use d-alpha-tocopherol form. *Caution:* Do not take this supplement for 2 weeks prior to surgery.
Important		
L-arginine and L-lysine	500 mg each daily, on an empty stomach. Take with water or juice. Do not take with milk. Take with 50 mg vitamin B$_6$ and 100 mg vitamin C for better absorption.	Essential amino acids important in recovery after surgery. Both are needed to avoid an imbalance in amino acids. (*See* AMINO ACIDS in Part One.)
Micellized Vitamin A and E from American Biologics	50,000 IU daily.	Important in immune function and to promote tissue repair. Use emulsion
plus carotenoid complex plus zinc	50 mg daily. Do not exceed a total of 100 mg daily from all supplements.	form for easier assimilation and greater safety at higher doses. Boosts the immune system. Use zinc gluconate lozenges or zinc methionate (OptiZinc) for best absorption.
Helpful		
Melatonin	As directed on label.	This hormone stimulates the immune system and is important in the production of estrogen, testosterone, and, possibly, other hormones.
Multiglandular complex (Cytozyme-F from Biotics Research)	As directed on label.	Aids in glandular function.
Multivitamin and mineral complex	As directed on label.	Restores the essential vitamins and minerals to balance.

Herbs

❏ Herbs that act as natural estrogen promoters include anise, dong quai, fennel, fenugreek, ginseng, licorice, red clover, sage, suma, and wild yam.

Cautions: Do not use ginseng if you have high blood pressure or are pregnant or nursing. Licorice root should not be used during pregnancy or nursing. It should not be used by persons with diabetes, glaucoma, heart disease, high blood pressure, or a history of stroke. Do not use sage if you suffer from any type of seizure disorder, or are pregnant or nursing.

❏ The following herbs may alleviate symptoms of ovarian cysts and uterine fibroids: black cohosh, black haw, blue cohosh, dandelion root, lady's mantle (yarrow), milk thistle, and pau d'arco.

Caution: Do not use blue or black cohosh if you are pregnant or have any type of chronic disease. Black cohosh should not be used by those with liver problems.

❏ St. John's wort is helpful for depression.

Caution: St. John's wort may cause increased sensitivity to sunlight. It may also produce anxiety, gastrointestinal symptoms, and headaches. It can interact with some drugs including antidepressants, birth control pills, and anticoagulants.

Recommendations

❏ Adopt a hypoglycemic diet; eat plenty of foods that are high in fiber, such as vegetables, whole grains, and high-fiber fruits, plus fish, skinless white turkey or chicken breast, soy products, and low-fat yogurt, kefir, and cottage cheese for protein. Eat starchy foods in moderation only. Do not consume any refined sugar, white flour, alcohol, processed foods, saturated fats, or foods containing artificial colors, preservatives, or other additives. Eat six to eight small meals spaced regularly throughout the day, rather than two or three larger meals. (*See* HYPOGLYCEMIA in Part Two for additional suggestions.)

❑ Add more fiber to your diet. Chronic constipation is a known and accepted complication of radical hysterectomy. In one study, women who had hysterectomies for treatment of cervical cancer and ate a high-fiber diet had more and softer bowel movements without pain or straining, compared to women who followed a low-fiber diet. The high-fiber diet contained 23 grams of fiber versus 12 grams for the low-fiber diet. To increase fiber in your diet eat lots of fruits and vegetables, whole grains, and use a fiber supplement to obtain at least 23 grams a day of fiber.

❑ Avoid caffeine, colas, dairy products (except for low-fat soured products), processed foods, red meat, and sugar.

❑ Use vitamin E to help prevent incisional scarring and relieve itching and discomfort in the area surrounding the stitches. Open a vitamin E capsule and apply the oil along the incision (but not on the stitches themselves).

❑ If you are considering a hysterectomy, give the matter close and careful consideration. Seek wise counsel and second opinions. Check into alternative treatments. Remember, once the operation has been performed, it is impossible to restore the uterus if you find the symptoms unacceptable or unbearable. The results of a hysterectomy are irreversible.

Considerations

❑ Women over forty who have hysterectomies performed often have their ovaries removed as well, supposedly as a precaution against the later development of ovarian cancer. However, many health care professionals question the logic of doing this; ovarian cancer is relatively rare.

❑ Estrogen replacement therapy is often recommended following a hysterectomy. For some women, it is, unfortunately, unavoidable, because of severe posthysterectomy symptoms. Not all women can tolerate estrogen replacement. In our opinion, synthetic estrogens are potentially dangerous because they are strongly linked to breast cancer and cardiovascular disease. Natural estrogens, on the other hand, are safe and effective. Natural estrogen-promoters include anise, dong quai, fennel, fenugreek, ginseng, licorice, primrose oil, red clover, sage, suma, and wild yam. (*See* MENOPAUSAL AND PERIMENOPAUSAL PROBLEMS in Part Two.)

Cautions: Do not use dong quai if you have a bleeding disorder or take drugs that increase the risk of bleeding. It may increase your sensitivity to sunlight. Do not use ginseng if you have high blood pressure, or are pregnant or nursing. Licorice root should not be used during pregnancy or nursing. It should not be used by persons with diabetes, glaucoma, heart disease, high blood pressure, or a history of stroke. Do not use sage if you suffer from any type of seizure disorder, or are pregnant or nursing.

❑ A hysterectomy usually requires four or five days in the hospital followed by approximately six weeks of at-home recuperation. Recovery can be more painful if the surgeon makes a vertical incision as opposed to a horizontal one. In addition, the scar that results from a vertical incision acts as a lifelong reminder of the surgery (a horizontal incision can be hidden below the pubic hairline).

❑ Evidence is mounting that there is a higher incidence of cardiovascular disorders, osteoporosis, and Alzheimer's disease among women who have undergone hysterectomies.

❑ Some doctors advocate performing hysterectomies on women with fibroid tumors because they say that the fibroids block access to the ovaries during pelvic exams, which might delay a possible diagnosis of ovarian cancer. This position is no longer valid, however, because technology allows the use of ultrasound to examine the ovaries for any abnormality. If fibroid tumors need to be removed, a myomectomy should be considered and opted for if at all possible. (*See* FIBROIDS, UTERINE, in Part Two.)

❑ There are instances in which hysterectomy proves advantageous. Some women manage to avoid the major hormonal changes that are so common after surgery, and in addition to no longer being bothered with monthly menses, they may feel liberated because they no longer need to fear becoming pregnant and have more fulfilling sex lives as a result. Others with major pain from fibroid disease have a greatly improved quality of life, and those with cancer live longer after a hysterectomy.

❑ While some women who have their ovaries left in place still experience drastic estrogen loss, this is not always permanent. A vitamin and mineral supplement regimen can reduce the risk of severe estrogen deprivation. Remember the natural estrogen promoters discussed in this section.

❑ If you do require hormone replacement to control symptoms after a hysterectomy, take the lowest dose possible. Ask your doctor for a combined hormone containing estrogen and progesterone to help reduce the risk of cancer.

❑ Dr. Betty Kamen, an expert in women's health problems, says that progesterone, not estrogen, should be the hormone of choice for replacement therapy.

❑ *See* MENOPAUSE-RELATED PROBLEMS in Part Two.

❑ *See also* SURGERY: PREPARING FOR AND RECOVERING FROM in Part Three.

IMMUNE SYSTEM, WEAKENED

See WEAKENED IMMUNE SYSTEM.

IMMUNE THROMBOCYTOPENIC PURPURA

See under RARE DISORDERS.

IMPOTENCE

See ERECTILE DYSFUNCTION and SEXUAL DYSFUNCTION IN WOMEN.

INCONTINENCE

Incontinence (loss of bladder control) is a common complaint. There are many factors that can cause this annoying problem. Incontinence can be either acute or persistent. Acute incontinence is most often caused by an infection. Persistent incontinence develops over time and tends to last longer. There are several different types of persistent incontinence, among them stress incontinence, urge incontinence, functional incontinence, reflex incontinence, and total incontinence.

Stress incontinence is the most common bladder control problem. This is leakage that occurs when a person coughs, sneezes, laughs, lifts a heavy object, or otherwise increases pressure in the lower abdomen. The bladder is rarely completely emptied. Dribbling is more common than complete evacuation of the bladder. This problem is a result of weakened pelvic muscles, which can be due to aging, obesity, and/or pregnancy.

Urge incontinence is the result of an overactive bladder. The detrusor muscle, which surrounds the bladder, may involuntarily contract and begin the flow of urine. Frequent urination is common with this type of incontinence, as is nocturnal urination, especially in men. Difficulty urinating may also be due to prostate inflammation. Possible underlying causes of urge incontinence include a history of pelvic inflammatory disease, abdominal surgery, stimulants such as alcohol and coffee, and bladder infection. It may also be due to prostate problems.

Functional incontinence is characterized by an uncontrollable urge to empty the bladder before you can reach the bathroom. It can be caused by stress; changes in environment, such as having to stay in the hospital and not being able to get to the bathroom in time; and mobility restrictions. Some individuals are not aware when their bladders are full, and this loss of sensation can lead to urine leakage. This is reflex incontinence, and it is most often due to spinal cord injury or other neurological impairment. Total incontinence is the unpredictable loss of urine at all times. It can be caused by neurological dysfunction, abdominal surgery, spinal cord injury, or an anatomical defect.

Incontinence is most common in people over fifty, but loss of bladder control can occur at any age, especially in pregnant women. It is wrong to assume that loss of bladder control is an inevitable part of getting older. It is also wrong to assume that nothing can be done about this problem.

Unless otherwise specified, the dosages recommended here are for adults. For children between the ages of twelve and seventeen, reduce the dose to three-quarters the recommended amount. For children between six and twelve, use one-half the recommended dose, and for children under the age of six, use one-quarter the recommended amount.

NUTRIENTS

SUPPLEMENT	SUGGESTED DOSAGE	COMMENTS
Very Important		
Free form amino acid	As directed on label.	Helps to strengthen bladder muscle. Use a product made from a vegetable source.
Important		
Calcium and	1,500 mg daily.	To aid in controlling bladder spasms.
magnesium	350 mg daily.	
Helpful		
Multivitamin and mineral complex with vitamin B complex	As directed on label.	Aids in relieving stress and supplies all needed nutrients.
Potassium	99 mg daily.	Aids in balancing sodium and potassium in the body.
Vitamin A and	As directed on label. If you are pregnant, do not exceed 10,000 IU daily.	To aid in normalizing bladder muscle function.
vitamin E	200 IU daily or 400 IU every other day.	Use d-alpha-tocopherol form.
Zinc	80 mg daily. Do not exceed a total of 100 mg daily from all supplements.	For improved bladder function. Also enhances the immune system.

Herbs

❏ Kidney Bladder Formula from Nature's Way and Kidney Blend SP-6 from Solaray are herbal formulas that have a diuretic effect and reduce bladder spasms. Take 2 capsules twice daily.

Recommendations

❏ Stay away from alcohol, caffeine, carbonated beverages, coffee, chocolate, refined or processed foods, and simple sugars. Chemicals in food, drugs, and impure water have an adverse effect on the bladder.

❏ If you are overweight, adopt a healthy weight-loss diet and exercise program to help you lose the excess pounds. Obesity is a common factor in incontinence. (*See* OBESITY in Part Two.)

Caution: If you are thirty-five or older and/or have been sedentary for some time, consult with your health care provider before beginning an exercise program.

❏ Do not delay emptying the bladder. Making sure that you urinate every two to three waking hours—"voiding by the clock"—can help.

❏ Do not use "feminine hygiene sprays," packaged douches, bubble baths, or tampons, sanitary pads, or toilet paper containing fragrance. The chemicals these products contain are potentially irritating.

❏ Do pelvic exercises such as Kegel exercises. (*See under* PROLAPSE OF THE UTERUS in Part Two.) These are useful because weak pelvic muscles are often involved in bladder control problems. Daily exercises can strengthen pelvic muscles and improve bladder control. Exercising your muscles for just five minutes three times a day can make a big difference. The National Kidney and Urologic Diseases Information Clearinghouse (*see* Health and Medical Organizations in the Appendix) can supply very useful information on all types of pelvic exercises.

Considerations

❑ Anyone who is experiencing bladder control problems should consult a physician to check for possible underlying causes and investigate the possibilities for treatment. The appropriate type of treatment depends on the type of bladder control problem.

❑ *Cantharis* is a homeopathic remedy for pain during urination and for frequent urination.

❑ Tolterodine (Detrol), an antispasmodic drug, may be prescribed for some types of incontinence. Muscle relaxers and calcium channel blockers may be tried as well.

❑ Local injections of Botulinum toxin (BoTox) are sometimes recommended for men who have bladder control difficulties related to prostate problems.

❑ For names and addresses of organizations that can provide additional information on incontinence and its treatments, *see* Health and Medical Organizations in the Appendix.

INDIGESTION (DYSPEPSIA)

Indigestion may be a symptom of a disorder in the stomach or the intestines, or it may be a disorder in itself. Symptoms can include abdominal pain, allergic symptoms, belching, a bloated feeling, a burning sensation after eating, chronic bowel irritation, chronic fatigue, constipation, diarrhea, gas, insomnia, joint and muscle pain, nausea, rumbling noises, skin disorders, sugar cravings, and vomiting. Heartburn often accompanies indigestion.

Swallowing air—by chewing with the mouth open, talking while chewing, or gulping down food—can cause indigestion. Drinking liquids with meals contributes to indigestion because it dilutes the enzymes needed for digestion (a lack of digestive enzymes can cause intestinal problems). Certain foods and beverages can cause indigestion because they are irritating to the digestive tract. These include alcohol; caffeine; greasy, spicy, or refined foods; and vinegar. Other factors that can cause or contribute to indigestion include intestinal obstruction, lack of friendly bacteria, malabsorption, peptic ulcers, and disorders of the gallbladder, liver, or pancreas. Food allergies and intolerances (such as lactose intolerance) also can cause indigestion.

If food is not digested properly, it ferments in the stomach and upper intestines, producing hydrogen, carbon dioxide, and organic acids. These acids do not help digestion, but are factors in gas and bloating. Foods high in complex carbohydrates, such as grains and legumes, are the primary foods responsible for gas because they are difficult to digest, and therefore are more likely to yield undigested particles on which the intestinal bacteria act. Some have postulated that the undigested food and bacteria present in the gut can produce toxins that can damage the mucosal lining, causing "leaky gut syndrome." This condition occurs when tiny particles of undigested food normally eliminated in the feces pass through tiny rips in the intestinal lining and get absorbed into the system, causing severe digestive distress. This is more likely to occur in inflammatory bowel syndrome. Contributing factors include abnormal intestinal flora (candida), food allergies, regular alcohol consumption, and parasites, chemicals, or drugs that irritate the small intestine. Psychological factors such as anxiety, stress, worry, or disappointment can disturb the nervous mechanism that controls the contractions of stomach and intestinal muscles.

Stomach Acid Self-Test

Hydrochloric acid (HCl), which is produced by glands in the stomach, is necessary for the breakdown and digestion of many foods. Insufficient amounts of HCl can lead to indigestion. HCl levels often decline with age.

You can determine if you need more hydrochloric acid with this simple test. Take a tablespoon of apple cider vinegar or lemon juice. If this makes your indigestion go away, then you need more stomach acid. If it makes your symptoms worse, then you have too much acid, and you should take care not to take any supplements that contain HCl.

Unless otherwise specified, the dosages recommended here are for adults. For children between the ages of twelve and seventeen, reduce the dose to three-quarters the recommended amount. For children between six and twelve, use one-half the recommended dose, and for children under the age of six, use one-quarter the recommended amount.

NUTRIENTS

SUPPLEMENT	SUGGESTED DOSAGE	COMMENTS
Very Important		
Glucomannan or ABC Aerobic Bulk Cleanse from Aerobic Life Industries	1 tbsp in a full glass of liquid upon arising. Take separately from other supplements and medications.	Colon cleansers that aid in normal stool formation.
Proteolytic enzymes or Inf-zyme Forte from American Biologics or pancreatin	As directed on label, with each meal. Take ½ the recommended dose with snacks.	To aid in the breakdown of protein for proper absorption. Important for combating gas and bloating. *Caution:* Do not give these supplements to a child.

Important		
Acidophilus (Kyo-Dophilus from Wakunaga or Probiotic All-Flora from New Chapter)	As directed on label, ½ hour before each meal.	Necessary for normal digestion. Use a nondairy formula.
Garlic (Kyolic from Wakunaga)	2 capsules 3 times daily, with meals.	Aids in digestion and destroys unwanted bacteria in the bowel.
Omega-3 fatty acids	As directed on label.	Maintains proper digestive function.
Vitamin B complex	100 mg of each major B vitamin 3 times daily, with meals (amounts of individual vitamins in a complex will vary).	Essential for normal digestion.
plus extra vitamin B$_1$ (thiamine) and	50 mg 3 times daily.	Enhances production of hydrochloric acid.
vitamin B$_6$ (pyridoxine) and	150 mg twice daily.	Digesting protein increases need for this vitamin, which is required for HCl production.
vitamin B$_{12}$	1,000 mcg twice daily.	Important for proper digestion. Use a lozenge or sublingual form.

Helpful		
AbsorbAid from Nature's Sources	As directed on label.	To prevent acid reflux.
Activated charcoal	As directed on label.	To absorb intestinal gas.
Alfalfa		See under Herbs, below.
Copper	2–3 mg daily.	Required for protein metabolism.
Hydrochloric acid (HCl)	As directed on label.	Required for protein digestion.
L-carnitine	As directed on label.	Carries fat into the cells for breakdown into energy.
Lecithin granules or capsules or phosphatidyl choline	1 tbsp 3 times daily, before meals. 1,200 mg 3 times daily, before meals. As directed on label.	Fat emulsifiers that aid in the breakdown of fats. Restores gastrointestinal mucosa by strengthening the mucosal lining.
L-methionine	As directed on label, on an empty stomach. Take with water or juice. Do not take with milk. Take with 50 mg vitamin B$_6$ and 100 mg vitamin C for better absorption.	A potent liver detoxifier. (See AMINO ACIDS in Part One.)
Manganese	3–10 mg daily.	Required for fat and carbohydrate metabolism.
Multienzyme complex	As directed on label. Take with meals.	To improve digestion. Caution: Do not use a formula containing HCl.
N-Acetylcysteine (NAC)	500–1,000 mg daily, on an empty stomach with a small amount of vitamin B$_6$ and vitamin C.	Essential for repair of the large, and especially the small, intestines. Also detoxifies harmful substances.
Selenium	100–300 mcg daily. If you are pregnant, do not exceed 40 mcg daily.	Required for proper pancreatic function.
Zinc	20–50 mg daily.	Required for proper digestion and protein metabolism.

Herbs

❏ Acid-Ease from Prevail Corporation is an herbal formula that aids in the breakdown and assimilation of foods, and also contains natural plant enzymes to ease heartburn. It can be taken between meals if needed.

❏ Alfalfa supplies needed vitamin K and trace minerals. It can be taken in liquid or tablet form.

❏ Aloe vera is good for heartburn and other gastrointestinal symptoms. Take ¼ cup of aloe vera juice on an empty stomach in the morning and again at bedtime.

❏ Anise seeds can help relieve a sour stomach. Chew the whole seeds or grind them and sprinkle on food.

❏ Catnip, chamomile, fennel, fenugreek, goldenseal, papaya, and peppermint are all good for indigestion.

Cautions: Do not use chamomile if you are allergic to ragweed. Do not use during pregnancy or nursing. It may interact with warfarin or cyclosporine, so patients using these drugs should avoid it. Do not take goldenseal internally on a daily basis for more than one week at a time. Do not use it during pregnancy or if you are breast-feeding, and use with caution if you are allergic to ragweed. If you have a history of cardiovascular disease, diabetes, or glaucoma, use it only under a doctor's supervision.

❏ Ginger is a time-honored remedy for nausea.

❏ A few sprigs of fresh parsley, or ¼ teaspoon of dried, taken with a glass of warm water, can help relieve indigestion.

Recommendations

❏ If you are prone to indigestion, consume well-balanced meals with plenty of fiber-rich foods such as fresh fruits, vegetables, and whole grains. Eat slowly and chew food well. Don't eat in a stressful environment or when you feel under stress.

❏ Include in your diet fresh papaya (which contains papain) and fresh pineapple (which contains bromelain). These are good sources of beneficial digestive enzymes.

❏ Add acidophilus to your diet. Acidophilus can be useful for indigestion because a shortage of the "friendly" bacteria is often the cause. Open 10 capsules or use 1 tablespoon of powdered formula. Kyo-Dophilus from Wakunaga is a nondairy product that can be used if you have a reaction to dairy products. Acidophilus used as an enema hardly ever results in a problem. You may experience some rumbling and slight disturbance for an hour or so, but it will subside. (See ENEMAS in Part Three.)

❏ For disorders such as gas, bloating, and heartburn, try brown rice and/or barley broth. Use 5 parts water to 1 part grain, and boil the mixture, uncovered, for ten minutes. Then put the lid on and simmer for fifty-five minutes more. Strain and cool the liquid. Sip this throughout the day.

❑ Limit your intake of lentils, peanuts, and soybeans. They contain an enzyme inhibitor.

❑ Avoid bakery products, beans, caffeine, carbonated beverages, citrus juices, fried and fatty foods, pasta, peppers, potato chips and other snack foods, red meat, refined carbohydrates (sugar), tomatoes, and salty or spicy foods.

❑ Do not eat dairy products, junk foods, or processed foods. These cause excess mucus formation, which results in inadequate digestion of protein.

❑ For upper gastrointestinal gas, take pancreatin; for lower gastrointestinal gas, take supplemental trace minerals. If you have gas, use the juice of one fresh lemon in a quart of lukewarm water as an enema to balance the body's pH. If gas is constant for days, use a *B. bifidus* enema. This should relieve the problem within hours. (*See* ENEMAS in Part Three.)

❑ For relief of occasional digestive difficulties, use charcoal tablets, available in health food stores. These are good for absorbing gas and toxins. Because they can interfere with the absorption of other medications and nutrients, they should be taken separately, and they should not be taken for long periods of time. Occasional use is not harmful and has no side effects.

❑ If stools are foul-smelling and are accompanied by a burning sensation in the anus, follow a fasting program. This is often a sign that the colon contains toxic material. (*See* ENEMAS and FASTING in Part Three.)

❑ If you have had abdominal surgery (such as a bowel shortened), take pancreatin to help digest foods. If you have hypoglycemia (low blood sugar), you also need pancreatin. After meals, if you have a stuffed feeling and a rumbling or gurgling with bloating and gas, use pancreatin.

❑ If the results of the stomach acid self-test showed that you need more hydrochloric acid, sip 1 tablespoon of pure apple cider vinegar in a glass of water with each meal to aid digestion.

❑ Chew your food thoroughly. Digestion starts in the mouth, and chewing signals the rest of the digestive system to prepare to break down the food for absorption.

❑ Do not eat when you are upset or overtired.

❑ Do not drink liquids while eating. This dilutes the stomach juices and prevents proper digestion.

❑ Find out which foods your body has trouble digesting, and stay away from foods that cause a reaction. (*See* ALLERGIES in Part Two.)

❑ If you are experiencing an excess of acid backup with heartburn symptoms, see your doctor to rule out gastroesophageal reflux disease (GERD) or heartburn.

❑ If you develop heartburn and the symptoms persist, consult your health care provider. If the pain begins to travel down your left arm, or if the sensation is accompanied by a feeling of weakness, dizziness, or shortness of breath, seek emergency medical help. The early symptoms of a heart attack can be very much like those of indigestion, particularly heartburn, and as a result, many people mistakenly dismiss them. (*See* HEART ATTACK in Part Two.)

Considerations

❑ Fructooligosaccharides (FOS) and galactooligosaccharides (GOS) have been clinically proven to promote the growth of friendly intestinal bacteria.

❑ Drinking the juice of a lemon in a cup of water first thing in the morning is good for healing and for purifying the blood.

❑ Exercise, such as brisk walking or stretching, aids the digestive process.

Caution: If you are thirty-five or older and/or have been sedentary for some time, consult with your health care provider before beginning an exercise program.

❑ Food combinations are important. Proteins and starches are a poor combination, as are vegetables and fruits. Milk should not be consumed with meals. Foods containing sugar, such as fruit, should not be consumed with proteins or starches.

❑ Older people often lack sufficient hydrochloric acid and pancreatin to digest foods properly.

❑ Many people take antacids to relieve the discomfort of indigestion and heartburn, but these medications may actually make matters worse. Antacids neutralize the acid in the stomach, preventing proper digestion and interfering with the absorption of nutrients. This only leads to continued indigestion. Antacids may not help with gas and bloating.

❑ Most antacids sold in the United States contain aluminum compounds, calcium carbonate, magnesium compounds, or sodium bicarbonate. Aluminum-based antacids can cause constipation. Calcium carbonate can cause a rebound effect in which the stomach produces more acid than before once the antacid's effects wear off. Although you may produce more acid for a short time, over the long term, continued use has been shown to be effective in treating ulcers, and the rebound effect will not make your ulcer worse. Magnesium compounds can cause diarrhea. Sodium bicarbonate can cause gas and bloating. However, these also are quite effective in treating ulcers, which can outweigh the uncomfortable side effects they may produce.

❑ Beano, available at most supermarkets and drugstores, is good for preventing gas. This product must be taken with the first bite of food to be effective.

❑ The *Johns Hopkins Medical Letter* reported that decreased sexual ability or breast enlargement may result from prolonged, excessive (more than 3 grams a day) use of the heartburn medication cimetidine (Tagamet).

❑ *See also* ENZYMES in Part One.

❑ *See also* ALLERGIES in Part Two and take the self-test.

☐ *See also* DIVERTICULITIS; FOODBORNE/WATERBORNE DISEASE; GALLBLADDER DISORDERS; HEARTBURN/GASTROESOPHAGEAL REFLUX DISEASE (GERD); IRRITABLE BOWEL SYNDROME; LACTOSE INTOLERANCE; MOTION SICKNESS; PANCREATITIS; PEPTIC ULCER; and/or ULCERATIVE COLITIS, all in Part Two.

INFERTILITY

Infertility is usually defined as the failure to conceive after a year or more of regular sexual activity during the time of ovulation. It may also refer to the inability to carry a pregnancy to term. Some 7.3 million American women between the ages of fifteen and forty-four are impaired in their ability to have children; 2.1 million of these women are infertile. Pinpointing the exact cause of the problem can be difficult. Ovulation, fertilization, and the journey of the fertilized ovum through the fallopian tube and finally into the uterus are highly intricate processes. Many events must work together perfectly for pregnancy to occur. In general, however, about one-third of the cases of infertility can be traced to the woman, another third to the man, and the remaining third can be attributed to both partners or no cause is found.

In about half of infertile couples, problems affecting the male partner are either partially or wholly the cause of infertility. For men, infertility is most often the result of a low sperm count or an anatomical abnormality. A variety of factors can result in a low sperm count, including alcohol consumption; endocrine disorders; exposure to toxins, radiation, or excessive heat; recent acute illness or prolonged fever; testicular injury; and, very rarely, mumps-induced wasting of the testicles. Obesity also reduces sperm count because estrogen levels increase in males who have excess body fat. Varicoceles, abnormal enlargements of veins that drain the testicles, can cause infertility in men because the veins of the testes no longer moderate the temperature of the testicles correctly, and this can negatively affect sperm.

For women, the most common causes of infertility include ovulatory failure or defect, blocked fallopian tubes, endometriosis, prior abdominal surgery, and uterine fibroids. Some women develop antibodies to their partners' sperm, in effect becoming allergic to them. Chlamydia is a sexually transmitted disease that causes many cases of infertility. Psychological issues, such as stress or fear of parenthood, may contribute to infertility as well, although stress is usually the result of infertility, not the cause of it. Some infertility cases are due to sperm abnormalities. The following are the most common reasons couples are unable to conceive:

- The woman has endometriosis.
- The man has abnormal sperm, a low sperm count, or erectile dysfunction.
- The woman's fallopian tubes are blocked.
- Ovulation takes place rarely or irregularly.

- The couple is unable to have complete sexual intercourse.
- The cervical mucous attacks and kills the sperm.
- The woman does not manufacture enough progesterone to carry a baby to term.
- The woman is over thirty-four (fertility declines rapidly after that age).
- One or both members of the couple eats a poor diet and experiences too much stress.

Often, more than one cause for infertility is found, and in approximately 20 percent of cases, nothing that would seem to inhibit conception can be found.

Ovulation Timing Self-Test

If you wish to become pregnant, there are a number of tests available over the counter that can help you determine the best time to attempt to conceive. These tests predict the time of ovulation by detecting the release of luteinizing hormone (LH), which in turn triggers the release of the egg.

A chemically treated dipstick detects the LH in urine samples. If the hormone has been released, the stick changes color. After a positive result, ovulation takes place within twelve to thirty-six hours. Remember, however, that no test is 100 percent accurate.

Unless otherwise specified, the following nutrients in this section are recommended for either or both partners.

NUTRIENTS

SUPPLEMENT	SUGGESTED DOSAGE	COMMENTS
Essential		
Selenium	200–400 mcg daily. If you become pregnant, cut back to no more than 40 mcg daily.	Deficiency leads to reduced sperm count and has been linked to sterility in men and infertility in women.
Vitamin C with bioflavonoids	2,000–6,000 mg daily, in divided doses.	Important in sperm production. Keeps the sperm from clumping and makes them more motile.
Vitamin E	200 IU daily or 400 IU every other day.	Needed for balanced hormone production. Has been known as the "sex vitamin" that carries oxygen to the sex organs and increases sperm count. Use d-alpha-tocopherol form.
Zinc	80 mg daily. Do not exceed a total of 100 mg daily from all supplements.	Important for the functioning of the reproductive organs. Zinc is found in high concentrations in semen.
Important		
Dimethylglycine (DMG) (Aangamik DMG from FoodScience of Vermont)	As directed on label.	Increases oxygen supply in the blood to all tissues. Use a sublingual form.

Octacosanol	As directed on label.	The heart of wheat germ. Aids in hormone production.
Phosphatidyl choline	1,000 mg daily.	Improves the transmission of messages from the brain to the genitals, thus increasing sex drive.
Helpful		
Essential fatty acids (Kyolic-EPA from Wakunaga)	As directed on label.	Essential for normal glandular function and activity, especially for the reproductive system.
L-arginine plus	As directed on label.	Increases sperm count and plays a role in sperm motility.
L-cysteine and	As directed on label.	Sulfur-containing amino acids that are effective free radical destroyers and chelating agents that protect glandular and hormonal function.
L-methionine plus	As directed on label.	
L-tyrosine	As directed on label. 500 mg daily, on an empty stomach. Take with water or juice. Do not take with milk. Take with 50 mg vitamin B$_6$ and 100 mg vitamin C for better absorption.	Alleviates stress and aids in stabilizing moods. (*See* AMINO ACIDS in Part One.) *Caution:* Do not take tyrosine if you are taking an MAO inhibitor drug.
plus acetylcholine	As directed on label.	Increases sexual pleasure.
Manganese	As directed on label. Take separately from calcium.	Maintains sex hormone production.
Proteolytic enzymes	As directed on label. Take between meals.	Aids in the breakdown of foods. Facilitates absorption of nutrients.
Pycnogenol or grape seed extract	As directed on label. As directed on label.	Powerful antioxidant bioflavonoids that may increase sperm count.
Raw orchic glandular	As directed on label.	For men. Supports testicular function. (*See* GLANDULAR THERAPY in Part Three.)
Raw ovarian glandular	As directed on label.	For women. Supports ovarian function. (*See* GLANDULAR THERAPY in Part Three.)
7-Keto DHEA	As directed on label.	Improves libido.
Vitamin A plus	15,000 IU daily.	Important in reproductive gland function.
carotenoid complex (Betatene)	As directed on label.	Antioxidants and vitamin A precursors.
Vitamin B complex plus extra	50 mg of each major B vitamin daily (amounts of individual vitamins in a complex will vary).	Important in reproductive gland function.
vitamin B$_5$ (pantothenic acid) and	As directed on label.	Maintains sex hormone production. Helpful for stress.
vitamin B$_6$ (pyridoxine) and	50 mg 3 times daily.	Needed for the synthesis of RNA and DNA.
para-aminobenzoic acid (PABA) and	50 mg daily.	Plays a role in restoring fertility in some women.
folic acid and	400 mcg daily.	Protects the egg, sperm, and genetic material.
vitamin B$_{12}$	2,000 mcg daily.	Maintains fertility. Use a sublingual form.

Herbs

❑ Astragalus extract has been reported to stimulate sperm motility. Damiana, ginseng, sarsaparilla, saw palmetto, and yohimbe enhance sexual function in men. Damiana, dong quai, false unicorn root, ginseng, gotu kola, licorice root, and wild yam root enhance sexual function in women.

Cautions: Do not use astragalus in the presence of a fever. Do not use ginseng if you have high blood pressure or are pregnant or nursing. Licorice root should not be used during pregnancy or nursing. It should not be used by persons with diabetes, glaucoma, heart disease, high blood pressure, or a history of stroke. Yohimbe should not be used by women who are pregnant or nursing. Do not use yohimbe if you have high blood pressure, heart disease, stomach ulcers, depression, or other psychiatric conditions. There have been cases of people dying from taking too much yohimbe.

❑ Green oat (*Avena sativa*) extract is an excellent aid if the reason for infertility is the man's inability to maintain an erection.

❑ Yin-yang-huo (*Aceranthus sagittatum*), a Chinese herb also known as horny goatweed, is a male aphrodisiac, and may increase sperm count and semen density.

❑ Heavy use of echinacea, ginkgo biloba, and St. John's wort may cause infertility in men, and should be avoided.

Cautions: Do not take echinacea for longer than three months. It should not be used by people who are allergic to ragweed. St. John's wort may cause increased sensitivity to sunlight. It may also produce anxiety, gastrointestinal symptoms, and headaches. It can interact with some drugs including antidepressants, birth control pills, and anticoagulants.

Recommendations

❑ Avoid all alcohol; it reduces sperm count in men and can prevent implantation of the fertilized egg in women.

❑ Lose weight if you are overweight. Infertility is more prevalent in obese men and women.

❑ Avoid douching, as this appears to reduce fertility.

❑ Do not take any drugs except those prescribed by your physician. Inform your physician if you are attempting to have a baby. He or she will be able to advise you if your medications may inhibit conception or may be dangerous for the fetus.

❑ Do not smoke, and avoid being around cigarette smoke.

❑ A balanced diet is important. Do not consume animal fats, fried foods, sugar, or junk foods. Do eat pumpkin seeds, bee pollen, or royal jelly.

Caution: Bee pollen may cause an allergic reaction in some people. Start with a small amount at first, and discontinue use if a rash, wheezing, discomfort, or other symptom occurs.

❑ Some artificial lubricants can prevent the sperm from reaching the cervix. Saliva may also have a detrimental effect on spermatozoa.

❑ Investigate the possibility of heavy metal intoxication, which may affect ovulation. A hair analysis can reveal heavy metal poisoning. (*See* HAIR ANALYSIS in Part Three.)

❑ Infertility is stressful, but do all you can to reduce the stresses in your life. Learn stress management techniques to help you deal with stresses that cannot be avoided. (*See* STRESS in Part Two.)

Considerations

❑ Because there are so many causes of infertility, in most cases the opinion of a qualified health care professional is needed.

❑ Sperm factors account for approximately 40 percent of all cases of infertility. Some causes of sperm inadequacy (recent illness, endocrine disorders) may be temporary or reversible, but others are not. Except for artificial insemination, orthodox drug therapy is ineffective in such cases.

❑ Varicoceles are sometimes treatable with surgery, and fertility can sometimes be restored.

❑ The ulcer medications cimetidine (Tagamet) and ranitidine (Zantac) may decrease the sperm count and even produce decreased sexual ability.

❑ Strict adherence to a gluten-free diet has enabled some previously sterile men to become fathers. A gluten-free diet has also enabled women who were previously unable to conceive to become pregnant. *See* CELIAC DISEASE in Part Two for more information about a gluten-free diet.

❑ In one study, 83 percent of infertile women with abnormal menses who lost weight on a 1,200- to 1,300-calorie diet, and exercised for one hour, three times a week, resumed normal menses and improved their estrone/estradiol ratio. Another study found that in men with poor semen quality, diet also had an effect. Compared to men with normal sperm counts, men with poor semen ate more processed meats, potatoes, and dairy. The men with normal sperm counts ate more fruits (apricots and peaches), vegetables (lettuce and tomatoes), shellfish, and skim milk.

Caution: If you are thirty-five or older and/or have been sedentary for some time, consult with your health care provider before beginning an exercise program.

❑ Marijuana and cocaine lower sperm count.

❑ The transdermal use of natural progesterone cream may benefit infertile women.

❑ Scientists are looking at gene abnormalities that may lead to new male infertility treatments and male contraception.

❑ If a woman has developed antibodies to her partner's sperm, it may help to have him use a condom for at least thirty days. The sperm antibodies should then decrease, and intercourse without the use of a condom during the time of ovulation may lead to conception.

❑ Conception is more likely if the woman is on the bottom during intercourse.

❑ Sperm count reaches its highest level after two or three days of abstinence from any sexual activity, but sperm that remains in a man's body for longer than a month is less effective at fertilizing an egg.

❑ A woman who suffers from such premenstrual symptoms as bloating and breast tenderness is probably ovulating, so if she is having difficulty becoming pregnant, the cause probably lies elsewhere.

❑ Increasingly, women are waiting to bear children until their later reproductive years. However, a woman's fertility begins to decrease when she reaches her thirties.

❑ Para-aminobenzoic acid (PABA) stimulates the pituitary gland and sometimes restores fertility to some women who cannot conceive.

❑ In one study, infertile men benefited from 225 micrograms of selenium and 400 IU of vitamin E. The men had better sperm motility and less oxidative damage to the sperm. In contrast, large doses (4.5 grams) of a B-vitamin complex had no effect.

❑ Caffeine consumption may prevent some women from becoming pregnant.

❑ Procedures known as transcervical balloon tuboplasty (TBT) and selective fallopian tube canalization have roughly 90-percent success rates in removing obstructions of the fallopian tubes. TBT is similar to the artery-clearing technique called angioplasty. A tiny balloon is inserted into the tube by means of a catheter; when the catheter reaches the blockage, the balloon is inflated to stretch and clear the blocked section of the tube. The procedure may be performed in about fifteen minutes under either local or general anesthesia. Because this procedure is relatively noninvasive (no incision is required), the risks involved are few. However, there is a chance that a tube may become blocked again. Fallopian tube canalization produces similar results to those of TBT.

❑ Assisted reproductive techniques (ART) may be tried if all other methods have been attempted. These techniques include the following:

- *Gamete intrafallopian tube transfer* (GIFT). In this technique, eggs and sperm are mixed and put into the fallopian tube immediately, without waiting to see if fertilization has taken place.

- *Intracytoplasmic sperm injection* (ICSI). In this procedure, which may be used if the man has a low sperm count or too many abnormal sperm, the woman is injected with healthy sperm extracted from the testes.

- *In vitro fertilization* (IVF). Here a woman's eggs are fertilized outside the womb and inserted into the uterus. This is usually done if the fallopian tubes are blocked.

Fertility Tests

There are a number of tests—some for men, some for women—that may be performed if conception does not occur within a twelve-month period. It is both easier and more cost-effective to test the male partner first before going on to the more invasive techniques needed to test the female partner. The following table lists some of the most frequently performed fertility tests.

TEST	DESCRIPTION
Tests Performed on Men*	
Anti-sperm antibody tests	These tests are used to check for immune cells (antibodies) that attack sperm and can affect their ability to function.
Genetic tests	These tests are used if your doctor suspects your fertility problems could be caused by an inherited sex chromosone abnormality. A blood test can reveal whether there are subtle changes in the Y chromosone.
Hormone test	A blood test is done to determine the level of testosterone and other male hormones that affect fertility.
Scrotal ultrasound	Uses high-frequency sound waves to produce images of structures within the body.
Semen analysis	This is the most important test for the male partner. A laboratory analyzes the physical characteristics of the semen and the number of sperm present, and looks for any abnormalities in the shape and structure (morphology) and movement (motility) of the sperm. The lab will also check semen for signs of problems, such as infections or blood. Often sperm counts fluctuate from one specimen to the next, so the doctor may want to evaluate a few different samples.
Specialized sperm function tests	A number of different tests can be used to evaluate how well the sperm survive ejaculation, how well they can penetrate the egg membrane, and whether there is any problem attaching to the egg.
Testicular biopsy	This test involves removing samples from the testicle with a needle. It may be used if the semen analysis shows no sperm at all. The results of the testicular biopsy will tell if sperm production is normal. If it is, the problem is likely caused by blockage or another problem with sperm transport.
Vasography	In some cases, contrast dye is injected into each vas deferens to see whether they are blocked.
Tests Performed on Women*	
Endometrial biopsy	A tiny sample of the endometrium (the lining of the uterus) is taken in the later part of the menstrual cycle and tested to see if there is enough progesterone in the lining as it matures. If not, the condition is called luteal phase defect. It can be treated with hormone therapy.
FSH test	A blood sample is taken on day three of the menstrual cycle and tested for FSH. FSH levels increase as a woman reaches menopause. If there is a high FSH level, pregnancy is unlikely.
Genetic testing	Genetic testing may be done to determine whether there is a genetic defect causing infertility.
Hysterosalpingo-gram (HSG)	Dye is inserted through the cervix into the fallopian tubes and uterus, and an X-ray is taken to determine whether the tubes are open and if the uterus is a normal shape.
Laparoscopy	A surgical procedure in which a physician examines the reproductive organs by means of a tiny scope. If scar tissue or endometrial buildup is found, it can be removed by means of the scope as well.
Postcoital test (PCT, Sims-Huhner test)	The partners have intercourse 2–8 hours before this test. A sample of cervical mucus and tissue is removed and examined to determine whether the mucus or the cervix is prohibiting fertilization. Undergoing a PCT is much the same as having a Pap smear.
Transvaginal ultrasound	A probe is inserted into the vagina to look for fibroid tumors or ovarian cysts. This can also be done to track early pregnancies.

**Source:* mayoclinic.com

- *Zygote intrafallopian tube transfer* (ZIFT). Eggs and sperm are combined, and if an egg is fertilized, it is inserted into the fallopian tube.

❏ A University of Michigan study indicated that intense exercise may result in a drop in the production of hormones involved in potency, fertility, and sex drive.

Caution: If you are thirty-five or older and/or have been sedentary for some time, consult with your health care provider before beginning an exercise program.

❏ The use of donor eggs to impregnate women who cannot conceive on their own is controversial and is extremely expensive.

❏ Your health care provider must get your consent before performing diagnostic tests to determine the cause of infertility. There may be risks involved any time you penetrate the body using a tube, needle, or viewing instrument, or expose the body to the radiation, drugs, anesthetics, and dye materials used in certain imaging techniques. The risks of any given procedure vary depending on your age and health status, and the skill of the practitioner.

INFLAMMATION

Inflammation is a natural reaction to injury or infection. The affected tissues swell, redden, become warm and tender, and may be painful. Proteins called cytokines attack the threatening germ and repair damaged tissues. Too much inflammation can do the body harm, however, leading to immobility, weight loss, and eroding of muscle tissue and the power to fight disease. Disorders that involve specific types and/or locations of inflammation include bursitis, carpal tunnel syndrome, fibromyalgia, osteoarthritis, and tendinitis, just to name a few. Cardiovascular disease also may be at least partially a result of inflammation in the linings of the arteries. Things that can trigger inflammation include a diet rich in omega-6 fatty acids, drug overuse, exposure to environmental toxins, free radical damage, infections, injury, trauma, and bacterial, fungal, or viral infection.

Any organ or tissue of the body, internal or external, can become inflamed. Internal inflammation is often caused by bacterial infection, but can also be caused by disorders such as allergies, anemia, arthritis, asthma, autoimmune diseases, Crohn's disease, osteoarthritis, peptic ulcer disease, or ulcerative colitis. External inflammation is most often the result of injury, but can also result from (or be aggravated by) allergies, infection, and other factors. Unfortunately, it is often difficult to identify the source or sources of inflammation.

Unless otherwise specified, the dosages recommended here are for adults. For children between the ages of twelve and seventeen, reduce the dose to three-quarters the recommended amount. For children between six and twelve, use one-half the recommended dose, and for children under the age of six, use one-quarter the recommended amount.

NUTRIENTS

SUPPLEMENT	SUGGESTED DOSAGE	COMMENTS
Essential		
Omega-3 fatty acids	As directed on label.	Flax oil and other plant omega-3s are not as potent as those from fish oil.
Vitamin B complex plus extra vitamin B$_{12}$	50 mg of each major B vitamin 3 times daily (amounts of individual vitamins in a complex will vary). 2,000 mcg daily.	Needed for tissue repair.
Vitamin C with bioflavonoids	3,000–6,000 mg daily, in divided doses.	Essential to the healing process and in reducing inflammation. Use a buffered form.
Very Important		
Carotenoid complex	As directed on label.	Strengthens the immune response.
Essential fatty acids (evening primrose oil, flaxseed oil)	As directed on label.	Reduces inflammation.
Grape seed extract	As directed on label.	Powerful antioxidant.
Proteolytic enzymes or Inf-zyme Forte from American Biologics	As directed on label, between meals and at bedtime, for 1 month. 2 tablets twice daily, between meals.	Aids in controlling inflammation.
Superoxide dismutase (SOD)	As directed on label.	A high-potency free radical scavenger that reduces infection and inflammation.
Zinc	50 mg daily. Do not exceed a total of 100 mg daily from all supplements.	Helps to control inflammation and promotes healing. Use zinc gluconate lozenges or OptiZinc for best absorption.
Important		
Bromelain	As directed on label. Take on an empty stomach with 100–500 mg magnesium and 500 mg L-cysteine to enhance results. Take separately from copper and iron.	Has anti-inflammatory activity and increases the breakdown of fibrin, which forms around the inflamed area, blocking the blood and lymphatic vessels.
Garlic (Kyolic from Wakunaga)	2 capsules 3 times daily, with meals.	Has natural anti-inflammatory properties.
Micellized Vitamin A and E from American Biologics	As directed on label.	Supplies vitamins A and E in easily assimilated emulsion form to destroy free radicals, boost the immune system, and help the body to use oxygen efficiently.
Multimineral complex	As directed on label.	Supplies important minerals. Needed to reduce stress. Use a formula high in calcium.
Silica	As directed on label, twice daily.	Supplies silicon, which aids in absorption of calcium and repair of connective tissues.
Helpful		
Beta-1,3-D-glucan	As directed on label.	Boosts immune function and fights inflammation.

Kelp or alfalfa	1,000–1,500 mg daily.	Contains a balance of essential minerals plus chlorophyll, which cleanses the blood. *See* under Herbs, below.
Raw thymus glandular	As directed on label.	Improves thymus function, which is important for immune function.
Selenium	200 mcg daily. If you are pregnant, do not exceed 40 mcg daily.	A powerful antioxidant and aid in inflammation reduction.
Vitamin E	200 IU daily or 400 IU every other day.	Effective antioxidant and reducer of inflammation. Use d-alpha-tocopherol form.

Herbs

❑ Alfalfa is a good source of minerals and chlorophyll.

❑ Aloe vera juice is helpful for inflammation.

❑ Bilberry contains flavonoids that reduce inflammation.

❑ Boswellia and turmeric (curcumin) help to reduce inflammation.

❑ Cat's claw is good for inflammation and healing.

Caution: Do not use cat's claw during pregnancy.

❑ Cayenne, curcumin, devil's claw, echinacea, ginger, goldenseal, pau d'arco, red clover, stinging nettle, white willow bark, and yucca are all good for inflammation.

Cautions: Do not take echinacea for longer than three months. It should not be used by people who are allergic to ragweed. Do not take goldenseal internally on a daily basis for more than one week at a time. Do not use it during pregnancy or if you are breast-feeding, and use with caution if you are allergic to ragweed. If you have a history of cardiovascular disease, diabetes, or glaucoma, use it only under a doctor's supervision.

❑ A poultice that combines fenugreek and flaxseed can be applied directly to the affected area to subdue inflammation. As an alternative, a goldenseal or mustard poultice can be used. *See* USING A POULTICE in Part Three.

❑ Olive leaf extract eases inflammation and is good for any bacterial infection.

Recommendations

❑ Eat a diet composed of 75 percent raw foods, and drink plenty of herbal teas and juices.

❑ Eat foods high in flavonoids, which are powerful antioxidants and useful for inflammation reduction. Spinach and blueberries are excellent sources of flavonoids. Strawberries contain smaller amounts. Quercetin, found in onions, is good for inflammation as well.

❑ Consume half of a fresh pineapple or fresh papaya daily. Pineapple contains bromelain and papaya contains papain, both enzymes that reduce swelling and inflammation. It should reduce the pain and swelling in two to six days. Only fresh pineapple or papaya (not canned) is effective. Bromelain is also available in pill form.

❑ Eat cold-water fish such as herring, mackerel, salmon, and sardines at least twice a week, as they are rich sources of essential fatty acids. Take fish oil capsules as well.

❑ Limit saturated fats and polyunsaturated fats that are rich in omega-6s like corn oil, cottonseed oil, and sunflower oil. For heart health, use other polyunsaturated fats such as canola, safflower, and soybean oil. Avoid packaged goods, because many contain omega-6-rich fats.

❑ Limit your intake of salt.

❑ Avoid cola, sugar, white flour products, and junk foods.

❑ For quick results, *see* FASTING in Part Three and follow the program.

Considerations

❑ Heart disease used to be associated only with an increase in cholesterol levels. Now it is thought to be related to inflammation, as evidenced by increases in homocysteine and C-reactive protein levels in many patients; these are markers of inflammation. Also, obesity causes an increase in blood cytokine levels, indicating that it too is causing increased inflammation in the body. Obese children as young as two and three years old have elevated cytokine levels.

❑ Bacterial arthritis, which causes painful inflammation of the joints, is usually associated with an infection elsewhere in the body, such as in the lungs, kidneys, or gallbladder.

❑ The complex sugar beta-1,3-D-glucan (found in the cell walls of baker's yeast, and a variety of fungi, such as maitake and reishi mushrooms) has proven to be a powerful immune booster. When beta-1,3-D-glucan attaches to the receptor site on macrophage cells, these immune cells are activated to attack and destroy invading organisms and reduce infection and inflammation.

❑ The traditional methods for relieving inflammation are positioning the affected part properly (including splinting, if necessary), applying heat and/or ice (heat and cold therapies), taking painkillers along with nutritional supplements, and getting plenty of rest. Nonsteroidal anti-inflammatory drugs (NSAIDs) are prescribed to 33 million people a year for chronic inflammation. However, NSAIDs increase the risk of stomach pain, intestinal bleeding, heart problems, and kidney failure.

❑ Goat's milk mineral whey is used to promote bone density as well as relieve aching, painful joints.

❑ *See* ABSCESS; ARTHRITIS; and SPRAINS, STRAINS, AND OTHER INJURIES OF THE MUSCLES AND JOINTS, all in Part Two.

❑ *See also* PAIN CONTROL in Part Three.

INFLUENZA

Influenza, better known as "the flu," is a highly contagious viral infection of the upper respiratory tract. There are two types of influenza viruses, designated type A and type B, that cause this acute infection of the throat, nose, bronchial tubes, lungs, and middle ear. The virus enters the body's airways through mucous membranes in the nose, eyes, or mouth. Because this illness can be spread easily by coughing and sneezing, influenza epidemics are very common, especially in winter. Every year in the United States, on average 5 to 20 percent of the population gets the flu. Up to 36,000 Americans die each year of influenza, with approximately 200,000 hospitalized. The flu is unpredictable and can strike anyone, at any age. More than two hundred different individual strains of virus can cause colds and flu, and strains of these viruses are constantly changing, so vaccinations against influenza have been only partly successful in preventing outbreaks of the disease.

Vaccines become available each year to try to reduce the likelihood of getting the flu. Most are safe and effective, if the strain targeted is actually the one that hits during the winter months. The vaccine decision is based on a best guess at the time the vaccine is manufactured. In April 2009, a new virus appeared and was called swine flu, because many genes in the virus were thought to be similar to flu viruses that normally occur in pigs in North America. Later it was learned that the genes really harbor two genes from flu viruses that are found in pigs in Europe and Asia, avian genes, and human genes. This is referred to as a quadruple reassortant virus, and the CDC renamed it H1N1. The H1N1 was declared a pandemic by the World Health Organization in June 2009. It was the first pandemic in forty-one years.

The symptoms of influenza begin much like those of the common cold—body aches, cough, fatigue, headache, and hot and cold sweats. In many cases, a fever develops, and you may feel unbearably hot one moment and chilled and shaking the next. Most influenza sufferers have a dry throat and cough. Nausea and vomiting may occur as well. Often, a person with the flu is so weak and so uncomfortable that he or she does not feel like eating or doing anything else. Colds last for about one week to ten days, on average, but the flu lasts longer—up to twelve days or more, followed by a week or more of residual coughing and fatigue.

Influenza is rarely dangerous in healthy adults sixty years of age or younger, but it does make a person more susceptible to pneumonia, ear infections, and sinus trouble. Among people sixty-five or older, serious respiratory infections such as influenza and pneumonia are the fifth leading cause of death, so the flu is clearly a serious infection for older people. High-risk flu groups also include those of any age with weakened immune systems or with chronic conditions such as heart or lung disease. The H1N1 virus of 2009 was particularly dangerous for young children and pregnant women.

Unless otherwise specified, the dosages recommended here are for adults. For a child between the ages of twelve and seventeen, reduce the dose to three-quarters of the recommended amount. For a child between six and twelve, use one-half of the recommended dose, and for a child under the age of six, use one-quarter of the recommended amount.

NUTRIENTS

SUPPLEMENT	SUGGESTED DOSAGE	COMMENTS
Essential		
ACES + Zn from Carlson Labs	As directed on label.	Contains vitamins A, C, and E, plus selenium and zinc. Take this supplement in addition to zinc lozenges as directed below.
Vitamin A	15,000 IU daily. If you are pregnant, do not exceed 10,000 IU daily.	A powerful antioxidant and immunity booster.
plus natural beta-carotene	15,000 IU daily.	Antioxidants and precursors of vitamin A.
or carotenoid complex (Betatene)	As directed on label.	
Vitamin C with bioflavonoids	5,000–20,000 mg daily, in divided doses. (*See* ASCORBIC ACID FLUSH in Part Three.)	Strengthens the immune system by increasing the number and quality of white blood cells. For a child, use buffered vitamin C or calcium ascorbate.
Zinc lozenges	Adults and children over 6 years: 1 15-mg lozenge every 2 hours for 2 days, starting at the first signs of the flu. Then reduce dosage to a total of 80 mg or less daily.	A potent immunostimulant that nourishes the cells. Keep these on hand and use them as soon as symptoms develop.
Important		
Free form amino acid	As directed on label.	Helps to repair tissue and control fever. Free-form amino acids are rapidly absorbed into the body.
Garlic (Kyolic from Wakunaga)	2 capsules 3 times daily.	Has antiviral and antibacterial properties.
L-lysine	500 mg daily, on an empty stomach. Take with water or juice. Do not take with milk. Take with 50 mg vitamin B_6 and 100 mg vitamin C for better absorption.	Aids in combating viral infection and preventing outbreaks of cold sores in and around the mouth, common when the body is under stress from illness. (*See* AMINO ACIDS in Part One.) *Caution:* Do not take lysine longer than six months at a time.
N-acetylcysteine (NAC)	As directed on label.	Thins mucus and aids in preventing respiratory disease.
Helpful		
Dioxychlor	10–20 drops sublingually, 1–2 times daily. Also, add 20 drops to 1 oz water and instill a dropperful in each nostril daily.	An important antibacterial, antifungal, and antiviral agent. Especially good for older adults.
Maitake extract	As directed on label.	Helps to boost immunity and fight viral infection.
or shiitake extract	As directed on label.	
or reishi extract	As directed on label.	

Multivitamin and mineral complex with	As directed on label.	All vitamins are needed for healing. Necessary in all cellular and enzyme functions.
vitamin B complex	100 mg of each major B vitamin daily (amounts of individual vitamins in a complex will vary).	Reduces stress caused by viral infection.
and selenium	200 mcg daily. If you are pregnant, do not exceed 40 mcg daily.	Boosts the immune response, enhancing the body's ability to fight infection.

Herbs

❑ Astragalus, black cherry, echinacea, ginger, goldenseal, pau d'arco, and yarrow tea are good for influenza. Combining peppermint tea with any of these herbal teas is effective for helping to open up the nasal passages. Echinacea is also good for children.

Cautions: Do not use astragalus in the presence of a fever. Do not take echinacea for longer than three months. It should not be used by people who are allergic to ragweed. Do not take goldenseal internally on a daily basis for more than one week at a time. Do not use it during pregnancy or if you are breast-feeding, and use with caution if you are allergic to ragweed. If you have a history of cardiovascular disease, diabetes, or glaucoma, use it only under a doctor's supervision.

❑ The herb boneset works as an expectorant and eliminates mucus from the lungs.

Caution: Do not use boneset on a daily basis for more than one week, as long-term use can lead to toxicity.

❑ If it is necessary to lower fever, take catnip tea enemas and ¼ to ½ teaspoon lobelia tincture every three to four hours until fever drops. This is good for children also.

Caution: Do not use this mixture if you are pregnant or breast-feeding, and do not give it to a child under one year old. Do not take lobelia internally on an ongoing basis.

❑ Cat's claw may cut the duration of the flu. Cold-X10 from Olympian Labs is a complex that contains cat's claw and many nutrients effective against flu and colds.

❑ Cayenne (capsicum) helps to keep mucus flowing, aiding in preventing congestion and headaches. Simply add a bit of cayenne powder to soups and other foods.

❑ ClearLungs from RidgeCrest Herbals is a Chinese herbal formula designed to provide nutrients to the lungs.

❑ The Chinese mushroom cordyceps is available in a tonic formula to support the lungs.

❑ At the first sign of a cough, place one dropperful of alcohol-free echinacea and goldenseal extract in your mouth and hold it there for five to ten minutes. Repeat this every hour for three to four hours. This stops the virus from multiplying.

Cautions: Do not take echinacea for longer than three months. It should not be used by people who are allergic to ragweed. Do not take goldenseal internally on a daily basis for more than one week at a time. Do not use it during pregnancy or if you are breast-feeding, and use with caution if you are allergic to ragweed. If you have a history of cardiovascular disease, diabetes, or glaucoma, use it only under a doctor's supervision.

❑ Alcohol-free echinacea and goldenseal combination extract is recommended for children. Give a child 4 to 6 drops of combination extract in water or juice every four hours for three days. Echinacea is very effective at enhancing the body's own natural defenses. Goldenseal is a natural antibiotic and helps to relieve congestion.

Cautions: Do not take echinacea for longer than three months. It should not be used by people who are allergic to ragweed. Do not take goldenseal internally on a daily basis for more than one week at a time. Do not use it during pregnancy or if you are breast-feeding, and use with caution if you are allergic to ragweed. If you have a history of cardiovascular disease, diabetes, or glaucoma, use it only under a doctor's supervision.

❑ Elderberry has antiviral properties and reduces flu symptoms.

❑ Elderflower tea promotes sweating and cleanses the body of toxins.

❑ Eucalyptus oil is beneficial for relieving congestion. Put 5 drops in a hot bath or 6 drops in a cup of boiling water, put a towel over your head, and inhale the vapors.

❑ Fenugreek breaks up phlegm and mucus, and slippery elm helps remove them from the body.

❑ Linden-flower tea suppresses cough and reduces fever.

❑ Lung Tonic Extract by Herbs Etc. is a mixture of herbs designed to protect the lungs.

❑ Maitake, shiitake, and reishi mushrooms possess beta-1,3-D-glucan, a type of polysaccharide that stimulates the immune cells. Their immune-boosting power makes them essential for fighting the flu.

❑ Olive leaf extract enhances immune function and fights all types of infection, including the flu virus.

❑ Wild pansy tea can treat colds accompanied by fever and respiratory congestion.

Recommendations

❑ Follow these basic tips for keeping flu away:

- Cover your nose and mouth with a tissue when you cough or sneeze.

- Wash your hands frequently, especially after coughing or sneezing, after using the bathroom, and before eating.

- Stay away from others who are sick.

- Maintain the best overall health possible to ward off germs by getting enough sleep, eating nutritiously, and exercising.

- Do not share glasses, cups, or utensils.
- Teach children not to touch their eyes or noses, or to put things into their mouths.
- Scrub your desk at work with a disinfecting wipe once a week.
- Spray your keyboard with disinfecting spray.
- Spray your telephone with disinfecting spray.

❏ If you do come down with the flu, consume plenty of fluids, especially fresh juices, herbal teas, soups, and filtered water, to prevent dehydration and help flush out the body. To shorten the length of the flu, go on a liquid diet emphasizing hot herbal teas and hot broth for one or two days.

❏ Eat plenty of hot chicken or turkey soup. This is grandmother's old remedy and it is still good today. Add a bit of cayenne pepper to help prevent and break up congestion. Avoid dairy products, mucus-forming foods, and sugar.

❏ Sleep and rest as much as possible.

❏ In treating a sore throat, *avoid* using aspirin chewing gum and aspirin gargles. Aspirin applied directly to mucous membranes does not reduce pain and can act as an irritant.

❏ Do not take zinc at the same time you eat or drink citrus fruits or juices. It will diminish the effectiveness of the zinc. Do consume a lot of other types of fruit.

❏ Do not take iron supplements while a fever exists.

❏ Do not give aspirin to a child who has the flu. The combination of aspirin and a viral illness has been linked to the development of Reye's syndrome, a potentially dangerous complication. (*See* REYE'S SYNDROME in Part Two.)

❏ Fever is one of the body's major defense mechanisms against the flu. Flu viruses do not survive well in a warmer environment. If you have a fever, do not try to suppress it, unless it is over 103°F.

❏ If you consume alcoholic beverages even occasionally, or if you have liver or kidney disease, be cautious about using the painkiller acetaminophen (Tylenol, Datril Extra Strength, and others). The combination of alcohol and acetaminophen has been associated with serious liver problems.

❏ If you are over sixty-five, see your health care provider. Influenza can cause serious complications for people in this age group.

❏ Since flu viruses are often transmitted by way of the hands, wash your hands frequently with an antibacterial soap. Rinse and dry your hands thoroughly and keep them away from your eyes, nose, and mouth. If you sneeze, use a disposable tissue.

❏ Buy a new toothbrush—toothbrushes can harbor viruses and prolong the illness.

❏ Try one or more of the following homeopathic remedies to ease flu symptoms:

- *Anas barbariae* (Oscillococcinum), a homeopathic treatment, works very well if taken at the first signs of the flu.
- *Aconitum napellus*, *Belladonna*, and *Eupatorium perfoliatum* help to ease flu symptoms.

Caution: You should not use this formula if you are pregnant.

Considerations

❏ Antibiotics are useless against viral illnesses like influenza. The best way to get rid of the flu or any other infectious illness is to attack it head-on by strengthening the immune system. The thymus and the adrenal glands are the power seat of the immune system. When the body is getting sick, or is already sick, it is under stress, and stress taxes the immune system. Researchers have linked vulnerability to colds and flu to psychological stress.

❏ Zanamivir (Relenza), an inhaled antiviral drug, battles flu symptoms and shortens the duration of the illness. It has also been shown to be effective in preventing the flu in both strains of influenza. Another medication, oseltamivir (Tamiflu) has shown comparable results. Both of these medications may be beneficial for people with immune system problems. The U.S. Centers for Disease Control and Prevention (CDC) recommends these two drugs specifically for the treatment and prevention of the H1N1 virus.

❏ Children who have the flu frequently should be checked for thyroid malfunctions. (*See* HYPOTHYROIDISM in Part Two.) Warning signs that need urgent medical attention in children include: fast breathing, bluish/gray skin color, not drinking fluids, severe vomiting, and not being able to be woken up when asleep.

❏ The term "stomach flu" is commonly used to refer to another condition, gastroenteritis. This is not influenza, but an acute inflammation of the lining of the stomach. Gastroenteritis is characterized by diarrhea, vomiting, and abdominal cramps that vary in severity, and may be accompanied by fever, chills, head and body aches, chest pain and cough, and extreme fatigue. It may be caused by a number of different factors, including food poisoning, viral infection, alcohol intoxication, sensitivity to drugs, and certain allergies. This type of illness usually runs its course in one or two days.

❏ *See also* COMMON COLD and PNEUMONIA, both in Part Two.

INSECT ALLERGY

There are only a few stinging insects in the United States that can cause an allergic reaction: honeybees, hornets, yellowjackets, bumblebees, wasps, and ants. Insects of the group known as *hymenoptera*, which includes bees, wasps, hornets, and ants, cause an allergic reaction in 10 to 20 percent of the population. This reaction is known as an insect venom allergy, and it can be dangerous, even life-threatening. The yellow jacket and honeybee are the cause of most allergic reactions to insects.

Allergic reactions to stings can cause wheezing, tightness in the throat, nausea, diarrhea, hives, itching, pain and swelling in the joints, respiratory distress, and vascular swelling. In a person with a mild allergy to venom, the reaction can occur within a few minutes, but when a person experiences a severe allergic reaction, the symptoms can take longer to appear (ten to twenty minutes). If the reaction to the venom is delayed, symptoms such as fever, hives, inflamed lymph glands, and joint pain can occur. In some circumstances, a person who is highly allergic to insect venom can go into shock (circulatory collapse) and die within minutes. Signs that a dangerous reaction is developing include confusion, difficulty swallowing, extreme drop in blood pressure, hoarseness, labored breathing, severe anxiety, severe swelling, weakness, and a feeling of impending disaster. A more severe reaction can also result in closing of the airway, producing unconsciousness.

Some biting insects, such as mosquitoes, can cause allergic skin reactions that appear as scaly and itchy eczema.

Unless otherwise specified, the dosages recommended here are for adults. For children between the ages of twelve and seventeen, reduce the dose to three-quarters the recommended amount. For children between six and twelve, use one-half the recommended dose, and for children under the age of six, use one-quarter the recommended amount.

NUTRIENTS

SUPPLEMENT	SUGGESTED DOSAGE	COMMENTS
Essential		
Quercetin (Activated Quercetin from Source Naturals)	As directed on label.	A unique bioflavonoid that reduces allergic reactions.
Vitamin C with bioflavonoids	5,000–20,000 mg daily, in divided doses. (*See* ASCORBIC ACID FLUSH in Part Three.)	Acts as an anti-inflammatory and helps fight the toxicity of insect venom. For a child, use buffered vitamin C or calcium ascorbate.
Helpful		
Aller Bee-Gone from CC Pollen	As directed on label.	A combination of herbs, enzymes, and nutrients designed to fight acute allergic symptoms.
Inf-zyme Forte from American Biologics	As directed on label.	A potent enzyme and powerful inflammatory inhibitor.

Herbs

❏ Calendula is an excellent topical cream to apply to skin irritations.

❏ Herbal flea-repellent pet collars contain oils of cedar, citronella, eucalyptus, pennyroyal, rosemary, and rue. These herbs may be effective insect repellents for humans as well.

Caution: Do not use pennyroyal or rue during pregnancy. Avoid excessive and/or prolonged use.

❏ Lavender may help relieve itching.

❏ Tea tree oil can be rubbed on exposed areas of skin to ward off insects. It can also be applied to bites. If pure tea tree oil is too strong, dilute it with canola oil or another low-fragrance vegetable oil until a tolerable strength is achieved.

Recommendations

❏ If you have ever had an allergic reaction to an insect sting, you should have access to an epinephrine (adrenaline) kit at all times. Have your physician prescribe an emergency treatment kit and instruct you in its proper use. Epinephrine raises the blood pressure and speeds the heart rate, counteracting the allergic response. It is best administered via a preloaded syringe found in injection kits. Your emergency kit should also include antihistamine tablets and an identification card listing your medical information.

❏ To avoid insect stings, wear plain, light-colored clothing when spending time outdoors—avoid wearing anything that is flowered or dark. Do not wear shiny jewelry, and do not use hair spray, perfume, scented soaps, or suntan lotion. Avoid wearing sandals or loose-fitting clothes.

❏ Avoid areas where bees are concentrated, such as orchards and flower gardens.

❏ If you are bothered by a yellow jacket, do not squash it; doing so releases a chemical that attracts other yellowjackets and wasps. It is best to leave these insects alone, or to find and destroy the nest after dark, when they are less active.

❏ Immediately after getting stung, *carefully* remove any stinger left in the skin. It is best not to pull the stinger out. Instead, gently and carefully scrape or tease it out with a sterilized knife. If no knife is readily available, you can use a fingernail or even the edge of a credit card instead. After a sting, be alert for signs that a reaction is developing. Reactions can occur in minutes or hours, and they can progress very quickly. If you have any doubts about your condition, seek treatment at once.

❏ Once the stinger has been removed and the area cleansed, try one or more of the following home remedies to ease pain and swelling:

• Make a paste by adding a bit of cool water to baking soda, a crushed aspirin, or a crushed papaya enzyme tablet, and apply the mixture to the sting.

• Use charcoal tablets, available in health food stores, to make a poultice. Crush 2 tablets, then add 6 drops of liquid alcohol-free goldenseal extract to make a paste. Smooth the mixture on a sterile gauze pad and place it on the sting area. This will absorb the poisons and prevent infection. Use only charcoal recommended for internal use.

- Apply an ice compress to the sting area a few minutes every two hours for the first day after you've been stung. Not only will you reduce the swelling and pain from the sting, but you will be stopping the spread of venom.

- Apply lavender oil to the sting area to reduce inflammation and pain.

- Crush plantain leaves and squeeze out the juice. Apply this extract directly to the sting. Within thirty minutes, the pain and swelling should be greatly reduced.

❑ Other remedies to consider include the following: rubbing toothpaste on the sting (its cooling effect can make the sting area feel better); applying calamine lotion to the area; or rubbing a meat tenderizer containing papain (an enzyme) on the sting can also ease the pain.

❑ *Apis mellifica,* a homeopathic remedy, is good for wasp or bee stings. When taken promptly after a bite, it helps to prevent severe swelling and anaphylactic shock. It works quickly and can be used while waiting for medical attention. Another homeopathic remedy, *Silica,* is useful if a stinger is embedded deep in the skin; it forces the object out of the body in a few hours.

Considerations

❑ Sometimes brewer's yeast or garlic rubbed on the skin deters insects. Eating garlic may help also.

Caution: Brewer's yeast can cause an allergic reaction in some individuals. Start with a small amount at first, and discontinue use if any allergic symptoms occur.

❑ Antihistamines given by injection or by mouth following a sting can reduce later-appearing symptoms.

❑ When a person has had a severe allergic reaction, the treatment usually involves an injection of adrenaline (epinephrine) and/or cardiopulmonary resuscitation. Corticosteroids may be prescribed to diminish swelling and reduce the hives.

❑ If you are diagnosed with an insect allergy, your physician may suggest immunotherapy, which involves building up tolerance to the venom. Small doses of the venom are introduced into the body over a period of time until your system can tolerate the toxin.

❑ *See also* BEE STING; INSECT BITE; and/or SPIDER BITES AND SCORPION STINGS in Part Two.

INSECT BITE

Many different insects bite, including mosquitoes, fire ants, fleas, gnats, no-see-ums, and ticks. Most insect bites are merely a nuisance. They cause localized itching and redness, but are relatively harmless. Others can be serious. Tick bites can spread diseases such as babesiosis, Lyme disease, or Rocky Mountain spotted fever. In some places (principally in developing countries), mosquito bites may transmit malaria and yellow fever, as well as viruses that cause encephalitis, an inflammation of the brain. Spiders, while not technically insects, can cause similar bites. The black widow and brown recluse are two of the most poisonous spiders, inflicting painful and serious bites. (*See* SPIDER BITES AND SCORPION STINGS in Part Two.) Bees, hornets, and yellow jackets may sting in self-defense or to subdue their prey. (*See* BEE STING in Part Two.) There are also stings that can be obtained from aquatic life such as jellyfish, sea anemones, and some types of coral.

Unless otherwise specified, the dosages recommended here are for adults. For children between the ages of twelve and seventeen, reduce the dose to three-quarters the recommended amount. For children between six and twelve, use one-half the recommended dose, and for children under the age of six, use one-quarter the recommended amount.

NUTRIENTS

SUPPLEMENT	SUGGESTED DOSAGE	COMMENTS
Essential		
Bromelain plus	400–500 mg 3 times daily.	Reduces inflammation, swelling, and pain.
curcumin	As directed on label.	Has anti-inflammatory properties.
Grape seed extract	75 mg daily.	An effective anti-inflammatory and powerful antioxidant.
Quercetin (Activated Quercetin from Source Naturals)	300–400 mg every 4 hours.	A unique bioflavonoid that reduces allergic reactions.
Vitamin C with bioflavonoids	5,000–20,000 mg daily, in divided doses. (*See* ASCORBIC ACID FLUSH in Part Three.)	An anti-inflammatory that is helpful for relieving the toxicity of bites. For a child, use buffered vitamin C or calcium ascorbate.

Herbs

❑ Calendula ointment is an excellent insect repellent and counterirritant. You can also try cedar, eucalyptus, and/or tea tree oils. These are available in oil, spray, and lotion forms.

❑ Citronella candles are good for repelling mosquitoes.

❑ Goldenseal and tea tree oil are natural insect repellants and are beneficial when applied to affected areas.

❑ Poultices made with lobelia and charcoal tablets (found in health food stores) are helpful for insect bites. (*See* USING A POULTICE in Part Three.)

❑ Pennyroyal oil helps to repel insects.

Caution: Do not use this herb during pregnancy. Avoid excessive and/or prolonged use.

❑ Apple cider vinegar diluted with water in a one-to-one ratio reduces skin irritations resulting from insect bites.

Recommendations

❑ For ant, mosquito, or chigger (mite) bites, wash the area thoroughly with soap and water. For chigger bites, use a brush and scrub. Then apply a paste made of baking soda and water. Use cloth-wrapped ice packs if swelling occurs and, if bitten on an arm or leg, elevate the affected limb to decrease swelling.

❑ For tick bites, remove the tick as quickly as you can. The sooner the tick is removed, the less chance there is of contracting any disease the tick may be carrying. Using tweezers, grasp the head of the tick firmly, as close to the skin as possible, and pull straight back with the tweezers. Try not to leave the head or any other part of the tick embedded in the skin. Do not touch the tick with your hands. Once it has been removed, scrub the bite with soap and water. *Do not* try to burn the tick out, or use home remedies like kerosene, turpentine, or petroleum jelly.

❑ Make a paste using a charcoal capsule and a few drops of goldenseal extract and place it on a piece of gauze. Apply the gauze to the bite and cover it with a bandage. This will draw out the poisons and aid in fast relief. Do this immediately after being bitten, if possible.

❑ Apply calamine lotion to help relieve itching.

❑ Rub a cut onion on an insect bite to provide a powerful antioxidant treatment.

❑ Take a dose of homeopathic *Apis mellifica* promptly after a bite. It works quickly to help prevent severe swelling.

❑ Dab a paste consisting of meat tenderizer and water directly on a bite or sting. Leave for thirty minutes, then rinse off. Enzymes in the tenderizer draw the poison out.

❑ If you have been bitten by a spider you suspect may be a black widow or a brown recluse, seek medical attention immediately. If possible, take the spider with you for identification. (*See* SPIDER BITES AND SCORPION STINGS in Part Two.)

❑ To avoid mosquito bites, eat fish, brown rice, brewer's yeast, blackstrap molasses, or wheat germ before spending time outside. These foods are rich in vitamin B_1 (thiamine). Mosquitoes appear to be repelled by the B vitamins, which are excreted through the skin, and especially by thiamine, so as an alternative, take thiamine supplements. Carbon dioxide, estrogens, moisture, sweat, and warmth attract mosquitoes.

Caution: Brewer's yeast can cause an allergic reaction in some individuals. Start with a small amount at first, and discontinue use if any allergic symptoms occur.

❑ To avoid many insect bites, try a very diluted chlorine bleach bath before going out. Add 1 cup of bleach per tub of water. Insects dislike the smell. Swimming in a pool treated with chlorine also works. Rubbing brewer's yeast or garlic on the skin may deter insects as well.

Caution: Brewer's yeast can cause an allergic reaction in some individuals. Start with a small amount at first, and discontinue use if any allergic symptoms occur.

❑ Avoid walking barefoot outside.

❑ Avoid all refined sugar, which causes the skin to give off a sweet smell that attracts mosquitoes.

❑ Avoid alcoholic drinks. Alcohol causes the skin to flush and the blood vessels to dilate, which attracts mosquitoes and horseflies.

❑ Avoid using perfume, hair spray, and other cosmetics. These attract insects.

❑ Avoid wearing bright colors—wear white clothing. Also, wear clothing that covers your arms and legs (although mosquitoes can bite through cotton clothing).

❑ Apply citrus juice to exposed areas to repel mosquitoes.

Considerations

❑ Diethyl-meta-toluamide (DEET) works to repel chiggers, ticks, and mosquitoes. It is probably the most effective insect repellent known, but it is also potentially quite toxic and it can destroy substances such as plastics and synthetic fabrics, so it must be used with care and only in accordance with package directions. Never apply a product that has more than 35 percent DEET to the skin. Children are especially at risk for problems due to this potentially hazardous chemical, so their skin exposure to it should be strictly limited. To be safe, apply DEET to clothing and use it sparingly, if at all, on the skin.

Caution: DEET is extremely toxic and can be deadly if ingested. However, when used according to the product directions, it does not pose a health concern because its use is expected to be brief. Be extremely careful when using it around small children. Do not use under clothing.

❑ If you are in the wilderness, or anywhere without access to the above remedies, the traditional remedy of immediately applying mud to a sting can help to neutralize the pain and swelling.

❑ We do not recommend using electric insect-repelling devices ("bug zappers"). They kill biting bugs, but not black flies and mosquitoes. Many of the insects they kill are an important part of the daily diet of birds. If you feel you must use one of these devices, do not place it near children's play areas, barbecue grills, or picnic tables. When insects like houseflies get zapped, the parts can spray as far as seven feet, spreading bacteria and viruses.

❑ Information on poisonings from insect bites can be obtained from the U.S. Centers for Disease Control and Prevention (CDC) in Atlanta (*see* Health and Medical Organizations in the Appendix).

❑ *See also* BEE STING; INSECT ALLERGY; LYME DISEASE; and/or SPIDER BITES AND SCORPION STINGS, all in Part Two.

INSOMNIA

Habitual sleeplessness is classified as insomnia. Failure to get an entire night's sleep on most nights over a one-month period can be considered chronic insomnia. Insomnia can take the form of being unable to fall asleep when you first go to bed or waking during the night and being unable to go back to sleep. It affects one out of ten Americans. Over half of those over the age of sixty-five experience disturbed sleep. Those over sixty-five make up about 13 percent of the U.S. population, but consume over 30 percent of prescription drugs and 40 percent of sleeping pills.

While insomnia can be very frustrating, it is usually only a temporary annoyance. In some cases, however, sleep-related problems can last for months or even years.

Chronic insomnia is often a symptom of a serious underlying medical disorder. At least 80 percent of depressed people experience insomnia. Insomnia cases can be attributed to other psychological disorders, such as anxiety, stress, or grief. Insomnia can also result from a wide variety of physical causes, including arthritis, asthma, breathing problems, hypoglycemia, hyperthyroidism, indigestion, kidney or heart disease, muscle aches, Parkinson's disease, or physical pain. Caffeine consumption, jet lag, and the use of certain drugs, including the antiseizure medication phenytoin (Dilantin), most appetite suppressants, the decongestant pseudoephedrine (found in many cold and allergy remedies), and thyroid hormone replacement drugs can also lead to insomnia.

A lack of the nutrients calcium and magnesium can cause you to wake up after a few hours and not be able to return to sleep. Systemic disorders involving the brain, digestive system, endocrine system, heart, kidneys, liver, lungs, and pancreas all may affect sleep, as can poor nutritional habits and eating too close to bedtime. A sedentary lifestyle can be a major contributor to sleep disorders.

While one or two sleepless nights can cause irritability and daytime sleepiness, with decreased ability to perform creative or repetitive tasks, most people can adapt to short-term periods of sleep deprivation. After more than three days, however, sleep deprivation begins to cause a more serious deterioration in overall performance and can even result in mild personality changes. If chronic, inadequate sleep compromises productivity, creates problems in relationships, and can contribute to other health problems.

Normal sleep consists of two main states, designated *rapid-eye-movement* (REM) and *non-rapid-eye-movement* (non-REM) sleep. It is REM sleep that is most often associated with dreaming. The stages of sleep are further broken down as follows:

- *Stage 1: Light sleep.* We drift in and out and can be awakened easily. Our eyes move slowly and muscle activity slows.
- *Stage 2: Light sleep.* Our eye movement stops and our brain waves become slower, with occasional bursts of rapid waves called *sleep spindles.*

- *Stage 3: Deep sleep.* Extremely slow brain waves called delta waves appear, interspersed with smaller, faster waves.
- *Stage 4: Deep sleep.* The brain produces mostly delta waves. There are no eye movements and no muscle activity.
- *Stage 5: REM sleep.* Breathing becomes more rapid, irregular, and shallow. The eyes jerk rapidly while limb muscles become temporarily paralyzed. Dreams almost always happen in this stage, but may occur in other sleep stages.

It takes about two hours to go through all five stages of sleep, after which they are normally repeated. REM sleep usually occurs about ninety minutes after we fall asleep. Adults spend half their sleep time in Stage 2 sleep, 20 percent in REM sleep, and 30 percent in the other stages. Infants start out spending about half their sleep time in REM sleep.

There are four stages to non-REM sleep, and the deepest two (stages three and four) are referred to as *delta sleep.* Older people spend less time in delta sleep, and some may not experience it at all.

There are no hard-and-fast rules about how much sleep is enough, because every individual's requirements are different. Some people can function on as little as five hours of sleep a night, while others seem to perform better with nine, ten, or even more hours of sleep. Most adults need about eight hours of sleep nightly in order to feel refreshed and function at peak efficiency during the day.

Children, especially very young children and adolescents, generally require more sleep than adults to be at their best. It is not uncommon for people to sleep less as they get older, especially after the age of sixty. The cardinal sign of a sleep problem requiring a doctor's attention is inappropriate sleepiness, such as dozing off at the dinner table, during conversation, or while driving. Even dozing off in front of the television can be a warning sign that something is amiss with the body's internal clock.

Millions of people have trouble getting to sleep due to a condition commonly known as restless leg syndrome (RLS). For reasons unknown, when these people are in bed, their legs jerk, twitch, and kick involuntarily. Restless leg syndrome has also been linked to the painful nighttime leg muscle cramps that afflict so many people. A deficiency of magnesium may be involved in RLS, and some research strongly suggests that anemia may play a major role in this annoying disorder.

Sleep apnea affects an estimated 12 million American adults. Of those who have sleep apnea, half are overweight. This condition is often found in overweight and obese patients because their diaphragm cannot fully exert itself to take a full breath, as it is hindered by excess abdominal body fat. This problem is commonly associated with snoring and extremely irregular breathing throughout the night. In sleep apnea, breathing actually stops for as long as two minutes at a time while the individual is asleep. When breathing stops, the level of oxygen in the blood drops, resulting in oxygen deprivation. The individual then awakens, startled and gasping. A person with sleep apnea may awaken as many as two hundred times throughout the night. The affected individual may not remember these awakenings, but anyone else who is awake at the time can naturally become alarmed when a person with sleep apnea stops breathing. In the less common form, central sleep apnea, breathing is stopped, not because the airway is closed, but because the diaphragm and chest muscles stop working.

Aside from disrupting normal sleep and causing extreme sleepiness during the day, sleep apnea is associated with other, more serious, health problems. People who have sleep apnea tend to have higher than normal blood pressure and are more likely to have strokes than the general population, and they also face an increased risk of heart disease, although the reason or reasons for these links are not known. People with sleep apnea also seem to have a higher-than-normal incidence of emotional and psychotic disorders. Experts attribute this to what they call a "dream deficit"—a lack of adequate rapid-eye-movement (REM) sleep, the stage of sleep in which dreaming occurs. A person with sleep apnea often cannot settle into REM sleep for even the eight to twelve seconds it takes to have a normal, healthy dream. While there is much about the phenomenon of dreaming that is not understood, it is known that prolonged periods of REM sleep deprivation can induce various psychoses and other serious emotional disorders.

Unless otherwise specified, the dosages recommended here are for adults. For children between the ages of twelve and seventeen, reduce the dose to three-quarters the recommended amount. For children between six and twelve, use one-half the recommended dose, and for children under the age of six, use one-quarter the recommended amount.

NUTRIENTS

SUPPLEMENT	SUGGESTED DOSAGE	COMMENTS
Important		
Calcium	1,500–2,000 mg daily, in divided doses, after meals and at bedtime.	Has a calming effect. Use calcium lactate or calcium chelate form (do not use lactate form if you are allergic to dairy products).
and magnesium	1,000 mg daily.	Needed to balance with calcium and relax the muscles.
Melatonin	Start with 1.5 mg daily, 30 minutes to 1 hour before bedtime. If this is not effective, gradually increase the dosage until an effective level is reached (up to 5 mg daily).	A natural hormone that promotes sound sleep. Use it only occasionally and do not give it to children.
Helpful		
Vitamin B complex plus extra	As directed on label.	Helps to promote a restful state.
vitamin B₅ (pantothenic acid) and	50 mg daily.	Good for relieving stress.
inositol and	100 mg daily, at bedtime.	Enhances REM sleep.
niacinamide	100 mg daily.	Promotes serotonin production.
Vitamin C with bioflavonoids	500 mg daily.	Very important for reducing stress.
Zinc	15 mg daily.	Aids in the recovery of body tissues while sleeping.

Herbs

❑ California poppy, hops, kava kava, lemon balm, passionflower, skullcap, and valerian root, taken in capsule or extract form, are all good for helping to overcome insomnia. Valerian root has become the favorite among many experts. It is best not to rely on one herb on a regular basis, but to rotate among several. Take these herbs before bedtime.

Caution: Kava kava can cause drowsiness. It is not recommended for pregnant women or nursing mothers, and it should not be taken with other substances that act on the central nervous system, such as alcohol, barbiturates, antidepressants, and antipsychotic drugs.

❑ The combination of California poppy, passionflower, and valerian promote sound sleep and beneficial REM sleep. California poppy and chamomile will strengthen the nervous system to calm you before bedtime.

Caution: Do not use chamomile if you are allergic to ragweed. Do not use during pregnancy or nursing. It may interact with warfarin or cyclosporine, so patients using these drugs should avoid it.

❑ Catnip and chamomile have mild sedative properties. These herbs are safe even for children if taken in tea form. For adults, drinking chamomile tea several times throughout the day helps to calm and tone the nervous system, promoting restful sleep.

Caution: Do not use chamomile if you are allergic to ragweed. Do not use during pregnancy or nursing. It may interact with warfarin or cyclosporine, so patients using these drugs should avoid it.

❑ Kava kava is a good relaxant. If stress or anxiety is the reason for your insomnia, this herb can help you develop better sleep patterns.

Caution: Kava kava can cause drowsiness. It is not recommended for pregnant women or nursing mothers, and it should not be taken with other substances that act on the central nervous system, such as alcohol, barbiturates, antidepressants, and antipsychotic drugs.

Recommendations

❑ In the evening, eat bananas, dates, figs, milk, nut butters, tuna, turkey, whole grain crackers, or yogurt. These foods are high in tryptophan, which promotes sleep. Eating a grapefruit half at bedtime also helps.

❑ Do not eat large meals within two hours of bedtime.

❏ Avoid caffeine, alcohol, and nicotine in the four to six hours before bedtime. A small amount can help induce sleep initially, but it invariably disrupts deeper sleep cycles later. While smoking may seem to have a calming effect, nicotine is actually a neurostimulant and can cause sleep problems.

❏ Avoid bacon, cheese, chocolate, eggplant, ham, potatoes, sauerkraut, sugar, sausage, spinach, tomatoes, and wine close to bedtime. These foods contain tyramine, which increases the release of norepinephrine, a brain stimulant.

❏ Avoid taking nasal decongestants and other cold medications late in the day. While many ingredients in these preparations are known to cause drowsiness, they can have the opposite effect on some people and act as a stimulant.

❏ Establish a set of habits and follow them consistently to establish a healthy sleep cycle. Among them:

- Go to bed only when you are sleepy.

- Do not stay in bed if you are not sleepy. Get up and move to another room and read, watch television, or do something quietly until you are really sleepy.

- Use the bedroom only for sleep and sex—not for reading, working, eating, or watching television.

- Keep a regular sleep-wake cycle. Try to go to bed and wake up at the same time every day.

- Set an alarm clock and get out of bed at the same time every morning, no matter how you slept the night before. Once normal sleep patterns are reestablished, most people find that they have no need for an alarm clock.

- Sleep in a dark, quiet room with a comfortable temperature.

- Do not nap during the day if this isn't a normal thing for you to do. Especially avoid napping later than 3:00 P.M.

- Exercise regularly in the late afternoon or early evening—but not within two hours of bedtime. Physical exertion is an excellent way to make your body tired so that sleep comes about more easily. Exercising five or six hours before bedtime may help you sleep more soundly.

Caution: If you are thirty-five or older and/or have been sedentary for some time, consult with your health care provider before beginning an exercise program.

- Take a hot bath (not a shower) an hour or two before bedtime. For further relaxation, put several drops of a soothing essential oil such as chamomile (if you are not allergic to ragweed) in the bathwater. (*See* AROMATHERAPY AND ESSENTIAL OILS in Part Three.)

Caution: Do not use chamomile if you are allergic to ragweed. Do not use during pregnancy or nursing. It may interact with warfarin or cyclosporine, so patients using these drugs should avoid it.

- Keep the bedroom comfortable and quiet. If *too much* quiet is the problem, try running a fan or playing a radio softly in the background. There are also devices available that generate "white noise" sounds like the ocean surf or a steady rain that help people who are "quiet-sensitive" to sleep.

- Learn to put worries out of your mind. If you have occasional trouble getting to sleep, concentrate on pleasant memories and thoughts. Re-create a pleasurable time or event in your life and relive it in your mind. Learning a relaxation technique such as meditation or the use of guided imagery is extremely helpful in getting sleep patterns back to normal for many people.

❏ For occasional sleeplessness, try using melatonin, Calcium Night from Source Naturals, or one of the herbs recommended above. These are effective and safe sleep promoters.

❏ One of the best remedies for insomnia is taking 5 milligrams of melatonin one hour before bedtime. If you feel groggy in the morning, reduce the dosage the next time you use it. Certain drugs frequently prescribed for older adults, including beta-blockers (for high blood pressure) and even aspirin, can lower melatonin levels.

Caution: Do not overuse melatonin. According to some recent reports, more than occasional use of melatonin can permanently stop the body's own production of this vital hormone.

❏ If you snore, try sleeping on your side. Sleep on a couch for a few nights to become accustomed to sleeping on your side.

Considerations

❏ During sleep, the body's systems are still controlling basic functions. Nutrients are essential for the body and are used during the sleep cycle.

❏ Sleep is needed to restore appetite hormones to their normal levels. Many obese people do not get at least eight hours of sleep a night. In one study, inadequate sleep was shown to increase calorie intake from snacks by 20 percent.

❏ A lack of sleep can encourage serious illness and cause premature aging. Experts recommend at least eight hours of sleep per night.

❏ Two of the most common sleep problems are not being able to fall asleep and waking in the middle of the night. It should take less than thirty minutes to get to sleep, but for many people it takes much longer. Others fall asleep, but wake up and can't get back to sleep. If you have either of these disturbances and feel tired in the morning, speak to your health care provider. You are not alone.

❏ An estimated 12 million Americans suffer from restless leg syndrome (RLS), a disorder marked by uncomfortable urges to move the legs, especially just before falling asleep.

Various treatments have been attempted for restless leg syndrome, but nothing seems to work consistently for everyone. The drug pramipexole (Mirapex) has shown positive benefits for some people with this condition. If you have restless leg syndrome, see your doctor to rule out anemia. We believe that taking the proper vitamin and mineral supplements is the best approach to this problem. The supplements that help this condition more than anything are calcium, potassium, magnesium, and zinc. The following nutrients may prevent restless leg syndrome and leg cramps: 400 milligrams of B complex, 1,000 milligrams of magnesium, and 200 international units of vitamin E (d-alpha-tocopherol) per day.

❑ Type 2 diabetes and sleep apnea are commonly seen together. In one study, patients who used a device called CPAP (continuous positive airway pressure) while sleeping experienced lower blood sugar levels and less fluctuations in blood sugar.

❑ Regardless of how many hours of sleep you get each night, if you wake up easily in the morning, and especially if you rarely (or ever) need the services of your alarm clock, and if you can make it through the entire day without seeming to run out of steam or feeling drowsy after sitting quietly or reading for a while, you are probably getting enough sleep.

❑ The hormonal shifts that occur during premenstrual syndrome and menopause may trigger insomnia. Estrogen affects the production and balance of the brain chemicals responsible for wakefulness.

❑ 5-hydroxy L-tryptophan (5-HTP) and the amino acid tryptophan are helpful for insomnia and depression. For more information, *see under* AMINO ACIDS and NATURAL FOOD SUPPLEMENTS in Part One.

❑ Dehydroepiandrosterone (DHEA) is a naturally occurring hormone that improves the quality of sleep. (*See* DHEA THERAPY in Part Three.)

❑ Anyone who snores excessively should be evaluated for sleep apnea. Many cases of sleep apnea respond to such measures as allergy treatment, weight reduction, or a simple laser surgery procedure to remove obstructions in the nasal passages.

❑ Mild cases of obstructional sleep apnea can sometimes be treated with lifestyle and diet changes. Oral devices are available for mild cases to prevent obstruction of the airway by holding the tongue or jaw forward.

❑ An effective treatment for snoring is the use of radio waves to reduce the soft palate tissue that obstructs the air passage in the mouth. In this technique, a health care practitioner inserts a probe into the back of the mouth and the radio waves are directed at the palate.

❑ Millions of Americans consciously choose to skimp on their sleep in the mistaken belief that sleeping fewer hours allows them to be more productive. Many people even look on the fact that they can "get by" on so few hours of sleep as a badge of honor. In fact, however, they are likely doing themselves a great deal of harm in the long run. Moreover, the night owls who sleep less to accomplish more are actually less creative and less productive than those who get adequate amounts of sleep. Dr. Richard Bootzin, professor of psychology and director of the insomnia clinic at the University of Arizona Sleep Disorders Center, conducted long-term research into normal sleep habits and patterns. He discovered that people who get seven to eight hours of sleep each night live longer, happier, healthier lives than those who skimp on their sleep.

❑ Sleep therapists and other experts are greatly divided about the virtues of napping. While some maintain that napping is not necessary for people who are well rested, others say it is a natural human tendency and should not be discouraged. There have been studies that seem to demonstrate that productivity is higher and the incidence of accidents lower in countries where napping is common.

❑ Consistency is probably the most important factor for healthy sleep. While it is usually most advisable to consolidate all sleeping into one time period, if you regularly take an afternoon nap and you do not suffer from any sleeping disorders, then giving up naps might actually cause a disruption in your sleeping habits. If you nap, keep your naps short—less than an hour—and make sure that they are a *regular* part of the daily routine, not a now-and-then proposition.

❑ Sleep experts advise that people with insomnia avoid caffeine, but many people who are accustomed to drinking coffee late in the day and in the evening hours have been known to have their sleep cycles disrupted if they give up drinking coffee. This seems to bear out the idea that maintaining a steady routine is the most important factor in establishing a healthy sleep pattern. Of course, this applies only to those who are not experiencing any difficulties with their sleeping habits. Anyone who develops a bout of insomnia should consider eliminating all caffeine from his or her diet.

❑ Many people who suffer from insomnia resort to taking sleeping pills, whether over-the-counter or prescription medications. Sleeping pills do not cure insomnia, and they can interfere with REM sleep. The continued use of pharmacological sleeping aids can eventually lead to disruption of all the deeper stages of sleep. Researchers have found that many people who take sleeping pills on a regular basis actually find that their insomnia becomes worse. The persistent use of sleeping pills also leads to dependency, either psychological or physical. The use of sleep medication should therefore be reserved for those whose insomnia has a physical basis, and then only as a temporary solution.

❑ Tranquilizers like the benzodiazepines and similar medications are being prescribed for insomnia because they pose a lower risk of overdose than sedatives. However, they become less effective after thirty days of use. The most prescribed include quazepam (Doral), estazolam

(ProSom), flurazepam (Dalmane), temazepam (Restoril), and triazolam (Halcion). Triazolam can cause mental confusion and even amnesia. There have also been reports that drugs such as temazepam, flurazepam, and diazepam (Valium) may lead to confusion, sluggishness, restlessness, and heightened anxiety, as well as prolonged sedation and drug dependency. Elderly people need a smaller dose than younger people. All of these products are dangerous if mixed with alcohol.

❑ Zolpidem (Ambien) and Eszopiclone (Lunesta) are a different type of prescription sleep-aid drug. Their manufacturers claim that they do not inhibit or disrupt the deep-sleep cycles, like REM.

❑ People over sixty-five years of age who use sleeping pills have four times the risk of suicide.

❑ Over-the-counter sleep aids can cause a wide range of side effects, including agitation, confusion, depression, dry mouth, and worsening of symptoms of enlarged prostate. Check with your doctor before using over-the-counter sleep medicines for short-term insomnia. These drugs use sedating antihistamines to make you drowsy. Examples include diphenhydramine (in Nytol and other products) and doxylamine (Unisom and others). People with breathing problems, glaucoma, or chronic bronchitis; women who are pregnant or nursing; and men who have difficulty urinating due to an enlarged prostate should not use these medicines. People with sleep apnea should not take sleep-promoting medicine because it could suppress their respiratory drive, making it harder to wake up when they experience episodes of interrupted breathing.

❑ *See also under* PREGNANCY-RELATED PROBLEMS.

IRRITABLE BOWEL SYNDROME

Irritable bowel syndrome (IBS) is the most common digestive disorder seen by physicians. It is estimated that approximately 10 to 15 percent of the U.S. population have symptoms of IBS, although fewer than half of them seek a physician's help for it. More than twice as many women suffer from the condition as men. IBS is also sometimes called *intestinal neurosis, mucous colitis, spastic colitis,* or *spastic colon,* but these are outdated terms. Irritable bowel syndrome is one of a range of conditions known as functional gastrointestinal disorders. In IBS, this disorder of functioning is with the way nerves and muscles are working. In the doctor's office nothing abnormal is seen on tests. The bowels look fine. Yet there is pain, discomfort, and other symptoms that won't go away or keep coming back.

In IBS, the normally rhythmic muscular contractions of the digestive tract become irregular and uncoordinated. This interferes with the normal movement of food and waste material, and leads to the accumulation of mucus and toxins in the intestine. This accumulated material sets up a partial obstruction of the digestive tract, trapping gas and stools, which in turn causes bloating, distention, and constipation. IBS may affect the entire gastrointestinal tract, from the mouth through the colon. There are no physical signs of disease in bowel tissue with this disorder, and its cause is unknown, but one theory is that irregularities in the intestinal hormones responsible for bowel motility, cholecystokinin (CCK), motilin, and vasoactive intestinal peptide (VIP), are behind this disorder. According to this theory, people with IBS have abnormal contractions of the smooth muscle of the digestive tract. Some scientists believe a virus or bacterium may play a role. Lifestyle factors such as stress and diet are probably common causes, as are food allergies. The overuse of antibiotics, antacids, or laxatives, which disturb the bacterial microflora of the bowel, may also be a factor.

Symptoms of IBS may include abdominal pain, anorexia, bloating, constipation and/or diarrhea (often alternating), flatulence, intolerances to certain foods, mucus in the stools, and nausea. Pain is often triggered by eating and may be relieved by a bowel movement. Because of the pain, diarrhea, nausea, and sometimes severe headaches and even vomiting, a person with IBS may dread eating. Whether or not an individual with IBS eats normally, malnutrition may result because nutrients often are not absorbed properly. As a result, people with IBS require as much as 30 percent more protein than normal, as well as an increased intake of minerals and trace elements, which can quickly be depleted by diarrhea.

Many other diseases can be related to IBS, including candidiasis, colon cancer, diabetes mellitus, gallbladder disease, malabsorption disorders, pancreatic insufficiency, ulcers, and the parasitic infections amebiasis and giardiasis. More than a hundred different disorders may be linked to the systemic effects of IBS. One disorder that is linked in about 25 percent of adults with IBS is arthritis, usually peripheral arthritis, which affects the ankles, knees, and wrists. Less frequently, the spine is affected. IBS can also be related to skin disorders, but this is unusual. Some people with IBS have abnormalities in the levels of liver enzymes in their blood.

Diagnosis of irritable bowel syndrome requires ruling out disorders that can cause similar symptoms, such as celiac disease, colon cancer or benign tumors, Crohn's disease, depression, diverticulitis, endometriosis, focal impaction, food poisoning, infectious diarrhea, ischemic or ulcerative colitis, and lactose intolerance. A physician may recommend one or more of a variety of procedures to do this, including barium enema, colonoscopy, rectal biopsy, sigmoidoscopy, and stool examination to check for the presence of bacteria, blood, and/or parasites.

Irritable bowel syndrome is painful, but not serious, and most people who have it can lead active, productive lives if they change their diets, get regular exercise, and replace needed nutrients.

Unless otherwise specified, the dosages recommended here are for adults. For children between the ages of twelve and seventeen, reduce the dose to three-quarters the recommended amount. For children between six and twelve, use one-half the recommended dose, and for children under the age of six, use one-quarter the recommended amount.

NUTRIENTS

SUPPLEMENT	SUGGESTED DOSAGE	COMMENTS
Very Important		
Acidophilus (Bio-Bifidus from American Biologics)	As directed on label.	To replenish the "friendly" bacteria. Needed for digestion and for the manufacture of the B vitamins. Use a nondairy formula.
Essential fatty acids (flaxseed oil or primrose oil)	As directed on label.	Needed to protect the intestinal lining.
L-glutamine	500 mg twice daily, on an empty stomach. Take with water or juice. Do not take with milk. Take with 50 mg vitamin B_6 and 100 mg vitamin C for better absorption.	A major metabolic fuel for the intestinal cells; maintains the villi, the absorption surfaces of the gut. (*See* AMINO ACIDS in Part One.)
Vitamin B complex	50–100 mg of each major B vitamin 3 times daily, with meals (amounts of individual vitamins in a complex will vary).	Needed for proper muscle tone in the gastrointestinal tract.
plus extra vitamin B_{12}	1,000–2,000 mcg daily.	Needed for proper absorption of foods, protein synthesis, and metabolism of carbohydrates and fats, and to prevent anemia. Use a lozenge or sublingual form.
Important		
Colostrum (Colostrum Plus from Symbiotics or Colostrum Prime Life from Jarrow Formulas)	As directed on label.	Heals intestinal lining and aids in nutrient absorption.
Fiber (oat bran, flaxseeds, psyllium seeds, or ABC Aerobic Bulk Cleanse from Aerobic Life Industries)	As directed on label. Take separately from other supplements and medications.	Has both a healing and cleansing effect. Avoid wheat bran, as it may be too irritating.
Free form amino acid	As directed on label.	Necessary for repair of mucous membranes of the intestines.
Garlic (Kyolic from Wakunaga)	As directed on label.	Aids in digestion and destruction of toxins in the colon. Liquid form is best.
Multivitamin and mineral complex	As directed on label.	Supplies those nutrients lost or not absorbed. Use a hypoallergenic formula.
N-Acetylglucosamine (N-A-G from Source Naturals)	As directed on label.	A major constituent of the intestinal lining and of the barrier layer that protects the intestinal lining from digestive enzymes and other potentially damaging intestinal contents.
Proteolytic enzymes with pancreatin	As directed on label.	To aid in protein digestion and prevention of "leaky gut syndrome." Also aids in reducing inflammation. Use a formula that is low in HCl and high in pancreatin.
Quercetin	As directed on label.	Helps control the allergic response to foods.
Ultra Clear Sustain from Metagenics	As directed on label.	A complex that provides nutritional support for gastrointestinal mucosa. Available only through health care professionals.
Helpful		
Calcium and magnesium	2,000 mg daily. 1,000 mg daily.	Help the "nervous stomach" and the central nervous system. Aid in preventing colon cancer. Use chelate forms.
Dioxychlor	As directed on label.	Destroys foreign bacteria in the digestive tract and carries oxygen to the tissues.

Herbs

❑ If you have IBS, it is wise to treat your liver as well as your digestive tract, preferably with silymarin (milk thistle extract). Licorice can also be used. Other beneficial herbs are burdock root and red clover, which are good for cleansing the bloodstream, and thereby the liver.

Caution: Licorice root should not be used during pregnancy or nursing. It should not be used by persons with diabetes, glaucoma, heart disease, high blood pressure, or a history of stroke.

❑ Alfalfa contains vitamin K, needed to build intestinal flora for proper digestion, and chlorophyll for healing and cleansing of the bloodstream. It can be taken in liquid or tablet form.

❑ Aloe vera is healing to the digestive tract. Used in combination with ABC Aerobic Bulk Cleanse from Aerobic Life Industries, it helps to keep the colon walls clean of excess mucus and slow down food reactions. Take ½ cup of aloe vera juice three times daily, on an empty stomach.

❑ Peppermint aids in healing and digestion, and also relieves upset stomach and gas or that "too-full" feeling. It must be taken in enteric-coated capsule form to prevent the oil from being released before it reaches the colon. Do not take any other form, or heartburn may result.

❑ Skullcap and valerian root are helpful for the nerves that regulate intestinal muscle function. These are good taken at bedtime or when an upset occurs.

❑ Other herbs that can be beneficial for irritable bowel syndrome include balm, chamomile, fenugreek, ginger, goldenseal, lobelia, marshmallow, pau d'arco, and rose hips.

Cautions: Do not use chamomile if you are allergic to ragweed. Do not use during pregnancy or nursing. It may interact with warfarin or cyclosporine, so patients using these drugs should avoid it. Do not take goldenseal internally on a daily basis for more than one week at a time. Do not use it during pregnancy or if you are breast-feeding, and use with caution if you are allergic to ragweed. If you have a history of cardiovascular disease, diabetes, or glaucoma, use it only under a doctor's supervision. Lobelia is only to be taken under supervision of a health care professional as it is potentially toxic. People with high blood pressure, heart disease, liver disease, kidney disease, seizure disorders, or shortness of breath should not take lobelia. Pregnant and lactating women should avoid lobelia as well.

❏ The Indian herb myrobalan (*Terminalia chebula*) alleviates diarrhea, dysentery, and many other digestive complaints.

Recommendations

❏ Eat a high-fiber diet including plenty of vegetables, whole grains (especially brown rice), and legumes. However, be careful of fruit; fructose and fructans may cause worsening of symptoms—limit intake of all fruit and juices to two servings per day. Eating less fruit may result in fewer symptoms with less severity.

❏ Use supplemental fiber. Psyllium powder regulates bowel movements and should be used daily. Also use oat bran and ground flaxseeds daily, on an alternating basis.

❏ Avoid animal fats, butter, all carbonated beverages, coffee and all other substances containing caffeine, candy, chocolate, all dairy products, fried foods, ice cream, all junk foods, the additives mannitol and sorbitol, margarine, nuts, orange and grapefruit juices, pastries, all processed foods, seeds, spicy foods, sugar, sugar-free chewing gum, and wheat bran and wheat products. These foods encourage the secretion of mucus by the membranes and prevent the uptake of nutrients.

❏ Limit your consumption of gas-producing foods such as beans, broccoli, and cabbage if they cause any problems.

❏ Avoid alcohol and tobacco; these irritate the linings of the stomach and colon.

❏ When an intestinal upset occurs, switch to a bland diet. Put vegetables and nonacidic fruits through a food processor or blender. Organic baby food is good. If you are on a soft diet, take some type of fiber and a protein supplement.

❏ To relieve occasional gas and bloating, use charcoal tablets (available in health food stores). Take 5 tablets as soon as this problem arises. Do not use charcoal daily, however, because it also absorbs needed nutrients, and do not take it at the same time as other supplements or medications.

❏ For excessive gas and bloating that lingers, read the section on ENEMAS in Part Three and follow the instructions for the retention enema. This will replace the "friendly" bacteria very quickly and resolve the problem. Exercise, such as stretching exercises, swimming, or walking, is also important.

Caution: If you are thirty-five or older and/or have been sedentary for some time, consult with your health care provider before beginning an exercise program.

❏ Check to see if you have food allergies; they are important factors in this disorder. Eliminating allergenic foods from the diet relieves symptoms in many cases. (*See* ALLERGIES in Part Two.)

❏ Chew your food well. Do not overeat or eat in a hurry.

❏ Practice deep-breathing exercises. Shallow breathing reduces the oxygen available for proper bowel function.

❏ Wear loose-fitting clothing. Do not wear anything that is tight around the waist.

❏ Do not eat right before going to bed. Wait one or two hours after eating before lying down.

❏ *See* ACID/ALKALI IMBALANCE in Part Two and take the self-test. Significant acidosis may occur with IBS.

Considerations

❏ Eating the correct diet, using supplemental fiber, and drinking plenty of quality water are very important in controlling IBS. Early recognition of the disease, good nutrition, and a positive outlook help minimize complications.

❏ It takes between twelve and fifteen hours for food to be completely processed. Food such as meat can take longer, whereas fresh foods, raw foods, or lightly steamed foods are processed much more quickly.

❏ Certain foods irritate the wall of the intestinal tract. Lactose (milk sugar) is a common culprit, as are all dairy products. Avoid grains, nuts, and seeds until symptoms subside. Always chew these types of foods until they are almost liquefied in the mouth.

❏ As with other chronic conditions, alternative therapies are popular for treating IBS symptoms. In one study, the most commonly tried alternative treatments included lifestyle modifications such as dietary changes, yoga, acupuncture, and using suppositories.

❏ IBS should not be confused with the more serious bowel disorders, such as Crohn's disease and ulcerative colitis. These are also inflammatory bowel diseases but, unlike IBS, they result in demonstrable lesions in the digestive tract. Crohn's disease affects the entire length and thickness of the wall of the large and/or small intestine; ulcerative colitis affects the lining of the large intestine, the last five to seven feet of the digestive tract. (*See* CROHN'S DISEASE and/or ULCERATIVE COLITIS, both in Part Two.)

❏ People with irritable bowel syndrome are also likely to have associated conditions such as dysphagia (difficulty swallowing), gastroesophageal reflux disease (GERD), globus sensation (a feeling of having a ball in the throat), gynecological problems, heartburn, noncardiac chest pain, and urologic dysfunction.

❏ An imbalance of gut flora is common for those with irritable bowel syndrome. Usually, the pathogenic flora outnumber the friendly bacteria. This can be corrected somewhat with probiotics (live microorganisms) and prebiotics (fiber).

❑ People with IBS should receive regular physical examinations. This disorder has been linked to a higher than normal incidence of colon cancer and diverticulitis.

❑ If IBS causes chronic diarrhea, electrolyte and trace mineral deficiencies are likely. (*See* DIARRHEA in Part Two for suggested mineral supplementation. *See also* MALABSORPTION SYNDROME in Part Two.)

❑ Certain drugs can aggravate the malabsorption problems often present with IBS. These include antibiotics, corticosteroids, cholestyramine (Questran), and sulfasalazine (Azulfidine), among others. These drugs increase the need for nutritional supplements.

❑ Antispasmodic drugs (Di-Spaz, Lomotil) and antidiarrheal drugs (Imodium) slow the function of the gastrointestinal tract and are regularly prescribed for irritable bowel syndrome. However, they have serious side effects and can induce dependency. Some health practitioners have also prescribed highly addictive tranquilizers and antidepressants. Consult a pediatrician before using any of these or any drugs for children.

❑ Many people with irritable bowel syndrome have experienced improvements in symptoms after using Chinese herbal medicine (CHM).

❑ In one study, children eight to eighteen years of age with IBS benefited from gut-directed hypnotherapy. After one year, the children in this study experienced less pain and less frequent attacks. The authors concluded that this was a highly effective therapy for children. This practice has also been shown to be effective for adults.

❑ Research and testing have found not only that breathing exercises can control IBS, but that people who practice stress management have fewer and less severe attacks. Stress management also relieves symptoms. (*See* STRESS in Part Two. *Also see* BREATHING EXERCISES *under* PAIN CONTROL in Part Three.)

❑ The symptoms of IBS are similar to those of many other disorders, including cancer. If dietary modification and natural remedies yield no relief, it is wise to consult a physician to rule out some other underlying problem. We recommend this only after natural remedies have been tried, however.

❑ *See also* DIVERTICULITIS; HEARTBURN; and/or INDIGESTION in Part Two.

JAUNDICE

Jaundice is a yellowing of the skin and eyes that is caused by a buildup of bilirubin in the blood. Bilirubin is a yellow-brown substance that results from the breakdown of old red blood cells. If this waste product is not removed from the bloodstream by the liver, as it should be, a backup of bilirubin in the blood occurs, producing a yellowing of the skin and the whites of the eyes. The urine may be darker than normal, while the stools may appear lighter. Jaundice may be accompanied by edema (fluid retention) in the trunk of the body, fatigue, generalized itching, nausea, rashes on the skin, and vomiting. If you suspect you have jaundice, seek medical attention.

Jaundice is not a disease in itself, but a sign of any one of several blood or liver disorders. Among the conditions that can cause jaundice are cirrhosis of the liver, pernicious anemia, hepatitis, and hemolysis (abnormal destruction of red blood cells). Jaundice can also be a sign of an obstruction in the path of the bile flow, from the liver through the bile ducts to the gallbladder, and then to the intestinal tract. If any part of the biliary tract is obstructed for some reason, the bile (which contains bilirubin) passes back into the bloodstream instead of into the digestive system, producing jaundice. Occasionally, jaundice is caused by some form of parasitic infestation such as tapeworm or hookworm, or a bite from a flea or mosquito that carries a viral, bacterial, or parasitic infection. It can also be caused by a tumor, a gallstone, or inflammation.

Some degree of jaundice is common in newborn babies, especially premature babies, and is not considered serious. It occurs because a new baby's liver is limited in its ability to process bilirubin, and in most cases soon resolves itself. Some babies are placed under a heating lamp to speed up the removal of the excess bilirubin.

Unless otherwise specified, the dosages recommended here are for adults. For children between the ages of twelve and seventeen, reduce the dose to three-quarters the recommended amount. For children between six and twelve, use one-half the recommended dose, and for children under the age of six, use one-quarter the recommended amount.

NUTRIENTS

SUPPLEMENT	SUGGESTED DOSAGE	COMMENTS
Very Important		
Coenzyme Q10 plus	As directed on label.	Promotes tissue oxygenation and removes toxic substances from the body.
Coenzyme A from Coenzyme-A Technologies	As directed on label.	Works with coenzyme Q10 to support the immune system's detoxification of many dangerous substances.
Colostrum (Colostrum Plus from Symbiotics)	As directed on label.	Improves immune function and protects the liver.
Grape seed extract	As directed on label.	A powerful antioxidant that aids the liver in removing toxic substances from the body.
Kyo-Dophilus from Wakunaga	As directed on label.	Protects the liver and the intestinal tract.
Kyolic from Wakunaga	As directed on label.	Potent immune enhancer.
L-glutathione and L-methionine	500 mg each daily, on an empty stomach. Take with water or juice. Do not take with milk. Take with 50 mg	Substances that work together to protect the liver. (*See* AMINO ACIDS in Part One.)

		vitamin B$_6$ and 100 mg vitamin C for better absorption.
Liquid Kyolic with B$_1$ and B$_{12}$ from Wakunaga	As directed on label.	An excellent liver detoxifier.
Raw liver extract	As directed on label.	Aids in building the liver. (*See* GLANDULAR THERAPY in Part Three.) Use liver from organically raised beef.
S-Adenosylmethio-nine(SAMe)	As directed on label.	Aids in relief of stress and depression, eases pain, and produces antioxidant effects that can improve the health of the liver. *Caution:* Do not use if you have bipolar mood disorder or take prescription antidepressants. Do not give to a child under twelve.
Vitamin B complex	50 mg of each major B vitamin three times daily (amounts of individual vitamins in a complex will vary).	The B vitamins are necessary for proper digestion, absorption of nutrients, and formation of red blood cells. They help to maintain the health of the eyes, liver, and skin. Use a high-potency formula.
Vitamin C with bioflavonoids	3,000–6,000 mg daily.	Vitamin C combines with toxic substances, renders them harmless, and removes them from the body.

Herbs

❏ Burdock root and red clover aid in cleansing the blood.

❏ Celandine, and dandelion aid in cleansing the liver.

❏ Oregano is good for relieving jaundice.

❏ Silymarin, an active flavonoid extracted from the herb milk thistle, is known to repair damaged tissues in the liver. Liv-R-Actin from Nature's Plus is a good source of silymarin.

Recommendations

❏ Eat only raw vegetables and fruits for one week. Then eat a diet consisting of 75 percent raw food for a month. Take fresh lemon enemas daily during this period. This is for adults only. (*See* ENEMAS in Part Three.)

❏ Use the spices coriander and turmeric in your cooking. These are good liver cleansers.

❏ Drink the following juices: lemon juice and water, beet and beet greens, and dandelion or black radish extract. All are good for rebuilding and cleansing the liver.

❏ Never consume raw or undercooked fish, meat, or poultry. All raw fish pose a risk of infection from bacteria, parasites, and viruses.

❏ Do not consume *any* alcohol. Alcohol places a great strain on the liver, which can aggravate the condition even further.

Considerations

❏ If jaundice is a result of a tumor or gallstone, surgery may be necessary to correct the problem.

❏ To diagnose the problem that is causing jaundice, your physician may perform a blood test, liver biopsy, or ultrasound scan of the liver.

❏ *See* CIRRHOSIS OF THE LIVER and HEPATITIS, both in Part Two, for additional nutritional and dietary suggestions.

JOB SYNDROME

See HYPERIMMUNOGLOBULIN E [HYPER-IGE] SYNDROME *under* RARE DISORDERS.

JOCK ITCH

See under FUNGAL INFECTION.

KAPOSI'S SARCOMA

See under SKIN CANCER.

KIDNEY DISEASE (RENAL FAILURE)

Kidneys remove waste products from the body, keep body chemicals in balance, and help maintain the body's water balance. There are a number of different renal (kidney) problems that may occur. The kidneys may be damaged by exposure to certain drugs or toxins, including heavy metals, solvents, chemotherapy agents, snake or insect venom, poisonous mushrooms, and pesticides. Renal failure can also accompany or result from many other disorders, such as congestive heart failure, diabetes, chronic hypertension, liver disease, lupus, and sickle-cell anemia. If you think your kidneys are not working properly, consult your health care provider.

Bright's disease is a kidney disease marked by the presence of blood protein in the urine, along with hypertension and edema (retention of water in the tissues). Glomerulonephritis is an inflammation of tiny blood vessels within the kidneys that filter out wastes from the blood. This may occur as a result of an immunological response to infection, such as a *Streptococcus* throat infection. Pyelonephritis is a kidney infection that may be caused by a birth defect. Both glomerulonephritis and pyelonephritis can be chronic or acute, and can be serious. Hydronephrosis is a condition in which the kidneys and the renal pelvis (the structure into which urine is discharged from the kidneys) become filled with urine due to an obstruction of urinary flow. Polycystic kidney disease (PKD) is an inherited disease in which cysts grow on the kidneys, rendering them incapable of functioning. Kidney stones are mineral accumulations (primarily calcium) in the kidneys. In renal tubular acidosis, the kidneys fail to reabsorb bicarbonate normally, causing impaired ammonia production and acid excretion. Severe acidosis, potassium depletion, and bone disorders may result. Nephrotic syndrome is not a disease in itself, but can be a sign of kidney disease. It is marked by edema and excess protein in the urine. It can be caused by lesions of glomeruli (small structures in the kidneys made of capillaries) that become inflamed, or by chronic diseases such as diabetes or lupus.

One important symptom of kidney problems is edema. Edema results when the kidneys produce less urine because they are unable to properly excrete salt and other wastes, and fluid builds up in the body. Ankles and hands may swell, and the person becomes short of breath. Toxic wastes may accumulate in the bloodstream due to kidney malfunction, a condition known as uremia. Symptoms of kidney problems include abdominal pain, appetite loss, back pain, chills, fever, fluid retention (bloating), nausea, urinary urgency, and vomiting. The urine may be cloudy or bloody. Back pain may be sudden and intense, occurring just above the waist and running down the groin.

The following supplements aid in controlling urinary tract infection, and help maintain proper kidney function. Unless otherwise specified, the dosages recommended here are for adults. For children between the ages of twelve and seventeen, reduce the dose to three-quarters of the recommended amount. For children between six and twelve, use one-half of the recommended dose, and for children under the age of six, use one-quarter of the recommended amount.

NUTRIENTS

SUPPLEMENT	SUGGESTED DOSAGE	COMMENTS
Very Important		
Acidophilus (Kyo-Dophilus from Wakunaga)	As directed on label, 3 times daily. Take on an empty stomach.	Especially important if you are taking antibiotics.
Coenzyme A from Coenzyme-A Technologies	As directed on label.	Acts as an antioxidant and removes harmful substances from the body.
Vitamin B$_6$ (pyridoxine)	50 mg 3 times daily.	To reduce fluid retention.
plus choline	50 mg daily.	
and inositol hexaphosphate (IP$_6$)	100 mg daily.	
Vitamin C with bioflavonoids	2,000–4,000 mg daily.	Acidifies the urine, boosts immune function, and aids healing.
Helpful		
Calcium	1,500 mg daily.	For proper mineral balance; calcium and magnesium should be in a 2-to-1 ratio in the body. Do not use bone meal, oyster shells, or dolomite as a source.
and magnesium	750 mg daily.	Important in water absorption.
L-arginine and L-methionine	500 mg 4 times daily.	For kidney disease.
	As directed on label, on an empty stomach. Take with water or juice. Do not take with milk. Take with 50 mg vitamin B$_6$ and 100 mg vitamin C for better absorption.	For improved kidney circulation. (*See* AMINO ACIDS in Part One.)
Lecithin granules or capsules	1 tbsp 3 times daily, before meals. 1,200 mg 3 times daily, before meals.	Needed for nephritis.
Multienzyme complex	As directed on label.	Necessary for digestion. *Caution:* Do not give this supplement to a child under sixteen years except as directed by physician.
plus hydrochloric acid (HCl)	As directed on label.	Particularly important for older adults, who tend to be deficient. *Caution:* Do not take HCl if you have a history of ulcers.
Multimineral complex	As directed on label.	Corrects mineral depletion, common with kidney disease. Use a high-potency formula.
Vitamin A with mixed carotenoids	100,000 IU daily for 3 days, then 50,000 IU daily for 5 days, then reduce to 25,000 IU daily. If you are pregnant, do not exceed 10,000 IU daily.	Important in healing of urinary tract lining and in immune function. Use emulsion form for easier assimilation and greater safety at high doses. Do not take this amount in pill form.
Vitamin B complex	100 mg of each major B vitamin daily (amounts of individual vitamins in a complex will vary).	B vitamins work best when taken together. Use a high-potency formula.
plus extra vitamin B$_2$ (riboflavin)	25 mg 3 times daily.	Needed for nephritis.
Vitamin E emulsion	200 IU daily or 400 IU every other day.	Promotes immune function. An important free radical destroyer. Use d-alpha-tocopherol form.
Zinc	50–80 mg daily. Do not exceed 100 mg daily from all supplements.	An immunostimulant necessary for healing and an important inhibitor of crystallization and crystal growth. Use zinc gluconate lozenges or OptiZinc for best absorption.
plus copper	3 mg daily.	Needed to balance with zinc.

Herbs

❑ Buchu tea is good. Do not boil it, however.

❑ Celery and parsley seeds are natural diuretics. Taken in combination, they are especially helpful if high uric acid levels are present in the blood. Eating large amounts of animal proteins makes one susceptible to high levels of uric acid. These two herbs help keep them in check.

❑ Cranberries contain substances that acidify the urine, destroy bacterial buildup, and promote healing of the bladder. Drink at least 8 ounces of cranberry juice three times daily. Use only pure, unsweetened juice (available at health food stores). Do not substitute a commercial cranberry juice cocktail product; these contain large amounts of sugar. If natural cranberry juice is not available, cranberry capsules can be used as a substitute. Cranberry supplements are also available, and work just as well.

❏ Dandelion root extract aids in excretion of the kidney's waste products and is very beneficial for nephritis.

❏ The herbs hydrangea and uva ursi are excellent natural diuretics. One of the best first steps in cleaning out the urinary tract and keeping it healthy is to help it flush itself. Voiding the urinary tract keeps harmful deposits of calcium or other mineral salts from forming obstructions. Uva ursi is also slightly germicidal, so if there are any bacteria present, they will likely be destroyed by it.

❏ Marshmallow tea helps to cleanse the kidneys. Drink 1 quart daily.

❏ Kidney Blend SP-6 from Solaray helps reduce water retention. Kidney Bladder Formula from Nature's Way is also a good herbal diuretic.

❏ Other herbs that are beneficial for kidney problems include goldenrod tea, juniper berries, marshmallow root, nettle, parsley, red clover, and watermelon seed tea.

Recommendations

❏ Consume a diet composed of 75 percent raw foods. Eat asparagus, bananas, celery, cucumbers, garlic, papaya, parsley, potatoes, and watercress. Watermelon and pumpkin seeds are also beneficial. Watermelon should be eaten by itself so that it passes through the system quickly; if it stays in the body too long, toxins begin to form. Also eat sprouts and most green vegetables. Raw foods tend to be high in potassium. Potassium may be difficult for the kidneys to clear from the blood in people with kidney disease. Check with your physician before following this recommendation.

❏ Include in the diet legumes, seeds, and soybeans. These foods contain the amino acid arginine, which is beneficial for the kidneys.

❏ Reduce your intake of potassium and phosphates if your levels of these are elevated. Do not use any salt or potassium chloride, a salt substitute. Also avoid beet greens, chocolate, cocoa, eggs, fish, meat, rhubarb, spinach, Swiss chard, and tea.

❏ If you have symptoms of kidney problems, especially blood in the urine or severe back pain, consult your health care provider promptly. You may need medical treatment.

❏ Drink 8 to 10 ounces of steam-distilled water every waking hour. Quality water is essential for urinary tract function.

❏ Reduce your intake of animal protein, or eliminate it altogether. A diet high in animal protein puts stress on the kidneys. Excess accumulation of protein can result in uremia. Protein is easiest to utilize if it has been broken down into free form amino acids. Other good protein sources include beans, lentils, millet, peas, soybeans, and whole grains.

❏ Avoid all dairy products except for those that are soured, such as low-fat yogurt, buttermilk, and cottage cheese.

❏ Try a raw goat's milk diet for two weeks, consuming nothing but 4 quarts of raw goat's milk, warmed to body temperature, each day. Add 1 tablespoon of crude blackstrap molasses to each quart. During this period, take 1,000 international units of vitamin E and 75,000 international units of vitamin A in emulsion form.

Caution: If you are pregnant, this diet is not recommended.

❏ Try a three-day cleansing and juice fast, and coffee or catnip tea enemas. (*See* ENEMAS and FASTING in Part Three.)

❏ If you are taking antibiotics for a kidney problem, do not take iron supplements as long as the problem exists.

Considerations

❏ To test for kidney failure, a doctor can test your urine for levels of albumin protein, creatinine (waste from muscle cells), hemoglobin (if the kidneys are not working properly, hemoglobin levels may fall), phosphorus, potassium, and urea (waste from protein you have eaten). The most common tests are BUN (blood urea nitrogen) and serum creatinine.

❏ Lead and other metallic poisons are very harmful to the kidneys. Anyone who works with lead, or who is exposed to lead regularly, should take precautions to protect his or her kidneys from damage. (*See* LEAD POISONING in Part Two.)

❏ If you have diabetes, high blood sugar, high blood pressure, or a family history of kidney disease, you may be at higher risk for kidney disease.

❏ A study reported in the *Journal of Nutritional and Environmental Medicine* found that treatment with coenzyme Q_{10} decreased the progression of kidney disease and also reversed renal dysfunction in a majority of patients with end-stage disease.

❏ Infectious diseases, such as measles, scarlet fever, and tonsillitis, can damage the kidneys if not treated properly and completely.

❏ A study at the pharmaceutical department of Chiba University in Japan found that spirulina reduced kidney poisoning caused by mercury and drugs. Researchers discovered that adverse effects of certain drugs on the kidneys also may be decreased by the use of spirulina.

❏ Human growth hormone treatment can improve kidney function. (*See* GROWTH HORMONE THERAPY in Part Three.)

❏ Recurrent urinary tract infections indicate the possibility of a serious underlying problem. See your health care provider.

❏ High doses of the painkiller ibuprofen (Advil, Nuprin, and others) can lead to kidney dysfunction.

❏ A home dialysis system is available for those requiring dialysis treatments.

❏ *See also* BLADDER INFECTION and KIDNEY STONES in Part Two.

KIDNEY STONES

Kidney stones, medically termed *renal calculi,* are accumulations of mineral salts that can lodge anywhere along the course of the urinary tract, and they can be one of the most painful of all health ailments. Human urine is often saturated to the limit with uric acid, phosphates, and calcium oxalate. Normally, due to the secretion of various protective compounds and natural mechanisms that control the pH of urine, these substances remain suspended in solution.

However, if the protective compounds are overwhelmed or immunity becomes depressed, the substances may crystallize and the crystals may begin to clump together, eventually forming stones large enough to restrict urinary flow. These stones can be jagged or smooth. Symptoms of kidney stones include pain radiating from the upper back to the lower abdomen and groin, profuse sweating, frequent urination, pus and blood in the urine, odorous or cloudy urine, absence of urine formation, nausea and vomiting, and, sometimes, chills and fever. In milder cases, the symptoms may mimic a bad case of stomach flu or other gastrointestinal ailment.

An estimated 1.5 percent of Americans develop kidney stones at some point in their lives. They are most common in white men between the ages of thirty and fifty, although if you are prone to kidney stones, they can occur as early as your twenties. Kidney stones are rare in children and in African-Americans. They are more prevalent in the southeastern United States (known to doctors as the "Stone Belt") than in other parts of the country. The reason for this is not known, but it is theorized that the hot climate, which promotes dehydration, and/or regional dietary habits may be to blame. Men are much more likely than women to suffer from this ailment (four out of five cases are in men). Adults have a 50 percent rate of recurrence.

Stones can range in size from microscopic specks to the size of a fingertip. There are four kinds of kidney stones: calcium stones (composed of calcium oxalate); uric acid stones; struvite stones (composed of magnesium ammonium phosphate); and cystine stones.

About 80 percent of all stones are calcium oxalate stones. High blood calcium levels lead to hypercalciuria—excessive absorption of calcium from the intestine—which increases the level of calcium in the urine. This excess calcium eventually forms a stone. High blood calcium levels can also result from malfunctioning parathyroid glands (tiny glands in the neck that regulate blood calcium levels), vitamin D intoxication, and multiple myeloma. The consumption of refined carbohydrates, especially sugar, can help precipitate kidney stones as well, because the sugar stimulates the pancreas to release insulin, which in turn causes extra calcium to be excreted in the urine. Mild chronic or recurrent dehydration can also be a factor in kidney stones; it concentrates the urine, increasing the likelihood of stone formation.

Uric acid stones form when the volume of urine excreted is too low and/or blood levels of uric acid are abnormally high. The latter condition is commonly associated with symptoms of gout. Unlike other types of kidney stones, struvite stones are unrelated to metabolism; these stones are caused by infection. Women often get them with recurrent urinary tract infections. Cystine stones are caused by a condition called cystinuria, a rare congenital defect that can cause stones composed of the amino acid cystine to form in the kidney or bladder.

Calcium stones often run in families because the tendency to absorb too much calcium is hereditary. Also, in people with a family history of kidney stones, there seems to be a stronger than normal correlation between the intake of either vitamin C or oxalic acid and the urinary excretion of oxalate. Apparently, such individuals either absorb more oxalate from their diets or metabolize greater amounts of oxalate precursors. People who have Crohn's disease or irritable bowel syndrome, or who eat diets high in oxalic acid, may have an increased risk of kidney stones as well, as these factors can cause the excretion of oxalate in the urine to increase. Other risk factors for kidney stones include low urine volume, low bodily pH, heredity, living in a tropical climate, and reduced production of natural urinary inhibitors of crystal formation.

Kidney stones are ten times as common now as they were at the start of the twentieth century. While the consumption of foods high in oxalic acid (mostly eggs, fish, and certain vegetables) has declined markedly in this country in that time, the amount of animal fats and protein in the average American's diet has increased significantly. The ratio of plant to animal protein in the typical diet at the beginning of the twentieth century was roughly 1 to 1. This ratio has since changed to 1 to 2. The consumption of animal protein is strongly associated with oxalate absorption.

Unless otherwise specified, the dosages recommended here are for adults. For children between the ages of twelve and seventeen, reduce the dose to three-quarters the recommended amount. For children between six and twelve, use one-half the recommended dose, and for children under the age of six, use one-quarter the recommended amount.

NUTRIENTS

SUPPLEMENT	SUGGESTED DOSAGE	COMMENTS
Very Important		
Inositol hexaphosphate (IP$_6$) with	As directed on label.	Has been shown in many studies to help prevent and treat kidney stones.
inositol	As directed on label.	
L-methionine	500 mg daily, on an empty stomach. Take with water or juice. Do not take with milk. Take with 50 mg vitamin B$_6$ and 100 mg vitamin C for better absorption.	Reduces the incidence of kidney stones by destroying free radicals associated with stone formation. (*See* AMINO ACIDS in Part One.)

Magnesium citrate	500 mg daily.	Reduces calcium absorption and can lower urinary oxalate, a mineral salt common in kidney stones.
Vitamin B complex	50 mg of each major B vitamin 3 times daily, with meals (amounts of individual vitamins in a complex will vary).	B vitamins work best when all are taken together.
plus extra vitamin B₆ (pyridoxine)	50 mg twice daily.	Taken with magnesium, reduces oxalate.
Zinc	50–80 mg daily. Do not exceed 100 mg daily from all supplements.	An important inhibitor of crystallization, which can lead to stone formation. Use zinc gluconate lozenges or OptiZinc for best absorption.
Helpful		
L-arginine	500 mg daily. If you are prone to herpes outbreaks, take with L-lysine.	Aids kidney disorders.
Multivitamin complex	As directed on label.	To maintain a balance of all nutrients.
Potassium	99 mg daily.	Inhibits crystallization, which can lead to stone formation. Use potassium citrate form.
Proteolytic enzymes	As directed on label. Take between meals.	Aids normal digestion.
Raw kidney glandular	500 mg daily.	Strengthens the kidneys. (*See* GLANDULAR THERAPY in Part Three.)
Vitamin A with mixed carotenoids	25,000 IU daily. If you are pregnant, do not exceed 10,000 IU daily.	Promotes healing of the urinary tract lining, which is often damaged by stones. If you are pregnant, use a natural carotenoid complex such as Betatene in place of vitamin A.
Vitamin E	200 IU daily or 400 IU every other day.	A powerful antioxidant. Use d-alpha-tocopherol form.

Herbs

❑ Aloe vera juice, taken at levels that do not produce a laxative effect, can be useful in preventing stone formation and in reducing the size of a stone during an acute attack.

❑ Ginkgo biloba and goldenseal, taken in extract form, aid circulation to the kidneys and have anti-inflammatory properties. They are also powerful antioxidants.

Cautions: Do not take ginkgo biloba if you have a bleeding disorder, or are scheduled for surgery or a dental procedure. Do not take goldenseal internally on a daily basis for more than one week at a time. Do not use it during pregnancy or if you are breast-feeding, and use with caution if you are allergic to ragweed. If you have a history of cardiovascular disease, diabetes, or glaucoma, use it only under a doctor's supervision.

❑ A combination of lobelia tincture (3 to 4 drops) and wild yam tincture (15 drops) in a glass of warm water helps to relax the ureters, relieve pain, and hasten the passing of stones. Sip this mixture throughout the day.

❑ Marshmallow root tea daily helps to cleanse the kidneys and to expel kidney stones. Drink 1 quart daily.

❑ Uva ursi helps to relieve pain and bloating.

❑ Other herbs that may aid in alleviating kidney stones include cleavers, gravel root, juniper berries, and pipsissewa (also called Prince's Pine).

Recommendations

❑ For pain relief, drink the juice of half a fresh lemon in 8 ounces of water every half-hour until the pain subsides. You can alternate between lemon juice and fresh apple juice.

❑ To maintain good kidney function, drink plenty of quality water—at least ten 8-ounce glasses daily. By far the single most important measure one can take to prevent kidney stones from forming is to increase water consumption. Water dilutes urine and helps prevent concentrations of the minerals and salts that can form stones. (Chronic dehydration is a major risk factor in kidney stone disease.) Also drink unsweetened cranberry juice to help acidify the urine (unless you are prone to uric acid stones). Drinking the juice of a fresh lemon in a glass of warm water first thing each morning can help prevent stones from forming. Lemon juice contains nearly five times the concentration of citric acid—a natural citrate source—in orange juice. One study showed people who consumed lemonade on a daily basis actually reduced stone recurrence.

❑ Increase your consumption of foods rich in vitamin A. Vitamin A is beneficial to the urinary tract and helps to discourage the formation of stones. Good sources of vitamin A include alfalfa, apricots, cantaloupes, carrots, pumpkin, sweet potatoes, and squash.

❑ Use only distilled water for drinking and cooking. Add trace mineral drops to your drinking water.

❑ Minimize your consumption of animal protein, or eliminate it from your diet altogether. A diet high in animal protein causes the body to excrete calcium, producing excessive amounts of calcium, phosphorus, and uric acid in the kidneys and often resulting in painful kidney stones.

❑ Reduce your intake of potassium and phosphates. Do not use any salt or potassium chloride, a salt substitute, and avoid carbonated soft drinks. Cola drinks are thought to be a risk factor for stone formation, while some other drinks containing citric acid may lessen stone activity. In one study, water was compared to caffeine-free Diet Coke and Fresca (citrate containing). The last two were chosen to prevent the known increase in calcium excretion promoted by caffeine and carbohydrates. With respect to stone formation, none of these three beverages differed. Thus, it seems that all sodas do not need to be removed from the diet in order to maintain healthy kidney function.

❑ Do not omit calcium from your diet—it is important in lowering your risk of developing osteoporosis, which is a much more common problem than kidney stones, especially for women. Getting extra magnesium can reduce the risk of kidney stones by increasing the solubility of calcium oxalate. Seafood, brown rice, tofu, and soybeans are naturally high in magnesium.

❏ Try drinking a large amount of liquid (preferably pure water), allow twenty minutes for digestion, and then run up and down stairs vigorously. This has been known to allow small, stubborn kidney stones to pass naturally.

❏ If you do not pass the lodged stone, see your physician. He or she may order a urine test and an X-ray for formal diagnosis and proper treatment.

❏ If you have a family history of kidney stones, take calcium supplements *with meals.* When you consume calcium-rich foods with oxalates, they bind together and are expelled in the stool, lessening your risk of kidney stones. Calcium supplements should be avoided only by those with a personal history of kidney stones.

❏ Avoid foods that contain or lead to the production of oxalic acid, including asparagus, beet greens, beets, blueberries, celery, eggs, fish, grapes, parsley, rhubarb, sorrel, spinach, Swiss chard, and vegetables of the cabbage family. Also avoid alcohol, black tea (green tea is a good substitute), chocolate, cocoa, dried figs, nuts, pepper, and poppy seeds.

Caution: Green tea contains vitamin K, which can make anticoagulant medications less effective. Consult your health care professional if you are using them. The caffeine in green tea could cause insomnia, anxiety, upset stomach, nausea, or diarrhea.

❏ Avoid all refined sugar and products that contain it. Sugar stimulates the pancreas to release insulin, which in turn causes extra calcium to be excreted in the urine.

❏ Stay active. People who are sedentary tend to accumulate high levels of calcium in the bloodstream. Exercise helps pull calcium from the blood into the bones, where it belongs.

Caution: If you are thirty-five or older and/or have been sedentary for some time, consult with your health care provider before beginning an exercise program.

❏ If you have a history of cystine stones, avoid the amino acid L-cystine. If you must take a supplement containing L-cystine, take at least three times as much vitamin C at the same time. Otherwise, cystine can crystallize in the kidneys and form large stones that fill the interior of the kidney.

Considerations

❏ A Harvard University study found that consuming dairy products may actually lower the risk of developing kidney stones, instead of increasing the risk, as was previously thought. They also found that calcium supplements raise the risk slightly unless they are taken with meals.

❏ Drinking coffee, tea, and wine may lower the risk of kidney stones, while grapefruit juice may increase it.

❏ Vitamin C at high doses poses a risk of stone formation. In one study, 40 percent of people with a history of calcium oxalate stones who took 2,000 milligrams of vitamin C a day had increased urinary oxalate levels and a higher risk of developing more stones, according to the Tiselius Risk Index (TRI). Get vitamin C from fruits and vegetables instead of supplements.

❏ In one study, people with idiopathic calcium stone formation who adhered to a low animal protein diet (less than 10 percent of total calories) had fewer kidney stones. Another group of patients in this study was assigned to a high-fiber group (greater than 25 grams per day), and this had no effect on stone formation.

❏ Some people avoid milk because they fear it may cause kidney stones. One study showed that substituting apple juice for one and a half cups of milk did not lower the risk of calcium oxalate stone formation in people with a history of kidney stones. The diet consumed in this study had moderate oxalate from whole grains, legumes, fruits, and vegetables. A healthy diet with some milk seems to not be harmful.

❏ In Japan, the incidence of kidney stones has been rising steadily since the middle of the last century, when dietary changes typical of an industrialized nation began to occur. People in Japan who develop kidney stones consume far more proteins, refined carbohydrates, fats, and oils than did their forebears.

❏ Most kidney stones eventually pass by themselves. Depending on the type and size of stone, your physician may recommend the use of electroshock wave lithotripsy (ESWL) to break up the stones, ureterscope calculus removal, or percutaneous nephrolithotomy (in which the surgeon creates a small tunnel through the skin and inserts an instrument to remove the stone), or the use of a laser or other tiny device that is threaded up the urinary tract to break up stones.

❏ Once kidney stones have formed and have been treated, the risk of recurrence increases; once a person has formed a stone, there is a 20 to 50 percent chance that he or she will form another in the next ten years. Once a second incidence has occurred, the risk increases markedly.

❏ Prescription medications containing sodium cellulose phosphate are effective on calcium-based stones. Potassium citrate (Urocit-K) is effective on stones not of calcium origin. Allopurinol (Lopurin, Zyloprim) is another medication that may help to prevent the occurrence of stones.

❏ Taking up to 100 milligrams of zinc daily can help inhibit the formation of crystals that later accumulate into stones.

Caution: While the recommended amount of zinc helps to enhance immune function, anything over 100 milligrams per day tends to depress immunity.

❏ To control calcium stones, the pH of the body should be raised, while to control uric acid stones, bodily pH should be lowered. (*See* ACID/ALKALI IMBALANCE in Part Two.)

❏ Diet alone cannot remove kidney stones, but it can be very effective at preventing them. Kidney stones are primarily an affliction of well-fed societies in which people consume large quantities of animal protein. A vegetarian diet can be of great benefit to anyone prone to kidney stones. A strict vegan diet that contains no animal proteins whatsoever, is almost entirely devoid of processed foods, and is low in sodium and high in fiber and water is generally considered conducive to kidney stone prevention.

❏ In one study, for children with intractable epilepsy who developed kidney stones, following a ketogenic diet and taking oral potassium citrate seemed to reduce the incidence of kidney stones.

❏ Measures used to treat kidney stones and to prevent recurrences depend on the nature of the stone, so it is important to take any stone you pass to your health care provider for analysis.

LACTOSE INTOLERANCE (LACTASE DEFICIENCY)

Lactose intolerance is the inability to digest lactose (milk sugar). It is caused by a lack or deficiency of lactase, an enzyme manufactured in the small intestine that splits lactose into glucose and galactose. When a person with lactose intolerance consumes milk or other dairy products, some or all of the lactose they contain remains undigested, retains fluid, and ferments in the colon, resulting in abdominal cramps, bloating, diarrhea, and gas. Symptoms usually begin between thirty minutes and two hours after consumption of dairy foods.

The degree of lactose intolerance varies from individual to individual. For most of the world's adults, lactose intolerance is actually a normal condition. Only Caucasians of northern European origin generally retain the ability to digest lactose after childhood. In the United States, an estimated 30 to 50 million people are lactose intolerant. Lactase deficiency can also occur as a result of a gastrointestinal disorder that damages the digestive tract, such as celiac disease, irritable bowel syndrome, regional enteritis, or ulcerative colitis. It can also develop on its own. There is no known way to prevent it.

Although far less common, lactose intolerance can occur in children as well as adults. In infants, lactose intolerance can occur after a severe bout of gastroenteritis, which damages the intestinal lining. Symptoms of lactose intolerance in an infant can include foamy diarrhea with diaper rash, slow weight gain and development, and vomiting.

Lactose intolerance can cause discomfort and digestive disruption, but it is not a serious threat to health and it can easily be managed through dietary modification. Unless otherwise specified, the dosages recommended here are for adults. For a child between the ages of twelve and seven-

teen, reduce the dose to three-quarters of the recommended amount. For a child between six and twelve, use one-half of the recommended dose and for a child under six years old, use one-quarter of the recommended amount.

NUTRIENTS

SUPPLEMENT	SUGGESTED DOSAGE	COMMENTS
Very Important		
Acidophilus (Kyo-Dophilis from Wakunaga)	1 tsp in distilled water twice daily, on an empty stomach.	Replaces lost "friendly" bacteria and promotes healthy digestion. Use a nondairy formula only.
Charcoal tablets	For an acute attack, take 4 tablets every hour with water until symptoms subside. Take separately from other medications and supplements.	Absorbs toxins and relieves diarrhea.
Helpful		
Bone Defense from KAL	As directed on label.	To supply necessary calcium and nutrients needed for calcium absorption.
LactAid from Lactaid, Inc.	As directed on label.	To supply the enzyme lactase, needed for digesting milk sugar.
Magnesium	1,000 mg daily.	Needed for calcium uptake. Promotes pH balance.
Multivitamin and mineral complex	As directed on label.	All nutrients are needed for optimal health.
Ultra Clear Sustain from Metagenics	As directed on label.	Promotes favorable bacteria in the digestive tract and provides additional nutritional support for the digestive system. Available only through health care professionals.
Vitamin D	400 IU daily.	Needed for calcium uptake.
Vitamin E	200 IU daily or 400 IU every other day.	Protects the cell membranes that line the colon wall. Use d-alpha-tocopherol form.
Zinc	30 mg 3 times daily. Do not exceed a total of 100 mg daily from all supplements.	To maintain immune system and proper mineral balance. Use zinc gluconate lozenges or OptiZinc for best absorption.
plus copper	3 mg daily.	Needed to balance with zinc.

Recommendations

❏ Avoid milk and all dairy products except yogurt. This is the most important dietary measure for anyone who is intolerant to lactose. Use soymilk in place of milk, and soy cheese instead of dairy cheese. Rice milk has no lactose, but is not a suitable substitute as it is often low in protein.

❏ Include yogurt in your diet. Yogurt is the one dairy product that can be good for a person with lactose intolerance. The cultures present in yogurt digest the lactose it contains, so it is no longer a problem. They also aid in overall digestion. Be sure to eat only yogurt that contains active live yogurt cultures. Homemade yogurt is best.

❏ Be sure to eat plenty of foods that are high in calcium. Good choices include apricots, blackstrap molasses, broccoli, collard greens, dried figs, kale, calcium-fortified orange juice, rhubarb, salmon, sardines, spinach, tofu, and yogurt. Calcium supplements may be beneficial.

❑ Check with your pharmacist before taking any medications. Many pills are formulated using lactose as filler. Some birth control pills and stomach medications contain lactose.

❑ During an acute attack, do not eat any solid food, but do drink plenty of quality water and replace lost minerals. *See* DIARRHEA in Part Two for dietary suggestions.

❑ Read food product labels carefully, and avoid any that contain lactose or "milk solids." Lactose is added to many different types of processed food, including breads, canned and powdered soups, cookies, pancake mixes, powdered drink mixes such as flavored coffees, processed breakfast cereals, processed meats, and salad dressings.

❑ If you are pregnant and have a family history of lactose intolerance, give serious consideration to breast-feeding your baby. If that is not possible, first see if the baby can tolerate regular formula. Then discuss with your pediatrician choosing a nondairy baby formula, such as a soy-based product.

Considerations

❑ There are several tests used to measure the absorption of lactose into the digestive system. The first test is known as the lactose tolerance test, in which the person drinks a liquid containing lactose after fasting overnight. Approximately one-half hour later, the amount of glucose (blood sugar) in the blood is measured and the presence of symptoms assessed. If the blood glucose does not rise by at least 20 points, and especially if there are symptoms such as bloating or discomfort, a diagnosis of lactose intolerance is confirmed. The hydrogen breath test measures the amount of hydrogen in the breath. Again, the person is given a drink containing a high level of lactose. When lactose is improperly digested in the colon, gases form and are carried through the bloodstream to the lungs and are exhaled. A higher level of hydrogen in the breath indicates faulty digestion of lactose. This test is given to adults and children, but is not recommended for infants and very young children. Young children and infants are tested by the stool acidity test, which measures the amount of acid in the stool. This test also assesses the levels of glucose and lactic acid present in the stool.

❑ Lactose intolerance is not the same as milk allergy. Lactose intolerance specifically refers to a syndrome caused by the failure to digest milk sugar; a person with a milk allergy may be able to digest milk normally, but his or her immune system then has an allergic response to one or more of the milk's components. (*See* ALLERGIES in Part Two.)

❑ Hard, aged cheeses, such as Parmesan cheese, are relatively low in lactose, and may be easier to tolerate than other dairy products.

❑ Many people can't tolerate much lactose at one sitting. Consuming small amounts of dairy products with meals may help improve the lactose tolerance level. The large intestine becomes more accustomed to digesting the lactose when it is introduced in small quantities on a regular basis. Ten grams of lactose a day is considered a low-lactose diet. Much less is found in a tablespoon of milk for coffee (about 2 grams), an ounce of cheese (about 2 grams), or ½ cup of ice cream (about 6 grams). If you want to see how much lactose you can tolerate, try one of these foods each day. Be careful with ice cream; not only is ice cream made from milk, but many brands add extra lactose to achieve the desired texture, and the cold temperature can be shocking to the digestive system as well. Also, a half-cup serving is smaller than you are likely to eat; be sure to try only 4 ounces to begin with and see how you do. More expensive ice creams may be easier to tolerate because they are higher in fat from cream and have less milk.

❑ The symptoms of lactose intolerance are similar to those of celiac disease, and the two disorders may occur together. (*See* CELIAC DISEASE in Part Two.)

❑ Lactose-free and lactose-reduced products are available in most supermarkets.

LEAD POISONING

Lead is one of the most toxic metal contaminants known. It is a cumulative poison that is retained in the body. Even at low levels, lead that is not excreted through the digestive system accumulates in the body and is absorbed directly from the blood into other tissues. When lead leaves the bloodstream, it is stored, along with other minerals, in the bones, where it continues to build up over a lifetime. Lead from the bones may then reenter the bloodstream at any time as a result of severe biologic stress, such as renal failure, pregnancy, menopause, or prolonged immobilization or illness.

Unlike some metallic elements, lead has no known functions or health benefits for humans. It is considered a metabolic poison, which means that it inhibits some basic enzyme functions. Lead reacts with selenium and sulfur-containing antioxidant enzymes in the cells, seriously diminishing the ability of these substances to protect against free radical damage. When present in toxic amounts, it can damage the heart, kidneys, liver, and nervous system.

The body cannot distinguish between calcium and lead. Once lead enters the body, it is assimilated in the same manner as calcium. Because young children and pregnant women absorb calcium more readily to meet their extra needs, they also absorb more lead than other people. Children absorb 25 to 40 percent more lead per pound of body weight than adults do. People with deficiencies of calcium are more susceptible to lead toxicity as well.

Symptoms of lead poisoning typically come on over the course of several weeks in adults and several days in children. Children's symptoms also tend to be more severe. People with lead poisoning commonly have days of severe gastrointestinal colic. Their gums often turn blue, and they may experience muscle weakness. Other possible symptoms include anxiety, arthritis, confusion, chronic fatigue, diarrhea, gout, insomnia, learning disabilities, loss of appetite, a metallic taste in the mouth, seizures, tremors, and vertigo. Lead poisoning can eventually lead to blindness, loss of memory, mental disturbances, mental retardation, paralysis of the extremities, and even coma and death. Chronic lead poisoning can also cause erectile dysfunction, infertility and other reproductive disorders, and liver failure.

Lead is one of the most widely used metals in the United States today, and it is estimated that a large number of people have high levels of lead in their bodies. Sources of lead exposure include lead-based paints, ceramic glazes, lead crystal dishes and glassware, leaded gasoline, lead-acid batteries used in automobiles, tobacco, liver, water, some domestic and imported wines, canned fruit (the lead from lead-soldered cans leaches out and is absorbed by fruits), garden vegetables (if grown in lead-contaminated soil), bone meal, and insecticides. Even such innocuous-seeming items as vinyl mini-blinds and porcelain-glazed sinks and bathtubs have been implicated in lead exposure.

Another potential source of lead poisoning is water supplied through lead piping. Lead piping was used in most homes built before 1930. Newer homes use copper pipes; however, even if you have copper pipes in your home, the chances are very good that they were assembled with lead solder, which is 50 percent lead. Solder can leach a significant amount of lead into the water supply, especially in the first few years after installation. Due to mounting concern over the amount of lead leaching into the water, the use of lead solder was banned in 1986.

Lead poisoning first gained widespread public attention when large numbers of children, especially children in inner cities, were found to have been poisoned by chips of lead-based paint that had peeled off the walls. Lead-based paints were banned for use in housing in 1978. All houses built before 1978 are likely to contain some lead-based paint. However, it is the deterioration of this paint that causes a problem. Approximately 24 million housing units have deteriorated leaded paint and elevated levels of lead-contaminated house dust. More than 4 million of these dwellings are homes to one or more young children. Newer buildings are required to use non-lead-based paints. Some children acquired high lead levels from playing in lead-contaminated dirt, which would get on their hands and then into their mouths.

Since then, it has been learned that pregnant women who have high levels of lead in their bodies can give birth to babies with high lead levels. Lead stored in the mother's body is free to cross the placenta to the fetus. Children born to women who have toxic amounts of lead in their bodies generally suffer from growth retardation and nervous system disorders. Even low-level lead exposure in young children may be associated with impaired intellectual development and behavioral problems.

In 2007, the U.S. Consumer Protection Commission began issuing recalls of many toys manufactured in China because unacceptably high levels of lead were found in the toys' paint. Still, average blood lead levels in the United States have declined dramatically in recent decades, but, according to the U.S. Centers for Disease Control and Prevention, about 250,000 American children under the age of five still have blood lead levels that exceed the acceptable norm.

Unless otherwise specified, the dosages recommended here are for adults. For children between the ages of twelve and seventeen, reduce the dose to three-quarters of the recommended amount. For children between six and twelve, use one-half of the recommended dose, and for children under the age of six, use one-quarter of the recommended amount.

NUTRIENTS

SUPPLEMENT	SUGGESTED DOSAGE	COMMENTS
Essential		
Alpha-lipoic acid (ALA)	As directed on label.	Helps to detoxify the body of metal pollutants and works as a powerful antioxidant.
Apple pectin	As directed on label.	Binds toxins and metals, removing them from the body.
Calcium	2,000 mg daily.	Prevents lead from being deposited in the body tissues. Use calcium chelate form. Do not obtain calcium from dolomite, bone meal, or cow's milk, which can contain lead.
and magnesium	1,000 mg daily.	Needed to balance with calcium. Use magnesium chelate form.
Garlic (Kyolic from Wakunaga)	2 tablets 3 times daily, with meals.	Protects the body's immune system. Helps to bind with and excrete lead.
Kelp and/or alfalfa	As directed on label.	Contains essential minerals, especially calcium and magnesium. Also removes unwanted metal deposits. *See* under Herbs, below.
L-lysine plus	500 mg daily, on an empty stomach.	Assists calcium absorption.
L-cysteine and L-cystine	500 mg each daily, on an empty stomach. Take with water or juice. Do not take with milk. Take with 50 mg vitamin B_6 and 100 mg vitamin C for better absorption.	Sulfur-containing amino acids that act as detoxifiers and remove heavy metals. (*See* AMINO ACIDS in Part One.)
Methylsulfonyl-methane (MSM)	As directed on label.	Helps the body detoxify toxic metals.
S-adenosylmethio-nine (SAMe)	As directed on label.	Has antioxidant effects and helps chelate heavy metals and remove them from the body.

		Caution: Do not use if you have bipolar mood disorder or take prescription antidepressants. Do not give to a child under twelve.
Vitamin C with bioflavonoids	5,000–20,000 mg daily, in divided doses. (See ASCORBIC ACID FLUSH in Part Three.)	Helps to neutralize the effects of lead.
Zinc	80 mg daily. Do not exceed a total of 100 mg daily from all supplements.	Can displace lead and lower the body burden. Low levels of zinc have been found in people with high lead levels.
Very Important		
Glutathione plus L-methionine	As directed on label, on an empty stomach. Take with water or juice. Do not take with milk. Take with 50 mg vitamin B$_6$ and 100 mg vitamin C for better absorption.	Powerful antioxidants that protect the liver, kidneys, heart, and central nervous system. (See AMINO ACIDS in Part One.)
Lecithin granules or capsules	1 tbsp 3 times daily, before meals. 1,200 mg 3 times daily, before meals.	Protects cell membranes.
Selenium	200 mcg daily. If you are pregnant, do not exceed 40 mcg daily.	A potent antioxidant.
Important		
Vitamin B complex plus extra vitamin B$_1$ (thiamine) and vitamin B$_6$ (pyridoxine)	100 mg of each major B vitamin 3 times daily, with meals (amounts of individual vitamins in a complex will vary). 100 mg daily. 50 mg daily.	B vitamins work best when taken together. These B vitamins are vital in cellular enzyme function and important in brain metabolism; they help to remove lead from the brain.
Helpful		
Vitamin A with mixed carotenoids plus vitamin E or Micellized Vitamin A and E from American Biologics	5,000 IU daily for 2 months. If you are pregnant, do not exceed 10,000 IU daily. 200 IU daily or 400 IU every other day. As directed on label.	Potent antioxidants that destroy free radicals and protect the cells from damage due to lead poisoning. Use d-alpha-tocopherol form. A form of vitamins A and E that enters the system rapidly.

Herbs

❑ Alfalfa is rich in vitamins, minerals, and other valuable nutrients, and has a detoxifying effect on the body.

❑ Try using aloe vera juice. Take ½ cup in the morning and ½ cup before bedtime. This softens bowel movements and aids in removing metals from the digestive tract.

❑ Chlorella and cilantro are helpful for absorbing toxic metals.

Recommendations

❑ Make sure that your diet is high in fiber and that you supplement it with pectin (found in apples).

Note: Always take supplemental fiber separately from other supplements and medications.

❑ Eat beans, broccoli, Brussels sprouts, cauliflower, eggs, garlic, kale, legumes, onions, and spinach. These help to rid the body of lead.

❑ Make sure your diet is low in fat and contains adequate amounts of iron and calcium. The body absorbs lead more easily if it is lacking in calcium or iron, or if it has been exposed to a high-fat diet.

❑ Drink steam-distilled water only.

❑ Do not smoke, and avoid secondhand smoke.

❑ If you suspect lead poisoning, have a hair analysis done to determine long-term accumulation of lead. Blood tests reveal only the most recent exposure. (See HAIR ANALYSIS in Part Three.)

❑ Always check the labels when purchasing foreign-made products such as eye makeup (kajal, surma, or kohl dyes from the Middle East) and over-the-counter remedies (Alarcon, Azarcon, Coral, Greta, Liga, Maria Luisa, or Rueda). Some of these products may contain as much as 99 percent lead oxide.

Considerations

❑ Succimer (Chemet) is a drug that may be prescribed to treat lead poisoning.

❑ Chelation with EDTA can help prevent accumulation of lead. Chelating agents work by binding to lead in the bloodstream and expediting its elimination from the body in urine. (See CHELATION THERAPY in Part Three.)

❑ In 1991, the Centers for Disease Control and Prevention (CDC) set a federal standard of 10 micrograms of lead per deciliter of blood. So the 8 percent of U.S. kids five and younger who have lead levels between 5 and 10 micrograms are considered safe. But recent Cornell University research in the journal *Environmental Health Perspectives* supports a stricter standard. The research team had previously followed kids from birth through age five. The current study looked again at the children at age six. The kids were divided into two groups: one with blood lead levels between 0 and 5, and the other with levels between 5 to 10—again, currently considered okay. It turned out that those in the 5 to 10 group had IQ scores about five points lower than those with the lowest lead levels.

❑ The CDC recommends routine blood testing for lead in all children at one and two years of age. When small children have blood lead levels above 10 micrograms per deciliter (mg/dL)—the highest level the CDC considers acceptable—

Tips for a Lead-Free Environment

Once lead accumulates in the body, it remains there. Prevention is therefore much better than treatment when it comes to lead poisoning. The following are simple measures you can take to avoid exposure to lead:

• Do not buy foods in cans sealed with lead solder, which leaches into foods. Lead-soldered cans often have remnants of solder and indentations along the seam. If you buy canned foods, look for lead-free cans that have no side seams. Be wary of imported canned foods. Other countries may have no regulations governing the use of lead solder.

• Make sure children's hands are clean before they eat.

• Keep painted surfaces in good repair, so that older layers of paint are not exposed, chipping, or peeling. Although lead-based paints have been banned for use in residences, numerous older homes and public housing units still contain these paints. Do not allow children to eat paint chips. Hire a professional to remove lead-based paint from any surface; people can poison themselves by burning or scraping off layers of paint.

• Have your water tested to ensure a safe level of lead and other minerals. National Testing Laboratories sells a kit for testing impurities in your water. (*See* Resource Organizations in the Appendix.) Your state health department may also conduct tests for water contaminants at a reasonable price. Culligan International provides a WaterWatch Hot Line that can put you in contact with a local Culligan dealer, who will provide a free water-testing service. (*See* Manufacturer and Distributor Information in the Appendix.) You can also request a free booklet entitled *Water Quality Answers* by writing to the Water Quality Association. (*See* Resource Organizations.)

• Never use the first water drawn from your tap in the morning. Let it run for at least three minutes before you use it. Better yet, use only steam-distilled, filtered, deionized water for drinking and cooking. If safe drinking water is not available, treat water with grapefruit seed extract (available in health food stores) before using it. Add 10 drops of extract per gallon of water and shake or stir vigorously.

• Never boil water longer than necessary. Five minutes is enough. Boiling concentrates contaminants in water, including lead.

• Be careful about buying imported ceramic products. The amount of lead allowable in ceramicware manufactured in the United States is strictly regulated, but there are often no rules governing the glazing techniques of foreign producers. Standards for acceptable lead levels are relatively strict in countries where many of our dishes are manufactured—Great Britain and Japan, for example—but they are often more lax in other countries, such as Mexico and China. The FDA is unable to check a significant number to ensure safety.

• Antiques and other collectibles may look attractive, but this type of dinnerware is more likely to leach lead than dishes made more recently. If you buy such items, use them for decorative purposes only.

• Do not store alcoholic beverages, or acidic foods or beverages such as vinegar, fruit juices, or foods made with tomatoes, in lead crystal glassware for any length of time. The lead that gives fine crystal its sparkle and brilliance leaches into foods and beverages served or stored in it. Babies and children should not be fed from crystal dishes or glassware at all.

• If you are pregnant, avoid drinking hot coffee or other hot acidic beverages, such as tomato soup, from lead-glazed ceramic cups or mugs.

• Do not turn bread bags inside out and use them to store other foods. The ink used to print labels on many bread bags contains considerable amounts of lead. While the lead on the labels doesn't get through the plastic to the bread inside, it can contaminate food if you turn the bags inside out and use them to store other foods.

• If you drink wine, always wipe the mouth of the bottle well (inside and out) with a damp cloth before pouring the wine. The foil wrappers around the corks of wine bottles can deposit lead around the mouth of a bottle and contaminate the beverage.

---

their intelligence suffers. Numerous studies show an average decrease of one-quarter point in intelligence quotient (IQ) for each 1-mg/dL increase in blood lead level.

❑ A portable, battery-operated testing system that can analyze lead levels in the blood within three minutes is available. The testing unit, called LeadCare II, was developed by ESA Biosciences Inc. (www.esainc.com) and Andcare Inc. of Durham, North Carolina (which has merged with ESA).

❑ Hair analysis is another method that can be used to detect heavy metal toxicity. However, results may not be accurate if the sample is contaminated, for example, by hair dye or other possible sources of lead. (*See* HAIR ANALYSIS in Part Three.)

❑ One way to get an indication if your child may be at risk of developing lead poisoning is to have a veterinarian check the lead level in your family dog. Long before children show symptoms of lead poisoning, dogs can get colic, then diarrhea or vomiting, and even seizures. Dogs ingest lead the way small children do—licking toys covered with lead-filled dust, chewing old paint on walls or furniture, or putting things covered with old lead paint flakes in their mouths.

❏ Children with above-average levels of lead in their blood are half an inch shorter, on average, than other children. According to one researcher, lead levels are significantly higher in infants who die of sudden infant death syndrome (SIDS) than in infants who die of other causes.

❏ A study reported in *The New England Journal of Medicine* suggested that even low levels of lead in children may lead to lifelong problems, such as severe reading difficulties, learning disabilities, poor eye-hand coordination, retarded growth, and slowed reflexes. High levels of lead in the body have also been implicated in autism, behavioral problems, hyperactivity, and juvenile delinquency.

❏ Even though leaded gasoline has been almost completely replaced with unleaded fuel, there is still an estimated 4 to 5 million metric tons of lead in American soil that accumulated as a result of leaded gasoline use in the past. Anyone who grows crops or garden produce near busy roads or highways or near a house painted with lead paint should check the lead level in the soil.

❏ Any building fifty years old or older should be inspected by a professional, and if there is lead-based paint on the walls, it should be removed by someone with the proper expertise and equipment. Simply painting over old lead-based paint can release tiny particles containing lead into the air, posing a possible lead hazard.

❏ A previously underreported source of lead poisoning may be lead-based hair colorings used by men. According to the Cosmetic, Toiletry, and Fragrance Association, 80 percent of the hair-coloring products designed for men use so-called progressive coloring agents, which are made of lead acetate. It is known that some lead is absorbed through the scalp, raising questions about the risk of lead poisoning.

❏ The U.S. Food and Drug Administration (FDA) considers children and pregnant women at highest risk for lead poisoning.

❏ An easy way to test dishes for lead is to use LeadCheck Swabs from Hybrivet Systems. The same company also makes a kit for testing for lead in water.

❏ More information about lead poisoning is available from the U.S. Environmental Protection Agency's National Lead Information Center. (*See* Health and Medical Organizations in the Appendix.)

LEG CRAMPS

See MUSCLE CRAMPS. *See also under* PREGNANCY-RELATED PROBLEMS.

LEG ULCERS

Ulcers are open sores that develop on deteriorated patches of skin. When poor circulation in the legs restricts blood flow, the skin tissue begins to erode; it is thus more suscep-

tible to the development of an open sore. The broken skin can be very slow to heal. Leg ulcers are more likely to develop in people with poor circulation, thrombophlebitis, and/or varicose veins. *Venous ulcers* are leg ulcers related to a condition known as venous stasis, in which leg veins cease to function as they should. Blood pools in the veins, resulting in inflammation of the overlying skin that leads to the development of ulcers. Venous ulcers are usually situated on the lower third of the leg. *Arterial ulcers* occur when an artery or arteries serving the leg fail to deliver an adequate blood supply, which in turn may be caused by atherosclerotic plaque or by an embolism blocking the proper flow of blood. These ulcers usually occur on bony areas around the feet and ankles. *Diabetic ulcers* can be a result of peripheral neuropathy or insufficient blood supply to the surface of the skin. (*See* DIABETES in Part Two.) They normally occur around the feet.

Unless otherwise specified, the dosages recommended here are for adults. For children between the ages of twelve and seventeen, reduce the dose to three-quarters the recommended amount. For children between six and twelve, use one-half the recommended dose, and for children under the age of six, use one-quarter the recommended amount.

NUTRIENTS

SUPPLEMENT	SUGGESTED DOSAGE	COMMENTS
Important		
Coenzyme Q10 plus	60 mg daily.	Increases resistance to leg ulcers by increasing tissue oxygenation.
Coenzyme A from Coenzyme-A Technologies	As directed on label.	Supports the immune system's detoxification of many dangerous substances.
Dimethylglycine (DMG) (Aangamik DMG from FoodScience of Vermont)	As directed on label.	Enhances utilization of oxygen to improve blood flow to the legs.
Garlic (Kyolic from Wakunaga)	2 capsules 3 times daily.	Improves circulation and aids the healing process.
Grape seed extract	As directed on label.	A powerful antioxidant that prohibits free radical damage.
Shark cartilage	As directed on label.	To improve blood vessel integrity.
Ultra Connexin from American Biologics	As directed on label.	Supports wound healing and blood vessel wall health.
Vitamin C with bioflavonoids	5,000–10,000 mg daily, in divided doses.	Improves circulation and aids in the healing process. Also keeps infection in check.
Vitamin E emulsion	200 IU daily or 400 IU every other day.	Helps the body use oxygen efficiently and speeds healing. Use d-alpha-tocopherol form. Emulsion is preferable to capsules; it provides for easier assimilation and greater safety at higher doses.

Helpful		
Colloidal silver	Apply topically to the affected area as directed on label.	A broad-spectrum antiseptic that promotes rapid healing and subdues inflammation.
Flaxseed oil or Ultimate Oil from Nature's Secret	2 tsp daily. As directed on label.	To minimize clot formation and help keep veins soft and pliable.
Free form amino acid (Amino Balance from Anabol Naturals)	As directed on label. Take on an empty stomach.	Promotes healing and tissue repair.
Iron or Floradix Iron + Herbs from Salus Haus	As directed by physician. Take with 100 mg vitamin C for better absorption. As directed on label.	Important for cell growth and healing. *Caution:* Do not take iron unless anemia is diagnosed. A natural and nontoxic source of iron.
Multivitamin and mineral complex	As directed on label, with meals.	Necessary for proper healing and to remedy and/or prevent nutritional deficiencies.
Vitamin A emulsion with mixed carotenoids	25,000 IU daily for 1 month. If you are pregnant, do not exceed 10,000 IU daily.	Necessary for healing and protection of tissues. Use emulsion form for more rapid and complete assimilation.
Vitamin B complex plus extra vitamin B$_{12}$ and folic acid	As directed on label. 1,000–2,000 mcg daily. 400 mcg 3 times daily, plus injections (under a doctor's supervision) twice weekly or as prescribed by physician.	B vitamins work best when taken together. Use a high-potency formula. Allows proper tissue enzyme function for healing. Helps to prevent anemia. Use a lozenge or sublingual form. Vital for proper utilization of protein during the healing process.
Vitamin K	As directed on label.	Needed for blood clotting and healing.
Zinc	50 mg daily. Do not exceed a total of 100 mg daily from all supplements.	Aids in the healing of ulcers and boosts immune function. Use zinc gluconate lozenges or OptiZinc for best absorption.

Herbs

❑ Alfalfa, taken in capsule or tablet form, is a good source of vitamin K. Red clover tea or capsules are also beneficial.

❑ Make comfrey tea and use it as a compress; soak a clean cloth in it and apply the cloth to aching, inflamed leg ulcers.

Caution: Comfrey is recommended for external use only.

❑ Echinacea improves immune function and aids healing.

Caution: Do not take echinacea for longer than three months. It should not be used by people who are allergic to ragweed.

❑ Goldenseal is a natural antibiotic and promotes healing.

It can be taken in tea or capsule form. It can also be used as a poultice. Moisten a piece of sterile gauze with alcohol-free goldenseal extract and use this to cover the ulcer.

Caution: Do not take goldenseal internally on a daily basis for more than one week at a time. Do not use it during pregnancy or if you are breast-feeding, and use with caution if you are allergic to ragweed. If you have a history of cardiovascular disease, diabetes, or glaucoma, use it only under a doctor's supervision.

Recommendations

❑ Go on a diet of raw foods with lightly steamed vegetables for one month to help the healing process.

❑ Eat dark green leafy vegetables to obtain vitamin K.

❑ Include plenty of fresh garlic and onions in your diet. These promote circulation and healing, and also contain the trace element germanium, which boosts the immune system and improves tissue oxygenation.

❑ *See* FASTING in Part Three and follow the program.

❑ To speed healing, apply vitamin E oil to the sore and bandage it lightly with a sterile gauze pad. Change the bandage daily until the sore is healed.

❑ Keep the ulcer clean and germ-free to prevent infection.

❑ See your physician if you have this medical problem. Sometimes antibiotics are necessary for the sores to heal.

❑ If you must take antibiotics, be sure to take acidophilus liquid or tablets. You can also obtain acidophilus from yogurt and soured milk products.

Considerations

❑ Dimethylsulfoxide (DMSO) can be applied topically to the sores. It helps to relieve pain and promote healing. In one study, DMSO powder produced significantly higher healing rates in venous leg ulcers than a placebo.

Caution: Only pure DMSO from a health food store should be used. Commercial-grade DMSO such as that found in hardware stores is not suitable for healing purposes. Any contaminants on the skin or in the product can be taken into the tissues by action of the DMSO.

Note: The use of DMSO may result in a garlicky body odor. This is temporary, and is not a cause for concern.

❑ Laser therapy has not proved beneficial for venous leg ulcers. There may be some benefit in combining laser and infrared light therapy, but more research is needed to prove this conclusively.

❑ CircAid Medical Products makes adjustable bands specifically for venous stasis and venous ulcer conditions. (*See* Manufacturer and Distributor Information in the Appendix.)

❑ Leg ulcers often do not cause much pain, so if you have

diabetes or circulatory problems, it is advisable to examine your lower legs and feet often.

❏ *See also* CIRCULATORY PROBLEMS and VARICOSE VEINS in Part Two.

LEGIONNAIRES' DISEASE

This is a serious lung and bronchial tube infection caused by bacteria of the genus *Legionella,* especially *Legionella pneumophila.* It was first identified following an outbreak that affected 182 people attending an American Legion convention in 1976—hence the name. The bacteria live primarily in water and are transmitted through airborne vapor droplets, although they are sometimes found in excavation sites and newly plowed soil. The incubation period is from two to ten days after exposure to the bacteria. The disease does not spread from one person to another.

The first signs of illness may resemble those of the flu—achiness, fatigue, headache, and moderate fever. The disease then progresses to include high fever (up to 105°F), chills, coughing, diarrhea, disorientation, nausea and vomiting, severe chest pain, shortness of breath, and, as a result of inadequate oxygen, a bluish tinge to the lips, nails, or skin. The coughing begins without sputum but eventually produces sputum that is gray or blood-streaked. Laboratory blood studies and cultures of sputum aid in diagnosis.

The risk of contracting Legionnaires' disease increases with chronic illness such as diabetes, emphysema, or kidney failure, and with immune-suppressing lifestyle habits such as smoking and alcohol consumption. Young adults usually recover fully from the disease, whereas elderly people, especially those in poor health, are at greater risk of developing respiratory failure.

Unless otherwise specified, the dosages recommended here are for adults. For children between the ages of twelve and seventeen, reduce the dose to three-quarters the recommended amount. For children between six and twelve, use one-half the recommended dose, and for children under the age of six, use one-quarter the recommended amount.

NUTRIENTS

SUPPLEMENT	SUGGESTED DOSAGE	COMMENTS
Essential		
Garlic (Kyolic from Wakunaga)	2 capsules 3 times daily, with meals.	Aids in destroying bacteria.
Natural beta-carotene or carotenoid complex (Betatene)	25,000 IU daily. As directed on label.	A precursor of vitamin A that protects the lungs.
Vitamin C plus bioflavonoids	3,000 mg 3 times daily. 100 mg twice daily.	Powerful antioxidants that help to kill bacteria. Intravenous treatment (under a doctor's supervision) may be beneficial.

Very Important		
Coenzyme Q10 plus Coenzyme A from Coenzyme-A Technologies	60 mg daily. As directed on label.	Increases and regulates immunity. Carries oxygen to the cells. Supports and boosts the body's immune system. Works well with coenzyme Q10.
Lactobacillus bulgaricus	As directed on label.	Aids digestion and destroys harmful bacteria.
L-carnitine plus L-cysteine	500 mg each daily, on an empty stomach. Take with water or juice. Do not take with milk. Take with 50 mg vitamin B6 and 100 mg vitamin C for better absorption.	Important in immune function. Protect lung tissues. (*See* AMINO ACIDS in Part One.)
Vitamin B complex	100 mg of each major B vitamin daily (amounts of individual vitamins in a complex will vary).	A complex of vital coenzymes needed for cellular function and protection.
Important		
Inf-zyme from Biotics Research	2 tablets 3 times daily, on an empty stomach.	Stimulates the immune system and reduces inflammation in the body.
Raw thymus glandular and raw lung glandular	As directed on label. As directed on label.	Glandulars that potentiate thymus and lung function and enhance immune function.
Vitamin A with mixed carotenoids	25,000 IU daily. If you are pregnant, do not exceed 10,000 IU daily.	Boosts the immune system and protects and repairs lung tissue. Use emulsion form for easier assimilation and greater safety at high doses.
Vitamin E emulsion or capsules	200 IU twice daily. 200 IU daily or 400 IU every other day.	An important antioxidant that protects lung tissue. Use d-alpha-tocopherol form. Emulsion form is easier to assimilate.
Zinc	80 mg daily. Do not exceed a total of 100 mg daily from all supplements.	Important for immune response. Zinc gluconate in lozenge form is best.
Helpful		
Aerobic 07 from Aerobic Life Industries or Dioxychlor	As directed on label. As directed on label.	To destroy infectious bacteria but not "good" bacteria. A potent antibacterial, antifungal, and antiviral agent.

Herbs

❏ Catnip tea is good for reducing fever.

❏ Clear Lungs from RidgeCrest Herbals is a Chinese herbal formula that protects the lungs. Take 2 capsules three times daily.

❏ Echinacea is a powerful immune stimulant.

Caution: Do not take echinacea for longer than three months. It should not be used by people who are allergic to ragweed.

❏ Eucalyptus helps to open up air passages.

❑ Goldenseal is a natural antibiotic.

Caution: Do not take goldenseal internally on a daily basis for more than one week at a time. Do not use it during pregnancy or if you are breast-feeding, and use with caution if you are allergic to ragweed. If you have a history of cardiovascular disease, diabetes, or glaucoma, use it only under a doctor's supervision.

❑ Olive leaf extract helps protect against bacterial and viral infections. It has proven effective against pneumonia and sore throat.

Recommendations

❑ Eat a diet consisting of 75 percent raw foods and very lightly steamed vegetables.

❑ Consume no alcohol, dairy products, fried foods, sugar, or tobacco.

❑ Use a cool mist humidifier to increase the amount of moisture in the air and to thin lung secretions.

❑ Keep warm—do not get chilled, as this will worsen the disease.

❑ Practice deep-breathing exercises. (*See* BREATHING EXERCISES *under* PAIN CONTROL in Part Three.)

❑ Use a heating pad or a hot water bottle on the chest to relieve pain.

❑ Be aware that recovery from Legionnaires' disease takes time. Allow yourself two to four weeks for recovery, and be sure to get adequate rest. Do not push yourself to resume normal activities prematurely.

Considerations

❑ Legionnaires' disease progresses rapidly and can be very dangerous. Hospitalization and aggressive treatment with intravenous antibiotics and oxygen may be necessary.

❑ *Legionella* bacteria may inhabit heating and cooling systems. It is wise to have the heating and cooling systems in both your home and workplace cleaned and inspected regularly, and to change the filters often.

LEUKODYSTROPHIES

See under RARE DISORDERS.

LEUKORRHEA

See VAGINITIS in Part Two.

LIVER DISEASE

See CIRRHOSIS OF THE LIVER *and* HEPATITIS *in* Part Two.

LUMBAGO

See under BACKACHE.

LUPUS

Lupus is a chronic inflammatory disease that can affect many of the body's organs. It is an autoimmune disease—that is, it occurs when the immune mechanism forms antibodies that attack the body's own tissues. Many experts believe that it is due to an as-yet-unidentified virus. According to this theory, the immune system develops antibodies in response to the virus that then attack the body's own organs and tissues. This produces inflammation of the skin, blood vessels, joints, and other tissues. Heredity and sex hormones are two other possible factors in the development of this illness.

This disease was named *lupus,* which means "wolf," because many people who got it developed a butterfly-shaped rash over the cheeks and nose that was considered to give them something of a wolflike appearance. In fact, rashes may appear elsewhere on the body as well, such as the chest, ears, hands, shoulders, and upper arms. At least 90 percent of lupus patients between the ages of fifteen and forty-five are women. However, after the age of fifty (approximately the age of the onset of menopause), the percentage of women with lupus falls to 75 percent and the percentage of men with the disease rises to 25 percent. African American women are two to three times more likely to get it than Caucasian women. Women of Asian, Hispanic, and Native American background also appear to be at greater risk of developing lupus than Caucasian women.

There are two main types of lupus: systemic lupus erythematosus (SLE) and discoid lupus erythematosus (DLE). Two others that are far less common are drug-induced lupus, which is caused by medications, and neonatal lupus, which is a rare disease that can occur in newborn babies of women with SLE, Sjögren's syndrome, or no disease at all. SLE is the form of the disease that most people are referring to when they say lupus. As the name implies, SLE is a systemic disease that affects many different parts of the body. The severity can range from mild to life-threatening. The first symptoms of many cases of SLE resemble those of arthritis, with swelling and pain in the fingers and other joints. The disease may also appear suddenly, with acute fever. The characteristic red rash may appear across the cheeks; there may also be red, scaling lesions elsewhere on the body. Sores may form in the mouth. Other symptoms can include abdominal and chest pains, blood in the urine, fatigue, hair loss, loss of appetite, low-grade fever, nausea, poor circulation in the fingers and toes, shortness of breath, ulcers, vomiting, and weight loss. The lungs and kidneys are often involved. Approximately one-third of those with lupus will develop the kind that needs treatment. In serious cases, the brain, lungs, spleen, and/or heart may be affected. SLE can cause anemia and inflammation of the surface membranes of the heart and lungs. It can also cause excessive bleeding and increased susceptibility to infection. If the central nervous system is involved, amnesia, deep depression, headaches, mania, paralysis, paranoia, psychosis, seizures, and stroke may be present. Patients with lupus are at greater risk of heart attacks, strokes, infections (sepsis), and kidney failure.

The discoid type of lupus is a less serious disease that primarily affects the skin. The characteristic butterfly rash forms over the nose and cheeks. There may also be lesions elsewhere, commonly on the scalp and ears, and these lesions may recur or persist for years. The lesions are small, soft yellowish lumps. When they disappear, they often leave scars. If these scars form on the scalp, permanent bald patches may result. While DLE is not necessarily dangerous to overall health, it is a chronic and disfiguring skin disease. Some experts have related it to a reaction to infection with the tubercle bacillus.

Both types of lupus follow a pattern of periodic flare-ups alternating with periods of remission. Exposure to the sun's ultraviolet rays can result in a flare-up of DLE and may even induce the first attack. Fatigue, pregnancy, childbirth, infection, some drugs, stress, unidentified viral infections, and chemicals may also trigger a flare-up. Drug-induced cases usually clear up when the drug is discontinued.

According to the American Rheumatism Association, four of the following eight symptoms must occur, either serially or at the same time, before a diagnosis can be made:

1. Abnormal cells in the urine.

2. Arthritis.

3. Butterfly rash on the cheeks.

4. Low white blood cell count, low platelet count, or hemolytic anemia.

5. Mouth sores.

6. Seizures or psychosis.

7. Sun sensitivity.

8. The presence in the blood of a specific antibody that is found in 50 percent of people with lupus.

A kidney biopsy may be needed to diagnose lupus-related nephritis.

Unless otherwise specified, the dosages recommended here are for adults. For children between the ages of twelve and seventeen, reduce the dose to three-quarters the recommended amount. For children between six and twelve, use one-half the recommended dose, and for children under the age of six, use one-quarter the recommended amount.

NUTRIENTS

SUPPLEMENT	SUGGESTED DOSAGE	COMMENTS
Very Important		
Calcium and magnesium	1,500–3,000 mg daily. / 750 mg twice daily.	Necessary for pH balance and for protection against bone loss due to arthritis.
Essential fatty acids (fish or flax oil)	As directed on label.	Aids in arthritis prevention.
L-cysteine and L-methionine plus L-lysine	500–1,000 mg each daily, on an empty stomach. Take with water or juice. Do not take with milk. Take with 50 mg vitamin B6 and 100 mg vitamin C for better absorption.	Assist in cellular protection and preservation; important in skin formation and in white blood cell activity. Aids in preventing mouth sores and offers protection against viruses. (*See* AMINO ACIDS in Part One.)
Proteolytic enzymes	As directed on label. Take with meals.	Powerful anti-inflammatory and antiviral agents.
Important		
Garlic (Kyolic from Wakunaga)	2 capsules 3 times daily, with meals.	An immune system enhancer that protects enzyme systems.
Glucosamine sulfate or N-acetylglucosamine (N-A-G from Source Naturals)	As directed on label. / As directed on label.	Important for healthy skin, bones, and connective tissue. May help to prevent lupus erythematosus.
Raw thymus glandular and raw spleen glandular	As directed on label. / As directed on label.	Glandulars that enhance thymus and spleen immune function. (*See* GLANDULAR THERAPY in Part Three.)
Zinc plus copper	50–100 mg daily. Do not exceed this amount from all supplements. / 3 mg daily.	Aids in normalizing immune function; protects the skin and organs and promotes healing. Use zinc gluconate lozenges or OptiZinc for best absorption. Needed to balance with zinc.
Helpful		
Acidophilus (Kyo-Dophilus from Wakunaga)	As directed on label. Take on an empty stomach.	Protects against intestinal bacterial imbalances. Use a nondairy formula.
Herpanacine from Diamond-Herpanacine Associates	As directed on label.	Contains a balance of antioxidants, amino acids, and herbs that promote skin health.
Kelp	1,000–1,500 mg daily.	Supplies commonly deficient minerals.
Multivitamin and mineral complex with vitamin B complex	50 mg of each major B vitamin 3 times daily, with meals (amounts of individual vitamins in a complex will vary).	To supply commonly deficient nutrients. Use a high-quality, hypoallergenic formula. Heals mouth sores, protects against anemia, and protects the skin tissues. Important for brain function and digestion.
Pycnogenol or grape seed extract	As directed on label. / As directed on label.	Powerful antioxidants and free radical scavengers that protect the cells.
Vitamin A with mixed carotenoids plus natural beta-carotene or carotenoid complex (Betatene)	25,000 IU daily. If you are pregnant, do not exceed 10,000 IU daily. / 15,000 IU daily. / As directed on label.	Potent antioxidant and free radical scavenger needed for tissue healing. Use emulsion form for easier assimilation. An antioxidant and vitamin A precursor.

Herbs

❑ Alcohol-free goldenseal extract is good for mouth sores or inflammation. Place a few drops on a small piece of gauze or cotton before bedtime and leave it on overnight for fast healing.

Caution: Do not take goldenseal internally on a daily basis for more than one week at a time. Do not use it during pregnancy or if you are breast-feeding, and use with caution if you are allergic to ragweed. If you have a history of cardiovascular disease, diabetes, or glaucoma, use it only under a doctor's supervision.

❑ Other herbs beneficial in treating lupus include burdock root, feverfew, pau d'arco, and red clover.

Caution: Do not use feverfew when pregnant or nursing. People who take prescription blood-thinning medications should consult a health care provider before using feverfew, as the combination can result in internal bleeding.

❑ Try using licorice root as a tea or dilute it to alleviate lupus symptoms. If you are taking immunosuppressive agents such as steroids, you may find licorice root to provide comparable results without being as harmful to your system.

Caution: Licorice root should not be used during pregnancy or nursing. It should not be used by persons with diabetes, glaucoma, heart disease, high blood pressure, or a history of stroke.

❑ Milk thistle cleanses and protects the liver.

❑ Yucca is good for arthritis-type symptoms.

❑ Many herbal remedies are being studied for use in patients with lupus. Herbs can both suppress and enhance various aspects of the immune system. For example, Cordyceps sinensis, reishi, and nettles have all been studied in lupus for immunosuppression and pain relief. The most studied herbs were thunder god vine and lei gong teng.

Recommendations

❑ Eat a diet low in fat, salt, and animal protein—this kind of diet keeps the immune system from being overly reactive and is easy on the kidneys. Use only canola or olive oil.

❑ Consume sardines often; they are a good source of omega-3 essential fatty acids. Other good sources are flax oil and any seafood. Include seafood twice a week in your diet and use fish oil supplements.

❑ Eat eggs, garlic, and onions. These foods contain sulfur, which is needed for the repair and rebuilding of bone, cartilage, and connective tissue, and aids in the absorption of calcium.

❑ Include in the diet brown rice, fish, green leafy vegetables, nonacidic fresh fruits, oatmeal, and whole grains.

❑ Eat fresh (not canned) pineapple frequently. Bromelain, an enzyme present in fresh pineapple, is excellent for reducing inflammation.

❑ Use some form of fiber daily.

❑ Do not consume milk, dairy products, or red meat. Also avoid caffeine, citrus fruits, paprika, salt, tobacco, and everything that contains sugar.

❑ Avoid the nightshade vegetables (eggplant, peppers, tomatoes, white potatoes). These foods contain a substance called solanine, which can contribute to inflammation and pain.

❑ Get your iron from food sources, not supplements, unless your doctor tells you that you need it. Taking iron in supplement form may contribute to pain, swelling, and joint destruction.

❑ Avoid eating alfalfa sprouts. They contain canavain, a toxic substance that is incorporated into protein in place of arginine.

❑ Get plenty of rest and regular moderate exercise that promotes muscle tone and fitness.

Caution: If you are thirty-five or older and/or have been sedentary for some time, consult with your health care provider before beginning an exercise program.

❑ Avoid strong sunlight and use protection from the sun. Protect your skin by applying a sunscreen product with an SPF of 15 or higher. Wear a wide-brimmed hat and clothing that will adequately cover exposed skin. Go out in the sun only when absolutely necessary.

❑ Use hypoallergenic soaps and cosmetics. Some deodorant soaps and other toiletry items may contain ingredients that will increase your sensitivity to light.

❑ Try to avoid fluorescent lighting in both the home and the workplace. Exposure to fluorescent lighting can aggravate lupus symptoms. If possible, remove all fluorescent and halogen lighting and replace them with incandescent bulbs.

❑ Avoid large groups of people and those with colds or other viral infections. Autoimmune diseases such as lupus render an individual more susceptible to viral infections.

❑ Avoid using birth control pills. They may cause lupus to flare up.

Considerations

❑ Some researchers believe that faulty genes are the ultimate culprit behind this disorder, but that outside factors can trigger it. Substances that are common contributing factors include chemicals, environmental pollutants, food additives, and some foods.

❑ A test for food allergies is helpful and often very revealing in cases of lupus. (*See* ALLERGIES in Part Two.)

❑ In one study, blood cholesterol was improved with fish oil and a healthy diet. This combination helps reduce the risk of heart attack. In another study, flax oil was shown to help maintain kidney function. Patients who followed their daily flax oil regimen over two years had a lowering of creatinine, a marker of worsening kidney function. Patients took 30 grams of ground flaxseeds each day, but many found it caused gastrointestinal distress and some thought it was inconvenient to prepare. Taking both fish oils and ground flaxseeds may lead to improved heart and kidneys.

❏ Ronenn Roubenoff, MD, a Senior Director of Immunology Medical Research at Biogen Idec, Inc. in Cambridge, Massachusetts, advises that lupus patients take a multivitamin as well as calcium and iron. However, he cautions that there is no proof that megavitamin therapy is effective.

❏ Up to 10 percent of lupus cases could be caused by drug reactions, according to an article that was published in *The New England Journal of Medicine.* Certain drugs, such as hydralazine (Apresoline), a blood pressure medication, procainamide (Pronestyl), used for irregular heartbeat, and quinidine (Quinaglute), seem to be able to initiate lupus in susceptible individuals. Drug-related lupus usually does not affect the kidneys or nervous system. It is likely to be milder, and the condition usually subsides when the drug is stopped.

❏ Many people with lupus also have Raynaud's disease. (*See* RAYNAUD'S DISEASE/RAYNAUD'S PHENOMENON in Part Two.) The condition can lead to false-positive blood test results for syphilis.

❏ Many different treatments are used for lupus. Anti-inflammatory drugs are usually used first. Antimalarial drugs such as hydroxychloroquine (Plaquenil) may alleviate the skin problems and joint problems that afflict those who have lupus. Corticosteroids, such as prednisone (Deltasone and others), are adrenal hormones that are considered important in the treatment of lupus. In severe cases, physicians may have to use cortisone and immunosuppressive agents to induce remission. Anticonvulsants, drugs used to control seizures, and warfarin (Coumadin), an anticoagulant used to prevent blood clotting and reduce the possibility of stroke or heart attack, may also be prescribed. All of these drugs, especially the corticosteroids, have potentially serious side effects.

❏ Dehydroepiandrosterone (DHEA) therapy has been found to help in treating lupus. (*See* DHEA THERAPY in Part Three.)

❏ Some research into experimental procedures and new drugs is under way. These include stem cell transplant, where your own adult stem cells are used to rebuild the immune system, and the drug rituximab (Rituxan), which decreases the number of B cells, a type of white blood cell involved in modulating immune function. Rituximab may help those patients who haven't responded to other therapies. However, it has been linked to fatal brain infections in two people with lupus.

❏ Mild cases of lupus respond well to supplements that build up the immune system. (*See* WEAKENED IMMUNE SYSTEM in Part Two.)

❏ Further information on lupus can be obtained from the Lupus Foundation of America. (*See* Health and Medical Organizations in the Appendix).

❏ *See also* ARTHRITIS in Part Two.

LYME DISEASE

This disease takes its name from the town of Old Lyme, Connecticut, where it was first identified in 1975. Since that time, the locations and the number of cases of Lyme disease have continued to increase. In 1983, the year after national surveillance began, 48 cases were reported to the national Centers for Disease Control and Prevention in Atlanta. More than 27,000 cases of Lyme disease were reported in the United States in 2007, according to the CDC, although they say the disease is greatly underreported. Most known cases in the United States have occurred in the northeastern, mid-Atlantic, and north-central states, and it is most common among persons five to fourteen and forty-five to fifty-four years of age. It also occurs in Europe, Russia, China, Japan, and Australia.

Lyme disease is the most common tick-borne illness in the United States. The bacteria that cause it, spirochetes called *Borrelia burgdorferi,* are transmitted by the deer tick (carried by deer and mice) in most places. In several counties along the northern Pacific coast of California, however, they are transmitted by the closely related black-legged tick, which is also carried by wood rats. Both deer ticks and black-legged ticks are very tiny; an adult tick is less than one-tenth of an inch long, and the nymph is the size of a pinhead. They are hard to spot because they are so much smaller than the common dog tick. Because they are so tiny, they often go undetected. The nymphs and larvae feed primarily on white-footed mice, and the adults on white-tailed deer, although they may feed on many other animals as well, including birds, chipmunks, cows, horses, cats, dogs, lizards, and jackrabbits. The ticks fall off one host animal into grasses in marshes or fields, or into brush in wooded areas, from which they can be picked up by an unsuspecting passerby, whether human or animal, who becomes the next host. Not surprisingly, those most likely to be affected are people who spend time outdoors in or near wooded areas, where the ticks are prevalent, and the majority of cases occur in the summer and fall. Household pets like dogs and cats can pick up ticks and carry them into the home, where they can be transmitted to humans.

After a tick bites, it waits several hours before it begins to feed on the host's blood, and once it does, it feasts for three or four days. As it feeds, it may deposit its infectious cargo in the host's bloodstream. The longer the tick remains attached, the greater the risk of disease.

The symptoms of Lyme disease are extremely variable, as is the incubation period, which may take anywhere from two to thirty-two days. The first sign may be the appearance of a red, circular lesion or rash on the skin, which is known as *erythema migrans* (EM). This is caused by the migration of the infecting organism outward through the skin, and it may appear anywhere from a few days to a few weeks after the bite. The lesion gradually expands in a circular pattern, while the center appears to clear up. For this reason, it is often referred to as a bull's-eye rash. In addition to the rash (or, in some cases, instead of the rash), achiness, backache, difficulty sleeping, fatigue, flulike symptoms, headache, muscle weakness, stiff neck, and, occasionally, nausea and vomiting may occur. The disease then usually progresses through the following three stages, although not everyone experiences all three:

1. Three days to three weeks after a tick bite, small raised bumps on the skin and/or a rash appears and may cover the entire torso, for as little as a day or two or as much as several weeks, and then fade. (If a rash appears immediately at the site of the tick bite, it may be a reaction to the bite itself and not to the bacteria that causes Lyme disease.) Chills, fever, nausea, sore throat, and vomiting may also occur.

2. Facial paralysis that mimics Bell's palsy may occur weeks to months later. An abnormal heart rhythm, enlargement of the heart muscle, enlargement of the spleen and lymph glands, and severe headaches may also occur about this time.

3. Over the long term, persistent backache, stiff neck, joint pains that attack the knees, swelling and pain in other joints, and even degenerative muscle disease may be caused by Lyme disease.

Because these tick bites are usually painless, the incubation period is so long, and the symptoms of Lyme disease are so varied, the disorder may go unrecognized for weeks or even months. A physician may fail to diagnose the disease before it is in its advanced stages. Be sure to go to the doctor right away if you have a red bull's-eye mark (darker red in the center). Don't guess; most doctors are familiar with what Lyme disease marks look like, so it is better to have it checked by a professional than to analyze it yourself. Lyme disease produces symptoms that resemble those of chronic fatigue syndrome, gout, lupus, and multiple sclerosis, and misdiagnosis is not uncommon. Once arthritis appears, the joint pain and stiffness can come and go, recurring even years later. An estimated 10 percent of those with Lyme disease arthritis are left with permanent stiffness in their joints.

Lyme disease is treatable and almost always curable if found in its early stages. If the disease is not treated in the early stages, however, arthritis, enlargement of the spleen and lymph nodes, eye inflammation, hepatitis, irregular heart rhythm, and damage to the cardiovascular and central nervous systems can occur. Some people find that their symptoms slowly subside over two to three years; others develop chronic problems. Often, symptoms leave and recur without another tick bite.

A simple test has been developed to identify Lyme disease. A blood sample is used to measure the levels of certain antibodies that usually increase in number from three days to three weeks after infection.

Unless otherwise specified, the dosages recommended here are for adults. For children between the ages of twelve

and seventeen, reduce the dose to three-quarters of the recommended amount. For children between six and twelve, use one-half of the recommended dose, and for children under the age of six, use one-quarter of the recommended amount.

NUTRIENTS

SUPPLEMENT	SUGGESTED DOSAGE	COMMENTS
Very Important		
Essential fatty acids (Kyolic-EPA from Wakunaga)	As directed on label.	Reduces inflammation and joint stiffness.
Pancreatin and bromelain or	As directed on label 2–3 times daily, between meals and at bedtime.	To aid protein digestion and reduce inflammation.
Inf-zyme Forte from American Biologics	As directed on label.	
Primrose oil	1,000 mg 2–3 times daily.	Helps to combat pain and inflammation by promoting the production of anti-inflammatory prostaglandins.
Helpful		
Garlic (Kyolic from Wakunaga)	2 capsules 3 times daily.	A powerful immune system stimulator; acts as an antibiotic.
Kelp	1,000–1,500 mg daily.	Contains essential vitamins and minerals and aids in detoxifying the body.
Multivitamin and mineral complex	As directed on label.	For necessary vitamins. Use a high-potency formula.
Selenium	200 mcg daily. If you are pregnant, do not exceed 40 mcg daily.	A free radical scavenger.
Taurine Plus from American Biologics	As directed on label.	An important antioxidant and immune system regulator necessary for white blood cell activation and neurological function. Use the sublingual form.
Vitamin A with mixed carotenoids	25,000 IU daily. If you are pregnant, do not exceed 10,000 IU daily.	An important antioxidant.
Vitamin C with bioflavonoids	6,000–10,000 mg daily, in divided doses.	Needed for adequate immune function.
Vitamin E	200 IU daily or 400 IU every other day.	An important antioxidant. Use d-alpha-tocopherol form.
Zinc lozenges	1 15-mg lozenge every 3 waking hours for 4 days. Do not repeat this regimen for at least 30 days.	Necessary for immune function.
plus copper	3 mg daily.	Needed to balance with zinc.

Herbs

❏ Alfalfa supplies needed minerals.

❏ Dandelion root, ginseng, hawthorn, and marshmallow root are all good for helping to rebuild the blood and damaged tissues.

Caution: Do not use ginseng if you have high blood pressure or are pregnant or nursing.

❑ Echinacea is an immune enhancer.

Caution: Do not take echinacea for longer than three months. It should not be used by people who are allergic to ragweed.

❑ Goldenseal is a natural antibiotic. Take ½ dropperful of alcohol-free goldenseal extract three times a day for one week. It can be taken under the tongue for fast results, or added to tea.

Caution: Do not take goldenseal internally on a daily basis for more than one week at a time. Do not use it during pregnancy or if you are breast-feeding, and use with caution if you are allergic to ragweed. If you have a history of cardiovascular disease, diabetes, or glaucoma, use it only under a doctor's supervision.

❑ Milk thistle extract protects the liver.

❑ Red clover cleanses the bloodstream.

Recommendations

❑ Include plenty of garlic in your diet or take garlic supplements. It is a natural antibiotic and immune-booster.

❑ Use barley grass, bee pollen, and/or royal jelly to supply nutrients needed to repair tissue and rebuild the blood.

Caution: Bee pollen may cause an allergic reaction in some people. Start with a small amount at first, and discontinue use if a rash, wheezing, discomfort, or other symptom occurs.

❑ Use "green drinks" to provide chlorophyll, which aids in detoxification, and other valuable nutrients and enzymes. Kyo-Green from Wakunaga is an excellent choice.

❑ If you develop a bull's-eye-type rash anywhere on your body, see your health care provider as soon as possible, even if you have no memory of being bitten by a tick. Early treatment is essential.

❑ If antibiotics are prescribed, be sure to take some form of acidophilus supplement daily.

❑ Take hot baths or whirlpool treatments. Heat relieves joint pain.

❑ Take precautionary measures to help prevent tick bites:

• When spending time in or near wooded areas, wear long pants and tuck them into your socks. Wear a long-sleeved shirt with a high neck or a scarf, plus a hat and gloves. Wear light-colored clothing so that any ticks will be more visible.

• Use an insect repellent containing diethyl meta-toluamide (DEET) on your clothing, your neck, and any other exposed area except your face. Deet lasts longer and is safer when applied to certain clothing (*see* Caution below) than on exposed skin, so cover as much of the body with clothing as you can. Do not use excessive amounts of DEET. Follow product label directions carefully, and wash the repellent off as soon as you go indoors.

Caution: DEET is extremely toxic and can be deadly if ingested. However, when used according to the product directions, it does not pose a health concern because its use is expected to be brief. Be extremely careful when using it around small children. Do not use under clothing.

• After spending time outdoors, check yourself carefully for any small raised bumps and for pinpoint-sized specks on clothing. Do this right away; the longer a tick is attached, the greater the risk of Lyme disease.

• Check children before they go to bed during the summer if they spend a lot of time outdoors. Look closely at their hair, ears, underarms, trunks, groins, and the backs of their knees. Have them shower when they come in from outdoors, and wash their clothes immediately.

• Dry your laundry in an electric clothes dryer for half an hour to kill any ticks that may be present. Washing clothes, even in hot water and bleach, will not necessarily kill ticks.

• Inspect pets before letting them indoors. They may carry ticks into the house that can fall off and bite family members.

• In a wooded or overgrown area, try to stay near the centers of trails and out of wooded areas, especially in May, June, and July.

• Keep your lawn mowed and remove leaf litter and brush. Move woodpiles away from the house during the summer.

❑ If you find a tick on your body, do the following:

1. Remove the tick with a pair of tweezers. Grasp the tick with the tweezers as close to the skin as possible and pull the tick straight out. Do not twist the tweezers as you pull, and do not squeeze the tick's body, or bacteria may be injected into the skin. If possible, save the tick in a small bottle or jar. *Do not* use a match to try to burn the tick out, or resort to other home remedies like kerosene or petroleum jelly.

2. Once the tick is removed, thoroughly wash your hands and the bite area, and apply rubbing alcohol or another topical antiseptic to the bite. If you suspect the tick may be a deer tick, see your health care provider promptly. Take the tick with you for identification.

3. For the three weeks following a tick bite, be alert for any of the symptoms described in this section. If you have any doubts about your condition, consult your health care provider.

❏ If you are being treated for Lyme disease but are not getting better, consider having yourself tested again. False positive results are possible, and you may actually have a different problem.

Considerations

❏ Pregnant women need to be especially careful to avoid ticks in Lyme disease areas. The infection can be transferred to the developing fetus and, in rare circumstances, can cause complications such as miscarriage or the birth of a stillborn baby.

❏ Prompt treatment with antibiotics can halt the course of Lyme disease. Many physicians do not like to prescribe antibiotics unless a person develops the characteristic symptoms of Lyme disease—a small red bump at the site of the tick bite, and a bull's-eye rash surrounding it, with flulike symptoms such as fatigue, chills, and joint pain. If treatment is deferred until the onset of more advanced symptoms, such as involvement of the brain, heart, or joints, antibiotic therapy is not as effective. One study found that with antibiotic treatment, patients felt better and were better able to care for themselves while recovering from Lyme disease compared to a group given a placebo. An intravenous drug also is available to treat Lyme disease. Speak to your health care provider about the latest treatment methods and best practices.

❏ The vaccine against Lyme disease was removed from the market in 2002 due to low demand. Because antibiotics are so effective at treating Lyme disease, the vaccine was considered no longer necessary.

❏ One study showed that of 788 people diagnosed with Lyme disease, over half had other health problems, not Lyme disease. Physicians blame current laboratory tests for the false-positive results.

❏ Pets can get Lyme disease, too. Call your veterinarian if your pet exhibits any of the following:

- Fever of 103°F to 106°F.

- One or more swollen, hot joints.

- A tendency to sit or lie in one place for longer periods of time than usual.

- Lameness that seems to come and go.

- Reluctance to move.

- Poor appetite.

- A hot, dry nose.

❏ The CDC provides information on Lyme disease to health professionals and the public. (*See* Health and Medical Organizations in the Appendix.) The CDC also works with state health departments to track cases of Lyme disease. Your state or local health department can tell you if Lyme disease has been reported in your area.

MACHADO-JOSEPH DISEASE (MJD)

See under ATAXIA in RARE DISORDERS.

MACULAR DEGENERATION

See under EYE PROBLEMS.

MALABSORPTION SYNDROME

Malabsorption is the failure of the body to properly absorb vitamins, minerals, and other nutrients from food. Even though his or her diet is adequate, an individual with malabsorption develops various nutritional deficiencies. This problem can result from impaired digestion, impaired absorption of nutrients into the bloodstream from the digestive tract (especially the small intestine), or both.

Common symptoms of malabsorption syndrome include constipation or diarrhea, dry skin, fatigue, gas, mental difficulties such as depression or an inability to concentrate, muscle cramps and/or weakness, premenstrual syndrome (PMS), steatorrhea (pale, bulky, fatty stools), a tendency to bruise easily, failure to grow normally, thinning hair, unexplained weight loss, and visual difficulties, especially problems with night vision. Abdominal discomfort may be present as well. A combination of anemia, diarrhea, and weight loss is typical. In addition, in an attempt to get the nutrients it needs but is not absorbing, the body may begin to crave more and more food, often leading to the consumption of many empty and/or fat calories.

Digestive disorders are among the most common health problems in America today. Impaired digestion leads to malabsorption because if food is not broken down properly, the nutrients it contains cannot be absorbed through the lining of the intestines. The intestinal tract, pancreas, liver, and gallbladder all have parts to play in the uptake of nutrients. Consequently, anything that interferes with the proper functioning of any of these can lead to impaired digestion. Some factors that can contribute to impaired digestion are a lack of adequate levels of digestive enzymes; food allergies; a diet deficient in nutrients, such as the B vitamins, that are needed to produce digestive enzymes; and diseases of the pancreas, gallbladder, liver, and bile ducts that result in a lack of bile and essential enzymes. Although any type of nutrient may be affected by poor digestion, lipids (fats) are affected most often. In addition to causing nutritional deficiencies, the failure to digest food properly causes gastrointestinal problems. Undigested food ferments in the intestinal tract, causing gas, bloating, and abdominal pain and discomfort.

Even if food is properly digested, there may be a problem that prevents nutrients from being taken up by the bloodstream and used to nourish the body tissues. Damage to the intestinal walls, through which nutrients are absorbed, is one such problem. Disorders such as celiac disease, colitis, Crohn's disease, diverticulitis, irritable bowel syndrome, lactose intolerance, parasitic infestation, and excessive consumption of alcohol, antacids, or laxatives can all cause intestinal damage. Chronic constipation and/or diarrhea can have the same result. Another problem is too-rapid intestinal transit time, which results in nutrients being passed out of the body as waste before they can be absorbed. Radiation therapy, digitalis treatment, and surgery that shortens the intestinal tract all reduce the absorptive area, and therefore the absorptive capacity, of the small bowel.

Other factors that can contribute to a malfunction of the absorption mechanism include a poor diet; excess mucus covering the intestinal lining (most commonly a result of the overconsumption of mucus-forming and processed foods); an imbalance in intestinal bacterial flora, such as in candidiasis; the use of certain medications, such as neomycin (an antibiotic), colchicine (an antigout drug), and cholestyramine (a cholesterol-lowering drug); food allergies; and illnesses such as cancer. Obstructions in the lymphatic system may also interfere with nutrient absorption.

Regardless of how good your diet is or how many supplements you take, if you suffer from malabsorption syndrome, you will have nutritional deficiencies. These in turn lead to other problems. The impaired absorption of protein can induce edema (swelling of the tissues due to fluid retention). A lack of potassium can result in muscle weakness and cardiovascular problems. Anemia results from a lack of needed iron and folic acid. Calcium and vitamin D deficiency result in bone loss and tetany, a condition characterized by painful muscular spasms and tremors. Bruising easily results from a lack of vitamin K, night blindness from a deficiency of vitamin A. Malabsorption is also self-perpetuating; the failure to absorb B vitamins and to transfer amino acids across the intestinal lining interferes with the production of needed digestive enzymes and causes further malabsorption, since these nutrients are essential in the absorption process itself. A vicious cycle results.

Besides being a serious condition in itself, malabsorption is a factor in other medical and physical problems. The body needs all nutrients in balance because they work in concert. If there is a deficiency in even a single nutrient, the body can no longer function as it should, and all kinds of things can go awry. The result is disease. Malabsorption is a common contributing factor to a wide range of disorders, including cancer, heart disease, osteoporosis, and—because immune function is damaged by a lack of necessary nutrients—all types of infection.

Malabsorption is also a significant factor in the overall aging process, and it may account for the fact that some people seem to age more rapidly than others. As we age, the intestinal tract gets "out of shape" and the lining becomes covered with hard fecal matter and mucus, which makes absorption of nutrients more difficult. This is one reason older people need to consume greater amounts of nutrients. It is also why it is so important to keep the colon clean. Fecal deposits can irritate the nerve endings in the colon, leading to spastic colon or inflamed colon. Both of these conditions interfere with bowel function and with the proper absorption of nutrients. In addition, the impacted deposits decay after a time, releasing toxins that can seep into the bloodstream, poisoning the organs and tissues.

People with malabsorption syndrome must take in more nutrients than the average person to compensate, and to treat and correct the problem. In supplying these nutrients, it is best to bypass the intestinal tract as much as possible. When choosing supplements, sustained-release and large, hard tablets should be avoided. Many people with malabsorption problems are unable to break down supplements taken in hard pill form; some even discharge pills whole in the stool. Injections, powders, liquids, and lozenges provide nutrients in forms that are more easily assimilated and therefore are preferred.

Unless otherwise specified, the dosages recommended here are for adults. For children between the ages of twelve and seventeen, reduce the dose to three-quarters of the recommended amount. For children between six and twelve, use one-half of the recommended dose, and for children under the age of six, use one-quarter of the recommended amount.

NUTRIENTS

SUPPLEMENT	SUGGESTED DOSAGE	COMMENTS
Very Important		
Acidophilus (Kyo-Dophilus from Wakunaga)	1 tsp 3 times daily, on an empty stomach.	Needed for uptake and manufacture of many nutrients. Use a nondairy formula.
Vitamin B complex injections	2 cc twice weekly, or as prescribed by physician.	To correct deficiencies. B vitamins must be replenished daily. Injections (under a doctor's supervision) are best. Needed for normal digestion and to prevent anemia. A good source of B vitamins and other valuable nutrients. If injections are not available, use a lozenge, sublingual, or spray form such as No Shot B-6/B-12/Folic from Superior Source.
plus extra vitamin B_{12} injections	1 cc twice weekly, or as prescribed by physician.	
and liver extract injections	1 cc twice weekly, or as prescribed by physician.	
or vitamin B complex plus extra	As directed on label.	
vitamin B_{12}	1,000 mcg 3 times daily, on an empty stomach.	
and vitamin B_6 (pyridoxine)	50 mg 3 times daily.	
and folic acid	400 mcg 3 times daily.	
Important		
Bioperine (Bioperine from Sabinsa or Bioperine 10 from Nature's Plus)	As directed on label.	Increases the absorption of nutrients and improves digestion.
Calcium	As directed on label.	Necessary for maintaining healthy bones. Use calcium citrate chelate form.
Free form amino acid (Amino Balance from Anabol Naturals)	As directed on label 3 times daily, on an empty stomach.	Needed because protein is not broken down properly into amino acids, which are needed for virtually all life functions.
Garlic (Kyolic from Wakunaga)	As directed on label. Take with meals.	Aids digestion and promotes healing of the digestive tract. Use the liquid form.

Supplement	Suggested Dosage	Comments
Inf-zyme Forte from American Biologics	2 tablets with each meal.	A balanced, potent enzyme and cofactor as a powerful inflammatory inhibitor.
Magnesium	As directed on label.	Important for energy production. Assists in calcium and potassium absorption. Use chelate form.
Vitamin C with bioflavonoids	2,000–8,000 mg daily, in divided doses. Take with juice.	Needed to stimulate immune system function and to aid uptake of nutrients. Use a buffered powder form.
Vitamin E	200 IU daily or 400 IU every other day.	An essential antioxidant, it improves circulation and is necessary for tissue repair. Use d-alpha-tocopherol form.
Helpful		
Essential Fatty Acid Complex	As directed on label.	To repair the cells along the intestinal walls and to assist in proper utilization of fats.
Multivitamin and mineral complex plus carotenoid complex	As directed on label. As directed on label.	To replace lost nutrients. Minerals are the key to protein and vitamin utilization. Use a powdered form that is yeast- and allergen-free.
Proteolytic enzymes or multienzyme complex with pancreatic enzymes	As directed on label 3–6 times daily. Take with meals and between meals. As directed on label, 3 times daily, with meals.	Needed for protein digestion and breakdown of carbohydrates and fats.
Zinc lozenges plus copper	1 15-mg lozenge 3 times daily for 1 month. Do not exceed a total of 100 mg daily from all supplements. 3 mg daily.	Aids in the manufacture of digestive enzymes and in protein uptake. Needed to balance with zinc.

Herbs

❑ Alfalfa, dandelion root, fennel seed, ginger, and nettle are rich in minerals and can aid the body in absorbing nutrients.

❑ Aloe vera and peppermint aid digestion.

❑ Black pepper contains piperine, which aids in the digestion and absorption of some nutrients.

❑ Buchu decreases inflammation of the colon and mucous membranes.

❑ Goldenseal promotes the functioning capacity of the colon, liver, and pancreas.

Caution: Do not take goldenseal internally on a daily basis for more than one week at a time. Do not use it during pregnancy or if you are breast-feeding, and use with caution if you are allergic to ragweed. If you have a history of cardiovascular disease, diabetes, or glaucoma, use it only under a doctor's supervision.

❑ Irish moss and rhubarb are good for colon disorders.

❑ Yellow dock improves colon and liver function.

Recommendations

❑ Follow the dietary recommendations in this section for at least thirty days to give the colon a chance to heal and to cleanse its walls of hard matter and mucus. After thirty days, you may gradually reintroduce the foods that you have eliminated back into your diet; however, do not add them back too quickly or all at once. Instead, add small amounts of these foods, one at a time, back into your diet.

❑ Eat a diet that is high in complex carbohydrates and low in fats. Include in the diet well-cooked brown rice, millet, oatmeal, and steamed vegetables.

❑ Eat plenty of fruits (except for citrus fruits).

❑ Consume fresh papaya and pineapple often. Chew four to six papaya seeds after meals.

❑ Eat broiled, steamed, or baked whitefish three times a week.

❑ Do not eat large meals, as this places too much stress on the digestive system. Instead, eat smaller portions of food throughout the day.

❑ Drink six to eight glasses of liquids daily, including juices, quality water, and herbal teas (*see* Herbs, above, for suggestions). Use barley malt, a small amount of honey, or nut or soymilk for sweeteners, if necessary.

❑ Do not consume wheat products until healing is complete.

❑ Avoid products containing caffeine, which interferes with iron absorption. These include teas, coffee, colas, chocolate, many processed foods, and some over-the-counter medications (read labels).

❑ Keep fats and oils to an absolute minimum. Do not consume any animal products (including butter), fried or fatty foods, or margarine. The fats these foods contain exacerbate malabsorption problems by coating the stomach and small intestine, blocking the passage of nutrients. For the same reason, avoid all dairy products and processed food products, which encourage the secretion of mucus. Make sure to take supplemental calcium and vitamin D, if you avoid all dairy products.

❑ Eliminate citrus fruits, shellfish, and white rice from the diet.

❑ Strictly avoid all junk foods, such as potato chips and candy, as well as other products containing sugar, salt, monosodium glutamate (MSG), and preservatives.

❑ *See* COLON CLEANSING in Part Three and follow the program.

❑ Follow the fasting program once monthly. (*See* FASTING in Part Three.)

❑ Avoid using mineral oil or other laxatives. Especially avoid using them for extended periods, as dependence and damage to the colon may result.

❑ If diarrhea or other symptoms of digestive disturbance occur for longer than three days, call your health care provider. Also consult a professional if you notice black and tarry or bright red stools, or if digestive problems are accompanied by severe abdominal pain or a fever of over 101°F.

❏ If a change of diet and the correct supplements do not improve your health status in a few months, consult your physician. You may have a malabsorption problem that requires medical attention.

Considerations

❏ Chronic pancreatic insufficiency is a condition in which the pancreas does not secrete enough enzymes for proper digestion. Serious pancreatic disease can lead to malabsorption severe enough to damage the nervous system. Gallbladder and/or liver problems can lead to trouble in the digestion and absorption of essential fatty acids, which are necessary for good health. Impaired absorption of fats in turn can lead to deficiencies of fat-soluble nutrients, such as beta-carotene and vitamins A, D, E, and K. A simple stool test can measure which nutrients you are excreting.

❏ Aging is associated with low levels of vitamins B_{12} and D. Levels are easily measured by a blood test. If you are over sixty years of age, you should have these measured at your yearly physical exam.

❏ Treatment of malabsorption requires recognition and, if possible, correction of the underlying cause of the problem, plus a healthful dietary regimen and supplementation. Appropriate medical consultation is needed in cases related to the use of cancer drugs, pancreatic insufficiency, and special problems associated with gastric or intestinal surgery. In some cases of severe malnutrition, intravenous nutrition may be needed.

❏ Certain drugs interfere with the absorption of nutrients. Examples include corticosteroids, cholestyramine (Questran), sulfasalazine (Azulfidine), and especially antibiotics. Corticosteroids depress protein synthesis, inhibit normal calcium absorption, and increase the amount of vitamin C lost through excretion. Cholestyramine interferes with the absorption of the fat-soluble vitamins A, D, E, and K. Sulfasalazine inhibits the transport of folate and iron, potentially causing anemia. Antibiotics disrupt the essential bacterial flora of the intestine. All of these drugs may increase the need for nutritional supplements.

MALNUTRITION

See MALABSORPTION SYNDROME; UNDERWEIGHT.

MANIC-DEPRESSIVE DISORDER

See BIPOLAR MOOD DISORDER.

MASTITIS

See under BREAST-FEEDING-RELATED PROBLEMS.

MEASLES

Measles, known to doctors as *rubeola,* is a viral infection that attacks the respiratory tract, eyes, and skin. Although it is typically a childhood disease, adults are also susceptible. This is not the same disease as rubella, or German measles, and is caused by a different virus.

Measles is very contagious and is easily spread through the nose, mouth, or throat; secretions on articles or surfaces; or by coughing and sneezing.

Illness usually sets in between seven and fourteen days after exposure to the virus. The first symptoms include fever (temperature of 103°F or higher), cough, sneezing, runny nose, and red eyes that may be sensitive to light. Several days later, Koplik's spots (tiny red spots with white centers) appear in the mouth and throat, the throat becomes sore, and a raised red rash erupts on the forehead and ears. Over a period of five to seven days, the rash spreads to all parts of the body.

In previously healthy children, measles usually runs its course in about ten days. However, measles is almost nonexistent in the United States because a vaccine is given to most children early in life. The measles vaccine (contained in MMR, MR, and measles vaccines) can prevent this disease. The MMR vaccine is a live, weakened combination vaccine that protects against the measles, mumps, and rubella viruses. It was first licensed in the combined form in 1971. It is made by taking the measles virus from the throat of an infected person and adapting it to grow in chick embryo cells in a laboratory. As the virus becomes better able to grow in the chick embryo cells, it becomes less able to grow in a child's skin or lungs. When this vaccine virus is given to a child, it replicates only a little before it is eliminated from the body. This replication causes the body to develop an immunity that, in 95 percent of children, lasts for a lifetime. A second dose of the vaccine is recommended to protect those 5 percent who did not develop immunity in the first dose and to give a booster effect to those who did develop an immune response.

If measles does develop, it can be followed by a number of complications, some of them potentially serious. These include middle ear infection (especially in children with a history of repeated ear infections), bronchitis, croup, pneumonia, strep throat, and even, in rare cases, encephalitis or meningitis. Adults who develop measles tend to suffer more serious cases of the disease than children do.

Unless otherwise specified, the dosages recommended here are for adults. For children between the ages of twelve and seventeen, reduce the dose to three-quarters the recommended amount. For children between six and twelve, use one-half the recommended dose, and for children under the age of six, use one-quarter the recommended amount.

NUTRIENTS

SUPPLEMENT	SUGGESTED DOSAGE	COMMENTS
Helpful		
Bio-Strath from Nature's Answer	As directed on label.	Acts as a tonic. Contains the vitamin B complex. Use the liquid form.
Calcium and magnesium	As directed on label.	Needed for tissue repair.
Micellized Vitamin A and E from American Biologics or vitamin A	As directed on label. If you are pregnant, do not exceed 10,000 IU daily. 10,000 IU twice daily for 1 week, then reduce to 10,000 IU once daily. Do not exceed this dosage.	For adults. Needed to reduce infection and to repair tissues. For children.
or cod liver oil	As directed on label.	For children unable to swallow capsules.
Proteolytic enzymes	As directed on label 2–3 times daily, between meals.	Reduces infection and aids digestion.
Raw thymus glandular	500 mg twice daily.	Stimulates the immune system.
Vitamin B complex	100 mg of each major B vitamin 3 times daily or as directed on label (amounts of individual vitamins in a complex will vary).	Important in all bodily functions, including immune response and proper healing. For a child under eight, use a formula designed specifically for children.
Vitamin C with bioflavonoids	Adults: 3,000–10,000 mg daily, in divided doses. Children: 1,000–3,000 mg daily, in divided doses.	Very important for immune function. Fights fever and infection. Has antiviral properties. Use an ascorbate or esterified form.
Vitamin E	200 IU daily or 400 IU every other day. Children's dosage should not exceed 200 IU daily.	Neutralizes harmful free radicals, which can destroy cell membranes. Use d-alpha-tocopherol form.
Zinc lozenges	1 15-mg lozenge 3 times daily for 4 days. Then reduce to 1 lozenge daily.	For immune response and tissue repair. Reduces symptoms and speeds healing. Also relieves itchy throat and coughing.

Herbs

❑ Catnip tea or garlic enemas can be used to help to lower fever if necessary. (*See* ENEMAS in Part Three.)

❑ Lobelia extract helps to relieve pain. Take ½ teaspoon of lobelia extract every four to five hours.

Caution: Lobelia is to be taken only under supervision of a health care professional, as it is potentially toxic. People with high blood pressure, heart disease, liver disease, kidney disease, seizure disorders, or shortness of breath should not take lobelia. Pregnant and lactating women should avoid lobelia as well.

❑ Spirulina is helpful for bolstering the immune system and can help slow replication of the virus.

Recommendations

❑ If you suspect that you or a member of your family has measles, see your health care provider. This is important for a correct diagnosis and to prevent serious complications.

❑ Drink plenty of fluids such as water, juices, herbal teas, and vegetable broths.

❑ Avoid processed foods.

❑ To help relieve coughing, mix 1 tablespoon lemon juice and 2 tablespoons honey with ¼ cup water. Take as needed.

Caution: Never give honey to an infant under one year of age.

❑ To alleviate itching, place ½ cup of baking soda in a bathtub filled with lukewarm water and soak in the bath until the itching decreases. Gently applying witch hazel to the affected area also will help to ease the discomfort and itching associated with the rash.

❑ Try homeopathic remedies to ease symptoms. *Aconitum napellus* (monkshood), a homeopathic version of vitamin C, is helpful in the initial stage of measles. *Ferrum phosphoricum* (homeopathic phosphate of iron) is beneficial for mild infections. These remedies may not have been tested on children. If considering giving these to a child, consult a homeopathic practitioner first.

❑ Rest until the rash and fever have disappeared.

❑ Keep the lights dim. Do not read or watch television while your eyes are sensitive to light.

❑ Do not send a child who has had measles to school until seven to nine days after the fever and rash have disappeared.

Considerations

❑ Doctors generally recommend that children receive two measles vaccinations, one at about fifteen months and one before entering school or at about age twelve. A second vaccination is considered necessary because measles outbreaks have occurred among college students who received a single immunization in childhood. Certain individuals should *not* be immunized against measles, including pregnant women and anyone who has cancer or a weakened immune system, is on cortisone or anticancer drugs, is undergoing radiation therapy, or has any type of illness with fever. People allergic to eggs should tell their physicians before having the vaccine. A person who has had and recovered from measles does not require immunization; a single attack of measles gives lifelong immunity.

❑ Short-term, high doses of vitamin A have been used to lessen the severity and complications of measles. Since high doses can be toxic, they should be taken only briefly (two weeks or less) and monitored very carefully. Ask the pediatrician before using vitamin A in excessive amounts.

❑ Antibiotics are useless against viruses, so they are not called for unless complications occur.

MELANOMA

See under SKIN CANCER.

MEMORY PROBLEMS

Memory is as natural to us as breathing. It is an ability we all have, yet rarely ever think of—unless we perceive that we are losing that ability. Memory lapses are an annoyance in themselves, but worse is the anxiety that often comes along with them. We begin asking ourselves if they are a symptom of some other problem, such as midlife depression or arteriosclerosis. Probably the greatest fear provoked by lapses in memory is that of Alzheimer's disease, a progressive and debilitating disease that usually starts in midlife with minor defects in memory and behavior. Although this is a fairly common disorder among older people, it is important to realize that most memory lapses have nothing to do with Alzheimer's disease.

It is generally believed that advancing age brings an increasing likelihood of developing memory loss. The mildest form of this malady is called mild cognitive impairment (MCI), and is characterized by one's perception of one's own memory loss. An estimated 1 percent of normal Americans over the age of sixty-five experiences MCI. Scientists have been interested in memory impairment in part because a significant percentage of people over the age of sixty-five with MCI eventually develops Alzheimer's disease—in some studies, approximately 12 to 15 percent per year (or about 40 percent after three years). As such, MCI is a risk factor for developing Alzheimer's disease. However, not all memory loss is attributable to aging. Occasional memory lapses, such as misplacing the car keys or forgetting something at the grocery store, are a natural, normal part of life at virtually any age, and are not likely to precede serious memory loss. In fact, with proper diet, nutrition, and memory use, the memory can remain sharp and active well into one's nineties or beyond.

One reason many people suffer from memory loss is an insufficient supply of necessary nutrients (especially the B vitamins and amino acids) to the brain. The life of the body is in the blood. It literally feeds and nourishes every cell within our bodies. The brain is surrounded by a protective envelope known as the blood-brain barrier, which allows only certain substances to pass from the bloodstream into the brain. If the blood is "thick" with cholesterol and triglycerides, the amount of nutrient-rich blood that can pass through the blood-brain barrier decreases. Over time, this can result in the brain becoming malnourished.

In addition, the functioning of the brain depends upon substances called neurotransmitters. Neurotransmitters are brain chemicals that act as electrical switches in the brain and, through the functioning of the nervous system, are ul-

timately responsible for all the functions of the body. If the brain does not have an adequate supply of neurotransmitters, or the nutrients from which to make them, it begins to develop the biochemical equivalent of a power failure or a short circuit. If your mind goes blank when you are trying to recall a specific fact or piece of information, or it begins to plug into some other, irrelevant memory instead, it is likely that such a "short circuit" has occurred.

There are numerous other factors involved in the deterioration of memory. One of the most important is probably exposure to free radicals, which can wreak enormous damage to the memory if unchecked. Alcoholics and drug addicts often suffer a great deal from memory loss. Alcoholics are notorious for "blackouts"—huge memory gaps that occur even though they are conscious. Allergies, candidiasis, stress, thyroid disorders, and poor circulation to the brain may also be contributing factors. Hypoglycemia (low blood sugar) can play a role in memory loss as well, because to function properly, the brain requires that the level of glucose in the blood fall within a very specific narrow range. Wide swings in blood sugar levels affect brain function and memory.

The dosages given below are for adults.

NUTRIENTS

SUPPLEMENT	SUGGESTED DOSAGE	COMMENTS
Essential		
Ginkgo biloba	As directed on label.	Has been shown to enhance memory. *Caution:* Do not take ginkgo biloba if you have a bleeding disorder, or are scheduled for surgery or a dental procedure.
Vitamin B complex	100 mg of each major B vitamin daily (amounts of individual vitamins in a complex will vary).	Needed for improved memory. Injections (under a doctor's supervision) may be necessary.
plus extra vitamin B₅ (pantothenic acid) and	50 mg 3 times daily.	Helps in transformation of the amino acid choline to the neurotransmitter acetylcholine.
vitamin B₆ (pyridoxine)	50 mg 3 times daily.	Needed for proper brain function.
Vitamin B₃ (niacin)	As directed on label.	To promote proper circulation to the brain and aid in brain function. *Caution:* Do not take niacin if you have a liver disorder, gout, or high blood pressure.
Very Important		
Acetylcholine	As directed on label.	Most important of the neurotransmitters. Maximizes mental ability and prevents memory loss in adults.
Boron	3–6 mg daily. Do not exceed this amount.	Improves brain and memory function.
Dimethylamino-ethanol (DMAE)	As directed on label.	Aids in learning and memory. *Note:* This supplement is not intended for everyday use. It is

Supplement	Suggested Dosage	Comments
		best reserved for days when you need to be more focused and alert.
Garlic (Kyolic from Wakunaga)	As directed on label.	May be useful for treating physiological aging and age-related memory deficits. Potent brain cell protector.
Huperzine A or vinpocetine	As directed on label. As directed on label.	Aid the effectiveness of acetylcholine in preventing memory loss.
Lecithin granules or capsules	1 tbsp 3 times daily, before meals. 1,200 mg 3 times daily, before meals.	Needed for improved memory. Contains choline.
Manganese	As directed on label. Take separately from calcium.	Helps nourish the brain and nerves. Aids in the utilization of choline.
Multivitamin and mineral complex with potassium	As directed on label. 99 mg daily.	All nutrients are necessary in balance. Use a high-potency formula. Needed for proper electrolyte balance.
Omega-3 fatty acid complex	As directed on label.	Low levels have been associated with impaired brain function.
Phosphatidylcholine	As directed on label.	Improves memory.
Superoxide dismutase (SOD)	As directed on label.	Known for its ability to eliminate free radicals.
Vitamin A plus carotenoid complex with beta-carotene	15,000 IU daily. If you are pregnant, do not exceed 10,000 IU daily. 25,000 IU daily.	Deficiencies of antioxidants expose the brain to oxidative damage.
Vitamin C with bioflavonoids	3,000–10,000 mg daily.	A powerful antioxidant that also improves circulation.
Vitamin E	200 IU daily or 400 IU every other day.	Causes dilation of blood vessels, improving blood flow to the brain. Use d-alpha-tocopherol form.
Zinc plus copper	50–80 mg daily. Do not exceed 100 mg daily from all supplements. 3 mg daily.	Important in binding toxic substances and removing them from the brain. Use zinc gluconate lozenges or OptiZinc for best absorption. Needed to balance with zinc.

Important

Supplement	Suggested Dosage	Comments
Acetyl-L-carnitine	500 mg twice daily.	May enhance brain metabolism. Slows deterioration of memory and reduces the production of free radicals.
L-glutamine and L-phenylalanine plus L-aspartic acid	As directed on label, on an empty stomach. Take with water or juice. Do not take with milk. Take with 50 mg vitamin B6 and 100 mg vitamin C for better absorption.	Amino acids necessary for normal brain function; serve as fuel for the brain and prevent excess ammonia from damaging the brain. Caution: Do not take phenylalanine if you are pregnant or nursing, or if you suffer from panic attacks, diabetes, high blood pressure, or PKU.
L-tyrosine	Up to 100 mg per kg of body weight daily. Take on an empty stomach with	Helps sharpen learning, memory, and awareness; elevates mood and motivation;

Supplement	Suggested Dosage	Comments
	1,000 mg vitamin C and 50 mg vitamin B6 for better absorption.	aids in preventing depression. Caution: Do not take this supplement if you are also taking an MAO inhibitor drug.

Helpful

Supplement	Suggested Dosage	Comments
Coenzyme Q10 plus Coenzyme A from Coenzyme-A Technologies	100 mg daily. As directed on label.	Improves brain oxygenation. Improves the effectiveness of coenzyme Q10.
Dehydroepiandrosterone (DHEA from Natrol) or 7-Keto DHEA	As directed on label. Take with vitamins C and E and selenium to prevent oxidative damage to the liver. As directed on label.	May help to improve memory. (See DHEA THERAPY in Part Three.) A metabolite of DHEA that has been found to be superior to DHEA in enhancing memory. Unlike DHEA, it is not converted into estrogen or testosterone in the body.
Diamond Mind from Diamond-Herpanacine Associates or Bacopin & Ginkgo Complex from America's Finest	As directed on label. As directed on label.	Combination supplements that can aid with memory-related functions.
Dimethylglycine (DMG) (Aangamik DMG from FoodScience of Vermont)	As directed on label.	Improves brain oxygenation.
Melatonin	2–3 mg daily, taken 2 hours or less before bedtime.	A powerful antioxidant that may prevent memory loss.
Nicotinamide adenine dinucleotide (NADH)	As directed on label.	A coenzyme form of niacin that is essential for the production of certain neurotransmitters and energy. Natural levels decline with age. Supplemental NADH can improve energy production in the brain and nervous system.
Pregnenolone from TriMedica	As directed on label.	May improve brain function and enhance memory.
RNA and DNA	As directed on label.	Increases energy production for memory transfer in the brain. Caution: Do not take this supplement if you have gout.

Herbs

❏ Brahmi, an Ayurvedic herb related to gotu kola, increases circulation in the brain and has been found to improve both short- and long-term memory.

❏ Garlic has been found to possess memory-enhancing properties.

❏ Ginkgo biloba has been attracting attention from researchers because of its ability to increase blood flow to the brain and central nervous system, thereby enhancing memory and brain function. Ginkgo is available in capsule or extract form at most health food stores. For memory enhancement, take capsules as directed on the product label, or place 6 drops of an alcohol-free extract under your tongue, hold them there for a few minutes, then swallow. Do this twice daily.

Caution: Do not take ginkgo biloba if you have a bleeding disorder, or are scheduled for surgery or a dental procedure.

❑ Other herbs that are helpful for memory include anise, ginseng, gotu kola, and rosemary.

Caution: Do not use ginseng if you have high blood pressure or are pregnant or nursing.

Recommendations

❑ Eat a diet high in raw foods. Consume the following often: brewer's yeast, brown rice, farm eggs, fish, legumes, millet, nuts, soybeans, tofu, wheat germ, and whole grains.

Caution: Brewer's yeast can cause an allergic reaction in some individuals. Start with a small amount at first, and discontinue use if any allergic symptoms occur.

❑ Combine complex carbohydrates with foods containing 10 percent protein and 10 percent essential fats.

❑ Avoid dairy and wheat products (except for wheat germ) for one month. If there is no memory improvement, slowly add these foods back to your diet.

❑ Eat more blueberries and spinach. Some researchers believe that flavonoids found in these foods may aid in memory retention.

❑ Make certain that you are getting the correct amounts of amino acids, antioxidants, B vitamins, choline, coenzyme Q_{10}, iron, and pregnenolone, either from the diet or through supplementation.

❑ Avoid refined sugars—these "turn off" the brain.

❑ Practice holding your breath for thirty seconds every hour for thirty days. This improves mental alertness.

❑ Consider having a hair analysis done to rule out intoxication by metals such as aluminum and lead. Either of these conditions can lead to impaired mental functioning. (*See* HAIR ANALYSIS in Part Three.)

❑ Use the following tips to help minimize age-related memory loss:

• Reduce stress.

• Keep active mentally.

• Eat a healthy brain diet.

• Get regular physical exercise.

• Get plenty of sleep.

• Limit sugar intake.

• Avoid tobacco.

• Avoid excessive use of alcohol.

❑ Make sure to focus on things that you may wish to remember, and be sure to give them meaning. Often, we blame our inability to recall something on a failing memory when the problem is that we did not really pay attention in the first place.

❑ Keep yourself active mentally by using your brain on a daily basis. Pursue activities such as reading, doing crossword puzzles, surfing the Internet, or playing a mentally challenging game. Research has shown that the more you put your memory to use, the more vital it will be.

❑ Keep yourself physically active. This increases blood flow to the brain. One study of older women indicated that those who engaged in moderate exercise, such as walking at least six hours per week, had a 20 percent decrease in risk of cognitive impairment as compared with those who were inactive. They also demonstrated cognitive functioning of someone three years younger, on average, than their actual age.

Caution: If you are thirty-five or older and/or have been sedentary for some time, consult with your health care provider before beginning an exercise program.

❑ Be sure to get the proper amount of rest to avoid fatigue, which can have a direct effect on the ability to focus.

Considerations

❑ In Europe, ginkgo is the principal therapeutic treatment of cerebral dysfunction or cerebral insufficiency. An extract standardized to 22 to 27 percent flavonoid glycosides and 5 to 7 percent terpene lactones has been tested in normal individuals and shown to enhance memory and working memory in postmenopausal women. Similarly, in one study, elderly individuals improved their speed in processing information, working memory, and executive processing. When you buy your ginkgo, be sure that the brand you are buying has the right mixture of flavonoids (22 to 27 percent) and terpenes (5 to 7 percent). These results were based on taking 120 milligrams per day.

Caution: Do not take ginkgo biloba if you have a bleeding disorder, or are scheduled for surgery or a dental procedure.

❑ Human growth hormone (HGH) has been shown to improve brain function. But this therapy is not the first line of treatment. (*See* GROWTH HORMONE THERAPY in Part Three.)

❑ Some medications may have an adverse effect on memory, including beta-blockers, benzodiazepines (prescribed for anxiety), some painkillers and antihistamines, and anticholinergics (prescribed for incontinence or depression).

❑ Occasional memory loss or forgetfulness is common. However, if you begin to notice certain memory-related problems happening, such as forgetting things much more often than you did before, forgetting how to do something that was commonplace to you before, getting lost in familiar surroundings, or repeating the same conversation over and over again to the same person, there may be cause for concern. Seek medical help. Early treatment with Alzheimer's medications can slow the progression of the disease.

❑ Absent a disease such as Alzheimer's, the keys to having a good memory often are in attitude and approach. As we age, our attitudes change. Our ability to remember isn't affected as much as we think. It is the change in our motivation to remember things that is probably the larger factor.

❑ According to a study conducted at the University of Toronto, Canada, potatoes, pasta, and bread boost memory. The natural sugars found in these foods apparently enhance the brain's ability to store memories.

❑ Studies from the 1990s showed that phosphatidyl serine improved memory. This supplement was once made from cow brains. However, after the mad cow (in humans it is called Creutzfeldt-Jakob disease) scare, dietary supplement companies began making it from soybean oil, and there are no studies to show whether it still works.

❑ *See also* AGING; ALZHEIMER'S DISEASE; ARTERIOSCLEROSIS; HYPOGLYCEMIA; and/or SENILITY, all in Part Two.

MÉNIÈRE'S DISEASE

Ringing in the ears, variable loss of hearing, loss of balance, vertigo or dizziness, tinnitus (buzzing or ringing in the ears), and a sensation of fullness or pressure are symptoms of the inner ear disturbance known as Ménière's disease. The condition may affect one or both ears.

Ménière's disease is rare and the exact cause or causes are unknown, but many experts believe it results from a condition known to researchers as *endolymphatic hydrops,* an excessive swelling of the small, fluid-filled chambers of the inner ear. Eventually, the pressure and severe disruptions within the inner ear cause periodic attacks of vertigo. The attacks can last from ten minutes to several hours. During a severe attack, symptoms can include nausea, sweating, vomiting, and loss of balance. Unsteadiness may last for several days after the attack. Impaired blood flow to the brain from clogged arteries and poor circulation may also be involved. Allergies, consumption of alcohol or caffeine, stress, barometric changes, pregnancy, visual stimuli, experiencing orgasm, sugar, exposure to loud noises, and excessive salt intake may trigger this disorder. Other factors, such as obesity and high blood cholesterol, may contribute to this syndrome. Allergies, spasms of the blood vessels that supply the inner ear, and, for women, fluid retention during the premenstrual period may also be related to Ménière's disease. Drug use, smoking, trauma, and temporomandibular joint (TMJ) syndrome may be involved as well.

Ménière's disease usually affects adults (men more often than women) between the ages of thirty and sixty. For many individuals, Ménière's disease is an unpredictable disorder and the attacks only occur occasionally; for others is it severe and can cause complete deafness and repeated, debilitating vertigo.

Unless otherwise specified, the dosages recommended here are for adults. For children between the ages of twelve and seventeen, reduce the dose to three-quarters of the recommended amount. For children between six and twelve, use one-half of the recommended dose, and for children under the age of six, use one-quarter of the recommended amount.

NUTRIENTS

SUPPLEMENT	SUGGESTED DOSAGE	COMMENTS
Essential		
Manganese	5 mg daily. Take separately from calcium.	Deficiency may be the cause of Ménière's disease.
Very Important		
Bio-Strath from Nature's Answer	As directed on label.	A natural source of the B vitamins. Acts as a tonic and enhances brain function.
Chromium picolinate	200 mcg daily.	Aids in controlling blood sugar levels, which are often high in people with this disorder.
Coenzyme Q10 plus	100 mg daily.	Improves circulation.
Coenzyme A from Coenzyme-A Technologies	As directed on label.	Supports and boosts the immune system.
Vitamin B3 (niacin)	100 mg twice daily. Do not exceed this amount.	Improves circulation. If you are uncomfortable with the flush caused by niacin, use part niacinamide. *Caution:* Do not take niacin if you have a liver disorder, gout, or high blood pressure.
Important		
Vitamin B complex plus extra vitamin B6 (pyridoxine)	As directed on label. 100 mg twice daily.	Important for the nervous system. Use a high-stress formula. Reduces fluid retention.
Vitamin C with bioflavonoids	3,000–6,000 mg daily, in divided doses.	Boosts immune function. Use an esterified or buffered form.
Helpful		
Calcium and magnesium	1,500 mg daily. 1,000 mg daily.	Needed for stability of the nervous system and for muscle contraction. Chelated forms are the most effective.
Essential fatty acids (primrose oil, salmon oil, or Kyolic-EPA from Wakunaga)	As directed on label 3 times daily, with meals.	To correct metabolic disturbances.
Lecithin granules or capsules	1 tbsp 3 times daily, before meals. 1,200 mg 3 times daily, before meals.	For cellular protection and brain function.
Vitamin E	200 IU daily or 400 IU every other day.	Promotes efficient oxygen use. Use d-alpha-tocopherol form.

Herbs

❑ Butcher's broom combats fluid retention and improves circulation.

❑ Ginger is helpful for nausea.

❑ Ginkgo biloba, taken in extract or tablet form, increases circulation to the brain.

Caution: Do not take ginkgo biloba if you have a bleeding disorder, or are scheduled for surgery or a dental procedure.

❏ St. John's wort can relieve anxiety and depression.

Caution: St. John's wort may cause increased sensitivity to sunlight. It may also produce anxiety, gastrointestinal symptoms, and headaches. It can interact with some drugs including antidepressants, birth control pills, and anticoagulants.

Recommendations

❏ Limit your intake of salt. Under normal conditions, the body needs about 2 grams of salt a day; most Americans eat 10 grams. Over time, restricting the amount of salt you eat should help to decrease the fluid in the inner ear and reduce any pressure on nerve endings that may be affecting your balance and hearing.

❏ Try a hypoglycemic diet for two weeks. If you experience an improvement, remain on the diet. (*See* HYPOGLYCEMIA in Part Two.)

❏ Do not consume any fats, fried foods, added salt, monosodium glutamate (MSG), alcohol, sugar (in any form), or anything containing caffeine. Caffeine excessively stimulates nerve endings.

❏ Stop smoking. Smoking constricts and reduces blood flow to the tiny blood vessels that nourish the inner ear nerve endings.

❏ Check for food allergies. (*See* ALLERGIES in Part Two.)

❏ To help with vertigo attacks, restrict your head movement and keep your eyes fixed on a stationary object at a good distance from you. Also, you can lie down with your unaffected ear against the floor, and look in the direction of the affected ear.

❏ As much as possible, reduce the anxiety in your life. Stress is a major trigger in Ménière's disease.

❏ Reasonable exercise such as a daily brisk walk will stimulate circulation and help blood flow.

Considerations

❏ Some doctors recommend a high-protein, low-refined-carbohydrate diet because they have found that people with this disorder have high blood insulin levels. High insulin levels impair circulation. (*See* ARTERIOSCLEROSIS and CIRCULATORY PROBLEMS, both in Part Two.)

❏ Doctors prescribe a variety of medications to combat the symptoms of vertigo and nausea. Promethazine (Phenergan) is usually prescribed to treat the nausea, vomiting, and vertigo symptoms. To reduce fluids in the system, diuretics may be prescribed. A low-salt diet may accompany this plan. Diazepam (Valium) is frequently prescribed to lessen anxiety and to sedate the vestibular system. For some people, physicians prescribe antihistamines, and in some cases, steroids.

❏ If symptoms are severe and interfere drastically with daily life, surgery may be recommended. Surgical procedure options for Ménière's disease include the insertion of a small tube into the eardrum (a tympanostomy tube), enlarging the endolymphatic sac by drilling the bone surrounding it or draining the fluid to reduce pressure (endolymphatic sac decompression), placing a small tube into the endolymphatic sac to drain excess fluid (endolymphatic sac shunt), removal of the labyrinth or a portion of the labyrinth (surgical labyrinthectomy), cutting the vestibular nerve to destroy the balance function of the ear (vestibular nerve section surgery), placing ototoxic drugs (toxic antibiotics like gentamicin) in the ear to destroy the balance portion of the ear (chemical labyrinthectomy), or inserting drugs into the eardrum with a syringe by laser.

❏ A Meniett device has been shown to help treat and control acute attacks of vertigo in patients with unilateral cochleo-vestibular disease who had tympanostomy tubes inserted. These patients also followed a low-salt diet, and 67 percent had reduced symptoms—80 percent of these had reduced symptoms for as long as a year after treatment.

❏ *See also* HEARING LOSS in Part Two.

❏ For the name and address of an organization that can provide more information about Ménière's disease, *see* American Academy of Otolaryngology *under* Health and Medical Organizations in the Appendix.

MENINGITIS

Meningitis is an infection of the three membranes, called the meninges, that lie between the brain and the skull. The thin membranes that cover the spinal cord may also be involved. This disorder is more common in children than in adults.

The most common type of meningitis is viral meningitis. This disease causes comparatively mild symptoms, such as headache and malaise, and usually improves on its own in a week or two. Also called *aseptic meningitis,* viral meningitis usually occurs in conjunction with other diseases. Almost 50 percent of cases of viral meningitis infections are caused by intestinal viruses. This condition may also accompany mumps or a herpes outbreak, and it can be carried by mosquitoes as well. The early symptoms of viral meningitis include sore throat, fever, headache, stiff neck, fatigue, and, possibly, a rash and vomiting.

Bacterial meningitis is the more serious infection, and it requires prompt, aggressive medical treatment. The bacteria responsible for most outbreaks of bacterial meningitis are *Neisseria meningitidis* (meningococcus), *Streptococcus pneumoniae* (pneumococcus), *Haemophilus influenzae* type B, and group B *Streptococcus*. *Neisseria* and *Streptococcus* are the leading causes of infection since, after 1990, routine immunization curbed the outbreaks of *H. influenzae* type B (Hib). In the case of *N. meningitidis,* at any one time, some 5 to 20 percent of the population carry this bacteria in their saliva without feeling any ill effects—but it can be transmitted through the saliva to other people. The *Streptococcus pneumoniae* bacteria is commonly found in the throat and is not contagious. The symptoms of bacterial meningitis include stiff neck, headache, irritability, high fever, chills, nausea, vomiting, delirium, and sensitivity to light. A blotchy, red skin rash may appear. In infants, the signs include fever, vomiting, poor muscle tone, difficulty feeding, irritability, a high-pitched cry, and a bulging fontanel (soft spot). Changes in temperament and extreme sleepiness signal dangerous changes in the cerebrospinal fluid (the fluid that surrounds and cushions the brain). Meningococcal meningitis kills 10 to 12 percent of those affected; among the survivors, 10 to 15 percent suffer hearing loss, diminished intellect, kidney disease, or need to have limbs amputated because of blood poisoning (septicemia).

Children with cochlear implants to treat hearing loss have a greater risk of developing bacterial meningitis than children in the general population. A study conducted by the U.S. Centers for Disease Control and Prevention, the U.S. Food and Drug Administration, and state and local health departments, and published in *The New England Journal of Medicine,* found that children with a specific type of cochlear implant that had an extra piece called a positioner had 4.5 times the risk of developing meningitis compared with those who had other types of implants. It is possible that individuals who are candidates for implants may have factors that increase their risk of meningitis.

The recommendations in this section are designed to support medical treatment, not replace it. Meningitis can progress very quickly and become life-threatening in a matter of twenty-four hours for adults, much less for children. If untreated, this disease can cause permanent brain damage and paralysis, even coma and death.

Unless otherwise specified, the dosages recommended here are for adults. For children between the ages of twelve and seventeen, reduce the dose to three-quarters the recommended amount. For children between six and twelve, use one-half the recommended dose, and for children under the age of six, use one-quarter the recommended amount.

NUTRIENTS

SUPPLEMENT	SUGGESTED DOSAGE	COMMENTS
Helpful		
Acidophilus (Kyo-Dophilus from Wakunaga)	As directed on label. Take on an empty stomach.	Needed to replenish the friendly bacteria antibiotics destroy. Use a nondairy formula.
Dimethylglycine (DMG) (Aangamik DMG from FoodScience of Vermont)	125 mg twice daily.	Carries oxygen to the cells, relieving many symptoms. Use a sublingual form.
Free form amino acid (Amino Balance from Anabol Naturals)	As directed on label.	Needed for tissue repair and protection of membranes.
Garlic (Kyolic from Wakunaga)	2 capsules 3 times daily, with meals.	An immune system stimulant that also acts as a natural antibiotic.
Geoxy-132 from American Biologics	As directed on label.	An antioxidant and immune system stimulator.
Maitake extract or reishi extract or shiitake extract	As directed on label. As directed on label. As directed on label.	To help to build immunity and fight viral infection.
Multivitamin and mineral complex	As directed on label.	All nutrients are needed for tissue protection and healing. Use a high-potency formula.
Raw thymus glandular	500 mg twice daily.	Enhances immune response.
Taurine Plus from American Biologics	As directed on label.	An antioxidant and immune system regulator necessary for white blood cell activation and neurological function. Use the liquid form.
Vitamin A emulsion or capsules	50,000 IU daily. 25,000 IU daily for 7 days, then reduce to 15,000 IU daily. If you are pregnant, do not exceed 10,000 IU daily.	A powerful antioxidant and immune system booster. Needed for protection and healing of all membranes. Emulsion form is recommended for easier absorption and greater safety at higher doses.
Vitamin C with bioflavonoids	3,000–10,000 mg daily.	Reduces infection and aids in cleansing the bloodstream.
Zinc lozenges	1 15-mg lozenge 3 times daily. Do not exceed a total of 100 mg daily from all supplements.	An immune system booster.

Herbs

❑ For fever, use catnip tea enemas. (*See* ENEMAS in Part Three.) Catnip tea is also good for sipping.

❑ Echinacea boosts the immune system.

Caution: Do not take echinacea for longer than three months. It should not be used by people who are allergic to ragweed.

❑ Goldenseal is a natural antibiotic.

Caution: Do not take goldenseal internally on a daily basis for more than one week at a time. Do not use it during pregnancy or if you are breast-feeding, and use with caution if you are allergic to ragweed. If you have a history of cardiovascular disease, diabetes, or glaucoma, use it only under a doctor's supervision.

❑ Olive leaf extract helps fight viral infections.

❑ St. John's wort is good for viral infections.

Caution: St. John's wort may cause increased sensitivity to sunlight. It may also produce anxiety, gastrointestinal symptoms, and headaches. It can interact with some drugs including antidepressants, birth control pills, and anticoagulants.

Recommendations

❏ If you develop symptoms characteristic of meningitis, see a physician or go to the emergency room of the nearest hospital immediately.

❏ Avoid drinking out of the same glass or container as someone else, and avoid sharing cigarettes, food, lipstick, and eating utensils.

❏ Avoid heavy use of alcohol.

❏ Avoid passive smoking (secondhand smoke).

❏ Avoid aspirin, which increases bleeding tendencies.

❏ Once the acute phase of the illness has passed and recovery has begun, eat a well-balanced diet including fresh fruits and vegetables (50 percent of them raw), grains, nuts, seeds, and yogurt and other soured products.

❏ Consume fresh pineapple and papaya frequently. Pineapple reduces inflammation; papaya is good for digestion. Only the fresh forms are effective.

❏ Avoid the following foods, which encourage the formation of mucus: animal protein and its by-products, caffeine, dairy products (except for yogurt), processed foods, salt, sugar, and white flour products.

❏ Rest in bed in a dimly lit room. Drink plenty of high-quality liquids.

❏ Take cool sponge baths.

Considerations

❏ Diagnosis of meningitis requires microscopic analysis and culture of the cerebrospinal fluid.

❏ If there are no complications, recovery from viral meningitis generally takes three weeks under a physician's care.

❏ Antibiotics do not fight viruses, so they are not appropriate treatment for viral meningitis. Only strains of *bacterial* meningitis can be treated with antibiotics.

❏ For bacterial meningitis, aggressive treatment with antibiotics is necessary. For viral meningitis, antibiotics are ineffective and therefore inappropriate. If meningitis is caused by a fungal infection, treatment with an antifungal drug is used.

❏ Pain medication may be needed such as nonsteroidal anti-inflammatory drugs (Advil, Aleve) and acetaminophen (Tylenol).

❏ It is wise to seek prompt treatment for a bacterial infection anywhere in the body, such as strep throat or an ear infection.

❏ Antibiotics may be prescribed as a preventive for those who have been in close contact with a person who has bacterial meningitis.

❏ Adults tend to be immune to *H. influenzae* type B, and the Hib vaccine protects most young children. However, if you have been in close contact with someone who has this infection, you may need to see your physician to inquire about antibiotic treatment. The vaccine is sometimes given to those over five years of age with sickle cell disease or HIV/AIDS, as well as those who have had their spleens removed, had bone marrow transplants, or are taking cancer-treatment drugs.

❏ If you are a parent contemplating the placement of a cochlear implant in your child, discuss with your physician all of the potential risks and benefits, and whether or not the child has certain medical conditions that might make meningitis more likely. If you do opt for the implant, make sure your child is up to date on vaccines at least two weeks before the procedure. If the implant has already been done, check with the child's doctor to ensure that vaccines are updated. (Current vaccines protect against the most common strains of meningitis-causing bacteria, but not all.) Watch for possible signs and symptoms of meningitis: high fever, headache, stiff neck, nausea or vomiting, discomfort looking into bright lights, sleepiness, or confusion. A young child or infant may be sleepy or cranky or eat less. Contact a doctor promptly if these symptoms are present. Also watch for signs and symptoms of an ear infection, which can include ear pain, fever, and decreased appetite. Seek prompt medical attention for these symptoms.

MENOPAUSAL AND PERIMENOPAUSAL PROBLEMS

Menopause is the point at which a woman stops ovulating and menstruation ceases, indicating the end of fertility. It is important to remember that menopause is *not* a disease. It is as natural a progression in life as puberty.

Many years before a woman stops ovulating, her ovaries slow their production of the hormones estrogen, progesterone, and testosterone. Estrogen and progesterone are commonly thought of as sex or reproductive hormones. While estrogen is indeed essential for reproduction, it also acts on many nonreproductive organs and systems in the body. Cells in the vagina, bladder, breasts, skin, bones, arteries, heart, liver, and brain all contain estrogen receptors, and require this hormone to stimulate these receptors for normal cell function. Estrogen is needed to keep the skin smooth and moist, and the body's internal thermostat operating properly. It is also necessary for proper bone formation. Although estrogen levels drop sharply after menopause, the hormone does not disappear entirely. Other organs take over from the ovaries and continue to produce a less potent form of estrogen. The organs known as endocrine glands secrete some hormones from fatty tissue to maintain bodily functions.

Progesterone works as a counterpart to estrogen. During the second half of the menstrual cycle, it stimulates changes in the lining of the uterus to complete its preparation to act as a "home" for a fertilized egg. If no egg is fertilized, the uterine lining is broken down and expelled. The cycle then begins again. Progesterone too has effects beyond the reproductive system. It has a calming effect on the brain and appears to affect other aspects of nervous system function as well.

Testosterone is the hormone that is most important for sex drive. Women produce much less of this hormone than men do—about 80 percent less—but it is the driving force for maintaining a healthy libido (sexual appetite).

Perimenopause is the period when a woman's body is preparing for menopause. For most women, hormone production begins to slow down when they reach their thirties, and continues to diminish as they age. Many women experience few if any symptoms during this time, but others may suffer from some, or all, of the following: anxiety, dry skin, fatigue, feelings of bloating, headaches, heart palpitations, hot flashes, insomnia, irritability, decreased interest in sex, loss of concentration, mood swings, night sweats, reduced stamina, urinary incontinence, vaginal dryness and itching, weight gain, cold hands and feet, joint pain, hair loss, and skin changes. Some women experience none of these symptoms; others may have some of these symptoms, but find that they are not related to hormonal changes.

Menopause is the time when a woman stops menstruating altogether. By this stage, most of the acute problems a woman may have experienced are actually over and a new balance between all hormones should be established. However, this is the time women become increasingly vulnerable to other, potentially serious health problems. Over the long term, the diminished supply of estrogen increases the likelihood of cardiovascular disease, osteoporosis, and vaginal atrophy. Osteoporosis in particular is a major problem for women after menopause. An estimated 45 to 50 percent of the 1.5 million hip fractures that occur in the United States every year are due to osteoporosis in women over fifty years of age.

With a proper diet, nutritional supplements, and exercise, most of the unpleasant side effects of menopause can be minimized, if not eliminated.

The dosages given below are for adults.

NUTRIENTS

SUPPLEMENT	SUGGESTED DOSAGE	COMMENTS
Very Important		
Beta-1,3-D-glucan	As directed on label.	Boosts bone marrow production and acts as a powerful stimulant for the immune system.
Cerasomal-cis-9-cetylmyristoleate	As directed on label.	Acts like a lubricant for joints and reduces inflammation. *Caution:* Do not take this supplement if you have liver problems.
Coenzyme Q10 plus Coenzyme A from Coenzyme-A Technologies	As directed on label. As directed on label.	To support the immune system's detoxification of many dangerous substances, streamline metabolism, ease depression and fatigue, increase energy, support adrenal glands, process fats, boost the immune system, and
Dehydroepiandrosterone (DHEA) or 7-keto DHEA	As directed on label. As directed on label.	improve overall physical and mental processes. Increases memory function, reduces stress, and enhances sex drive. *Note:* DHEA is converted into testosterone and estrogens in the body. Use with caution if you are taking HRT. A metabolite of DHEA that is not converted into sex hormones. Some studies have shown benefit for short-term use, but data for long-term use is not available.
Essential fatty acids (primrose oil, black currant seed oil, or Kyolic-EPA from Wakunaga)	As directed on label.	Act as sedatives and diuretics. Good for hot flashes. Important for production of estrogen.
Lactobacillus rhamnosus and *L. reuteri*	2.5 million cells of each daily.	Restores normal vaginal flora.
Lecithin granules or capsules	1 tbsp 3 times daily, before meals. 1,200 mg 3 times daily, before meals.	Important as an emulsifier for vitamin E, which reduces hot flashes and related symptoms.
Multienzyme complex with hydrochloric acid (HCl)	As directed on label. Take with meals.	To aid digestion. HCl production declines with age. *Caution:* Do not use HCl if you have a history of ulcers.
Soy protein	30 grams daily.	Soybeans contain a form of estrogen. Helps relieve hot flashes and protect against heart disease and osteoporosis.
Ultra Osteo Synergy from American Biologics	As directed on label.	Nutritional support for bone renewal.
Vitamin B complex	As directed on label.	For improved circulation and cellular function. Use a sublingual form for best absorption. Or consider injections (under a doctor's supervision).
plus extra vitamin B5 (pantothenic acid) and	100 mg 3 times daily.	A powerful antistress vitamin needed for adrenal function.
vitamin B6 (pyridoxine) and	50 mg 3 times daily	Minimizes water retention and eases symptoms.
folic acid	As directed on label.	Helps to protect against heart disease.
Vitamin E	200 IU daily or 400 IU every other day.	Reduces hot flashes and many other symptoms. Use emulsion form for easier assimilation. Use d-alpha-tocopherol form.
Important		
Boron	3 mg daily. Do not exceed this amount.	Enhances calcium absorption.
Calcium and magnesium	1,000–2,000 mg daily. 1,000 mg daily.	To relieve nervousness and irritability, and to protect against bone loss. Use chelate forms.
Quercetin Plus from Nature's Plus or Nutrition Now	2 mg daily.	An antioxidant flavonoid that may help with hot flashes.

Silica	As directed on label.	Supplies silicon, needed for connective tissue and for calcium uptake.
Vitamin D	400–600 IU daily.	Regulates calcium within the body. Calcium (1,000 mg) and vitamin D (400 IU) may reduce mortality in postmenopausal women.
Zinc plus copper	50 mg daily. Do not exceed a total of 100 mg daily from all supplements. 3 mg daily.	Aids in protecting against bone loss and reducing symptoms. Use zinc gluconate lozenges or OptiZinc for best absorption. Needed to balance with zinc.
Helpful		
L-arginine and L-lysine	500 mg twice daily. 500 mg daily, on an empty stomach. Take with water or juice. Do not take with milk. Take with 50 mg vitamin B$_6$ and 100 mg vitamin C for better absorption.	Detoxifies the liver. Aids liver function. (*See* AMINO ACIDS in Part One.)
Multiglandular complex	As directed on label.	For hormonal stability. (*See* GLANDULAR THERAPY in Part Three.)
Multivitamin and mineral complex with potassium and selenium	As directed on label. Take with meals. 99 mg daily. 200 mcg daily.	All nutrients are needed for normal hormone production and function. To replace potassium lost through perspiration during hot flashes. Potassium protects the nervous system and encourages a regular heart rhythm. An important trace mineral linked to normal hormonal balance.
Vitamin C plus mixed bioflavonoids	3,000–10,000 mg daily. 1,000 mg daily.	For hot flashes. Also for heart health.

Herbs

❑ A paste made from aloe vera gel, mixed to the consistency of toothpaste and inserted into the vagina at night, can relieve vaginal dryness.

❑ Amaranth, chickweed, dandelion greens, nettle, seaweed, and watercress are rich in calcium and can help prevent osteoporosis.

❑ Anise, black cohosh, fennel, licorice, raspberry, sage, unicorn root, and wild yam root are natural estrogen promoters, as are soybean products. Black cohosh has received the most attention, and the results of the studies are mixed. The biggest study, paid for by the National Institutes of Health (NIH), did not find black cohosh to be of benefit in relieving hot flashes or night sweats. Studies on soy and hot flashes have had both positive and negative results.

Cautions: Do not use black cohosh if you are pregnant or have any type of chronic disease. Black cohosh should not be used by those with liver problems. Licorice root should not be used during pregnancy or nursing. It should not be used

by persons with diabetes, glaucoma, heart disease, high blood pressure, or a history of stroke. Do not use sage if you suffer from any type of seizure disorder, or are pregnant or nursing.

❑ Damiana enhances sexual desire and pleasure.

❑ Hops and valerian root help to calm the body and promote restful sleep. Ginseng has been shown to help improve mood and sleep during menopause. Kava kava decreases anxiety but has no effect on hot flashes.

Cautions: Do not use ginseng if you have high blood pressure, or are pregnant or nursing. Kava kava can cause drowsiness. It is not recommended for pregnant women or nursing mothers, and it should not be taken together with other substances that act on the central nervous system, such as alcohol, barbiturates, antidepressants, and antipsychotic drugs.

❑ Gotu kola, black cohosh, red clover, and dong quai relieve hot flashes, vaginal dryness, and depression.

Cautions: Do not use black cohosh if you are pregnant or have any type of chronic disease. Black cohosh should not be used by those with liver problems. Dong quai enhances the action of the blood thinner warfarin, so the two should not be used together.

❑ Seaweed and soy foods are commonly consumed in Japan, where 10 to 20 percent of women experience hot flashes compared to 70 to 80 percent in Western countries. In one study, soy protein containing 60 milligrams of isoflavones reduced hot flashes by 57 percent and night sweats by 43 percent.

❑ St. John's wort is valuable if you suffer from anxiety or depression.

Caution: St. John's wort may cause increased sensitivity to sunlight. It may also produce anxiety, gastrointestinal symptoms, and headaches. It can interact with some drugs, including antidepressants, birth control pills, and anticoagulants.

❑ Siberian ginseng aids in relieving depression and in the production of estrogen.

Caution: Do not use this herb if you have hypoglycemia, high blood pressure, or a heart disorder.

Recommendations

❑ Eat a diet consisting of 50 percent raw foods and take a protein supplement to help stabilize blood sugar. Add blackstrap molasses, soybean products, broccoli, dandelion greens, kelp, salmon with bones, sardines, and whitefish to your diet.

❑ Eat foods high in phytoestrogens, such as soybeans, flaxseeds, nuts, whole grains, apples, fennel, celery, parsley, and alfalfa. Soy and soy isoflavones may help to alleviate hot flashes associated with menopause. A high intake of phytoestrogens is thought to explain why hot flashes and other menopausal symptoms rarely occur among women in Asian cultures. If you have breast, uterine, or

Hormones, Hormone Therapy, and Menopause

Menopause is something all women experience, and as it approaches, they are faced with the decision as to whether or not to opt for some sort of hormone therapy, whether it is hormone replacement therapy (HRT) with estrogen and progesterone, or estrogen replacement therapy (ERT) only. In order to make an informed decision, it is necessary first to understand something about different types of hormones.

Broadly speaking, there are two types of hormone products available: natural and synthetic. Natural hormones are hormones whose molecular structures most closely resemble those of the hormones made by the body. Some doctors argue that natural hormone replacement therapy is not regulated sufficiently. Because the hormones are considered natural, some say, they have not been exposed to the rigorous tests that the synthetic variety has had to undergo. Yet other physicians argue that synthetic hormones carry an additional risk to the health of some, if not all, women. There are no simple answers at present. However, if hormones are recommended, the lowest dose should be used for the least amount of time. Much more research into this controversial topic is needed.

ESTROGEN

Three estrogens are naturally made by the body: estradiol, estrone, and estriol. Estradiol is the dominant estrogen produced by the ovaries. Levels of estriol are highest during pregnancy, and this form of estrogen has been shown to have a protective effect against breast cancer. Estrone is formed from estradiol, and appears to be the estrogen responsible for estrogen-dependent breast cancer. Estradiol is available for replacement therapy. Climara, Estrace, Estraderm, Estring, Menostar, and Vagifem are some of the brand names under which replacement estradiol is sold. Some are taken orally or as vaginal creams, and others are absorbed from skin patches. Both estriol and estrone are also available for replacement therapy.

There are also synthetic versions of estrogen that may be prescribed. These are compounds that have estrogen-like effects in the body, but they are less similar, on a molecular level, to the body's own estrogens. Conjugated or esterified estrogen is manufactured from the purified urine of pregnant mares. Premarin is the synthetic estrogen most prescribed for HRT.

PROGESTERONE

Estrogen dominance is an important concept to understand if you are perimenopausal and/or thinking of hormone replacement. This is a situation that can occur if the correct balance between estrogen and progesterone is not maintained. Symptoms of estrogen dominance can include flagging energy, fluid retention and bloating, and weight gain. Estrogen dominance can also increase certain types of cancer, notably endometrial cancer. This is why, unless you have undergone hysterectomy, HRT regimens usually include both estrogen and progesterone. There are many natural progesterone creams that may be prescribed by your doctor. Despite wild yam being touted as a source of estrogen, sometimes synthetic progesterone (medroxyprogesterone acetate) is added to wild yams. The resulting product is no longer natural. Furthermore, when the two are combined, the product is not effective for treating menopausal symptoms, and it can cause side effects including headache, breast tenderness, and upset stomach.

TESTOSTERONE

Testosterone is the essential hormone for continuing sexual desire in both sexes. It also supports the skin, muscles, and bones. If sexual desire diminishes, women may want to add this hormone to their replacement therapy. Natural testosterone or methyltestosterone is available for use as part of hormone therapy. It is sold as a combination (estrogen and testosterone) called Estratest.

TYPES OF REPLACEMENT THERAPY

There are two basic approaches to hormone replacement therapy: single hormone therapy and combination hormone therapy. Single hormone therapy usually involves estrogen only. Thus, it has been referred to as estrogen replacement therapy (ERT). ERT was and still is the most frequently prescribed treatment for women who have had a hysterectomy, or women without an intact uterus. ERT treatment should *not* be used by a woman who has an intact uterus, as it may increase her risk of developing cancer of the uterus or the endometrium (the uterine lining) by as much as six to eight times. Estrogen is available in tablets, patches, vaginal creams, vaginal rings, and intervaginal gels. The vaginal creams, rings, and gels are used for vaginal dryness or itchiness only, or for urinary problems. In addition to coming in various forms, estrogen products come in various doses. You must discuss the appropriate dose with your doctor.

Combination hormone therapy, or HRT, uses both estrogen and progesterone (usually in the form of progestin, a synthetic form of this hormone). HRT is normally prescribed for women who have a uterus and ovaries and who are approaching, or have reached, menopause. Progestin is believed to protect against the increased risk of uterine cancer posed by taking estrogen alone. There are many different doses and different methods of taking these hormones. You and your doctor need to decide what is right for you.

In addition to ERT and HRT, there is combination estrogen and testosterone therapy (see above). If tests indicate that levels of estrogen and testosterone are low, these hormones are available in combination formulas.

RISKS AND BENEFITS

A study conducted by the Women's Health Initiative (WHI) and sponsored by the National Institutes of Health (NIH), beginning in 1993 and involving 16,600 women aged fifty to seventy-nine, examined the benefits and risks associated with HRT. Two distinct groups were studied, those using ERT and those using HRT.

In July 2002, the study involving women prescribed HRT was halted due to the increased risks of breast cancer, heart attack, stroke, and blood clots that were observed during the study. In March 2004, women with intact uteruses stopped taking ERT due to increased risk of stroke. However, data was inconclusive as to whether ERT increased risk of blood clots. The data also suggested that the risk of developing ovarian cancer increased with the length of time ERT was used. Hormone replacement is now recommended for two groups of women:

1. Women who are going through menopause and women who have already gone through it (called postmenopausal) and are experiencing symptoms such as hot flashes, night sweats, vaginal dryness, and sleep disorders.

2. Women with certain health conditions such as premature ovarian failure, where their bodies don't produce normal amounts of the hormone estrogen.

Overall, as with any type of treatment, hormone therapy promises certain benefits but also poses risks. Some of the risks and benefits that have been most studied concern the following:

• *Aging.* Most research shows that HRT keeps the skin more supple and the sex organs better lubricated, with less atrophy (thinning of tissues).

• *Alzheimer's disease.* A study editorialized in the *Journal of the American Medical Association* indicates that HRT, once thought to prevent dementia and Alzheimer's disease, now seems to cause thinking and memory impairment.

• *Blood clots.* According to the WHI study released in July of 2002, women taking combined hormone therapy, HRT, had twice the risk of developing blood clots as compared with those who did not take HRT.

• *Breast cancer.* According to the WHI study, data demonstrated a compelling link between combined hormone replacement, HRT, and invasive (infiltrating) lobular breast cancer and ductal breast cancer. In fact, the study showed a 26 percent increase in breast cancer cases.

• *Colorectal cancer.* Studies suggest that women taking HRT are better protected against colorectal cancer than those who are not taking HRT. All women over forty should have regular colorectal examinations to test for cancer.

• *Heart disease.* According to the WHI study, taking combined hormone therapy, HRT, was associated with a 29 percent increase in the risk of heart disease. Heart disease kills more women than all types of cancer put together, so it is important to take measures to protect yourself against heart disease whether you opt for hormone therapy or not. (*See* HEART ATTACK in Part Two.)

• *Hot flashes and mood swings.* Hormone therapy, whether ERT or HRT, should eliminate hot flashes. It may also alleviate mood swings—although that depends on exactly what causes them.

• *Osteoporosis.* Estrogen replacement does appear to protect women from severe bone loss and osteoporosis. For osteoporosis prevention, experts recommend taking estrogen with about 1,000 milligrams of calcium a day. (*See* OSTEOPOROSIS in Part Two.)

• *Stroke.* The WHI study concluded that women who took combined hormone therapy, HRT, had a 41 percent increase in their risk for stroke.

• Summarized by the type of hormone therapy, certain known risks can be described as follows.

• *ERT (estrogen only).* This is associated with an *increased* risk of osteoporosis and, possibly, an increase in the risk of dementia or memory loss; and a *decreased* risk of hip fracture. It has not been found to have any effect on the risk of breast cancer or heart disease.

• *HRT (estrogen plus progestin).* This is associated with an *increased* risk of breast cancer, blood clots, stroke, and dementia (including Alzheimer's disease); and a *decreased* risk of hip fracture, colorectal cancer, and endometrial cancer as compared with women who did not take hormones.

MAKING THE DECISION

This decision to take—or not to take—hormone therapy is not an easy one for many women, and there are no easy answers. Researchers are only beginning to really understand the biological effects of estrogen replacement. A woman's age when she begins taking HRT, the duration of treatment, and the method—whether patch or pill—could all have an effect on her risk.

Everyone must weigh her own particular risk factors and decide whether the potential benefits outweigh those risks. You also need to decide whether to use synthetic or natural hormones, or approach any discomfort you may have with a more holistic approach that makes use of the nutrients and other remedies outlined elsewhere in this section.

There are also the questions of when to begin hormone therapy and how long to continue. Some doctors think that women should be introduced to HRT during perimenopause, but there are many others who think that this is unnecessary and, with the correct diet, stress management, and exercise, women do not need to opt for replacement therapy at this early stage unless there are profound reasons for doing so. Discuss this issue with your doctor. Also discuss how long you should continue taking HRT. The uncomfortable symptoms of menopause and perimenopause often last for only a short time, so you may not need to remain on the therapy for a prolonged period. In fact, many women are opting for low-dose HRT for a short period of time when menopausal symptoms are interfering with their quality of life. On the other hand, if you are taking hormone therapy because of long-term concerns such as osteoporosis prevention, a different duration may be necessary. Consult your physician.

Male Menopause

The term "male menopause" is often used in a joking way, sometimes as a dismissive substitute for "midlife crisis." But while men do not face the end of fertility in midlife as women do, they too undergo important physical and hormonal changes at that time. Men should not take male menopause—sometimes called andropause—lightly.

During male menopause, sex drive may weaken, anxiety may increase, and depression and moodiness may accompany a sense of failure. These symptoms can occur because of falling levels of testosterone. Men's testosterone levels begin to decline by the age of forty—earlier in some cases—and this may cause a loss of sexual desire,

mood swings, and irritability, and may even increase the risk of heart disease. If low testosterone levels are a problem, testosterone replacement therapy may be prescribed. Before a man makes a decision about testosterone replacement, he should undergo a prostate specific antigen (PSA) test to look for signs of prostate cancer, and he should have a frank discussion with his physician about potential side effects. It is advisable also to check DHEA and estrogen levels (estrogen is a male as well as a female hormone) so that if therapy is needed, it can be tailored to the individual's particular needs.

---

ovarian cancer, or have had or are at risk for any of these, you may want to speak to your health care professional about the risks of increasing your dietary soy intake.

❏ Do not consume any animal products except for those recommended in this section. Avoid dairy products—limit your consumption to small amounts of low-fat yogurt or buttermilk. Dairy products and meat promote hot flashes.

❏ Make sure you take calcium and vitamin D as supplements to reduce your risk of osteoporosis.

❏ Avoid alcohol, caffeine, sugar, spicy foods, and hot soups and drinks; they can trigger hot flashes, aggravate urinary incontinence, and make mood swings worse. They also make the blood more acidic, which prompts the bones to release calcium to act as a buffering agent. This is an important factor in bone loss.

❏ Get regular moderate exercise.

❏ Avoid stress as much as possible.

❏ Substitute garlic or onion powder for salt when cooking. Consuming salt increases urinary excretion of calcium.

❏ Drink 2 quarts of quality water each day to help prevent drying of the skin and mucous membranes.

❏ For itching in the vaginal area, use vitamin E cream (with no fragrance added) or open a vitamin E capsule and apply the oil.

❏ If sexual intercourse is painful, try using vitamin E oil or aloe vera gel to lubricate the vagina.

Considerations

❏ Gamma-oryzanol, a nutrient derived from rice bran, has been shown to be effective in treating symptoms of menopause. A daily dose of 20 milligrams reduced symptoms by 50 percent in 67 percent of the women studied.

❏ In one study, taking soy isoflavones (40 to 80 milligrams per day) seemed to be effective at reducing the number of

hot flashes in women who experience hot flashes frequently—ten or more a day. Most of the women had a 22 percent reduction in hot flashes. In another study, 60 milligrams of isoflavones from soy each day reduced hot flashes by 57 percent and night sweats by 43 percent. Check with your doctor before taking soy isoflavones as a supplement.

❏ Red clover has been the subject of five controlled studies, with mixed results as to their effectiveness in reducing hot flashes. Red clover contains phytoestrogens. Women should speak to their doctors before using red clover.

❏ Smoking is associated with early menopause.

❏ Frequent sexual intercourse can help relieve vaginal dryness.

❏ Some physicians recommend hormone replacement therapy (HRT) to control severe symptoms caused by estrogen deficiency in menopausal and postmenopausal women. Although hormone therapy appears to be effective, it does have possible serious risks, which should be carefully considered. Investigators in the Women's Health Initiative announced that estrogen increases the risk of stroke and might even raise the likelihood of developing dementia, although the hormone had no effect on breast cancer or heart disease. Be aware that research is ongoing in all aspects of replacement hormones—there is probably more conflicting information on this medical topic than there is about any other condition. It is essential to work with a good physician who can advise you about which of the vast array of products available may help you overcome any discomforts you may be experiencing. (*See* Hormones, Hormone Therapy, and Menopause on page 580.)

❏ Conventional treatment for a problematic perimenopause is to prescribe a low-dose contraceptive. However, natural progesterone is a precursor to make estrogen in the body, and may be the answer during this period, rather than supplemental estrogen, because symptoms are often a result of estrogen dominance. (See the discussion of estrogen dominance in Hormones, Hormone Therapy, and Menopause on page 580.)

❑ After menopause, a reduction in the amount of the sex hormone estrogen can cause shrinkage of urethral and vaginal membranes, promoting incontinence. There may be a continuous dribbling of urine. Urethral dilation helps stretch a contracted urethra.

❑ It may be more important to replace progesterone than estrogen. Natural progesterone cream is a good way to do this.

❑ Some of the bioidentical hormones on the market are custom-mixed formulas containing various hormones that are chemically identical to those made naturally by the body. Saliva testing is often used to determine your particular need. They may offer some benefit, according to the North American Menopause Society, but they are not regulated for purity, potency, safety, or efficacy by the FDA. Other bioidentical hormones are made by drug companies and are sold in standard doses, and are approved by the FDA. FDA-approved bioidentical hormone therapies are:

• Estradiol (Estrace, Climara Patch, Vivelle-Dot Patch)

❑ Hypothyroidism is common in menopausal women. Many symptoms ascribed to menopause may be due to improper thyroid function. (*See* HYPOTHYROIDISM in Part Two.)

❑ Symptoms of perimenopause are often mistaken for those of premenstrual syndrome (PMS). Both PMS and perimenopausal symptoms are a result of an imbalance between estrogen and progesterone—specifically, rising estrogen and diminishing progesterone. If your menstrual cycles have changed—for example, if your periods are lasting for a longer or shorter time than they used to, or if they are irregular when they were not irregular before—it is more likely that you are perimenopausal rather than premenstrual. A blood test to determine your level of a hormone called follicle-stimulating hormone (FSH) is also helpful in determining whether you are experiencing perimenopause. FSH levels increase as estrogen diminishes.

❑ It is important for menopausal and postmenopausal women to take measures to protect themselves against heart disease. (*See* HEART ATTACK in Part Two.) Many women have been led to believe that taking estrogen protects against this disease, but there is very reasonable doubt about the protective benefits of synthetic estrogen against heart attacks. (*See* Hormones, Hormone Therapy, and Menopause on page 580.)

❑ *See also* HYPOGLYCEMIA and HYSTERECTOMY-RELATED PROBLEMS in Part Two.

MENSTRUAL CRAMPS

See under PREMENSTRUAL SYNDROME.

MERALGIA PARESTHETICA

See under RARE DISORDERS.

MERCURY TOXICITY

Mercury is one of the most toxic metals—even more so than lead. This poison is found in our soil, water, and food supply, as well as in sewage sludge, fungicides, and pesticides. Some grains and seeds are treated with methyl mercury chlorine bleaches, which seep into the food supply. Because methyl mercury contaminates our waters, large amounts are found in fish, particularly larger ones that are farther up in the food chain. An estimated one-third (or possibly more) of America's lakes and one-fourth of its rivers now contain fish that may be contaminated with mercury. Mercury is also present in a wide variety of everyday products, including cosmetics, dental fillings, fabric softeners, batteries, industrial instruments, inks used by printers and tattooists, latex, some medications, some paints, plastics, polishes, solvents, and wood preservatives.

Mercury is a cumulative poison. There is no barrier that prohibits mercury from reaching the brain cells, and it is retained in the pain center of the brain and in the central nervous system. Its presence there can prevent both the normal entry of nutrients into the cells and the removal of wastes from the cells. It can bind to immune cells, distorting them and interfering with normal immune responses. This may be one factor behind autoimmune disorders. Mercury can cause permanent kidney, cardiac, and respiratory problems. Significant amounts of mercury in the body can produce arthritis, depression, dermatitis, dizziness, fatigue, gum disease, nausea, vomiting, hair loss, insomnia, headaches, joint pain, slurred speech, memory loss, diarrhea, muscle weakness, and excessive salivation. High levels can also interfere with enzyme activity, resulting in blindness and paralysis. The symptoms of mercury poisoning can mimic those of multiple sclerosis and amyotrophic lateral sclerosis (ALS, also known as Lou Gehrig's disease). Many food and environmental allergies may be directly attributable to mercury poisoning. The U.S. Environmental Protection Agency has linked exposure to mercury vapor to menstrual disorders and spontaneous abortion (miscarriage) as well. Mercury exposure in pregnant women can cause neurological damage, such as lowered intelligence and delayed development in infants. In addition, the mortality rate for infants is significantly increased when mothers are exposed to mercury. Children who have severe mercury poisoning can experience acrodynia, a syndrome characterized by peeling and pinkness of the skin on the hands, nose, and feet; blindness; increased heart rate; agitation; and pain in the arms and legs.

Signs that indicate the presence of toxic mercury levels include behavioral changes, depression, confusion, irritability, and hyperactivity. People with this toxicity may also experience allergic reactions or asthma. They may complain about a metallic taste in the mouth, and their teeth may loosen. These symptoms can occur within a few minutes, or they can take as long as thirty minutes to appear.

People get most of their mercury from eating fish. Microorganisms in the environment can convert inorganic mercury to the organic form methylmercury. This form can build up in the environment and accumulate in certain freshwater and saltwater fish and marine mammals. Methylmercury is the form of mercury that is most likely to cause adverse health effects in the general population. It is particularly damaging to developing embryos, which are five to ten times more sensitive than adults.

Although concerns have been raised over the years about the safety of mercury in dental amalgams, researchers have shown these concerns to be unfounded. Previous estimates of how much mercury is absorbed from fillings were too high. The measured levels in the brain, blood, and urine from an amalgam are about 1 to 3 micrograms per day. Toxic amounts are considered to be 30 micrograms per gram of creatinine (a protein in the urine) a day. You would need to have 450 to 530 fillings to achieve this level. According to the American Dental Association, fewer than 100 cases of allergic reactions to mercury in the amalgams have been reported. Furthermore, in two major studies in children, no effect was seen on kidney function, behavior, or IQ from mercury in fillings.

Unless otherwise specified, the dosages recommended here are for adults. For children between the ages of twelve and seventeen, reduce the dose to three-quarters of the recommended amount. For children between six and twelve, use one-half of the recommended dose, and for children under the age of six, use one-quarter of the recommended amount.

NUTRIENTS

SUPPLEMENT	SUGGESTED DOSAGE	COMMENTS
Essential		
Glutathione plus L-methionine and L-cysteine	As directed on label, on an empty stomach. Take with water or juice. Do not take with milk. Take with 50 mg vitamin B₆ and 100 mg vitamin C for better absorption.	Needed for sulfur. Also helps to detoxify harmful metals and toxins. (*See* AMINO ACIDS in Part One.)
Selenium	200 mcg daily, in divided doses. If you are pregnant, do not exceed 40 mcg daily.	Neutralizes the effects of mercury.
Vitamin E	200 IU daily or 400 IU every other day.	Works with selenium to neutralize mercury. Use d-alpha-tocopherol form.
Very Important		
Apple pectin	As directed on label.	Aids in removing toxic metals from the body.
Garlic (Kyolic from Wakunaga)	2 capsules 3 times daily.	Acts as a detoxifier.
Kelp or alfalfa	1,000–1,500 mg daily.	Aids the body in removing toxins. See under Herbs, below.
Vitamin A plus carotenoid complex with beta-carotene	25,000 IU daily. If you are pregnant, do not exceed 10,000 IU daily. 15,000 IU daily.	A powerful antioxidant; destroys free radicals. Powerful free radical scavengers.
Vitamin C with bioflavonoids	4,000–10,000 mg daily.	Helps remove metals and strengthens the immune system.
Important		
Vitamin B complex	100 mg of each major B vitamin twice daily (amounts of individual vitamins in a complex will vary).	Important for the functioning and protection of the brain.
Helpful		
Brewer's yeast	As directed on label.	A good source of B vitamins.
Hydrochloric acid (HCl)	As directed on label.	To aid digestion. Take this supplement if you are over forty and deficient in HCl (see INDIGESTION in Part Two).
Lecithin granules or capsules	1 tbsp 3 times daily, before meals. 1,200 mg 3 times daily, before meals.	Protects brain cells from mercury poisoning.

Herbs

❑ Alfalfa contains valuable nutrients and helps the body to eliminate toxins.

Recommendations

❑ Eat organically grown foods, especially beans, onions, and garlic, for added sulfur, which helps protect the body against toxic substances.

❑ Drink water only if it is steam-distilled. Drink plenty of pure fresh fruit and vegetable juices.

❑ Supplement your diet with plenty of fiber (oat bran is a good source) and pectin (found in apples).

Note: Always take supplemental fiber separately from other supplements and medications.

❑ Eat fish in moderation (two 6-ounce servings a week), and always broil it; do not baste it in its juices. While some fish may contain mercury, fish also contains compounds called alkylglycerols, which help to remove mercury from the body. If there is mercury in the fish, it is primarily stored in the fat. By broiling the fish and draining the juices, you will get rid of much of the fat and retain the beneficial alkylglycerols. Rarely eat high-mercury fish such as tilefish, swordfish, king mackerel, shark, and albacore tuna. Good seafood choices include canned light tuna, salmon, shrimp, catfish, and pollock.

❑ If you suspect mercury toxicity, have a hair analysis performed. This can detect toxic levels of mercury. A urine mercury test also can give you this information. (*See* HAIR ANALYSIS in Part Three.)

Considerations

❑ Maintain regular dental check-ups for yourself and your children to avoid having fillings in the first place. Regular brushing and flossing helps as well. Have decayed teeth treated.

❑ In a study published in *The New England Journal of Medicine,* high mercury levels in the body predicted heart attack risk. The investigators measured toenail mercury levels and found those with the highest amounts were at greater risk. In addition, these same people had the highest levels of DHA, an omega-3 fatty acid from fish. High mercury intake from fish may diminish the cardioprotective effect of fish. Another article in the same issue of the journal found that toenail mercury did not predict heart attack risk. Given the conflicting data, it seems prudent to avoid high-mercury seafood and choose mostly low-mercury fish. However, because low-mercury fish tend to have lower amounts of omega-3 fats, take high-quality omega-3 supplements to increase your omega-3 intake without the mercury.

❑ Chelation therapy removes toxic metals from the body. (*See* CHELATION THERAPY in Part Three.)

❑ High mercury levels have been linked to candidiasis. (*See* CANDIDIASIS in Part Two.)

❑ The U.S. Consumer Product Safety Commission (CPSC) has issued a warning to consumers to inform them of the dangers of inhaling mercury vapors. Certain ethnic and religious customs involve using a product called *azogue,* which in reality is metallic mercury. This product is sold in herb shops, or *botanicas.* Azogue is sprinkled throughout the home for religious purposes. The CPSC suggests *immediate* removal of the mercury if it has been sprinkled in the home, but removal must be done in the proper way to avoid making the danger worse. Call your local health department for information on the correct procedure for mercury removal.

❑ *See also* CHEMICAL ALLERGIES and ENVIRONMENTAL TOXICITY in Part Two.

MIGRAINE

Migraines are severe, throbbing headaches that may or may not be accompanied by nausea, visual disturbances, and other symptoms. The incidence of migraine headaches has increased by 50 percent within the last twenty years. An estimated 28 million people in the United States—17 percent of women and 6 percent of men—suffer from them. Migraines are one of the most severe types of headache.

Traditional research has described migraines as vascular headaches involving excessive dilation or contraction of the brain's blood vessels. More current research gives other clues. Single photon emission computerized tomography (SPECT) scanning indicates that the inflammation involved in migraines is most noticeable in the meninges. These are three membranes—the dura, the arachnoid, and the very inner layer of membrane, called the pia, which is separated from the other two by cerebrospinal fluid. These membranes surround the brain and the spinal cord.

However, it is not the inflammation of the meninges that leads to the pain of migraine, but rather abnormal nerve activity. Stimulation of the trigeminal nerve, which goes from the brain to the head and face, appears to trigger the release of substances known as calcitonin gene-related peptides (CGRP), which both induce inflammation and send messages to pain receptors in the meninges. Some researchers liken migraines in many ways to meningitis, another condition affecting the meninges, noting that with meningitis, the symptoms are very similar—headache, nausea, and sensitivity to light. Meningitis, however, is caused by viral or bacterial infection.

Migraines may occur anywhere from once a week to once or twice a year, and they often run in families. One factor behind the higher incidence of migraines in women may be fluctuations in the level of the hormone estrogen; women typically get migraines around the time of menstruation, when estrogen levels are low. Migraines occur most often in people between the ages of twenty and thirty-five, and tend to decline with age. However, children too can suffer from migraines. In children, migraine pain tends to be more diffuse, rather than localized. Migraines can first show up in childhood not as headaches, but as colic, periodic abdominal pains, vomiting, dizziness, and severe motion sickness. There are usually five phases in a migraine:

1. A day or so before the onset of a headache, there may be detectable changes in mood, problems with memory, an alteration in one or all of the five senses, or speech problems.

2. Just before the headache begins, some people see flashes or patterns of light and/or experience numbness of the hands or mouth. This is called an *aura,* much like the auras that affect many people with epilepsy before a seizure. A migraine preceded by an aura is called a *classic migraine.* Migraines without auras are called *common migraines.*

3. The headache starts, with severe, throbbing pain. It may occur on one side or on both sides of the head. The pain can also move from side to side. Nausea may set in, along with tenderness in the neck and scalp. The eyes may be very sensitive to light, and the person may be almost immobilized by the pain.

4. The headache dissipates. Nausea may linger, however.

5. The person may feel tired and lethargic and may simply want to sleep.

Any number of things can trigger a migraine in a susceptible individual, including allergies, constipation, stress, liver malfunction, too much or too little sleep, emotional changes, hormonal changes, sun glare, flashing lights, lack of exercise, and changes in barometric pressure. Dental problems may also be a factor. Low blood sugar is frequently associated with migraine; studies have shown that blood sugar

Distinguishing Migraine Headaches

Just because a headache is very painful, that does not mean it is a migraine. Migraines have certain distinct characteristics that set them apart from other types of headaches.

The following table will help you to determine whether you have a true migraine or one of the two types most commonly confused with migraine—a tension or cluster headache.

Characteristic	Migraine	Tension Headache	Cluster Headache
Site of pain	One or both sides of the head	Both sides of the head	One side of the head
Duration of pain	4–72 hours	2 hours–days	30–90 minutes per episode, but episodes can recur multiple times daily
Severity of pain	Usually severe, but may be moderate	Mild or moderate	Very severe
Accompanied by nausea, sensitivity to light, sound, or smells	Common	No	No
Accompanied by fatigue and dizziness	Sometimes	No	No

levels are low during a migraine attack, and the lower the blood sugar level, the more severe the headache. Underlying causes of migraines that render an individual susceptible to various immediate triggers can include genetic factors, chemical imbalances in the brain, poor nutrition, and the overuse of painkillers.

Unless otherwise specified, the dosages recommended here are for adults. For children between the ages of twelve and seventeen, reduce the dose to three-quarters the recommended amount. If a child under twelve experiences severe headache pain, especially if it is accompanied by nausea or visual disturbances, contact a physician promptly. (*See* MENINGITIS in Part Two.)

NUTRIENTS

SUPPLEMENT	SUGGESTED DOSAGE	COMMENTS
Very Important		
Calcium and magnesium	2,000 mg daily. 1,000 mg daily.	Minerals that help to regulate muscular tone and to transmit nerve impulses throughout the body and to the brain. Use chelate forms.
Coenzyme Q$_{10}$ plus Coenzyme A from Coenzyme-A Technologies	60 mg daily. As directed on label.	Increases blood flow to the brain and improves circulation. Works with coenzyme Q$_{10}$.
Dimethylglycine (DMG) (Aangamik DMG from FoodScience of Vermont) and trimethylglycine (TMG)	125 mg twice daily. As directed on label.	Improve brain oxygenation.
DL-phenylalanine (DLPA)	As directed on label.	Taken with care, and after consulting a physician, DLPA can relieve pain and elevate mood.
Essential fatty acid complex or primrose oil	As directed on label. As directed on label.	Needed for brain cells and for fat metabolism. An anti-inflammatory agent to keep the blood vessels from constricting.
5-hydroxytryptophan (5-HTP)	As directed on label.	Increases the body's production of serotonin, a neurotransmitter involved in blood vessel regulation.
Multivitamin and mineral complex	As directed on label.	All nutrients are necessary in balance.
Rutin	200 mg daily.	Removes toxic metals, which may cause migraines.
Vitamin B complex plus extra vitamin B$_2$ (riboflavin) and vitamin B$_3$ (niacin) and niacinamide and vitamin B$_5$ (pantothenic acid) or royal jelly and vitamin B$_6$ (pyridoxine)	As directed on label. 400 mg daily. 200 mg 3 times daily. Do not exceed this amount. 800 mg daily. 100 mg twice daily. 1 tsp twice daily. As directed on label.	Needed for a healthy nervous system. Use a hypoallergenic form. Injections (under a doctor's supervision) may be necessary. Necessary for cell respiration and growth. Increases blood flow to the brain. *Caution:* Do not take niacin if you have a liver disorder, gout, or high blood pressure. Needed by the adrenal glands when the body is under stress. Royal jelly is high in pantothenic acid. Use royal jelly from a natural source. Required for normal brain function. Use a hypoallergenic form.

Helpful		
Garlic (Kyolic from Wakunaga)	2 capsules 3 times daily, with meals.	A potent detoxifier.
Quercetin and bromelain or Activated Quercetin from Source Naturals	500 mg daily, before meals. As directed on label.	Helps control food allergies. Needed for a variety of enzyme functions. Contains quercetin plus bromelain and vitamin C to aid absorption.
Taurine Plus from American Biologics	10–20 drops daily.	An important antioxidant and immune system regulator, needed for white blood cell activation and neurological function. Use the sublingual form.
Vitamin C with bioflavonoids	3,000–6,000 mg daily.	Aids in producing antistress adrenal hormones and enhances immunity. A buffered or esterified form is best.

Herbs

❑ Cordyceps is a Chinese herb that may, through its ability to reduce anxiety and stress and promote sound sleep, help people who suffer from migraines.

❑ Feverfew helps to alleviate pain.

Caution: Do not use feverfew when pregnant or nursing. People who take prescription blood-thinning medications should consult a health care provider before using feverfew, as the combination can result in internal bleeding.

❑ Ginkgo biloba extract enhances cerebral circulation.

Caution: Do not take ginkgo biloba if you have a bleeding disorder, or are scheduled for surgery or a dental procedure.

❑ Other herbs effective for the treatment of migraines include cayenne (capsicum), chamomile, fumitory, ginger, peppermint, rosemary, valerian, willow bark, and wormwood.

Cautions: Do not use chamomile if you are allergic to ragweed. Do not use during pregnancy or nursing. It may interact with warfarin or cyclosporine, so patients using these drugs should avoid it. Consult with your physician before using fumitory. Do not use wormwood in high doses or for extended periods because it contains the chemical compound thujone that can be poisonous. Do not use wormwood if you suffer from any type of seizure disorder or are pregnant.

Recommendations

❑ Adopt a diet that is low in simple carbohydrates and high in protein. *See* HYPOGLYCEMIA in Part Two and follow the dietary guidelines.

❑ Include almonds, almond milk, watercress, parsley, fennel, garlic, cherries, and fresh pineapple in the diet.

❑ Omit from the diet foods that contain the amino acid tyramine, including aged meats, avocados, bananas, beer, cabbage, canned fish, dairy products, eggplant, hard cheeses, potatoes, raspberries, red plums, tomatoes, wine, and yeast. Also avoid alcoholic beverages, aspirin, chocolate, monosodium glutamate (MSG), and nitrites (preservatives found in hot dogs and luncheon meats). Through the process of elimination, try to see if you have a particular allergy to some, or all, of these foods.

❑ Get regular moderate exercise.

❑ Massage your neck and the back of your head daily.

❑ Avoid salt and acid-forming foods such as meat, cereal, bread, and grains. Also avoid fried foods and fatty and greasy foods.

❑ Eat small meals, and eat small, nutritious snacks between meals if needed, to help stabilize wide swings in blood sugar that may precipitate a migraine. Especially avoid missing meals.

❑ Take only hypoallergenic supplements.

❑ See your dentist for treatment of any tooth problems, such as gum disease, tooth decay, bacterial infection, temporomandibular joint (TMJ) syndrome, or tooth-grinding, that may be contributing to the problem.

❑ Do not smoke, and avoid secondhand smoke.

❑ Avoid loud noises, strong odors, and high altitudes.

❑ Call a doctor if you have a headache that is triggered by, accompanied by, or linked to, any of the following:

• Exertion (including sexual exertion), bending, or coughing.

• Stiff neck and fever.

• Head injury.

• Vomiting.

• Slurred speech, distorted vision, or numbness or tingling in part of the body.

These can be signs of more serious disorders.

Considerations

❑ Some researchers believe many migraine attacks are caused by chemical imbalances in the brain. Serotonin levels in the brain drop during a headache. This triggers an impulse along the trigeminal nerve to blood vessels in the meninges, the brain's outer covering. In the meninges, the blood vessels become inflamed and swollen. The result is a headache.

❑ Among the natural remedies that can provide safe relief of migraine include omega-3 fatty acids, magnesium, vitamin B_6 (pyridoxine), probiotics like *Acidophilus* and *Bifidus* bacteria, feverfew, ginkgo, black cohosh, proper diet, and regular exercise.

Cautions: Do not use feverfew when pregnant or nursing. People who take prescription blood-thinning medications should consult a health care provider before using feverfew, as the combination can result in internal bleeding. Do not use black cohosh if you are pregnant or have any type of chronic disease. Black cohosh should not be used by those with liver problems.

❏ Migraine headaches in women may result from hormonal changes during the menstrual cycle. After menopause, the headaches usually decrease.

❏ Women who suffer from migraines may benefit from the use of natural progesterone cream.

❏ There is a relationship between food ingestion and migraines that is in part based on allergic mechanisms. Testing for IgE-specific food allergies appears helpful in selecting which people would likely benefit from diet therapy involving eliminating trigger foods. In one study, people with migraines who eliminated some foods had a 66 percent reduction in headaches.

❏ A study reported in the British medical journal *The Lancet* found that when allergenic foods were eliminated from the diets of migraine sufferers, as many as 93 percent of them found relief. (*See* ALLERGIES in Part Two.)

❏ In one study, subjects were tested to see whether red wine was a cause of headaches. In nine out of eleven subjects the wine provoked a headache, even though the wine did not contain tyramine (a natural substance formed from the breakdown of protein as food ages). Moreover, this group did not experience a headache following a drink of vodka.

❏ Researchers in France have identified a gene linked to a rare, severe type of migraine called *familial hemiplegic migraine.*

❏ Music has a calming effect and can help to relieve migraines. (*See* MUSIC AND SOUND THERAPY in Part Three.)

❏ Some find migraine relief by taking lecithin (a soybean derivative). In one study, those who took between three and six 1,200-milligram capsules when they felt a headache coming on had fewer, milder migraine attacks.

❏ Acupuncture and acupressure have helped many people control the pain of migraines.

❏ A study on the herb feverfew conducted at the University of Nottingham in England found that participants who took the herb got an average of 24 percent fewer migraines than those who did not, and they also found that vomiting was reduced, with no side effects.

Caution: Do not use feverfew when pregnant or nursing. People who take prescription blood-thinning medications should consult a health care provider before using feverfew, as the combination can result in internal bleeding.

❏ The FDA has approved three over-the-counter medications to treat migraines: Excedrin Migraine (a combination aspirin, acetaminophen, and caffeine); Advil Migraine; and Motrin Migraine Pain. (The last two are ibuprofen-based.)

❏ Prescription medications for treating the pain of a migraine include: Dihydroergotamine (DHE) injection and as a nasal spray (Migranal); a combination product containing DHE plus isometheptene (Midrin) is not very effective. Triptans (5-hydroxytryptamine [5-HT], serotonin, agonists) are a class of medications used to treat migraines that are categorized as acute. They include: Sumatriptan (Imitrex), an injection, nasal spray, and rapid-dissolving tablet; almotriptan (Axert); naratriptan (Amerge); rizatriptan (Maxalt); zolmitriptan (Zomig); frovatriptan (Frova); and eletriptan (Relpax). These migraine-specific therapies are most effective when taken early in an attack. The goal is to relieve the pain and associated symptoms. Triptans should not be used by those who have a past history of, or risk factors for, heart disease, high blood pressure, high cholesterol, angina, peripheral vascular disease, impaired liver function, stroke, or diabetes.

❏ The FDA has approved four drugs for migraine prevention: propranolol (Inderal); timolol (Blocadren); topiramate (Topamax); and divalproex sodium (Depakote). Amitriptyline (Elavil) is also sometimes used. If patients have frequent migraine attacks, attacks that do not respond consistently to the treatments above, or if the migraine-specific medications are ineffective or contraindicated because of other medical problems, then these preventive medications should be given to reduce the migraine frequency and improve the response to the acute migraine medicines.

❏ Antidepressants are sometimes prescribed for people who get migraines. Most effective are tricyclic antidepressants such as nortriptyline (Pamelor) and protriptyline (Vivactil). Other classes of drugs such as selective serotonin reuptake inhibitors (SSRIs) and serotonin and norepinephrine reuptake inhibitors (SNRIs) haven't proved effective, with the exception of venlafaxine (Effexor), which may be helpful in preventing migraines.

❏ Some women who experience migraines also have eating disorders such as bulimia nervosa.

❏ For names and addresses of organizations that offer information about how to deal with headaches, see Health and Medical Organizations in the Appendix.

❏ *See also* HEADACHE in Part Two and PAIN CONTROL in Part Three.

MISCARRIAGE

See under PREGNANCY-RELATED PROBLEMS.

MONONUCLEOSIS

Mononucleosis ("mono") is an infectious viral disease. The vast majority of cases (85 percent) are caused by the Epstein-Barr virus (EBV). More rarely, it may be caused by cytomegalovirus (CMV). Both of these viruses are members of the herpes family. Once the virus enters the body, it multiplies in lymphocytes (white blood cells). Mono affects the respiratory system, the lymphatic tissues, and glands in the neck, groin, armpits, bronchial tubes, spleen, and liver.

Symptoms include depression, extreme fatigue, fever, generalized aching, headache, jaundice, loss of appetite, sore throat, pain on the upper left side of the abdomen, puffy eyelids, swollen glands, and, sometimes, a bumpy red rash. The spleen may become enlarged, and liver function may be affected. Meningitis, encephalitis (inflammation of the brain), or rupturing of the spleen are very rare complications that can develop from mono.

The viruses that cause mono are contagious and can be transmitted from person to person by close contact such as kissing (mono is often referred to as the "kissing disease") or by sharing food or utensils, although they can also spread during sexual contact or through respiratory droplets. The incubation period is about ten days in children and thirty to fifty days in adults. Many of the cases occur in the military and in colleges, where living conditions are crowded and sleeping patterns are inadequate. High school students also have a high incidence of this disease. Mono is most common among children and adolescents. As many as 95 percent of people over age thirty-five have mono antibodies in their blood, indicating that they had the disease at some point in their lives—although many do not even know they had it.

Because the symptoms are often so similar to those of influenza, mononucleosis is often mistaken for it. However, with mono, the symptoms tend to be more persistent. The acute symptoms usually last from two to four weeks, and fatigue can persist for three to eight weeks after the other symptoms disappear. In some individuals, the disease lingers for a year or more, producing recurring, but successively milder, attacks. If the immune system is weakened due to an organ transplant or other viruses, the mononucleosis symptoms can be serious and chronic.

A diagnosis of mono is made through a blood test called a mononucleosis spot test. This reveals the presence of specific viral antibodies and confirms the presence of mono. A liver function test may aid in diagnosis. If you have been exposed to the virus or feel unusually fatigued, get tested.

Unless otherwise specified, the dosages recommended here are for adults. For children between the ages of twelve and seventeen, reduce the dose to three-quarters of the recommended amount. For children between six and twelve, use one-half of the recommended dose, and for children under the age of six, use one-quarter of the recommended amount.

NUTRIENTS

SUPPLEMENT	SUGGESTED DOSAGE	COMMENTS
Very Important		
Acidophilus (Kyo-Dophilus from Wakunaga or Bio-Dophilus from American Biologics)	As directed on label.	"Friendly" bacteria are important. Use a nondairy formula.
Proteolytic enzymes	As directed on label 3–4 times daily on an empty stomach, between meals and at bedtime.	Reduces inflammation and aids in absorption of nutrients.
Vitamin A with mixed carotenoids and vitamin E	25,000 IU daily for 2 weeks, then slowly reduce to 15,000 IU daily. If you are pregnant, do not exceed 10,000 IU daily. 200 IU daily or 400 IU every other day.	Essential for the immune system. Use emulsion forms for easier assimilation and greater safety at high doses. Use d-alpha-tocopherol form.
Vitamin C with bioflavonoids	5,000–10,000 mg daily, in divided doses.	Destroys the virus and boosts the immune system. A buffered esterified form is best.
Important		
Dimethylglycine (DMG) (Aangamik DMG from FoodScience of Vermont)	125 mg twice daily.	An immune stimulant that enhances oxygenation.
Free form amino acid	¼ tsp 2–3 times daily, on an empty stomach.	To provide protein, necessary for healing and to rebuild tissues. Use a powdered form.
Garlic (Kyolic from Wakunaga)	2 capsules 3 times daily, with meals.	A powerful immune booster. Acts as a natural antibiotic.
Vitamin B complex plus extra vitamin B12	100 mg of each major B vitamin 3 times daily, with meals (amounts of individual vitamins in a complex will vary). 2,000 mcg twice daily.	B vitamins increase energy and are needed for every bodily function, including proper digestion and brain function. Use a high-stress, hypoallergenic formula. A sublingual form is recommended. Injections (under a doctor's supervision) may be necessary. Required for proper digestion and to prevent anemia. Use a lozenge or sublingual form.
Zinc lozenges	As directed on label.	A powerful antioxidant that helps fight free radicals.
Helpful		
Maitake extract or reishi extract or shiitake extract	As directed on label. As directed on label. As directed on label.	Mushroom extracts with immune-boosting and antiviral properties.
Multivitamin and mineral complex with calcium and magnesium and potassium	As directed on label. 1,000 mg daily. 75–1,000 mg daily. 99 mg daily.	All nutrients are necessary for normal cellular function and repair. Use a high-potency formula.
Raw thymus glandular plus multiglandular complex (Multi-Glandular from American Biologics)	500 mg 3 times daily. As directed on label.	To enhance immune response. (See GLANDULAR THERAPY in Part Three.)

Herbs

❏ Astragalus and echinacea boost the immune system.

Cautions: Do not take astralagus in the presence of a fever. Do not take echinacea for longer than three months. It should not be used by people who are allergic to ragweed.

❏ Cat's claw has immune-enhancing properties and acts against viral infection.

Caution: Do not use cat's claw during pregnancy.

❏ Dandelion and milk thistle protect the liver.

❏ Goldenseal fights infection. If a sore throat is present, place a dropperful of alcohol-free goldenseal extract in the mouth and hold it there for a few seconds, then swallow. Do this every four hours for three to five days.

Caution: Do not take goldenseal internally on a daily basis for more than one week at a time. Do not use it during pregnancy or if you are breast-feeding, and use with caution if you are allergic to ragweed. If you have a history of cardiovascular disease, diabetes, or glaucoma, use it only under a doctor's supervision.

❏ Olive leaf extract appears to help inhibit the growth of viruses that cause diseases such as mononucleosis.

❏ Pau d'arco balances the bacteria in the colon.

❏ Spirulina contains phytonutrients that appear to boost the immune system.

Recommendations

❏ Eat a diet composed of at least 50 percent raw foods. Consume as much of your food raw as possible. Also emphasize wholesome soups, root vegetables, and whole grains, including brown rice.

❏ Each day, drink ten 8-ounce glasses of distilled water, plus fresh juice.

❏ Do not consume any coffee, fried foods, processed foods, soft drinks, stimulants, sugar, tea, or white flour products. These depress immune function. Any omega-6-rich fat—found in most vegetable oils—is immunosuppressive and should be avoided or limited.

❏ Eat four to six small meals daily. Avoid overeating at any one meal.

❏ Get plenty of rest. Round-the-clock bed rest is a good idea during the acute phase of the disorder.

❏ Gargle with a glass of warm salt water to relieve sore throat. Add ½ teaspoon of salt to a glass of warm water and gargle several times a day.

❏ Use a protein supplement from a vegetable source. Spiru-tein from Nature's Plus is a good protein drink for between meals.

❏ Use chlorophyll in tablet form, or in a liquid form such as "green drinks" made from leafy green vegetables or wheatgrass. Kyo-Green from Wakunaga is a highly concentrated natural barley and wheatgrass source of amino acids, vitamins, minerals, carotene, chlorophyll, and enzymes. It is also available in powder form containing chlorella, kelp, and brown rice.

❏ Do not strain when having a bowel movement, as this may injure an enlarged spleen.

❏ Do not give aspirin to a child or adolescent with mononucleosis, as it may lead to complications such as Reye's syndrome. (*See* REYE'S SYNDROME in Part Two.)

❏ Avoid close physical contact with others as much as possible. Flush all tissues after use, and do not share food, eating utensils, or towels. Wash your hands frequently.

❏ Avoid strenuous exercise and competitive sports until you are completely recovered.

❏ If you have a fever over 102°F, or if you develop severe pain in the upper left abdomen that lasts for five minutes or more, or if breathing and/or swallowing becomes difficult as a result of throat inflammation, consult your health care provider promptly. These can be signs that a more serious condition is developing.

Considerations

❏ Once contracted, both EBV and CMV remain in the body for life, but the acute illness eventually runs its course in nearly all cases. Because there is no cure for mononucleosis, a proper diet and supplements, plus adequate rest, are especially important for this disorder.

❏ Antibiotics are of no use unless there is a secondary infection such as ear infection or strep throat.

❏ Adequate rest, exercise, and nutrition are essential for the maintenance of general health and the prevention of mononucleosis.

❏ Protein is needed to stimulate the formation of antibodies that protect against complications such as hepatitis and jaundice.

❏ *See also* CHRONIC FATIGUE SYNDROME in Part Two.

MORNING SICKNESS

See under PREGNANCY-RELATED PROBLEMS.

MOTION SICKNESS

Motion sickness occurs when motion causes the eyes, the sensory nerves, and the vestibular apparatus of the ear to send conflicting signals to the brain, causing a loss of equilibrium or a sense of vertigo. It usually is experienced in a car, airplane, train, boat, elevator, or swing. Anxiety, genetics, over eating, poor ventilation, and traveling immediately after eating are common contributing factors. A susceptibility to things such as offensive odors, sights, or sounds can often precede an attack of motion sickness. Women are affected by this condition more frequently than men are. Elderly people and children under the age of two usually are not affected.

People suffering from motion sickness experience symptoms that range from severe headache to queasiness to nausea and vomiting while flying, sailing, or traveling in automobiles or trains. Other symptoms of motion sickness include cold sweats, dizziness, excessive salivation and/or yawning, fatigue, loss of appetite, pallor, severe distress, sleepiness, weakness, and, occasionally, breathing difficulties that can make you feel as though you are suffocating. If severe, an attack can make you completely uncoordinated, and sometimes injury can occur from loss of balance. Once the stimulus is removed, the motion sickness usually goes away; however, it can persist for hours or days. If you suffer from motion sickness for a prolonged amount of time, you may experience depression, dehydration, or low blood pressure. It can also worsen any other illness you may already have.

Natural remedies have been used with great success for motion sickness. Prevention is the key; motion sickness is far easier to prevent than it is to cure. Once excessive salivation and nausea set in, it is often too late to do anything but wait for the trip to be over so recovery can begin.

Unless otherwise specified, the dosages recommended here are for adults. For children between the ages of twelve and seventeen, reduce the dose to three-quarters of the recommended amount. For children between six and twelve, use one-half of the recommended dose, and for children under the age of six, use one-quarter of the recommended amount.

NUTRIENTS

SUPPLEMENT	SUGGESTED DOSAGE	COMMENTS
Important		
Charcoal tablets	5 tablets 1 hour before travel. Take separately from other medications and supplements.	A detoxifier.
Magnesium	500 mg 1 hour before trip.	Acts as a nerve tonic.
Vitamin B$_6$ (pyridoxine)	100 mg 1 hour before trip, then 100 mg 2 hours later.	Helps to relieve nausea.

Herbs

❑ Black horehound can reduce nausea.

❑ Butcher's broom, kudzu, and motherwort help to relieve vertigo.

❑ Ginger suppresses nausea and therefore is an excellent treatment and preventive for nausea and upset stomach. Studies have shown that it may be more effective than dimenhydrinate (Dramamine) without the side effects. Take 2 ginger capsules (approximately 1,000 milligrams) every three hours, starting one hour before the beginning of the trip.

❑ Peppermint tea soothes and calms the stomach. A drop of peppermint oil on the tongue provides excellent relief from nausea and motion sickness. Peppermint can also be taken in lozenge form.

Recommendations

❑ When traveling, take whole-grain crackers with you on trips. Olives can help ward off nausea because they have the effect of decreasing salivation.

❑ Try sipping green or ginger tea during long trips. Sucking on a fresh lemon may also calm the stomach.

❑ Pay special attention to your diet. If a certain dish disagrees with you at home, it will most certainly disagree with you on the road.

❑ Do not eat spicy, salty, sugary, heavy, or fatty foods, especially fried foods, before or during travel. Also avoid dairy products and processed and junk foods. These can contribute to nausea or cause digestive imbalances.

❑ Also avoid large meals when traveling. Instead, eat smaller, more frequent meals so that your stomach is never empty.

❑ Avoid alcohol. Alcohol disrupts the delicate operations that occur in the inner ear. If you are prone to motion sickness, alcohol consumption will only aggravate the problem by further disrupting communication between the eyes, the inner ears, and the brain.

❑ Avoid odors and aromas that can bring about nausea. Aside from obvious things such as smoke and engine exhaust, certain food odors can make you ill, as can paint fumes, nail polish, or animal waste. Even otherwise pleasant smells, such as those from perfume or aftershave, can cause a problem if you are prone to motion sickness.

❑ Sit still and breathe deeply. Your brain is already thoroughly confused without extra motion on your part. Especially try to keep your head still. Rest in a reclined position in an area where there is the least amount of motion (in the center of a ship or in the wing area of an airplane). Focus your eyes on a distant object and try not to allow your eyes to drift to either side. Or close your eyes and take deep breaths. If possible, lie down in a dark place with a cool, damp cloth over your eyes.

❑ Stay cool, if possible. Fresh air can assist in battling motion sickness. If in a car, roll down a window. If on a ship, standing on deck and taking in the sea breezes may help. In an airplane, open the overhead vent.

❑ When you begin to feel sick, rub or press on your wrist, about three fingers' width down from the line that separates the hand from the arm. Massaging this acupressure point often stops motion sickness.

❑ Do not read while traveling in a car.

❑ Limit or eliminate visual input. This will cut down on the conflicting information assaulting the brain. Traveling at night helps many people, simply because visual acuity is diminished, so that they do not perceive motion to the same degree as during the day.

Considerations

❑ Symptoms of nausea may indicate that the liver needs attention.

❑ A homeopathic liver remedy may help reduce nausea.

❑ Chewable papaya tablets can be helpful.

❑ There are numerous over-the-counter products available that may help to prevent motion sickness, including cyclizine (Marezine), dimenhydrinate (Dramamine), and meclizine (Antivert, Bonine). These drugs are not always effective, however, and can cause side effects, especially drowsiness. Motion sickness medication should not be taken with alcohol, sleep aids, or any type of tranquilizers. It is important to use extreme caution and carefully follow the dosage instructions for children.

❑ If motion sickness is debilitating, and herbal, homeopathic, and over-the-counter medications do not bring relief, a physician can prescribe scopolamine (which is a component of the herb belladonna) to be applied in a patch (Transderm Scop) that delivers the drug through the skin for up to three days. Possible side effects of scopolamine include dry mouth, drowsiness, blurred vision, and a dilated pupil on the side on which the patch is worn. This drug should not be used by anyone with glaucoma, as it raises pressure within the eye. If you are pregnant or nursing, talk to your doctor before using scopolamine. It is not recommended for use by children.

❑ To a certain extent, motion sickness is psychological. In many cases, it can be prevented if you consciously tell yourself that you *will not* get sick. If you travel frequently and are prone to motion sickness, you may benefit from psychotherapy or counseling.

MOUTH AND GUM DISEASE

See HALITOSIS; PERIODONTAL DISEASE. *See also* BLEEDING GUMS *under* PREGNANCY-RELATED PROBLEMS.

MULTIPLE SCLEROSIS

Multiple sclerosis (MS) is a progressive, degenerative disorder of the central nervous system, including the brain, the optic nerve, and the spinal cord. It is characterized by many areas of inflammation and scarring of the myelin sheaths in the brain and spinal cord. These are wrappings, composed of a fatty substance, that insulate the nerve fibers throughout the body. *Sclerosis* means hardening of tissue; *multiple* simply indicates many regions of tissue hardening. It seems that the body's immune system malfunctions and produces antibodies that attack the myelin sheaths. Consequently, the sheaths are damaged, and the damaged areas develop scarring that leads to either distorted communication or lack of communication between the nerve endings. This may produce a multiplicity of symptoms, from slurred speech to vision problems to loss of mobility.

At least 400,000 people in the United States have multiple sclerosis. Symptoms vary from individual to individual, depending on which portion or portions of the nervous system are most affected. In the earlier stages, the primary symptoms may include episodes of dizziness; extreme fatigue; eye problems such as blurred or double vision; a feeling of tingling and/or numbness, especially in the hands and feet; loss of balance and/or coordination; mus-

cular stiffness; slurred speech; tremors; or bowel and bladder dysfunction. Secondary symptoms, which are problems that arise because of the primary symptoms rather than because of the underlying illness itself, may include bone loss, muscle wasting, paralysis, sexual dysfunction, urinary tract infections, and weak respiration. Many of these secondary conditions occur as a result of decreased mobility if the disease progresses.

The disease typically follows a pattern of periodic flare-ups, called *exacerbations*, followed by periods in which symptoms diminish or even disappear called *remissions*. MS is variable in its rate of progression. It can be relatively benign, with only a few minor attacks spread over decades, or it can be rapidly and completely disabling. Most commonly, it progresses slowly, disappearing for periods of time but returning intermittently, often in progressively more severe attacks.

The underlying cause of MS is not known, but it is widely believed to be an autoimmune disease in which white blood cells attack the myelin sheaths as if they were a foreign substance. Stress and malnutrition, whether from poor absorption or poor diet, often precede the onset of the disease. Some experts suspect that an as-yet-unidentified virus may be involved. Heredity may also be a factor. Another theory is that this condition may be caused by food intolerances or allergies, especially allergies to dairy products and gluten.

Chemical poisoning of the nervous system by pesticides, industrial chemicals, and heavy metals may also play a part in the development of MS. Environmental toxins can cause disturbances in the body's normal metabolic pathways that result in damage to the nerves' protective myelin sheaths. Even substances that are not necessarily toxic to everyone can be a problem for susceptible individuals. Toxins such as those produced by bacteria and fungi in the body have been known to produce symptoms like those of MS.

Finally, diet may play a key role in the development of MS. This is suggested by the fact that MS is fairly common in the United States and Europe and almost unheard-of in some other countries, such as Japan, Korea, and China. The consumption of saturated fats, cholesterol, and alcohol, so common in Western countries, promotes the inflammatory response and worsens symptoms of multiple sclerosis. People in Asian countries typically consume much less fat than people in North America and northern Europe do. Their diets are also rich in marine foods, seeds, and fruit oils, which are high in essential fatty acids, including the omega-3 essential fatty acids, which have an inhibitory effect on the inflammatory response. Our American diet in contrast is rich in oils from grains that promote inflammation.

MS is usually diagnosed between the ages of twenty and fifty. Women are affected two to three times more than men; the rate is higher in younger women compared to men (3.2 to 1). MS is rarely diagnosed in children and in people over sixty years of age. In the United States, MS occurs much more often in states north of the thirty-seventh parallel (an imaginary line stretching approximately from Newport News, Virginia, to Santa Cruz, California) than in other parts of the country. It also appears in clusters in places including El Paso, Texas; De Pue, Illinois; and Galion, Ohio.

Diagnosing MS is not a simple task, so the illness often goes undiagnosed for some time. Tests that can be used to detect the disease include magnetic resonance imaging (MRI), to look for signs of plaques or lesions; lumbar puncture (spinal tap), to detect abnormalities in the levels of white blood cells and/or immune system proteins in the cerebrospinal fluid; a visual evoked potential (VEP) test, done to assess the connection between the retina and the visual area of the brain; an audio evoked potential (AEP) test, which may help to detect lesions in the brain; and electrodiagnostic tests that measure the rate at which nerve impulses travel (this may be slower than normal in people with MS).

There is no known cure for this disease, but the supplement and dietary programs outlined in this section have been shown to be helpful. Long-term sufferers of MS may not benefit as much, but younger people who are just starting to exhibit symptoms may find that the correct supplements slow or even stop the progression of the disease.

Unless otherwise specified, the dosages recommended here are for adults. For children between the ages of twelve and seventeen, reduce the dose to three-quarters the recommended amount. For children between six and twelve, use one-half the recommended dose, and for children under the age of six, use one-quarter the recommended amount.

NUTRIENTS

SUPPLEMENT	SUGGESTED DOSAGE	COMMENTS
Very Important		
Calcium	2,000–3,000 mg daily.	Deficiency may create a predisposition to developing MS. Use chelate form for best assimilation.
and magnesium	1,000–1,500 mg daily.	Needed for calcium absorption and for proper muscular coordination.
Coenzyme Q10	90 mg daily.	Needed for improved circulation and tissue oxygenation. Strengthens the immune system.
plus Coenzyme A from Coenzyme-A Technologies	As directed on label.	Supports the immune system's detoxification of many dangerous substances. Can ease depression and fatigue, increase energy, process fats, remove toxins from the body, and boost the immune system.
Gamma-linolenic acid (GLA)	As directed on label 3 times daily, with meals.	An essential fatty acid needed to control symptoms. Deficiency is common in people with MS.
or flaxseed oil or	As directed on label 3 times daily, with meals.	If GLA is not available, use one of these supplements
primrose oil or omega-3 essential fatty acid complex	As directed on label 3 times daily, with meals. As directed on label 3 times daily, with meals.	for essential fatty acids.
Garlic (Kyolic from Wakunaga)	2 capsules 3 times daily.	An excellent source of sulfur.
Methylsulfonyl-methane (MSM)	As directed on label.	Helps to keep cell walls permeable, allowing water and nutrients to freely flow into cells and allowing wastes and toxins to properly flow out. With vitamin C, is used by the body to build healthy new cells.
Oxy-5000 Forte from American Biologics	As directed on label.	A potent nutritional antioxidant formula.
Vitamin B complex	100 mg of each major B vitamin 3 times daily (amounts of individual vitamins in a complex will vary).	Aids immune system function and maintains healthy nerves. Use hypoallergenic formulas for all the B vitamins.
plus extra vitamin B6 (pyridoxine)	50 mg 3 times daily.	Promotes red blood cell production; aids the nervous system and immune function. Deficiency may cause MS in susceptible persons.
and vitamin B12	1,000 mcg twice daily.	Aids in cellular longevity and helps to prevent nerve damage by maintaining the protective myelin sheaths. Use a lozenge or sublingual form.
and choline and inositol	As directed on label.	To stimulate the central nervous system and aid in protecting the myelin sheaths from damage.
Vitamin D	800 IU daily.	Aids in calcium absorption.
Important		
Acidophilus (Kyo-Dophilus from Wakunaga)	1 tsp twice daily, on an empty stomach.	Helps to detoxify harmful substances, enhances absorption of nutrients, and aids digestion. Use a powdered nondairy form.
Amino-VIL from Carlson Labs	¼ tsp twice daily, on an empty stomach.	A combination of the branched-chain amino acids, which aid in use of nutrients by the muscles. (*See* AMINO ACIDS in Part One.)
plus L-glycine	500 mg twice daily, on an empty stomach.	Aids in supporting the myelin sheaths.
Creatine	As directed on label. Do not take with fruit juice, as this combination produces creatinine, which is difficult for the kidneys to process. Do not exceed the recommended dose.	May help counteract muscle depletion. Should be used in combination with a balanced diet.
Free form amino acid	As directed on label 3 times daily, between meals.	Helps to maintain good absorption of nutrients needed for proper brain function.
Grape seed extract	As directed on label.	A powerful antioxidant and anti-inflammatory.

Multienzyme complex or Inf-zyme Forte from American Biologics	As directed on label. Take with meals. As directed on label.	For proper breakdown of foods. To reduce inflammation and aid digestion.
Multiglandular complex	As directed on label.	Needed for the endocrine, hormonal, and enzyme systems. (See GLANDULAR THERAPY in Part Three.)
Nicotinamide adenine dinucleotide (NADH)	As directed on label.	Important in the creation and transfer of chemical energy, especially during breathing.
Parasitin from Växa International	As directed on label.	To detoxify the body of parasites.
Potassium	300–1,000 mg daily.	Needed for normal muscle function. Check with your health care provider before taking these amounts.
Raw thymus glandular	500 mg twice daily.	Enhances immune function.
Selenium	150–300 mcg daily.	An antioxidant and immune system stimulant.
7-Keto DHEA	As directed on label.	Slows overall body deterioration. Enhances fat loss and lean muscle mass development. Preferable to ordinary DHEA because it is not converted into sex hormones in the body.
Ultra Osteo Synergy from American Biologics	As directed on label.	To provide nutritional support for bone renewal.
Vitamin A plus carotenoid complex (Betatene)	25,000 IU daily. If you are pregnant, do not exceed 10,000 IU daily. As directed on label.	Important antioxidants. Use emulsion forms for easier assimilation.
Vitamin C with bioflavonoids	3,000–5,000 mg daily.	Promotes production of the antiviral protein interferon in the body. Also an antioxidant and immune system stimulant. Use buffered ascorbic acid or an esterified form.
Vitamin E	200 IU daily or 400 IU every other day.	Important for circulation, destroys free radicals, and protects the nervous system. Use d-alpha-tocopherol form. Emulsion form is recommended for easier assimilation and greater safety at high doses.
Vitamin K or alfalfa	200 mcg 3 times daily, with meals.	Helps to prevent nausea and vomiting. See under Herbs, below.
Helpful		
Brewer's yeast	Start with ¼ tsp daily and slowly increase to 2 tsp daily.	Improves blood sugar metabolism when taken with chromium. Aids in lowering cholesterol and improving HDL/LDL ratio.

Kyo-Green from Wakunaga	1 tsp in liquid 3 times daily.	A good source of organic chlorophyll, live enzymes, vitamins, and minerals plus amino acids.
Lecithin granules or capsules	1 tbsp 3 times daily, before meals. 1,200 mg 3–4 times daily, before meals.	Protects the cells. Needed for normal brain function.
Manganese	5–10 mg daily. Take separately from calcium.	An important mineral often deficient in people with MS.
Multimineral complex	As directed on label.	Needed for all enzyme systems in the body and to supply needed nutrients. Use a high-potency formula.
Phosphorus	900 mg daily.	Needed for transfer of energy within cells.

Herbs

❑ Alfalfa is a good source of vitamin K. It can be taken in liquid or tablet form.

❑ Burdock, dandelion, echinacea, goldenseal, pau d'arco, red clover, St. John's wort, sarsaparilla, and yarrow are effective detoxifiers.

Cautions: Do not take echinacea for longer than three months. It should not be used by people who are allergic to ragweed. Do not take goldenseal internally on a daily basis for more than one week at a time. Do not use it during pregnancy or if you are breast-feeding, and use with caution if you are allergic to ragweed. If you have a history of cardiovascular disease, diabetes, or glaucoma, use it only under a doctor's supervision. St. John's wort may cause increased sensitivity to sunlight. It may also produce anxiety, gastrointestinal symptoms, and headaches. It can interact with some drugs including antidepressants, birth control pills, and anticoagulants.

❑ Cordyceps is a Chinese herb that improves memory, helps you assimilate nutrients more efficiently, and increases energy.

❑ Lobelia, skullcap, and valerian root relax the nervous system. Taken at bedtime, they aid in preventing insomnia. Lobelia is good for daytime use also.

Caution: Lobelia is to be taken only under supervision of a health care professional, as it is potentially toxic. People with high blood pressure, heart disease, liver disease, kidney disease, seizure disorders, or shortness of breath should not take lobelia. Pregnant and lactating women should avoid lobelia as well.

Recommendations

❑ Eat only organically grown foods with no chemical treatments or additives, including eggs, fruits, gluten-free grains, raw nuts and seeds, vegetables, and cold-pressed vegetable oils. The best diet for people with this disorder is totally vegetarian. Make sure that you study up on what following a well-balanced vegetarian diet entails. Missing out on essential nutrients will only worsen your condition.

❑ Eat plenty of raw sprouts and alfalfa, plus foods that contain lactic acid, such as sauerkraut and dill pickles. Also good are "green drinks" that contain plenty of chlorophyll.

❑ Eat plenty of dark leafy greens. These are good sources of vitamin K.

❑ Drink at least ten 8-ounce glasses of quality water each day to prevent toxic buildup in the muscles.

❑ Do not consume any alcohol, barley, chocolate, coffee, dairy products, fried foods, highly seasoned foods, meat, oats, refined foods, rye, salt, spices, sugar, tobacco, wheat, or processed, canned, or frozen foods.

❑ Take a fiber supplement. Fiber is important for avoiding constipation. Periodically take warm cleansing enemas with the juice of a fresh lemon. A clean colon is important for keeping toxic waste from interfering with muscle function. (*See* COLON CLEANSING and ENEMAS in Part Three.)

❑ Never consume saturated fats, processed oils, oils that have been subjected to heat (either in processing or in cooking), or oils that have been stored without refrigeration.

❑ Have yourself tested for possible food allergies. (*See* ALLERGIES in Part Two.) We believe that food allergies are a major factor in the development and progression of multiple sclerosis. Unfortunately, all too often the allergies are not discovered until irreversible nerve damage has occurred. Early detection is therefore vital. Eliminating offending foods from your diet may slow down the progression of the disease and help you avoid further damage.

❑ Avoid stress and anxiety. Attacks of MS are often precipitated by a trauma or a period of emotional distress.

❑ Avoid exposure to heat, such as hot baths, showers, sunbathing, and overly warm surroundings, and avoid becoming overheated when working or exercising. Avoid exhaustion and viral infections. All of these may trigger an attack or worsen symptoms.

❑ Get periodic massages and regular exercise, and keep mentally active. These are extremely valuable in maintaining muscle function and bringing about remission of symptoms. However, exercises that may increase body temperature can decrease the function of the nerves involved and make symptoms worse. Swimming is the best activity. Doing other exercises in cool water is good as well because body temperature is kept lower and the body's weight is supported by the water. Stretching exercises help to prevent muscle contractures. Physical therapy is often needed.

❑ When an exacerbation begins, take at least two days of complete bed rest. This can often stop a mild attack.

❑ Educate yourself and your family about the disease, and seek out sources of emotional support. For names and addresses of organizations that can help, *see* Health and Medical Organizations in the Appendix.

Considerations

❑ A strong immune system may help to prevent multiple sclerosis by helping the body avoid infection, which often precedes the onset of this disease.

❑ While the effects of MS on pregnancy seem to be minimal, slightly more flare-ups occur during the six months following childbirth. During the reproductive years, there is a preponderance of autoimmune disorders in women, including MS.

❑ Gluten intolerance may make a person more susceptible to MS.

❑ Recent studies point to a possible link between MS and candida infection. A significant proportion of people with MS show evidence of imbalanced bowel flora, which is characteristic of candidiasis. Further, chronic fatigue is a symptom of candidiasis, and it is also one of the most common complaints of people with multiple sclerosis. Treatments to reduce candida activity have been found to reduce the fatigue experienced by many people with MS. (*See* CANDIDIASIS in Part Two.)

❑ The symptoms of Lyme disease may mimic those of multiple sclerosis. (*See* LYME DISEASE in Part Two.)

❑ *Chlamydia pneumoniae,* a very common type of bacteria, has been cited as a possible cause of MS. In an article in the July 1999 issue of *Annals of Neurology,* researchers reported that *C. pneumoniae* were found in all MS patients in their study group. (It may be that this was a result of MS, not a cause.)

❑ One recent study concentrated on the ability of hypericin, a chemical found naturally in St. John's wort, to destroy viruses and cancer cells when exposed to light. Hypericin has shown promise as a disease-fighting agent, and research is continuing.

Caution: St. John's wort may cause increased sensitivity to sunlight. It may also produce anxiety, gastrointestinal symptoms, and headaches. It can interact with some drugs including antidepressants, birth control pills, and anticoagulants.

❑ Researchers in Scandinavia have long studied the use of essential fatty acid supplementation to treat MS and to reduce the frequency of new events. A low-fat, high-fish-oil diet has been shown to be moderately effective in patients with relapsing-remitting MS.

❑ Some people with MS have experienced relief of symptoms by using honeybee venom. Bee venom apparently acts as an anti-inflammatory and immune system stimulant.

❑ Although its use is considered controversial by many physicians in the United States, hyperbaric oxygen therapy has been used with success for people with multiple sclerosis in some other countries. (*See* HYPERBARIC OXYGEN THERAPY in Part Three.)

❑ Drugs that are commonly used for multiple sclerosis include:

- Corticosteroids. The most common treatment for multiple sclerosis, corticosteroids reduce the inflammation that spikes during a relapse. Examples include oral prednisone and intravenous methylprednisolone. Side effects may include mood swings and weight gain.

- Interferons. These types of drugs—Betaseron, Avonex, and Rebif—appear to slow the rate at which multiple sclerosis symptoms worsen over time. But interferons can cause serious liver damage.

- Glatiramer (Copaxone). Doctors believe that glatiramer works by blocking the immune system's attack on myelin. This drug must be injected subcutaneously once daily. Side effects may include flushing and shortness of breath after injection.

- Mitoxantrone (Novantrone). This immunosuppressant drug can be harmful to the heart, so it's usually used only in people who have advanced multiple sclerosis.

- Natalizumab (Tysabri). This drug is designed to work by interfering with the movement of potentially damaging immune cells from the bloodstream to the brain and spinal cord. Tysabri is generally reserved for people who see no results from or can't tolerate other types of treatments. This is because Tysabri increases the risk of progressive multifocal leukoencephalopathy—a brain infection that is usually fatal.

❑ Always ask your physician about all available medications, and especially about possible side effects, so that you can make informed decisions about which (if any) to take.

❑ In one study, men with relapsing-remitting MS who were given 100 milligrams of testosterone showed improved cognition and slowed brain atrophy. They also had increased lean body mass, and there were no side effects.

❑ Epidemiological data suggests that there is a link between vitamin D deficiency and increased prevalence rates of MS. In one study, the use of oral calcitriol (1,25-dihydroxy vitamin D_3), in combination with a diet that provided 800 milligrams of calcium, reduced the symptoms in about one-third of the patients with MS. In another study, high doses of vitamin D—beyond the Upper Limits of Safety—and calcium reduced the number of lesions in patients with MS. This sort of treatment requires regular blood monitoring and close physician supervision, but these early results seem promising in terms of slowing the progression of the disease.

❑ According to the New Jersey College of Medicine, X-ray irradiation to the lymph glands and the spleen may halt the progress of MS in some cases. However, radiation exposure depresses the immune system.

❑ Because there are so many conditions that can occur over time with MS—including bowel and bladder problems, chronic fatigue, depression, headaches, impotence, pain, problems with vision and hearing loss, seizures, uri-

nary tract infections, and vertigo—it is advisable to read the sections that cover these individual conditions in this section of this book. Consult the Table of Contents to look for sections that may be relevant for you.

MUMPS

Before the routine vaccination program was introduced in the United States, mumps was a common viral illness, mostly of childhood, caused by a type of virus known as a paramyxovirus that infects the parotid glands—the salivary glands located at the jaw angles below the ears. Mumps vaccine (usually MMR) is the best way to prevent mumps. Children should be given the first dose of MMR vaccine at twelve to fifteen months of age. The second dose is recommended before the start of kindergarten. One dose of mumps vaccine prevents approximately 80 percent of mumps and two doses about 90 percent of cases. Although mumps are rare in the United States, small outbreaks do occur; the first recent cases of mumps-like illness were reported from Iowa in December 2005. More cases have been occurring since then in Iowa, and in several other states. There are on average 265 mumps cases reported each year in the United States.

Of those people who do get mumps, up to half have very mild or no symptoms, and therefore do not know they were infected with mumps. The most common symptoms include swelling of one or both glands plus headache, fever, chills, decreased appetite, sore throat, and pain when swallowing or chewing, especially when swallowing acidic substances such as citrus juices. Often, one of the parotid glands swells before the other, and as swelling in one gland subsides, the other begins to swell.

Symptoms typically appear sixteen to eighteen days after infection, but this period can range from twelve to twenty-five days after infection. Mumps is transmitted from person to person by means of infected droplets of saliva or direct contact with contaminated materials. It can be contracted through sneezing, coughing, kissing, talking, breathing, drinking out of the same glass as an infected person, and sharing utensils. A person with mumps is contagious any time from forty-eight hours before the onset of symptoms to six days after the symptoms have started. This illness is not as contagious as measles or chickenpox, and one attack usually affords lifetime immunity. Mumps is most common in children between the ages of three and ten, although it can occur through teenage years and, in rare cases, in adulthood. If it does occur after puberty, the ovaries or testes may become involved and sterility may result. If the testicles are affected, they become swollen and painful; if the ovaries or pancreas is affected, abdominal pain results. Other organs that can be affected in rare, severe cases include the brain, and kidneys—possibly with serious complications.

Unless otherwise specified, the dosages recommended here are for adults. For children between the ages of twelve and seventeen, reduce the dose to three-quarters the recommended amount. For children between six and twelve, use one-half the recommended dose, and for children under the age of six, use one-quarter the recommended amount.

NUTRIENTS

SUPPLEMENT	SUGGESTED DOSAGE	COMMENTS
Very Important		
Bifidobacterium bifidus	As directed on label.	"Friendly" bacteria contain antibiotic substances that inhibit pathogenic organisms.
Vitamin C with bioflavonoids	500 mg every 2 hours until improvement is noted, up to 3,000–10,000 mg daily.	Destroys the virus and eliminates toxins. For children, use sodium ascorbate form to lessen diarrhea.
Zinc lozenges (ImmunActinZinc lozenges from Nature's Plus)	1 15-mg lozenge every 4 to 6 hours. Do not exceed a total of 100 mg daily from all supplements.	Aids healing. Lozenges are fast acting. Do not chew them, but allow them to dissolve slowly in the mouth.
Important		
Acidophilus (Kyo-Dophilus from Wakunaga or Bio-Dophilus from American Biologics)	As directed on label.	For adults and children. Contains antibiotic substances that inhibit pathogenic organisms. Use a nondairy formula.
Free form amino acid	As directed on label.	Important for tissue repair and healing.
plus vitamin B complex	100 mg of each major B vitamin 3 times daily (amounts of individual vitamins in a complex will vary).	Needed for healing.
plus potassium	99 mg daily.	To restore electrolytes depleted by fever. Potassium levels are depressed by fever over 101°F.
Vitamin A with mixed carotenoids	Children under twelve: 14,000 IU daily. Adults and children over twelve: 50,000 IU daily. If you are pregnant, do not exceed 10,000 IU daily.	Vitamins A and E potantiate immune function. Use emulsion forms for easier assimilation.
and vitamin E	200 IU daily or 400 IU every other day for adults and children	Use d-alpha-tocopherol form.
Helpful		
Kelp	1,000–1,500 mg daily.	Contains essential minerals, iodine, and vitamins.

Herbs

❑ Catnip and chamomile teas are good calming agents and help to induce sleep. Catnip tea enemas help reduce fever. (*See* ENEMAS in Part Three.)

Caution: Do not use chamomile if you are allergic to ragweed. Do not use during pregnancy or nursing. It may interact with warfarin or cyclosporine, so patients using these drugs should avoid it.

❑ Taken as a tea, dandelion cleanses and supports the liver. Ground into a powder and combined with a little aloe vera gel in a poultice, it helps to reduce swelling.

❑ Echinacea helps to reduce swelling and cleanses the blood and lymphatic system. Take it in tea form, mixed with a little juice, four times a day or more.

Caution: Do not take echinacea for longer than three months. It should not be used by people who are allergic to ragweed.

❑ Elderflower tea helps to reduce fever.

❑ Lobelia extract is good for pain. Take ½ teaspoon every three to four hours.

Caution: Lobelia is to be taken only under supervision of a health care professional, as it is potentially toxic. People with high blood pressure, heart disease, liver disease, kidney disease, seizure disorders, or shortness of breath should not take lobelia. Pregnant and lactating women should avoid lobelia as well.

❑ Mullein poultices are good for relieving pain and swelling of the salivary glands. (*See* USING A POULTICE in Part Three.)

❑ Peppermint tea soothes an upset stomach and helps to flush infection from the body.

❑ Adding powdered slippery elm bark to barley water makes a drink that is nourishing and soothing to the throat and digestive tract. (*See* THERAPEUTIC LIQUIDS in Part Three.)

❑ Yarrow reduces fever and inflammation and is a good lymphatic cleanser.

Recommendations

❑ As long as the glands are swollen, eat mostly raw fruits and vegetables that are juiced or softened. Sticking to a diet of soft foods helps to minimize the pain of chewing.

❑ Drink plenty of pure water and fresh juices to keep the body well hydrated and to flush the system clean.

❑ Do not consume coffee, dairy products, tobacco, or white flour or sugar. Avoid acidic foods, such as pickles and citrus fruits or juices, as they are likely to cause discomfort.

❑ Follow a fasting program to detoxify the body. (*See* FASTING in Part Three.)

❑ Stay warm and dry, and get plenty of rest.

❑ Intermittently apply warmth or cold, whichever feels best, to the swollen glands and around the neck. Use hot towels, hot water bottles, and ice packs with caution.

❑ If testicular swelling and pain occur, support the scrotum by means of an adhesive tape "bridge" between the thighs and use cool compresses to help relieve pain.

Considerations

❑ Complete recovery from mumps usually can be expected in about ten days if no complications occur. If any of the following symptoms develop, you should see your doctor as soon as possible: tenderness or swelling of the testicles, severe vomiting (this may indicate infection that has spread to the pancreas), a fever over 104°F, lethargy, or a stiff neck accompanied by a severe headache (this may be a sign of developing meningitis).

❏ Because complications are more common when this disease is contracted in adulthood, immunization should be considered for any adult who has not had mumps or who has not already been vaccinated against it.

❏ The mumps virus may be contagious even during incubation. Anyone who has come in contact with a person who had or who developed mumps should be on the lookout for symptoms for a twelve to twenty-five-day period following exposure, and should minimize his or her contact with persons who may be susceptible during this period.

❏ There is no medication that can cure mumps. Treatment focuses on bed rest and measures to support the body as the virus runs its course. Your doctor may recommend acetaminophen (Tylenol, Datril Extra-Strength, and others) or ibuprofen (Advil, Nuprin, and others) if fever causes significant discomfort.

❏ A doctor may advise the use of corticosteroids to diminish testicular pain and swelling. These are powerful drugs, and should be used with caution.

❏ If nausea and/or pain on swallowing is so severe that a person with mumps becomes unable to eat, intravenous administration of dextrose and fluids may be required.

❏ Swelling of the parotid and/or other salivary glands can also be caused by a number of other factors, including cirrhosis of the liver; bulimia; a bacterial infection such as strep throat; poor oral hygiene; a salivary gland tumor or a calcium-based stone in one of the salivary ducts; and Mikulicz's syndrome, which is characterized by swelling (usually painless) of the parotid glands and, sometimes, the tear glands, and which can occur in people with a number of different diseases, including leukemia, lupus, non-Hodgkin's lymphoma, and tuberculosis. Swollen salivary glands can also be related to the use of certain drugs. Consequently, an isolated case of mumps (a case not associated with a local outbreak of the disease) warrants extra care in diagnosis.

❏ In most U.S. states, immunization against mumps is required before a child can be admitted into public kindergarten. Infections like mumps can cause infertility in males if the virus occurs during puberty. Not vaccinating a baby boy could increase the chances of sterility in adulthood.

MULTIPLE SYSTEM ATROPHY WITH ORTHOSTATIC HYPOTENSION

See ORTHOSTATIC HYPOTENSION *under* RARE DISORDERS.

MUSCLE CRAMPS

Ordinarily, a muscle contracts when it is used, then stretches out when the motion is completed or another muscle moves it in the opposite direction. If a muscle contracts with great intensity without stretching out again, you feel the pain of a muscle cramp. Many people experience muscle cramps during the night. This type of cramp generally affects the legs, especially the calf muscles, and the feet. They occur more frequently in older adults than in younger people. Children sometimes experience a type of crampy muscle and leg pain often called "growing pains."

Muscle cramping is often caused by an imbalance in the body's levels of electrolytes—minerals such as potassium, calcium, and magnesium, which in turn can be due to illness or exercise. A deficiency of vitamin E also may be involved. Another common cause is unaccustomed physical overexertion, overuse, or strain. Sitting, standing, or lying for a long time in one position; anemia; the use of tobacco; inactivity; fibromyalgia; hormone imbalances; allergies; arthritis; and even arteriosclerosis can also result in cramping, as can dehydration, heat stroke, hypothyroidism, or varicose veins, or, more rarely, the early stages of amyotrophic lateral sclerosis (ALS, or Lou Gehrig's disease).

Some medications can cause muscle cramping as a side effect. The use of diuretic drugs for high blood pressure or heart disorders may lead to electrolyte imbalances, causing muscle cramps. People using statins to lower blood pressure and those who take anti-osteoporosis medications such as alendronate (Fosamax) may also experience muscle cramps. Poor circulation also contributes to leg cramps.

Unless otherwise specified, the dosages recommended here are for adults. For a child between the ages of twelve and seventeen, reduce the dose to three-quarters of the recommended amount. For a child between six and twelve, use one-half of the recommended dose, and for a child under the age of six, use one-quarter of the recommended amount.

NUTRIENTS

SUPPLEMENT	SUGGESTED DOSAGE	COMMENTS
Essential		
Calcium and magnesium	1,500 mg daily. / 750 mg and up daily.	Deficiencies are most often the cause of cramping in the legs and feet at night. Use chelate or citrate forms.
Vitamin D	400 IU daily.	Needed for calcium uptake.
Vitamin E	200 IU daily or 400 IU every other day.	Improves circulation. Deficiency may cause leg cramps while standing or walking. Especially good if cramping is related to varicose veins. Use d-alpha-tocopherol form.
Very Important		
Malic acid and magnesium	As directed on label.	Malic acid is involved in the production of energy in muscle cells; magnesium is a cofactor in cellular energy production.
Potassium	99 mg daily.	Needed for proper calcium and magnesium metabolism; aids in relieving muscle cramps.

Silica	As directed on label.	Supplies silicon, which aids in calcium absorption.
Ultra Osteo Synergy from American Biologics	As directed on label.	Provides nutritional support for bone renewal.
Vitamin B complex	50 mg of each major B vitamin 3 times daily, with meals (amounts of individual vitamins in a complex will vary).	For improved circulation and cellular function.
plus extra vitamin B₁ (thiamine)	50 mg 3 times daily, with meals.	Enhances circulation and may aid in maintaining proper muscle tone.
and vitamin B₃ (niacin)	50 mg 3 times daily, with meals.	Increases circulation. Caution: Do not take niacin if you have a liver disorder, gout, or high blood pressure.
Vitamin C with bioflavonoids	3,000–6,000 mg daily.	Improves circulation.

| **Important** | | |
| Dimethylglycine (DMG) (Aangamik DMG from FoodScience of Vermont) | As directed on label. | Improves tissue oxygenation. |

Helpful		
Coenzyme Q₁₀	100 mg daily.	Improves heart function and circulation. Lowers blood pressure.
plus Coenzyme A from Coenzyme-A Technologies	As directed on label.	Improves the effectiveness of coenzyme Q₁₀.
Lecithin granules or capsules	1–2 tbsp 3 times daily, before meals. 1,200–2,400 mg 3 times daily, before meals.	Reduces cholesterol levels.
Multivitamin and mineral complex	As directed on label.	All nutrients are necessary for healthy muscles.
Zinc	50 mg daily. Do not exceed a total of 100 mg daily from all supplements.	Needed for absorption of calcium and action of B vitamins. Use zinc gluconate lozenges or OptiZinc for best absorption.

Herbs

Alfalfa, bayberry, blessed thistle, cayenne, dong quai, echinacea, elderflower, elderberry extract, garlic, ginkgo biloba, and saffron are good for circulation.

Caution: Do not take echinacea for longer than three months. It should not be used by people who are allergic to ragweed. Do not take ginkgo biloba if you have a bleeding disorder, or are scheduled for surgery or a dental procedure.

❏ Meadowsweet, valerian, and skullcap help to relieve muscle cramps.

❏ Rubbing lobelia extract on the affected area helps to relieve muscle spasms.

❏ Taking valerian root at bedtime helps to relax the muscles.

Recommendations

❏ Getting adequate calcium and vitamin D is important. You can get these from dairy products and/or supplements.

❏ Eat alfalfa, brewer's yeast, plenty of dark green and leafy vegetables, cornmeal, and kelp.

Caution: Brewer's yeast can cause an allergic reaction in some individuals. Start with a small amount at first, and discontinue use if any allergic symptoms occur.

❏ Drink plenty of fluids to stave off dehydration. Take a large glass of quality water (preferably steam-distilled) to flush out toxins stored in the muscles every three hours throughout the day.

❏ Warm up before intense exercise, and cool down and stretch afterward.

❏ Rub pure, unprocessed olive or flaxseed oil into your muscles before and after strenuous exercise. Add 25 drops of oil to a hot bath and soak. Canola oil is also good for this purpose.

❏ Avoid overworking your muscles.

❏ Massage cramping muscles and use heat to relieve pain.

❏ Take a hot bath using mineral salts before bedtime to increase blood flow to the muscles.

❏ Before going to bed, gently stretch the muscles that tend to cramp during the night.

❏ If you are on diuretic medication for high blood pressure or a heart disorder, be sure to take supplemental potassium daily.

Note: Do not take supplemental potassium if you are taking a potassium-sparing diuretic (discuss this with your doctor).

❏ If you have cramps during the day, while you are active, consult your health care provider. This can be a sign of impaired circulation or arteriosclerosis. (*See* CIRCULATORY PROBLEMS in Part Two.)

❏ If cramping occurs after walking and is relieved when you stop, suspect impaired circulation. *See* ARTERIOSCLEROSIS/ATHEROSCLEROSIS in Part Two and take the artery function self-test. (*See also* CIRCULATORY PROBLEMS in Part Two.)

Considerations

❏ Using creatine, actually creatine monohydrate, a popular supplement with athletes and body builders, may increase the likelihood of muscle cramps.

Caution: Using creatine along with cimetidine (Tagamet), NSAIDs such as ibuprofen, and/or diuretics also can cause kidney damage.

❏ Hydrotherapy (the therapeutic use of water, steam, and ice) or massage therapy (manipulation of muscles and other soft tissue) may be useful in controlling muscle cramps. (*See* HYDROTHERAPY and MASSAGE *under* PAIN CONTROL in Part Three.)

❑ Gabapentin (Neurontin), a drug that is used in the treatment of epilepsy, and may be used for bipolar mood disorder by some doctors, is under study for its ability to relieve muscle cramps. Oddly, however, documented side effects of this drug can include muscle ache or pain (in addition to blurred or double vision; dizziness; drowsiness; swelling of hands, feet, or lower legs; trembling or shaking; and unusual tiredness or weakness). Until the results are known, we recommend steering clear of this drug.

MUSCLE INJURIES

See SPRAINS, STRAINS, AND OTHER INJURIES OF THE MUSCLES AND JOINTS.

MYOCARDIAL INFARCTION

See HEART ATTACK.

NAIL PROBLEMS

The nails protect the nerve-rich fingertips and tips of the toes from injury. Nails are a substructure of the epidermis (the outer layer of the skin) and are composed mainly of keratin, a type of protein. The nail bed is the skin on top of which the nails grow. Nails grow from 0.05 to 1.2 millimeters (approximately 1/500 to 1/20 inch) a week. If a nail is lost, it takes about seven months to grow out fully.

Healthy nail beds are pink, indicating a rich blood supply. Changes or abnormalities in the nails are often the result of nutritional deficiencies or other underlying conditions. The nails can reveal a great deal about the body's internal health. Nail abnormalities on either the fingers or the toes can indicate an underlying disorder.

The following are some of the changes that nutritional deficiencies can produce in the nails:

• A lack of protein, folic acid, and vitamin C causes hangnails. White bands across the nails are also an indication of protein deficiency.

• A lack of vitamin A and calcium causes dryness and brittleness.

• A deficiency of the B vitamins, especially biotin, causes fragility, with horizontal and vertical ridges.

• Insufficient intake of vitamin B_{12} leads to excessive dryness, very rounded and curved nail ends, and darkened nails.

• Iron deficiency may result in "spoon" nails (nails that develop a concave shape) and/or vertical ridges.

• Zinc deficiency may cause the development of white spots on the nails.

• A lack of sufficient "friendly" bacteria (lactobacilli) in the body can result in the growth of fungus under and around nails as well as discoloration of the nails.

• A lack of sufficient hydrochloric acid (HCl) contributes to splitting nails.

The Nutrients table, below, lists supplements that promote healthy nail growth.

Unless otherwise specified, the dosages recommended here are for adults. For children between the ages of twelve and seventeen, reduce the dose to three-quarters the recommended amount. For children between six and twelve, use one-half the recommended dose, and for children under the age of six, use one-quarter the recommended amount.

NUTRIENTS

SUPPLEMENT	SUGGESTED DOSAGE	COMMENTS
Very Important		
Acidophilus (Kyo-Dophilus from Wakunaga)	As directed on label.	Taken internally, inhibits the harmful bacteria that cause fungal infection. Use a nondairy formula.
Free form amino acid (Amino Balance from Anabol Naturals) plus extra L-cysteine and L-methionine	As directed on label, on an empty stomach. Take with water or juice. Do not take with milk. Take with 50 mg vitamin B₆ and 100 mg vitamin C for better absorption.	The building materials for new nails. Also supplies sulfur, which is necessary for skin and nail growth. (*See* AMINO ACIDS in Part One.)
Silica or oat straw	As directed on label.	Supplies silicon, needed for hair, bones, and strong nails. *See under* Herbs, below.
Vitamin A emulsion or capsules plus carotenoid complex	50,000 IU daily. If you are pregnant, do not exceed 10,000 IU daily. 25,000 IU daily. As directed on label.	The body cannot utilize protein without vitamin A. Emulsion form is recommended for easier assimilation and greater safety at higher doses.
Helpful		
Black currant seed oil	500 mg twice daily.	Helpful for weak, brittle nails.
Calcium and magnesium and vitamin D	As directed on label. As directed on label. As directed on label.	Necessary for nail growth. Needed to balance with calcium. Enhances calcium absorption.
Iron (Floradix Iron + Herbs from Salus Haus)	As directed by physician. Take with 100 mg vitamin C for better absorption.	Deficiency produces "spoon" nails and/or vertical ridges. *Caution:* Do not take iron unless anemia is diagnosed. A natural, nontoxic source of iron.
Ultimate Oil from Nature's Secret	As directed on label.	A combination of essential fatty acids necessary for the health of skin, hair, and nails.
Ultra Nails from Nature's Plus	As directed on label.	Contains calcium, gelatin, amino acids, magnesium, iron, and other nutrients important for healthy nails.

Vitamin B complex plus extra	As directed on label.	Deficiencies result in fragile nails.
vitamin B$_2$ (riboflavin) and	50 mg 3 times daily.	
vitamin B$_{12}$ and	1,000 mcg 3 times daily.	
biotin and	300 mg 3 times daily for 9 months.	Useful for treating brittle nails.
folic acid	400 mcg 3 times daily.	Reduces splitting and other nail irregularities.
Vitamin C with bioflavonoids	3,000–6,000 mg daily.	Hangnails and inflammation of the paronychia (the tissue surrounding the nail) may be linked to vitamin C deficiency.
Zinc	50 mg daily. Do not exceed a total of 100 mg daily from all supplements.	Affects absorption and action of vitamins and enzymes. Use zinc gluconate lozenges or OptiZinc for best absorption.
plus copper	3 mg daily.	Needed to balance with zinc.

Herbs

❑ Alfalfa, black cohosh, burdock root, dandelion, gotu kola, and yellow dock are rich in minerals, including silica and zinc, as well as B vitamins—all of which strengthen the nails. Oat straw also is a good source of silica.

Caution: Do not use black cohosh if you are pregnant or have any type of chronic disease. Black cohosh should not be used by those with liver problems.

❑ Borage seed, flaxseed, lemongrass, parsley, primrose, pumpkin seed, and sage are all good sources of essential fatty acids, which nourish the nails.

Caution: Do not use sage if you suffer from any type of seizure disorder, or are pregnant or nursing.

❑ Butcher's broom, chamomile, ginkgo biloba, rosemary, sassafras, and turmeric are good for circulation, which nourishes the nails.

Caution: Do not use chamomile if you are allergic to ragweed. Do not use during pregnancy or nursing. It may interact with warfarin or cyclosporine, so patients using these drugs should avoid it. Do not take ginkgo biloba if you have a bleeding disorder, or are scheduled for surgery or a dental procedure.

Recommendations

❑ For healthy nails, be sure to get plenty of quality protein, and take a protein supplement. Eat grains, legumes, oatmeal, nuts, and seeds. Eggs also are a good source of protein, as long as your blood cholesterol levels are not too high.

❑ Avoid refined sugars and simple carbohydrates.

❑ Eat a diet composed of 50 percent fresh fruits and raw vegetables to supply necessary vitamins, minerals, and en-

zymes. Eat foods that are rich in sulfur and silicon, such as broccoli, fish, onions, and sea vegetables. Also include in the diet plenty of foods that are high in biotin, such as brewer's yeast, soy flour, and whole grains.

Caution: Brewer's yeast can cause an allergic reaction in some individuals. Start with a small amount at first, and discontinue use if any allergic symptoms occur.

❑ Drink plenty of quality water and other liquids. Cuts and cracks in the nails may indicate a need for more liquids.

❑ Drink fresh carrot juice daily. This is high in calcium and phosphorus and is very good for strengthening the nails.

❑ Consume citrus fruits, salt, and vinegar in moderation, if at all. Excessive intake of these foods can result in a protein/calcium imbalance that may adversely affect the health of the nails.

❑ Supplement your diet with royal jelly, a good source of essential fatty acids, and spirulina or kelp, which are rich in silica, zinc, and B vitamins, and help to strengthen nails. Be sure the B vitamins have biotin in the mix.

❑ For splitting nails and/or hangnails, take 2 tablespoons of brewer's yeast or wheat germ oil daily.

Caution: Brewer's yeast can cause an allergic reaction in some individuals. Start with a small amount at first, and discontinue use if any allergic symptoms occur.

❑ To restore color and texture to brittle, yellowed nails, make a mixture of equal parts of honey, avocado oil, and egg yolk, and add a pinch of salt. Rub the mixture into your nails and cuticles. Leave it on for half an hour, then rinse it off. Repeat this treatment daily. You should begin to see results after about two weeks.

❑ To strengthen the nails, try soaking them in warm olive oil or apple cider vinegar for ten to twenty minutes daily.

❑ Treat your nails gently. Using them to pry, pick, scrape, or perform tasks such as removing staples can damage them.

❑ Keep your nails relatively short. Nails longer than one-quarter inch beyond the fingertip break and bend easily.

❑ Do *not* cut the cuticles. Uncovering the nails this way is harsh and irritating, and may cause infection. Use baby oil or cream and gently push the cuticles back.

❑ Soak your nails before trimming them. Nails are most likely to split and peel when they are dry. Apply hand cream each morning and evening to prevent nails from drying out.

❑ Do not repeatedly immerse your hands in water that contains detergents or chemicals such as bleach or dish soap; this results in split nails. Wear cotton-lined gloves when doing housework such as dishes and laundry or when using furniture polish. This protects your hands and nails from harsh chemicals. Wearing gloves is especially important for people who work in jobs where their hands are exposed to chemicals. Not only does this damage the nails, but it causes the skin surrounding the nail bed to dry out and crack. This can lead to bleeding and can be quite painful.

Disorders That Show Up in the Nails

Nail changes may signify a number of disorders elsewhere in the body. These changes may indicate illness before any other symptoms do. Seek medical attention if any of the following symptoms are suspected.

• *Black, splinterlike bits under the nails* can be a sign of infectious endocarditis, a serious heart infection; other heart disease; or a bleeding disorder.

• *Black bands* from the cuticle outward to the end of the nail can be an early sign of melanoma.

• *Brittle, soft, shiny nails without a moon* may indicate an overactive thyroid.

• *Brittle nails* signify possible iron deficiency, thyroid problems, impaired kidney function, and circulation problems.

• *Crumbly, white nails near the cuticle* are sometimes an indication of AIDS.

• *Dark nails and/or thin, flat, spoon-shaped nails* are a sign of vitamin B_{12} deficiency or anemia. Nails can also turn gray or dark if the hands are placed in chemicals such as cleaning supplies (most often bleach) or a substance to which one is allergic.

• *Deep blue nail beds* show a pulmonary obstructive disorder such as asthma or emphysema.

• *Downward-curved nail ends* may denote heart, liver, or respiratory problems.

• *Flat nails* can denote Raynaud's disease.

• *Greenish nails,* if not a result of a localized fungal infection, may indicate an internal bacterial infection.

• *A half-white nail with dark spots at the tip* points to possible kidney disease.

• *An isolated dark-blue band in the nail bed,* especially in light-skinned people, can be a sign of skin cancer.

• *Lindsay's nails* (sometimes known as *half-and-half nails*), in which half of the top of the nail is white and the other half is pink, may be a sign of chronic kidney disease.

• *Nail beading* (the development of bumps on the surface of the nail) is a sign of rheumatoid arthritis.

• *Nails raised at the base with small white ends* show a respiratory disorder such as emphysema or chronic bronchitis. This type of nail may also simply be inherited.

• *Nails separated from the nail bed* may signify a thyroid disorder (this condition is known as onycholysis) or a local infection.

• *Nails that broaden toward the tip and curve downward* are a sign of lung damage, such as from emphysema or exposure to asbestos.

• *Nails that chip, peel, crack, or break easily* show a general nutritional deficiency and insufficient hydrochloric acid and protein. Minerals are also needed.

• *Nails that have pitting resembling hammered brass* indicate a tendency toward partial or total hair loss.

• *Pitted red-brown spots and frayed and split ends* indicate psoriasis; vitamin C, folic acid, and protein are needed.

• *Red skin around the cuticles* can be indicative of poor metabolism of essential fatty acids or of a connective tissue disorder such as lupus.

• *Ridges* can appear in the nails either vertically or horizontally. Vertical ridges indicate poor general health, poor nutrient absorption, and/or iron deficiency; they may also indicate a kidney disorder. Horizontal ridges can occur as a result of severe stress, either psychological or physical, such as from infection and/or disease. A horizontal indentation in the nail (Beau's line) can occur as a result of a heart attack, major illness, or surgery. Ridges running up and down the nails also indicate a tendency to develop arthritis.

• *Spooning (upward-curling) or pitting nails* can be caused by disorders such as anemia or problems with iron absorption. This can also be caused by poor lung function due to smoking or exposure to something that damaged the lungs' ability to properly oxygenate the blood such as smoke from a fire.

• *Thick nails* may indicate that the vascular system is weakening and the blood is not circulating properly. This may also be a sign of thyroid disease.

• *Thick toenails* can be a result of fungal infection.

• *Thinning nails* may signal lichen planus, an itchy skin disorder.

• *Two white horizontal bands that do not move as the nail grows* are a sign of hypoalbuminemia, a protein deficiency in the blood.

• *Unusually wide, square nails* can suggest a hormonal disorder.

• *White lines* show possible heart disease, high fever, or arsenic poisoning.

• *White lines across the nail* may indicate a liver disease.

• *If the white moon area of the nail turns red,* it may indicate heart problems.

• *If the white moon area of the nail turns slate blue,* it can indicate either heavy metal poisoning (such as silver poisoning) or lung trouble.

• *White nails* indicate possible liver or kidney disorders and/or anemia.

• *White nails with pink near the tips* can be a sign of cirrhosis.

• *Yellow nails or an elevation of the nail tips* can indicate internal disorders long before other symptoms appear. Some of these are problems with the lymphatic system, respiratory disorders, diabetes, and liver disorders.

❑ Do not pull at hangnails. Cut them with sharp clippers or scissors. Keep your hands moisturized to help prevent hangnails.

❑ If you have diabetes, see your health care provider if your cuticles become inflamed, because the infection can spread.

❑ If you wear nail polish, use a base coat underneath it to prevent yellowing.

❑ Use nail polish removers as little as possible. They contain solvents that leach lipids from the nails and make them brittle. These solvents are also potentially highly toxic and can be absorbed through the skin. If you need to use a polish remover, use one that contains acetate instead of acetone.

❑ Never apply polycrylic or other artificial nails over your own. They may look nice for a while, but they destroy the underlying nail. The chemicals and glue used are dangerous to the body, and are readily absorbed through the damaged nail and nail bed. The use of artificial nails also has been known to contribute to the development of fungal infection of the fingernails.

❑ Many professional manicure businesses have been cited for not meeting health codes. If you have professional manicures, always insist on sterile instruments or bring your own to ensure they are free from bacteria and disease. Use isopropyl alcohol to sterilize your instruments.

Considerations

❑ If you expose your hands to too much water and soap, the nail may become loose from the nail bed. Water causes the nails to swell. They then shrink as they dry, resulting in loose and brittle nails.

❑ Discolored nails can be caused by prolonged illness, stress, nicotine, allergies, or diabetes. If your nails are green, you may have a bacterial infection or a fungal infection between the nail and the nail bed. If you have a fungal or bacterial infection, and especially if you are taking antibiotics, acidophilus is needed.

❑ Fungal infections can be treated by using a cotton swab to apply a mixture of equal parts of vinegar and water.

❑ Physicians often prescribe a regimen of 250 milligrams of griseofulvin (Fulvicin), four times daily, for a fungal infection of the nails. The white blood cell count must be monitored during this treatment. Other effective oral drugs include: Itraconazole (Sporanox), Fluconazole (Diflucan), and Terbinafine (Lamisil). Doctors may not recommend these for people with liver disease or congestive heart failure or for those taking certain medications. Another prescription antifungal agent is ketoconazole (Nizoral), which is available as a cream or shampoo, as well as in tablet form. These drugs are highly effective against nail fungus, so if you are worried about the appearance of your nails, seek medical help.

❑ Anticancer medications can cause bands and streaks of color to appear on the nails. These conditions disappear when the medication is stopped.

❑ A recent study found that hospital nurses with artificial nails had twice as much bacteria on their hands as those nurses who had natural nails. The area around and underneath the fingernails is one of the easiest places for germs to collect. The best way to prevent this is to thoroughly wash your hands for at least fifteen seconds using antiseptic soap under hot water. Make sure you wash the area underneath the nail and around the cuticle area. Use a clean towel to dry your hands. Use disposable towels if they are available.

❑ Poor thyroid function may be reflected in the nails. (*See* HYPOTHYROIDISM in Part Two.)

NARCOLEPSY

Narcolepsy is a neurological disorder that is estimated to affect as many as 1.5 million Americans. However, fewer than 10 to 25 percent have all of the components of the disease to make a firm diagnosis. There are four classic symptoms that define this syndrome: sleep attacks, cataplexy, sleep paralysis, and hypnagogic (sleep-related) hallucinations. A person with narcolepsy may experience any or all of these classic phenomena.

The best-known symptom of narcolepsy is the sleep attack. A person with narcolepsy can suddenly fall into a sleep state with almost no warning whatsoever. Sleep attacks can occur at any time, even in midconversation, as many as ten times a day (even more, in some cases). These periods of sleep usually last only a matter of minutes, but in some cases sleep can continue for an hour or more. Afterward, the person may feel refreshed, yet he or she may fall asleep again in a few minutes.

While the sleep that results from narcolepsy looks like ordinary sleep, researchers have found at least one key difference. Normal sleep is a cyclical process that alternates between periods of rapid-eye-movement (REM) and non-rapid-eye-movement (NREM) sleep. During the NREM part of the cycle, the entire body slows down—pulse, breathing, blood pressure, and brain wave activity are all lowered. When the REM cycle begins, the body remains asleep, but the brain becomes significantly active; brain waves as recorded by an electroencephalograph (EEG) more closely resemble those of the waking brain. It is during REM sleep that most dreaming occurs.

In healthy individuals, sleep begins with the NREM phase. After sixty minutes or so of NREM sleep, REM sleep begins. A short time later, the entire cycle begins again. In a narcoleptic sleep attack, in contrast, researchers have found that REM sleep begins almost instantly, with no introductory NREM sleep. The precise significance of this is not yet understood, but it does provide a useful diagnostic tool as well as a clue for researchers to pursue in trying to understand this mysterious disorder.

The second classic symptom of narcolepsy is cataplexy. This is a type of paralysis that usually occurs in response to some type of heightened emotion, such as anger, fear, or excitement. The individual does not lose consciousness, but experiences a sudden and temporary loss of muscle tone. Often, only the legs and/or arms are affected. These episodes normally last less than a minute, and they seem to be most likely to occur if the person is surprised in some way.

Sleep paralysis is the third classic symptom of narcolepsy. Just as you are falling asleep, or as you are beginning to awaken, you try to move or say something but find that you cannot, even though you are fully conscious. This lasts for only a second or two, but it can be frightening, especially the first time it happens. These episodes usually end either on their own or when someone touches or speaks to you. Many doctors feel that sleep paralysis is similar to cataplexy and to the state that accompanies REM sleep, in which motor activity is inhibited even though the brain is active. This phenomenon is not strictly limited to people with narcolepsy; many otherwise healthy people may experience it occasionally.

Like sleep paralysis, sleep-related hallucinations—medically termed *hypnagogic phenomena*—usually occur just prior to sleep, or sometimes upon awakening. The affected individual may hear sounds that aren't there and/or see illusions. These visual and auditory illusions are very vivid. This phenomenon also can occur in individuals who do not suffer from narcolepsy, particularly in children.

Because the symptoms of narcolepsy vary from individual to individual (it is estimated that only 20 to 25 percent of people with narcolepsy experience all four of the classic symptoms), this disorder is frequently misdiagnosed. There is strong evidence that narcolepsy may run in families; 8 to 12 percent of people with narcolepsy have a close relative with the disorder. Further compounding the problem is the fact that other sleep disorders, such as sleep apnea, also can produce spells of marked daytime drowsiness. Narcolepsy is not a particularly dangerous problem, unless one experiences a sleep attack while operating a motor vehicle or other machinery. It can, however, be embarrassing and extremely inconvenient. The cause or causes of this disorder are unknown, but brain infection, head trauma, or brain tumors may be behind some cases. It is known that narcolepsy is almost never the result of insomnia or sleep deprivation. There is currently no cure for this disorder, so the focus must be on treating the symptoms.

Unless otherwise specified, the dosages recommended here are for adults. For children between the ages of twelve and seventeen, reduce the dose to three-quarters the recommended amount. For children between six and twelve, use one-half the recommended dose, and for children under the age of six, use one-quarter the recommended amount.

NUTRIENTS

SUPPLEMENT	SUGGESTED DOSAGE	COMMENTS
Essential		
Calcium and magnesium	2,000 mg daily, at bedtime. 400 mg twice during the day and again at bedtime.	Needed for energy production and the nervous system.
Choline or lecithin granules or capsules	300 mg daily. 1 tbsp 3 times daily, before meals. 1,200 mg 3 times daily, before meals.	Acts as a neurotransmitter and is important for brain function. A good source of choline.
Chromium picolinate	100 mcg daily.	Boosts energy and regulates sugar metabolism.
Coenzyme Q$_{10}$ plus Coenzyme A from Coenzyme-A Technologies	As directed on label. As directed on label.	Promotes circulation to the brain. Works with coenzyme Q$_{10}$.
Free form amino acid (Amino Balance from Anabol Naturals)	As directed on label.	Increases energy levels; needed for proper brain function. Use a formula that contains all the essential amino acids.
L-glutamine	As directed on label, on an empty stomach. Take with water or juice. Do not take with milk. Take with 50 mg vitamin B$_6$ and 100 mg vitamin C for better absorption.	Promotes mental ability. Known as brain fuel because it can pass the blood-brain barrier freely. (*See* AMINO ACIDS in Part One.)
L-tyrosine	As directed on label. Take at bedtime.	Important in thyroid function. Low levels have been associated with narcolepsy. *Caution:* Do not take tyrosine if you are taking an MAO inhibitor drug.
Multivitamin and mineral complex	As directed on label.	All nutrients are needed to balance body functioning.
Nicotinamide adenine dinucleotide (NADH)	As directed on label.	Important in the creation and transfer of chemical energy, especially during breathing.
Octacosanol	100 mg daily.	Increases oxygen utilization and boosts endurance.
Omega-3 essential fatty acids (fish oil or flaxseed oil)	As directed on label.	To protect cell membranes.
Vitamin B complex (Coenzymate B Complex from Source Naturals) plus extra vitamin B$_6$ (pyridoxine)	150 mg of each major B vitamin daily (amounts of individual vitamins in a complex will vary). 200 mg daily.	B vitamins boost metabolism and are essential for increased energy levels and normal brain function.
Vitamin C with bioflavonoids	2,000–6,000 mg daily, in divided doses.	Increases energy and promotes production of interferon in the body to protect against free radical damage.
Vitamin D	400 IU daily.	Essential for calcium absorption.

Vitamin E	200 IU daily or 400 IU every other day.	Increases circulation and protects heart functioning and brain cells. Use d-alpha-tocopherol form.

Herbs

❑ Gotu kola and St. John's wort boost energy levels and possess antioxidant properties as well.

Caution: St. John's wort may cause increased sensitivity to sunlight. It may also produce anxiety, gastrointestinal symptoms, and headaches. It can interact with some drugs including antidepressants, birth control pills, and antico-agulants.

❑ Ginkgo biloba improves circulation to the brain and is a powerful antioxidant for protecting cells.

Caution: Do not take ginkgo biloba if you have a bleeding disorder, or are scheduled for surgery or a dental procedure.

Recommendations

❑ Eat a low-fat diet high in cleansing foods such as leafy green vegetables and sea vegetables. Also eat foods high in the B vitamins, such as brewer's yeast and brown rice.

Caution: Brewer's yeast can cause an allergic reaction in some individuals. Start with a small amount at first, and discontinue use if any allergic symptoms occur.

❑ Eat foods high in protein (meats, poultry, cheese, nuts, seeds, and soy products) in the middle of the day, and save the complex carbohydrates (fresh fruits and vegetables, legumes, natural whole grains, and pasta) for the evening meal. High-protein foods increase alertness, whereas carbohydrates have a calming effect and can promote sleepiness.

❑ Include in the diet foods rich in the amino acid tyrosine. Good choices include eggs, oats, poultry, and wheat germ.

❑ One MAO inhibitor drug, selegiline, was shown to help with sleep issues in patients with narcolepsy. This drug is usually given to patients with Parkinson's disease, but in patients with narcolepsy who were given 20 to 40 milligrams a day, 43 to 89 percent had fewer narcoleptic symptoms such as longer periods of REM sleep.

Caution: If you are taking an MAO inhibitor drug, *avoid* foods containing tyrosine, as drug and dietary interactions can cause a sudden, dangerous rise in blood pressure. Discuss food and medicine limitations thoroughly with your health care provider or a qualified dietitian.

❑ Avoid alcohol and sugar. They may seem stimulating initially, but will only make you tired later.

❑ Exercise daily to improve circulation and oxygenate tissues.

Caution: If you are thirty-five or older and/or have been sedentary for some time, consult with your health care provider before beginning an exercise program.

❑ Napping can rejuvenate you when you have lost sleep. Take up to a forty-five-minute nap in the early afternoon.

❑ Make sure your home and workplace are well lit, either by natural sunlight or overhead lighting. Light suppresses the production of melatonin, which is the hormone that produces drowsiness. Full-spectrum light bulbs are best.

Considerations

❑ Narcolepsy and sleep apnea are the leading causes of tiredness during the day.

❑ A diagnosis of narcolepsy may involve a *multiple sleep latency test* (MSLT), usually conducted in a sleep disorders clinic.

❑ Irregular sleep patterns are just as likely to cause drowsiness as lack of sleep. Jet lag, shift work, inconsistent bedtimes, and weekend partying can all disturb our natural sleep/wake cycles. America is a nation of sleep-starved yawners fighting a daily battle against the sandman. We live in a world where people drive themselves on relentless schedules that leave insufficient time for quality sleep.

❑ There have been some documented cases in which persons who suffered from narcolepsy were cured by eliminating allergenic foods from the diet. One person, for instance, was found to have an allergy to potatoes. When he removed potatoes from his diet, he no longer experienced the symptoms. (*See* ALLERGIES in Part Two.)

❑ There is some evidence that the immune systems of people who suffer from narcolepsy may react abnormally to the chemical processes in the brain that cause sleep.

❑ Certain dogs, mainly Doberman pinschers, have been observed to sleep excessively and to collapse when overstimulated. Research has revealed a withering away of axons (the "communication cables" that convey signals between nerve cells) in the brains of these animals, especially in three regions of the brain that have been linked to sleep inhibition, motor control, and the processing of emotions. If similar degeneration can be demonstrated in human brains, this may offer further clues as to the causes of narcolepsy.

❑ Doctors have traditionally prescribed stimulants (amphetamines) and antidepressants for people with narcolepsy. A newer drug, modafinil (Provigil), acts on the hypothalamus, a part of the brain responsible for wakefulness, and may reduce sleep attacks. This drug should not be used by people with heart conditions, liver dysfunction, or a history of mental illness, and it can reduce the effectiveness of certain birth control methods. Doctors also prescribe antidepressant medications, which suppress REM sleep, to alleviate symptoms of cataplexy, hypnagogic hallucinations, and sleep paralysis. These medications include tricyclic antidepressants such as protriptyline (Vivactil) and imipramine (Tofranil) and selective serotonin reuptake inhibitors (SSRIs) such as fluoxetine (Prozac, Sarafem) and sertraline (Zoloft).

❑ *See also* the discussion of sleep apnea *under* INSOMNIA in Part Two.

NAUSEA AND VOMITING

See under FOODBORNE/WATERBORNE DISEASE and INDIGESTION. *See also under* INFLUENZA.

NEPHRITIS

See under KIDNEY DISEASE.

NERVOUSNESS

See ANXIETY DISORDER and STRESS.

NICKEL TOXICITY

Nickel is a silver-white metal used to produce steel, nickel-cadmium batteries, nickel plating, heating fuel, and ceramics. It has been described as a trace mineral, and is present in many cells within the human body. Small amounts of nickel are useful in certain bodily functions. For example, minute amounts of nickel are important in DNA and RNA stabilization. Nickel may play a role in the metabolism of glucose and hormonal functions. It also helps to activate certain important enzymes, such as trypsin and arginase. A nickel deficiency may affect iron and zinc metabolism.

Too much nickel can be toxic, however. Nickel carbonyl is the most toxic form of this metal. Lethal exposure to nickel through inhalation causes nausea, dizziness, diarrhea, headache, vomiting, chest pain, weakness, and coughing. Contact with the vapor can lead to brain and liver swelling; degeneration of the liver; irritation to the eyes, throat, and nose; and cancer. Although toxic levels of nickel have not been established, it is known that the presence of excess amounts of nickel can cause dermatitis (skin rash and inflammation), also called "nickel itch," and respiratory illness, and can interfere with the Kreb's cycle, a series of enzymatic reactions necessary for cellular energy production. Significant levels of nickel may also contribute to thyroid malfunction or myocardial infarction (heart attack). Environmental exposure to nickel can occur by contact with automobile exhaust, cigarette smoke, manufacturing emissions, and airborne dust. Skin absorption can come from coins, hairpins, jewelry, prosthetic joints and heart valves, and nickel plating.

Many foods naturally contain some amount of nickel. These include bananas, barley, beans, buckwheat, cabbage, hazelnuts, legumes, lentils, oats, pears, soybeans, and walnuts. Nickel can also be present in hydrogenated fats and oils, refined and processed foods, baking powder, cocoa powder, superphosphate fertilizers, and tobacco smoke. Using cooking utensils containing nickel may add unnecessarily to your dietary intake of nickel.

Unless otherwise specified, the dosages recommended here are for adults. For children between the ages of twelve and seventeen, reduce the dose to three-quarters the recommended amount. For children between six and twelve, use one-half the recommended dose, and for children under the age of six, use one-quarter the recommended amount.

NUTRIENTS

SUPPLEMENT	SUGGESTED DOSAGE	COMMENTS
Important		
Apple pectin	As directed on label.	Binds toxic metals and removes them from the body.
Garlic (Kyolic from Wakunaga)	As directed on label.	Acts as a detoxifier and aids in removing harmful metals.
Kelp	1,000–1,500 mg daily.	Supplies minerals and iodine to aid in removing toxic metals.
L-cysteine and L-methionine	As directed on label, on an empty stomach. Take with water or juice. Do not take with milk. Take with 50 mg vitamin B_6 and 100 mg vitamin C for better absorption.	Helps to detoxify the body, including the liver, of harmful metals. (*See* AMINO ACIDS in Part One.)
Selenium	200 mcg daily. If you are pregnant, do not exceed 40 mcg daily.	A powerful free radical destroyer.
Vitamin A with mixed carotenoids plus	25,000 IU daily. If you are pregnant, do not exceed 10,000 IU daily.	A powerful antioxidant that destroys free radicals.
natural beta-carotene	15,000 IU daily.	A free radical scavenger.
Vitamin C with bioflavonoids including rutin	4,000–10,000 mg daily.	Helps to remove metals from the body and strengthens immunity.
Vitamin E	200 IU daily or 400 IU every other day.	A powerful free radical scavenger that also improves circulation. Use d-alpha-tocopherol form.

Recommendations

❑ If you suspect you may have symptoms of metal toxicity, have a hair analysis done to detect toxic levels of nickel and other minerals. (*See* HAIR ANALYSIS in Part Three.)

❑ Avoid processed food products, as well as any products containing hydrogenated fats and oils.

❑ Do not smoke, and avoid those who do.

❑ Beware of metal cookware, especially when preparing acidic foods, such as tomato sauce. Use glass cookware instead. Also avoid using metal cooking utensils. Use utensils made from plastic or wood instead (wood is best).

❑ Ask your dentist about the metal content of the materials he or she uses. Nickel toxicity can result from nickel alloys used in dental surgery and appliances.

❑ If your job or hobby involves using nickel to plate metals, use a face mask while working. Inhalation of nickel can cause pulmonary edema (accumulation of fluid in the lungs).

Considerations

❑ Chelation can remove toxic metals from the body. (*See* CHELATION THERAPY in Part Three.)

❑ In one study, Antabuse, a nickel-chelating agent and drug used in the treatment of alcoholism, was tested in patients with hand eczema and nickel allergy, but it did not have an appreciable effect on scaly skin and flare-ups. However, in another study, a low-nickel diet combined with oral disulfiram (Antabuse) produced much better outcomes. Ninety percent of the patients experienced healing of their hand eczema.

❑ Aside from being potentially toxic, nickel is often allergenic. The nickel in watchbands, zippers, bra closures, pierced earrings, and other everyday items has been associated with many allergic reactions. A high incidence of allergic reactions to nickel in pierced earrings has been reported among children. Many earrings and posts contain nickel. Gold (14-karat or higher) is probably the safest metal for pierced earrings. (*See* CHEMICAL ALLERGIES in Part Two.)

NOSEBLEED

Any injury to the tissues inside the nose can cause a nosebleed. Injury can result from a blow to the nose; the intrusion of foreign objects (including fingers); a sudden change in atmospheric pressure; or simply blowing the nose too forcefully. Winter often brings about nosebleeds because heated air tends to be dry. Excessive dryness can cause the nasal membranes to crack, form crusts, and bleed.

In some cases, nosebleeds—medically termed *epistaxis*—can be associated with an underlying illness. Arteriosclerosis, high blood pressure, malaria, scarlet fever, sinusitis, and typhoid fever are all known to cause nosebleeds, some of which can be serious and result in significant blood loss. Conditions that cause increased bleeding tendencies, such as hemophilia, leukemia, thrombocytopenia (a below-normal concentration of platelets in the blood), aplastic anemia, or liver disease, also may be implicated in nosebleeds.

Nosebleeds are much more common in children than in adults. This is no doubt largely due to the fact that children are prone to inserting their fingers and other objects into their nostrils. In addition, children's tissues, including the mucous membranes lining the nose, are thinner than those of adults and therefore more susceptible to damage.

There are two classifications of nosebleeds, depending on where in the nose the blood is coming from. *Posterior nosebleeds* primarily afflict elderly people and those with high blood pressure. In this type of nosebleed, blood comes from the rear of the nose and runs down the back of the mouth into the throat, no matter what position the person

is in. The blood is usually dark red in color, although it can be bright red. If the bleeding is severe, blood can flow from the nostrils as well.

The overwhelming majority of nosebleeds are *anterior nosebleeds,* in which bright-red blood flows from the front part of the nose. Most often they are the result of some type of trauma to the nasal tissues. If the person stands or sits, the flow of blood comes out of one or both nostrils. If the person lies on his or her back, the blood may flow backward, into the throat. This type of nosebleed can be frightening, and it may look as if there is a lot of blood, but in reality it is not usually serious and very little blood is actually lost.

Unless otherwise specified, the dosages recommended here are for adults. For children between the ages of twelve and seventeen, reduce the dose to three-quarters the recommended amount. For children between six and twelve, use one-half the recommended dose, and for children under the age of six, use one-quarter the recommended amount.

NUTRIENTS

SUPPLEMENT	SUGGESTED DOSAGE	COMMENTS
Helpful		
Bioflavonoid complex with rutin	As directed on label.	Deficiencies have been linked to nosebleeds.
Vitamin C with bioflavonoids	3,000 mg when bleeding starts and 1,000 mg every hour thereafter until bleeding has completely stopped.	Promotes healing.

Herbs

❑ If your nasal membranes become sore from dryness, use aloe vera gel, calendula ointment, or comfrey ointment as needed.

Caution: Comfrey is recommended for external use only.

❑ A snuff made from finely ground oak bark is soothing and healing.

❑ To promote healing, rub a small amount of Calendula Cream from Natureworks into each nostril once the bleeding subsides. Repeat as needed.

Recommendations

❑ To stop an anterior nosebleed, do the following:

1. Sit up in a chair and lean forward (*do not* tilt your head back). Do not put your head between your legs or lie flat on your back.

2. Pinch all the soft parts of the nose together between your thumb and index finger for approximately ten minutes. The pressure should be firm but not painful. Breathe through your mouth.

3. Apply crushed ice or cold washcloths to your nose, neck, and cheeks. This can be done both as you apply pressure (*see* 2, above) and afterward.

4. Keep your head higher than your heart until the bleeding subsides. Refrain from any energetic physical activity for a few hours and any vigorous exercise for at least two days.

5. If the bleeding does not stop, place a cloth or piece of cotton moistened with water or an over-the-counter decongestant spray into the nasal cavity. Hold your nostrils together tightly for about five minutes.

❑ To help stop a nosebleed, try rolling a piece of cotton or gauze and place it in the top part of your upper lip, under the gum. An artery supplying blood to the nose is located in this region. Applying pressure in this manner may help constrict the blood flow.

❑ If you suspect a posterior nosebleed, consult your doctor. This type of nosebleed requires the care of a physician.

❑ Do not blow your nose for at least twelve hours after a nosebleed stops. Doing so may dislodge the blood clots that stanch bleeding.

❑ Once bleeding is controlled and healing has begun, apply a small amount of vitamin E to the affected tissues—open a capsule and *gently* apply the oil inside the nose. If vitamin E is unavailable, use a little petroleum jelly or A&D Ointment. If you wish, pack the nose with gauze to prevent leakage.

❑ While healing, eat plenty of foods high in vitamin K, which is essential for normal blood clotting. Good sources include alfalfa, kale, and all dark green leafy vegetables.

❑ Avoid foods high in salicylates, which are aspirin-like substances found in tea, coffee, most fruits, and some vegetables. Foods to avoid include almonds, all berries, apples, apricots, bell peppers, cherries, cloves, cucumbers, currants, grapes, mint, oil of wintergreen, peaches, pickles, plums, raisins, tangelos, and tomatoes.

❑ To counteract dryness in the nasal passages, especially during the winter, use nasal irrigation. Spray inside the nostrils with plain warm water or a saline mist spray from time to time.

❑ To prevent nosebleeds, increase the environmental humidity, especially in winter. Use a cool mist humidifier, a vaporizer, or even a pan of water placed near a radiator.

❑ When you sneeze, keep your mouth open.

❑ If you have frequent nosebleeds, see your doctor. The cause of frequent nosebleeds is often an underlying problem such as hypertension, which should be treated.

❑ If you are prone to nosebleeds, an iron supplement may help to rebuild the blood. Iron is an important component in hemoglobin, which is a vital element in red blood cells.

Caution: Check with your physician before taking iron supplements.

Considerations

❑ If packing the nose with gauze or cotton is necessary to stem the flow of blood, some medical authorities recommend moistening the packing material with white vinegar. They contend that the acid in white vinegar gently cauterizes broken blood vessels and aids in stopping the bleeding.

❑ Be careful about inserting any substance that contains zinc into your nose. Zicam, a cold prevention medicine that contains zinc, was removed from sale by the FDA because people lost their sense of smell.

❑ Sometimes the use of drugs that thin the blood, such as the anticoagulants warfarin (Coumadin) or heparin, may cause nosebleeds. Even aspirin can act as an anticoagulant and interfere with blood clotting, which is necessary in stopping nosebleeds.

❑ High estrogen levels increase the flow of blood from the mucous membranes in the nose. This is why nosebleeds are more common during pregnancy. Oral contraceptives also can contribute to nosebleeds.

❑ The risk of serious nosebleeds increases with hemophilia, Hodgkin's disease, rheumatic fever, vitamin C deficiency, or the prolonged use of nose drops or nasal sprays.

❑ Nosebleeds are common among alcoholics. As alcohol dilates blood vessels, including those in the nasal cavities, the vessels bleed more easily. Heavy alcohol use can also create problems with blood clotting because of the toxic effects of alcohol on the liver and bone marrow.

❑ People with hypertension are especially prone to nosebleeds. A low-fat, low-cholesterol diet is recommended for keeping blood pressure under control. (*See* HIGH BLOOD PRESSURE in Part Two.)

❑ If you have recurring nosebleeds, your doctor may recommend surgical or chemical treatment. In some situations, topical chemical solutions are applied to the blood vessels to constrict the blood flow. If topical applications are unsuccessful, nasal blood vessels can be constricted through cauterization (surgical burning of tissues), using either a chemical solution or an electrical heating tool. If all of the above measures fail, both sides of the nasal cavity may be packed with a spongelike or gauze material. Nasal packing is almost always a standard procedure when an anterior nosebleed will not stop bleeding. Your physician may not remove the packs for two to five days.

❑ *See also under* PREGNANCY-RELATED PROBLEMS in Part Two.

OBESITY

Obesity is, quite simply, an excessively high proportion of body fat. Health professionals commonly use a measurement called the *body mass index,* or BMI, to classify an adult's weight as healthy, overweight, obese, and extremely obese. Calculate BMI by dividing weight in pounds by height in inches squared and multiplying by 703. (Formula: (weight (lb)/[height (in)]^2 × 703). (*See* Body Mass Index on page 610.) Basically, according to this index, a BMI from 18.5 to 24.9 is considered healthy; from 25 to 29.9, overweight. Obesity class I is a BMI of 30 to 34.9, obesity class II is a BMI of 35 to 39.9, and extreme obesity class III is a BMI of 40 and above. A BMI below 18.5 is considered underweight and unhealthy. Generally, the higher your BMI, the greater your risk of developing other obesity-related problems. However, BMI does not tell the entire story.

In addition to the BMI number, excessive *abdominal* body fat can pose a health risk. Men with a waist size greater than 40 inches, or women with a waist size of 35 inches or more, are more at risk.

Americans are eating less fat, but are getting fatter. More than 66 percent of adults in the United States are either overweight or obese, according to the U.S. Centers for Disease Control and Prevention. Excess weight and inactivity account for more than 300,000 premature deaths each year in the United States. This is second only to deaths related to smoking, according to the CDC. People who are overweight or obese are more likely than those of normal weight to develop heart disease, stroke, high blood pressure, diabetes, gallbladder disease, joint pain (gout), sleep apnea, and osteoarthritis. In addition, carrying excess weight means a higher risk for cancer. At the American Institute for Cancer Research (AICR), researchers have concluded that obesity increases the risk for many of the most common cancers worldwide, and perhaps for cancer generally. Obesity is consistently linked to postmenopausal breast cancer, colon cancer, endometrial (uterine) cancer, prostate cancer, and kidney cancer.

Being overweight is a contributing cause of many preventable illnesses. How much a person weighs is only part of the story, however. Perhaps more important than weight is the percentage of fat in the body. For healthy women, fat can account for as much as 25 percent of body weight; 17 percent is a healthy percentage for men. Women's bodies are designed to carry a higher proportion of fat tissue to ensure that there is plenty of fuel for pregnancy and nursing, even if food is scarce. It is also important to know where the fat is stored—for example, abdominally or on the rear end.

The average human body has 30 to 40 billion fat cells. Most of the extra calories we eat that we do not need for immediate energy are stored as fat. If we were still "hunter/gatherers" like our early ancestors, the fat would provide a needed food store for times when no food is readily available. Today, however, instead of being a valuable survival mechanism, the body's ability to store fat is more likely to have a profoundly negative effect on health. Most people today still have this gene for fat storage, which in part explains why there is an obesity epidemic. Lean people are really genetic mutations and would not have survived tens of thousands of years ago. As fat accumulates, it crowds the space occupied by the internal organs. Obesity—even moderate overweight—puts an undue stress on the back, legs, and internal organs, and this can eventually exacerbate many physical problems and compromise health. Obesity increases the body's resistance to insulin and susceptibility to infection, and puts one at a higher risk for developing coronary artery disease, diabetes, gallbladder disease, high blood pressure, kidney disease, stroke, and other serious health problems that can result in premature death. Complications of pregnancy and liver damage also are more common in overweight individuals. Obese persons suffer psychologically as well as physically, because our society tends to equate beauty, intelligence, and even success with thinness.

The most common causes of obesity are poor diet and/or eating habits (eating too many calories) and a lack of exercise (burning too few calories). Other factors that can lead to obesity include glandular malfunctions, diabetes, hypoglycemia, or hyperinsulinemia. Obesity has also been linked to food sensitivities and/or allergies.

It has always been traditional wisdom that heredity is a causal factor for obesity. The discovery of the "obesity gene" in 2001 was a major breakthrough in the study of obesity. However, there are many more genes than just this one tied to obesity, and researchers are looking for these as well. What is certain is that carriers of the gene have a *tendency* toward obesity, assuming that other factors, not all now known, fall into place. Also known is that people of certain ethnic backgrounds are more likely to carry this gene than members of other groups (for the curious, North Africans and central Europeans more often have the gene).

Obesity is a serious health problem. Once thought to be a moral failing, it is now classified as a disease. The National Heart, Lung, and Blood Institute calls it a complex chronic disease involving social, behavioral, cultural, physiological, metabolic, and genetic factors. Obesity has reached epidemic proportions in the United States, Australia, and Europe, and in many developing countries in South America and Asia. For the statistics buffs, in the United States there are 76.5 million overweight people, 72 million obese people, and some 18 million with what is categorized as extreme obesity, defined as being 100 pounds or more over the ideal body weight or having a BMI of 40 or greater. Australia is rapidly catching up, and although Australians take no pride in it, they soon may surpass the United States as number one. Meanwhile, dieters are spending billions of dollars to get slim. Some 15 percent of American men and 26 percent of American women are on a diet on any given day. Americans spend over $100 billion on dieting and diet-related products each year.

Experts have different theories on how and why people become overweight, but they generally agree that the key to losing weight is simple: Eat less and move more. The body has to burn more calories than it takes in. Weight loss involves two distinct phases: active weight loss and weight maintenance. During the active weight loss phase, you

Body Mass Index

The body mass index (BMI) is a figure that represents the percentage of your body weight that is due to fat. It is determined by looking at your weight in combination with your height. The following table will give you a rough idea of your BMI.

Height (inches) BMI	19–24 normal	25–29 overweight	30–39 obese	40–54 extreme obesity
58"	91–115	119–138	143–186	191–258
59"	94–119	124–143	148–193	198–267
60"	97–123	128–148	153–199	204–276
61"	100–127	132–153	158–206	211–285
62"	104–131	136–158	164–213	218–295
63"	107–135	141–163	169–220	225–304
64"	110–140	145–169	174–227	232–314
65"	114–144	150–174	180–234	240–324
66"	118–148	155–179	186–241	247–334
67"	121–153	159–185	191–249	255–344
68"	125–158	164–190	197–256	262–354
69"	128–162	169–196	203–263	270–365
70"	132–167	174–202	209–271	278–376
71"	136–172	179–208	215–279	286–386
72"	140–177	184–213	221–287	294–397
73"	144–182	189–219	227–295	302–408
74"	148–186	194–225	233–303	311–420
75"	152–192	200–232	240–311	319–431
76"	156–197	205–238	246–320	328–443

Source: National Heart, Lung and Blood Institute, National Institutes of Health

should lose 10 percent of your body weight in about twelve to sixteen weeks (three to four months). This can be achieved in a variety of ways. Most diets—low-carbohydrate, low-fat, or other—have the same weight-loss potential as long as you are eating fewer calories. During the weight maintenance phase, which should last for the remaining eight to nine months of the year, the goal is to keep weight stable by exercising and eating only the amount of calories necessary so you don't gain weight. Every year the same two-phase program should be followed. This is how you achieve successful weight loss for the long term. The reason most people fail to lose weight on a diet is that they don't like the program they are on, or they try to lose more weight than they should to begin with and then can't adhere to the program because it is too rigid. Try to choose a diet that appeals to you in terms of the kinds of foods you will be eating; this will make it easier to stay with it.

Unless otherwise specified, the dosages recommended here are for adults. For children between the ages of twelve and seventeen, reduce the dose to three-quarters the recommended amount. For children between six and twelve, use one-half the recommended dose, and for children under the age of six, use one-quarter the recommended amount.

NUTRIENTS

SUPPLEMENT	SUGGESTED DOSAGE	COMMENTS
Very Important		
ABC Aerobic Bulk Cleanse from Aerobic Life Industries	As directed on label. Always take supplemental fiber separately from other supplements and medications.	Especially good for high or low blood sugar problems and also provides fiber. Gives a full feeling, cutting down hunger pangs.
or psyllium husks	1 tbsp ½ hour before meals with a large glass of liquid. Drink it quickly.	

Obesity-Related Health Risks

Obesity is a major health concern in great part because it can dramatically increase your risk of developing other serious disorders. The following table summarizes the effect of obesity on other conditions.

High Risk Associated with Obesity	Moderate Risk Associated with Obesity	Slightly Increased Risk Associated with Obesity
Diabetes mellitus	Arthritis	Accidents
Insulin resistance	Fibromyalgia	Breast cancer
High blood pressure (hypertension)	Heart disease	Colon cancer
High blood fat levels (including cholesterol)	Lower back pain	Congenital defects in offspring
Gallstones	Medical complications with surgery	Depression
Sleep apnea	Peripheral vascular disease	Hormone (especially sex hormone) disorders
Decreased aerobic fitness potential	Polycystic ovary syndrome	Infertility
Kidney cancer	Stroke	Uterine cancer
		Social isolation

Chromium picolinate	200–600 mcg daily.	Reduces sugar cravings by stabilizing the metabolism of simple carbohydrates (sugars).
Dimethylaminoethanol (DMAE)	As directed on label.	Increases vitality.
Essential fatty acids (flaxseed oil, primrose oil, or salmon oil)	As directed on label.	Use these with a low-fat diet to provide essential fatty acids, needed by every cell in the body and for appetite control.
Kelp	1,000–1,500 mg daily.	Contains balanced minerals and iodine. Aids in weight loss.
Lecithin granules or capsules	1 tbsp 3 times daily, before meals. 1,200 mg 3 times daily, before meals.	A fat emulsifier; breaks down fat so it can be removed from the body.
Spirulina or Spiru-tein from Nature's Plus	As directed on label 3 times daily. Take between meals.	Excellent sources of usable protein. Contains needed nutrients and stabilizes blood sugar. Can replace a meal.
Vitamin C with bioflavonoids	3,000–6,000 mg daily.	Necessary for normal glandular function. Speeds up a slow metabolism, prompting it to burn more calories.

Helpful

Calcium	1,500 mg daily.	Involved in activation of lipase, an enzyme that breaks down fats for utilization by the body.
Choline and inositol	As directed on label.	Helps the body burn fat.
Coenzyme Q_{10} plus	As directed on label.	Necessary for energy.

Coenzyme A from Coenzyme-A Technologies	As directed on label.	Improves the effect of coenzyme Q_{10}, metabolizes fat, and may aid in weight loss.
Dehydroepiandros- terone (DHEA)	As directed on label.	Inhibits an enzyme that is involved in fat production.
5-hydroxy L-tryptophan (5-HTP)	As directed on label.	Suppresses appetite. *Caution:* Do not use if you are pregnant or nursing.
Gamma-amino- butyric acid (GABA)	As directed on label.	Suppresses cravings and has antidepressant qualities. (*See* AMINO ACIDS in Part One.)
L-arginine and L-ornithine plus L-lysine	500 mg each or as directed on label, before bedtime. Take on an empty stomach with water or juice. Do not take with milk. Take with 50 mg vitamin B_6 and 100 mg vitamin C for better absorption.	These amino acids decrease body fat. (*See* AMINO ACIDS in Part One.) *Caution:* Do not take these supplements if you have diabetes. Do not take arginine or ornithine without lysine.
L-carnitine	500 mg daily.	Has the ability to break up fat deposits and aids in weight loss by giving you more energy.
L-glutamine	As directed on label.	Lessens carbohydrate cravings.
L-methionine	As directed on label.	Assists in the breakdown of fat.
L-phenylalanine	As directed on label, on an empty stomach.	An appetite suppressant that tells the brain you are not hungry. (*See* AMINO ACIDS in Part One.) *Caution:* Do not take this supplement if you are pregnant or nursing, or suffer from panic attacks, diabetes, high blood pressure, or PKU.

L-tyrosine	As directed on label. Take at bedtime.	Suppresses cravings and has antidepressant qualities. (*See* AMINO ACIDS in Part One.) *Caution:* Do not take tyrosine if you are taking an MAO inhibitor drug.
Maitake extract	As directed on label.	Aids in weight loss.
Multivitamin and mineral complex with potassium	As directed on label. 99 mg daily.	Obesity and nutritional deficiency are parts of the same syndrome. Important in the production of energy. Sodium and potassium levels must be balanced.
Pyruvate	As directed on label.	Promotes weight loss and may aid in reducing body fat.
Taurine	As directed on label.	Taurine is a building block for all other amino acids; aids in the digestion of fats.
Vitamin B complex	50 mg of each major B vitamin 3 times daily (amounts of individual vitamins in a complex will vary.)	Needed for proper digestion.
plus extra vitamin B$_2$ (riboflavin) and	50 mg 3 times daily.	Required for efficiency in burning calories.
vitamin B$_3$ (niacin)	50 mg 3 times daily. Do not exceed this amount.	Lessens sugar cravings. *Caution:* Do not take niacin if you have a liver disorder, gout, or high blood pressure.
and vitamin B$_6$ (pyridoxine) and	50 mg 3 times daily.	Boosts metabolism.
vitamin B$_{12}$	1,000 mcg 3 times daily.	Needed for proper digestion and absorption. A sublingual form is best.
and para-aminobenzoic acid (PABA)	As directed on label.	Aids in carbohydrate and protein utilization.
Zinc	80 mg daily. Do not exceed a total of 100 mg daily from all supplements.	Enhances the effectiveness of insulin and boosts immune function. Use zinc gluconate lozenges or OptiZinc for best absorption.
plus copper	3 mg daily.	Needed to balance with zinc.

Herbs

❑ Alfalfa, corn silk, dandelion, gravel root, hydrangea, hyssop, juniper berries, oat straw, parsley, seawrack, thyme, uva ursi, white ash, and yarrow can be used in tea form for their diuretic properties.

❑ Aloe vera juice improves digestion and cleanses the digestive tract.

❑ Amla is an Ayurvedic herb that helps to increase lean body mass and reduce fat.

❑ Astragalus increases energy and improves nutrient absorption.

Caution: Do not use astragalus in the presence of a fever.

❑ Borage seed, hawthorn berry, licorice root, and sarsaparilla stimulate the adrenal glands and improve thyroid function.

Caution: Licorice root should not be used during pregnancy or nursing. It should not be used by persons with diabetes, glaucoma, heart disease, high blood pressure, or a history of stroke.

❑ Butcher's broom, cardamom, cayenne, cinnamon, *Garcinia cambogia,* ginger, green tea (which has gained a great deal of attention for its ability to aid in weight loss), and mustard seed are thermogenic herbs that improve digestion and aid in the metabolism of fat.

Caution: Do not use cinnamon in large quantities during pregnancy. Green tea contains vitamin K, which can make anticoagulant medications less effective. Consult your health care professional if you are using them. The caffeine in green tea could cause insomnia, anxiety, upset stomach, nausea, or diarrhea.

❑ Chlorella, gudmar, schizandra, and suma aid in glucose utilization, hormone production, neural regulation, and digestion.

❑ Fennel removes mucus and fat from the intestinal tract and is a natural appetite suppressant.

❑ Fenugreek is useful for dissolving fat within the liver.

❑ Gotu kola aids in reducing body mass and aids in adrenal processes that facilitate carbohydrate metabolism. It also increases energy.

❑ Guarana and kola nut are appetite suppressants.

Caution: These contain caffeine; those who are sensitive to caffeine should avoid them.

❑ Guggul, an ancient Ayurvedic herbal remedy, helps to normalize blood cholesterol and triglyceride levels. It also has a mildly stimulating effect on the thyroid.

❑ Siberian ginseng aids in moving fluids and nutrients throughout the body and reduces the stress of adjusting to new eating habits.

Caution: Do not use this herb if you have hypoglycemia, high blood pressure, or a heart disorder.

❑ Trifala is an Ayurvedic herbal remedy that rejuvenates glandular balance and stimulates thyroid hormones with long-term use.

❑ Turmeric strengthens digestion, increases energy, and cleanses the blood.

Recommendations

❑ Consuming fewer calories than you burn in a day is the only way to lose weight. But consuming the right types of foods is important as well. Rotate your foods, and be sure to eat a variety of foods, especially an assortment of fruits and vegetables. Eat meals that consist of a balance of proteins, complex carbohydrates, and some fat. Proteins can increase your metabolic rate slightly and help to balance the release of insulin by prompting secretion of the pancreatic hormone glucagon. Protein-induced glucagon mobilizes fats from the tissues in which it is stored, thus aiding in weight loss. By eating balanced meals you get steadier blood sugar levels and the ability to burn stored body fat for long-term weight loss. Make sure that you have some protein at each meal and snack to keep you feeling full until the next meal.

❑ Eat more complex carbohydrates that also offer protein, such as tofu, lentils and other legumes, plain baked potatoes (no toppings, except for vegetables), and sesame seeds. Other foods that are good to include in your diet are brown rice, whole grains, skinless turkey or chicken breast, and seafood. Poultry and fish should be broiled or baked, never fried. Fish is particularly important for overweight people who have high blood pressure. In one study, those who ate fish once a day lost more weight and had lower blood pressure compared to those who did not eat fish.

❑ Eat fresh fruits and an abundance of raw vegetables. Use low-calorie vegetables such as broccoli, cabbage, carrots, cauliflower, celery, cucumbers, green beans, kale, lettuce, onions, radishes, spinach, and turnips. Low-calorie, low-carbohydrate fruits include apples, cantaloupe, grapefruit, strawberries, and watermelon. The following are higher in calories and should be consumed in moderation: bananas, cherries, corn, figs, grapes, green peas, hominy, pears, pineapple, sweet potatoes, white rice, and yams.

❑ In one study, a low-carbohydrate diet that was also high in vegetable proteins from soy, nuts, fruits, vegetables, cereals, and vegetable oils was shown to promote weight loss as well as lower total cholesterol and bad-cholesterol levels compared to the typical high-carbohydrate, heart-healthy diet, which is based on low-fat and whole-grain products. The low-carbohydrate plant-based diet produced similar weight loss to an Atkins-like diet, which is also low in carbohydrates but high in animal protein and fats.

❑ Eat foods raw, if possible. If foods are heated, they should be baked, broiled, steamed, or boiled. Never consume fried or greasy foods.

❑ Eat a healthful assortment of foods that includes vegetables, fruits, grains (especially whole grains), fish, beans, seeds, nuts, and soy products. Soy is a good source of protein if you are looking to lose weight, and it may have additional benefits beyond other protein sources. Soy may specifically promote the loss of body fat, reduce the risk of heart disease, and minimize bone loss.

❑ If you drink alcoholic beverages, do so in moderation only. Alcohol provides lots of calories, but few nutrients. Wine and beer or a spirit with soda water are better choices than a Mai Tai, for example, which is made with juice and other ingredients that add additional calories.

❑ Limit your intake of foods and beverages that contain added sugar. So-called fat-free and low-fat foods are not calorie-free. To add taste, food manufacturers often add sugars. You should always check the Nutrition Facts label on products before purchasing them. (*See* page 5 in Part One for how to interpret the Nutrition Facts label.)

❑ Try a Mediterranean diet—high in fish, whole grains, fruit, nuts, vegetables, and olive oil; low in meat, dairy products, and polyunsaturated fat.

❑ Drink ten 8-ounce glasses of liquids daily. Herbal teas and steam-distilled water with trace minerals (such as ConcenTrace from Trace Minerals Research) added are good. Taken before meals, they help to reduce your appetite. They are nonfattening fillers that also help to dilute toxins and flush them out of the body. Herbal teas mixed with unsweetened fruit juice are very satisfying low-calorie drinks and are also very filling. Use these between meals and when a desire for sweets hits you. Drink sparkling water mixed with fruit juice in place of sodas.

❑ Pay particular attention to the fat in your diet. Some fat is necessary, but it must be the right kind. Avocados, olives, olive oil, raw nuts and seeds, and wheat and corn germ are sources of "good" fats that contain essential fatty acids. Use these foods in moderation—no more than twice a week. Eliminate saturated fats from the diet completely. Avoid animal fat, found in butter, cream, gravies, ice cream, mayonnaise, meat, rich dressings, and whole milk. Do not eat any fried foods.

❑ Focus on eating low-glycemic-load foods. These include any meat, fish, or poultry, fats (in reasonable amounts), low-fat dairy products, and fruits and non-starchy vegetables. Anything with a grain or rice in it can increase blood sugar levels and insulin levels. Insulin is the storage hormone, so what you eat quickly turns to fat. People who adopt a low-glycemic-load diet weigh less, have less heart disease and diabetes, and have lesser incidences of fatty liver compared to those who eat a typical American diet, which tends to be high-glycemic load. It is easy to follow a low-glycemic-load diet. You can still have some bread, as long as you choose whole-grain bread and only eat one piece at a time. A baked potato is fine, but don't have it at the same meal with another starchy vegetable such as corn.

❑ If you must eat snacks occasionally to ward off hunger, make sure they are healthy. Good choices include:

• Celery and carrot sticks; in fact, any nonstarchy vegetable is fine.

• Low-fat cottage cheese topped with fresh applesauce and walnuts.

• Unsweetened gelatin made with fruit juice in place of sugar and water.

• Freshly made unsalted popcorn.

• Rice cakes topped with nut butter (but not peanut butter).

• Watermelon, fresh fruit, or frozen fruit popsicles.

• Unsweetened low-fat yogurt topped with granola or nuts and fresh fruit.

❑ Do not eat any white flour products, salt, white rice, or processed foods. Also, avoid fast food restaurants and all junk foods.

❑ Do not consume sweets such as soda, pastries, pies, cakes, doughnuts, or candy. These are high-glycemic-load foods. Omit all forms of refined sugar (including white sugar, brown sugar, and corn sweetener) from the diet. Sugar triggers the release of insulin, which then activates enzymes that promote the passage of fat from the bloodstream into the fat cells.

❑ Follow a fasting program once monthly. (*See* FASTING in Part Three.)

❑ Spirulina aids in fighting obesity. Take it thirty minutes before meals to decrease your appetite. Spirulina also sustains energy, aids in detoxification, and aids in maintaining proper bowel function.

❑ Avoid eating before bedtime and during the night. Supplementation with melatonin may help with this. "Night eaters" often have low melatonin levels.

❑ Use wheatgrass to calm the appetite. This is a very nutritious fuel from whole food that assists metabolic functions. Kelp is also beneficial.

❑ Use powdered barley malt sweetener (found in health food stores) instead of sugar. This is highly concentrated but not dangerous. It contains only 3 calories per gram (approximately 2 teaspoons). This sweetener is also beneficial for people with diabetes or hypoglycemia.

❑ Increase your intake of fiber. Dietary fiber intake prevents obesity by filling up your stomach and thus making you less hungry, decreasing the absorption of excess nutrients, and changing your body's hormones so that you feel full naturally. The best way to get fiber is from fruits, vegetables, and whole grains. In addition, a fiber supplement is useful. Women need 25 grams and men 38 grams of fiber a day.

❑ Guar gum and psyllium husks are good sources of supplemental fiber. Take fiber with a large glass of liquid one-half hour before meals.

Note: Always take supplemental fiber separately from other supplements and medications.

❑ Move your bowels daily. A clean colon is important in stabilizing your weight. (*See* COLON CLEANSING in Part Three.)

❑ Keep a diet diary to help you keep track of what you eat, the caloric and fat content of what you eat, and what triggers your eating. This can help you to pinpoint and eliminate trigger factors (such as allergies or depression), as well as let you see if you are eating too much of the wrong types of foods. (*See under* ALLERGIES in Part Two.)

❑ Be active. Take a brisk walk every day before breakfast or dinner to burn off fat. Make a habit of using the stairs instead of the elevator. Walk or ride a bicycle instead of driving whenever possible. Exercise increases the metabolic rate as well as burning off calories.

❑ Be sure to get regular aerobic exercise, such as walking, running, bicycling, or swimming, *and* do exercises for strength and flexibility, such as yoga or stretching exercises. Exercise is better than an overly strict diet for maintaining your health and controlling your weight. It is the best way to rid the body of fat and to maintain good muscle tone. Be sure to drink water during exercise to prevent dehydration and muscle cramps.

Caution: If you are over thirty-five and/or have been sedentary for some time, consult your health care provider before beginning an exercise program.

❑ If you have been sedentary for some time, try exercising in water. Water aerobics is excellent for those who are overweight or who find running or walking difficult. It is also good for arthritis sufferers. Water aerobics tones the body and strengthens the heart without straining the joints. Start by taking a class at a local fitness center or YMCA.

❑ Change your eating habits. This is extremely important not only for losing weight, but for maintaining weight loss. Begin with the following:

• Always eat breakfast. It jump-starts the metabolism at the beginning of the day. Eat small but nutrient-dense meals every three to four hours throughout the day to keep your metabolism stable, to maintain a full feeling, and to avoid wide swings in blood sugar. Good choices might include a 2-ounce portion of protein food (beans, an egg, poultry) with ½ cup fresh salad dressed with apple cider vinegar; or ½ cup of a steamed vegetable with some type of grain (½ cup brown rice or a piece of whole- or multigrain bread). If you can't limit yourself to small meals or are not hungry, go back to the traditional three-meal-a-day plan.

• Don't skip meals. This only intensifies hunger and food cravings.

• Make your main meal lunch, not dinner. Some people have had excellent results consuming no food after 3:00 P.M.

• At meals, put less food on your plate. Chew slowly. Stop eating as soon as you are no longer hungry—don't wait until you feel full. If you eat at a restaurant, stop eating when you are full. Take the leftovers home or leave them.

❑ If you get the urge to eat, put on a tight belt. This will make you uncomfortable and remind you that you want to lose that excess fat.

❑ Learn to ride out your food cravings. They peak and subside like ocean waves. When you get an urge to eat, tell yourself that you can satisfy the craving if you *really* want to. Then wait ten minutes. This ensures that your eating is conscious, not compulsive. Keep in mind that most cravings last only a few minutes. Try doing something to distract yourself. Also remember that food addiction is the same as any other addiction: That first bite only makes you want more. If you ultimately decide that you really do want that food, then decide how much is reasonable and enjoy it. *Really* enjoy it. Take one bite and savor the taste. Eat slowly.

❑ Find out what causes your cravings. A craving for salt, chocolate, or sugar may actually be an indication of an underlying condition such as a mineral deficiency, food allergy, hypoglycemia, or hypothyroidism. If you get a strong urge to snack while you're watching television, try reading a book, drinking a large glass of liquid, or taking a walk instead. If your cravings are triggered by where you are, move. If you're in the kitchen, go outside to relax, take a walk, or do yard work. If you're in the mall, avoid the food court.

❑ If you are always tired in midmorning or midday, are always craving carbohydrates, and are always hungry, you may be consuming too many simple carbohydrates. Simple carbohydrates include refined sugars and sweet fruits; complex carbohydrates, which include whole grains, peas, and beans, provide more long-term energy. (*See* Carbohydrates *under* NUTRITION, DIET, AND WELLNESS in Part One.) Protein is another long-term source of energy. Think of interesting protein choices you can have for breakfast. It doesn't always have to be bacon and eggs. In some countries people eat thin slices of cheese and meat and small amounts of fish for breakfast. A little protein goes a long way to sustain you until lunch. Be sure to have a piece of fruit and one high-glycemic-index food like a slice of bread or half of a bagel as well.

❑ Frequent bloating and water retention may be a result of excess insulin production, which makes it almost impossible to burn fat. Try lowering your carbohydrate intake and increasing your consumption of protein and fat. Excess sodium intake can also cause water retention.

❑ Consider being tested for food allergies. Many people who have eliminated allergenic foods from their diets have stabilized their weight quickly.

❑ Do not grocery shop on an empty stomach. You will be tempted to buy forbidden foods and will often buy more food than you need or can use before it loses its freshness.

❑ Read labels. A bottle of juice or a salty snack package may look like one serving, but often is more—sometimes two or three times more. You also may have noticed the new 100-calorie snack packages. While these may be convenient, when you see how small the portions are, you may be tempted to have more than one. But the calories add up quickly, so avoid them if you can't limit yourself to one.

❑ Avoid crash dieting. A very low-calorie diet causes the metabolism to slow down, resulting in fewer calories being burned. Instead, increase your activity level. This will raise your metabolic rate, burn fat, and help prevent the loss of lean tissue.

❑ To maintain weight loss, calculate how many calories you need daily by multiplying your weight by 10. Then add 30 percent (about one-third) of that amount to the result. Assuming a moderate activity level, consuming anything less than that number of calories should allow you to lose weight. This is the number of calories you can consume daily without gaining the weight back. Most diet plans allow for a 500-calorie reduction per day, which would produce one pound per week of weight loss. This is a healthy approach to losing weight. Remember, you didn't gain it all in one week; it likely took years. It should come off at the same pace to avoid rebounding to your starting weight.

❑ Losing weight sensibly and safely requires setting reasonable weight-loss goals, changing eating habits, and getting adequate exercise. Women and inactive men *generally* need to consume approximately 1,700 to 2,000 calories to maintain weight; men and very active women may consume up to 2,000 to 2,500 calories per day.

Considerations

❑ Dieting may conjure up visions of eating little but fruits and vegetables, but you can enjoy all foods as part of a healthy diet so long as you don't overdo it on fat (especially saturated fat and meat), sugars, salt, and alcohol. Portion sizes must be limited. Some foods high in calories—such as cookies, cakes, french fries, whole milk, whole milk cheese, cream, butter, ice cream, fatty fresh and processed meats, poultry skin and fat, lard, palm oil, coconut oil, miscellaneous fats, oils, and spreads—must be eliminated.

❑ The best way to lose weight—and virtually the only way to maintain weight loss—is to adopt a healthier, more active lifestyle. A lifestyle that includes a natural, healthy diet and regular exercise will keep you healthy; give you more energy; lower your risk of heart disease, stroke, and cancer; and still allow you to lose weight. Those who choose fad diets over such a lifestyle can count on gaining back their lost weight and more. Almost 95 percent of all dieters regain their lost weight within a year and have to diet all over again.

❑ If you do one form of exercise, walking seems to be the best. In one study, those who walked just 15 minutes a day (not counting regular walking for normal activities) gained less weight compared to a group of non-walkers. Walking is easy, convenient, and only requires a good pair of shoes. It can be done outdoors, or if the climate is too cold, shopping malls offer the perfect venue. Increasing your time will afford greater benefits.

❑ Dieting may be dangerous for people older than sixty, as malnutrition may result. Exercise if you want to lose weight, but don't stop eating essential foods that you need, such as proteins, fruits, and vegetables. The best thing to do is eat nutrient-dense foods; that is, those that have a lot of nutrition in every bite. You can't eat junk foods and expect to lose weight.

❑ Fad diets may produce some results, but the fact is that not only can these diets be unhealthy (particularly if you jump from one diet to the next), but once you go off the diet, the weight often returns—along with some added pounds. Much of the rapid weight loss you see with some of the diets and/or products available can be attributed to loss of water weight. However, using a reasonable fad diet for twelve weeks won't do any harm and, if it helps you to lose weight, it may be a good incentive for further weight loss. Regardless of which diet you choose, allow yourself to lose no more than one to two pounds a week.

❑ To ensure good health, any type of diet you follow should be closely monitored by a health care professional and/or a nutritionist.

❑ Repeated crash dieting is not healthy and can increase the risk of heart disease. Quick weight loss tends to come back rapidly. This rapid weight gain often results in elevated cholesterol levels and can also damage vital organs. In one study, a third of people who had gone on crash diets of 500 calories or less per day were found to have developed gallstones. The fourteen-year Framingham Heart Study showed that those whose weight changed a lot or changed often had higher death rates than other people. They also ran a greater risk of coronary heart disease. The study showed that weight fluctuation seemed to pose as great a risk of heart disease and premature death as being overweight.

❑ A weight cycler is someone who has lost ten pounds more than three times and gained it back. Although there appears to be no increased risk of heart disease or death from weight cycling, data from weight cyclers showed that it is fairly easy to lose weight but hard to keep it off. If you do lose weight, try to keep it off for one year. This will be harder than losing it in the first place. It requires a commitment to lifestyle change such as increasing the amount of exercise you do in addition to dietary modifications.

❑ Thermogenesis is a term used to describe the body's natural process for burning calories. Scientists studying thermogenesis are focusing on understanding and improving the thermogenic process, which may aid in weight loss. Many new weight-loss products focus on thermogenesis.

❑ A study conducted by the U.S. Department of Agriculture showed that one of every four teenagers carries enough excess weight to put him or her at high risk of heart attack, stroke, colon cancer, gout, and other health problems later in life—regardless of whether the individual slims down as an adult. The prevalence of obesity among children aged six to eleven years more than doubled in the past twenty years, going from 6.5 percent to 17 percent. The rate among adolescents aged twelve to nineteen years more than tripled, increasing from 5 percent to 17.6 percent. In a group of children aged five to seventeen years, 70 percent had at least one heart disease risk factor, such as high cholesterol levels.

❑ The thinking once was that people who regularly use artificial sweeteners tend to gain, not lose, weight. However, newer data suggests otherwise. If you are overweight, it may be better to choose the low-calorie food or beverage that contains artificial sweeteners than to choose the higher caloric options. If you would rather use a low-calorie sweetener from a natural source, try stevia, which is derived from a plant.

❑ A person whose body has a high ratio of muscle to fat will have a higher metabolic rate than a person of the same weight with a lower muscle-to-fat ratio, and therefore will require more calories. This is because it takes more calories to maintain muscle tissue than fat tissue. Conversely, obese persons tend to have lower than normal metabolic rates.

❑ Calories derived from fat are more easily converted into body fat than calories from other sources. Only 3 percent of fat calories are burned in the digestive process. By contrast, 25 percent of calories from complex carbohydrates (fruits, vegetables, whole grains) are burned in the course of digestion.

❑ An omega-6 fatty acid known as gamma-linolenic acid (GLA) has been shown to stimulate the body's metabolic ability to burn fat. GLA, an active ingredient found in black currant seed oil, flaxseed, and evening primrose oil, helps to control the metabolism of fats. In particular, it mobilizes the metabolically active fat called brown adipose tissue (BAT).

❑ Many people feel the need to eat something sweet after meals, but this is an acquired habit and it *can* be broken. In many cultures, sweetened foods are reserved only for rare special occasions (and even then are less sweet tasting than many of the foods Americans eat every day).

❑ Eating a low-fat diet that is high in complex carbohydrates does *not* mean eating tasteless, bland foods. There are many delicious and healthy foods available that can be eaten. The goal is to reduce the total fat, saturated fat, and cholesterol in the diet and to increase the amount of complex carbohydrates. Potatoes, pasta, bread, corn, rice, and other complex-carbohydrate-rich foods are not the cause of obesity, as some people think. They are the cure. The exception to this rule involves people who are addicted to carbohydrates. (See Are You a Carbohydrate Addict? on page 617.)

❑ A study sponsored by the U.S. Department of Agriculture revealed that the trace mineral boron may speed the burning of calories. Raisins and onions are good food sources of boron.

❑ In human studies, the hormone dehydroepiandrosterone (DHEA) has led to a loss of body fat by blocking an enzyme that is known to produce fat tissue. (See DHEA THERAPY in Part Three.)

❑ Researchers have found that weight reduction can be improved with the use of a combination of the amino acids L-ornithine and L-arginine, enhanced by L-lysine (see the Nutrients table in this section for recommended dosages). L-ornithine helps to release growth hormone, normally lacking in adults, which burns fat and builds muscle. This combination works best while the body is at rest.

Note: Never take an amino acid that contains L-arginine but not L-lysine. Too much L-arginine without L-lysine can

Are You a Carbohydrate Addict?

Carbohydrate addicts respond to carbohydrates in a way that can be compared to the way alcoholics respond to alcohol. When they consume carbohydrates, it results in a release of insulin that is even greater than is needed, which in turn leads to even less of a feeling of satisfaction, so the urge to eat sets in again. Because of this, carbohydrate addicts end up trying to satisfy their hunger by eating more and more carbohydrates.

People who are addicted to carbohydrates should limit their intake of foods high in complex carbohydrates (or high-glycemic-load foods) to one serving per meal and avoid *all* simple carbohydrates (very high-glycemic-load foods). The carbohydrates from fruits and vegetables don't count, as they have virtually no effect on insulin production. Chromium picolinate has been shown to reduce carbohydrate cravings. In addition, be sure to include a protein at each meal. Keeping a daily record of what you eat and when, and how you feel afterward, is a simple way to reveal possible carbohydrate addiction.

cause an imbalance of amino acids, possibly causing an outbreak of cold sores or previously dormant herpes.

❑ Gastric bypass surgery may be recommended for extreme obesity. You are a candidate for this surgery if you are twice your ideal body weight. Your doctor may recommend this surgery even if you don't meet the weight criteria but you have one or more comorbidities that may improve by losing weight, such as diabetes or heart disease. The surgery is done by restricting the amount of food consumed by creating a small pouch using part of the stomach. This small pouch is then hooked up to the lower part of the intestine. This reduces the amount of food absorbed into the body. Obviously, this is a drastic measure. However, the complication rate for gastric bypass surgery is small. Death rates were 0.1 percent to 2.0 percent and complications (such as an inability to digest food) after surgery were 13 percent. Other devices, such as a gastric-band (LAP-BAND), which makes you feel sated, are available, and pose less surgical risk, but still pose some risk. Given the many health risks that come with remaining obese, some people decide it makes sense to have a surgical procedure. This, of course, is something to discuss with a skilled health care professional. If you do decide on surgery, be sure to choose a surgeon who has performed many of these procedures and that the hospital has an experienced support team of nurses and dietitians to help you recover and go back to eating sensibly.

❑ The U.S. Food and Drug Administration has approved the use of a synthetic fat called olestra in certain foods. A synthetic compound of fatty acids and sugar, olestra is neither absorbed nor digested by the body and therefore contributes no calories. For the same reason, however, it can cause indigestion, gas, and diarrhea, and possible anal leakage or loose stools. Scientists have also raised concerns because it may inhibit the absorption of necessary fat-soluble vitamins. A warning label had been added to olestra-containing foods that stated "Olestra inhibits the absorption of some vitamins and other nutrients. Vitamins A, D, E and K have been added." If you are trying to adjust your intake of vitamins in accordance with a therapeutic plan,

you should probably steer well clear of olestra-containing foods. The FDA dropped its requirement for the label in August 2003. The product, however, has not changed. All of the products that contain olestra seem to be snack-type foods, in any case—foods that should be avoided on any sensible diet plan. However, if you are overweight, it may still be better to use these products than to eat the full-fat version of other foods.

❑ There are many drugs, such as sibutramine (Meridia) and orlistat (Xenical), on the market today that doctors may prescribe to fight obesity. All of these drugs have potential side effects. If you are considering prescription weight-loss medication, do as much research as possible on the drugs available, and discuss with your doctor how these medications could affect your health. Scientists also are studying hormones and other compounds in the blood that regulate food intake, such as ghrelin, leptin, and adiponectin, in hopes of coming up with a new generation of drugs to treat obesity. In addition to new drugs, scientists are exploring different diets and how they can be used to change hormone levels and promote weight loss. For example, a high-protein diet (30 percent protein) increases energy expenditure (how many calories the body burns during sleep and wake), satiety, fat burning, and ghrelin levels.

❑ There are many nutritional products available today that may aid in weight reduction, including the following:

- CelluRid from BioTech Corporation is an herbal product intended to reduce the appearance of cellulite. Ingredients include kelp, uva ursi, juniper berries, lecithin, milk thistle, and cayenne.

- Cravex from Natrol contains the herb *Gymnema sylvestre,* chromium picolinate, L-glutamine, and other nutrients intended to reduce food cravings, especially cravings for sweets.

- Ripped Fuel from Twinlab contains a blend of bitter orange and St. John's wort and has been shown to reduce body weight when used with a sensible diet.

Caution: St. John's wort may cause increased sensitivity to sunlight. It may also produce anxiety, gastrointestinal symptoms, and headaches. It can interact with some drugs including antidepressants, birth control pills, and anti-coagulants.

- Ripped Fuel Extreme from Twinlab contains a blend of *Acacia catechu* and *Scutellaria baicalensis* with green tea extract. It has been shown to reduce body weight.

Caution: Green tea contains vitamin K, which can make anticoagulant medications less effective. Consult your health care professional if you are using them. The caffeine in green tea could cause insomnia, anxiety, upset stomach, nausea, or diarrhea.

- Everslender from Twinlab contains conjugated linoleic acid, shown to reduce body fat.

- Carb Intercept from Natrol has white bean extract, shown to promote weight loss. It is thought to work by blocking the absorption of carbohydrates.

- Chromium picolinate such as the one from Nature's Way has been shown to reduce body fat.

OILY SKIN

Oily skin occurs when the sebaceous (oil-secreting) glands produce more oil than is needed for proper lubrication of the skin. This excess oil can clog pores and cause blemishes. Oily skin is probably largely a matter of heredity, but it is known to be affected by factors such as diet, hormone levels, pregnancy, birth control pills, and the cosmetics you use. Humidity and hot weather both stimulate the sebaceous glands to produce more oil. Because skin tends to become dryer with age, and because of the hormonal shifts of adolescence, oily skin is common in teenagers, but it can occur at any age. Many people have skin that is oily only in certain areas and dry or normal in others, a condition known as combination skin. In general, the forehead, nose, chin, and upper back tend to be oilier than other areas.

Oily skin has its positive aspects. It is slow to develop age spots and discoloration, fine lines, and wrinkles. It often doesn't freckle or turn red in the sun—on the contrary, it tans evenly and beautifully. On the negative side, oily skin is prone to "breakouts" well past adolescence and has a chronically shiny appearance, an oily or greasy feeling, and enlarged pores.

Unless otherwise specified, the dosages recommended here are for adults. For children between the ages of twelve and seventeen, reduce the dose to three-quarters of the recommended amount.

NUTRIENTS

SUPPLEMENT	SUGGESTED DOSAGE	COMMENTS
Very Important		
Flaxseed oil capsules or	1,000 mg daily.	Supplies needed essential fatty acids. A good healer for most skin disorders.
liquid or	1 tsp daily.	
primrose oil	Up to 500 mg daily.	Contains linoleic acid, which is needed by the skin.
Vitamin A with mixed carotenoids	25,000 IU daily for 3 months, then reduce to 15,000 IU daily. If you are pregnant, do not exceed 10,000 IU daily.	Necessary for healing and construction of new skin tissue.
Vitamin B complex plus extra vitamin B$_{12}$	As directed on label. 1,000–2,000 mcg daily.	B vitamins are important for healthy skin tone.
Important		
Kelp	1,000–1,500 mg daily.	Supplies balanced minerals needed for good skin tone.
Vitamin E	200 IU daily or 400 IU every other day.	Protects against free radicals. Use d-alpha-tocopherol form.
Zinc plus copper	50 mg daily. Do not exceed a total of 100 mg daily from all supplements. 3 mg daily.	For tissue repair. Enhances immune response. Use zinc gluconate lozenges or OptiZinc for best absorption. Needed to balance with zinc.
Helpful		
Grape seed extract	As directed on label.	A powerful antioxidant that protects skin cells.
Herpanacine from Diamond-Herpanacine Associates	As directed on label.	Contains antioxidants, amino acids, and herbs that promote overall skin health.
L-cysteine	500 mg daily, on an empty stomach. Take with water or juice. Do not take with milk. Take with 50 mg vitamin B$_6$ and 100 mg vitamin C for better absorption.	Contains sulfur, needed for healthy skin. (*See* AMINO ACIDS in Part One.)
Lecithin granules or capsules	1 tbsp 3 times daily, before meals. 1,200 mg 3 times daily, before meals.	Needed for better absorption of the essential fatty acids.
Superoxide dismutase (SOD)	As directed on label.	A free radical destroyer.
Tretinoin (Retin-A)	As prescribed by physician.	Acts as a gradual chemical peel; unclogs pores and speeds up sloughing off of top layers of skin, exposing new, fresh skin. Available by prescription only.

Herbs

❏ Aloe vera has excellent healing properties. Apply aloe vera gel topically, as directed on product label or as needed.

❏ Burdock root, chamomile, oat straw, and thyme nourish the skin.

Caution: Do not use chamomile if you are allergic to ragweed. Do not use during pregnancy or nursing. It may interact with warfarin or cyclosporine, so patients using these drugs should avoid it.

❑ Lavender is very good for oily skin. Mist your skin with lavender water several times daily.

❑ A facial sauna using lemongrass, licorice root, and rosebuds is good for oily skin. Two or three times a week, simmer a total of 2 to 4 tablespoons of dried or fresh herbs in 2 quarts of water. When the pot is steaming, place it on top of a trivet or thick potholder on a table, and sit with your face at a comfortable distance over the steam for fifteen minutes. You can use a towel to trap the steam if you wish. After fifteen minutes, splash your face with cold water and allow your skin to air-dry or pat it dry with a towel. After the sauna, you can allow the herbal water to cool and save it for use as a toning lotion to be dabbed on your face with a cotton ball after cleansing.

Caution: Licorice root should not be used during pregnancy or nursing. It should not be used by persons with diabetes, glaucoma, heart disease, high blood pressure, or a history of stroke.

❑ Witch hazel applied to the skin is excellent for absorbing oil.

Recommendations

❑ Drink plenty of quality water to keep the skin hydrated and flush out toxins.

❑ Reduce the amount of fat in your diet. Consume no fried foods, animal fats, or heat-processed vegetable oils such as those sold in supermarkets. Do not cook with oil, and do not eat any oils that have been subjected to heat, whether in processing or cooking. If a little oil is necessary, such as in salad dressing, use cold-pressed canola or olive oil only.

❑ Do not drink soft drinks or alcoholic beverages. Avoid sugar, chocolate, and junk food.

❑ Keep your skin very clean. Wash your face two or three times in the course of a day—but no more, because too much washing will stimulate your skin to produce more oil. Use your hands instead of harsh scrubs or washcloths. Sterile gauze pads are also good for cleaning the skin. (Do not use a pad more than once.) Do not use harsh soaps or cleansers. Use a pure soap with no artificial additives, such as E-Gem Skin-Care Soap from Carlson Laboratories. Do not use cleansers or lotions that contain alcohol. After cleansing, apply a natural *oil-free* moisturizer to keep the skin supple.

❑ Use hot water when washing your face. Hot water dissolves skin oil better than lukewarm or cold water.

❑ Try using a clay or mud mask. White or rose-colored clays are best for sensitive skin.

❑ Choose cosmetic and facial care products specifically designed for oily skin.

❑ Alpha-hydroxy acids are a group of naturally occurring acids (found mostly in fruits) that help to stimulate cell renewal, aid the skin in retaining water, and give it a smoother, less oily appearance. Oily skin can benefit from the use of products containing alpha-hydroxy acids because they aid in removal of the top layer of dead skin cells, which stimulates healthy skin growth and may diminish large pores. Glycolic acid is probably the best of the alpha-hydroxy acids for this purpose. If you decide to try an alpha-hydroxy acid product, begin with a product containing 5 percent alpha-hydroxy acid (not more), and apply it at night only. First wash your face, then wait five minutes before applying a small amount of the product. After two or three weeks of nighttime application, you can begin applying the product in the morning as well. As your skin becomes accustomed to the effects of alpha-hydroxy acids, you may wish to work your way up to higher-concentration products.

❑ Products containing benzoyl peroxide are effective for oily skin. Start with a mild-strength formula to minimize possible irritation.

❑ Choose an astringent that contains acetone, which is known for dissolving oil.

❑ Two or three times a week, use a loofah sponge and warm water for the face to boost circulation, remove dead skin cells, and remove many of the impurities found in oily skin. Avoid using the loofah around your eyes, and do not use it on areas with open sores.

❑ To clear away excess oil, use a clay or mud mask. Blend together well 1 teaspoon green clay powder (available in health food stores) and 1 teaspoon raw honey. Apply the mixture to your face, avoiding the eye area. Leave it on for fifteen minutes, then rinse well with lukewarm water. Do this at least three times a week—or more often if necessary. White or rose-colored clays are best for sensitive skin.

❑ Once or twice daily, mix equal parts of lemon juice and water. Pat the mixture on your face and allow it to dry, then rinse with warm water. Follow with a cool-water rinse.

❑ Look for facial powder that contains talcum powder. It is oil-free and blots the oil on your skin.

❑ For combination skin, simply treat the oily areas as oily skin and the dry areas as dry skin. (*See* DRY SKIN in Part Two.)

❑ Do not smoke. Smoking promotes enlargement of the pores and impairs the overall health of the skin.

Considerations

❑ Caring for oily skin does *not* mean trying to dry the skin out. Despite having excess oil, skin may still lack moisture. Moisture is a term that is used to refer to the amount of water inside the skin cells, not the amount of oil on the surface of the skin. While oil and moisture levels are related (the oil helps prevent loss of moisture through evaporation), the two are not the same. There are products available that help to supply and protect moisture without adding oil. Vitamin E 12,000 IU Deep Moisturizing Crème from Derma-E Skin Care is a good nongreasy moisturizer.

❑ Many companies that specialize in skin care have developed foil-wrapped packets of wipes saturated in alcohol for skin care away from home. These can be placed in your briefcase or purse for cutting through the oil and freshening up the skin.

❑ Although it is a common myth, oily skin doesn't actually cause acne. Although there is an association between the severity of acne and the amount of oil a person's skin produces, not all people with oily skin have acne.

❑ *See also* ACNE in Part Two.

ORTHOSTATIC HYPOTENSION

See under RARE DISORDERS.

OSTEOARTHRITIS

See under ARTHRITIS.

OSTEOMALACIA

See RICKETS/OSTEOMALACIA.

OSTEOPOROSIS

Osteoporosis is a progressive disease in which the bones gradually become weaker and weaker, causing changes in posture and making the individual extremely susceptible to bone fractures. The term *osteoporosis,* derived from Latin, literally means "porous bones." Because of the physiological, nutritional, and hormonal differences between males and females, osteoporosis affects many more women than men. However, men also suffer from bone loss, often as a side effect of certain medications, such as chemotherapy drugs, thyroid hormone, corticosteroids, and anticonvulsants, or as a result of other illnesses. Fifty-six percent of women and eighteen percent of American men fifty years of age and older show signs of some degree of osteopenia (low bone mass) or osteoporosis.

Bone is constantly restoring itself. Cells called osteoblasts are responsible for making bone, and other cells, called osteoclasts, are needed to remove old bone as its minerals are absorbed for use elsewhere in the body. If the osteoclasts break down the bone more quickly than it is replaced, then bone tends to become less dense and is therefore likely to break more easily.

Bone is at its strongest when a person is around age thirty, and thereafter begins to decline. In women, this decline begins to accelerate at menopause. If you have not accumulated sufficient bone mass during those formative times in childhood, adolescence, and early adulthood, or if you lose it too quickly in later years, you are at increased risk of osteoporosis.

A diagnosis of osteoporosis is reached by measuring bone density. The standard of measurement for that diagnosis has been determined by the World Health Organization and was obtained by measuring the bone mass of people who have not had fractures related to low bone mass. The standard measurement is therefore the bone density of a thirty-year-old premenopausal woman. The bone density measurement is referred to as a T-score or an SD (standard deviation) score. T-scores of less than 1 standard deviation (SD) indicate a low risk of fracture, T-scores of 1 to 2 are considered to indicate osteopenia, and T-scores of more than 2.5 standard deviation from the norm confirm a diagnosis of osteoporosis. But the T-score alone is not the only determinant of fracture risk. Heavy women are less likely to fracture a bone in a fall than thin women; women taking medications that may cause disturbances in balance are more likely to fall and suffer from a fracture. So two women with the same T-score may have a different fracture risk.

Many women, then, can be diagnosed with osteoporosis yet suffer few, if any, ill effects from the condition. The T-score is based on a comparison with the bone of a thirty-year-old, so the standard is set very high. Moreover, it is possible to have osteoporosis in one area of the skeleton and not in another. The spine and hips are the areas that cause most concern because hip fractures in older adults take a long time to heal and osteoporosis in the spine may lead to loss of height and curvature of the spine. With the techniques now being used to diagnose this condition early, so that treatment can begin before fractures occur, many people will probably discover the beginnings of osteoporosis before it is diagnosed due to a fracture. Osteoporosis is not a curable condition as yet, but there are various methods that may slow down the process of bone loss.

Many people have the impression that osteoporosis is caused solely by a dietary calcium deficiency and that it therefore can be remedied by taking calcium supplements. This is not quite correct. It is the way calcium is absorbed and used by the body that seems to be the important factor, not necessarily the amount of calcium consumed. Also, the *type* of calcium consumed is important.

While calcium supplementation is important in dealing with osteoporosis, there are other considerations as well. The correct balance of magnesium, boron, potassium, folic acid, and vitamins C, D, E, and K all play vital roles in battling osteoporosis, as does protein. Of these, vitamin D, K, and boron have been shown to be the most useful. There is some debate on the subject of osteoporosis and dietary protein. Some research has indicated that consuming large quantities of protein may cause an acid imbalance in the body, which the body attempts to counteract by releasing minerals from the bone—including calcium. A contrary point of view holds that protein consumption increases the production of insulin-like growth factor-1 (IGF-1), which is responsible for maintaining muscle and bone strength. What we do know is that all protein-containing foods leave an acid residue in the blood, which is capable of causing bone erosion. However, if it is balanced with alkaline-producing foods such as fruits and vegetables, then the acidity is neutralized and protein has no effect.

In the United States alone, 44 million people are affected by osteoporosis—68 percent of whom are women. Of that total, 10 million people have osteoporosis already and 34 million more have low bone mass. Osteoporosis can appear at any age. It is responsible for more than 850,000 fractures annually. In those sixty-five years of age or older, 74 percent were fractures of the hip, 38 percent of the wrist, 22 percent of the shoulder, and 19 percent of the ankle. Hospitals and nursing homes in the United States spend an estimated $14 billion each year in direct costs for osteoporosis and related fractures.

There are three basic types of osteoporosis. Type I is believed to be caused by hormonal changes, particularly a loss of estrogen, which causes the loss of minerals from the bones to accelerate. Type II is linked to dietary deficiency, especially a lack of sufficient calcium and of vitamin D, which is necessary for the absorption of calcium. Type III occurs in men and women at any age and is caused by drug treatment for other illnesses or other diseases unconnected with osteoporosis. Many women mistakenly believe that osteoporosis is something they need to be concerned about only after menopause. However, recent evidence indicates that osteoporosis often begins early in life and is *not* strictly a postmenopausal problem. Although bone loss accelerates after menopause as a result of the drop in estrogen levels, it begins much earlier. A number of factors are known to influence an individual's risk of developing osteoporosis. The first, and probably the most important, is the peak bone mass achieved in adulthood; the larger and denser the bones are to begin with, the less debilitating bone loss is likely to be. Small, fine-boned women therefore have more reason for concern than women with larger frames and heavier bones. Race and ethnicity also appear to play roles. Women of northern European or Asian ancestry are more likely to develop osteoporosis, while women of African descent are less likely to be affected.

Dietary and lifestyle habits are important as well. Insufficient calcium intake is one factor, but equally important are other dietary practices that affect calcium metabolism. Caffeine, alcohol, and many other drugs appear to have a detrimental effect on calcium absorption. Bone density also depends on exercise. When the body gets regular weight-bearing exercise (such as walking), it responds by depositing more mineral in the bones, especially the bones of the legs, hips, and spine. Conversely, a lack of regular exercise accelerates the loss of bone mass. Other factors that make one more likely to develop osteoporosis include smoking, late puberty, early menopause (natural or artificially induced), a family history of the disease, hyperthyroidism, chronic liver or kidney disease, and the long-term use of corticosteroids, antiseizure medications, or anticoagulants.

The dosages given below are for adults.

NUTRIENTS

SUPPLEMENT	SUGGESTED DOSAGE	COMMENTS
Essential		
Bone Defense from KAL	As directed on label.	Contains calcium, magnesium, phosphorus, and other valuable bone-reinforcing nutrients.
or JCTH from Right Foods	As directed on label.	A combination formula that contains almost all of the nutrients mentioned in this table.
or Osteo-B Plus from Biotics Research	As directed on label.	Contains calcium, magnesium, zinc, and other vitamins and minerals.
Boron	3 mg daily. Do not exceed this amount.	Improves calcium absorption. *Note:* If you are taking a complex containing boron, omit this supplement.
Calcium	Women under 50 and men under 65: 1,200 mg daily. Women over 50 and men over 65: 1,500–2,000 mg daily.	Necessary for maintaining strong bones. Injections (under a doctor's supervision) may be needed. (*See* Calcium and Osteoporosis on page 623.)
Copper	3 mg daily.	Aids in the formation of bone.
Floradix Iron+ Herbs from Salus Haus	As directed on label.	Provides organic iron and other nutrients needed for optimum health. Postmenopausal women usually do not need supplemental iron. *Caution:* Only use after checking with your health care provider.
Glucosamine plus chondroitin	As directed on label.	Nutrients necessary for the development of bone and connective tissue.
Magnesium	1,000 mg daily.	Important in calcium uptake.
Phosphorus	As directed on label.	Works with calcium to increase bone strength.
Potassium	300–1,000 mg daily.	Needed to counteract high-acid diet. Shown to increase bone matrix, reduce calcium loss in the urine, and lower blood pressure. *Caution:* Check with your health care provider before using these amounts.
Silica	As directed on label.	Supplies silicon, for calcium utilization and bone strength.
Soy isoflavones	As directed on label.	They have an estrogenic effect on the body. Estrogen promotes bone mass.
Ultra Osteo Synergy from American Biologics	As directed on label.	To support bone renewal.
Vitamin B complex plus extra vitamin B_6 (pyridoxine) and vitamin B_{12}	As directed on label. 200 mg daily. Do not exceed this amount. 1,000–2,000 mcg daily.	Provides strength to protein in bone tissue and promotes the production of progesterone.
Vitamin D	As directed on label.	Needed for the absorption of calcium.
Vitamin K	As directed on label.	Essential for the production of bone protein.

Very Important

L-lysine and L-arginine	As directed on label, on an empty stomach. Take with water or juice. Do not take with milk. Take with 50 mg vitamin B$_6$ and 100 mg vitamin C for better absorption.	Aid in calcium absorption and connective tissue strength. (*See* AMINO ACIDS in Part One.)
Methylsulfonyl-methane (MSM) (OptiMSM from Cardinal Nutrition)	As directed on label. Do not exceed the recommended dose.	A natural sulfur compound found in foods and present in body tissues. It is used by the body to build healthy new cells. MSM provides the flexible bond between the cells and provides support for tendons, ligaments, and muscles. Use a capsule form for easier absorption.
Multienzyme complex with betaine hydrochloride (HCl) plus proteolytic enzymes	As directed on label. Take with meals. As directed on label. Take between meals.	Needed for proper absorption of calcium and all nutrients. *Note:* Do not use a formula containing HCl if you have an ulcer or suffer from stomach acidity.
Vitamin A with mixed carotenoids and vitamin E	25,000 IU daily. If you are pregnant, do not exceed 10,000 daily. 200 IU daily or 400 IU every other day.	Important in retarding the aging process. Use emulsion forms for easier assimilation. Aids in the use of vitamin A and protects it from destruction by oxygen. Use d-alpha-tocopherol form.
Zinc plus copper	50 mg daily. Do not exceed a total of 100 mg daily from all supplements. 3 mg daily	Important for calcium uptake and immune function. Use zinc gluconate lozenges or OptiZinc for best absorption. Needed to balance with zinc.

Helpful

Chromium picolinate	400–600 mcg daily.	Improves insulin efficiency, which improves bone density.
DL-phenylalanine (DLPA)	As directed on label, on an empty stomach. Take with water or juice. Do not take with milk. Take with 50 mg vitamin B$_6$ and 3,000 mg vitamin C for better absorption.	Good for bone pain. (*See* AMINO ACIDS in Part One.) *Caution:* Do not take this supplement if you suffer from panic attacks, diabetes, high blood pressure, or PKU.
Kelp	2,000–3,000 mg daily.	A rich source of important minerals.
Manganese	As directed on label. Take separately from calcium.	Vital in mineral metabolism.
Multivitamin and mineral complex	As directed on label.	To supply essential minerals. Use a high-potency formula.
Trace mineral complex (Trace Supreme from International Health Products)	As directed on label.	Trace (also called micro) minerals are important for healthy bone formation.
Vitamin C with bioflavonoids	3,000 mg and up daily.	Important for collagen and connective tissue formation

Herbs

☐ Alfalfa, barley grass, black cohosh, boneset, dandelion root, nettle, parsley, poke root, rose hips, and yucca help to build strong bones.

Cautions: Do not use black cohosh if you are pregnant or have any type of chronic disease. Black cohosh should not be used by those with liver problems. Do not use boneset on a daily basis for more than one week, as long-term use can lead to toxicity.

☐ Feverfew is good for pain relief and acts as an anti-inflammatory.

Caution: Do not use feverfew when pregnant or nursing. People who take prescription blood-thinning medications should consult a health care provider before using feverfew, as the combination can result in internal bleeding.

☐ Oat straw contains silica, which helps the body absorb calcium.

☐ Red clover isoflavones may mimic the effects of estrogen by slowing the degenerative breakdown of bone mass.

☐ Common herbs such as sage, rosemary, and thyme can inhibit the breakdown of bone that contributes to osteoporosis.

Caution: Do not use sage if you suffer from any type of seizure disorder, or are pregnant or nursing.

Recommendations

☐ Eat plenty of foods that are high in calcium and vitamin D. The most potent sources are dairy products, but not all dairy has vitamin D. Check the label, as calcium and vitamin D should be consumed at the same time. Other good sources of easily assimilated calcium include broccoli, chestnuts, clams, dandelion greens, most dark green leafy vegetables, flounder, hazelnuts, kale, kelp, molasses, oats, oysters, salmon, sardines (with the bones), sea vegetables, sesame seeds, shrimp, soybeans, tahini (sesame butter), tofu, turnip greens, and wheat germ.

☐ Consume whole grains and calcium foods at different times. Whole grains contain a substance that binds with calcium and prevents its uptake. Take calcium at bedtime, when it is best absorbed and also aids in sleeping.

☐ Include garlic and onions in the diet, as well as eggs (if your cholesterol level is not too high). These foods contain sulfur, which is needed for healthy bones.

☐ If you are a menopausal or postmenopausal woman with osteoporosis, include plenty of soy products in your diet. Soy is rich in phytoestrogens, which may, to some extent, substitute for your body's own estrogen if it is manufacturing too little. The latter effect is very important for osteoporosis. Estrogen depletion is strongly associated with osteoporosis.

☐ Avoid phosphate-containing drinks and foods such as soft drinks and alcohol. Avoid smoking, sugar, and salt.

Calcium and Osteoporosis

People in the United States consume more dairy products and other foods high in calcium per capita than the citizens of any other two nations on earth put together. We even have orange juice and antacids that are fortified with calcium. Yet we eat far less total food, take in less calcium, and get less exercise that stimulates bone growth than our grandparents did. At the same time, we consume more animal protein and phosphate-containing foods such as soft drinks. Perhaps not surprisingly, therefore, we also have the world's highest rates of osteoporosis and bone fractures among elderly people. Obviously, we need to eat more of the right foods and take high-quality supplements in some form as well.

If you are depending on your diet to supply your calcium requirements, it is useful to know that you can get about 300 milligrams of calcium from the following foods: 1 cup of low-fat yogurt, 2¼ cups of broccoli, 1½ ounces of cheese, 8 cups of spinach, and 1½ cups of kale. Green vegetables, sardines, salmon (including the bones), beans, and almonds also contain calcium. In addition to supplying enough calcium, your diet needs to be balanced with the correct amounts of other vitamins and minerals that allow the calcium to be absorbed and used to nourish bone. Among these are magnesium, potassium, and vitamin K. Magnesium and potassium are found in all fruits and vegetables. Vitamin K is found in dark green leafy vegetables, including broccoli, collard greens, kale, and spinach. If you find that you cannot meet the suggested requirements and other nutrients from your diet, then you should consider a supplement.

Drugstores and health food stores carry a bewildering array of vitamin and mineral supplements in a variety of brands and forms. There can be significant nutritional differences between the various supplements available.

Where calcium is concerned, the number on the label does not necessarily reflect the amount of calcium you can expect to absorb from the product. For example, if a label says "calcium lactate 600 milligrams," this may mean that each tablet weighs 600 milligrams—but out of 600 milligrams of calcium lactate, only 13 percent is actually calcium that is available for absorption. This is because minerals cannot be turned into tablets in their pure state; they must be combined with some other substance or substances to make a stable compound.

The important information to look for is the amount of *elemental* calcium that is present in the supplement. It is the elemental calcium that is absorbed by the body. Then, too, some supplements may contain large amounts of calcium, but in a form that is not absorbed, or is not well absorbed, by the body. The letters *USP* (U.S. Pharmacopeia) on the label are an indication that the standard for absorbability has been met.

The following are some of the common forms of calcium found in calcium supplements:

• *Calcium carbonate* usually contains a relatively large percentage of elemental calcium, and is as easily absorbed by the body as milk calcium. It contains 40 percent elemental calcium by weight. It is the lowest cost supplement as well.

• *Calcium citrate* is absorbed by the body more quickly. However, many calcium citrate products contain about half as much elemental calcium. Calcium citrate can be used if you have low stomach acid levels, which is common in postmenopausal women and people who take antacid medications. This type of supplement contains 21 percent elemental calcium by weight. You will have to take many more pills to get the same amount of calcium.

• *Calcium gluconate* contains 9 percent elemental calcium. This form of calcium can sometimes cause diarrhea and nausea.

• *Calcium lactate* contains 13 percent elemental calcium, along with lactic acid.

• *Calcium lactate gluconate* contains 13 percent elemental calcium.

• *Calcium phosphate* contains phosphorus and vitamin D in addition to calcium. This helps the body absorb the calcium. This type of supplement contains 38 or 31 percent elemental calcium (depending on whether it is tricalcium or dicalcium phosphate). (Tums contains calcium phosphate.)

For men, problems with calcium appear to be more complex than was originally thought. Research conducted over ten years by the Physicians' Health Study—the group that discovered aspirin's effect on heart attack risk—found that men who consumed two and a half servings of dairy products per day were 30 percent more likely to develop prostate cancer than men who did not. Calcium is known to lower body levels of 1,25-dihydroxy vitamin D. This is the most active form of vitamin D and is not the same form of vitamin D that is sometimes added to milk. Low levels of this vitamin may protect men against prostate cancer. In a previous study, the same group of researchers found that men who consumed high amounts of dairy foods had 70 percent increased risk of prostate cancer, and that calcium supplements increased the risk of prostate cancer by 30 percent. For now, men can continue to get calcium from foods, but taking calcium supplements is something that should be discussed with a health care provider. Calcium increases the risk of prostate cancer. Ask about this as well if you are concerned.

❑ Limit your consumption of citrus fruits and tomatoes; these foods may inhibit calcium intake.

❑ Avoid yeast products. Yeast is high in phosphorus, which competes with calcium for absorption by the body.

❑ If you are over fifty-five years old, include a calcium supplement in your daily regimen, and take hydrochloric acid (HCl) supplements. In order for calcium to be absorbed, there must be an adequate supply of vitamin D as well as sufficient HCl in the stomach. Older people often lack sufficient stomach acid.

❑ If you take thyroid hormone or an anticoagulant drug, increase the amount of calcium you take by 25 to 50 percent.

❑ Vitamin K_1, found in dark green vegetables like kale, cooked greens, spinach, Brussels sprouts, broccoli, asparagus, and some lettuces, retards bone loss. A three-year study in the *Journal of Clinical Endocrinology and Metabolism* found that taking the Upper Limit of vitamin K (500 micrograms per day) with 600 milligrams of calcium and 400 IU of vitamin D did not aid in additional bone health of the spine or hip. Do not take more vitamin K than 500 micrograms without consulting your health care professional. Continue to eat foods high in vitamin K.

❑ If you take a diuretic, consult your physician before beginning calcium and vitamin D supplementation. Thiazide-type diuretics increase blood calcium levels, and complications may result if these drugs are taken in conjunction with calcium and vitamin D supplements. Other types of diuretics increase calcium requirements, however.

❑ Keep active, and exercise regularly. A lack of exercise can result in the loss of calcium, but this can be reversed with sensible exercise. Walking is probably the best exercise for maintaining bone mass. Other activities that strengthen bones include dancing, tennis, stair climbing, aerobics, skating, and weight lifting. Although swimming and cycling are good for your cardiovascular system, they are not weight-bearing and do not affect bone density. If you are overweight, inflammatory proteins called cytokines are released due to excess body fat. These increase the loss of bone. Weight loss increases bone loss as well. However, engaging in aerobic exercise while losing weight reduces inflammation and increases bone mineral density.

Considerations

❑ In a study published in the *American Journal of Clinical Nutrition,* women in the early stages of menopause did not reduce postmenopausal bone loss by including isoflavone-enriched foods in their diet. These women consumed 110 milligrams of isoflavone aglycones a day from the foods. It is possible that this amount was too low to show an effect. However, long-term trials using soy extracts have shown conflicting results. Women who have breast cancer or are at risk for it should consult their health care provider before using soy or isoflavone-enriched foods.

❑ In one study, taking 1,200 milligrams of calcium per day for four years was shown to reduce the risk of fractures by 72 percent. However, the participants in the study were followed for six more years; they did not get this much calcium, and the risk of fractures increased again.

❑ Some studies have reported an adverse effect on bones with high vitamin A intakes. It appears that vitamin A is safe if vitamin D intake is adequate. Be sure to take vitamin D with vitamin A supplements.

❑ Getting at least 400 micrograms per day of folic acid was shown to improve bone density, but riboflavin and vitamin B_{12} had no effect over a five-year study.

❑ Women are about four times more likely than men to develop osteoporosis, or weak, porous bones. But a study links vitamin B_{12} deficiency with low bone mineral density in men, and confirms similar, previously reported findings in women. Researchers funded by the Agricultural Research Service (ARS) reported the findings in the *Journal of Bone and Mineral Research*. While vitamin B_{12} deficiency has been linked with low levels of markers of bone formation, the mechanism behind the relationship is not known. The scientists examined the relationship between vitamin B_{12} blood levels and indicators of bone health measured in 2,576 men and women, aged thirty to eighty-seven, participating in the Framingham Osteoporosis Study. They found that those with vitamin B_{12} levels lower than 148 picomoles per liter (pM/L) were at greater risk of osteoporosis than those with higher levels. Plasma B_{12} levels below 185 pM/L are considered "very low," according to some experts. The study found that those with vitamin B_{12} concentrations below 148 pM/L had significantly lower average bone mineral density—at the hip in men, and at the spine in women—than those with concentrations above this level. This study suggests adequate vitamin B_{12} intake is important for maintaining bone mineral density. Animal protein foods, such as fish, liver, beef, pork, milk, and cheese are good sources of vitamin B_{12}.

❑ A study conducted by the *Journal of Clinical Nutrition* reported that women who are vegetarians experience significantly less bone loss than women who consume meat. Soy, beans, peas, and lentils supply proteins, and green vegetables are all very rich in calcium, as well as containing abundant amounts of other vitamins and minerals.

❑ Klinefelter's syndrome, which results in low testosterone levels in men, also leads to osteoporosis.

❑ A study reported in the *Journal of the American Medical Association* revealed that senior citizens who took tranquilizers suffered 70 percent more hip fractures than did other people their age. Very often, medications can affect balance. You should discuss this particular side effect with your physician before taking any medication.

❑ One study purports to have identified a link between osteoporosis and high blood levels of the amino acid homocysteine. Homocysteine is involved in methionine metabolism, and is normally recycled into methionine or converted into cysteine in the body. High levels result in possible increased risk of heart disease and stroke.

❑ Caffeine has been linked to calcium loss. In one study, adults given 300 milligrams of caffeine excreted more than the normal amount of calcium in their urine. Another study revealed that caffeine is associated with decreased bone minerals in women.

❑ Carbonated soft drinks contain high amounts of phosphates. These cause the body to eliminate calcium as the phosphates themselves are excreted, even if calcium must be taken from the bones to do this.

❑ Bone disintegration with pain in the hips, lower back, or legs and vertebral fractures (usually affecting people over fifty years old) is common.

❑ A balloon kyphoplasty, in which a balloon is inserted into a spinal fracture, inflated, and injected with a bone cement, can provide support and pain relief for people with some spinal fractures.

❑ The use of sodium fluoride, which was once thought to be helpful in building bone, has been shown to be ineffective for the treatment of osteoporosis. While sodium fluoride does increase bone mass in the vertebral column, the bone itself is of inferior quality. Women participating in a study at the Mayo Clinic in Rochester, Minnesota, were three times as likely to suffer from a fracture of the arm, leg, or hip if they took sodium fluoride than if they took a placebo. Some of the participants also suffered from unusual lower leg pain, perhaps due to stress fractures.

❑ A number of different prescription drugs are sometimes prescribed for people with osteoporosis, including:

• Alendronate (Fosamax) is a type of drug known as a bisphosphonate. It inhibits the resorption of bone. Other drugs in this class are risedronate (Actonel) and ibandronate (Boniva), which are taken orally one or more times a month. A newer option is an intravenous drug (Reclast), which can be taken just once a year.

• Calcitonin (sold under the brand names Cibacalcin and Miacalcin) is said to prevent further loss of bone mass in 70 percent of the people who take it. It should not be taken by anyone with a history of kidney stones.

• Raloxifene (Evista) is a selective estrogen receptor modulator (SERM)—a drug that acts *like* an estrogen in some respects but is not estrogen.

• Teriparatide (Forteo) is a new drug that is a synthetic version of parathyroid hormone and works by increasing the action of osteoblasts, the body's bone-building cells. This causes bones to become denser and more resistant to fractures. It is the first drug to stimulate new bone growth, but it requires giving yourself daily injections, and the drug can only be used for up to two years.

All of these drugs have potential side effects. They are not suitable for everyone. If bone mass is still decreasing after two years on the same medication, doctors usually prescribe another drug.

❑ Hormone replacement therapy is often prescribed for people who have osteoporosis. There are risks attached to this treatment. Before agreeing to it, you need to consider whether the risks outweigh the benefits. (*See* Hormones, Hormone Therapy, and Menopause on page 580.)

❑ The FDA has approved three drugs for men with osteoporosis—alendronate (Fosamax), risedronate (Actonel), and zoledronic acid (Reclast). These are all bisphosphonates. Teriparatide (Forteo) has also been approved for men.

❑ Dehydroepiandrosterone (DHEA) and human growth hormone (HGH) are two hormones whose production progressively declines with age. Research suggests that supplementation with either of these hormones may help increase bone strength and treat osteoporosis. However, these hormones should be used only by those with true growth hormone deficiencies. (*See* DHEA THERAPY and GROWTH HORMONE THERAPY in Part Three.)

❑ Research conducted by the World Health Organization concluded that people who were given a protein supplement recovered more quickly from hip fractures than those who were not. In addition, they found that people who took protein supplements were less likely to suffer a hip fracture in the first place.

❑ A study reported in the March 2000 issue of *The Journal of Family Practice* found that taking vitamin C can help to prevent nerve pain after a fracture.

❑ Tests for bone loss are very easy and noninvasive. Dual energy x-ray absorptiometry (DEXA) is probably the most reliable method of determining osteoporosis. It is easier to fix bone problems before too much loss has occurred. So, women should be tested in their mid-thirties and then every five to ten years until menopause and more frequently after menopause. Exposure to radiation from this test is less than in other methods used to detect this condition. Another type of test, the collagen cross-linked N-telopeptide (NTx) test, is particularly useful for women in that it shows how fast you are losing bone mass. It is performed on a urine sample.

❑ See also RICKETS in Part Two.

PAGET'S DISEASE OF BONE

Paget's disease of bone (named for Sir James Paget, who first described it) is a chronic disorder characterized by excessive bone degeneration combined with the creation of new bone that is deficient in calcium and therefore more fragile than normal bone. The result is enlarged and deformed bones in one or more sections of the skeleton, bone degeneration, bone pain, arthritis, noticeable deformities, and an increased susceptibility to fractures.

Paget's disease most often affects the bones of the pelvis, the spine, the thighs, the skull, the hips, the shins, and the upper arms. It affects more than 3 to 5 percent of Americans over the age of fifty and about 10 percent of those over the age of eighty, although in rare instances it has been reported in young adults. It affects men and women nearly equally.

In the early stages, the disease usually causes no symptoms, although there may be mild pain in the affected bones. As it progresses, bone pain tends to become more severe and persistent, especially at night, and to worsen with exertion. Paget's disease can also lead to neck and/or back pain; pain and/or stiffness in affected joints; warming of the skin over the area of the affected bones; unexplained bone fractures; hearing loss; headaches; dizziness; ringing in the ears; and impaired mobility. If the pelvis or a thighbone is involved, there may be hip pain. The disease follows a pattern of alternating remissions and flare-ups. Over time, the flare-ups gradually become worse. Sometimes joints adjacent to the affected bone become involved, and osteoarthritis may develop. Over time, deformities such as bowed legs, an increasingly barrel-shaped chest, a bent spine, and/or an enlarged forehead may develop as well.

Other possible late complications include kidney stones (caused by immobilization), congestive heart failure, deafness or blindness (caused by the skull pressing on the brain), high blood pressure, and gout. In approximately 5 percent of cases, the affected bone undergoes malignant changes, leading to osteosarcoma (bone cancer). High-output cardiac failure can occur from prolonged increased blood flow. The life expectancy of individuals with Paget's disease is somewhat reduced, but most live with the disease for at least ten to fifteen years.

Because this disease usually does not cause significant symptoms, especially in the early stages, most cases go undetected unless discovered accidentally when X-rays or blood tests are taken for another reason. The cause is unknown, although some researchers suspect a slowly progressing viral infection of the bone is involved. Multiple cases of the disease within families have been reported. However, Paget's disease does not appear to be transmitted from one generation to another, a finding more consistent with an infectious disorder than with a hereditary condition.

Paget's disease is often confused with hyperthyroidism and other disorders that cause bone lesions, such as bone cancer, fibrous dysplasia, and multiple myeloma. To diagnose Paget's disease, doctors may use bone scans or X-rays to detect bone changes characteristic of the disease. Blood tests may detect elevated levels of alkaline phosphatase, an enzyme produced by bone-building cells. Urine tests and CT scans also may be used to arrive at a diagnosis of Paget's disease.

Unless otherwise specified, the dosages recommended here are for adults. For children between the ages of twelve and seventeen, reduce the dose to three-quarters the recommended amount. For children between six and twelve, use one-half the recommended dose, and for children under the age of six, use one-quarter the recommended amount.

NUTRIENTS

SUPPLEMENT	SUGGESTED DOSAGE	COMMENTS
Essential		
Calcium plus	1,500 mg daily.	For the formation of strong bones. Use a chelate form.
boron and	3 mg daily. Do not exceed this amount.	Nutrients that are needed for calcium absorption.
magnesium and	750 mg daily.	
vitamin D	400 IU daily.	
Copper	3 mg daily.	Aids in the formation of bone.
Glucosamine Plus from FoodScience of Vermont plus	As directed on label.	Contains nutrients necessary for healthy development of bone and connective tissues.
chondroitin and	As directed on label.	Helpful for pain.
methylsulfonyl-methane (MSM)	As directed on label.	
Kyolic-EPA from Wakunaga	As directed on label.	Supplies essential fatty acids, vital for proper growth and cell formation.
Liquid Kyolic with B$_1$ and B$_{12}$ from Wakunaga	As directed on label.	Aids in red blood cell formation and energy production.
Manganese	2 mg daily.	Required for normal bone growth.
Phosphorus	1,200 mg daily.	Required for bone formation.
Primrose oil or	As directed on label.	To supply essential fatty acids vital for proper growth and cell formation.
Ultimate Oil from Nature's Secret	As directed on label.	
Silica	As directed on label.	Necessary for bone formation.
Vitamin A with mixed carotenoids including natural beta-carotene	10,000 IU daily.	To improve immune function and promote proper bone growth.
Vitamin B complex	50 mg of each major B vitamin 3 times daily, with meals (amounts of individual vitamins in a complex will vary).	Involved in energy production.
plus extra vitamin B$_{12}$	1,000–2,000 mcg daily.	Assists in nutrient absorption and aids in cell formation.
and folic acid	400 mcg daily.	Needed for energy production.
Vitamin C with bioflavonoids	3,000–6,000 mg daily, in divided doses.	Enhances immunity and aids in proper bone growth.
Zinc	30 mg daily. Do not exceed a total of 100 mg daily from all supplements.	Promotes a healthy immune system. Use zinc gluconate lozenges or OptiZinc for best absorption.
Helpful		
Bone Builder from Ethical Nutrients	As directed on label.	Contains minerals and the organic matrix that makes up bone.
DL-phenylalanine (DLPA)	As directed on label.	Alleviates chronic pain. *Caution:* Do not take this supplement if you are pregnant or nursing, or suffer

		from panic attacks, diabetes, high blood pressure, or PKU.
Floradix Iron + Herbs from Salus Haus	As directed on label.	Provides organic iron and other nutrients needed for optimum health and fitness. Ask your health care provider about your need for iron.
Reishi extract or shiitake extract	As directed on label. As directed on label.	To help reduce inflammation.

Herbs

❑ Alfalfa contains minerals needed for proper bone formation and that help to reduce inflammation.

❑ Angelica, cayenne (capsicum), feverfew, hops, passionflower, skullcap, valerian root, and white willow bark work well for pain.

Caution: Do not use feverfew when pregnant or nursing. People who take prescription blood-thinning medications should consult a health care provider before using feverfew, as the combination can result in internal bleeding.

❑ Black cohosh and St. John's wort help both to reduce inflammation and to alleviate pain.

Cautions: Do not use black cohosh if you are pregnant or have any type of chronic disease. Black cohosh should not be used by those with liver problems. St. John's wort may cause increased sensitivity to sunlight. It may also produce anxiety, gastrointestinal symptoms, and headaches. It can interact with some drugs including antidepressants, birth control pills, and anticoagulants.

❑ Boneset, dandelion root, nettle, parsley, poke root, rose hips, and yucca help to build strong bones.

Caution: Do not use boneset on a daily basis for more than one week, as long-term use can lead to toxicity.

❑ Echinacea, goldenseal, and licorice aid in reducing inflammation.

Cautions: Do not take echinacea for longer than three months. It should not be used by people who are allergic to ragweed. Do not take goldenseal internally on a daily basis for more than one week at a time. Do not use it during pregnancy or if you are breast-feeding, and use with caution if you are allergic to ragweed. If you have a history of cardiovascular disease, diabetes, or glaucoma, use it only under a doctor's supervision. Licorice root should not be used during pregnancy or nursing. It should not be used by persons with diabetes, glaucoma, heart disease, high blood pressure, or a history of stroke.

Recommendations

❑ Eat plenty of calcium-rich foods. These include brewer's yeast, buttermilk, carob, goat's milk and other dairy products containing vitamin D, all leafy greens, salmon, sardines, seafood, tofu, whey, and yogurt.

Caution: Brewer's yeast can cause an allergic reaction in some individuals. Start with a small amount at first, and discontinue use if any allergic symptoms occur.

❑ Include plenty of garlic in the diet. Garlic is beneficial for circulation and helps to keep inflammation down.

❑ Eat fresh papaya and pineapple frequently. These fruits contain enzymes that help to reduce inflammation.

❑ Avoid nightshade vegetables. These include tomatoes, potatoes, eggplant, cayenne peppers, chili peppers, sweet peppers, paprika, and pimiento. These vegetables are high in alkaloids, chemical substances with strong physiological effects. They affect the metabolism of calcium and, through a mechanism not yet understood, cause calcium from the bones to be deposited in other areas of the body where it does not belong, such as the arteries, joints, and kidneys.

❑ Use barley grass and/or kelp to supply valuable minerals and other nutrients needed for bone formation.

❑ Use heat to alleviate pain. Hot soaks, hot compresses, and heat lamps are all effective.

❑ Follow an exercise program recommended by your health care provider to combat immobility.

❑ Sleep on a very firm mattress or use a bed board. This will lessen the chance of developing spinal deformities.

❑ During active phases of the disease, rest in bed and move or turn often to prevent pressure sores.

❑ Accident-proof your home to help prevent fractures. Remove throw rugs and avoid slippery flooring. Install handrails next to the bathtub and toilet.

❑ Avoid placing extreme physical stress on the bones.

❑ Get regular medical checkups to screen for early bone cancer and to detect hearing loss. If hearing loss occurs, consider a hearing aid.

Considerations

❑ There is no known cure for Paget's disease. However, most patients never develop symptoms and so do not require treatment. For those who do, drug treatment can relieve and manage symptoms. Drug therapy for Paget's disease may include:

- *Analgesics or nonsteroidal anti-inflammatory drugs (NSAIDs)* can be useful in relieving pain.

- *Bisphosphonates* increase bone density and also slow the progression of Paget's disease. These include: alendronate (Fosamax), etidronate (Didronel), pamidronate (Aredia), risedronate (Actonel), and zoledronic acid (Zometa).

- *Calcitonin* (Cibacalcin, Fortical, Miacalcin) is a natural hormone given by injection or through the nose for bone metabolism.

- *Pliamycin* (Mithracin), an antitumor drug, can produce a remission of symptoms within two weeks, and further improvement in two months. However, this drug can also cause kidney damage and destruction of red blood cells.

❑ For names and addresses of organizations that can provide more information on Paget's disease, *see* Health and Medical Organizations in the Appendix.

PAGET'S DISEASE OF THE NIPPLE

See under BREAST CANCER.

PANCREATITIS

Pancreatitis is an inflammation of the pancreas, a five- to six-inch-long leaf-shaped gland situated behind the lower part of the stomach and extending downward toward the spleen and left kidney. It has two primary functions: to produce digestive enzymes that break down proteins, fat, and carbohydrates in the small intestine; and to release the hormones glucagon and insulin, which regulate blood sugar levels. The pancreas can become inflamed if digestive enzymes build up inside it and begin to attack it.

The disease can be either acute or chronic. The leading cause of acute pancreatitis is excessive alcohol use over many years. This condition can also come about as a result of infection (such as with hepatitis A or D or Epstein-Barr virus) or the use of certain drugs (such as divalproex [Depakote], used to prevent seizures and treat bipolar mood disorder; azathioprine [Imuran], sometimes used for rheumatoid arthritis; and 6-MP [Purinethol], a cancer chemotherapy agent). In very rare cases, acute pancreatitis may be caused by injury to the abdomen.

Acute pancreatitis usually causes severe pain that comes on suddenly, starting in or around the area of the navel and radiating to the back. The pain is typically exacerbated by movement and relieved by sitting, and may be accompanied by nausea and vomiting, sometimes severe. Other symptoms include upper abdominal swelling and distension, excessive gas, upper abdominal pain described as burning or stabbing, fever, sweating, hypertension, muscle aches, and abnormal, fatty stools. The incidence of this acute form is increasing by 5 percent per year, mainly owing to an increase in biliary pancreatitis. Infectious complications are a major concern. The infections are thought to be started by small-bowel bacterial overgrowth that eventually crosses the intestinal tract into the bloodstream.

Chronic pancreatitis is a condition in which the inflammation has caused irreversible changes in the microscopic structure of the gallbladder tissue. Repeated episodes of gallbladder infection and gallstones are often involved. (*See* GALLBLADDER DISORDERS in Part Two.) The symptoms of chronic pancreatitis may be hard to distinguish from those of acute pancreatitis, except that the pain tends to be chronic rather than coming on suddenly. In addition, chronic pancreatitis may be punctuated with periodic episodes of acute

disease. In the majority of cases, chronic pancreatitis is caused by long-term alcohol use.

Because the pancreas is the gland that produces the hormones insulin and glucagon, which regulate blood sugar levels, pancreatitis—especially if chronic—often leads to glucose intolerance (diabetes) and digestive difficulties.

Unless otherwise specified, the dosages recommended here are for adults. For children between the ages of twelve and seventeen, reduce the dose to three-quarters the recommended amount. For children between six and twelve, use one-half the recommended dose, and for children under the age of six, use one-quarter the recommended amount.

NUTRIENTS

SUPPLEMENT	SUGGESTED DOSAGE	COMMENTS
Essential		
Chromium picolinate	300–600 mcg daily.	Important in maintaining stable blood sugar levels.
Garlic (Kyolic from Wakunaga)	As directed on label.	Powerful antiviral and antioxidant.
Very Important		
Calcium and magnesium	1,500 mg daily. 1,000 mg daily.	Works closely with magnesium. Counteracts glandular disorders. Use chelate forms.
Digestive enzymes with ox bile (Digestive Aid #34 from Carlson Labs)	As directed on label.	Needed for proper digestion and gallbladder function. Important if gallbladder has been removed.
Kyo-Dophilus from Wakunaga	As directed on label.	To replace the "friendly" bacteria and aid in digestion.
Pancreatin	As directed on label. Take with food.	Pancreatic enzyme deficiency is common in people with pancreatitis.
Proteolytic enzymes	As directed on label. Take between meals and at bedtime, on an empty stomach.	Aids in reducing inflammation; reduces strain on the pancreas by aiding protein digestion. *Caution:* Do not give this supplement to a child.
Raw pancreas glandular	As directed on label.	Contains certain proteins needed to repair the pancreas. (*See* GLANDULAR THERAPY in Part Three.)
Vitamin B complex plus extra vitamin B₃ (niacin) and vitamin B₅ (pantothenic acid)	50 mg of each major B vitamin 3 times daily (amounts of individual vitamins in a complex will vary). 50 mg 3 times daily. Do not exceed this amount. 100 mg 3 times daily.	Antistress vitamins. Niacin and pantothenic acid are important in fat and carbohydrate metabolism. *Caution:* Do not take niacin if you have a liver disorder, gout, or high blood pressure.
Important		
Choline and inositol	As directed on label. As directed on label.	Fat emulsifiers that aid in fat digestion.

and/or lecithin and/or lipotropic factors	As directed on label. As directed on label.	
Vitamin C with bioflavonoids	1,000 mg 4 times daily.	Potent free radical scavengers. Use a buffered form.
Helpful		
Coenzyme Q10 plus Coenzyme A from Coenzyme-A Technologies	75 mg daily. As directed on label.	A powerful antioxidant and oxygen carrier. Works well with coenzyme Q10 and increases energy, supports adrenal glands, processes fats, removes toxins from the body, and boosts the immune system.
CTR Support from PhysioLogics	As directed on label.	Helps diminish damage caused by inflammation and protects against future damage.
DL-phenylalanine (DLPA)	As directed on label.	To relieve pain in acute cases. *Caution:* Do not take this supplement if you are pregnant or nursing, or if you suffer from panic attacks, diabetes, high blood pressure, or PKU.
Grape seed extract	As directed on label.	A powerful anti-inflammatory and antioxidant.
L-cysteine	As directed on label.	Protects the liver.
Vitamin E	200 IU daily or 400 IU every other day.	A powerful antioxidant and oxygen carrier. Important in tissue repair. Use d-alpha-tocopherol form.
Zinc	50 mg daily. Do not exceed a total of 100 mg daily from all supplements.	Facilitates proper enzyme activity for cell division, growth, and repair. Plays a role in the manufacture of insulin. Use zinc gluconate lozenges or OptiZinc for best absorption.

Herbs

❑ Burdock root, milk thistle, and red clover aid in cleansing the bloodstream and liver, reducing the burden on the pancreas.

❑ Cedar berries, echinacea, gentian root, and goldenseal stimulate and strengthen the pancreas.

Cautions: Do not take echinacea for longer than three months. It should not be used by people who are allergic to ragweed. Do not take goldenseal internally on a daily basis for more than one week at a time. Do not use it during pregnancy or if you are breast-feeding, and use with caution if you are allergic to ragweed. If you have a history of cardiovascular disease, diabetes, or glaucoma, use it only under a doctor's supervision.

❑ Dandelion root stimulates bile production and improves the health of the pancreas.

❑ Detoxygen from Nature's Plus is an herbal formula that detoxifies the body and oxygenates cells.

❑ Licorice root supports all glandular functions.

Caution: Licorice root should not be used during pregnancy or nursing. It should not be used by persons with diabetes, glaucoma, heart disease, high blood pressure, or a history of stroke.

❑ Olive leaf extract acts as an anti-inflammatory agent and is helpful if you have an infection.

Recommendations

❑ If you develop symptoms of pancreatitis, call your physician. This is an extremely serious condition that requires medical attention.

❑ Eat a diet low in fat and sugar. This is very important for recovery. High levels of sugar and fats in the blood are common in pancreatitis. *See* DIABETES in Part Two and follow the dietary guidelines. Sometimes intravenous feeding is needed, which quiets the pancreas down. Alternatively, a feeding tube may be inserted in the nose or through the abdomen to supply a highly digested formula.

❑ Consume no alcohol in any form.

❑ Never use probiotics, even if you are taking antibiotics. In a study of patients with acute pancreatitis, there was no difference in the number of infections between those taking probiotics and those who were given a placebo. However, those taking probiotics had twice the death rate as the placebo group. The probiotics used in this study included: *Lactobacillus acidophilus, L. casei, L. salivarius, L. lactis, Bifidobacterium bifidum,* and *B. lactis.*

❑ If you smoke, stop, and try to avoid secondhand smoke. Recent studies point to a distinct link between chronic pancreatitis and cigarette smoking.

❑ *See* FASTING in Part Three and follow the program. Fasting can improve the health of all organs, including the pancreas.

Considerations

❑ Pancreatic cancer is the fourth leading cause of cancer deaths in the United States, causing about 35,000 deaths every year. Pancreatitis can lead to the development of this type of cancer. Improving the health of the pancreas may help to prevent it. In one study, the incidence of pancreatic cancer was higher in those with low vitamin D intakes (less than 600 IU per day). Another study found a connection between pancreatic cancer and high intakes of sugars (fructose, sucrose, and high-fructose corn syrup). In another study, taking folic acid and vitamin B6 and B12 supplements did not reduce the risk of pancreatic cancer. However, those who got these vitamins from foods had a modest protection against developing pancreatic cancer.

❑ A high level of triglycerides (fat) in the blood is a factor in pancreatitis.

PANIC ATTACK

See under ANXIETY DISORDER.

PARKINSON'S DISEASE

Parkinson's disease (PD) is a degenerative disease affecting the nervous system. The underlying cause is unknown, but symptoms appear when there is a lack of dopamine in the brain. Dopamine is a neurotransmitter that carries messages from one nerve cell to another. In healthy persons, it exists in balance with another neurotransmitter, acetylcholine. In people with what is called primary Parkinson's disease, the *substantia nigra*—the area of the brain containing cells that manufacture dopamine, noradrenaline, and serotonin—are damaged or dying, and the brain loses the ability to manufacture these chemicals.

The disease may start almost imperceptibly, with a mild to moderate tremor of the hand or hands while at rest, a general slow and heavy feeling, muscular stiffness, bradykinesia (slowness of movement), and a tendency to tire more easily than usual. Later symptoms may include muscular rigidity; drooling; loss of appetite; a stooped, shuffling gait; tremors, including a characteristic "pill rolling" movement in which the thumb and forefinger rub against each other; impaired speech; and a fixed facial expression. The body gradually becomes rigid and the limbs stiffen. Depression and/or dementia may accompany the physical symptoms.

While tremors can be a sign of Parkinson's disease, not all tremors can be attributed to it. Hand tremors are common in middle age and later. There are different types of tremors. Parkinsonian tremors are most pronounced during rest, can be aggravated by tension or fatigue, and disappear during sleep. Intention tremors occur only when a muscle is being used, rather than at rest. Essential tremor is a condition characterized by more or less continuous up-and-down tremors that seems to run in families. Essential tremors usually affect both hands and become milder with rest, more severe with activity and/or stress. Attempts to stop this type of tremor through willpower often seem to make the trembling worse. Any persistent or recurrent tremor deserves investigation, especially if it interferes with normal activity, but it should be kept in mind that most tremors are *not* an indication of Parkinson's disease.

Parkinson's disease is one of the most common debilitating diseases in North America. There are approximately 1 million people with the disease throughout the United States and Canada. It affects men more often than women. Recent statistics indicate that 3 percent of the population over sixty-five years of age has the disease. For those between sixty and seventy years of age, about 15 percent of adults have it, and for those between seventy-five and eighty-four years it rises to 30 percent. There is no known cure. Treatment is focused on relieving the symptoms and maintaining independence as long as possible. Drug therapy, physical therapy, and surgery are among the treatment methods used.

While the cause of the loss of brain cells that causes Parkinson's disease remains unknown, a number of different theories have been developed. One is that oxidative stress plays a prominent role in the degeneration of the nerves that secrete dopamine and that this causes the tremors that are a common symptom of Parkinson's disease. High homocysteine levels cause oxidative stress. It's customary to give all three B vitamins (B_{12}, B_6, and folic acid) to lower homocysteine levels in patients with heart disease. However, in those with Parkinson's disease, it turns out that only B_6 is effective at lowering homocysteine levels. This is because B_6 is the major driver required to convert homocysteine to cysteine, which in turn allows for the increased production of glutathione. Glutathione is a major antioxidant that seems to protect the nerve endings.

Others have hypothesized that the cells are destroyed by toxins within the body that the liver is unable to filter out, metabolize, or detoxify because as the body ages, the liver loses its ability to work as effectively and as efficiently as it once did. Another theory is that exposure to environmental toxins, such as herbicides and pesticides that leach into groundwater, is responsible.

The dosages given below are for adults.

NUTRIENTS

SUPPLEMENT	SUGGESTED DOSAGE	COMMENTS
Essential		
Calcium	As directed on label.	People with Parkinson's disease often develop porous bones and are in danger of fractures. Calcium also supports the nervous system. Use calcium citrate form.
and magnesium	As directed on label.	Important for the function of nerves and muscles.
and potassium	As directed on label.	Aids nerve impulse transmission and muscle contraction.
Coenzyme Q_{10}	As directed on label.	Allows cells to produce energy. May slow brain cell death and slow progression of the disease.
plus Coenzyme A from Coenzyme-A Technologies	As directed on label.	Works well with coenzyme Q_{10} to streamline metabolism, ease depression and fatigue, and increase energy.
Creatine	As directed on label. Never exceed the recommended dose.	Often used by body builders to increase muscle stamina. Research is ongoing in the use of creatine in muscle-depleting illnesses.
5-hydroxy L-tryptophan (5-HTP)	As directed on label.	Increases serotonin levels in the brain, which helps overcome insomnia and depression.
Glutathione	As directed on label.	Often depleted in people with Parkinson's disease. Found in

Supplement	Suggested Dosage	Comments
		the substantia nigra in the brain, where cells are dying.
L–phenylalanine and L–tyrosine	As directed by physician. / As directed by physician.	Amino acids that are converted into dopamine. *Caution:* Do not take these supplements if you are pregnant or nursing; if you take an MAO inhibitor drug or levodopa; or if you suffer from panic attacks, diabetes, high blood pressure, or PKU.
Vitamin B complex	50 mg of each major B vitamin 3 times daily, with meals (amounts of individual vitamins in a complex will vary).	Extremely important in brain function and enzyme activity. Use a high-potency sublingual formula. Consider injections (under a doctor's supervision).
plus extra vitamin B$_2$ (riboflavin)	50 mg 3 times daily, with meals.	A lack of this vitamin causes depression, nerve damage, and a reduction in neurotransmitter levels.
and vitamin B$_3$ (niacin) or niacinamide	50 mg 3 times daily, with meals. Do not exceed this amount.	Helps to maintain a strong immune system and overcome depression and irritability. Flushing may occur from niacin use—this is normal. Niacinamide does not cause flushing. *Caution:* Do not take niacin if you have a liver disorder, gout, or high blood pressure.
and vitamin B$_6$ (pyridoxine)	50–75 mg 3 times daily, with meals.	Dopamine production depends on adequate supplies of this vitamin. Consider injections (under a doctor's supervision). *Caution:* Do not take this supplement if you are taking a levodopa preparation.
Vitamin C and vitamin E plus selenium	3,000–6,000 mg daily, in divided doses / 200 IU daily or 400 IU every other day. / 200 mcg daily. Do not exceed this amount.	Antioxidants that may slow progression of the disease and postpone the need for drug therapy. A powerful antioxidant.

Very Important

Supplement	Suggested Dosage	Comments
Dimethylamino-ethanol (DMAE)	As directed on label.	Stimulates the production of choline for brain function. Improves memory and learning ability.
Dimethylglycine (DMG) (Aangamik DMG from Food-Science of Vermont)	50 mg twice daily.	Enhances tissue oxygenation.
Floradix Iron + Herbs from Salus Haus	As directed on label.	Contains iron derived from natural food sources, beneficial in the treatment of Parkinson's disease. Ask your health care provider if you should take iron.
Gamma-aminobutyric acid (GABA)	As directed on label.	Functions as a neuro-transmitter that stabilizes neuron activity. (*See* AMINO ACIDS in Part One.)
Grape seed oil	As directed on label.	Contains a high level of vitamin E as well as the essential fatty acid linoleic acid.

Supplement	Suggested Dosage	Comments
Lecithin granules or capsules and/or phosphatidylcholine	1 tbsp 3 times daily, before meals. / 1,200 mg 3 times daily, before meals. / As directed on label.	To supply choline, important in transmission of nerve impulses.
Nicotinamide adenine dinucleotide (NADH)	10 mg daily.	A form of vitamin B$_3$ that is important in the creation and transfer of chemical energy, especially during breathing.
Pycnogenol or grape seed extract	As directed on label. / As directed on label.	Potent bioflavonoids and free radical scavengers.
Superoxide dismutase (SOD)	As directed on label.	An enzyme that retards oxidation, protecting neurons and sparing neurotransmitters like dopamine.
Trimethylglycine (TMG)	As directed on label.	A natural phytochemical extracted from sugar beets that has been shown in laboratory tests to increase muscle mass, reduce body fat, and increase bone density. Reduces levels of homocysteine.

Helpful

Supplement	Suggested Dosage	Comments
Multienzyme complex (Novenzyme from International Health Products)	As directed on label.	To aid digestion and assimilation of all nutrients, especially the B vitamins.
Multivitamin and mineral complex with potassium	As directed on label. / 99 mg daily.	To correct nutritional deficiencies, common in people with Parkinson's disease.
Primrose oil or omega-3 essential fatty acid complex	2,000–4,000 mg daily, in divided doses. / As directed on label.	May reduce the severity and frequency of tremors.
Raw brain glandular	As directed on label.	A glandular extract that improves brain function. (*See* GLANDULAR THERAPY in Part Three.)

Herbs

Degenerative disease is often facilitated by the accumulation of toxins in the body. The following herbs have detoxifying properties.

❑ Burdock root, dandelion root, ginger root, and milk thistle detoxify the liver.

❑ Cayenne (capsicum), goldenseal, mullein, Siberian ginseng, and yarrow stimulate the thymus and lymphatic system.

Cautions: Do not take goldenseal internally on a daily basis for more than one week at a time. Do not use it during pregnancy or if you are breast-feeding, and use with caution if you are allergic to ragweed. If you have a history of cardiovascular disease, diabetes, or glaucoma, use it only under a doctor's supervision. Do not use Siberian ginseng if you have hypoglycemia, high blood pressure, or a heart disorder.

❏ Hawthorn, licorice, red clover, and sarsaparilla cleanse the blood.

Caution: Licorice root should not be used during pregnancy or nursing. It should not be used by persons with diabetes, glaucoma, heart disease, high blood pressure, or a history of stroke.

❏ Yellow dock cleanses the blood and detoxifies the liver.

❏ Black cohosh, catnip, lemon balm, passionflower, skullcap, and valerian root have antistress properties and can help nourish the nervous system.

Caution: Do not use black cohosh if you are pregnant or have any type of chronic disease. Black cohosh should not be used by those with liver problems.

❏ Ginkgo biloba helps to improve memory and brain function. Source Naturals offers an excellent extract.

Caution: Do not take ginkgo biloba if you have a bleeding disorder, or are scheduled for surgery or a dental procedure.

❏ To reduce inflammation, use holy basil, also known as tulsi or bai gka-prow (*Ocimum sanctum*), or thunder god vine (*Tripterygium wilfordii*).

Caution: Use only the roots of thunder god vine. The stems and leaves are highly toxic.

Recommendations

❏ Eat a diet consisting of 75 percent raw foods, with seeds, grains, nuts, and raw milk.

❏ Include in the diet foods containing the amino acid phenylalanine, such as almonds, Brazil nuts, fish, pecans, pumpkin seeds, sesame seeds, lima beans, chickpeas, and lentils.

Caution: Brazil nuts contain high levels of selenium, over 500 mg per ounce of nuts. If you eat Brazil nuts, adjust your supplement dosages accordingly.

❏ Reduce your intake of protein, especially if you are taking levodopa (*see under* Considerations, below). This can help with control of coordination and muscle movements. You still need protein to stay healthy; a minimum of about 60 grams (about 0.36 gram of protein per pound) a day from high-biological proteins is best. These include tofu, yogurt, beans and lentils and other legumes, meat, fish, and poultry. Try to consume your protein at times that you are not taking this medicine. Fat interferes with absorption of levodopa, so limit its intake as well.

❏ Fiber is important; those with Parkinson's disease need about 25 to 35 grams a day.

❏ If your work or a hobby exposes you to chemicals or metals such as lead or aluminum, always wear protective clothing, including gloves and a face mask.

Considerations

❏ Some people with Parkinson's disease have been found to have high levels of lead in their brains. Chelation ther-apy is the only way to remove lead from the body. (*See* CHELATION THERAPY in Part Three.)

❏ Because there are no definitive tests for Parkinson's disease, people with hypoglycemia are sometimes misdiagnosed as having the condition. (*See* HYPOGLYCEMIA in Part Two.)

❏ Fasting and chelation are both beneficial and may help to halt the progression of Parkinson's disease. (*See* FASTING and CHELATION THERAPY in Part Three.)

❏ Physical therapy, including active and passive range-of-motion exercises, plus daily moderate exercise like walking, can help to maintain normal muscle tone and function.

❏ A study conducted by the National Institute on Aging using rhesus monkeys shows a long-term low-calorie diet may offer protection from Parkinson's disease.

❏ In one study, high intakes of vitamin B_6 (greater than 1.74 milligrams per day) led to a 31 percent reduction in the risk of developing Parkinson's disease. No effect was seen for B_{12} or folic acid.

❏ Patients with Parkinson's disease who suffer from depression were shown to benefit from taking fish oil capsules, regardless of whether the fish oil was taken with or without antidepressants.

❏ "Green drinks" may significantly reduce symptoms. (*See* JUICING in Part Three.)

❏ Octacosanol, a substance found in wheat germ oil, has been shown to have beneficial effects on neuron membranes, and may make it possible to reduce the dosage of levodopa required.

❏ Iron supplementation appears to be beneficial to some people with Parkinson's disease. The production of tyrosine hydroxylase, an enzyme involved in the production of dopa (the precursor of dopamine), apparently can be stimulated by iron supplementation. Check with your physician before taking iron supplements.

❏ A study published in *The New England Journal of Medicine* concluded that when the drug selegiline (Eldepryl), also known as deprenyl, is taken in the early stages of the disease, the onset of the more disabling symptoms seems to be delayed. The drug's mechanism of action is to prevent the breakdown of a chemical in the brain called dopamine; low levels are associated with Parkinson's disease. Selegiline needs to be taken with other Parkinson's medications. Talk to your doctor about which prescription medicines and over-the-counter preparations you are using. This drug produces side effects when combined with alcohol or foods containing tyramine, such as avocados, bananas, fava beans, chocolate, aged cheeses, sausage/pepperoni, sauerkraut, soy sauce, tap beer, and red wine. It has not been proved that selegiline can actually delay or slow the disease process, as opposed to easing symptoms.

❏ Treatment with the hormone dehydroepiandrosterone (DHEA) may help to prevent Parkinson's disease. (*See* DHEA THERAPY in Part Three.)

❏ The use of antioxidant supplements may delay the need for the levodopa therapy in people with Parkinson's disease, in some cases by as much as two to three years. In one study, people with Parkinson's disease were given 3,000 milligrams of vitamin C and 3,200 international units of vitamin E daily. The results strongly suggested that the progression of the disease can be slowed significantly by the administration of high dosages of antioxidants. If Parkinson's disease is related to free radical damage of dopamine-producing brain cells, in theory, a person who takes antioxidants while still healthy might never develop Parkinson's disease. Other research is exploring the role of a naturally occurring substance, glial-cell-line-derived neutrotrophic factor (GDNF), which nourishes the neurons that produce dopamine.

❏ The first line of defense in treating Parkinson's disease is levodopa (sold under the brand names Dopar and Larodopa). However, as the disease progresses, the benefit from levodopa may wear off. A combination of levodopa and a drug called carbidopa (Parcopa, Sinemet) is also used. This drug also reduces stiffness. Other drugs that may be prescribed for people with Parkinson's disease are bromocriptine (Parlodel), pramipexole (Mirapex), and ropinirole (Requip). Some of these drugs can be used either on their own or with levodopa; others must be used with levodopa. All of these medications can cause side effects.

❏ Another drug class is anticholinergics. These drugs, which include trihexyphenidyl (Artane), benztropine (Cogentin), and biperiden (Akineton), dampen acetylcholine, a neurotransmitter that works in conjunction with dopamine to produce smooth movement. Some of the nerve cells in the brain are specialized to use either dopamine or acetylcholine to send different messages, depending on their purpose. Smooth muscle control requires a balance of dopamine and acetylcholine. In Parkinson's, there is an imbalance between the two.

❏ A treatment for episodes of hypomobility, or "off-periods," in which a person with Parkinson's disease becomes immobile or unable to perform daily activities, is apomorphine (Apokyn). Because of possible side effects and drug interactions, it should only be used under the guidance of a physician. It is the first and only prescription medication that reverses off-episode motor symptoms.

❏ Pallidotomy is a surgical procedure sometimes recommended for people with Parkinson's disease. In this technique, the surgeon uses targeted electrical current to destroy the area in the brain that is causing involuntary movements. Although this has become safer and more accurate, it is still a high-risk operation.

❏ The transplantation of brain tissue from an animal that is still manufacturing dopamine into the brains of people with Parkinson's disease has proved successful in relieving symptoms in some cases.

❏ Brain stimulators to curb involuntary movements are much like pacemakers for the heart. They can be implanted in the brain and operated by the individual when needed. A device called the Activa Tremor Control System stimulates targeted cells in the thalamus via electrodes that are implanted in the brain and connected to a neurostimulator implanted near the collarbone. The electrical stimulation can be adjusted for each person's needs. These devices require the services of a physician to obtain, implant, and maintain. Information about Activa Parkinson's Control System is available from the manufacturer, Medtronic. (*See* Manufacturer and Distributor Information in the Appendix.)

❏ Additional information on Parkinson's disease and its management is available from the National Parkinson's Foundation. (*See* Health and Medical Organizations in the Appendix).

PEPTIC ULCER

A peptic ulcer is a spot where the lining of the stomach or small intestine and the tissues beneath—and sometimes part of the stomach muscle itself—have been eroded, leaving an internal open wound. The surrounding tissue is usually swollen and irritated. Ulcers can occur anywhere along the gastrointestinal tract, but are most common in the stomach (gastric ulcers) and duodenum (duodenal ulcers), the portion of the small intestine closest to the stomach. Peptic ulcers affect approximately 4.5 million Americans each year, and it is estimated that they will affect approximately 10 percent of Americans at some point in their lives. The incidence of peptic ulcers has declined in the United States in part due to the increased use of proton-pump inhibitor drugs like omeprazole (Prilosec).

The symptoms of a peptic ulcer include chronic burning or gnawing stomach pain that usually begins forty-five to sixty minutes after eating or at night, and that is relieved by eating, taking antacids, vomiting, or drinking a large glass of water. The pain may range from mild to severe. It may cause the individual to awaken in the middle of the night. Other possible symptoms include lower back pain, headaches, a choking sensation, itching, and possibly nausea and vomiting.

An ulcer results when the lining of the stomach fails to provide adequate protection against the effect of digestive acids and enzymes, which, in effect, start to digest the stomach itself.

It was once believed that stress and anxiety were the main causes of ulcers. However, evidence has shown ulcers to be the result of infection with *Helicobacter pylori* bacteria combined with the presence of stomach acid. *H. pylori* can live on the lining of the stomach and small intestine, where it can cause damage to the lining and also to the mucous layer that protects the lining from digestive acids. Many health care professionals believe that the bacteria are transmitted from person to person through close contact. However, many health care professionals still consider stress to be a risk factor for peptic ulcers, as it increases stomach acid production. Certain drugs and supplements also may increase acid production. Taking aspirin or nonsteroidal anti-inflammatory drugs (NSAIDs), especially over a long period of time, can increase stomach acidity and lead to ulcers. Steroids, such as those taken for arthritis, can contribute to stomach ulcers. Those who consume alcohol and heavy smokers are more prone to developing ulcers, and have greater trouble getting ulcers to heal. African-Americans and Latinos are twice as likely as Caucasians to have ulcers. If left untreated, ulcers can cause internal bleeding or perforation of the stomach or small intestine.

Unless otherwise specified, the dosages recommended here are for adults. For children between the ages of twelve and seventeen, reduce the dose to three-quarters the recommended amount. For children between six and twelve, use one-half the recommended dose, and for children under the age of six, use one-quarter the recommended amount.

Stomach Acid Self-Test

If you suffer from stomach pain, you can determine whether the problem is caused by excess stomach acid with this simple test. When you have the pain, swallow a tablespoon of apple cider vinegar or lemon juice. If this makes the pain go away, you most likely have too little stomach acid, not too much. If it makes your symptoms worse, then you may have an overly acidic stomach. The suggestions in this section should help to correct the problem. If your pain is significant and has continued for several days, seek medical care.

NUTRIENTS

SUPPLEMENT	SUGGESTED DOSAGE	COMMENTS
Important		
Acid-Ease from Enzymatic Therapy	As directed on label.	Balances acidity in the body, reducing symptoms. For some people, may be able to replace ulcer medications such as ranitidine (Zantac).
L-glutamine	500 mg daily, on an empty stomach. Take with water or juice. Do not take with milk. Take with 50 mg vitamin B$_6$ and 100 mg vitamin C for better absorption.	Important in the healing of peptic ulcers. (*See* AMINO ACIDS in Part One.)
Pectin	As directed on label.	Helps relieve duodenal ulcers by creating a soothing protective coating in the intestines.
Vitamin E	200 IU daily or 400 IU every other day.	A potent antioxidant that aids in reducing stomach acid and in relieving pain. Helps promote healing. Use d-alpha-tocopherol form.
Helpful		
Acidophilus (Kyo-Dophilus from Wakunaga)	2–3 capsules, 1 to 3 times daily.	To provide flora for the small intestine that improve assimilation of nutrients and aid in digestion. Use a nondairy formula that requires no refrigeration.
Bromelain	250 mg 3 times daily.	An enzyme from pineapple that improves digestion and relieves symptoms. Chewable papaya tablets are also good.
Curcumin	250–500 mg 2 to 3 times daily, between meals.	Promotes healing.
Essential fatty acids (MaxEPA, primrose oil, or salmon oil)	As directed on label.	Protects the stomach and intestinal tract from ulcers.
Iron	As directed by physician. Take with 100 mg buffered or esterified vitamin C for better absorption.	Helps to prevent anemia, which may occur with bleeding ulcers. Use ferrous chelate or ferrous fumarate form. *Caution:* Do not take iron unless anemia is diagnosed.
or Floradix Iron + Herbs from Salus Haus	As directed on label.	A nontoxic form of iron from food sources.
Multivitamin and mineral complex	As directed on label.	To provide a balance of essential nutrients.
Proteolytic enzymes or Inf-zyme Forte from American Biologics	As directed on label. Take between meals. As directed on label.	Works on undigested food remaining in the colon, and helps to reduce inflammation. *Caution:* Do not use a formula containing HCl.
Pycnogenol or grape seed extract	As directed on label. As directed on label.	Powerful free radical scavengers that also act as anti-inflammatories and strengthen tissues.
S-Adenosylmethionine (SAMe)	200 mg twice a day, in the morning and in the evening.	Aids in relief of stress and depression, eases pain, and produces antioxidant effects. *Caution:* Do not use if you have bipolar mood disorder or take prescription antidepressants. A very small number of people taking high doses have reported gastrointestinal disturbances. If this happens, discontinue the supplement. Do not give to a child under twelve.
Vitamin A emulsion or capsules	50,000 IU daily for 1 month; then 25,000 IU daily for 1 month; then reduce to 10,000 IU daily. 25,000 IU daily. If you are pregnant, do not exceed 10,000 IU daily.	Needed for healing. Protects the mucous membranes of the stomach and intestines. Emulsion form is recommended for easier assimilation and greater safety at high doses. One study found that higher intakes of vitamin A, retinol, and provitamin A carotenoids (beta-carotene) were associated with 40 to 60 percent lower rates of gastric cancer.
Vitamin B complex	50 mg of each major B vitamin 3 times daily (amounts of individual	Needed for proper digestion. A sublingual type is best.

plus extra vitamin B$_6$ (pyridoxine)	vitamins in a complex will vary.) Do not exceed a total of 25 mg vitamin B$_3$ (niacin) daily from all sources. 50 mg 3 times daily.	Needed for enzyme production and wound healing.
Vitamin C	3,000 mg daily.	Promotes wound healing and protects against infection. Use a buffered or esterified form.
Vitamin K	100 mcg daily.	Needed for healing and to prevent bleeding; promotes nutrient absorption and has a neutralizing effect on the intestinal tract. Deficiency is common in those with digestive disorders.
Zinc	50–80 mg daily. Do not exceed a total or 100 mg daily from all supplements.	Promotes healing. Use zinc gluconate lozenges or OptiZinc for best absorption.

Herbs

❏ Alfalfa is a good source of vitamin K.

❏ Aloe vera aids in pain relief and speeds healing. Take 4 ounces of aloe vera juice or gel daily. Be sure to buy a food-grade product.

❏ Bupleurum, used in combination with angelica and licorice root, is good for treating ulcers.

Caution: Licorice root should not be used during pregnancy or nursing. It should not be used by persons with diabetes, glaucoma, heart disease, high blood pressure, or a history of stroke.

❏ Cat's claw is cleansing and healing to the digestive tract. Cat's Claw Defense Complex from Source Naturals is a combination of cat's claw and other herbs, plus antioxidant nutrients such as beta-carotene, N-acetylcysteine, vitamin C, and zinc.

Caution: Do not use cat's claw during pregnancy.

❏ Comfrey is beneficial for treating ulcers.

Caution: Do not take this herb internally for more than one month, and use it only under the close supervision of a health care professional.

❏ Garlic is an antimicrobial and may aid in eradicating ulcers.

❏ Hops, passionflower, skullcap, and valerian root are good for promoting a restful sleep. These supplements can be found in a single complex.

❏ Kava kava and St. John's wort have calming effects and reduce stress.

Cautions: Kava kava can cause drowsiness. It is not recommended for pregnant women or nursing mothers, and it should not be taken with other substances that act on the central nervous system, such as alcohol, barbiturates, antidepressants, and antipsychotic drugs. St. John's wort may cause increased sensitivity to sunlight. It may also produce anxiety, gastrointestinal symptoms, and headaches. It can interact with some drugs, including antidepressants, birth control pills, and anticoagulants.

❏ Licorice promotes healing of gastric and duodenal ulcers. Take 750 to 1,500 milligrams of deglycyrrhizinated licorice (DGL) two to three times daily, between meals, for eight to sixteen weeks. Studies have shown that DGL may be as effective as the pharmaceutical drug cimetidine (Tagamet) or ranitidine (Zantac) in treating peptic ulcers.

Caution: Do not substitute ordinary licorice root for the deglycyrrhizinated variety. Ordinary licorice can elevate blood pressure if used on a daily basis for more than seven days in a row, and should be avoided completely by persons with high blood pressure. Deglycyrrhizinated licorice has had a component known as glycyrrhizinic acid removed, which should eliminate this side effect.

❏ Malva tea calms the stomach and reduces intestinal irritation.

❏ Marshmallow root soothes irritated mucous membranes.

❏ Rhubarb, taken in juice or tablet form, is good for treating intestinal bleeding, which sometimes accompanies peptic ulcers.

❏ Other beneficial herbs include bayberry, catnip, chamomile, goldenseal, myrrh, and sage. All of these can be taken in tea form.

Cautions: Do not use chamomile if you are allergic to ragweed. Do not use during pregnancy or nursing. It may interact with warfarin or cyclosporine, so patients using these drugs should avoid it. Do not take goldenseal internally on a daily basis for more than one week at a time. Do not use it during pregnancy or if you are breast-feeding, and use with caution if you are allergic to ragweed. If you have a history of cardiovascular disease, diabetes, or glaucoma, use it only under a doctor's supervision. Do not use sage if you suffer from any type of seizure disorder, or are pregnant or nursing.

Recommendations

❏ Eat plenty of dark green leafy vegetables. These contain vitamin K, which is needed for healing and is likely to be deficient in people with digestive problems.

❏ Do not consume coffee (even decaffeinated) or alcoholic beverages.

❏ Drink freshly made cabbage juice daily. Drink it immediately after juicing. (*See* JUICING in Part Three.)

❏ If symptoms are severe, eat soft foods such as avocados, bananas, potatoes, squash, and yams. Put vegetables through a blender or food mill. Eat harder vegetables like broccoli and carrots occasionally—well steamed.

❏ Eat frequent small meals; include well-cooked millet, well-cooked rice, goat's milk, and soured milk products such as yogurt, cottage cheese, and kefir. Drink barley, wheat, and alfalfa juice. They contain chlorophyll, making them potent anti-ulcer treatments.

❑ If you have a bleeding ulcer, consume organic baby foods or steamed vegetables blended in a blender or mashed. Add nonirritating fiber such as guar gum and/or psyllium seed. These foods are easy to digest and nutritious, and they contain no chemicals.

❑ For rapid relief of pain, drink a large glass of water. This dilutes the stomach acids and flushes them out through the stomach and duodenum.

❑ Avoid fried foods, tea, caffeine, chocolate, animal fats of any kind, and carbonated drinks. Instead of drinking soda, sip distilled water with a bit of lemon juice added.

❑ Avoid salt and sugar. They have been linked to increased stomach acid production.

❑ Reduce your intake of refined carbohydrates, as they have been linked to peptic ulcers.

❑ Do not drink cow's milk. Even though it neutralizes existing stomach acid, the calcium and protein it contains actually stimulate the production of more acid, and it is known to be associated with the occurrence of ulcers. Soymilk is a good substitute.

❑ Chew your food thoroughly. This improves digestion. Taking bitters also improves digestion. Place 10 to 15 drops under your tongue before meals.

❑ Allow teas and other hot beverages to cool before drinking them. Otherwise, they may trigger gastric discomfort.

❑ Keep the colon clean. Make sure the bowels move daily, and take cleansing enemas periodically. (*See* COLON CLEANSING and ENEMAS in Part Three.)

❑ Do not smoke. Smoking can delay or even prevent healing, and makes relapse more likely.

❑ Avoid painkillers such as aspirin and ibuprofen (Advil, Nuprin, and other products) that can aggravate the ulcer.

❑ Try to avoid stressful situations. Learn stress-management techniques. (*See* STRESS in Part Two and Meditation *under* PAIN CONTROL in Part Three.) Music therapy may be helpful. (*See* MUSIC AND SOUND THERAPY in Part Three.)

Considerations

❑ Physicians can use two procedures to locate a peptic ulcer: an upper gastrointestinal (GI) series, in which you drink a chalky barium liquid and have a series of X-rays taken of the stomach and duodenum; and an endoscopy, in which a physician inserts a thin lighted tube attached to a camera down through your throat and into the stomach or duodenum.

❑ Infection with *H. pylori* is very common. About one out of six infected people develops ulcers. There are several tests available to test for *H. pylori*. They include: a direct biopsy of the stomach lining, a blood antibody test, a urea breath test, or a stool antigen test. A blood test is the most common.

❑ Because many ulcers stem from *H. pylori* bacteria, doctors use a two-pronged approach to peptic ulcer treatment: Kill the bacteria and reduce the level of acid in your digestive system to relieve pain and encourage healing. Accomplishing these two goals may require the use of at least two, and sometimes three or four, of the following medications: antibiotics to kill the organism; acid blockers to relieve ulcer pain and encourage healing; antacids to neutralize stomach acid; proton pump inhibitors to reduce acid; and cytoprotective agents that protect the tissues that line your stomach and small intestine.

❑ Acid blockers—also called histamine (H-2) blockers—reduce the amount of hydrochloric acid released into your digestive tract, which relieves ulcer pain and encourages healing. Acid blockers are available by prescription or over the counter and include: ranitidine (Zantac), famotidine (Pepcid), cimetidine (Tagamet), and nizatidine (Axid). People who take cimetidine (Tagamet) or ranitidine (Zantac) for ulcers should be cautious about ingesting alcohol. These drugs can magnify the effects of alcohol on the brain.

❑ Antacids are often recommended for people with ulcers. An antacid may be taken in addition to an acid blocker or in place of one. Instead of reducing acid secretion, antacids neutralize existing stomach acid and can provide rapid pain relief. If you must take antacids, avoid products containing aluminum, which has been linked to Alzheimer's disease. (*See* ALZHEIMER'S DISEASE in Part Two.) Maalox has been known to cause a gray film on the tongue in rare instances. Discontinue use if this occurs.

❑ Another way to reduce stomach acid is to shut down the "pumps" within acid-secreting cells. Proton pump inhibitors reduce acid by blocking the action of these tiny pumps. These drugs include the prescription and over-the-counter medications omeprazole (Prilosec), lansoprazole (Prevacid), rabeprazole (Aciphex), and esomeprazole (Nexium). However, long-term use of proton pump inhibitors, particularly at high doses, may increase your risk of hip fracture. Ask your doctor if you need a calcium supplement while taking these medications.

❑ In some cases, your doctor may prescribe cytoprotective medications that help protect the tissues that line your stomach and small intestine. They include the prescription medications sucralfate (Carafate) and misoprostol (Cytotec). A nonprescription cytoprotective agent is bismuth subsalicylate (Pepto-Bismol).

❑ Peptic ulcers were once thought to be a chronic illness that one "just has to live with." However, it is now known that 90 percent of peptic ulcers can be cured with appropriate treatment.

❑ If an ulcer does not heal, your physician may perform a biopsy to rule out cancer.

❑ The combination of two prescription medications, omeprazole (Prilosec) and clarithromycin (Biaxin, an antibiotic), may be prescribed for people with *H. pylori* infection and duodenal ulcer.

❑ Gastroesophageal reflux disease (GERD) and peptic ulcers cause very similar symptoms. However, GERD is both more common and, usually, less serious than a peptic ulcer. (*See* HEARTBURN/GASTROESOPHAGEAL REFLUX DISEASE [GERD] in Part Two.)

❑ Some believe that food allergies may be a cause of ulcers. *See* ALLERGIES in Part Two and follow the self-test program to identify possible problem foods.

PERIODONTAL DISEASE

Periodontal disease is second only to the common cold as the most prevalent infectious ailment in the United States. It affects 75 percent of Americans over the age of thirty-five and is responsible for 70 percent of adult tooth loss. The rate of periodontal disease increases with age; it is only 50 percent in adolescents.

Periodontal means "located around a tooth." Periodontal disease therefore can refer to any disorder of the gums or other supporting structures of the teeth. Gingivitis (inflammation of the gums) is the early stage of periodontal disease. It is caused by plaque—sticky deposits of bacteria, mucus, and food particles—that adheres to the teeth. The accumulation of plaque causes the gums to become infected and swollen. As the gums swell, pockets form between the gums and the teeth that act as a trap for still more plaque. Other factors that contribute to the development of gingivitis include breathing through the mouth, badly fitting fillings and prostheses that irritate surrounding gum tissue, and a diet consisting of too many soft foods that rob the teeth and gums of much-needed "exercise." Genetics also may be a factor, as a tendency toward periodontal disease seems to run in families. The gums become red, soft, and shiny, and they bleed easily. In some cases, there is pain, but gingivitis can also be essentially painless.

If left untreated, gingivitis can lead to a condition called *pyorrhea* or *periodontitis*. This is an advanced stage of periodontal disease in which the bone supporting the teeth begins to erode as a result of the infection. Abscesses are common. Pyorrhea causes halitosis, with bleeding and often painful gums. Poor nutrition, improper brushing, wrong foods, sugar consumption, chronic illness, glandular disorders, blood disease, smoking, drugs, and excessive alcohol consumption make an individual more likely to develop pyorrhea. It is often related to a deficiency of vitamin C, bioflavonoids, calcium, folic acid, or niacin. Smokers are more susceptible than nonsmokers to periodontitis and tooth loss. Periodontal disease can be made worse by missing teeth, food impaction, malocclusion, tongue thrusting, teeth grinding, and toothbrush trauma.

Stomatitis is inflammation of the oral tissues, and may affect the lips, palate, and insides of the cheeks. It often occurs as part of another disease. Stomatitis produces swollen gums that bleed easily. Sores may develop in the mouth and eventually become blisterlike lesions that can affect the gums. Two common types of stomatitis are acute herpetic stomatitis (better known as oral herpes) and aphthous stomatitis (canker sores).

Problems in the mouth often are reflections of deficiencies or underlying disorders in the body. Bleeding gums may signal a vitamin C deficiency; dryness and cracking at the corners of the mouth may indicate a deficiency of vitamin B_2 (riboflavin). Both conditions may also signal a generalized nutritional deficiency. Dry or cracked lips can be the result of an allergic reaction. Raw, red mouth tissue may be a sign of stress; a smooth, reddish tongue can indicate anemia or poor diet. Sores under the tongue can be an early warning sign of mouth cancer. Regular dental checkups can help detect these conditions early.

Warning signs of potentially severe periodontal disease include the following:

• Loose teeth.

• A change in the way your teeth fit together.

• A change in the fit of partial dentures.

• Red, swollen, or tender gums.

• Gums that bleed when you brush or floss.

• Gums that have pulled away from the teeth.

• Constant bad breath.

• Dry mouth.

• Bruxism (teeth grinding).

Unless otherwise specified, the dosages recommended here are for adults. For children between the ages of twelve and seventeen, reduce the dose to three-quarters the recommended amount. For children between six and twelve, use one-half the recommended dose, and for children under the age of six, use one-quarter the recommended amount.

NUTRIENTS

SUPPLEMENT	SUGGESTED DOSAGE	COMMENTS
Essential		
Coenzyme Q_{10} plus	100 mg daily.	Provides energy needed for gum cell growth and healing of gum tissue.
Coenzyme A from Coenzyme-A Technologies	As directed on label.	Works effectively with coenzyme Q_{10} to support the immune system's detoxification of many dangerous substances.
Vitamin C with bioflavonoids	4,000–10,000 mg daily, in divided doses throughout the day.	Promotes healing, especially of bleeding gums. Bioflavonoids retard the growth of plaque.

Vitamin A	25,000 IU daily for 1 month, then reduce to 10,000 IU daily. If you are pregnant, do not exceed 10,000 IU daily.	Needed for healing of gum tissue. Emulsion form is recommended for easier assimilation and greater safety at high doses.
plus carotenoid complex (Betatene)	As directed on label.	Antioxidants used by the body to manufacture vitamin A as needed.
Vitamin E	200 IU daily or 400 IU every other day. Also open a capsule and rub the oil on the gums 2–3 times daily.	Needed for healing of gum tissue. Use d-alpha-tocopherol form. Do *not* use the dl-form.
plus selenium (E-Sel from Carlson Labs)	200 mcg daily. If you are pregnant, do not exceed 40 mcg daily.	A powerful antioxidant that works with vitamin E.

Important

Grape seed extract	As directed on label.	A powerful antioxidant and anti-inflammatory.
Proteolytic enzymes with pancreatin	As directed on label. Take between meals and also at bedtime.	Aids in keeping down inflammation and aids proper digestion.
Quercetin	As directed on label.	Has anti-inflammatory properties.
Vitamin B complex	50 mg of each major B vitamin 3 times daily, with meals (amounts of individual vitamins in a complex will vary).	Needed for proper digestion and healthy mouth tissues.
Zinc	50–80 mg daily. Do not exceed a total of 100 mg daily from all supplements.	Enhances immune function. Needed to prevent infection and promote healing. Use zinc gluconate lozenges or OptiZinc for best absorption.
plus copper	3 mg daily.	Needed to balance with zinc.

Herbs

❏ Applying aloe vera gel directly to inflamed gums eases discomfort and soothes the tissues.

❏ Strained chamomile tea and calendula flower tea are both soothing and help to heal gum tissues.

Caution: Do not use chamomile if you are allergic to ragweed. Do not use during pregnancy or nursing. It may interact with warfarin or cyclosporine, so patients using these drugs should avoid it.

❏ Clove oil is good for temporary relief of tooth and/or gum pain. Simply rub a drop or two of clove oil on the affected area. If the oil is too strong in its pure form, it can be diluted with a drop or two of olive oil.

❏ Echinacea, hawthorn berries, myrrh gum, and rose hips all help to keep down inflammation and enhance immune function. You can apply these herbs directly to the inflamed areas as a poultice or drink them in tea form.

Caution: Do not take echinacea for longer than three months. It should not be used by people who are allergic to ragweed.

❏ Goldenseal destroys the bacteria that cause periodontal disease. Take 3,000 milligrams daily. Or place a dropperful of alcohol-free goldenseal extract in your mouth, swish it around for three minutes, then swallow. For inflamed gums, place 5 drops of alcohol-free goldenseal extract on a piece of gauze or pure cotton and place this on the inflamed area. Do this immediately whenever mouth sores or inflammation starts, and you will be amazed at the results. In severe cases, it may take three to five nights for sores to heal. Be sure to pack the gauze or cotton tightly up under the inside of the front of the mouth between the lips and gums.

Caution: Do not take goldenseal internally on a daily basis for more than one week at a time. Do not use it during pregnancy or if you are breast-feeding, and use with caution if you are allergic to ragweed. If you have a history of cardiovascular disease, diabetes, or glaucoma, use it only under a doctor's supervision.

❏ Sage is good for its anti-inflammatory properties. Boil 2 tablespoons of dried, crushed sage leaves in one cup of water, steep for twenty minutes, strain, and rinse your mouth several times daily.

Caution: Do not use sage if you suffer from any type of seizure disorder, or are pregnant or nursing.

❏ Tea tree oil, rubbed on the gums, helps to prevent and treat gum disease.

Caution: Do not take tea tree oil internally.

❏ Thyme is a natural antiseptic that reduces the level of bacteria in the mouth.

Recommendations

❏ Eat a varied diet of fresh fruits, green leafy vegetables, meat, and whole grains to provide the teeth and gums with needed exercise and supply the body with the vitamins and minerals that are essential for dental health. Although all vitamins and minerals are essential for the proper formation and continued health of the teeth, adequate vitamin C intake is particularly important for the prevention of gingivitis and pyorrhea. Vitamin A seems to control the development and general health of the gums; a lack of this vitamin often results in gum infection. Vitamin A is also necessary for healthy tooth development in children. Minerals important for healthy teeth include sodium, potassium, calcium, phosphorus, iron, and magnesium.

❏ Eat plenty of high-fiber foods, such as whole grains, vegetables, and legumes.

❏ Avoid sugar and all refined carbohydrates. Sugar causes plaque buildup and inhibits the ability of white blood cells to fight off bacteria.

❏ Brushing after every meal is best. Avoid snacking unless you can brush afterward. Especially avoid sugar-containing gum, candy, or other foods that are nibbled on throughout the day.

❑ Brush your teeth with goldenseal powder every day for at least one month. You can open up a capsule of goldenseal and mix the contents with toothpaste, or use a liquid extract in the same way. Make sure not to swallow the powder and rinse your mouth thoroughly. After one month, change brands of toothpaste. Don't stay with the same brand; some brands may irritate the gums.

Caution: Do not take goldenseal internally on a daily basis for more than one week at a time. Do not use it during pregnancy or if you are breast-feeding, and use with caution if you are allergic to ragweed. If you have a history of cardiovascular disease, diabetes, or glaucoma, use it only under a doctor's supervision.

❑ Change toothbrushes every month to keep the disease in check, and keep your toothbrush clean between uses. Bacteria live on toothbrushes. There are special devices that kill bacteria that you can keep your toothbrush in when not in use.

❑ Floss your teeth at least once a day. Unwaxed dental floss is good for getting under the gum line.

❑ Scrape your tongue each morning after you brush. Use a tongue scraper (available in health food stores and some pharmacies), the back of a spoon, or your toothbrush to brush your tongue. This is important because bacteria thrive on a moist tongue.

❑ Stim-U-Dent, found in drugstores, is beneficial for keeping the gums massaged and clean between brushing. Make sure you soak it in water or hold it in the mouth until it softens, so as not to damage the gums. Massage between each tooth between meals. This also helps to remove plaque and should be used daily after eating.

❑ Use your fingertips to massage your gums to increase circulation. Make sure your hands are clean.

❑ Interdental-space brushes are good for cleaning the spaces between teeth.

❑ Try using a dental rinse called Plax to help loosen plaque. Unlike mouthwashes, this is designed to be used before brushing.

❑ Use a *very* soft natural bristle toothbrush. Be sure to brush your gums and tongue as well as your teeth at least twice a day, but after each meal or snack is best. The most effective way to get under the gum line is to tilt the toothbrush so that the bristles are at a 45-degree angle to the gum, and brush in a forward and backward motion using short strokes across the gums to remove bacteria.

❑ If inflammation is present, run very hot water over the toothbrush to soften it before brushing, and be gentle until healing is complete.

❑ Open a capsule of vitamin E and rub the oil on inflamed gums. This is very healing and helps to alleviate soreness.

❑ For relief of toothache pain until you can get to your dentist, apply ice to the gums. Clove oil can also be helpful (*see under* Herbs, above).

❑ Avoid taking antibiotics. The mouth is the hardest place for them to work, and they destroy needed friendly bacteria in the colon. Try goldenseal first (*see under* Herbs, above).

Caution: Do not take goldenseal internally on a daily basis for more than one week at a time. Do not use it during pregnancy or if you are breast-feeding, and use with caution if you are allergic to ragweed. If you have a history of cardiovascular disease, diabetes, or glaucoma, use it only under a doctor's supervision.

❑ In addition to the products described above, we recommend the following tooth and gum products. Most of these can be bought at health food stores:

- Dentargile (Pierre Cattier). Contains a clay base for healing.

- Peelu Dental Chewing Gum. Contains a natural tooth whitener derived from the small peelu tree, native to the Middle East and Asia. People have chewed its branches for centuries to keep their teeth white. Also contains natural flavor, fruit pectin, sodium lauryl sulfate (from coconut oil), and vegetable glycerine. Unlike many over-the-counter tooth-whitening products, this does not irritate or damage gums.

- Healthy Teeth and Gums Toothpaste from the Natural Dentist. Fights plaque and gingivitis.

- Herbal Crème de Anise from Nature's Gate. Another good product found in health food stores.

- Herbal Mouth and Gum Therapy Mouth Wash from the Natural Dentist. Good for rinsing the mouth between brushes.

- Tom's Natural Toothpaste. Offers several different kinds of toothpaste.

- Weleda Salt Toothpaste. Contains baking soda and salt formulation with medicinal herbs and silica.

- Vicco Pure Herbal Ayurvedic Toothpaste. Contains extracts from plants, bark, roots, and flowers used in Ayurvedic medicine.

❑ See a dentist every six months. Be sure your dentist is taking the proper steps to avoid transmitting disease. The dentist's office and waiting room should be clean. Dentists, hygienists, and dental assistants should wash their hands and change gloves between patients. Every reusable instrument should be sterilized between patients, and large equipment and all surfaces in the treatment room should be cleaned and disinfected periodically. If you have questions about your dentist's procedures, do not hesitate to ask.

Considerations

❑ Periodontal disease should ideally be treated by a periodontist, a dentist who specializes in this area of dentistry. Your dentist should be able to refer you to one.

❏ The process of periodontal disease is easier to reverse if it is caught early. It is important to know the symptoms and get regular dental checkups for periodontal disease.

❏ Severe cases of periodontal disease may necessitate surgery to remove the infected tissue from the gum and reshape the bone.

❏ Certain illnesses, such as diabetes and several kinds of blood disorders, create a higher risk for developing gum disease.

❏ Research suggests that people who have severe periodontal disease are at greater risk of heart disease, lung disease, stroke, ulcers, poor control of diabetes, and giving birth prematurely. Studies are ongoing regarding the effect periodontal disease has on the health of the body. It is suspected that bacteria that exist in periodontal pockets may easily enter the bloodstream. So by caring for your teeth, you may also be caring for whole-body health.

❏ Regular intimate contact with an infected person can transmit the bacteria that cause periodontal disease.

❏ Smoking is a major factor in irritating the gums and mouth. It has also been linked to mouth and esophagus cancer.

❏ Some people appear to be more susceptible than others to the bacteria that cause gum disease because of a genetic predisposition.

❏ Dry mouth, a condition in which there is not enough saliva in the mouth, can promote tooth decay and periodontal disease. Saliva is essential for ridding the mouth of plaque, sugar, and debris. Dry mouth problems increase with age; more than half of people over the age of fifty-five are affected by it. It can also be caused by alcohol consumption or by prescription or over-the-counter drugs, especially those for high blood pressure, depression, colds, and allergies. Diabetes is also associated with dry mouth. The best treatment for dry mouth is to draw more moisture from the salivary glands by chewing carrots, celery, or sugar-free gum; drinking 8 to 10 cups of water a day; chewing ice chips; and/or breathing through the nose.

❏ Dental implants look more natural than dentures, and many people are opting for them. Unfortunately, improperly inserted dental implants can cause or exacerbate periodontal disease. If you are interested in implants, consult an implant specialist. Often the gum disease can be treated first, and then the implants can be done.

❏ Researchers are studying a possible link between hormone replacement therapy (HRT) and a decrease in tooth loss. Researchers at Harvard Medical School and Brigham and Women's Hospital in Boston found a 24 percent decrease in tooth loss among woman using HRT. It is suspected that this may be because HRT aids in protecting against loss of bone-mineral density in the jaw. HRT is not without its risks, however, some of them potentially serious (*see* MENOPAUSAL AND PERIMENOPAUSAL PROBLEMS in Part Two).

❏ Air abrasion technology, a dental technique that painlessly removes tooth decay without drilling, allows dentists to make smaller fillings and save more of the natural tooth. The new technique, considered to be a major breakthrough, does not necessitate numbing drugs or anesthesia.

❏ Regular dental checkups are important in detecting oral cancer, a disease that strikes 35,000 Americans each year. If oral cancer is caught early, nine out of ten people survive.

❏ One advantage (perhaps the only one) to having allergies is that people who suffer from allergies are less likely to lose teeth to periodontal disease. The reason apparently is that the allergy sufferer's overactive immune system is better at fighting off the bacteria that cause periodontal disease.

❏ There is a tablet you can purchase at most drugstores that shows areas your toothbrush missed. Chew a tablet after brushing, then brush until the color is gone.

❏ Electric toothbrushes, such as the Braun or Oral B systems, help to remove plaque.

❏ An automatic toothbrush sanitizer has been proven effective in keeping toothbrushes free of bacteria. The device automatically turns on every half-hour for two minutes to sanitize the bristles twenty-four hours a day. As an alternative, you can store your toothbrush in hydrogen peroxide or grapefruit seed extract to kill germs (if using hydrogen peroxide, rinse it well before brushing).

❏ Fluoride is a mineral that strengthens the underlying structure supporting the teeth—especially important for menopausal women who have lost density in their jawbones. Fluoride also helps to protect from decay root surfaces that become exposed as gums recede with age. There is debate among health care professionals regarding the use of fluoride. Some believe in using it, while others cite claims of immune system damage and increased cancer risk as reasons not to.

❏ Premalignant oral lesions may occur and are usually caused by tobacco. However, certain nutrients may also have an effect. In a study of 42,000 men (the Health Professionals Follow-Up Study), the risk of this type of cancer was lower in those who had high intakes of vitamin C from foods and not supplements. In contrast, men were at increased risk when they took high doses of vitamin E and beta-carotene, and this was particularly a problem for men who smoked. Taking close to the DRI for vitamin E and about 3,500 micrograms of beta-carotene posed the lowest risk.

❏ *See also* CANKER SORES and HERPES INFECTION, both in Part Two.

❏ *See also* BLEEDING GUMS *under* PREGNANCY-RELATED PROBLEMS in Part Two.

PHENYLKETONURIA

See under RARE DISORDERS.

PHLEBITIS

See THROMBOPHLEBITIS.

PHOTOPHOBIA

See under EYE PROBLEMS.

PINKEYE

See under EYE PROBLEMS.

PIRIFORMIS SYNDROME

See under RARE DISORDERS.

PKU

See PHENYLKETONURIA under RARE DISORDERS.

PLANTAR FASCIITIS

See under HEEL OR BONE SPUR.

PMS

See PREMENSTRUAL SYNDROME.

PNEUMONIA

Pneumonia is a serious infection of the lungs that can be caused by any of a number of different infectious agents, including viruses, bacteria, fungi, protozoa, and mycoplasma. The infection causes tiny air sacs in the lung area to become inflamed and filled with mucus and pus, inhibiting oxygen from reaching the blood. Lobar pneumonia affects only a section, or lobe, of one lung. Bronchial pneumonia affects portions of both lungs. Although symptoms can vary in intensity, they usually include fever, chills, cough, bloody sputum, muscle aches, fatigue, sore throat, enlarged lymph glands in the neck, cyanosis (a bluish cast to the skin and nails), pain in the chest, and rapid, difficult respiration.

Pneumonia is typically preceded by an upper respiratory tract infection such as a cold, influenza, or measles. Factors that increase the risk of pneumonia include being either under one year or over sixty years of age, a weakened immune system, cardiovascular disease, diabetes, HIV infection, seizure or stroke, aspiration under anesthesia, alcoholism, smoking, kidney failure, sickle cell disease, malnutrition, foreign bodies in the respiratory passages, exposure to chemical irritants, and even allergies.

Bacterial pneumonia can be very dangerous and may come on either suddenly or gradually, usually as a complication of some other health problem such as respiratory disease, a weakened immune system, or viral infection. Older adults, young children, alcoholics, and people who

have just undergone surgery are also at risk. *Streptococcus pneumoniae* is the most common cause of bacterial pneumonia. Symptoms usually include shaking, chills, and a high temperature. The cough is dry at first. Then a rust-colored sputum is produced, and breathing becomes rapid and labored. Chest pain that worsens upon inhalation, abdominal pain, and fatigue are also common. This type of pneumonia is unlikely to spread from one person to another.

Viral pneumonia is more variable in course and severity. It can come on suddenly or gradually, and symptoms—which are much the same as those of bacterial pneumonia—can be mild, severe, or anywhere in between. It is less serious than bacterial pneumonia, but if not cared for properly, a second, bacterial pneumonia infection can set in.

Fungal pneumonia, especially *Pneumocystis carinii* pneumonia (PCP), is much less common than either the bacterial or viral variety, and is often associated with a weakened or suppressed immune system. People with HIV or AIDS or certain types of cancer, or people who are taking immunosuppressive drugs following organ transplantation, are most likely to be affected.

Mycoplasma pneumonia, or "walking pneumonia," is caused by an agent that is unclassified but appears to be both bacterium and virus. This form of pneumonia usually affects people under forty. The symptoms tend to be less severe than those of viral or bacterial pneumonia and include a cough that is spasmodic, along with chills and a fever. Infants can contract pneumonia due to a *Chlamydia trachomatis* infection transferred to the child during birth. Childhood pneumonia can also be caused by the same bacteria that cause whooping cough.

Young children (especially infants), older adults, and people who have compromised immune systems are very vulnerable to the potentially life-threatening effects of this illness. Pneumonia is now the sixth leading cause of death in the United States. This is a condition that requires immediate medical attention. No matter what the cause, pneumonia usually leaves the sufferer with weakness that persists for four to eight weeks after the acute phase of the infection has resolved.

Unless otherwise specified, the dosages recommended here are for adults. For children between the ages of twelve and seventeen, reduce the dose to three-quarters the recommended amount. For children between six and twelve, use one-half the recommended dose, and for children under the age of six, use one-quarter the recommended amount.

NUTRIENTS

SUPPLEMENT	SUGGESTED DOSAGE	COMMENTS
Essential		
Garlic (Kyolic from Wakunaga)	As directed on label.	Protects against respiratory infections and destroys unwanted bacteria in the body.
Liquid oxygen supplement	As directed on label.	Increases oxygen intake and aids the body in eliminating toxins.

Nicotinamide adenine dinucleotide (NADH)	10 mg daily.	Important in the creation and transfer of chemical energy, especially during breathing.
Vitamin A with mixed carotenoids	Up to 25,000 IU daily. If you are pregnant, do not exceed 10,000 IU daily.	Enhances immunity and promotes repair of lung tissue. Use emulsion form for easier assimilation and greater safety at high doses. Do not take such high doses in capsule form.
Vitamin C plus bioflavonoids	5,000–20,000 mg daily, in divided doses. (*See* ASCORBIC ACID FLUSH in Part Three.) 100 mg twice daily.	Very important for immune response and for reducing inflammation. Needed to activate vitamin C.

Very Important

Free form amino acid (Amino Balance from Anabol Naturals)	As directed on label.	To supply protein, important in tissue repair.
L-carnitine plus L-cysteine plus glutathione	As directed on label, on an empty stomach. Take with water or juice. Do not take with milk. Take with 50 mg vitamin B_6 and 100 mg vitamin C for better absorption.	To protect the lungs from free radical damage and break down mucus in the respiratory tract.
Pycnogenol and/or grape seed extract	50 mg 4 times daily. As directed on label.	Boosts the immune system and protects lung tissue; reduces the frequency and severity of colds, flu, and their complications.
Vitamin B complex	100 mg of each major B vitamin 3 times daily (amounts of individual vitamins in a complex will vary).	Needed for normal digestion, production of antibodies, and formation of red blood cells, and for healthy mucous membranes. Use a sublingual form.

Important

Raw thymus glandular and raw lung glandular	500 mg each twice daily.	Stimulates immune response and promotes healing of lung tissue. (*See* GLANDULAR THERAPY in Part Three.)
Vitamin E emulsion	200 IU daily or 400 IU every other day.	A potent antioxidant that protects the lung tissues and enhances oxygen utilization. Emulsion form is recommended. Use d-alpha-tocopherol form.
Zinc	80 mg daily. Do not exceed a total of 100 mg daily from all supplements.	Needed for tissue repair and immune function. Zinc gluconate lozenges are very effective.

Helpful

Coenzyme Q_{10} plus Coenzyme A from Coenzyme-A Technologies	100 mg daily. As directed on label.	Enhances cellular oxygen utilization. Works well with coenzyme Q_{10} and supports the immune system's detoxification of many dangerous substances.

Essential fatty acids (flaxseed oil, primrose oil, salmon oil, or Ultimate Oil from Nature's Secret)	As directed on label.	Needed to build new lung tissue and to reduce inflammation. Improves stamina, speeds recovery, and boosts immunity.
Maitake extract or reishi extract or shiitake extract	As directed on label. As directed on label. As directed on label.	Mushroom extracts that help to build immunity and fight infection.
Melatonin	1.5–5 mg daily, taken 2 hours or less before bedtime.	To improve sleep. This is a natural hormone produced by the pineal gland that controls the body's sleep/wake cycle. *Caution:* This supplement is not suitable for children.
Multivitamin and mineral complex	As directed on label.	To maintain a balance of all necessary nutrients in the body.
Proteolytic enzymes (Novenzyme from International Health Products)	As directed on label 3 times daily, on an empty stomach.	Aids in absorption of nutrients and reduces inflammation.

Herbs

❑ Astragalus enhances the immune system.

Caution: Do not use astragalus in the presence of a fever.

❑ ClearLungs from RidgeCrest Herbals is an herbal combination that helps provide relief from shortness of breath, tightness in the chest, and wheezing due to bronchial congestion.

❑ Echinacea enhances immunity.

Caution: Do not take echinacea for longer than three months. It should not be used by people who are allergic to ragweed.

❑ Ginger is an effective antimicrobial agent and is helpful for fever.

❑ Goldenseal and licorice root are natural antibiotics.

Cautions: Do not take goldenseal internally on a daily basis for more than one week at a time. Do not use it during pregnancy or if you are breast feeding, and use with caution if you are allergic to ragweed. If you have a history of cardiovascular disease, diabetes, or glaucoma, use it only under a doctor's supervision. Licorice root should not be used during pregnancy or nursing. It should not be used by persons with diabetes, glaucoma, heart disease, high blood pressure, or a history of stroke.

❑ Lung Tonic from Herbs, Etc. contains a variety of herbs that support the lungs.

Recommendations

❑ See your health care provider if you suspect pneumonia. This is a potentially dangerous disease.

❑ Eat a diet consisting of raw fruits and vegetables.

❑ Take a protein supplement from a vegetable source; soy is an excellent source of nondairy protein. In addition, a free form amino acid complex may be helpful. Amino acids are the building blocks of proteins.

❑ Drink plenty of fresh juices. Liquids help to thin the lung secretions. Fast on pure juices, fresh lemon juice, and distilled water. (*See* FASTING and JUICING, both in Part Three.)

❑ Include "green drinks" in your diet or take chlorophyll in tablet form. Earth Source Greens & More from Solgar is a good green drink product.

❑ If you are taking antibiotics, take acidophilus in capsule or liquid form three times each day.

❑ Exclude dairy products, sugar, and white flour products from your diet. Make sure to get your calcium, vitamin D, and magnesium from other foods or from supplements.

❑ Do not smoke.

❑ Use a cool mist from a humidifier or vaporizer to help ease breathing.

❑ Place a heating pad or a hot water bottle on your chest to relieve pain.

❑ Consider using a device called Air Supply from Wein Products. This is a personal air purifier that is worn around the neck. It kills and deactivates airborne viruses, bacteria, molds, and spores.

❑ To avoid passing the infection along to others, dispose of secretions properly. Sneeze and/or cough into disposable tissues. Flush used tissues to discard them.

❑ Children with pneumonia have to be carefully monitored. If you suspect that your child might have pneumonia, seek medical advice immediately.

Considerations

❑ Vitamin A is necessary for maintaining the health of the lining of the respiratory passages. A deficiency of this vitamin increases susceptibility to respiratory infections, which in turn can lead to pneumonia. Deficiencies of this vitamin are almost nonexistent in the United States.

❑ Pneumococcal vaccine provides protection against more than twenty different strains of microorganisms that can cause pneumonia. It is recommended for anyone without a spleen, anyone with a chronic disease (especially diseases that affect the lungs), and everyone over the age of sixty-five.

❑ A urine test for *Streptococcus pneumoniae* takes fifteen minutes to perform. It is more efficient than diagnosis from mucus, blood, or saliva.

❑ The use of antibiotics for minor infections such as colds may lead to the development of antibiotic-resistant bacteria in the upper airway, which can cause pneumonia.

❑ *See also* INFLUENZA and COMMON COLD, both in Part Two.

POISON IVY/POISON OAK/POISON SUMAC

Poison ivy, poison oak, and poison sumac are probably the most common allergenic plants in the United States. These plants grow in every state except Alaska and are common along roadsides, in forests and pastures, and along streams—even, in the case of poison ivy, in suburban backyards.

Poison ivy and poison oak are members of the same botanical family. Poison ivy is more prevalent east of the Rocky Mountains; poison oak is more common to the west and southwest. Poison sumac is common in southern swamps and northern wetlands. All three plants produce similar symptoms, and as a result all three are often referred to simply as poison ivy.

More than half the population is allergic to one of these three plants. About 15 percent of the 120 million Americans who are allergic to poison oak, poison ivy, and poison sumac are so highly sensitive that they break out in a rash and begin to swell in four to twelve hours, instead of the usual twenty-four to forty-eight hours. Sensitivity to poison ivy is acquired and is at its peak during childhood. Most susceptible are people who are sensitive to sunlight. The irritating substance in poison ivy is urushiol, a substance present in the oily sap in the leaves, flowers, fruit, stem, bark, and roots. Urushiol is one of the most potent toxins on earth; less than 1 ounce would be enough to affect every living person. The blisters, swelling, and itching are caused by an immune system response to this poisonous sap. The plant is poisonous even long after it has dried out, but it is particularly irritating in the spring and early summer, when it is full of sap. Every part of these plants is toxic.

The first symptom of poison ivy is a burning and itching sensation. This is followed by the development of a red, intensely itchy rash, often accompanied by swelling, oozing, and crusting blisters. A mild case may involve only a few small blisters, while a severe case may cause many large blisters, acute inflammation, fever, and/or inflammation affecting the face or genitals. Symptoms can appear anywhere from a few hours to seven days after contact and tend to be at their worst between the fourth and seventh days. The rash often forms a linear pattern. Exposed parts of the body, such as the hands, arms, and face, are the areas most likely to be affected. Scratching can then spread the inflammation to other parts of the body. Itching, redness, and swelling begin to heal by the second day after the appearance of the rash, and most people are completely healed within seven to fourteen days.

Direct contact with the plant is the most common means of contracting poison ivy, but the poisons can be conveyed to the skin in other ways. Some people have contracted poison ivy by petting an animal that has been in contact with it. It can also be transmitted by clothing or objects that have come in contact with the plant. People who are highly sensitive to poison ivy can develop a reaction if the plant is burned and they inhale the smoke. Severe cases of mouth poisoning have occurred in children who have eaten the plant's leaves or grayish berries.

Unless otherwise specified, the dosages recommended here are for adults. For children between the ages of twelve and seventeen, reduce the dose to three-quarters the recommended amount. For children between six and twelve, use one-half the recommended dose, and for children under the age of six, use one-quarter the recommended amount.

NUTRIENTS

SUPPLEMENT	SUGGESTED DOSAGE	COMMENTS
Important		
Vitamin C with bioflavonoids	3,000–8,000 mg daily.	To prevent infection and spreading of the rash. A natural antihistamine that reduces swelling.
Helpful		
Calamine lotion	Apply topically as directed on label.	Contains calamine, phenol, and zinc oxide. Has drying properties for faster healing.
Shark cartilage	1 gram per 15 lbs of body weight daily, divided into 3 doses.	Reduces inflammation.
Vitamin A with mixed carotenoids	25,000 IU daily. If you are pregnant, do not exceed 10,000 IU daily.	Needed for healing of skin tissue. Also boosts the immune system.
Vitamin E oil or cream	Apply topically as directed on label. Apply topically as directed on label.	To aid in healing and prevent scarring.
Zinc	80 mg daily. Do not exceed a total of 100 mg daily from all supplements.	Needed for repair of skin tissues. Use zinc gluconate lozenges or OptiZinc for best absorption.

Herbs

❑ Aloe vera gel helps relieve burning and itching. Apply pure aloe vera gel as directed on the product label or as needed.

❑ A strong tea made of equal parts lime water and white oak bark is very good for poison ivy, poison oak, or poison sumac. Apply a compress wet with this solution. Replace the compress with a fresh one as often as it becomes dry.

❑ Marshmallow root both soothes and heals skin.

❑ Tea tree oil disinfects and heals skin conditions. Melagel, an ointment that contains tea tree oil, is very effective.

❑ Witch hazel helps stop itching and aids in healing.

❑ The following herbs can be used topically as remedies for poison ivy, poison oak, or poison sumac: black walnut extract, bloodroot, echinacea, goldenseal, and myrrh. Black walnut has antiseptic properties and helps to fight infection; bloodroot reduces swelling; echinacea promotes healing of skin wounds; goldenseal is good for skin inflammation; myrrh is a powerful antiseptic. Echinacea can also be taken internally to boost the immune system.

Cautions: Do not use bloodroot during pregnancy. Do not take echinacea for longer than three months. It should not be used by people who are allergic to ragweed. Do not take goldenseal internally on a daily basis for more than one week at a time. Do not use it during pregnancy or if you are breast-feeding, and use with caution if you are allergic to ragweed. If you have a history of cardiovascular disease, diabetes, or glaucoma, use it only under a doctor's supervision.

Recommendations

❑ Treat a mild case of poison ivy with one or more of the following:

• Apply compresses made with very hot plain water for brief intervals.

• Apply compresses soaked in a diluted Burow's solution (use 1 pint to 15 pints of cool water). You can purchase Burow's solution at most drugstores.

• Soak the affected skin in cool water with colloidal oatmeal (Aveeno) added, available at most drugstores.

• For relief of itching, apply a paste made from water, cornstarch, baking soda, oatmeal, or Epsom salts. Use 1 teaspoon of water to 3 teaspoons of the dry ingredient.

• Apply aloe vera juice, tofu, or watermelon rind to the area for cooling relief. Using 1 pint of buttermilk with 1 tablespoon of sea salt added may be helpful.

• Use an herbal preparation suggested under Herbs, above.

• Try homeopathic remedies. *Rhus toxicodendron* is the classic homeopathic remedy for poison ivy. It relieves itching and promotes healing. Poison Ivy/Oak Tablets from Hyland's is a homeopathic combination remedy for poison ivy.

❑ If alternative therapies are not working, try some over-the-counter remedies. Commonly used over-the-counter medications include IvyBlock, which reduces the severity of the rash; Tecnu Skin Cleanser; Ivy Stat; Benadryl; calamine lotion; Burt's Bees Poison Ivy Soap; Ivy-Dry; and low-dose steroids.

❑ For a severe case of poison ivy, consult a physician. Symptoms that warrant medical attention include an extensive rash that covers more than half of the body; extreme swelling and redness; and fever. You should also consult your health care provider if poison ivy occurs near the eyes, mouth, or genitals.

❑ Stay cool. Sweating and heat can make itching worse.

Considerations

❑ Oral prednisone is sometimes prescribed to relieve itching and reduce swelling. However, this treatment should be reserved only for very severe cases involving fever, difficulty urinating, dangerous facial or genital swelling, or other symptoms of acute illness. Oral steroids are extremely powerful drugs and can cause serious side effects, when misused.

❑ The toxin urushiol does not affect dogs or cats, but they can bring the irritating substance home on their fur and pass it to you. If you suspect your pet may have walked through poison ivy or poison oak, wash the animal thoroughly (wear rubber gloves and protective clothing).

❑ Prevention is better than treatment when it comes to poison ivy, poison oak, and poison sumac. When spending time outdoors, keep the following in mind:

- Lightweight fabrics do not provide adequate protection against poison ivy or oak, because the sap can easily penetrate them. Wear gloves and heavier clothing if you might be exposed to these plants.

- Everyone, even children, should learn to recognize, and avoid, these harmful plants. Poison ivy usually grows as a vine, but it can also take the form of a shrub, growing anywhere from two to seven feet high. Its leaves always grow in clusters of three, one at the end of the stalk, the other two opposite each other. Poison oak grows as a shrub exclusively, and its leaves are lobed, like oak leaves. Like those of poison ivy, they grow in threes. Poison sumac grows as a shrub or small tree that has multiple leaflets growing on both sides of a stem. The number of leaflets may range from seven to thirteen, but it is always an odd number.

- Appropriate protective clothing should be worn for activities that take you into forests or through thick underbrush—long pants, a long-sleeved shirt, shoes, socks, and gloves. These items should be washed after they are worn; if they come into contact with poison ivy, they are not safe to wear again until they have been laundered or dry-cleaned.

- If you know or suspect that you may have come in contact with poison ivy, remove all clothing and shoes, and *immediately* scrub your skin using brown or yellow laundry soap (such as Fels Naptha) and water or alcohol to remove the irritating oil. Lather several times and rinse in running water after each sudsing. This procedure is useless if not done within ten minutes; after that time, the oil will have penetrated the skin and cannot be washed off. Wash clothing, gear, or pack material in plenty of hot, soapy water, with chlorine bleach added, if possible. Stubborn cases of poison ivy that do not respond to proper treatment are often due to repeated contact with contaminated clothing.

POISONING

There are literally thousands of substances, both natural and synthetic, that can cause poisoning. Many of these are present in everyday items and products, including drugs,

---

Poison Control Center

It is a good idea to post the number of the American Association of Poison Control Centers somewhere accessible, especially if you have young children. If you can program your telephone for automatic dialing, you may wish to add the number to your phone's programming as well. The operator at this general number will immediately forward you to your local Poison Control Center for emergency guidance.

UNITED STATES

www.dorway.com/poisons.html
800-222-1222

---

cleaning products, pesticides, paints and varnishes, hobby and art supplies, batteries, cosmetics, and houseplants. Some are poisonous only if ingested; others can cause problems if inhaled or absorbed through the skin or eyes.

Most cases of accidental poisoning involve young children, especially children under the age of five. Young children are very curious, and their preferred method of exploring often involves putting things in their mouths. However, there are also many cases of poisoning every year among elderly people and hospital patients (most commonly the result of overmedication or drug mix-ups), as well as adolescents, who may experiment with the ingestion of toxic substances, including recreational drugs. Other causes of poisoning include exposure to environmental pollutants and toxic substances used in the workplace. Toxins in food can also cause poisoning. (*See* FOODBORNE AND WATERBORNE DISEASE in Part Two.)

Recommendations

❑ If you suspect that you or another person has been poisoned, call the American Association of Poison Control Centers (see phone number listed above) and follow its directions. The appropriate measures to take depend on the toxin involved and the method of ingestion. The professionals who staff these centers will be able to tell you what to do.

Keep a bottle of syrup of ipecac and charcoal tablets, available in drugstores and health food stores, on hand at all times. However, *do not* use syrup of ipecac unless specifically directed to do so by a physician or your Poison Control Center. For some poisonous substances, it is not advisable to take anything by mouth—for example, if the poison contains an acid that will create more internal burning. If advised to do so by the Poison Control Center, take 5 charcoal tablets immediately. This will help to absorb the poison. Do not use charcoal tablets that are not made for internal use.

❏ Childproofing your house is essential if children or grandchildren are around. Keep cleaning items up in high cupboards and not under the sink. Drain cleaner (lye) is particularly caustic if ingested, so make sure this is out of reach of children.

❏ If you are directed to go to the nearest hospital emergency room, take the container of the suspected poison with you, if possible. This can help medical personnel to deal with the situation and save precious time.

Considerations

❏ When dealing with suspected poisoning, it is better to rely on the advice of a Poison Control Center staff member rather than the information on product packaging. Poison Control Centers keep up-to-date with the latest knowledge and practices; information provided by manufacturers may not be as current or reliable.

❏ *See also* ALUMINUM TOXICITY; ARSENIC POISONING; CADMIUM TOXICITY; CHEMICAL POISONING; COPPER TOXICITY; ENVIRONMENTAL TOXICITY; FOODBORNE/WATERBORNE DISEASE; LEAD POISONING; MERCURY TOXICITY; and/or NICKEL TOXICITY, all in Part Two.

POLYPS

Polyps are benign (noncancerous) growths of various sizes that are found on stalk-like structures growing from the epithelial lining of the large intestine, cervix, bladder, nose, and other body structures. They are most common in the rectum and sigmoid colon, and usually occur in groups.

Most polyps of the colon and/or rectum cause no symptoms at all and are discovered only during routine physical examinations that include examination of the colon (colonoscopy), or during examination or treatment of other disorders. If they are very large, however, they may cause rectal bleeding, cramping, or abdominal pain. The relationship between polyps and cancer is not fully understood. Some physicians believe most colon cancers begin as polyps. However, most polyps probably do not turn into cancer. On the other hand, it is true that many people who have a cancerous growth in the colon also have multiple polyps surrounding that growth, and it does appear that the larger a polyp grows, the greater the chance that it will become malignant.

Familial polyposis is a hereditary disease in which large numbers of growths (one hundred or more) develop in the colon. If removed, they grow back. Rectal bleeding and mucous drainage are common symptoms. This disorder is more closely linked to cancer than ordinary polyps are; unless it is treated, it virtually always leads to colon cancer.

Cervical polyps line the inside of the cervix, the passage from the vagina into the uterus. Symptoms indicative of cervical polyps include a heavy, watery, bloody discharge from the vagina. Bleeding may occur after sexual intercourse, between periods, and after menopause. The growth of cervical polyps may be caused by infection, injury to the cervix, or hormonal changes during pregnancy. Polyps are more common in women who have not had children. Women with diabetes also have a higher than normal chance of developing polyps. A Pap smear may or may not detect cervical polyps. They rarely return once removed.

Bladder polyps produce blood in the urine. Unless they are removed, cancer of the bladder may follow.

Nasal polyps usually form in the back of the nose, near the openings into the sinuses. They too can bleed and can interfere with normal breathing. People with hay fever and other nasal allergies are most prone to nasal polyps, as are people who overuse nose drops and nasal sprays.

Polyps on the vocal cords are caused by abuse (such as from repeated and prolonged episodes of screaming or, among singers especially, improper vocal technique), usually in the presence of an infection. People who smoke or have allergies are more susceptible. Vocal cord polyps usually cause painless hoarseness.

Unless otherwise specified, the dosages recommended here are for adults. For children between the ages of twelve and seventeen, reduce the dose to three-quarters the recommended amount. For children between six and twelve, use one-half the recommended dose, and for children under the age of six, use one-quarter the recommended amount.

NUTRIENTS

SUPPLEMENT	SUGGESTED DOSAGE	COMMENTS
Essential		
Multivitamin and mineral complex plus extra	As directed on label.	Provides a balance of necessary nutrients.
calcium and	1,000–1,500 mg daily.	Protects against colorectal polyps and colon cancer.
magnesium	750 mg daily.	Assists in the absorption of calcium.
Vitamin A with mixed carotenoids	25,000 IU daily. If you are pregnant, do not exceed 10,000 IU daily.	Protects the membranous linings. Use emulsion form for easier assimilation.
Vitamin C with bioflavonoids	5,000–10,000 mg daily, in divided doses.	Can reduce the number of polyps, and may eliminate them altogether.
Very Important		
Vitamin E	200 IU daily or 400 IU every other day.	A potent antioxidant. Protects against the effects of lipid peroxidation; if deficiency occurs, cells are vulnerable to damage. Use d-alpha-tocopherol form.
Important		
ABC Aerobic Bulk Cleanse from Aerobic Life Industries	As directed on label. Take with aloe vera juice.	Cleanses the colon, assisting in normal stool formation to aid in removing harmful toxins.

Helpful		
Coenzyme Q$_{10}$ plus	60 mg daily.	An important antioxidant. Increases cellular oxygen levels.
Coenzyme A from Coenzyme-A Technologies	As directed on label.	Works well with coenzyme Q$_{10}$ to support adrenal glands and boost the immune system.
ConcenTrace trace mineral drops from Trace Minerals Research	As directed on label.	Normalizes electrolytes after bowel cleansing.
Garlic (Kyolic from Wakunaga)	2 capsules 3 times daily, between meals.	Acts as a natural antibiotic and enhances immune function.
Superoxide dismutase (SOD) or	As directed on label.	An important antioxidant and free radical destroyer.
Cell Guard from Biotec Foods	As directed on label.	An antioxidant complex that contains SOD.

Herbs

❑ Aloe vera juice improves digestion and cleanses the digestive tract.

❑ Butcher's broom, cardamom, cayenne, cinnamon, *Garcinia cambogia*, ginger, green tea, and mustard seed are thermogenic herbs that improve digestion.

Cautions: Do not use cinnamon in large quantities during pregnancy. Green tea contains vitamin K, which can make anticoagulant medications less effective. Consult your health care professional if you are using them. The caffeine in green tea could cause insomnia, anxiety, upset stomach, nausea, or diarrhea.

❑ Cascara sagrada is a colon cleanser and laxative.

❑ Coloklysis from PhysioLogics contains herbs and a blend of soluble and insoluble fiber to support healthy digestion.

Recommendations

❑ A high-fiber diet with no animal fats is important. Include in your diet apricots, broccoli, brown rice, cabbage, cantaloupe, carrots, cauliflower, garlic, oatmeal, onions, green peppers, sweet potatoes, sesame seeds, spinach, sunflower seeds, and whole grains. Fruits with edible seeds, such as figs, raspberries, strawberries, and even bananas, tend to contain lots of fiber. *See* CANCER in Part Two and follow the diet recommended there.

❑ Take some form of supplemental fiber daily. Barley, legumes, oat bran, psyllium husks (in Aerobic Bulk Cleanse), and rice bran are good sources of fiber.

Note: Always take supplemental fiber separately from other supplements and medications.

❑ Be sure to increase your water intake when increasing fiber consumption. If you do not, it may result in bloating, gas, pain, and constipation. Increase fiber intake slowly over several weeks.

❑ Exclude from your diet fried foods, highly processed foods, caffeine, and alcohol. Do not use tobacco.

❑ Regular physical examinations are important, particularly after age forty. A digital rectal exam is easily performed in the physician's office and can quickly determine if there are any abnormalities along the colon wall. Beyond age fifty, a colonoscopy is recommended.

❑ If you experience rectal bleeding, or if blood appears in the stool, consult your physician. A fecal occult blood test (FOBT) should be done to identify the source of the blood. Bleeding can be a symptom of polyps, but it also can be a sign of cancer.

Considerations

❑ The treatment of choice for most polyps, regardless of location, is surgical removal. In most cases this is a relatively minor procedure, often performed on an outpatient basis.

❑ Vocal cord polyps may be treated with humidification, speech therapy, and rest. Surgical removal of the polyps may be necessary.

❑ For familial polyposis, a surgical procedure called a colectomy (removal of the colon) may be necessary. In some cases, the rectum is left in place and connected to the small intestine to allow for bowel evacuation. However, in most cases, polyps return in the rectum.

❑ Research has found that men with the highest consumption of saturated fat were twice as likely to develop potentially malignant polyps as men who limited their fat intake.

POSTURAL TACHYCARDIA SYNDROME

See under RARE DISORDERS.

PREGNANCY-RELATED PROBLEMS

Many women find being pregnant a thoroughly enjoyable experience and suffer very few unpleasant symptoms, but there are those who discover that being pregnant can lead to some uncomfortable effects. Very few of these incidental discomforts threaten either the fetus or the expectant mother—but the more enjoyable a pregnancy, the better for both mother and child.

Pregnancy lasts for approximately forty weeks. This time is commonly divided into three periods, or trimesters: from the first day of the last menstrual period to week 12; from week 12 to week 28; from week 28 until delivery.

Most of the discomforts that occur during pregnancy are the result of hormonal changes within the body, nutritional deficiencies, and profound anatomical changes. This section addresses some of the most common pregnancy-related problems and offers natural remedies as well as helpful hints and suggestions for maintaining maximum health during pregnancy. For a healthy pregnancy and birth, it is necessary to consult and work with a qualified health care professional, be it a physician, nurse practitioner, or midwife. It is also wise to work with your health care practitioner on a birth plan. (*See* Birth Plan on page 660.) This allows you to decide in advance what you want and what you would choose from among your options before, during, and after labor.

PREGNANCY SELF-TEST

Over-the-counter pregnancy test kits are sold in most drugstores. You should always see your health care provider to confirm a positive result.

ANEMIA

During pregnancy, blood volume (the amount of blood circulating in the body) increases by as much as 50 percent. The increase in volume is largely due to an increase in plasma (the liquid part of blood) rather than in red (or white) blood cells. Plasma volume, then, is increasing faster than red blood cell volume. The protein hemoglobin, which carries oxygen to the body's cells, inhabits red blood cells. Because there is a decreased proportion of red blood cells in the blood, there is also a decreased proportion of hemoglobin, and the result can be anemia.

Anemia is most likely to develop in the second trimester of pregnancy. It can cause fatigue, a rapid heartbeat, and paleness of the skin, gums, and around the inside of the eye. There may also be cravings to eat substances other than food, such as coal, dirt, ice, starch, or hair. This is called *pica* and is normally the sign of a nutritional deficiency.

Anemia is unlikely to affect the developing baby. The fetus depletes the mother's iron resources and does not suffer any deficiency itself.

Recommendations

❑ Make sure you have enough folic acid, vitamin B_{12}, and the other B-complex vitamins in your diet.

❑ Eat foods rich in iron, such as organically raised red meat and liver. Other foods that have lesser amounts include green leafy vegetables, prunes, raisins, and bread and pastas made from whole-grain flour.

❑ If your health care provider prescribes iron supplements, take them with vitamin C to help the absorption of this mineral. Iron supplements can also cause constipation, so eat plenty of high-fiber foods and increase your fluid intake.

Note: Do not take iron supplements unless anemia has been diagnosed.

ASTHMA

Many women who have asthma reduce their use of asthma medication when they become pregnant to avoid harming the fetus—and as a result, their asthma symptoms become worse. It currently appears that there is more danger to a developing fetus from frequent asthma attacks than from taking asthma medications. Inhaled medications are normally preferred during this time because they are more localized in action. Asthma sufferers should be checked at least every four to six weeks by a physician during pregnancy. You should discuss your medication in detail with your physician.

Recommendations

❑ Avoid anything that might trigger an attack. Keep your bedroom, at least, as a place you can go to relax and get away from any airborne pollutants that can trigger an attack.

❑ The Air Supply personal air purifier from Wein Products is a miniature unit that is worn around the neck. It sets up an invisible, pure air shield against microorganisms (such as viruses, bacteria, and mold) and microparticles (including dust, pollen, and pollutants) in the air. It also eliminates vapors, smells, and harmful volatile compounds in the air.

BACKACHE

Backache is common during pregnancy due to the considerable anatomical changes and stresses in the body. The increase in body weight, the muscle-relaxing effects of the hormone progesterone, and the shift in one's center of gravity contribute to the problem.

Recommendations

❑ To minimize back pain during pregnancy, do not stay in any one position for a long period of time.

❑ Pay attention to your posture. Keep your shoulders relaxed and your back as straight as possible at all times.

❑ Swimming is a good way to relieve the strain on the back and on all other parts of the body.

❑ Include two to three minutes of gentle stretching exercises in your daily routine. Do not strain—stretch only to your comfort level.

❑ Make sure your mattress is firm enough to support you, and sleep with a pillow supporting your back. Sleep on your side, not on your back.

❑ Do not wear high-heeled shoes. High heels throw your body off balance and put extra strain on your back. Instead, wear well-fitting, well-padded flat or low-heeled shoes that support your feet and provide ample room for your toes. Be aware that you may require larger shoes than normal while you are pregnant.

❏ Teach your partner or friends how to massage your back. You can use liniments or herbal oils.

❏ Learn how to lift correctly, putting less pressure on the back.

❏ When your back hurts, try soaking a small towel in apple cider vinegar. Squeeze out any excess and lie down on your side in bed. Spread the towel directly across your back. Relax this way for fifteen to twenty minutes.

❏ *See also* BACKACHE in Part Two.

BLADDER DISCOMFORT/INFECTION

During pregnancy, the bladder is pressed upon by an expanding uterus and must, in general, deal with far more fluids. You may need to urinate more frequently. However, the bladder may not always empty fully, so infections of the bladder are very common. These should always be treated.

Recommendations

❏ Avoid sugary foods. Infectious bacteria thrive on sugar.

❏ Increase your fluid intake. Drink quality bottled or filtered water rather than tap water. *Do not* cut back on liquids because of urinary frequency.

❏ Eat plain natural yogurt every day. This helps to maintain the correct balance of natural "friendly" bacteria in the system.

❏ Wear cotton underwear, or at least underwear that is cotton-lined. Avoid wearing anything tight or containing synthetic material next to your skin.

❏ Do not douche.

❏ *See also* BLADDER INFECTION (CYSTITIS) and CANDIDIASIS in Part Two.

BLEEDING GUMS

During pregnancy, increasing estrogen levels cause the gums to swell and become somewhat softer than normal, and the circulation of blood to them increases. This makes the gums more prone to bleeding and infection, especially if good oral hygiene is not maintained.

Recommendations

❏ Be sure your diet contains enough calcium and high-quality, complete proteins such as soy products.

❏ Increase your intake of foods rich in vitamin C, as a deficiency in this vitamin can contribute to bleeding gums.

❏ If you smoke, quit—preferably *before* you get pregnant. Cigarette smoking reduces the oxygen supply to the developing fetus and also drains vitamin C from the body.

❏ Brush your teeth three to four times daily (remembering to rinse your mouth well), and massage your gums with clean fingers when necessary. Floss your teeth daily.

❏ See your dentist at least once during the pregnancy, and be sure to inform the dentist that you are pregnant. *Do not* permit him or her to take any dental X-rays while you are pregnant.

CONSTIPATION

Hormonal changes during pregnancy have a relaxing effect on the muscles, including those of the digestive tract. The increasing level of progesterone in your system makes the bowels less efficient. The normal rhythmic contractions of the intestines slow down, and the result can be constipation. This happens most often in the third trimester.

Recommendations

❏ Eat fresh and dried fruit such as prunes, raisins, and figs.

❏ Eat fresh vegetables and salads containing a variety of raw green and colored vegetables daily.

❏ Increase the amount of fiber in your diet. Whole-grain breads, cereals, and bran are helpful. Begin by taking 2 teaspoons of bran in a glass of apple juice twice daily. The bran may cause some gas until your system is used to it, but after that you should not have any difficulty.

❏ Drink ten 8-ounce glasses of liquid, including water, each day.

❏ Walk at least a mile a day.

❏ Set a regular time each day for a bowel movement. This is very helpful for digestion and elimination. Elevate your feet and legs during elimination to relax the anal muscles.

❏ If your health care provider prescribes iron supplements, be aware that they can cause constipation. Increase your fluid intake and eat a diet high in fiber. Some iron supplements have a stool softener added to them; if you are having trouble with the iron supplements, ask your health care provider about them.

❏ *Do not* take over-the-counter laxatives unless specifically recommended by your health care provider.

❏ *See* HEMORRHOIDS later in this section.

❏ *See also* CONSTIPATION in Part Two.

COUGHS AND COLDS

Coughs and colds are more common during pregnancy and are often more difficult than usual to shake off. Once you have a cold, there is little you can do but let it run its course, so prevention is most important.

Recommendations

❑ Eat a healthy diet and increase your consumption of foods containing vitamin C.

❑ For congestion, make a steam inhaler using essential oil of eucalyptus, lavender, or lemon.

❑ *See* COMMON COLD in Part Two for additional recommendations. You can use any of the external remedies mentioned, but consult your health care provider before taking any nutrients or other supplements internally.

DEPRESSION

Depression is fairly common during pregnancy. It can come and go, but because of shifting hormone levels, it is not uncommon to experience at least one bout of depression at some point during the forty weeks of pregnancy. Mood swings are common too. It is not unusual to find that you are more emotional and volatile during pregnancy. It helps if people around you are sympathetic to this and know what to expect.

Recommendations

❑ Do not continue to feel depressed without seeking help. Having someone to talk to and knowing that you are not alone in experiencing these feelings can help you to cope during times of depression.

❑ Acupuncture has been used successfully for hundreds of years to treat depression.

❑ Exercise can help to lessen depression.

❑ Be open about your fears and concerns relating to having a child. Pregnancy and childbirth are profound experiences, and many women experience feelings of anxiety about the responsibilities attached to this event. Pregnancy is a complicated emotional experience, and you should be aware that it is normal not to be happy all the time.

❑ If you become pregnant while taking antidepressants, consult your physician about the possible effect on the development of the fetus. You should not stop taking your medication without discussing it with your physician.

DIABETES, GESTATIONAL

This is a form of diabetes that occurs only during pregnancy. It affects about 4 percent of pregnant women and about 135,000 cases occur each year in the United States. It occurs because insulin, which regulates blood sugar, does not work as efficiently during pregnancy due to hormones secreted by the placenta. Blood sugar can become high, and although this condition rarely causes harm to the mother, the baby's birth weight often increases, and the baby may be born with a low blood sugar level. A problem may arise if the baby's birth weight is excessive enough to make delivery complicated. *Macrosomia* (heavy birth weight), a poten-

tial complication, is defined as a birth weight over 9 pounds 14 ounces.

Women are normally tested for blood sugar levels around the twenty-eighth week of pregnancy. The 50-gram screen (gestational diabetes screening) involves drinking a glass of very sweet liquid containing 50 grams of sugar and testing the blood sugar level one hour later to see how your body has processed the sugar. Symptoms of gestational diabetes may include frequent urination, excessive thirst, and increased fatigue, but it is also likely that there will be no symptoms at all.

Recommendations

❑ Eat a little at a time, but frequently. Do not miss meals, even if you are experiencing nausea.

❑ Discuss your dietary intake with your health care provider. Try to keep to the recommended schedule for weight gain.

❑ Avoid foods rich in sugar, and remember that some carbohydrates increase blood sugar levels more than sugar. (*See* DIABETES in Part Two.)

Considerations

❑ If a baby is born with low blood sugar, sweet drinks can alleviate the condition; these are to be administered by your health care team. The baby's blood sugar level should return to normal within hours. The mother's blood sugar level also should return to normal after delivery.

❑ If the baby is too large, your health care provider may recommend delivering the baby early, possibly by cesarean section.

DIZZINESS

During pregnancy, especially during the second trimester, blood pressure often drops as the expanding uterus presses on major blood vessels. The blood supply also has extra work to do, and at times the blood may pool in the lower part of the body, leaving the brain a bit short of oxygen for brief moments. These factors can cause dizziness.

Recommendations

❑ Do not change positions quickly. Always go from lying down to sitting to standing slowly. Take your time and focus on what you are doing.

❑ If you have to stand for long periods, keep moving and flexing your muscles to make sure the blood is circulating properly.

❑ Do not take hot baths.

❑ If you feel dizzy, sit down somewhere safe. Try lowering your head to your knees until the feeling passes.

❑ If you have diabetes, make sure your blood sugar level is well controlled. (*See* DIABETES in Part Two.)

ECLAMPSIA AND PREECLAMPSIA

Preeclampsia is a complication of pregnancy characterized by high blood pressure, edema (swelling due to fluid retention), and an excess of protein in the urine. It may develop in the second half of pregnancy or later. The cause is not known, but if you have suffered from this complaint during a prior pregnancy, you are at increased risk of having it again in following pregnancies. Other risk factors include multiple births, kidney disease, diabetes, lupus, long-term high blood pressure, and heredity. A small percentage of women who develop preeclampsia go on to develop eclampsia, with seizures and/or coma.

It was once thought that eclampsia and preeclampsia were a result of toxemia—the presence of some sort of toxin or poison in the bloodstream—but it is now known that this is not the case. If you develop *any* of the symptoms of preeclampsia, you must be monitored constantly by your health care provider.

The dosages given below are for adults.

NUTRIENTS

SUPPLEMENT	SUGGESTED DOSAGE	COMMENTS
Essential fatty acids (black currant seed oil, flaxseed oil, Kyolic-EPA from Wakunaga, olive oil, or primrose oil)	As directed on label or by your physician.	Improves circulation, lowers blood pressure, and thins the blood. *Caution:* If you have blood-clotting problems, do not take this supplement.
Garlic (Kyolic from Wakunaga)	As directed on label.	Effective in lowering blood pressure.
Vitamin E	200 IU daily or 400 IU every other day.	Improves circulation. Use d-alpha-tocopherol form.

Recommendations

❑ Get adequate rest. Rest is vitally important if you develop this condition.

❑ Make sure that your physician or midwife is aware of any risk factors you may have for preeclampsia.

Considerations

❑ If you develop high blood pressure without any of the other symptoms of preeclampsia, your physician may recommend treatment for high blood pressure.

❑ Because the cause is not known, there is no specific treatment for eclampsia except delivery of the baby.

ECTOPIC PREGNANCY

An ectopic pregnancy, sometimes called a tubal pregnancy, is a situation in which a fertilized egg becomes implanted in a fallopian tube rather than in the uterus. The result is that the pregnancy is not viable because there is not room for the fetus to grow. This can happen if the fallopian tube is blocked due to inflammation, scar tissue, or endometriosis, making it impossible for the egg to pass into the uterus. Other possible causes for ectopic pregnancy include anatomical abnormalities such as a misshapen fallopian tube.

The easiest way to diagnose an ectopic pregnancy, after a pelvic examination, is to measure levels of human chorionic gonadotropin (hCG), a hormone produced by the placenta that increases in quantity until the end of the first trimester. If the hCG level is *not* increasing, a physician may decide that the pregnancy is not proceeding as it should and order more tests, such as an ultrasound, to find out where the fetus is growing.

Considerations

❑ There is no known way to salvage an ectopic pregnancy. The fetus must be removed to preserve the life of the woman. This is usually done surgically and laparoscopically.

❑ You are more at risk for this condition if you have had a previous ectopic pregnancy. Discuss this risk with your health care provider.

EDEMA (SWELLING) OF THE HANDS AND FEET

The rise in estrogen in the body during pregnancy increases the tendency to retain fluids. This can cause some swelling of the hands and feet, and is considered normal—but it must be monitored continually because it may be an indication of a more serious condition called preeclampsia.

Recommendations

❑ Early in the pregnancy, remove any rings you wear on a regular basis. Do not wait, or the rings may have to be cut off.

❑ As soon as you notice your hands, legs, or feet getting puffy or larger than usual, tell your health care provider. While some swelling is acceptable, the condition should nevertheless be evaluated by a professional, as edema can also be the first sign of preeclampsia, a potentially serious complication of pregnancy.

❑ Avoid salt and all highly processed foods, while maintaining a well-balanced high-protein diet. *Do not* take diuretics (water pills).

❑ Wear loose, comfortable clothing and properly fitting shoes. You may require larger shoes than normal. Once the baby arrives, your feet will return to normal.

❑ When you are relaxing, sit with your feet elevated.

❑ Walk one mile each day. This helps to keep edema under control.

❑ *See also* EDEMA in Part Two.

GAS (FLATULENCE)

Gas, like other digestive upsets, is a common complaint during pregnancy. Even foods that cause no difficulties at other times may begin to cause trouble.

Recommendations

❏ Keep a food diary to help you determine which foods, or combinations of foods, seem to be causing the gas. Avoid any suspect foods.

❏ You may have to adapt your usual diet during pregnancy. Many foods you liked before may suddenly seem unappealing.

❏ Eat four to five small meals a day, instead of three big meals. Chew your food slowly and well. Do not overtax your digestive system. Be careful not to increase your caloric intake so much that weight gain becomes excessive.

❏ Eat four or more servings of fresh fruits and vegetables every day.

❏ Cook vegetables quickly using a perforated steamer instead of boiling them for long periods of time.

❏ Drink as much quality water (not tap water) as you can.

❏ Get adequate exercise. Walking is an excellent way to alleviate gas.

❏ To reduce gas-causing sulfur compounds in beans (garbanzo, pinto, navy, and so on), use the following cooking method: Place 1 cup of beans in 5 cups of water and bring them to a boil. Boil the beans for one minute. Then drain them and add 5 cups of fresh water. Bring the water to a boil and continue cooking the beans according to directions. Cabbage, cauliflower, and broccoli can also cause flatulence.

❏ When eating potentially gas-inducing foods, take the enzyme product Beano with the first bite. This should help to eliminate the problem.

GROIN SPASM, STITCH, OR PRESSURE

When the round ligaments connecting the corners of the uterus to the pubic area kink and go into spasm, it feels like a "stitch" on the right side. In the later months of pregnancy, lower groin pressure may develop.

Recommendations

❏ Exercise daily, using exercises recommended by your health care provider. This can help alleviate this condition.

❏ During spasms, breathe deeply and bend toward the point of pain in order to allow the ligament to relax. Rest in bed on one side until the spasm is over.

HEARTBURN

Heartburn occurs more often than normal during pregnancy. This is because the expanded size of the uterus pro- motes the reentry of stomach fluids into the esophagus, and hormones present during pregnancy tend to soften the sphincter muscles.

Recommendations

❏ To prevent heartburn, do not consume spicy or greasy foods, alcohol, coffee, baking soda, or antacids containing sodium bicarbonate (such as Alka-Seltzer).

❏ Remain active and upright, especially after meals.

❏ When heartburn strikes, try drinking a glass of warm soymilk.

❏ Do not eat or drink anything except water for a few hours before going to bed or taking a nap.

Considerations

❏ A high-carbohydrate diet can help if heartburn is a problem.

❏ See also HEARTBURN/GASTROESOPHAGEAL REFLUX DISEASE (GERD) in Part Two.

HEMORRHOIDS

Hemorrhoids are common during pregnancy. A number of factors contribute to the development of hemorrhoids, including constipation and the pressure exerted by the uterus as the fetus gains in size and weight.

Recommendations

❏ Increase your intake of roughage. Eat plenty of raw vegetables, fruits, dried fruits, bran, and whole-grain breads. These fiber-rich foods help to soften stools and make elimination easier. Hard stools can be very painful to pass and can cause bleeding.

❏ Drink ten 8-ounce glasses of liquid each day, including water, juices, and herbal teas.

❏ Use cold witch hazel compresses to help shrink hemorrhoids.

❏ Walk one mile a day to help digestion and elimination.

❏ Do not strain to have a bowel movement if you are constipated. (See CONSTIPATION in Part Two.)

❏ See also HEMORRHOIDS in Part Two.

INFERTILITY

See INFERTILITY.

INSOMNIA

Insomnia is very common during the last weeks of pregnancy when finding a comfortable sleeping position is difficult. Needing to get up to urinate can disrupt a night's sleep. Deficiencies of the B vitamins also may cause insomnia. The emotional changes that accompany pregnancy often contribute to sleep difficulties as well.

Recommendations

❏ Increase your intake of foods rich in the B vitamins. (*See* VITAMINS in Part One.)

❏ Take a warm (not hot) bath with a soothing oil (such as lavender) added to the water.

❏ Consider taking up yoga or some form of meditation. These can help you to relax and may be useful during and after labor. (*See* BREATHING EXERCISES; GUIDED IMAGERY; MEDITATION; and RELAXATION TECHNIQUES *under* PAIN CONTROL in Part Three. *Also see* YOGA in Part Three.)

❏ Do not force yourself to sleep if you are not really tired. Read, meditate, or do something else nonstrenuous until you feel sleepy.

❏ Try drinking a cup of hot herbal tea with honey or lemon before bed or in the middle of the night. Herbal teas such as chamomile, marjoram, lemon balm, and passionflower are known for their sleep-inducing qualities.

Caution: Do not use chamomile if you are allergic to ragweed. Do not use during pregnancy or nursing. It may interact with warfarin or cyclosporine, so patients using these drugs should avoid it.

❏ Avoid stimulants.

❏ Do not eat heavy meals before bedtime.

❏ Arrange pillows behind or under your abdomen to relieve breathlessness.

❏ *See also* INSOMNIA in Part Two.

LEG CRAMPS

Leg cramps during pregnancy are often a result of nutritional deficiencies, electrolyte imbalances, and/or circulatory changes, in addition to the strain placed on the legs by the extra weight.

Recommendations

❏ Increase your calcium and potassium intake by eating foods such as almonds, bananas, grapefruit, low-fat cottage cheese, oranges, salmon, sardines, sesame seeds, soy products (such as tofu), and low-fat yogurt and other calcium-rich dairy products to help avert leg cramps. Adequate calcium is also needed to help prevent high blood pressure and for fetal development.

❏ While sleeping or sitting, elevate your legs so that they are higher than your heart.

❏ Do not stand in one place for too long. Shift your weight from one leg to the other every few minutes.

❏ Do not point your toes.

❏ Walk at least a mile every day to stimulate the circulation of blood through the legs.

❏ Make sure your levels of calcium, magnesium, and potassium are correctly balanced. It is often easier to take a single formula that contains all three minerals in the correct proportions.

❏ To relieve cramps, flex your feet, with your toes pointing upward.

❏ When experiencing a cramp, apply a hot water bottle or heating pad to the cramping area and apply pressure with your hands.

❏ *See also* MUSCLE CRAMPS in Part Two.

MISCARRIAGE (SPONTANEOUS ABORTION)

Some pregnancies are not carried to full term, resulting in a miscarriage. About 15 to 20 percent of pregnancies are miscarriages and occur in the first thirteen weeks of pregnancy. *Spontaneous abortion* is the technical term for a miscarriage. It is defined as the loss of a pregnancy before twenty weeks. The most likely reason for a miscarriage is a chromosomal abnormality in the fetus that makes it unlikely the fetus would survive. Other reasons for a miscarriage include cervical incompetence (the cervix opens and thins before the pregnancy has reached full term), ectopic pregnancy (implantation of the fertilized egg outside the uterine cavity, most commonly in one of the fallopian tubes), infection, glandular disorders, diabetes, and pregnancy-induced hypertension (high blood pressure). Miscarriages generally are *not* caused by exercise, sexual activity, heavy lifting, or falls.

Herbs

❏ Taking raspberry leaf tea during the last few months of pregnancy is thought to help strengthen the uterus and minimize the risk of miscarriage.

Recommendations

❏ If you experience bleeding or cramping during pregnancy, contact your health care provider immediately and follow his or her advice.

❏ Do not minimize any feelings of grief, depression, or guilt you may experience after having a miscarriage. Your health care provider can refer you to a grief counselor or someone who will understand how you feel. It is also important to talk to your doctor about the possible reason for the miscarriage so that he or she can reassure you about the outcome of a following pregnancy. It is also quite normal to be able to cope with a miscarriage without experiencing any emotional trauma.

Considerations

❑ Bleeding is not necessarily a sign of impending miscarriage, but it should always be taken seriously. A pelvic examination will probably be necessary to determine if your cervix has started to dilate and if the membranes surrounding the fetus have broken. If both of these conditions are present, it is certain that you will have a miscarriage.

❑ Premature labor is the onset of rhythmic uterine contractions before fetal maturity. It usually occurs between the twentieth and thirty-seventh weeks of gestation.

❑ Decaffeinated coffee, rather than caffeinated coffee, is thought to be a contributing cause of spontaneous abortion during the first trimester.

❑ Women with either of two genetic irregularities that make them prone to blood clots may be at increased risk of multiple miscarriages. Women who have at least two miscarriages can be tested for the flaws. It has been suggested that certain blood-thinning medications might increase the chances for a healthy pregnancy. A doctor should be consulted before taking any medications while pregnant.

MORNING SICKNESS

Approximately 50 percent of all pregnant women experience some degree of nausea and vomiting between the sixth and twelfth weeks of pregnancy. This is normal. Although it is commonly called morning sickness, it can occur at any time of day.

Abnormal vomiting—severe, continual nausea and vomiting after the twelfth week—occurs in approximately 1 percent of all pregnancies. This is called *hyperemesis gravidarum*, and it can result in dehydration, acidosis, malnutrition, and substantial weight loss. If the condition persists, it can endanger the fetus. Sometimes intravenous feeding (parenteral nutrition) is given until the nausea and vomiting subside. The reason for abnormally severe nausea is not clear, but an association has been made between it and very high levels of the hormones estrogen and human chorionic gonadotropin (hCG), a hormone produced by the placenta that increases in quantity until the end of the first trimester.

Other possible causes of abnormal vomiting include bile duct disease, drug toxicity, pancreatitis, low blood sugar, a molar pregnancy (a rare condition in which an abnormal mass rather than a fetus grows inside the uterus), problems with the thyroid, and inflammatory bowel disorders.

NUTRIENTS

SUPPLEMENT	SUGGESTED DOSAGE	COMMENTS
L-methionine	1,000 mg daily.	Effective in preventing nausea.
Vitamin B₆ (pyridoxine) plus	50 mg 2 times daily.	A combination of nutrients that helps to prevent and alleviate nausea.
magnesium	400 mg daily, upon arising.	*Caution:* Do not take this combination for longer than six weeks.

Herbs

❑ Ginger, taken in capsule or tea form, is helpful for relieving nausea. Other beneficial herbs include catnip, dandelion, peppermint, and red raspberry leaf.

Recommendations

❑ Keep crackers or whole wheat toast near your bed and eat some before arising.

❑ Eat small, frequent meals and snack on whole-grain crackers with nut butters (but not peanut butter) or cheese. It helps to keep some food in the stomach at all times.

❑ Do not go without food or drink because of the nausea.

❑ Do not sit up or get out of bed too quickly.

❑ Try using *Nux vomica*, a homeopathic remedy that is good for nausea.

❑ Keep in mind that morning sickness usually does not last beyond the first thirteen weeks of pregnancy. If you suffer from persistent nausea or vomiting later in pregnancy, consult your health care provider. With appropriate treatment, the prognosis is good.

NOSEBLEEDS AND NASAL CONGESTION

During pregnancy, increased blood volume often causes some of the tiny capillaries in the nasal passages to rupture, causing a nosebleed. Inner nasal passages normally swell as well. A lack of vitamin C and the bioflavonoids may be a contributing factor. These conditions disappear with the birth of the baby.

Recommendations

❑ Increase your intake of foods rich in vitamin C, including broccoli, cabbage, grapefruits, lemons, oranges, peppers, and strawberries.

❑ If congestion is a problem, eat fewer dairy products and supplement your diet with calcium and magnesium. Dairy products tend to stimulate the secretion of mucus.

❑ Use a humidifier to help keep nasal tissues moisturized.

❑ Do not use nasal sprays or nose drops. Instead, use an empty nasal spray container filled with warm water to spray into the nostrils. This helps to moisten the nose and shrink the membranes.

❑ *See also* NOSEBLEED in Part Two.

PREMATURE BIRTH

An infant is classified as premature when it is delivered before thirty-seven weeks of pregnancy. Premature birth is a major public health concern because underdeveloped babies are at increased risk of death in the first year of life and are more likely to develop heart, lung, and brain disorders if they survive. There are more than a half million babies born prematurely in the United States each year.

Women who take more than a year to get pregnant have a slightly higher than normal chance of giving birth prematurely.

Considerations

❑ Scientists have taken a big step toward developing an earlier, safer, and simple test that might make it possible to prevent many of the premature births that occur in the United States each year. Researchers say they have identified certain proteins that can indicate imminent premature birth. Now widely available, the test is performed between the twenty-fourth and thirty-fourth weeks of pregnancy on women who are considered to be at high risk. It checks for the presence of fetal fibronectin, a protein found in the uterus when the placenta begins to separate from the uterine wall. The presence of this protein signals that a woman is at high risk for giving birth within seven days, and intervention can be started.

SCIATICA

The sciatic nerve is the longest nerve in the body. It arises from the sacral plexus, in the lower back, threads downward through the pelvis through an opening called the greater sciatic foramen, and runs through the hip joint and down the back of the thigh. Irritation of this nerve is common during pregnancy and usually disappears with the birth of the baby.

Recommendations

❑ Ask your health care provider to recommend a registered physical therapist or a chiropractor who has been specially trained to deal with pregnancy problems. A competent practitioner is best able to deal with this problem.

SKIN PROBLEMS

Common skin problems during pregnancy include pimples, acne, red marks, and mask of pregnancy (dark blotches on the skin of the face). These skin changes usually disappear with the birth of the baby.

Recommendations

❑ Keep your skin clean.

❑ If you wear makeup, use only water-based, hypoallergenic cosmetics if your skin is broken out.

Considerations

❑ Folic acid, one of the most essential nutrients during pregnancy, should also help with skin problems.

❑ *See also* ACNE and OILY SKIN, both in Part Two.

SORENESS IN THE RIB AREA

Soreness in the rib area during pregnancy is common. It is caused by the pressure of the expanding uterus.

Recommendations

❑ Change positions frequently.

❑ Keep in mind that this problem is temporary. It often disappears in the last six weeks of pregnancy, once the baby drops into position to be born.

STRETCH MARKS

Stretch marks are wavy stripes appearing on the abdomen, buttocks, breasts, and thighs. They start out reddish in color and gradually turn white. They are caused by rapid weight gain such as that typically associated with pregnancy, and appear when the skin becomes overstretched and the fibers in the deep layers tear. Once they appear, they are permanent, but they do become much less noticeable with time.

Recommendations

❑ Try the following recipe for preventing stretch marks:

> ½ cup virgin olive oil
> ¼ cup aloe vera gel
> liquid from 6 capsules vitamin E
> liquid from 4 capsules vitamin A

1. Mix all the ingredients together in a blender.

2. Pour the mixture into a jar and store it in the refrigerator.

Once a day, apply the oil externally all over the abdomen, hips, and thighs—the places where stretch marks commonly appear. If you do this diligently, every day, you may be able to prevent stretch marks.

❑ Apply cocoa butter and/or elastin cream topically as directed on the product label. These substances are very good for stretch marks.

❑ To prevent stretch marks during pregnancy, rub your breasts and abdomen every day with a massage oil made of ½ cup sweet almond oil with 50 drops of mandarin essential oil added.

SWEATING

While you are pregnant, your body makes sure that its temperature is perfect for your baby's development. In addition, as your size increases, the amount of effort it takes to walk, climb stairs, and do many everyday things also increases. As a result, you may find yourself sweating more than you did before.

Recommendations

❑ Wear loose, light, comfortable clothing. Choose clothing made of "breathable" natural fibers such as cotton or linen.

❑ Do not use a hot tub during pregnancy. This increase in body temperature can cause fetal distress. For the same reason, be careful about strenuous exercise, especially in hot weather.

VARICOSE VEINS

Varicose veins are enlarged veins close to the surface of the skin that often emerge during pregnancy. In some cases they disappear after the baby's birth.

Recommendations

❑ As often as possible, sit with your feet elevated, higher than your heart.

❑ Change positions frequently. Do not stand for long periods of time or sit in cross-legged positions.

❑ Wear support hose if your health care provider recommends them. Keep them near your bed and put them on before you get out of bed.

❑ Walk one mile each day to promote circulation.

❑ Do not wear elastic-topped knee socks, garters, belts, or high-heeled shoes.

❑ *See also* VARICOSE VEINS in Part Two.

NUTRITIONAL HEALTH IN PREGNANCY

During pregnancy, it is more important than ever to have a balanced diet that is high in nutrients and fiber and low in bad fats and cholesterol. A prenatal multivitamin has the right mix of nutrients that you need to support your own health and that of your unborn child's. Taking a prenatal vitamin should be done throughout your childbearing years, so that upon becoming pregnant, your body is full of essential nutrients. The following are other recommendations for maintaining health in pregnancy. Speak with your health care provider (obstetrician, midwife, etc.) before using anything on this list.

NUTRIENTS

SUPPLEMENT	SUGGESTED DOSAGE	COMMENTS
Very Important		
Iron	30 mg daily, or as directed by physician. Take with 100 mg vitamin C for better absorption.	Extra iron is needed during pregnancy. Increase fiber consumption, as iron supplements may cause constipation.
or		
Floradix Iron + Herbs from Salus Haus	As directed on label.	A natural, nontoxic source of iron.
Multivitamin (prenatal) with folic acid	As directed on label. 1.0–1.1 mg daily.	For women who have a hard time being compliant with taking pills, larger amounts of folic acid are sometimes prescribed (5 mg per day). Taking folic acid is key to avoiding having a baby with neural tube problems.
Protein supplement	As directed on label.	A lack of protein has been linked to birth defects. Use protein from a vegetable source, such as soy.
Quercetin	500 mg daily.	A valuable bioflavonoid that promotes proper circulation.
Vitamin B complex plus extra folic acid	As directed on label. 400 mcg daily.	To prevent deficiencies. Adequate levels of folic acid reduce the chance of birth defects such as spina bifida. Recommended for women throughout the childbearing years, and especially in the first six weeks of pregnancy.
Vitamin C with bioflavonoids	Up to 2,000 mg daily, in divided doses.	Larger doses taken before delivery may help to reduce labor pain.
Zinc	15–25 mg daily. Do not exceed 40 mg daily from all supplements.	Insufficient zinc intake may be a cause of low birth weight. Use zinc gluconate lozenges or OptiZinc for best absorption.
Helpful		
Acidophilus or Kyo-Dophilus from Wakunaga	As directed on label. Take on an empty stomach. As directed on label.	To provide necessary "friendly" bacteria to prevent candidiasis (yeast infection), protect the baby at birth, and ensure proper assimilation of nutrients. The most benefit was for babies born by cesarean delivery. Using a combination of probiotics such as *lactobacillus* and bifidobacteria seems preferable.
Calcium and magnesium	1,500 mg daily. 750 mg daily.	Necessary for formation of healthy bones and teeth. May prevent hypertension and premature birth. Needed to balance with calcium.
Carotenoid complex with beta-carotene	10,000 IU daily.	Precursor of vitamin A. *Caution:* Do not substitute vitamin A for beta-carotene. Excessive intake of vitamin A during pregnancy has been linked to birth defects.

Coenzyme Q$_{10}$	As directed on label.	Helps the body convert food to energy, enhances circulation, and protects the heart. CoQ$_{10}$ (200 mg/day) was shown to cut the chance of preeclampsia in half.
Kelp	As directed on label.	Rich in necessary minerals.
Multimineral and trace mineral complex	As directed on label.	For optimal health and to provide a balance of nutrients needed for fetal development.
Vitamin D	1,000 IU daily.	Needed for calcium absorption and bone formation.
Vitamin K or alfalfa	As directed on label.	Take for excessive bleeding. *See* under Herbs, below.

Herbs

❑ Alfalfa is a good source of vitamins and minerals, especially vitamin K, which is essential for normal blood clotting.

❑ Red raspberry leaf tea helps the uterus contract more effectively. It also helps to enrich the mother's milk. Drink no more than 1 cup per day until the last four weeks of pregnancy. Then drink 1 quart daily.

❑ Avoid the following herbs during pregnancy: aloe vera (internally), angelica, arnica, barberry, black cohosh, bloodroot, cat's claw, celandine, cottonwood bark, dong quai, feverfew, ginseng, goldenseal, lobelia, myrrh, Oregon grape, pennyroyal, rue, sage, saw palmetto, tansy, and turmeric. Use caution when taking any herbs during pregnancy, especially in the first twelve weeks.

Recommendations

❑ Eat a well-balanced, nutritious diet and be sure to get moderate exercise, fresh air, and plenty of rest. Pregnant women need an additional 100 to 300 calories a day. This is not a lot of food, and if you are slowing down on your regular activities, don't increase your caloric intake. The two (lack of usual movement and increased caloric need) will cancel each other out. Three hundred calories is one tablespoon of nut butter—such as almond or soy butter—and jelly on one slice of whole-wheat bread and a glass of low-fat milk. Try to include the following foods in your diet each day:

Food Group	Amount Needed Per Day
Grains	6 servings (whole wheat and other grains)
Vegetables	2–4 cups (not cooked in oil)
Fruit	1–3 servings
Meat and beans	5–7 ounces protein (½ cup of legumes/beans is about 2 ounces of protein)
Milk	3 cups (dairy or soy; rice and almond milk do not have the right mix of nutrients, especially protein)

❑ Stick to a weight gain schedule. Below is what is recommended by the American College of Obstetricians and Gynecologists and depends on the starting weight of the mother.

Weight Status	Weight Gain (pounds)
Underweight	28–40
Normal weight	25–35
Overweight	15–25
Obese	At least 15
Carrying twins	35–45

❑ Eating vegetables has been found to be particularly important to assure a healthy baby weight and length. Eating a lot of vegetables increases the chances of a healthy-sized baby four- to fivefold. Vegetables are low in calories and rich in fiber, two good things a pregnant woman needs.

❑ Do not consume junk food, fried foods, or too much coffee.

❑ Avoid eating rare, undercooked, or raw meat, poultry, or fish. Do not eat grilled meats. Grilling has been shown to produce carcinogens in meat. In addition, to avoid a bacterial infection (listeriosis), avoid unpasteurized milk and soft cheese and prepared meats like hot dogs or deli meats unless they are reheated or steamed first, and wash fruits and vegetables well.

❑ Fish and fish oil have been associated with improved fetal brain function and birth weight. However, a recent study found no increased birth size in all of the women studied who consumed a lot of seafood. For overweight women, a higher consumption of seafood before pregnancy resulted in larger babies. Seafood is a good source of protein, but should be limited to twice a week to avoid consuming high levels of mercury. To be safe, try to stick with low-mercury fish.

❑ Do not use any medications while you are pregnant without consulting your health care provider. The first trimester is arguably the most important stage of development for your child. There are many drugs that may affect that development, so if you are planning to become pregnant—or if you are already pregnant—consult your physician about the possible consequences of any drug, prescription or otherwise, that you may be taking. If it is possible and does not harm your health, you should not take *any* medications during the first trimester of pregnancy.

❑ Do not smoke, consume alcohol in any form, or use drugs, except as prescribed by your health care provider.

❑ Do not take supplements containing the amino acid phenylalanine. Phenylalanine may alter brain growth in the fetus. Also avoid food products containing the sweetener aspartame (found in Equal, NutraSweet, and other products), which contains high levels of phenylalanine. (*See* Is Aspartame a Safe Sugar Substitute? on page 15.)

❑ Do not take mineral oil, which blocks the absorption of the fat-soluble vitamins. Consult your health care provider about the use of any supplements and over-the-counter medications.

Tests Performed During Pregnancy

Your health care provider may do a number of different tests when you become pregnant—or before pregnancy, if you are planning to have a child. If you believe that some of these tests are inappropriate or unnecessary, you can, of course, decline to have them. Discuss this with your physician.

There are also tests that can be performed during pregnancy to assess the health and development of the fetus. However, some of these tests involve an element of risk for both mother and child. Therefore, they should be done only when medically indicated and should not be used routinely or for the mother's or the health care provider's convenience. If a test is suggested, be sure that you are fully aware of why it is needed and of any dangers that may be involved before deciding to have it done. Some tests are required by the admitting hospital. If you refuse to get a test, you may have to decide whether to give birth at another hospital.

ROUTINE TESTS

The routine tests most health care providers recommend during pregnancy include the following:

- Blood pressure. This is taken to test for preeclampsia. It is usually taken at each visit.
- Blood sugar level. This is a urine test for gestational diabetes. It is usually taken at the first visit and on further visits if you are considered to be at high risk for the condition.
- Blood type. This is taken in case a blood transfusion becomes necessary and to see if there are blood type incompatibilities (Rh factor) between you and your baby. It is usually done during your first visit.
- Drug test. This is a urine test for illicit drug use. It may be taken on your first visit.
- Hemoglobin level. This is a blood test to check for anemia. It is usually done at your first visit.
- Pap smear. This is an internal swab test of the cervix to check for cancer cells. It is usually done on the first visit.
- Protein (albumin). This is another urine test for preeclampsia. It is usually done at each visit.
- Rubella antibody test. This is done to determine whether you have achieved immunity to rubella (German measles), which can be dangerous to a developing fetus in the first twelve weeks of pregnancy. It is usually taken on the first visit.
- Sexually transmitted disease testing. Genital swabs may be taken to test for signs of diseases such as chlamydia, gonorrhea, and syphilis. This is usually done during the first visit and, possibly, in later visits.
- Urinalysis. This is done to test for urinary tract infection. It is usually done at the first visit and, possibly, on subsequent visits.

AMNIOCENTESIS

This medical procedure is sometimes performed during pregnancy to determine the health of the fetus. It is rarely carried out unless there is a possibility of fetal abnormality. Routine amniocentesis is recommended only for women over the age of thirty-five, women who are more at risk for having a Down syndrome child, or for couples who have an increased risk of passing on a genetic abnormality to their child. A local anesthetic is administered and then a long, hollow needle is inserted through the mother's abdomen into the uterus to remove amniotic fluid for cellular analysis. The needle can be seen on ultrasound, which allows a three-dimensional real-time view of the uterus and fetus.

The amniotic fluid contains fetal cells that can be cultivated and tested. Although it has become fairly common as women are choosing to have children in later years, this procedure entails risks for both the pregnant woman and the fetus. There may be some danger of blood exchange between the mother and the fetus, infection of the amniotic fluid, peritonitis, the development of blood clots, placental hemorrhage, and premature labor. Therefore, great care must be taken in recommending, and then in performing, amniocentesis.

Amniocentesis is usually done only during the sixteenth to eighteenth week of pregnancy, and the results are not known for two weeks. This test should be performed only if you plan to terminate the pregnancy if an abnormality is found or if knowledge of any problem is necessary for proper prenatal care. Before the test, discuss with your partner and health care provider how you will handle the results if they are unfavorable.

CHORIONIC VILLUS SAMPLING (CVS)

This test carries a slightly greater risk than amniocentesis. The chorionic villi are fingerlike projections of the embryonic sac that contain cells with the same genetic composition as the embryo. In this test, a small sample of this chorionic tissue is taken and analyzed to determine genetic abnormalities in the fetus. It can be performed earlier than amniocentesis, usually in the tenth to twelfth week of pregnancy, and takes about a half-hour to complete.

Possible dangers from CVS include infection, maternal or fetal bleeding, spontaneous abortion, Rh immunization, birth defects, and perforation of the membrane surrounding the embryo. The chief advantage is that it can be performed earlier in pregnancy, when termination, if deemed necessary, is a simpler and less dangerous procedure. As with all tests, you should weigh all the pluses and minuses carefully before making a decision.

ESTRIOL EXCRETION STUDIES, NONSTRESS TEST, OXYTOCIN CHALLENGE TEST

These tests also are used to determine the health of the fetus. The estriol excretion study determines the best time for delivery of the baby in cases of diabetes or other difficulties in pregnancy. The nonstress test determines fetal well-being, and the oxytocin challenge test helps to predict how well the baby will fare during the stress of labor.

If it is determined that any of these tests is necessary, your health care provider should discuss it with you in depth. When considering any type of prenatal testing, always remember that it is your body and your baby. You should be fully informed of all the advantages and all the risks of any procedure before agreeing to it.

ULTRASOUND

Ultrasound imaging is a common diagnostic medical procedure that uses high-frequency sound waves to produce dynamic images (sonograms) of organs, tissues, or blood flow inside the body. Prenatal ultrasound examinations are performed by trained professionals, such as sonographers, radiologists, and obstetricians. The procedure involves using a transducer, which sends a stream of high-frequency sound waves into the body and then detects their echoes as they bounce off internal structures. The sound waves are then converted into electrical impulses, which are processed to form an image, which is displayed on a computer monitor. It is from these images that videos and portraits are made.

Ultrasound is a form of energy, and even at low levels laboratory studies have shown it can produce physical effects in tissue, such as jarring vibrations and a rise in temperature. Although there is no evidence that these physical effects can harm a fetus, the fact that they exist means that prenatal ultrasound cannot be considered completely innocuous. Legitimate uses for ultrasound imaging include: diagnosing pregnancy, determining fetal age, diagnosing congenital abnormalities, evaluating the position of the placenta, and determination of multiple pregnancies.

❑ Avoid activities that may endanger the abdomen, or that involve jarring, bouncing, or twisting movements. Also avoid activities involving rapid starts and stops, because the body's center of gravity changes during pregnancy and it is easy to lose your balance.

❑ Do not use an electric blanket. Several experts warn that the invisible electromagnetic field emanating from an electric blanket may increase the risk of miscarriage and developmental problems.

❑ Take warm, rather than hot, showers or baths. Anything that increases the core body temperature for any length of time may cause neural tube defects in babies such as anencephaly and spina bifida. Anencephalic babies do not develop a brain and rarely survive. Spina bifida is a defect of the spinal column that can affect the baby to varying degrees, depending on the severity of the condition.

Considerations

❑ Preventing malnutrition and hunger in pregnant women and children might help to prevent obesity later in life.

❑ Lack of zinc, manganese, and folic acid, as well as amino acid imbalances, have been linked to fetal deformities and mental retardation.

❑ All women of childbearing age who are thinking of becoming pregnant should take a daily supplement of iron (at least 18 milligrams per day), 400 to 800 micrograms of folic acid, and a B-vitamin complex. Iron maintains stores in the body, which are lost during monthly menses. Folic acid deficiency is linked to such neurologic birth defects as spina bifida and anencephaly. To prevent these disorders, this B vitamin must be present in the body during the first six weeks following conception, a crucial early phase in fetal neurological development. Approximately 1 in every 1,000 pregnancies is affected by neural tube defect. Since most women do not know they have conceived until several weeks afterward, the best way to prevent these birth defects is for women who are planning to become pregnant to have an adequate supply of folic acid at all times. Supplementation is recommended because many women do not get enough folic acid from dietary sources, although all flours in the United States are now supplemented with it, so the population intakes are increasing. Folic acid also helps alleviate hemorrhaging in childbirth and improves milk production. Men too should be as healthy as they possibly can before they conceive children.

❑ Both partners should give up alcohol, cigarettes, and drugs—legal or otherwise—at least three to six months before they decide to conceive. Marijuana, heroin, morphine, and tobacco all reduce levels of male sex hormones and increase the risks of birth defects.

❑ Men should make sure to have an adequate intake of selenium, zinc, vitamins C and E, and the carotenoids.

❑ Taking the drug phenytoin (Dilantin) or phenobarbital, used to control epileptic seizures, creates four times the usual risk of producing a baby with heart defects. In addition, the antibiotics ampicillin (Omnipen, Polycillin) and tetracycline may cause heart malformations. Ask your physician for a *detailed* list of teratogenic agents and drugs (chemicals that cause birth defects). These include, but are not limited to, the following:

• Some ACE inhibitors.

• Some acne medications.

• Some antibiotics.

• Some blood-thinning medications.

• Some cancer drugs.

• Some hormone preparations.

Birth Plan

Formulating a birth plan while you are pregnant is a good way to ensure that your wishes regarding labor and child-birth are clearly stated and respected. It allows you to decide in advance what you want and what you would choose from among the options you may face during the birth of your child. It is a good idea to work with your health care provider and your partner in drawing up the plan. The following are a number of things you should ask about, and decide upon, in developing a birth plan:

• Where will you have your child, and what options are open to you in that facility? For example, do you wish to simply stay in a bed during labor, or would you rather walk around or take a shower or sit in a tub? One study has shown that sitting in the warm water of a birth pool during the first stage of labor can soothe a woman's pain and reduce the likelihood she will need an epidural. Researchers from the University of Southampton in England had forty-nine women sit in an oval-shaped, acrylic pool during the early stages of their slowly progressing labors. The water temperatures were about 98 degrees Fahrenheit. The outcomes were compared with those of fifty women who received standard care for slow labor. Those who labored in water were less likely to need drugs to aid their contractions and said they had less pain and higher satisfaction with their freedom of movement than did those receiving standard care. Discuss all of your options for labor with your midwife or physician.

• If you have chosen to have the baby in a private home, who will be there and what additional facilities might you need?

• If you are in the hospital, can you wear your own clothes? Listen to music? Watch a video?

• How many people will be allowed to stay with you? How many people do you want to be with you? Do you want them to take photographs or videotape the birth?

• Do you want an intravenous (IV) line inserted during labor? In many places, this is considered routine procedure. However, it often is not necessary.

• Do you want to be given drugs (usually oxytocin [Pitocin]) to speed up labor? Oxytocin is often given through the IV and can make labor more painful.

• What type of medication (if any) do you want? If you decide against any pain medication at the time you write your birth plan, will it still be available should you change your mind at any time during labor?

• If you do decide to use drugs for any pain you might experience, what are the potential side effects? Is it safe for the baby if you breast-feed immediately after using pain medication? Does your physician or midwife use homeopathic and/or natural remedies for pain?

• What methods will be used to monitor the baby during labor?

• Do you have to have your baby in the lithotomy position (flat on your back with your feet in stirrups)?

• Will you have an episiotomy? (This is an incision made to enlarge the vaginal opening either so that forceps can be used or to hasten delivery or to prevent tearing in this area, which takes longer to heal than an incision does.)

• Probably the most important question: Are you willing to have a cesarean section, and under what emergency circumstances do they perform this operation? If you had a cesarean for a previous delivery, will you be supported through a vaginal birth after cesarean (VBAC) this time? Over 32 percent of American women who give birth in hospitals undergo cesarean sections. The World Health Organization has stated that no area in the world is justified in having a cesarean rate greater than 5 to 15 percent. Cesarean births cost more than twice as much as vaginal births. It often takes longer for the mother to recover, and she has to remain in the hospital for an extra two days, on average. The most common reason for performing a cesarean is that the mother had one for a previous delivery. But VBAC is possible, and this is something you should discuss with your physician or midwife. The risk of rupturing the previous incision is very small. The reasons for *emergency* cesarean usually relate to the health of the baby. Babies that appear distressed on the fetal monitors need to be removed at once. Sometimes the mother becomes too fatigued due to a long labor and the baby is removed. Other reasons fall into the following categories: the umbilical cord presents before the baby; the baby is a breech presentation (coming down the birth canal feet first, buttocks first, or sideways, instead of head down); the placenta breaks up before the baby is born; or the baby's head is too big to fit through the pelvis (a very unusual event). Many problems can be corrected before or during labor without resorting to a major operation such as a cesarean section.

• Some seizure medications.

• Some thyroid treatment drugs.

• Chronic (long-term) alcohol intake. (Any alcohol intake increases the risk of problems.)

• Cocaine.

These teratogens that affect the development of the baby include drugs taken by men during the time of conception.

❑ Excessive intake of vitamin A has been linked with cleft palate, heart defects, and other congenital defects. Foods rich in vitamin A may also cause problems. Foods containing natural beta-carotene, however, are not harmful because the body converts beta-carotene to vitamin A only as needed, and not in amounts that may be toxic to the body.

❑ One of the best things you can do for your child is to breast-feed your baby for at least the first three months of life—longer if possible. Mother's milk is not only the most nutritious food for a baby, but it also provides crucial disease-fighting agents. However, modern-day infant formulas are closer to mother's milk than they were just a few years ago. A new mother who breast-feeds may need to consume extra calories (up to 500 more calories per day) when nursing than she did during pregnancy. However, to lose weight gained from pregnancy, try not to eat the extra calories. Your diet must include mostly nutrient-dense foods and a substantial amount of liquids and extra portions of calcium-rich foods. Low-fat milk is a liquid that is both nutrient-dense and calcium-rich. Do not give your baby anything other than breast milk or infant formula; cow's milk does not have the right mix of macronutrients (protein, fat) and micronutrients (iron or vitamin E). Babies who are fed cow's milk may have a greater chance of developing allergies to milk and dairy products later in life.

PREMENSTRUAL SYNDROME

Premenstrual syndrome (PMS) is a disorder that affects many women during the seven to ten days before menstruation begins. Symptoms can include any or all of the following: abdominal bloating, acne, anxiety, backache, breast swelling and tenderness, cramps, depression, fainting spells, fatigue, food cravings, headaches, insomnia, joint pain, nervousness, skin eruptions, water retention, and personality changes such as drastic mood swings, outbursts of anger, violence, and, sometimes, even thoughts of suicide. The symptoms are so numerous and various that diagnosing and treating this condition is often difficult.

While there are no hard statistics, it is estimated that as many as 75 percent of all women experience some premenstrual symptoms at one time or another. Approximately 3 to 8 percent of women have symptoms so severe as to be incapacitating (called premenstrual dysphoric disorder). Most women report symptoms severe enough to interfere with their day-to-day lives.

For many years, PMS was dismissed as a psychological problem. We now know that this is a physically based problem, although it is still far from clear what causes all the symptoms. It is possible, of course, that there is more than one cause of PMS and that there may be different causes of symptoms in different people. One of the reasons for PMS may be hormonal imbalance—excessive levels of estrogen and inadequate levels of progesterone—as well as sensitivity to fluctuating hormones. Diet may be an important contributing factor for some women. Unstable blood sugar levels are an important factor as well. PMS has also been linked to food allergies, changes in carbohydrate metabolism, hypoglycemia, and malabsorption. Other suspected causes of PMS symptoms include serotonin dysfunction (a problem with the brain's mood regulator), erratic levels of beta-endorphin (a narcotic-like substance produced by the body), vitamin and/or mineral deficiencies (especially calcium deficiency), and an inability to metabolize fatty acids. All of these may play a part in PMS.

Unless otherwise specified, the dosages recommended here are for adults. For girls between the ages of twelve and seventeen, reduce the dose to three-quarters of the recommended amount.

NUTRIENTS

SUPPLEMENT	SUGGESTED DOSAGE	COMMENTS
Very Important		
Acidophilus (Kyo-Dophilus from Wakunaga)	As directed on label.	Breaks down metabolites of estrogen.
Calcium	1,500 mg daily.	Studies have shown that calcium supplements can reduce many symptoms of PMS by as much as 30 percent. Use a citrate or chelate form.
and magnesium	1,000 mg daily.	Deficiency may be associated with PMS. Should be taken with calcium. Use magnesium chloride or chelate form.
and vitamin D	As directed on label.	Needed for the uptake of calcium and magnesium.
Gamma-amino-butyric acid (GABA)	750 mg daily.	Assists in controlling anxiety and restlessness by increasing levels of serotonin in the brain.
Melatonin	As directed on label.	Important for regulating hormone levels. Helps combat insomnia.
Natural progesterone cream	As directed on label.	A progesterone supplement that has proved helpful for some women.
Pregnenolone	10–100 mg daily (increase the dose for the 5 days before your period, but never exceed more than 100 mg daily for 5 days).	Made from diosgenin, a compound found in some plants, this is a precursor to DHEA. In the body, it is converted into progesterone, cortisone, testosterone, DHEA, and estrogen.
or DHEA	10 mg daily.	Is converted into estrogen and testosterone.
or 7-keto DHEA	As directed on label.	Enhances memory and the immune system. Unlike ordinary DHEA, is not converted into hormones.
S-Adenosylmethio-nine (SAMe)	200 mg twice daily.	Aids in prevention of depression. *Caution:* Do not use if you have bipolar mood disorder or take prescription antidepressants. Do not give to a child under twelve.
Ultimate Cleanse from Nature's Secret	As directed on label.	A cleansing program that enhances the liver's ability to metabolize estrogen.

Vitamin B complex	100 mg of each major B vitamin 3 times daily (amounts of individual vitamins in a complex will vary).	B vitamins work best when taken together.
plus extra vitamin B₅ (pantothenic acid) and	100–200 mg daily.	Reduces stress and is needed by the adrenal gland.
vitamin B₆ (pyridoxine)	50 mg 3 times daily.	Reduces water retention and increases oxygen flow to the female organs. Also aids in restoring estrogen levels to normal.
and vitamin B₁₂	1,000–2,000 mcg daily.	Reduces stress, prevents anemia, and is needed for all bodily functions. Use a lozenge or sublingual form.
Vitamin E	200 IU daily or 400 IU every other day.	Good for sore breasts and other PMS symptoms; improves oxygen utilization and limits free radical damage. Also helps to relieve nervous tension, irritability, and depression. Use d-alpha-tocopherol form.

Helpful

Choline and	1,000 mg each daily.	To aid in nerve impulse transmission.
inositol or	As directed on label.	
lecithin	As directed on label.	
Chromium picolinate	200 mcg daily.	Stabilizes blood sugar levels.
DL-phenylalanine (DLPA)	375 mg 3 to 4 times daily.	Helpful for alleviating headaches and pain. *Caution:* Do not take this supplement if you suffer from panic attacks, diabetes, high blood pressure, or PKU.
Floradix Iron + Herbs from Salus Haus	As directed on label. Do not take at the same time as vitamin E; iron depletes vitamin E in the body. Check with your doctor before taking iron.	To supply iron in easily assimilated natural formula. Women with heavy menstrual flow are often anemic.
Kelp	1,000–1,500 mg daily.	A good source of needed minerals. Helps to protect thyroid function.
L-tyrosine	500 mg twice daily, on an empty stomach. Take with water or juice. Do not take with milk. Take with 50 mg vitamin B₆ and 100 mg vitamin C for better absorption.	Reduces anxiety, depression, and headache. *Caution:* Do not take this supplement if you are taking an MAO inhibitor drug.
Multivitamin and mineral complex	As directed on label.	All nutrients are needed for relief of symptoms.
Vitamin A plus	10,000 IU daily.	Deficiency has been linked to PMS.
carotenoid complex with natural beta-carotene	15,000 IU daily.	Antioxidants and precursors of vitamin A.
Vitamin C with bioflavonoids	3,000–6,000 mg daily, in divided doses.	Aids in relief of discomfort and breast swelling. Also boosts the immune system.

Zinc	50 mg daily. Do not exceed a total of 100 mg daily from all supplements.	Needed for proper immune function. Diuretics deplete zinc. Use zinc gluconate lozenges or OptiZinc for best absorption.
plus copper	3 mg daily.	Needed to balance with zinc.

Herbs

❑ Angelica root, cramp bark, kava kava, and red raspberry have antispasmodic properties and may alleviate cramps.

Caution: Kava kava can cause drowsiness. It is not recommended for pregnant women or nursing mothers, and it should not be taken together with other substances that act on the central nervous system, such as alcohol, barbiturates, antidepressants, and antipsychotic drugs.

❑ Black cohosh, blessed thistle, dong quai, false unicorn root, fennel seed, sarsaparilla root, and squawvine are hormone-balancing herbs effective in the treatment of PMS.

Caution: Do not use black cohosh if you are pregnant or have any type of chronic disease. Black cohosh should not be used by those with liver problems.

❑ Black haw and rosemary are good for cramps and help to calm the nervous system.

❑ Feverfew is good for migraines. (*See* MIGRAINE in Part Two.)

Caution: Do not use feverfew when pregnant or nursing. People who take prescription blood-thinning medications should consult a health care provider before using feverfew, as the combination can result in internal bleeding.

❑ Milk thistle cleanses the liver and helps improve liver function, thus enhancing the liver's ability to metabolize estrogen. For best results, this herb should be taken on a daily basis for a period of three months.

❑ Peppermint, strawberry leaf, and valerian root help to stabilize mood swings and tone the nervous system.

❑ Wild yam extract contains natural progesterone and has proved effective in alleviating many symptoms of PMS, including cramps, headache, mood swings, depression, irritability, and insomnia.

Recommendations

❑ Eat plenty of fresh fruits and vegetables, whole-grain cereals and breads, beans, peas, lentils, nuts and seeds, and broiled chicken, turkey, and fish. Have high-protein snacks between meals.

❑ Include in your diet foods that are high in complex carbohydrates and rich in fiber. These can help the body to get rid of excess estrogen if high estrogen levels are your problem.

❑ Drink 1 quart of distilled water daily, starting a week before the menstrual period and ending one week after.

❑ Do not consume salt, red meats, processed foods, or junk or fast foods. At the very least, omit these foods from the diet for at least one week before the expected onset of symptoms. Reducing sodium (principally salt and foods that contain it) is especially important for preventing bloating and water retention. Salt reduction is particularly important during the luteal phase before menses.

❑ Eat fewer dairy products. Dairy products block the absorption of magnesium and increase its urinary excretion. Refined sugars also increase magnesium excretion. Be sure to get calcium and vitamin D from other foods or supplements.

❑ Avoid caffeine and xanthine-containing foods and beverages such as coffee, tea, cola, and chocolate. Caffeine is linked to breast tenderness, and is a central nervous system stimulant that can make you anxious and jittery. It also acts as a diuretic and can deplete many important nutrients.

❑ Eat foods that are high in phytoestrogens such as soy products, flaxseeds, nuts, whole grains, apples, fennel, celery, parsley, and alfalfa.

❑ Do not consume alcohol or sugar in any form, especially during the week before symptoms are expected. These foods cause valuable electrolytes, particularly magnesium, to be lost through the urine.

❑ Fast on fresh juices and spirulina for several days before the anticipated onset of menstruation to help minimize symptoms. (See FASTING in Part Three.)

❑ Get regular exercise. Walking, even if only one-half to one mile per day, can be very helpful. Exercise increases the oxygen level in the blood, which helps in nutrient absorption and efficient elimination of toxins from the body. It also helps to keep hormone levels more stable. Stress management practices are also helpful, such as a cognitive behavioral therapy program.

❑ See a physician to rule out an underlying medical condition that may be causing symptoms, such as abnormal thyroid function, endometriosis, or a genuine psychological problem such as clinical depression. A food allergy test and a hair analysis to rule out heavy metal intoxication are also recommended. (See ALLERGIES in Part Two and HAIR ANALYSIS in Part Three.)

❑ Do not smoke.

Considerations

❑ PMS is a syndrome with many causes, and the problem may not have one solution that fits every woman. It may be best to experiment with altering your diet, using natural progesterone cream, avoiding certain foods and drinks, taking up meditation, or trying acupuncture, and seeing which one suits you best and gives you optimum relief from your particular symptoms. Some women experience PMS coupled with depression. If you are one of these women and are not benefiting from lifestyle changes such as those mentioned here, speak to your health care professional about other treatments such as antidepressants (SSRIs or others) and ovulation suppressants. The most important thing you can do is to get an accurate diagnosis of your condition so you can be treated effectively. Find a sympathetic health care provider. PMS is classified as a real disorder and requires the same attention as any other chronic condition.

❑ Premenstrual depression may be due to a miscue of the biological clock that results in lower than normal levels of certain brain chemicals. Research at the University of California–San Diego suggests that some women who suffer from PMS may be deficient in melatonin, a hormone secreted at night by the pineal gland.

❑ Studies have shown that women who regularly consume caffeine are four times more likely than others to have severe PMS.

❑ One study showed that calcium and magnesium supplements are effective for managing symptoms of PMS. The optimal amount for women in this study was 1,000 to 1,200 milligrams of calcium and 200 milligrams of magnesium daily.

❑ Some physicians recommend oral contraceptives for women with PMS, especially if they also are interested in reliable birth control. If you take oral contraceptives, be aware that their effectiveness at preventing pregnancy can be sharply reduced if you also take antibiotics. Oral contraceptives and other preparations containing estrogen-type substances should *not* be used if you are pregnant or if you have breast cancer, abnormal vaginal bleeding, or phlebitis (inflammation of leg veins).

❑ Proper diet is extremely important in treating PMS. Meals high in complex carbohydrates have been found to help in dealing with stress. Researchers speculate that such a diet may increase the body's production of serotonin, a brain chemical with antidepressant properties. Conversely, eating red meat and dairy products promotes the type of hormonal imbalance that causes PMS—excessive estrogen levels and inadequate progesterone levels.

❑ For about 20 to 25 percent of women with PMS, dietary and lifestyle changes are not enough to relieve PMS symptoms and they will need to use other treatments. Wild yam cream, which contains a natural form of the hormone progesterone, has been helpful for many women. You rub the cream into the skin on your chest, inner arms, thighs, and abdomen just after ovulation, and the active ingredient is absorbed through the skin. Progesterone creams such as those made from wild yam are prostaglandin inhibitors, which have been shown to produce some relief from symptoms of PMS. However, the American Cancer Society says that wild yam supplies a substance called diosgenin, which the human body cannot convert into progesterone. This finding is likely the reason for the lack of human studies on using wild yam to relieve symptoms of PMS.

❑ The amino acid L-glutamine, either alone or in combination with DL-phenylalanine (DLPA), may help to reduce food cravings.

☐ Research has discovered that many women with PMS also suffer from some form of immune system disorder or frequently suffer from some variety of yeast infection. (*See* CANDIDIASIS in Part Two.)

☐ A significant number of women who suffer from PMS have some sort of thyroid dysfunction. (*See* HYPOTHYROIDISM in Part Two.)

☐ Clinics specializing in the treatment of PMS are springing up all over the country. Experience and expertise can vary greatly among these establishments, however. Ask your health care provider for a referral or recommendation, or look for a clinic that is affiliated with a major local hospital. Beware of clinics that promote only one type of treatment or a quick-fix approach to this complicated disorder.

PROLAPSE OF THE UTERUS

Uterine prolapse (sometimes called a pelvic floor hernia or a pudendal hernia) is a condition that develops when muscular support for the uterus is lost. The uterus is normally held in place by the pelvic muscles and supporting ligaments. When these muscles become weakened or injured, uterine prolapse can occur. In mild cases, a portion of the uterus descends into the top of the vagina. In more serious cases, the uterus may even protrude through the vaginal opening and can be accompanied by a cystocele (a bladder that bulges into the front wall of the vagina) or a ureterocele (a urethra that does the same). In some instances, the rectum may bulge into the back wall of the vagina, a condition known as rectocele.

Symptoms of prolapse of the uterus can include backache, abdominal discomfort, a feeling of heaviness, and urinary incontinence, especially stress incontinence (the involuntary passage of urine when straining, sneezing, or otherwise putting pressure on the abdomen). Other symptoms can include excessive menstrual bleeding, abnormal vaginal discharge or bleeding, painful intercourse, and constipation. However, a woman with a prolapsed uterus may not exhibit any symptoms at all.

Women who have borne several children and/or who have gone through difficult and prolonged labor are more prone to prolapse. Other factors that can increase the likelihood of uterine prolapse include obesity, uterine cancer, diabetes, chronic bronchitis, asthma, heavy lifting or straining (particularly if the pelvic muscles are already weakened), and a retroverted uterus (a uterus that is tilted toward the back of the body).

NUTRIENTS

SUPPLEMENT	SUGGESTED DOSAGE	COMMENTS
Important		
Calcium and magnesium	1,500 mg daily. 1,000 mg daily.	Essential minerals needed for muscle tone and metabolism.
L-carnitine plus	500 mg twice daily, on an empty stomach.	Improves muscle strength in the uterus.
L-glycine	500 mg twice daily, on an empty stomach. Take with water or juice. Do not take with milk. Take with 50 mg vitamin B$_6$ and 100 mg vitamin C for better absorption.	Retards muscle degeneration.
branched-chain amino acid complex	As directed on label.	Promotes healing of muscle tissue.
Methylsulfonyl-methane (MSM) (OptiMSM from Bergstrom Nutrition)	As directed on label.	A natural sulfur compound found in foods and present in body tissues that is used by the body to build healthy new cells. MSM provides the flexible bond between the cells and provides support for tendons, ligaments, and muscles.
Multivitamin and mineral complex with mixed carotenoids and vitamin B complex	As directed on label.	All nutrients work together for healing and tissue repair.
Vitamin C with bioflavonoids	3,000–5,000 mg daily, in divided doses.	Important for keeping bladder infections under control and to enhance immune function. Use an esterified form for best absorption.
Zinc	50 mg daily. Do not exceed a total of 100 mg daily from all supplements.	Needed for proper immune function, bone support, and all bodily enzyme systems. Use zinc gluconate lozenges or OptiZinc for best absorption.

Herbs

☐ Buchu has anti-inflammatory properties and aids in controlling bladder problems.

☐ Cranberry aids in bladder function and helps to prevent urgency incontinence. It can be taken in capsule form. Pure, unsweetened cranberry juice is good also.

☐ Damiana helps provide oxygen to the genital area and balances female hormones.

☐ Ginger can help with bowel disorders.

Recommendations

☐ Eat a diet consisting of 75 percent raw fruits and vegetables plus whole grains such as brown rice and millet.

☐ Use a fiber supplement daily to prevent constipation.

☐ Do not strain during bowel movements or urination.

☐ Drink ten 8-ounce glasses of quality water daily.

☐ Try to achieve or maintain a normal weight.

Considerations

☐ Doing Kegel exercises to tone the pelvic floor muscles when prolapse is beginning may prevent the condition from getting worse. These exercises can be done in two ways:

1. Tighten and squeeze the vagina and rectum by drawing the muscles inward and upward. Hold this position for five to ten seconds, then relax. Repeat as many times as possible, preferably at least 100 times a day.

2. When urinating, start and stop the flow of urine as many times as possible. This form of the exercise is particularly useful for stress incontinence.

❏ If the prolapse causes no symptoms, no treatment is needed, other than perhaps adopting an exercise program designed for the individual problem and situation.

❏ Natural progesterone replacement may be more beneficial than estrogen therapy.

❏ A vaginal device (a ring-shaped pessary) can be inserted to hold the uterus in place. This approach can have undesirable results, however. It can interfere with sexual intercourse and may also cause an irritating discharge with an unpleasant odor and even infection.

❏ Adult diapers may be necessary in extreme cases. If so, speak to your health care professional about other options such as surgery.

❏ It is possible to surgically re-suspend the uterus into its normal position. This procedure is usually performed on women who wish to bear children in the future. For women who have completed childbearing, or who do not wish to have children, vaginal hysterectomy is a viable option for this condition. Women pondering a hysterectomy should give the matter close and careful consideration. (*See* HYSTERECTOMY-RELATED PROBLEMS in Part Two.)

PROSTATE CANCER

The prostate is a walnut-sized gland at the base of the bladder that encircles the urethra, the tube through which urine is voided. The prostate produces prostatic fluid, which makes up the bulk of the male ejaculate and nourishes and transports the sperm. Cancer of the prostate gland is the second leading cause of cancer death among men. It is primarily a disease of aging. Men in their thirties and forties rarely develop prostate cancer, but the incidence increases steadily after the age of fifty. Prostate cancer is most likely to be diagnosed between the ages of sixty-five and seventy-four. The American Cancer Society estimates that nearly 200,000 new cases of prostate cancer are diagnosed annually, and over 28,000 men die from the disease, making it the second leading cause of cancer deaths in the United States. Many experts feel that every man will eventually develop prostate cancer if he lives long enough. It is good news that prostate cancer deaths have been declining for the past ten years, which many experts believe to be the result of better screening and earlier diagnosis. Survival is improved if the disease is diagnosed early, which means regular screening is important. Five-year survival rates are 100 percent if the tumor is localized and regional, 31 per-cent for distant tumors, and 75 percent for unstaged tumors.

Although it is relatively common, in most cases prostate cancer is, fortunately, a slow-growing cancer. Most prostate cancers arise in the rear portion of the prostate gland; the rest originate near the urethra. Lymphatic vessels leading from the prostate gland to the pelvic lymph nodes provide a route for prostate cancer to spread to other areas of the body. Prostate cancers double in mass every six years, on average (by comparison, breast cancers commonly double every three and a half years). Possible symptoms of prostate cancer can include one or more of the following: pain or a burning sensation during urination, frequent urination, a decrease in the amount and force of urine flow, an inability to urinate, blood in the urine, and continuing lower back, pelvic, or suprapubic discomfort. However, the disease often causes no symptoms at all until it reaches an advanced stage and/or spreads outside the gland. In addition, these symptoms most often are caused not by cancer, but by an enlarged prostate, benign prostatic hyperplasia (BPH).

The exact cause or causes of prostate cancer are not known. However, there are certain risk factors that have been linked to its development. Men aged sixty-five and older, African-American men, and men who have a first-degree relative (parent or sibling) with prostate cancer are at increased risk. The incidence is higher among married men than it is among unmarried men. Also at increased risk are men who have had recurring prostate infections, those with a history of sexually transmitted disease, and those who have taken testosterone. Exposure to cancer-causing chemicals increases risk as well. Having a genetic variation of the cyclooxygenase-2 (COX-2) gene also may increase your risk for prostate cancer. This gene is involved with regulating inflammation, and too much inflammation is found to increase the risk of prostate cancer. Researchers have also found a link between a high-fat diet that is low in fruits and vegetables and prostate cancer. This may be due to the fact that heavy fat consumption raises testosterone levels, which could then stimulate growth of the prostate, including any cancer cells it may be harboring. Some studies have suggested that vasectomy may increase the risk of developing prostate cancer, although other studies contradict this hypothesis.

There is no known way to prevent this disease, but early detection can make it possible to catch the cancer before it spreads to other sites in the body. A careful digital rectal exam of the prostate is the simplest and most cost-effective approach for detecting prostate cancer. The American Cancer Society recommends that every man have an annual exam beginning at age forty; the American Urological Association suggests beginning at age fifty.

Prostate-specific antigen (PSA) is a protein produced by cells of the prostate gland. The PSA test measures the level of PSA in the blood. The doctor takes a blood sample, and the amount of PSA is measured in a laboratory. Because PSA is produced by the body and can be used to detect disease, it is sometimes called a biological marker or a tumor marker. A PSA test result between 0 and 4 is considered within the normal range. Numbers between 4 and 10 indicate a 25 percent chance of cancer and numbers higher than 10 indicate a 50 percent chance. PSA levels rise with age even if you don't have cancer. It is important to get regular screening and to discuss with your doctor what your numbers mean. A man's PSA level alone does not give doctors enough information to distinguish between benign prostate conditions and cancer. However, the doctor will take the result of the PSA test into account when deciding whether to check further for signs of prostate cancer.

High PSA levels can be caused by factors other than cancer, including benign enlargement or inflammation of the prostate, an activity as innocuous as bicycle riding, or even the rectal exam itself. Having the test repeated every year may help a physician to better interpret the results; in healthy men, PSA levels tend to remain relatively stable, rising only gradually from year to year, while cancer causes the levels to rise more dramatically. The U.S. Food and Drug Administration (FDA) has approved the use of the PSA test along with a digital rectal exam (DRE) to help detect prostate cancer in men fifty years of age or older. Doctors often use the PSA test and DRE as prostate cancer screening tests; together, these tests can help doctors detect prostate cancer in men who have no symptoms of the disease.

Ultrasound scanning of the prostate is often done to follow up on an abnormal rectal exam or PSA test. Other diagnostic tests, including computerized tomography (CT) scans, bone scans, and magnetic resonance imaging (MRI) may be necessary, but are costly. Ultimately, if test results point consistently to the presence of cancer, a tissue diagnosis must be done to confirm it. This can be done only by microscopic examination of a needle biopsy, preferably directed under ultrasound control. Repeated biopsies may be needed in some cases. This invasive procedure may itself cause complications. Bleeding, urinary retention, impotence, and sepsis ("blood poisoning") have been reported.

Another important measure, the Gleason score, gauges the probable aggressiveness of a tumor based on the cellular characteristics of the cancer. If you develop prostate cancer, your doctor will discuss your score and its implications for survival. Tumor cells that look more similar to normal cells tend to be less aggressive, while those that are distributed randomly with uneven edges are likely to spread rapidly. The dosages given below are for adults.

NUTRIENTS

SUPPLEMENT	SUGGESTED DOSAGE	COMMENTS
Essential		
Coenzyme Q10 plus	100 mg daily.	Improves cellular oxygenation.
Coenzyme A from Coenzyme-A Technologies	As directed on label.	Works effectively with coenzyme Q10 to support the immune system's detoxification of many dangerous substances.
Colostrum (Colostrum Plus from Symbiotics or Colostrum Prime Life from Jarrow Formulas)	As directed on label.	Has been shown to boost the immune system, burn fat, build lean muscle, and have an anti-aging effect.
Dimethylglycine (DMG) (Aangamik DMG from Food-Science of Vermont)	As directed on label.	Enhances oxygen utilization.
Garlic (Kyolic from Wakunaga)	2 capsules 3 times daily.	Enhances immune function. Helps to break down testosterone. Has been shown to slow cancer cell growth.
Proteolytic enzymes	As directed on label. Take with meals.	To keep down inflammation and destroy free radicals.
Selenium	200 mcg daily.	Needed for proper prostate function. The incidence of prostate cancer has been shown to be substantially lower in men with higher selenium levels.
Superoxide dismutase (SOD)	As directed on label.	Destroys free radicals. Consider injections (under a doctor's supervision).
Vitamin A plus carotenoid complex with extra lycopene plus vitamin E	50,000–100,000 IU daily for 10 days or as long as you are on the program. As directed on label. 200 IU daily or 400 IU every other day.	Powerful antioxidants that destroy free radicals. Use emulsion forms for easier assimilation, and greater safety at higher doses. Lycopene has been shown to lower the risk of developing prostate cancer. Protects against prostate cancer. Use d-alpha-tocopherol form.
Vitamin B complex plus extra vitamin B3 (niacin) and choline and folic acid plus vitamin B6 (pyridoxine) and vitamin B12	100 mg of each major B vitamin daily (amounts of individual vitamins in a complex will vary). 100 mg daily. Do not exceed this amount. 500–1,000 mg daily. 400 mcg daily. 100 mg daily. 2,000 mcg daily.	B vitamins necessary for normal cell division and to improve circulation, build red blood cells, and aid liver function. *Caution:* Do not take niacin if you have a liver disorder, gout, or high blood pressure. Enhances the efficacy of zinc. Prevents anemia. Use a lozenge or sublingual form. Consider injections (under a doctor's supervision).
Vitamin C with bioflavonoids	5,000–20,000 mg daily, in divided doses. (*See* ASCORBIC ACID FLUSH in Part Three.)	Powerful anticancer agents. Have been shown in laboratories to inhibit the spread of prostate cancer.
Vitamin D	As directed on label.	Low levels may be linked to higher prostate cancer incidence.
Important		
Maitake extract	4,000–8,000 mg (4–8 gm) daily.	Inhibits the growth and spread of cancerous tumors. Also boosts immune response.

Helpful		
Acidophilus (Kyo-Dophilus from Wakunaga)	As directed on label. Take on an empty stomach.	Has an antibacterial effect on the body. Use a nondairy formula that requires no refrigeration.
Aerobic 07 from Aerobic Life Industries	As directed on label.	An antimicrobial agent.
Berry seeds complex	1–2 tablets after each meal.	Has a regulating effect on cell function and a suppressive effect on cancer cells.
Glutathione plus L-cysteine and L-methionine	As directed on label. As directed on label, on an empty stomach. Take with water or juice. Do not take with milk. Take with 50 mg vitamin B_6 and 100 mg vitamin C for better absorption.	Protects against environmental toxins. Sulfur-containing amino acids that act as detoxifiers and protect the liver and other organs. (*See* AMINO ACIDS in Part One.)
Kelp or seaweed	1,000–1,500 mg daily. As directed on label.	For mineral balance.
L-carnitine	As directed on label.	Protects against free radical damage and toxins. Use a form from fish liver (squalene).
Multienzyme complex	As directed on label. Take with meals.	To aid digestion.
Multiglandular complex plus raw thymus glandular	As directed on label. As directed on label.	To stimulate glandular function, especially that of the thymus, site of T lymphocyte production. (*See* GLANDULAR THERAPY in Part Three.)
Multivitamin complex	As directed on label.	Many nutrients in this table may be found in a combination multivitamin. Do not use a sustained-release formula. Choose a product that is iron-free.
Taurine	As directed on label.	An amino acid that functions as a foundation for tissue and organ repair.

Herbs

❏ Black radish, dandelion, milk thistle, and red clover are good for cleansing the liver and the blood.

❏ Buchu, capsicum (red pepper), Carnivora, echinacea, goldenseal, pau d'arco, and suma have all shown anticancer properties. Take them in tea form, using two at a time and alternating among them.

Cautions: Do not take echinacea for longer than three months. It should not be used by people who are allergic to ragweed. Do not take goldenseal internally on a daily basis for more than one week at a time. Do not use it during pregnancy or if you are breast-feeding, and use with caution if you are allergic to ragweed. If you have a history of cardiovascular disease, diabetes, or glaucoma, use it only under a doctor's supervision.

❏ Damiana and licorice root have the ability to balance hormones and glandular function.

Caution: Licorice root should not be used during pregnancy or nursing. It should not be used by persons with diabetes, glaucoma, heart disease, high blood pressure, or a history of stroke.

❏ Gravel root, hydrangea, oat straw, parsley root, uva ursi, and yarrow are diuretics that also dissolve sediment.

❏ Green tea and lycopene may prevent tumor growth.

Caution: Green tea contains vitamin K, which can make anticoagulant medications less effective. Consult your health care professional if you are using them. The caffeine in green tea could cause insomnia, anxiety, upset stomach, nausea, or diarrhea.

❏ Modified citrus pectin has been shown to substantially inhibit the growth of cancer cells and is especially effective in combating prostate cancer.

❏ Resveratrol is a phytochemical derived from grapes that helps to maintain a healthy prostate.

❏ Turmeric is a spice that contains curcumin, an antioxidant that may be effective in controlling prostate cancer cells.

Recommendations

❏ Maintain a whole-foods diet. Eat plenty of whole grains, raw nuts and seeds, and unpolished brown rice. Millet cereal is a good source of protein. Eat wheat, oats, and bran. Also eat plenty of cruciferous vegetables, such as broccoli, Brussels sprouts, cabbage, and cauliflower, and yellow and deep-orange vegetables, such as carrots, pumpkin, squash, and yams. This type of diet is important for the prevention of cancer as well as for healing.

❏ Include in the diet apples, fresh cantaloupe, all kinds of berries, especially blueberries and strawberries; Brazil nuts; cherries; grapes; legumes, including chickpeas, lentils, and red beans; plums; and walnuts. All of these foods help to fight cancer.

❏ Consume freshly made vegetable and fruit juices daily. Carrot and cabbage juices are good choices.

❏ Eat plenty of grapefruit, watermelon, and tomatoes and tomato products such as tomato juice and tomato-based sauces. These contain lycopene, which has been shown to protect against prostate cancer.

❏ Include in your diet foods that are high in zinc, such as mushrooms, pumpkin seeds, seafood, spinach, sunflower seeds, and whole grains. Zinc nourishes the prostate gland and is vital for proper immune function.

❏ Eat salmon, mackerel, sardines, or herring. Regular consumption of these sources of omega-3 fatty acids may lower the risk of prostate cancer. One study found that eating fish more than three times a week was associated with a reduced risk of prostate cancer compared to infrequent fish consumption.

❏ Drink at least ten 8-ounce glasses of water a day. This hydrates the body, keeps the prostate working efficiently, and helps to eliminate toxins from the body.

❏ Restrict your intake of dairy products. Moderate consumption of soured products such as low-fat yogurt and kefir is acceptable.

❏ If you experience difficulty urinating or notice an increasing trend toward waking up to urinate during the night, consult your health care provider. This may indicate prostatic obstruction.

❏ Do not eat red meat. There is a definite correlation between high red meat consumption (five servings a week or more) and the development of prostate cancer.

❏ Eliminate from the diet alcoholic beverages, coffee, and all teas except for caffeine-free herbal teas. A study conducted at the Fred Hutchinson Cancer Research Center in Seattle suggested that drinking one glass of red wine per day may reduce the risk of prostate cancer by 50 percent. We still believe that alcohol consumption is not necessarily good for the body, and until more conclusive evidence becomes available we believe abstinence to be the best practice. If there is a compound in red wine that might help, it certainly isn't the alcohol.

❏ Strictly avoid the following foods: junk foods, processed refined foods, salt, saturated fats, polyunsaturated vegetable oils, sugar, and white flour. Instead of salt, use a kelp or potassium substitute. If necessary, a small amount of blackstrap molasses or pure maple syrup can be used as a natural sweetener in place of sugar. Use whole wheat or rye instead of white flour.

❏ Try to avoid *all* known carcinogens. Eat only organic foods, if possible. Avoid tobacco smoke, polluted air, polluted water, noxious chemicals, and food additives. Use only distilled water or reverse-osmosis filtered water. Municipal and well water can contain chlorine, fluoride, and agricultural chemical residue.

❏ Try following a macrobiotic diet.

❏ Get regular physical activity. Active men maintain better health and have lower risk of developing prostate cancer.

❏ Enjoy regular sexual activity. Regular ejaculation activates the prostate gland, keeping it from getting stagnant and inflamed.

❏ Do not take any drugs except those that are prescribed by your physician. Always seek counsel and alternative opinions before deciding which treatments, if any, you will pursue.

Considerations

❏ Some nutrients, such as vitamin C and E and selenium, have been thought to reduce the risk of certain cancers, or at least delay them, because they are potent antioxidants. Two earlier studies—the Nutritional Prevention of Cancer Study Group and the Alpha-Tocopherol, Beta-Carotene Cancer Prevention Study—showed prostate cancer risk reductions of 63 percent for selenium and 32 percent for alpha-tocopherol (vitamin E). In addition, the combination of selenium, vitamin E, and beta-carotene reduced overall cancer mortality. However, there are two newer studies, both published in the *Journal of the American Medical Association (JAMA)*; one found no benefit from supplemental selenium and vitamin E, and the other found no benefit from vitamin C and E. Both were randomized, placebo-controlled, and lasted at least seven years. There were over 50,000 men in the two studies. Keep in mind that the science of nutrition evolves, and it is considered best practice to think about all of the evidence to date and not just the recent studies. It seems safe and reasonable to take a multivitamin with all nutrients in balanced proportions. However, even doing that was shown to be ineffective at reducing the risk of early or localized prostate cancer in another study. Furthermore, these authors found that taking high single doses of selenium, beta-carotene, and zinc increased the chances of developing advanced and fatal prostate cancer. Based on this finding and the other studies, it seems prudent to avoid these nutrients in single, high-dose forms. Vitamin E from supplements appeared to not affect prostate cancer risk, but gamma-tocopherol, the form of vitamin E found in many American foods, such as margarine, butter, salad dressing, potatoes fried in corn oil, cookies, and brownies, did reduce the risk. Even though these foods are particularly unhealthy, as they lead to over-consumption and obesity, they still may help to reduce the risk of prostate cancer if eaten in moderation and occasionally.

❏ An eight-year study published in the *British Journal of Cancer* found a 22 percent increase in risk of prostate cancer with a high intake of dairy products in men living in Europe. American studies confirmed both a higher rate of the disease and a higher mortality from dairy products. It is thought that a high intake of dairy protein may increase the production of insulin-like growth-factor-1 (IGF-1), which in turn promotes the development of prostate cancer. In addition, others think that too much calcium from dairy products suppresses the body's ability to synthesize vitamin D. Vitamin D is thought to be protective against prostate cancer. The European collaborators found that for every increase of 35 grams of dairy protein (a cup of milk has 8 grams), there was a 32 percent increase in the risk of developing prostate cancer. Calcium from foods, other than dairy products like milk and yogurt, had no effect on disease risk.

❏ Eating fish that are rich in omega-3s (such as salmon, herring, and mackerel) once or more a week is helpful at reducing cancer risk. In one study, 2 servings a week reduced cancer risk by 26 percent; 3 to 4 servings reduced the risk by 36 percent, and more than 5 servings reduced the risk by 61 percent. This study was done in Sweden, where fish intake is already higher than in the United States. However, later researchers at the University of California–

San Francisco found that men who ate dark, fatty fish one to three times a week had a 36 percent reduction in the risk of prostate cancer compared to those who did not eat fish. Both studies looked at men who did and did not have a COX-2 gene variant. In both studies, having this gene increased the risk of prostate cancer, and eating fish regularly reduced it more than in those without the genetic variant.

❑ Diet and nutrition are important not only for treatment, but for prevention. An anticancer diet is composed primarily of brown rice, fresh raw fruits and vegetables, fresh juices, legumes, raw nuts and seeds, and whole grains, and *excludes* alcohol, coffee, refined carbohydrates, and strong tea. Regular intake of zinc (50 milligrams daily) and essential fatty acids (in supplement form or from cold-pressed sesame, safflower, or olive oil) in later life also may help to prevent the development of problems.

❑ A high-fat, low-fiber diet is linked not just to heart disease, but also to prostate cancer. Chemical reactions occur when fat is cooked, leading to the production of free radicals, which play a major role in certain cancers. Researchers theorize that a diet high in fat raises the levels of testosterone and other hormones in the body, which stimulates the prostate—and any cancerous cells in it—to grow. A high intake of milk and coffee may also increase the risk of developing prostate cancer. In addition, maintaining a normal weight during adulthood (age fourteen to fifty-nine years) reduces the risk of developing prostate cancer, and if you do get it, you get it at a later age.

❑ Research has shown that soybeans and soy products, such as tofu, tempeh, soy flour, and soymilk, have cancer-fighting powers due to the presence of a protein called genistein. Genistein apparently retards tumor growth by preventing the growth of new blood vessels to feed the tumor. It appears to be particularly effective against prostate cancer, but also works against breast cancer in women and colon cancer in both sexes.

❑ Berries help protect DNA from damage and mutation that may result in cancer.

❑ Green tea extract (200 milligrams per day) was shown to reduce the recurrence of tumors in men with high-grade prostatic intraepithelial neoplasia. Although PSA levels did not change, men randomized to the tea group developed one new tumor (out of thirty men) and those in the placebo group developed nine (out of thirty men). Moreover, men taking the tea reported reduced lower urinary tract symptoms, suggesting that this compound may benefit those with benign prostatic hyperplasia (BPH).

Caution: Green tea contains vitamin K, which can make anticoagulant medications less effective. Consult your health care professional if you are using them. The caffeine in green tea could cause insomnia, anxiety, upset stomach, nausea, or diarrhea.

❑ Lycopene from many plant-based foods like tomatoes is a potent quencher of free radicals and an immune-modulator. In one study, patients with metastatic prostate cancer were randomized to lycopene twice daily. The men getting the lycopene experienced a significant reduction in PSA levels and primary and secondary tumors shrank, providing better relief from bone pain and lower urinary tract symptoms, compared to men who did not get lycopene.

❑ The herbs pygeum and saw palmetto are mostly used for the management of benign prostatic hyperplasia (BPH). BPH is characterized by the enlargement of the prostate gland sufficient to cause obstruction of the urethra. With age, there is a build-up of dihydrotestosterone (DHT), which increases prostate size. There is also a shift in the normal balance of hormones in the body (less testosterone and more estrogens). These plants can inhibit 5-alpha-reductase, which slows the change of testosterone to DHT.

❑ Men who have higher levels of the enzyme 5-alpha reductase may be at greater risk for prostate cancer. This is an enzyme that transforms testosterone into dihydrotestosterone (DHT), a form of the hormone that promotes the growth of prostate cells.

❑ Prolactin is another hormone that may alter the cells of the prostate gland. Studies have shown that it may promote the growth of prostate cancer. If you have prostate cancer, you may want to consider having your prolactin levels checked. If they are elevated, the drugs bromocriptine (Parlodel), cabergoline (Dostinex), and pergolide (Permax) are effective in suppressing the release of prolactin from the pituitary gland.

❑ Researchers are looking into the role of angiogenesis (the formation of new blood vessels from existing microvessels) in prostate cancer.

❑ Research is ongoing on genes that may be related to inherited prostate cancer. Some researchers believe that mutated BRCA genes (the gene implicated in some cases of breast cancer) may slightly increase the risk of prostate cancer.

❑ With the numerous treatment methods available today, if you are diagnosed with prostate cancer, it is imperative to be educated about your treatment options. You should include your partner in your decisions.

❑ "Watchful waiting," an option that involves no specific treatment, but close monitoring plus nutritional support and lifestyle changes, is becoming the preferred approach if the cancer is in the early stages. If symptoms develop or if tests indicate that symptoms are likely to develop, treatment is usually started. The primary benefit of watchful waiting is that the adverse effects of the existing treatment options are avoided. This may be advantageous for older men who have other serious health problems and for men who have nonaggressive, early-stage cancers. The doctor will continue to observe you, and you will probably need a PSA blood test and a digital rectal examination every six months and, possibly, a yearly biopsy of the prostate.

❑ If the cancer has not spread outside the gland, surgical options include a radical prostatectomy (removal of the entire gland and some tissue around it) or a transurethral resection of the prostate (TURP). In the latter procedure, a device is inserted through the end of the penis, and a wire loop is used to cut away the cancerous tissue. This is far less radical than a prostatectomy; however, there is some risk of leaving some cancer cells in place. Radiation treatment is sometimes used if the cancer has not spread outside the gland, or has spread only to nearby tissue. Now there is a robot-assisted procedure for removing the prostate gland using a laparoscope, which reduces postoperative pain. The surgeon sits at a console and guides the instruments through a viewing device to perform surgery. So far, outcomes in terms of survival rates, urinary continence, and sexual function are the same as with conventional open prostatectomies.

❏ The Clinical Practice Guidelines in Oncology for prostate cancer state that additional treatment may be necessary for: men in a watching phase whose PSA has doubled or increased rapidly; men who have had a radical prostatectomy and their PSA levels have not fallen below detectable limits after surgery; or men who have had other initial therapy for prostate cancer such as radiation therapy, and the PSA levels have increased by 2 ng/mL or more after having no detectable PSA level.

❏ Hormone treatment is aimed at trying to block production of testosterone, which fuels the cancer. This can be done by means of orchiectomy (surgical removal of the testes) or through the use of hormone therapy to suppress the production and action of hormones. For the latter, either goserelin (Zoladex) or leuprolide (Lupron) is given by monthly injections (they are fundamentally the same drug). In addition, bicalutamide (Casodex) or nilutamide (Nilandron), which block your body's ability to use testosterone, can be taken orally. Together, these agents effectively shut down testosterone production and use by the body. In 2001, the FDA approved abarelix (Plenaxis), which lowers testosterone more quickly, but some people are allergic to the drug, which is given by injection. In 2009, the FDA approved degarelix, an injectable drug that is the first class of drugs called gonadotropin-releasing hormone receptor antagonists. This drug acts by blocking the body's production of testosterone. Both orchiectomy and hormone suppression result in impotence in nearly 100 percent of cases. Side effects of hormone therapy can include loss of sex drive, hot flashes, sexual dysfunction, and weight gain.

❏ Men whose cancer does not respond to hormone therapy may benefit from a docetaxel (Taxotere) injection in combination with the steroid prednisone.

❏ Cryosurgery (also called cryotherapy or cryoablation) is a treatment method for localized prostate cancer. In this technique, the cancerous cells are frozen by means of a metal probe. This type of treatment is less invasive than radical surgery and there is less blood loss. Brachytherapy (a form of radiation treatment in which tiny pellets containing radioactive material are implanted directly into the prostate) and neoadjuvant therapy (a combination of radi-

ation and hormonal treatment) are other approaches that may be recommended for fighting prostate cancer.

❏ Another drug, finasteride (Proscar), is sometimes used to treat moderate prostate enlargement. It blocks an enzyme that converts the male hormone testosterone into dihydrotestosterone, which promotes the growth of prostate tissue. It also reduces the amount of prostate tissue, which can skew the results of the blood test used to detect prostate cancer.

❏ Estrogens have been used for the treatment of prostate cancer for sixty years. However, they can cause breast growth and other feminizing effects, as well as cardiac complications. Because of these side effects, they are rarely used today.

❏ Fresh cabbage and carrot juice have also been used in alternative clinics worldwide in prostate cancer therapy.

❏ Several immunotherapies have been approved by the FDA for cancer treatment. Others are still under study. Regarding prostate cancer, in one therapy researchers remove dendritic cells, which regulate the immune system, from the individual's bloodstream and treat them with prostate cancer antigens. These are then infused back into the person's body, where the cells are now better equipped to deal with and attack cancer cells. In other studies, researchers are using a protein that is part of PSA as the basis for a vaccine. Monoclonal antibody research and DNA vaccines are also being explored.

❏ *See* PROSTATITIS/ENLARGED PROSTATE in Part Two.

❏ *See also* PAIN CONTROL in Part Three.

❏ For names and addresses of organizations that can provide more information on prostate cancer, *see* Health and Medical Organizations in the Appendix.

PROSTATITIS/ENLARGED PROSTATE

The prostate is a doughnut-shaped male sex gland, positioned beneath the urinary bladder. It encircles the urinary outlet, or urethra. Contraction of the muscles in the prostate squeezes fluid from the prostate into the urethral tract during ejaculation. Prostatic fluid makes up the bulk of semen.

The prostate is the most common site of disorders in the male genitourinary system. Generally speaking, there are three conditions that can cause problems with the prostate: prostatitis, which is inflammation of the prostate; benign prostatic hypertrophy (BPH), which is an enlarged prostate with no signs of cancer; and prostate cancer.

Prostatitis, common in men of all ages, is the inflammation of the prostate gland. The usual cause is infectious bacteria that invade the prostate from another area of the body.

Hormonal changes associated with aging may also be a cause. The inflammation can result in urine retention. This causes the bladder to become distended, weak, tender, and itself susceptible to infection. Infection in the bladder is in turn easily transmitted up the ureters to the kidneys.

There are three types of prostatitis: acute infectious prostatitis, chronic infectious prostatitis, and noninfectious prostatitis. Acute infectious prostatitis is usually caused by bacteria. The onset is sudden. Symptoms may include pain between the scrotum and rectum, fever, frequent urination accompanied by a burning sensation, a feeling of fullness in the bladder, and blood or pus in the urine. Chronic (long-term) prostatitis is also a bacterial infection. Symptoms may include nothing more than a recurring bladder infection.

Noninfectious prostatitis is, as the name suggests, not caused by a bacterial infection. The cause for this inflammation is not known. Symptoms can include frequent urination possibly accompanied by pain; pain after ejaculation; and lower abdominal pain. All types of prostatitis, if untreated, can lead to impotence and difficulty with urination.

Benign prostatic hyperplasia (BPH) is the gradual enlargement of the prostate, which usually starts to occur after age forty. Fifty percent of men over sixty years of age and ninety percent of men over seventy have it. After the age of fifty or so, a man's testosterone and free testosterone levels decrease, while the levels of other hormones, such as prolactin and estradiol (a type of estrogen), increase. This creates an increase in the amount of dihydrotestosterone—a very potent form of testosterone—within the prostate. This causes a hyperplasia (overproduction) of prostate cells, which ultimately results in prostate enlargement.

While not cancerous, an enlarged prostate can nevertheless cause problems. If it becomes too large, it obstructs the urethral canal, interfering with urination and the ability to empty the bladder completely. Because the bladder cannot empty completely, the kidneys also may not empty as they should. Dangerous pressure on the kidneys can result. In severe cases, the kidneys may be damaged both by pressure and by substances in the urine. Bladder infections are associated with both prostatitis and enlarged prostate.

The major symptom of enlargement of the prostate is the need to pass urine frequently, with frequency increasing as time passes. A man may find himself rising several times during the night to urinate. There can also be pain, burning, and difficulty in starting and stopping urination. The presence of blood in the urine is not uncommon.

Testing for prostatitis and enlarged prostate usually involves a digital rectal exam plus a blood test that screens for levels of prostate-specific antigen (PSA), a protein secreted by the prostate.

The dosages given below are for adults.

NUTRIENTS

SUPPLEMENT	SUGGESTED DOSAGE	COMMENTS
Essential		
Acidophilus (Kyo-Dophilus from Wakunaga)	As directed on label.	Breaks down metabolites of estrogen. Use a nondairy source.
Quercetin	1,200–2,000 mg daily.	An anti-inflammatory and antitumor flavonoid.
Selenium	As directed on label. Do not take more than the prescribed amount.	Has antioxidant properties that help protect cells from toxin damage linked to prostatitis.
	Overdoses can cause toxicity.	Particularly effective when taken with vitamin E.
Vitamin B complex	50 mg of each major B vitamin 3 times daily (amounts of individual vitamins in a complex will vary).	Necessary for all cellular functions. Antistress vitamins.
plus extra vitamin B₆ (pyridoxine)	50 mg twice daily.	Has anticancer properties.
Zinc	80 mg daily. Do not exceed a total of 100 mg daily from all supplements.	Deficiency has been linked to BPH, prostatitis, and even prostate cancer. Use zinc gluconate lozenges or OptiZinc for best absorption.
plus copper	3 mg daily.	Needed to balance with zinc.
Very Important		
Essential fatty acids (fish oil or flaxseed oil)	As directed on label 3 times daily.	Important in prostate function.
Garlic (Kyolic from Wakunaga)	2 capsules 3 times daily.	Acts as a natural antibiotic.
L-alanine and L-glutamic acid and L-glycine	As directed on label, on an empty stomach. Take with water or juice. Do not take with milk. Take with 50 mg vitamin B₆ and 100 mg vitamin C for better absorption.	Amino acids needed for maintaining normal prostate function. (See AMINO ACIDS in Part One.)
Methylsulfonyl-methane (MSM)	As directed on label.	Relieves pain and inflammation.
Raw prostate glandular	As directed on label.	To normalize prostate function.
Vitamin A plus carotenoid complex	5,000–10,000 IU daily.	Potent antioxidants and immune system enhancers.
Vitamin E	200 IU daily or 400 IU every other day.	Potent antioxidant and immune system enhancer. Use d-alpha-tocopherol form.
Helpful		
Berry seeds complex	1–2 tablets after each meal.	Has shown anti-inflammatory effects on benign prostatic hyperplasia.
Kelp	1,000–1,500 mg daily.	Supplies necessary minerals for improved prostate function.
Lecithin granules or capsules	1 tbsp 3 times daily, before meals. 1,200 mg 3 times daily, before meals.	For cellular protection.
Magnesium plus calcium	As directed on label. As directed on label.	Necessary minerals for improved prostate function.
Vitamin C with bioflavonoids	1,000–5,000 mg daily.	Promotes immune function and aids healing.

Herbs

❑ Teas made from the diuretic herbs buchu and corn silk are helpful. Juniper berries, parsley, slippery elm bark, and uva ursi are also natural diuretics and urinary tract tonics.

❑ Bilberry and birch are urinary tract antiseptics.

❑ Chinese ginseng is beneficial for prostate health and sexual vitality

Caution: Do not use ginseng if you have high blood pressure, or are pregnant or nursing.

❑ Echinacea and goldenseal have antiviral and antibacterial properties that can help to alleviate infection.

Cautions: Do not take echinacea for longer than three months. It should not be used by people who are allergic to ragweed. Do not take goldenseal internally on a daily basis for more than one week at a time. Do not use it during pregnancy or if you are breast-feeding, and use with caution if you are allergic to ragweed. If you have a history of cardiovascular disease, diabetes, or glaucoma, use it only under a doctor's supervision.

❑ Goldenseal root is a diuretic and antiseptic.

❑ A decoction of equal quantities of gravel root, hydrangea root, and sea holly helps to ease inflammation and reduce the discomfort of urination. Take 3 to 4 teaspoonfuls three times daily. Marshmallow leaves may be added to this mixture for their demulcent properties if burning persists.

❑ Olive leaf extract contains anti-inflammatory agents.

❑ Nettle and turmeric are anti-inflammatory agents. Combined extracts of nettle root and saw palmetto have proved effective for BPH.

❑ Pygeum (*Pygeum africanum*) has been proven effective in the treatment and prevention of BPH and prostatitis in many worldwide studies. It has become a primary therapy for these conditions in Europe.

❑ Saw palmetto has been used to treat prostate enlargement and inflammation, painful ejaculation, difficult urination, and enuresis (the inability to control urination). It reduces prostatic enlargement by reducing the amount of hormonal stimulation of the prostate gland.

❑ Siberian ginseng is a tonic for the male reproductive organs.

Caution: Do not use Siberian ginseng if you have hypoglycemia, high blood pressure, or a heart disorder.

❑ Other herbs beneficial for the prostate include cayenne (capsicum) and false unicorn root.

Recommendations

❑ Drink more cranberry juice. This can protect against urinary tract infections, which have been linked to some forms of prostatitis.

❑ *See* Herbs, above, and try one or more of the recommended combinations. Acute inflammation or enlargement of the prostate gland often responds to certain herbal teas. If no improvement takes place or if the symptoms recur, consult a urologist.

❑ Take steps to reduce your blood cholesterol level. (*See* HIGH CHOLESTEROL in Part Two.) Studies have shown a connection between high cholesterol and prostate disorders. Cholesterol has been shown to accumulate in enlarged or cancerous human prostates.

❑ Use hydrotherapy to increase circulation in the prostate region. One method involves sitting in a tub that contains the hottest water tolerable for fifteen to thirty minutes once or twice a day. Another form of hydrotherapy involves spraying the lower abdomen and pelvic area with warm and cold water, alternating between three minutes of hot water and one minute of cold. Still another technique involves sitting in hot water while immersing the feet in cold water for three minutes, and then sitting in cold water while immersing the feet in hot water for one minute.

❑ Eat 1 to 4 ounces of raw pumpkin seeds every day. Pumpkin seeds are helpful for almost all prostate troubles because they are rich in zinc. As an alternative, pumpkin seed oil can be taken in capsule form.

❑ Eliminate from your lifestyle such items as tobacco, alcoholic beverages (especially beer and wine), caffeine (especially coffee and tea), chlorinated and fluoridated water, and spicy and junk foods. Try to reduce your weight if you are overweight. Limit your exposure to pesticides and other environmental contaminants.

❑ If you have prostatitis, increase your fluid intake. Drink two to three quarts of spring or distilled water daily to stimulate urine flow. This helps to prevents cystitis and kidney infection as well as dehydration.

❑ Get regular exercise. Do not ride a bicycle with a standard seat, however; this may put pressure on the prostate. Special bicycle seats are available that have a central opening so that pressure is not put on the prostate. Walking is good exercise.

❑ If your prostate is enlarged, be cautious about using over-the-counter cold or allergy remedies. Many of these products contain ingredients that can inflame the condition and cause urinary retention.

❑ Avoid exposure to very cold weather.

Considerations

❑ It is important that prostatitis be diagnosed correctly because the appropriate treatment depends on the cause. For bacterial prostatitis, the conventional treatment involves antibiotics. Antibiotics do not work with the noninfectious type of this condition.

❑ Prostate Rx from Biotec Corporation and Prost-Actin from Nature's Plus are complexes designed to promote prostate health.

❑ If the prostate is infected, treatment with antibiotics and analgesics may be necessary.

❑ Enlarged prostate may be treated surgically with a procedure called transurethral resection of the prostate (TURP). This procedure is twice as likely to provide long-term relief than drugs or other treatments are. Side effects of the procedure include retrograde ejaculation (in which the semen is pumped back up into the bladder) and, in some cases, impotence or incontinence. About 2 to 3 percent of men who have the procedure need another operation within three years. Prostatron is a transurethral procedure that uses microwaves to destroy excess prostate tissue. In addition, another microwave procedure, Targis System, protects the urethra using a cooling system. Both procedures are done in about an hour on an outpatient basis without general anesthesia. The microwave procedures do not cure benign prostatic hyperplasia (BPH), but they reduce urinary frequency, urgency, straining, and intermittent flow.

❏ The drugs finasteride (Proscar) and dutasteride (Avodart) may be used to treat moderate prostate enlargement. They both block an enzyme that converts the male hormone testosterone into dihydrotestosterone, which promotes the growth of prostate tissue. These increase urine flow and reduce the size of the prostate. Side effects are rare and mild and are mostly related to sexual dysfunction. Sexual performance is recovered when the drug is stopped. In addition, because it reduces the amount of prostate tissue, it can skew the results of the blood test used to detect prostate cancer.

❏ Alpha-blockers such as terazosin (Hytrin) and doxazosin (Cardura) can be used to reduce the size of an enlarged prostate.

❏ Engaging in sexual intercourse while the prostate is infected and irritated may further irritate the prostate and delay recovery.

❏ Some people believe that prostatitis is caused by an inability to process uric acid, a condition that can lead to gout. (*See* GOUT in Part Two.)

❏ Vasectomy for sterilization has been linked to prostate disorders and even cancer.

❏ Zinc deficiency is linked to enlargement of the prostate. Soil used for farming is often deficient in zinc, and unless you eat husks of cereals or brewer's yeast, it is difficult to get enough zinc in the diet. Alcohol causes a deficiency of zinc and other serious nutritional deficiencies. However, too much zinc (over 100 milligrams a day) can depress immune function.

Caution: Brewer's yeast can cause an allergic reaction in some individuals. Start with a small amount at first, and discontinue use if any allergic symptoms occur.

❏ All men aged forty or over should have a yearly rectal examination, during which the prostate gland is checked.

PSORIASIS

Psoriasis is a chronic skin disease that affects 7 million Americans, and 150,000 cases are diagnosed each year. It appears as patches of skin on the legs, knees, arms, elbows, scalp, ears, and back that are red to brown in color and covered with silvery-white scales. Toes and fingernails can lose their luster and develop ridges and pits.

Often hereditary, this condition is linked to a rapid growth of cells in the skin's outer layer. These growths on the epidermis never mature. Whereas a normal skin cell matures and passes from the bottom layer of the skin to the epidermis in about twenty-eight days, psoriatic cells form in about eight days, causing scaly patches that spread to cover larger and larger areas. The result of this disorder is the production of excessive numbers of skin cells in a very short time. The condition is not contagious.

Psoriasis generally follows a pattern of periodic flare-ups alternating with periods of remission, most commonly beginning between the ages of fifteen and thirty. About 75 percent of those with psoriasis develop it before turning forty years of age. Among other things, attacks can be triggered by nervous tension, stress, illness, injury, surgery, cuts, poison ivy, viral or bacterial infection, sunburn, cold weather, overuse of drugs or alcohol, smoking, or the use of nonsteroidal anti-inflammatory drugs, lithium, chloroquine (Aralen), and beta-blockers, a type of medication frequently prescribed for heart disease and high blood pressure. Some people experience an associated arthritis (psoriatic arthritis) that is similar to rheumatoid arthritis and difficult to treat.

The underlying cause of the condition is not known, but it may result from a faulty utilization of fat; psoriasis is rare in countries where the diet is low in fat. Current research points also to an immune system role in psoriasis. The buildup of toxins in an unhealthy colon also has been linked to the development of psoriasis.

The dosages given below are for adults.

NUTRIENTS

SUPPLEMENT	SUGGESTED DOSAGE	COMMENTS
Essential		
Flaxseed oil or primrose oil or Ultimate Oil from Nature's Secret	As directed on label 3 times daily. As directed on label 3 times daily. As directed on label.	To supply essential fatty acids, important for all skin disorders. Aid in preventing dryness.
Vitamin A with mixed carotenoids plus natural beta-carotene	25,000 IU daily. If you are pregnant, do not exceed 10,000 IU daily. As directed on label.	Protects the skin tissue. *Note:* If you have diabetes, omit these supplements. People with diabetes often cannot utilize beta-carotene.
Vitamin D	As directed on label.	A hormone vital for healthy skin.
Zinc plus copper	50–100 mg daily. Do not exceed this amount. 3 mg daily.	Protein metabolism depends on zinc. Protein is needed for healing. Use zinc gluconate lozenges or OptiZinc for best absorption. Needed to balance with zinc.
Very Important		
Proteolytic enzymes	As directed on label. Take between meals.	Stimulates protein synthesis and repair.
Selenium	200 mcg daily. Do not exceed this amount. If you are pregnant, do not exceed 40 mcg daily.	Has powerful antioxidant properties.

Shark cartilage	1 gm per 15 lbs of body weight daily, divided into 3 doses. If you cannot tolerate taking it orally, it can be administered rectally, in a retention enema.	Inhibits the growth of blood vessels to stop the spread of psoriasis. Itching and scaling clear first, then redness gradually fades. Allow two to three months to see results.
Vitamin B complex	50 mg of each major B vitamin 3 times daily. (amounts of individual vitamins in a complex will vary).	Necessary for all cellular functions; antistress vitamins that help to maintain healthy skin.
plus extra vitamin B₁ (thiamine) and	50 mg 3 times daily.	Needed for repair and healing of skin tissue.
vitamin B₅ (pantothenic acid) and	100 mg 3 times daily.	Aids in proper adrenal function, relieving stress on this organ.
vitamin B₆ (pyridoxine) and	50 mg 3 times daily.	Aids in reducing fluid retention, keeping down infection.
vitamin B₁₂ and	2,000 mcg daily.	Use a lozenge or sublingual form.
folic acid	400 mcg daily.	
Vitamin C with bioflavonoids	2,000–10,000 mg daily.	Important for formation of collagen and skin tissue, and for enhancing the immune system.
Vitamin E	200 IU daily or 400 IU every other day.	Neutralizes free radicals that damage the skin. Use an emulsion form for easier assimilation. Use d-alpha-tocopherol form.
Important		
Kelp	1,000–1,500 mg daily.	Supplies balanced minerals. A good source of iodine.
Methylsufonyl-methane (MSM)	As directed on label.	Needed for tissue repair. Often deficient in people with this disorder.
Helpful		
Glutathione	500 mg twice daily, on an empty stomach.	A powerful antioxidant that inhibits the growth of psoriatic cells.
Herpanacine from Diamond-Herpanacine Associates	As directed on label.	Contains antioxidants, amino acids, and herbs that promote overall skin health.
Lecithin granules or capsules or lipotropic factors	1 tbsp 3 times daily, with meals. 1,200 mg 3 times daily, with meals. 200–500 mg daily	Fat emulsifiers. Lecithin also protects the cells.
Multivitamin and mineral complex with calcium and magnesium	As directed on label. 1,500 mg daily. 750 mg daily.	Needed for basic vitamins and minerals.

Herbs

❏ Burdock root and red clover cleanse the blood.

❏ Poultices made from dandelion, and yellow dock can help psoriasis. (*See* USING A POULTICE in Part Three.)

❏ Add 2 teaspoons of ginger to bathwater.

❏ To reduce redness and swelling, lightly brush off scales with a loofah and apply alcohol-free goldenseal extract.

❏ Lavender is good to use in a sauna or steam bath. It fights inflammation and soothes and heals irritated skin.

Note: If you are pregnant or have heart disease or high blood pressure, do not use heat treatments.

❏ Sarsaparilla and yellow dock are good detoxifiers.

❏ Silymarin (milk thistle extract) increases bile flow and protects the liver, which is important in keeping the blood clean. Take 300 milligrams three times daily.

❏ Wild pansy is used to treat psoriasis.

Recommendations

❏ Eat a diet that is composed of 50 percent raw foods and includes plenty of fruits, grains, and vegetables. Include fish in the diet as well.

❏ Get plenty of dietary fiber. Fiber is critical for maintaining a healthy colon. Many fiber components, such as apple pectin and psyllium husks, are able to bind to bowel toxins and promote their excretion in the feces. Also follow the program for colon cleansing. (*See* COLON CLEANSING in Part Three.) A clean colon is very important.

❏ Use fish oil, flaxseed oil, or primrose oil supplements. They contain ingredients that interfere with the production and storage of arachidonic acid (AA), a natural substance that promotes the inflammatory response and makes the lesions of psoriasis turn red and swell. Red meat and dairy products contain small amounts of AA, so you may want to avoid these foods. The biggest source of AA is vegetable oils found in most baked goods, salty snacks, margarine, and salad dressings. Using flaxseed and olive oil for salads and canola and soy oils for cooking rather than oils such as corn and cottonseed reduces your AA intake.

❏ Apply seawater to the affected area with cotton several times a day.

❏ Use cold-pressed flaxseed, sesame, or soybean oils.

❏ Do not consume citrus fruits, fried foods, processed foods, saturated fats (found in meat and dairy products), sugar, or white flour.

Considerations

❏ There is no known cure for psoriasis. Treatment is aimed at reducing the symptoms, and includes the use of topical corticosteroids, ointments, and creams to soften the scales combined with gentle scrubbing to remove them, which reduces the itching. Sometimes ultraviolet light (UVL) therapy is used to retard the production of new skin cells. UVL therapy is sometimes combined with tar therapy; tar is applied to the scaly patches, which are then exposed to the UV light. Another treatment involves using a drug called anthralin (Drithocreme, Dritho-Scalp). This drug can also remove some of the scalp, making the skin smoother. It stains very badly, so its use is usually short-term.

❑ Outbreaks of psoriasis seem to lessen during the summer months. It may even go away on its own, but once you have had psoriasis, it is always possible that it will return.

❑ The freezing of moderately sized psoriatic lesions using liquid nitrogen has been tested with good results.

❑ Cortisone creams, which discourage skin cells from multiplying, are often prescribed for psoriasis, but long-term use makes the skin thin and delicate.

❑ The drug methotrexate (also sold as Rheumatrex) is effective for severe psoriasis. However, this drug can cause liver damage, especially with long-term use. Drugs called retinoids such as tazarotene (Tazorac, Avage) are related to vitamin A. This group of drugs may reduce the production of skin cells in severe psoriasis that doesn't respond to other therapies. These products make the skin dry and cause itching. Since this class of products can cause birth defects, they should not be used by pregnant women. Cyclosporine (Sandimmune) therapy has been tested with good results because it suppresses the immune system, which with psoriasis is in overdrive.

❑ A skin patch, Actiderm, manufactured by ConvaTec, can be applied over most topical psoriasis medications, especially steroid (cortisone) ointments, to make them more effective. The patch allows one to achieve better results with milder steroids and fewer doses.

❑ Activated vitamin D_3 ointment (Dovonex), available by prescription only, has produced good results for many people with mild to moderate forms of psoriasis. It is a cream and may be used with other topical medications or phototherapy.

❑ Ultraviolet light has been effectively used to treat severe psoriasis along with a drug called methoxsalen (Oxsoralen-Ultra). The drug makes the skin more sensitive to the light therapy. This combination effectively clears or improves severe, recalcitrant, disabling psoriasis in 84 percent of patients.

❑ The FDA has approved several biological therapies for psoriasis. These include alefacept (Amervive), etanercept (Enbrel), and infliximab (Remicade). These drugs are given intravenously, intramuscularly, or subcutaneously, and are reserved for those who have failed to respond to traditional therapies. The drugs have strong effects on immune function and may cause infections.

❑ For names and addresses of organizations that can provide more information about psoriasis, *see* Health and Medical Organizations in the Appendix.

PURPURA

See under IDIOPATHIC THROMBOCYTOPENIC PURPURA in RARE DISORDERS.

PYELONEPHRITIS

See under KIDNEY DISEASE.

PYORRHEA

See under PERIODONTAL DISEASE.

RADIATION EXPOSURE

Radioactive pollution from nuclear reactors, plutonium disposal, and uranium mining is a great concern today. Cellular telephones, X-rays, nuclear medicine, computer monitors, television sets, smoke detectors, and microwave ovens are among the common items that are sources of radiation exposure. Radiation is around us all the time in both natural and artificially introduced forms. The sun is a natural source of radiation exposure, and so is radon, a naturally occurring radioactive gas that is reported to be the second leading cause of lung cancer in the United States and claims about 20,000 lives annually. The human body itself is a source of some radiation.

Radioactive elements are made up of unstable atoms that give off energy as the result of spontaneous decay of their nuclei. If the energy released by a radioactive element is strong enough to dislodge electrons from other atoms or molecules in its path, it can damage or even kill living tissue.

This type of radiation is called ionizing radiation. Even if only one cell is exposed to radiation, the radiation can destroy, damage, or alter the makeup of that cell. The alteration of cell structure by radioactive particles can lead to the development of cancer. If a cell's DNA is damaged, this can cause genetic mutations that can be passed down to offspring.

Radiation exposure in the United States comes primarily from the following sources, in order:

- Radon: 79 percent.
- Other natural sources: 11 percent.
- Medical sources: 6 percent.
- Other man-made sources: 4 percent.

Radiation exposure is measured in units called *rems*. The average American is exposed to about 360 millirem (a millirem is equal to 1/1,000 rem) of radioactivity per year. Our bodies naturally produce about 40 millirem of radiation per year from potassium 40. A chest X-ray exposes you to about 10 millirem.

The risk of dying from radiation-induced cancer increases by 8 percent for each exposure exceeding 10 rem (or 10,000 millirem). Comparing estimated years of life lost from different causes is probably the best way to see how radiation affects our lives.

Health Risk	Estimated Time Lost
Smoking 20 cigarettes/day	6 years
Overweight by 15%	2 years
Alcohol	1 year
Natural hazards	7 days
Occupational dose at 1 rem/year	51 days
Occupational dose of radiation (300 millirem/year)	15 days

Radioactive elements are structurally similar to their nonradioactive counterparts, differing only in the number of neutrons the atoms contain. This is why nutrition is important in preventing or blocking damage from exposure to radioactive elements. If you do not obtain sufficient amounts of calcium, potassium, and other minerals in your diet, your body may absorb radioactive elements that are similar in structure to these nutrients. For example, if you do not obtain enough calcium, your body will absorb radioactive strontium 90 (Sr-90) or other elements that are similar in structure to calcium, if they are available. Similarly, if you obtain sufficient potassium from your diet, your body will be less likely to retain any radioactive cesium 137 it encounters, as this element is similar to potassium.

If the cells are able to obtain all nutrients they need from your diet, they will be less likely to absorb radioactive substitutes, which are then more likely to be discarded from the body.

The effects of radiation exposure can be acute, following a single, relatively high-intensity exposure, or they can be delayed or chronic. Acute reactions to radiation are extremely dangerous. They cause symptoms of listlessness, nausea, vomiting, weakness, and loss of coordination, leading to dehydration, convulsions, shock, and even death.

Fortunately, the amount and type of exposure that causes such serious reactions are extremely rare.

Radiotherapy treatment for cancer involves the administration of fairly high doses of radiation specifically targeted at cancerous cells. The idea underlying this treatment is that the radiation kills the cancer, but healthy tissue, which is not targeted, is only minimally affected. Not surprisingly, the major side effect of this type of treatment is radiation sickness, with the classic symptoms of nausea, vomiting, headache, weakness, loss of appetite, and hair loss.

Dental checkups today often include X-rays to locate cavities. Physicians take X-rays to determine whether a bone is broken, to check cardiovascular and respiratory health, and to locate tumors and areas of dysfunction.

Women are urged to have regular mammograms, or breast X-rays, for early detection of breast cancer. Cancer research indicates that a significant percentage of women in the United States have inherited a gene, dubbed *oncogene AC*, that is sensitive to X-ray exposure. For these women, even short periods of X-ray exposure can lead to the development of cancer.

Fruits and vegetables—in fact, all foods—contain some level of radioactive material. Milk is checked in some states for the presence of strontium 90 (Sr-90), an element that is present as a result of aboveground nuclear testing (though aboveground testing is now banned in the United States). Sr-90 has a half-life of about twenty-eight years.

There is nothing that can protect a person against radioactive substances such as radon except detection and eradication of the problem. If radon is detected in your home, you need to hire trained experts to have it removed. But good nutrition and a good supplement program will provide support and protection for your immune system. It is advisable to buy your fruit, vegetables, meat, and grains from sources that employ organic methods of farming to exclude further toxins from your diet.

Unless otherwise specified, the doses recommended here are for persons age eighteen and over. For children between twelve and seventeen, use three-quarters the recommended dose; for children between six and twelve, use one-half the recommended dose; and for children under six, use one-quarter the recommended dose.

NUTRIENTS

SUPPLEMENT	SUGGESTED DOSAGE	COMMENTS
Very Important		
Calcium and magnesium	1,500 mg daily. / 750 mg daily.	To help prevent the body from absorbing radioactive materials.
Coenzyme Q10 plus	100 mg daily.	Protects the body from harmful radiation.
Coenzyme A from Coenzyme-A Technologies	As directed on label.	Works with coenzyme Q10 to support the immune system and detoxify the bloodstream.
Glutathione plus L-cysteine and L-methionine	500 mg each daily, on an empty stomach. Take with water or juice. Do not take with milk. Take with 50 mg vitamin B6 and 100 mg vitamin C for better absorption.	To detoxify harmful substances and protect against the harmful effects of radiation.
Kelp	1,000–1,500 mg daily.	Protects against radiation. Take kelp in tablet form or eat sea vegetables.
Important		
Garlic (Kyolic from Wakunaga)	2 capsules 3 times daily.	Stimulates and protects the immune system.
Grape seed extract	As directed on label.	A powerful antioxidant.
Oxy-5000 Forte from American Biologics	As directed on label.	This antioxidant is high in superoxide dismutase (SOD), a powerful antioxidant.
Selenium	200 mcg daily. If you are pregnant, do not exceed 40 mcg daily.	A free radical scavenger that protects against cancer.
Vitamin B5 (pantothenic acid)	200 mg before and after X-ray exposure; 50 mg daily thereafter.	Protects against the harmful effects of radiation.
Vitamin C with bioflavonoids including rutin	5,000–20,000 mg daily in divided doses. (*See* ASCORBIC ACID FLUSH in Part Three.)	A powerful free radical scavenger. A vitamin C complex that contains 200 mg of rutin per capsule is best.
Helpful		
Brewer's yeast	As directed on label.	A natural source of pantothenic acid, as well as the other B vitamins.
Lecithin granules or capsules	1 tbsp 3 times daily, with meals. / 1,200 mg 3 times daily, with meals.	Protects cell membranes from radiation.

Vitamin A with mixed carotenoids including beta-carotene	25,000 IU daily. If you are pregnant, do not exceed 10,000 IU daily.	Protects and strengthens the immune system, especially in combination with vitamin E.
Vitamin B complex plus extra inositol	50 mg of each major B vitamin 3 times daily (amounts of individual vitamins in a complex will vary). 100 mg daily.	Helps to protect against the harmful effects of radiation.
Vitamin E	200 IU daily.	Protects and strengthens the immune system, especially in combination with vitamin A. Use d-alpha-tocopherol form.
Zinc	50–80 mg daily. Do not exceed a total of 100 mg daily from all supplements.	Helps to increase immunity. Use zinc gluconate lozenges or OptiZinc for best absorption.

Recommendations

❏ Include apples in the diet; they are a good source of pectin, which binds with radioactive particles. Pectin is also available in supplement form.

❏ Eat buckwheat, which is high in rutin, a bioflavonoid that protects against the effects of radiation.

❏ Consume avocados, lemons, and cold-pressed safflower and olive oils. These supply essential fatty acids.

❏ Drink plenty of steam-distilled water.

❏ If you use a cellular telephone, guard against possible contamination by purchasing an earpiece. Or buy one with a speaker and use that. No link between brain cancer and cell phone use has yet been proved, but it makes sense to be cautious. The electromagnetic waves from a cell phone are supposed to meet government guidelines, but this is uncharted territory. It is best to err on the side of caution. There are numerous products on the market that contain an earpiece and attached microphone allowing you to keep the telephone itself some distance from your body.

❏ If you use a computer and sit in front of a monitor all day, use a radiation/glare filter screen. Monitors are much better than they used to be, but it is wise to be cautious.

❏ Have your home tested for radon. This is a radioactive gas that occurs naturally in the soil in some places. It has no smell. The biggest danger is from exposure to radon inside the home, where the gas can accumulate and escape detection. People who smoke are at even greater risk from the damaging effects radon has on the lungs. Radon detection kits are available in most hardware stores and home centers. They may also be available from your local department of health and some drugstores. If the levels are too high, you can contact an expert company that can remove the radon.

❏ If there is even a chance you might be pregnant, do not let your doctor or dentist do any X-ray testing. Women exposed to X-rays in the first three to five weeks of pregnancy are at a higher risk of having a miscarriage or delivering a baby with birth defects. Exposure between the eighth and fifteenth week can cause the baby to suffer brain damage. Childhood leukemia can occur if a fetus is exposed to X-rays during the first trimester of pregnancy.

Considerations

❏ As technology improves and more becomes known about how cancer cells work, the part that radiation therapy has to play in cancer treatment has been reduced. Radiation exposure is also more carefully monitored than it was in the past.

❏ A study conducted at the University of Medicine and Dentistry of New Jersey in Newark showed that rats given orange juice before exposure to low-level radiation (1 to 50 rems) suffered two times less damage than rats given water before exposure.

❏ *See also* WEAKENED IMMUNE SYSTEM in Part Two.

RARE DISORDERS

Jumping Frenchmen of Maine sounds like an uproarious, modern-day stage show or a new music group of some kind. But it is neither. It is actually the name of an unusual disorder that causes an extreme startle reaction to unexpected noises or sights. Though little is known about Jumping Frenchmen of Maine, the disorder and more than 6,000 other rare, or "orphan," diseases are receiving increasing attention from the government, patient groups, and the pharmaceutical industry.

In the United States, an orphan disease is defined as a condition that affects fewer than 200,000 people nationwide; there are more than 5,000 such disorders. This includes diseases as familiar as cystic fibrosis, Lou Gehrig's disease, and Tourette syndrome, and as unfamiliar as hamburger disease, Job syndrome, and acromegaly (or gigantism). For some diseases, there are fewer than one hundred known cases. Collectively, however, rare disorders affect as many as 25 million Americans, according to the National Institutes of Health (NIH), and that makes these diseases—and finding treatments for them—a serious public health concern.

New rare diseases are discovered every year. Most are inherited and caused by alterations or genetic mutations (defects in genes). Genes are pieces of DNA, part of the code that determines the traits and individual characteristics of all living things. Each human cell contains around 30,000 genes. Besides influencing features such as eye and hair color, genes also can play a role in the development of diseases and in their transmission from parent to child. In addition to those with genetic causes, there are some rare diseases that can be acquired as a result of environmental and toxic conditions.

Rare Disorders and the Internet

New online support groups for people with various health problems continue to proliferate. Not only are people receiving comfort from others with the same conditions, but they are learning from each other's experiences as well. By the late 1990s, most nonprofit organizations had websites where people could ask questions and get immediate answers.

Nevertheless, people diagnosed with rare disease often are vulnerable to misguided assistance. While the National Institutes of Health's Office of Rare Diseases encourages people to use the Internet to find information, it also warns that it is dangerous to rely solely on the computer for medical advice. It is especially important to exercise caution when claims are made for unproven remedies and "miracle" cures. Too often, misleading or inaccurate information is given out that can do more harm than good. In addition, one person's experience may vary greatly from another's. The best way to use the Internet is to complement the communication between doctor and patient, not to replace it.

Be wary also of advertisements, newsletters, and books that offer "medical or natural cures." Always keep in mind, anything that sounds too good to be true probably is.

As disparate as rare diseases are, the people who have them share many common frustrations. For example, for one-third of people with a rare disease, getting an accurate diagnosis can take one to five years. And people often are so isolated that they may never know anyone else with the same disease. They often must travel long distances to visit the few doctors knowledgeable about their illnesses, and the costs involved with diagnosis, treatment, and other related expenses can be exorbitant. Finally, they have trouble obtaining health and life insurance coverage, and if they do manage to get it, it is very expensive.

Many rare diseases or conditions can be difficult to diagnose and manage because in their early stages, the symptoms may be absent or masked, misunderstood, or confused with those of other diseases. One disease that was originally misdiagnosed as multiple sclerosis (MS) led to delayed and inappropriate treatment of the individual's true problem—adrenomyeloneuropathy (AMN). AMN is a milder form of adrenoleukodystrophy (ALD), one of a group of genetically determined progressive disorders, known collectively as *leukodystrophies*, which affect the brain, spinal cord, and peripheral nerves. This one case raised a red flag for the individual's doctor when his patient mentioned that not only had his grandfather been diagnosed with MS—and in fact had died from it—but also that he had lost two brothers and several cousins to the same disease.

Because MS is not hereditary, the doctor in this case suspected that the disease that had befallen his patient's family members, and now him, was not MS because of its genetic pattern of inheritance. An in-depth family history revealed that he and his brothers had had a 50 percent chance of having either ALD or AMN because their mother was a carrier of the defective gene involved. Following his diagnosis of AMN, two more of his brothers died of the disease.

ALD affects only 1 in about 100,000 people. This was enough, however, to form an organization, the United Leukodystrophy Foundation (ULF), a voluntary health organization. According to the ULF, the leukodystrophies are often misdiagnosed as MS because diagnosis of neurological conditions relies on subtle and circumstantial evidence, and even the most experienced clinicians may have difficulty distinguishing between the two.

For people with rare disorders there may be no cures, but treatments of the symptoms can help. Having the support of family and friends, patient advocacy groups, and disease associations like ULF is also helpful. Participating in clinical trials may be a way to receive the most advanced care for some diseases. People who experience unexplained symptoms, recurrent infections, and pain that has gone undiagnosed for a long period of time might want to visit a referral center that is experienced in diagnosing those with rare diseases. Some rare diseases do not have clearly defined treatment guidelines and require the specific skills of an expert physician. Be sure to go to a hospital that is familiar with treating people with multiple problems.

Before the passage of rare disease laws in the United States, people diagnosed with rare diseases were denied access to effective medicines because prescription drug manufacturers rarely could make a profit from marketing drugs to such small groups. Consequently, the prescription drug industry did not adequately fund research for the development of so-called orphan products. Other potential sources, such as research hospitals and universities, also lacked the capital and business expertise to develop treatments for small patient groups. Despite the urgent health need for these medicines, they came to be known as orphans because companies were not interested in "adopting" them.

This changed in 1983 when Congress passed the Orphan Drug Act (ODA). Since 1983, the ODA has resulted in the development of nearly 325 orphan drugs, which now are available to treat a potential population of more than 17 million Americans. In contrast, the decade prior to 1983 saw fewer than ten such products developed without government assistance. As a result, treatments are available to people with rare diseases who once had no hope for survival.

Congress also approved funding for several regional Centers of Excellence on rare diseases. Support groups such as the National Organization for Rare Disorders (NORD; *see* Health and Medical Organizations in the Appendix) have worked aggressively in the last twenty years to draw attention to people with rare diseases, especially their lack of treatment options. Paramount in NORD's ongoing cause are efforts to promote legislation, such as the ODA, that encourages further research and continuing development of products that are necessary—and often lifesaving—and to provide easier access to such treatments.

Individuals suffering from these various rare diseases and their caregivers would be well advised to stay abreast of new research as it is reported in hopes of being able to wisely choose the best combination of therapy and nutritional supplementation. Unfortunately, our knowledge on the subject of orphan diseases is limited at this time, as the research to date is also limited. We look forward to information breakthroughs that we can share in future editions of this book.

In thinking about nutritional guidelines for rare orphan diseases, it may be helpful to consider the baffling symptoms, suspected causes, and possible nutritional supports appropriate for late-onset autism. Due to the multifaceted nature of late-onset autism and the successes and failures associated with attempted treatments, it is a disease that, when studied carefully, can give hints as to the factors influencing other rare diseases.

Late-onset autism is a rare neurological condition that afflicts young children, usually between their first and fifth years. The majority of affected families report normal development during the first year or so, but these skills then disappear and new skills fail to develop. The child ceases to socialize, and verbal abilities are usually completely lost. Temper tantrums become quite common and more severe as the child no longer has the ability to communicate his or her needs. An autistic child usually becomes intolerant of certain foods as his or her digestive system becomes less functional. His or her stool and sometimes urine can become unusually putrid, and his or her movements usually become repetitive and disassociated from surroundings. The resulting stress takes its toll on the entire family.

Most clinicians believe that a cure is impossible, but some disagree and believe that a cure will soon be found. The causes of late-onset autism are debated among researchers, clinicians, and informed parents. A few believe that the mercury compound used in some vaccines is to blame. In addition, there is often a history of frequent ear infections with much antibiotic use. Some believe that an overuse of antibiotics has killed off the friendly intestinal bacteria, leaving the gut vulnerable to the antibiotic-resistant, neurotoxin-producing bacterium clostridium. Other researchers suggest that, much like typical autism, there is a genetic component. In many cases, both mercury and clostridium are present. Perhaps all of these observations are correct to one degree or another. Hopefully, time and study will reveal the answers. For now, we can only guess which factors are to blame.

The afflicted children, whose blood tests high for mercury, may be treated with chelation therapy by licensed health care professionals. Many are reporting positive results though not a complete cure. Other practitioners are concentrating on the digestive system and are attempting to bring the overgrowth of clostridium bacteria under control and, again, are reporting improvement though not a cure. Most are making dietary and nutritional changes, administering antioxidants as well as many other supplements, and are reporting improvement but still no cure. As the body of evidence grows that making nutritional and dietary changes affects this form of autism, the argument for a genetic cause weakens. If external factors are to blame, avoidance of the disease, if not a cure, is probable. (For nutritional recommendations that may be of help in late-onset autism, *see* the recommendations *under* AUTISM, page 234.)

Late-onset autism is a disease where there are, in addition to chelation therapy, four primary areas of support that have shown some degree of success and perhaps can be applied when fighting other very difficult and rare diseases.

- Gastrointestinal support.

- Neurological support.

- Cardiovascular support.

- Immune system support.

Some general rules to consider when combating many diseases:

1. *Start with the gastrointestinal tract.* This should include digestive enzymes and probiotics. Care must be taken when giving digestive enzymes. Too much can result in a partial digestion of the stomach lining itself, resulting in severe inflammation, especially with small children. Digestive enzymes and probiotics and guidance for their use are available from:

   Healthy Alternatives, Inc.
   10458 Moe Hall Road NW
   Garfield, MN 56332
   888-362-0401
   www.healthyalternativesinc.com

2. *Provide the necessary nutritional supplements for neurological support.* Neurological stress consumes excessive quantities of gamma-aminobutyric acid (GABA). GABA acts as a stabilizer by inhibiting neurological overreaction. Vitamin B_{12}, in the methylcobalamin form, aids in the rebuilding and healing of nerve cells.

   The following formula includes precursors for the production of GABA, serotonin, and other supporting nutrients, and is available under the brand name GabaMax from:

   NeuroScience Inc.
   373 280th Street
   Osceola, WI 54020
   888-342-7272
   www.neurorelief.com

GabaMax includes the following ingredients:
- N-acetyltyrosine
- 5-hydroxy L-tryptophan (5-HTP)
- Theanine
- Glutamine
- Taurine
- Vitamin B$_6$
- Folic acid
- Vitamin C
- Magnesium

GabaMax should be taken as directed on the bottle.

The addition of 5,000 mcg (1,000 mcg for small children) of vitamin B$_{12}$ in the form of methylcobalamin works well with the above formula to help heal nerve damage.

3. *Provide support for the cardiovascular system.* There are many rare diseases where the circulatory system is so compromised that nutrients have great difficulty finding their way to the areas in desperate need of them. Therefore, supplements that target the circulatory system may help. (*See* CARDIOVASCULAR DISEASE, page 306.)

4. *Strengthen the immune system to help combat microbes that may attack during times of weakness.* There is also some suspicion that a few of the orphan diseases are virally induced. (*See* WEAKENED IMMUNE SYSTEM, page 774.)

Many rare diseases are known to be of genetic origin, and in many such cases there is evidence that even they may respond positively to sound nutrition. The diseases that follow may be caused by problems in some or all of the above areas. You'll find notes for each that suggest different combinations of treatment that could help to alleviate their symptoms and/or severity.

ACUTE DISSEMINATED ENCEPHALOMYELITIS

Acute disseminated encephalomyelitis (ADE) is characterized by inflammation of the brain and spinal cord caused by damage to the myelin sheath—the fatty insulator of the brain's nerve fibers. Both viral and bacterial infection can be associated with ADE. It can also arise as a complication of inoculation or vaccination. The onset of ADE is sudden and symptoms vary from person to person. They can include headaches, delirium, lethargy, coma, seizures, stiff neck, fever, ataxia, optic neuritis, transverse myelitis, vomiting, and weight loss. In some cases, a limb or an entire side of the body can become paralyzed. ADE strikes children more often than adults.

Considerations

❑ The treatment of ADE typically includes the use of corticosteroid medications plus symptom-relieving and supportive measures.

❑ The prognosis for people with ADE varies. Some patients achieve complete or nearly complete recovery, while others continue to suffer residual symptoms. In severe cases, the disorder can prove fatal. If diagnosed early and treated promptly, however, the prognosis for ADE disorder is generally good.

❑ For nutritional recommendations, *see* Neurological Support, page 679; CARDIOVASCULAR DISEASE, page 306; and WEAKENED IMMUNE SYSTEM, page 774.

AGNOSIA

Agnosia is a rare disorder characterized by the inability to recognize familiar objects or people. Agnosia can be limited to one sense such as hearing or vision. For example, a person may have difficulty identifying a sound as a cough or recognizing an object as a cup. The case made famous in neurologist Oliver Sacks's popular book *The Man Who Mistook His Wife for a Hat* (Touchstone, 1998) was one of a man with visual agnosia.

This disorder can be caused by stroke, dementia, or other neurological disorders. It can become debilitating and compromise the quality of life. Agnosia typically affects specific brain areas in the occipital or parietal lobes, areas of the brain that are important for processing and integrating information received through vision and other senses. People with agnosia may retain cognitive abilities in other areas.

Considerations

❑ The primary cause of agnosia must first be established in order to determine how best to treat symptoms.

❑ For nutritional recommendations, *see* CARDIOVASCULAR DISEASE, page 306; and WEAKENED IMMUNE SYSTEM, page 774.

ALPHA-1 ANTITRYPSIN DEFICIENCY

Alpha-1 antitrypsin deficiency is a genetic disease characterized by a lack of the protein alpha-1 antitrypsin in the liver. This substance is used to break down enzymes in various organs of the body. The disease can lead to hepatitis and cirrhosis, or scarring, of the liver. In addition, alpha-1 antitrypsin also protects the lungs from irritants in conjunction with an enzyme released by white blood cells. A person deficient in alpha-1 antitrypsin is therefore much more susceptible to lung disease, especially emphysema.

Alpha-1 antitrypsin deficiency most commonly appears in newborn infants and is characterized by jaundice, swelling of the abdomen, and poor feeding. However, the disease may also develop in late childhood or even in adulthood. In such cases, symptoms may include fatigue, poor appetite, swelling of the abdomen and legs, or abnormal results on liver tests.

Considerations

❑ Prolastin is used for alpha-1 antitrypsin deficiency in adults with emphysema. Other treatment aims to control abnormalities and to provide the liver with essential nutrients. Multiple vitamin supplements plus vitamins E, D, and K are typically prescribed.

❑ Avoid consuming too much salt or protein, and get protein from vegetable sources. Avoid large doses of vitamin A, niacin, and iron from supplements. However, it is fine to get these nutrients from food.

❑ Phenobarbital or cholestyramine is prescribed for jaundice.

❑ For nutritional recommendations, *see* CARDIOVASCULAR DISEASE, page 306.

ATAXIA

People with ataxia experience a failure of muscle control in their arms and legs, resulting in a lack of balance and coordination or a disturbance of gait. This can occur if parts of the nervous system that control movement are damaged. While the term *ataxia* is primarily used to describe this set of symptoms, it is sometimes also used to refer to a family of disorders.

Most disorders that result in ataxia cause cells in the part of the brain called the cerebellum to degenerate, or atrophy. Sometimes the spine is also affected. While the phrases *cerebellar degeneration* and *spinocerebellar degeneration* are used to describe changes that have taken place in a person's nervous system, neither term constitutes a specific diagnosis. Cerebellar and spinocerebellar degeneration can have many different causes. The age of onset of any resulting ataxia varies depending on the underlying cause of the degeneration. Among the more common inherited ataxias are Friedreich's ataxia and Machado-Joseph disease.

Friedreich's ataxia is an inherited disease that causes progressive damage to the nervous system, resulting in symptoms ranging from muscle weakness and speech problems to heart disease. Symptoms usually begin between the ages of five and fifteen, but can appear as early as eighteen months or as late as thirty years of age. The first symptom is usually difficulty in walking. The ataxia gradually worsens and slowly spreads to the arms and then the trunk. Foot deformities such as clubfoot, flexion (involuntary bending) of the toes, hammertoes, or foot inversion (turning in of the foot) may be early signs. Rapid, involuntary rhythmic movements of the eyeball are common. Most people with Friedreich's ataxia develop scoliosis (a sideways curvature of the spine), which, if severe, may impair breathing. Other symptoms include chest pain, shortness of breath, and heart palpitations.

Machado-Joseph disease (MJD), also called *spinocerebellar ataxia type 3*, is a rare hereditary ataxia. The disease is characterized by clumsiness and weakness in the arms and legs, spasticity, a staggering lurching gait easily mistaken for drunkenness, difficulty with speech and swallowing, involuntary eye movements, double vision, and frequent urination. Some people suffer form dystonia, or sustained

muscle contractions that cause twisting of the body and limbs, repetitive movements, abnormal postures, and/or rigidity—symptoms similar to those of Parkinson's disease. Others have twitching of the face or tongue, or peculiar bulging eyes. In Machado-Joseph disease, degeneration of cells in an area of the brain called the hindbrain leads to deficits in movement. The hindbrain includes the cerebellum, the brain stem, and the upper part of the spinal cord. MJD is an inherited, autosomal dominant disease, which means that if a child inherits one copy of the defective gene from either parent, the child will develop symptoms of the disease. People with a defective gene have a 50 percent chance of passing the mutation on to their children. The severity of the disease is related to the age of onset, with earlier onset associated with a more severe form of the disease. Symptoms can begin any time between early adolescence and about seventy years of age. MJD is also a progressive disease, meaning that symptoms get worse with time. Life expectancy ranges from the midthirties for those with severe forms of MJD to a normal life expectancy for those with mild forms. For those who die early from the disease, the cause of death is often aspiration pneumonia, which can occur if fluids or other materials are inhaled into the lungs and cannot be cleared away.

In addition to being a result of heredity, ataxia also can be acquired. Conditions that can cause acquired ataxia include stroke, multiple sclerosis, tumors, alcoholism, peripheral neuropathy, metabolic disorders, and vitamin deficiencies.

Considerations

❑ There is no cure for hereditary ataxias. If the ataxia is caused by another condition, that underlying condition is treated first. For example, ataxia caused by a metabolic disorder may be treated with medications and a controlled diet. Vitamin deficiency is treated with vitamin therapy. A variety of drugs may be used to treat gait and swallowing disorders. Foods mixed with thickening agents may help a person to swallow better. Physical therapy can strengthen muscles to improve gait, while devices or appliances can assist in walking and other activities of daily life. The prognosis for individuals with ataxia and cerebellar/spinocerebellar degeneration varies depending on its underlying cause. Most people with ataxia have had a stroke and may go to a nursing home until they are able to care for themselves.

❑ There is currently no effective cure or treatment for Friedreich's ataxia. However, many symptoms and accompanying complications can be treated to help individuals maintain optimal functioning as long as possible. Diabetes and heart problems can be treated with medications. Orthopedic problems such as foot deformities and scoliosis can be treated with braces or surgery. Physical therapy may prolong the use of the arms and legs. Generally, however, a person with Friedreich's ataxia requires a wheelchair, and in later stages of the disease, he or she is likely to become completely incapacitated. If significant heart disease is involved, a person with Friedreich's ataxia is likely to die in early adulthood, but some who have less severe symptoms live much longer.

❏ MJD is incurable, but some symptoms of the disease can be treated. Treatment with antispasmodic drugs, such as baclofen (Lioresal), can help reduce spasticity. Physiotherapy can help people to cope with disability associated with gait problems; and physical aids, such as walkers and wheelchairs, can assist with everyday activities. Other problems, such as sleep disturbances, cramps, and urinary dysfunction, can be treated with medications and medical care.

❏ For nutritional recommendations, *see* Neurological Support, page 679; and CARDIOVASCULAR DISEASE, page 306.

BELL'S PALSY

Bell's palsy is the result of damage to the seventh cranial nerve and is characterized by weakness and paralysis of one side of the face. Currently, 40,000 Americans develop Bell's palsy each year. Although it can strike anyone at any age, pregnant women and people who have diabetes, influenza, or a cold or other respiratory ailment are particularly susceptible to the disorder. The facial paralysis usually leads to an inability to close the eye on the affected side. Other symptoms may include pain, tearing, drooling, hypersensitivity to sound in the affected ear, and even impairment in taste. Many cases of Bell's palsy are believed to be caused by viruses, especially those in the herpes family such as the herpes simplex virus, which causes cold sores.

Considerations

❏ Sometimes steroid drugs (prednisone) are combined with the antiviral medication acyclovir (Zovirax) to treat this condition. However, as of 2001, the American Academy of Neurology concluded that steroids are safe but do not promote faster recovery, and that there is no conclusive evidence that the combination therapy (steroid and antiviral) actually works.

❏ Decompression surgery also has not been shown to be effective, and side effects like permanent hearing loss have been reported.

❏ The prognosis for people with Bell's palsy is very good. Although the condition is troublesome and even possibly alarming, 50 percent of those with the condition improve within a few weeks to a few months. Another 35 percent usually have full recovery within a year.

❏ For nutritional recommendations, *see* Neurological Support, page 679, and add 500–1,000 mg L-lysine daily.

BINSWANGER'S DISEASE

Binswanger's disease is a rare form of dementia, a loss of certain types of brain function. This disorder is sometimes known as *subcortical dementia*. It begins late in the fourth decade of life and increases in severity with age.

The mental disability characteristic of Binswanger's disease includes memory loss caused by the presence of cerebrovascular lesions in the deep white matter of the brain, cognitive problems, and mood changes. These problems are associated with tiny areas of tissue damage or death—multiple strokes, in effect—that occur deep within the brain's white matter (nerve cells) and that are probably due to severe high blood pressure and blood vessel disease in the head and neck.

In addition to mental symptoms, people with Binswanger's disease are often found to have blood abnormalities and heart valve disorders, and they can become incontinent, experience clumsiness, and develop difficulty with walking, speech, and physical activity in general. The ability to show normal facial expressions may become limited as well. For some people, symptoms progress steadily once they start; for others, symptoms may seem to come and go as people experience strokes followed by partial recovery.

Considerations

❏ There is no known cure and no specific treatment recommended for all people with Binswanger's disease. Drug therapy may be used to control blood pressure, depression, and heart arrhythmias.

❏ For nutritional recommendations, *see* Gastrointestinal Support, page 679; Neurological Support, page 679; and CARDIOVASCULAR DISEASE, page 306.

BROWN-SEQUARD SYNDROME

This is a rare neurological condition that leads to weakness or paralysis affecting one side of the body, accompanied by a loss of sensation on the opposite side. These problems are associated with a lesion in the spinal cord that in turn may be the result of a spinal cord tumor, injury to the neck or back, a blocked blood vessel causing ischemia (oxygen deprivation) to the area, or an underlying disease such as tuberculosis or multiple sclerosis.

Considerations

❏ The prognosis for people with Brown-Sequard syndrome depends on the underlying cause. Treatment therefore usually focuses on identifying and, if possible, removing the cause. Early treatment with high doses of steroids may be beneficial as well.

❏ For nutritional recommendations, *see* Neurological Support, page 679; and CARDIOVASCULAR DISEASE, page 306.

DYSTONIA

People with dystonia experience sustained, simultaneous muscle contractions that force affected body parts into abnormal and sometimes painful postures and movements. Dystonia is actually not a single disorder, but a category of them, usually divided into two types: primary dystonia, which occurs on its own and has no known cause; and secondary dystonias, which are caused by some underlying problem, such as Parkinson's disease, a brain tumor, or stroke.

Considerations

❑ A variety of treatments, among them drug therapy, surgery, and physical therapy (including biofeedback), have been used for dystonias. These measures are useful for some people, helping to reducing pain and muscle spasms, although overall the results are decidedly mixed and a certain amount of trial and error can be involved.

❑ A relatively new treatment for dystonia involves the use of a brain implant. A system called the Activa Dystonia Therapy system, which had already been used to treat Parkinson's disease and essential tremor, consists of electrodes and a deep brain neurostimulator. The electrodes are implanted into the brain and connected by wires under the skin to the neurostimulator, which is implanted in the chest. The neurostimulator sends a constant stream of tiny electrical pulses to the brain to suppress symptoms. If both sides of the brain are affected, it is necessary to use two separate systems, one in each side of the brain. A person with the implant touches a handheld magnet over the neurostimulator to switch the device on and off. This system is manufactured by Medtronic Inc. (*See* Manufacturer and Distributor Information in the Appendix.)

❑ For nutritional recommendations, *see* Neurological Support, page 679; and CARDIOVASCULAR DISEASE, page 306.

FABRY'S DISEASE

Fabry's disease is a lipid storage disorder resulting from a deficiency of the enzyme ceramide trihexosidase that is involved in the biodegradation of fats. Because of the enzyme deficiency, there is an insufficient breakdown of lipids, which build up in the body. This leads to a number of problems. Symptoms include burning sensations in the hands and feet that progressively worsen with hot weather and exercise, and reddish purple, raised blemishes on the skin. Eye manifestations like cloudiness of the cornea are found in some boys who suffer from the disorder. As people with Fabry's disease grow older, they become susceptible to heart attack and stroke due to impaired arterial circulation. Eventually, the kidneys are affected, and dialysis or transplantation may be required. Some people also develop gastrointestinal difficulties in which frequent bowel movements occur shortly after eating.

This serious genetic metabolic disorder affects about 1 in 40,000 to 1 in 60,000 men. Although it is believed that fewer women suffer the most serious consequences of the disease, they also can be seriously affected. People with Fabry's disease usually survive into adulthood. However, they have a higher than normal risk of heart attack, stroke, and kidney damage.

Considerations

❑ Treatment includes therapy with antiseizure medications such as carbamazepine (Tegretol) and phenytoin (Dilantin) for pain in the hands and feet, and nutritional replacement products such as Lipisorb or digestive medications such as metoclopramide (Reglan) to control gastrointestinal hyperactivity.

❑ Recent studies have shown that enzyme replacement is effective therapy. Agalsidase beta (Fabrazyme), a version of the human form of the missing enzyme produced by recombinant DNA technology, has now been approved to treat Fabry's disease. When given intravenously, this replacement enzyme reduces a particular type of fat accumulation in many types of cells, including blood vessels in the kidneys and other organs. It is believed that this reduction of fat deposition will prevent the development of life-threatening organ damage.

❑ For patients with this condition, the Fabry Registry (www.fabrycommunity.com) is an excellent resource to learn about new treatments and developments for this condition.

❑ For nutritional recommendations, *see* Gastrointestinal Support, page 679; and CARDIOVASCULAR DISEASE, page 306.

HEMORRHAGIC COLITIS (HAMBURGER DISEASE)

Hemorrhagic colitis is a gastrointestinal illness caused primarily by a particular strain of bacteria known as *Escherichia coli (E. coli)* O157:H7. It is actually a type of food poisoning. (*See* FOODBORNE AND WATERBORNE ILLNESS in Part Two.) In fact, it is also known as "hamburger disease" or "barbecue season syndrome" because outbreaks often are due to consuming grilled hamburger and other beef products that have not been thoroughly or properly cooked or handled. *E. coli* has been shown to come from fruits and vegetables (especially lettuce, alfalfa sprouts, and unpasteurized apple cider and other juices), and has even been found in a refrigerated cookie dough.

While other types of *E. coli* are common in the gastrointestinal tract of healthy people, the O157:H7 strain normally is not. This strain of bacteria produces extremely potent toxins that are the main cause of the symptoms related to the gastrointestinal illness. The most common symptoms of *E. coli* O157:H7 colitis include:

- Diarrhea (often with blood in the stools).

- Severe abdominal cramps.

- Vomiting.

These symptoms usually start within twenty-four hours of consuming contaminated food, but can take as long as two days to appear, and can continue for as long as two weeks. Some individuals develop fever as well with this infection.

People can get hamburger disease at any age; however, young children, older adults, and those with weakened immune systems tend to develop severe symptoms. Thousands of people become infected each year, with many local outbreaks reported in Canada, Japan, the United States, and Europe.

E. coli O157:H7 bacteria infect the intestines of cattle and, less frequently, the gastrointestinal tracts of other animals. Typically carried in feces, they can contaminate the meat during and after slaughtering. In addition to beef, these bacteria are associated with consuming unpasteurized milk and cheese and using contaminated water sources. The infection is highly contagious. Once someone has eaten contaminated food, hamburger disease can pass from person to person by hand-to-mouth contact. Poor hand-washing and improper food handling are factors that lead to the spread of these bacteria.

Considerations

❑ While *E. coli* bacteria can be killed with antibiotics, the toxins they produce—and that cause the illness—remain unaffected, and there is no evidence that these drugs do anything to relieve symptoms or shorten the illness in most cases. Treatment for hemorrhagic colitis therefore focuses on supporting the affected individual, trying to ease symptoms, and taking measures to prevent the spread of the infection.

❑ If complications develop, hospitalization may be required so that proper care can be administered. Especially for small children and older people who cannot adequately hydrate themselves, receiving an intravenous fluid replacement in the emergency room may speed recovery and avoid major dehydration.

❑ Once hemorrhagic colitis is contracted, antibiotics must be taken. However, a nutritional and probiotic regimen can help prevent contraction and/or restore friendly bacteria after completing antibiotics and once the intestine is healed

❑ For nutritional recommendations, *see* Gastrointestinal Support, page 679; and WEAKENED IMMUNE SYSTEM, page 774.

HEREDITARY FRUCTOSE INTOLERANCE

Hereditary fructose intolerance (HFI) is an inherited disorder characterized by the inability to digest fructose, or fruit sugar. In people with HFI, the enzyme fructose-1-phosphate aldolase is deficient, resulting in an accumulation of fructose-1-phosphate in the liver, kidneys, and small intestine. Symptoms include severe abdominal pain, vomiting, dehydration, convulsions due to low blood sugar,

extreme thirst, excessive urination and sweating, loss of appetite, and stunted growth. Acute symptoms are made worse by the consumption of anything containing fruit sugar. If untreated, HFI can result in coma or death.

Considerations

❑ Early treatment, primarily the adoption of a fructose-free diet, leads to a normal length and quality of life. Otherwise, the disorder can lead to serious and permanent damage to the liver and kidneys, and, eventually, death.

❑ Adhering to a diet with *no* fructose in it can be difficult in today's world. We encounter fructose not only in natural fruits, fruit juices, and some vegetables, but also in a vast array of processed food products. High-fructose corn syrup, for example, is one of the most common additives listed on food product labels, and it is present not only in foods that taste sweet. It may be worthwhile to consult a qualified nutritionist or dietitian who can help with this task.

❑ For nutritional recommendations, *see* Gastrointestinal Support, page 679.

HYPERIMMUNOGLOBULIN E [HYPER-IgE] SYNDROME (JOB SYNDROME)

Hyper-IgE syndrome, or Job syndrome, is an immunodeficiency syndrome characterized by recurrent bacterial (staphylococcal) infections, particularly of the skin, and markedly elevated levels of a natural immune-system protein, immunoglobulin E (IgE). Experts suspect that the origin is genetic. The term Job syndrome—named for the Biblical figure who was afflicted with boils—arose because one of the symptoms of this syndrome is recurrent skin abscesses. The staphylococcal infection may involve the skin, lungs, joints, and other sites. Decreased bone density and frequent fractures are common. Signs of allergies, such as eczema, asthma, and runny nose, are sometimes present.

Considerations

❑ There is no known cure for Job syndrome. The mainstay of treatment is bacterial infection control. Treatment consists of intermittent or continuous antibiotics. Long-term trimethoprim/sulfamethoxazole, a combination antibiotic, is not particularly effective in treating infection.

IDIOPATHIC THROMBOCYTOPENIC PURPURA

Idiopathic thrombocytopenic purpura (ITP) is a disorder of the blood that leads to low levels of platelets, which are essential for normal clotting activity. This can be due to problems with platelet production, abnormal destruction of platelets, or other factors. The main symptom is abnormal bleeding, which can be manifested as ecchymosis (bruising) and petechiae (tiny red dots on the skin or mucous membranes). In some instances, bleeding from the nose, gums, or digestive or urinary tracts may also occur. In rare cases, there is bleeding within the brain.

Some cases of ITP are caused by drugs. Others are associated with infection, pregnancy, or immune disorders such as systemic lupus erythematosus. (*See* LUPUS in Part Two.) About half of all cases are classified as idiopathic, meaning that there is no known underlying cause.

Acute, or temporary, thrombocytopenic purpura is most commonly seen in young children and first diagnosed between two and four years of age. Boys and girls are equally affected. Symptoms often, but do not necessarily, follow a viral infection. About 80 percent of children recover within six months. Thrombocytopenic purpura is considered chronic if it lasts for more than six months. Adults more often have the chronic form of the disorder and females, in this case, are affected two to three times more than males.

Considerations

❑ If use of a drug is the cause of the thrombocytopenia, standard treatment involves discontinuing the drug's use. Infection, if present, is treated vigorously, since control of the infection can return the platelet count to normal.

❑ The treatment of idiopathic thrombocytopenic purpura is determined by the severity of the symptoms. In some cases, no therapy is needed. In most cases, drugs that alter the immune system's attack on the platelets are prescribed. These include corticosteroids such as prednisone (Deltasone and others) and/or intravenous infusions of immune globulin. Another treatment that usually results in an increased number of platelets is removal of the spleen, the organ that destroys antibody-coated platelets. A splenectomy is needed if prednisone doesn't work.

❑ Except in certain situations, such as internal bleeding and preparation for surgery, platelet transfusions usually are not beneficial and are seldom performed. Because all therapies can have risks, it is important that overtreatment based solely on platelet counts rather than symptoms be avoided.

❑ In some instances, lifestyle adjustments may help to prevent bleeding due to injury. These would include using protective gear such as helmets and avoiding contact sports if there are symptoms or if platelet counts are less than 50,000 mm^3. Downhill skiing or any other activity where you can significantly hurt yourself is not advised. Otherwise, most people can carry on normal activities, but final decisions about activity should be made in consultation with a hematologist (a physician who specializes in blood disorders).

❑ For nutritional recommendations, *see* CARDIOVASCULAR DISEASE, page 306; and WEAKENED IMMUNE SYSTEM, page 774.

LEUKODYSTROPHIES

Leukodystrophy refers to progressive degeneration of the white matter of the brain due to imperfect growth or development of the myelin sheath, the fatty covering that acts as an insulator around nerve fiber. Myelin is a complex substance made up of at least ten different compounds. The leukodystrophies are a group of disorders that are caused by genetic defects in how myelin produces or metabolizes these chemicals. Each of the leukodystrophies is the result of a defect in the gene that controls only one of these chemicals.

The most common symptom of a leukodystrophy disease is a gradual decline in the functioning of an infant or child who previously appeared well. There may be a progressive loss in body tone, movements, gait, speech, ability to eat, vision, hearing, and behavior. There is often a slowdown in mental and physical development. Symptoms vary according to the specific type of leukodystrophy, and may be difficult to recognize in the early stages of the disease.

The prognosis and recommended treatment for most of the leukodystrophies is symptomatic and supportive, and may include medications; physical, occupational, and speech therapies; and nutritional, educational, and recreational programs. Bone-marrow transplantation is showing promise for some of these diseases, such as ALD. The prognosis for leukodystrophies varies according to the specific type of leukodystrophy. Some important types of leukodystrophy include adrenoleukodystrophy (ALD), Alexander disease, Canavan disease, Krabbe disease, metachromatic leukodystrophy (MLD), and Pelizaeus-Merzbacher disease (PMD).

Adrenoleukodystrophy

People with adrenoleukodystrophy, ALD, accumulate high levels of compounds known as saturated very-long-chain fatty acids (VLCFA) in the brain and parts of the adrenal glands because they do not produce the enzyme that breaks down these fatty acids in a normal manner. The loss of myelin and the progressive dysfunction of the adrenal glands are the primary characteristics of ALD.

There are main subtypes of ALD. The most common is the X-linked form (X-ALD), which involves an abnormal gene located on the X chromosome; and neonatal ALD, which is caused by defective genes that are not located on the X chromosome. The distinction between the two makes a significant difference because women have two X chromosomes while men have only one. Lacking the protective effect of a second, normal X chromosome (it is highly unlikely for both of a woman's X chromosomes to be defective), men are generally more severely affected by the disease—although a mild form of ALD is occasionally seen in women who are carriers of the disorder. Symptoms include progressive stiffness, weakness or paralysis of the lower limbs, ataxia, excessive muscle tone, mild peripheral neuropathy, and urinary problems. In contrast, neonatal ALD can affect either male or female babies, with symptoms including mental retardation, facial abnormalities, seizures, retinal degeneration, weak muscle tone, enlarged liver, and adrenal dysfunction. This form usually is present from birth and progresses rapidly.

The onset of X-ALD, on the other hand, can occur either in childhood or adulthood. The childhood form, with symptoms usually starting between the ages of two and ten years, is the more severe. The most common symptoms are usually behavioral changes such as abnormal withdrawal or aggression, poor memory, and poor school performance. Other symptoms include visual loss, learning disabilities, seizures, poorly articulated speech, difficulty swallowing, deafness, disturbances of gait and coordination, fatigue, intermittent vomiting, increased skin pigmentation, and progressive dementia.

In the milder adult-onset form, which typically begins between the ages of twenty-one and thirty-five, symptoms may include progressive stiffness, weakness or paralysis of the lower limbs, and ataxia (disturbances in coordination and motor function). Although adult-onset ALD progresses more slowly than the classic childhood form, it can also result in deterioration of brain function.

Considerations

❏ Adrenal function must be tested periodically in all patients with ALD. Treatment with adrenal hormones can be lifesaving.

❏ Symptomatic and supportive treatments for ALD include physical therapy, psychological support, and special education.

❏ Some evidence suggests that administering a mixture of oleic acid and euric acid, known as Lorenzo's oil (and made famous in the movie by that name) to boys with X-ALD can reduce or delay the appearance of symptoms in those who have not developed symptoms yet. It is important to eat a low-fat diet coupled with Lorenzo's oil.

❏ Bone marrow transplants can provide long-term benefit for boys who have early evidence of X-ALD, but the procedure carries substantial and serious risks, and is not recommended for those whose symptoms are already severe or who have the adult-onset or neonatal forms.

❏ The administration of the omega-3 essential fatty acid docosahexaenoic acid (DHA) may help some infants and children with neonatal ALD.

❏ The overall prognosis for people with ALD is generally poor because of the progressive neurological deterioration it causes. Death usually occurs within one to ten years after the onset of symptoms.

❏ For nutritional recommendations, *see* WEAKENED IMMUNE SYSTEM, page 774.

MERALGIA PARESTHETICA

Meralgia paresthetica is a disorder characterized by tingling, numbness, and burning pain in the outer side of the thigh. The disorder is also known as *Bernhardt-Roth syndrome* and *lateral femoral cutaneous nerve entrapment*.

Meralgia paresthetica is caused by compression of the lateral femoral cutaneous nerve, which transmits sensation from the outer thigh to nerves in the spinal cord, as it exits the pelvis. The disorder occurs in men more than women, and is generally found in middle-aged or overweight individuals. Affected individuals often complain that the symptoms worsen after walking or standing, and that the skin is sensitive to touch. Meralgia paresthetica disorder is associated with wearing clothing that is too tight, as well as with pregnancy, diabetes, and obesity.

Recommendations

❏ If you are overweight, lose the extra pounds. (*See* OBESITY in Part Two for recommendations.)

❏ Try wearing looser clothing.

❏ Avoid standing or walking for prolonged periods of time. Also avoid any position that places pressure on the outer thigh.

Considerations

❏ Treatments include acetaminophen, or other nonsteroidal anti-inflammatory drugs (NSAIDs) like Advil. In addition, steroid injections and tricyclic antidepressants are used. Gabapentin (Neurontin) or pregabalin (Lyrica) may be prescribed to help alleviate symptoms.

❏ In very few cases in which pain is persistent or severe, surgical intervention to relieve pressure may be needed. Surgery is not always successful, however.

❏ Meralgia paresthetica usually eases or disappears after treatment. In some cases, the disorder simply goes away on its own.

❏ For other nutritional recommendations, *see* Neurological Support, page 679; and CARDIOVASCULAR DISEASE, page 306.

MULTIPLE SYSTEM ATROPHY WITH ORTHOSTATIC HYPOTENSION

See ORTHOSTATIC HYPOTENSION in this section.

ORTHOSTATIC HYPOTENSION

Orthostatic hypotension is a sudden decrease in blood pressure when a person stands upright. Other known names for this disorder are *postural hypotension* and *Bradbury-Eggleston syndrome*. The condition may be caused by a decreased amount of blood in the body resulting from excessive use of diuretics, vasodilators, or other types of drugs. Dehydration and prolonged bed rest can also cause orthostatic hypotension. Symptoms appear upon standing (the more suddenly one stands, the more serious the problem) and generally include dizziness, light-headedness, blurred vision, and syncope or temporary loss of consciousness. Most people have experienced the dizzy feeling upon standing abruptly from a lying-down position; this is normal and is not to be confused with this condition.

Other diseases are sometimes associated with the disorder, including Addison's disease, atherosclerosis, diabetes, and certain neurological disorders like multiple system atrophy with orthostatic hypotension. Formerly known as Shy-Drager syndrome, multiple system atrophy with orthostatic hypotension is a progressive disorder of the central and autonomic nervous systems that is characterized by orthostatic hypotension—an excessive drop in blood pressure when standing up, causing dizziness and fainting. Multiple system atrophy can occur without orthostatic hypotension, but is very rare.

The disorder is classified into three types:

1. The Parkinsonian-type, which includes symptoms similar to those of Parkinson's disease such as slow movement, stiff muscles, and tremor.

2. The cerebellar-type, which causes problems with coordination and speech.

3. The combined-type, which includes symptoms of both Parkinsonism and cerebellar failure.

Problems with urinary incontinence, constipation, and sexual impotence in men occur early in the course of the disease. Other symptoms may include generalized weakness, double vision or other vision problems, difficulty breathing and swallowing, sleep disturbances, and decreased sweating. The disease can take years to diagnose because its features resemble those of so many other health problems.

Considerations

❏ If orthostatic hypotension is caused by hypovolemia (a decreased amount of blood in the body) due to medications, the disorder may be reversed by adjusting the dosage or by discontinuing the medication.

❏ If the condition is caused by prolonged bed rest, simply sitting up with increasing frequency each day may yield some improvement.

❏ In some cases, physical counterpressure such as elastic hose or whole-body inflatable suits may be required.

❏ Dehydration is treated with salt and fluids. The prognosis for most people with orthostatic hypotension depends on the underlying cause of the condition.

❏ There is no cure for multiple system atrophy with orthostatic hypotension. Treatment is aimed at controlling symptoms. Medications include fludrocortisone (Florinef), pyridostigmine (Mestinon), and epoetin (Procrit).

❏ People with multiple system atrophy with orthostatic hypotension should sleep with their heads elevated. Those who have breathing and swallowing difficulty may need to use an artificial breathing or feeding tube.

❏ The prognosis for individuals with multiple system atrophy with orthostatic hypotension is poor. People usually die within seven to ten years after the onset of symptoms. A problem with the respiratory system is the most common cause of death.

❏ For nutritional recommendations, *see* Neurological Support, page 679; and CARDIOVASCULAR DISEASE, page 306.

PHENYLKETONURIA

Phenylketonuria (PKU) is an inherited error of metabolism caused by a deficiency of the enzyme phenylalanine hydroxylase, which is responsible for processing the essential amino acid phenylalanine. Lack of the enzyme results in a buildup of phenylalanine in the body, which over time can lead to mental retardation, organ damage, abnormal posture, and in some cases, severely compromised pregnancy. Symptoms in affected infants include drowsiness, lethargy, difficulty feeding, and light eyes, as well as light pigmentation in skin and hair. A rash similar to eczema may develop.

If left untreated, PKU can develop into severe mental retardation, and also can cause neurological symptoms such as seizures, hyperactivity, clumsy walking, unusual posture, aggressive behavior, or psychiatric disturbances. Fortunately, the problem is detectable through blood tests within the first days of life. Screening for PKU has been a part of routine testing for newborns in the United States since 2008.

Considerations

❏ If treated properly with a carefully controlled, phenylalanine-restricted diet, mental retardation can be prevented. Among the things that people with PKU absolutely *cannot* consume are products containing the artificial sweetener aspartame (found in Equal, NutraSweet, and many processed food products), which has as one of its components the amino acid phenylalanine.

❏ For nutritional recommendations, *see* Neurological Support, page 679.

PIRIFORMIS SYNDROME

Piriformis syndrome is a rare neuromuscular disorder that occurs when the piriformis muscle (a narrow muscle located deep in the buttocks) compresses or irritates the sciatic nerve, the largest nerve in the body. As with sciatica, caused by a herniated or ruptured disc, compression of the sciatic nerve causes pain, frequently described as tingling or numbness, in the buttocks and along the nerve, often extending down the leg. The pain may worsen with prolonged periods of sitting, or by climbing stairs, walking, or running.

Considerations

❏ Treatment generally begins with stretching and massage. Anti-inflammatory drugs may be prescribed.

❏ It may be advisable to stop, or at least take a break from, physical activities that aggravate the problem.

❏ The prognosis for piriformis syndrome is good. Once symptoms are addressed, individuals can usually resume their normal activities. In some cases, exercise regimens may need to be modified in order to reduce the likelihood of recurrence or worsening symptoms.

❏ For nutritional recommendations, *see* Neurological Support, page 679.

POSTURAL TACHYCARDIA SYNDROME

People who suffer from postural tachycardia syndrome (POTS) experience a pulse rate that is too fast when they stand. Symptoms include rapid heartbeat, light-headedness with prolonged standing, headache, chronic fatigue, and chest pain. The underlying cause or causes of POTS usually cannot be identified, but the disorder is not thought to progress to heart disease.

Considerations

❏ The severity of symptoms usually determines the course of treatment for POTS. Individuals with the disorder are usually advised to increase their fluid and salt intake. Body stockings may provide some relief. Drug therapy, with fludrocortisone (for those on a high-salt diet), beta-blockers, or midodrine in low doses to increase blood volume and narrow blood vessels, can be beneficial. Physical exercise, especially calf muscle resistance training, also may help. Avoid heavy meals. Drinking 16 ounces of water before getting up can help raise blood pressure.

❏ Some people with postural tachycardia syndrome may require and benefit from insertion of a cardiac pacemaker.

❏ The prognosis for people with POTS varies. Many individuals improve with one or more of the treatments outlined above, although severe POTS can be disabling for years.

❏ For nutritional recommendations, *see* Neurological Support, page 679; and CARDIOVASCULAR DISEASE, page 306.

REFSUM DISEASE

Refsum disease is a hereditary disorder of fat metabolism caused by the deficiency of an enzyme that breaks down phytanic acid, a type of fatty acid. The result is an abnormal accumulation of phytanic acid in blood plasma and body tissues. Phytanic acid is not made in the human body; it comes from consuming dairy products, beef, lamb, and some seafood.

Symptoms of the disorder may include visual impairment, peripheral neuropathy (damage to nerves that can cause pain, tingling, burning, and other sensations in the extremities), ataxia (disturbances in coordination and motor function), impaired hearing, and bone and skin changes. Nystagmus (rapid, involuntary to-and-fro eye movements),

anosmia (loss of the sense of smell), and ichthyosis (dry, rough, scaly skin) may also occur.

The onset of Refsum disease usually occurs in early childhood, although some people will not develop symptoms until they are in their forties or fifties. The disorder affects both males and females.

Recommendations

❏ Strictly limit or avoid consumption of foods that contain phytanic acid, including dairy products; beef and lamb; and fatty fish such as tuna, cod, and haddock. The body also converts phytol, a substance found in green leafy vegetables, to phytanic acid, so limiting them may be helpful as well.

Considerations

❏ In addition to making dietary changes, plasmapheresis (the removal and reinfusion of blood plasma) may be required periodically to manage Refsum disease.

❏ The prognosis for individuals with Refsum disease varies. With treatment, symptoms of peripheral neuropathy and ichthyosis generally disappear. However, while treatment may forestall further deterioration of vision and hearing, it cannot undo damage to vision and hearing that may have occurred.

❏ For other nutritional recommendations, *see* Gastrointestinal Support, page 679.

TOURETTE SYNDROME

Tourette syndrome (TS) is an inherited neurological disorder distinguished by repeated involuntary movements and uncontrollable vocal sounds called *tics*. There may be facial tics and eye-blinking, head-jerking, neck-stretching, foot-stamping, body-twisting and -bending, throat-clearing, coughing, sniffing, and grunting, yelping, barking, or shouting noises. Tics can be suppressed for a short time, but when stress increases, eventually a tic will escape. In limited cases, such tics can include the compulsive use of inappropriate words and phrases.

The onset of TS generally appears before the age of eighteen, and the majority of cases are mild.

Considerations

❏ Medication is available to control tics that interfere with daily functioning, but the majority of people with TS require no medication.

❏ There is no cure for Tourette syndrome. However, while TS is generally a chronic lifelong condition, it does not get progressively worse. In fact, many people find that their symptoms improve as they mature.

❏ For nutritional recommendations, *see* Neurological Support, page 679; and CARDIOVASCULAR DISEASE, page 306.

RASH

See SKIN RASH.

RAYNAUD'S DISEASE / RAYNAUD'S PHENOMENON

Raynaud's disease is a circulatory disorder that results in the hands, and sometimes the feet, being hypersensitive to cold. When the hands are exposed to cold temperatures, the small arteries that supply the toes and fingers suddenly contract and go into spasm. As a result, the fingers and toes are deprived of adequate amounts of oxygenated blood, and become whitish or bluish in color. Over time, the condition may result in a general shrinkage of the affected area. Ultimately, ulcers may form, damaging the tissues and resulting in chronic infection under and around the fingernails and toenails. In severe cases, gangrene may result from prolonged and persistent contraction of the arteries. This condition is more common in women than in men. Raynaud's phenomenon is a condition similar to Raynaud's disease that is caused by complications of surgery, injury, frostbite, autoimmune diseases such as lupus or rheumatoid arthritis, or some other underlying condition. Dressing warmly and avoiding activities in the cold can eliminate many of the severe symptoms.

Certain drugs that affect the blood vessels—such as calcium channel blockers, ergot preparations, and alpha- and beta-adrenergic blockers—have been known to produce symptoms similar to those of Raynaud's as a side effect. Recent research has also linked Raynaud's with other conditions involving abnormal constriction of blood vessels, including migraine and Prinzmetal's angina, a type of angina caused by spasms in the coronary arteries. (*See* CIRCULATORY PROBLEMS in Part Two.)

Unless otherwise specified, the doses recommended here are for persons age eighteen and over. For children between twelve and seventeen, use three-quarters the recommended dose; for children between six and twelve, use one-half the recommended dose; and for children under six, use one-quarter the recommended dose.

NUTRIENTS

SUPPLEMENT	SUGGESTED DOSAGE	COMMENTS
Essential		
Coenzyme Q$_{10}$ plus	100–200 mg daily.	Improves tissue oxygenation.
Coenzyme A from Coenzyme-A Technologies	As directed on label.	Works well with coenzyme Q$_{10}$ in supporting the immune system's detoxification of many dangerous substances.
Vitamin E	200 IU daily.	Improves circulation; acts as an anticoagulant, dissolving clots in the legs, heart, and lungs. Use d-alpha-tocopherol form. Use emulsion form for easier assimilation and greater safety at higher doses.

Very Important		
Calcium and	1,500 mg daily, at bedtime.	To protect the arteries from stress caused by sudden blood pressure changes.
magnesium and	750 mg daily.	
zinc	50 mg daily. Do not exceed a total of 100 mg daily from all supplements.	
Chlorophyll or	As directed on label.	Helps to fight infection and enhance blood flow.
Kyo-Green from Wakunaga	As directed on label.	A fresh "green drink" made from leafy greens that supplies chlorophyll and other nutrients.
Choline and inositol	As directed on label.	Lowers cholesterol and helps circulation.
Dimethylglycine (DMG) (Aangamik DMG from FoodScience of Vermont	1 tablet 3 times daily.	Improves tissue oxygenation.
Lecithin granules or	1 tbsp 3 times daily, with meals.	Lowers blood lipid levels.
capsules	1,200 mg 3 times daily, with meals.	
Vitamin B complex	100 mg of each major B vitamin daily (amounts of individual vitamins in a complex will vary).	B vitamins are necessary for metabolism of fat and cholesterol. Use a high-potency formula.
plus extra vitamin B$_6$ (pyridoxine) and	50 mg daily.	
folic acid plus	400 mcg daily.	
vitamin B$_3$ (niacin)	100 mg daily. Do not exceed this amount.	Dilates small arteries, improving circulation. *Caution:* Do not take niacin if you have a liver disorder, gout, or high blood pressure.
Important		
Aerobic 07 from Aerobic Life Industries	As directed on label.	Improves tissue oxygenation.
Bee propolis or	As directed on label.	To strengthen the cardiovascular system and act as a natural antibiotic.
royal jelly	As directed on label.	
Flaxseed oil or	1,000 mg daily.	To supply essential fatty acids, which are necessary for circulation and help prevent hardening of the arteries.
primrose oil or	1,000 mg daily.	
salmon oil	As directed on label.	

Herbs

❑ Black cohosh aids circulation and lowers cholesterol levels.

Caution: Do not use black cohosh if you are pregnant or have any type of chronic disease. Black cohosh should not be used by those with liver problems.

❑ Butcher's broom, cayenne (capsicum), ginkgo biloba, and pau d'arco can be used separately or in combination to improve circulation and strengthen blood vessels.

Caution: Do not take ginkgo biloba if you have a bleeding disorder, or are scheduled for surgery or a dental procedure.

❑ Hyssop may prove helpful for problems affecting the circulation.

Recommendations

❑ Eat a diet composed of 50 percent raw foods. *See* NUTRITION, DIET, AND WELLNESS in Part One and follow the dietary guidelines.

❑ Avoid fatty and fried foods.

❑ Avoid caffeine. This stimulant constricts the blood vessels.

❑ Keep your hands and feet warm. A warm climate is best. Wear comfortable shoes and do not go barefoot outdoors. Always wear gloves and warm socks when you feel cold and not just when others do.

❑ Avoid stress as much as possible.

❑ Avoid drugs that constrict the blood vessels, such as birth control pills and migraine headache medicine.

❑ Do not smoke, and avoid exposure to secondhand smoke. Nicotine constricts the blood vessels.

Considerations

❑ The calcium channel blocker nifedipine (Adalat, Procardia) is a generally accepted treatment for Raynaud's phenomenon. Some people get relief from alpha blockers like prazosin (Minipress) or doxazosin (Cardura). Some doctors prescribe vasodilators such as nitroglycerine cream to relax blood vessels and eventually heal skin ulcers. Like all drugs, this can have side effects.

❑ *See also* CIRCULATORY PROBLEMS in Part Two.

REPETITIVE MOTION INJURY

See CARPAL TUNNEL SYNDROME.

RETINITIS PIGMENTOSA

See under EYE PROBLEMS.

REYE'S SYNDROME

Reye's syndrome is a rare, serious disease that affects many internal organs, particularly the brain and liver. It primarily strikes children between the ages of four and twelve. Most cases of Reye's syndrome occur in children who were given aspirin or aspirin-containing medications for a viral infection such as the flu or chickenpox. Reye's syndrome has also been associated with Epstein-Barr virus, influenza B, and enteroviruses (viruses that infect mainly the gastrointestinal tract).

Four to six days after the onset of the viral illness, the child suddenly develops a fever and severe vomiting. Other symptoms include mental and personality changes that may manifest themselves as confusion, drowsiness, lethargy, memory lapses, and/or unusual belligerence and irritability. In addition, the child may experience weakness and paralysis in the arms or legs, double vision, palpitations, speech impairment, impaired skin integrity, and/or hearing loss. Convulsions, coma, brain damage, and even death may follow, usually the result of cerebral edema or respiratory failure. Fortunately, due to increased awareness of the disease, and especially of the importance of early detection and prompt treatment, the mortality rate has declined in recent years. A high of 555 cases in 1980 has dwindled to about 37 cases a year. Forty percent of the cases were in children under five years of age; ninety percent were children under fifteen years.

The exact cause of Reye's syndrome is unknown, but as a result of research conducted in the early 1980s, it is known that the combination of aspirin and viral illness dramatically increases the risk of developing this dangerous disorder. This is why aspirin is no longer recommended for routine use as a pain reliever for children and acetaminophen (Tylenol) is recommended in its place.

The following supplements are designed for use once appropriate medical measures, including hospitalization, have been taken and recovery has begun. Discuss any supplements with a health care professional before using them. Unless otherwise specified, the recommended doses are for persons age eighteen and over. For children between twelve and seventeen, use three-quarters the recommended dose; for children between six and twelve, use one-half the recommended dose; and for children under six, use one-quarter the recommended dose.

NUTRIENTS

SUPPLEMENT	SUGGESTED DOSAGE	COMMENTS
Important		
Branched-chain amino acid complex	As directed on label.	Prevents muscle depletion. (*See* AMINO ACIDS in Part One.)
Flaxseed oil	As directed on label.	To supply essential fatty acids.
Garlic (Kyolic from Wakunaga)	As directed on label.	Increases energy and enhances immune function.
Lecithin granules or	1 tbsp 3 times daily.	To supply choline, important in transmission of nerve impulses and in energy production.
capsules or	1,200 mg 3 times daily.	
phosphatidyl choline	As directed on label.	
L-methionine plus	As directed on label.	Powerful antioxidants that protect and detoxify the liver.
glutathione	As directed on label.	
Raw brain glandular	As directed on label.	To improve brain function.
Vitamin A plus	5,000 IU daily.	Helps in formation of healthy skin cells.
carotenoid complex with beta-carotene	15,000 IU daily.	Used by the body to make vitamin A as needed.

Vitamin B complex	50–100 mg of each major B vitamin daily (amounts of individual vitamins in a complex will vary).	Needed for all enzyme systems and to support healing.
Vitamin E	200 IU daily.	To protect against free radical damage. Use d-alpha-tocopherol form.

Herbs

❑ The following are herbal remedies that can be useful once the acute phase of the illness has passed and recovery has begun:

• Alfalfa, hawthorn berry, hyssop, milk thistle, pau d'arco, Siberian ginseng, and wild yam help to rebuild and strengthen the liver.

   Caution: Do not use Siberian ginseng if you have hypoglycemia, high blood pressure, or a heart disorder.

• A lotion containing aloe vera, calendula, and/or chamomile can be used to nourish and heal the skin.

• Catnip or chamomile tea helps to reduce anxiety.

   Caution: Do not use chamomile if you are allergic to ragweed. Do not use during pregnancy or nursing. It may interact with warfarin or cyclosporine, so patients using these drugs should avoid it.

• Ginger and peppermint are good for relief of nausea.

• Gravel root, hydrangea, oat straw, parsley root, and uva ursi have diuretic properties.

• Korean (or Chinese) ginseng *(Panax ginseng)* helps to reduce fatigue.

   Caution: Do not use this herb if you have high blood pressure.

❑ Before administering them, discuss any herbal remedies you wish to use with your health care provider.

❑ Because the main component of the herbs meadowsweet and white willow bark are related to aspirin, these should *not* be given to a child with a fever that may be due to viral illness, including colds, flu, measles, or chickenpox.

Recommendations

❑ Be alert for the following warning signs any time your child is recovering from a viral infection such as a cold, the flu, an ear infection, or chickenpox:

• Prolonged and heavy vomiting, followed by drowsiness.

• Agitation, disorientation, and delirium.

• Fatigue, lethargy, and lapses in memory.

If you have *even a suspicion* that you (or your child) may be developing the disease, seek professional help at once.

Reye's syndrome progresses rapidly and is extremely dangerous. Go to the nearest hospital emergency room immediately and explain the situation.

❑ Be sure that any supplements your child is taking *do not* contain glutamine, as it can lead to an accumulation of ammonia in the blood. Be aware that although the names glutamine, glutamic acid (also sometimes called glutamate), glutathione, gluten, and monosodium glutamate sound similar, these are all different substances.

❑ If Reye's syndrome is diagnosed, follow your health care provider's recommendations regarding treatment and care, both during the period of hospitalization and afterward, at home.

❑ *Never* give aspirin to a child with a fever or other sign of viral illness. To be safe, many experts recommend against giving children aspirin for any reason. Use acetaminophen (Tylenol, Datril, and others).

Considerations

❑ There is no cure for Reye's syndrome. Treatment focuses on balancing chemical levels in the blood, while monitoring and supporting the functions of the lung, liver, heart, and brain. The measures that may be taken depend upon the stage of the disease, but treatment almost always involves hospitalization. Typical hospital care includes the administration of intravenous fluids to restore blood electrolytes and glucose levels, and sometimes a diuretic to help eliminate waste and excess fluid. In some cases, surgery may be performed to reduce swelling and pressure on the brain.

❑ One way that Reye's syndrome can be detected is through a spinal tap, a procedure that involves inserting a needle into the spinal canal, usually at the lower back, to withdraw a sample of cerebrospinal fluid for examination.

❑ If a person with Reye's syndrome receives an intravenous solution of glucose (sugar) and electrolytes (mineral salts) within twelve to twenty-four hours after the heavy vomiting starts, the chance of recovery is excellent. This treatment is safe.

❑ The British aspirin industry withdrew all children's aspirin products from the British market a number of years ago in response to the discovery of the link with Reye's syndrome.

❑ A study done by the U.S. Centers for Disease Control and Prevention found that 100 percent of the children who had Reye's syndrome had been given aspirin in the presence of a viral illness (chickenpox or flu). The study also indicated a direct correlation between the amount of aspirin taken and the severity of the disease. The makers of aspirin are now required to alert users to the link between aspirin and this potentially life-threatening condition.

❑ *See also* CHICKENPOX; COMMON COLD; and INFLUENZA, all in Part Two.

RHEUMATIC FEVER

Rheumatic fever is a complication of a streptococcal infection. It typically develops following strep throat, tonsillitis, scarlet fever, or ear infection. It most often affects children aged five to eighteen. Rheumatic fever develops as a result of the buildup of antibodies that have been produced to fight off the strep infection—only the antibodies end up attacking the body's own tissues. This disorder may affect one or several parts of the body, among them the heart, brain, and joints. If the heart is affected, permanent damage to one or more heart valves may result.

The first signs of rheumatic fever are typically pain, inflammation, and stiffness in a large joint such as the knee, accompanied by fever. The pain and swelling can travel from one joint to another. There may be an accompanying skin rash. Other symptoms may include bumps or nodules over a joint or joints, fatigue, and uncontrollable jerky movements of the arm, leg, or facial muscles. After one occurrence, the disease tends to recur.

Long-term effects of rheumatic fever can include heart failure, skin disorders, anemia, endocarditis (inflammation of the heart lining), heart arrhythmias, pericarditis (inflammation of the sac surrounding the heart), Sydenham's chorea (a disorder of the nervous system), and arthritis.

Unless otherwise specified, the following recommended dosages are for persons over the age of eighteen. For children between twelve and seventeen years old, reduce the dose to three-quarters the recommended amount. For children between six and twelve, use one-half the recommended dose, and for children under six years old, use one-quarter the recommended amount.

NUTRIENTS

SUPPLEMENT	SUGGESTED DOSAGE	COMMENTS
Important		
Acidophilus (Kyo-Dophilus from Wakunaga)	As directed on label.	Especially important if antibiotics are prescribed. Use a nondairy formula.
Chondroitin sulfate	500–1,000 mg daily.	To provide nutritional support for strengthening joints, ligaments, and tendons.
Garlic (Kyolic from Wakunaga)	2 capsules 3 times daily.	A natural antibiotic that boosts immune function and fights infection. Destroys free radicals.
L-carnitine	500 mg twice daily, on an empty stomach.	Protects the heart.
L-methionine	500 mg daily, on an empty stomach. Take with water or juice. Do not take with milk. Take with 50 mg vitamin B6 and 100 mg vitamin C for better absorption.	An important free radical fighter. (See AMINO ACIDS in Part One.)
Vitamin C with bioflavonoids	5,000–20,000 mg daily, in divided doses. (See ASCORBIC ACID FLUSH in Part Three.)	Boosts immune function and aids in reducing pain and swelling.
Helpful		
Calcium plus magnesium	1,500 mg daily. 1,000 mg daily.	Important nutrients that work together. Use chelate forms.
Coenzyme Q10 plus Coenzyme A from Coenzyme-A Technologies	100 mg daily. As directed on label.	Boosts immune function. Enhances the effectiveness of coenzyme Q10.
ConcenTrace from Trace Minerals Research	As directed on label.	To supply trace minerals needed for bone and joint health. Increases energy.
Dimethylsulfoxide (DMSO)	Apply topically as directed on label.	To relieve joint pain. Should be used by adults only. Note: Use only DMSO from a health food store. Products from hardware and other stores are not suitable for use in healing.
Flaxseed oil	As directed on label.	Reduces pain and inflammation.
Free form amino acid (Amino Balance from Anabol Naturals)	As directed on label.	To supply protein, needed to strengthen the body and for tissue repair. Use a formula containing all essential amino acids.
Kelp	1,000–1,500 mg daily.	Contains essential nutrients.
Multivitamin and mineral complex	As directed on label.	To maintain a balance of all necessary nutrients.
Proteolytic enzymes	As directed on label. Take between meals.	An important antioxidant.
Raw thymus glandular	As directed on label.	An important antioxidant. Stimulates the immune response.
S-Adenosylmethionine (SAMe) (SAMe Rx-Mood from Nature's Plus)	As directed on label.	Deficiency results in inability to maintain cartilage properly. Aids in reducing pain and inflammation. Caution: Do not use if you have bipolar mood disorder or take prescription antidepressants. Do not give this supplement to a child under twelve.
Vitamin A plus carotenoid complex with beta-carotene	10,000 IU daily. As directed on label.	Important antioxidants. Use emulsion forms for easier assimilation.
Vitamin B complex	50 mg of each major B vitamin 3 times daily (amounts of individual vitamins in a complex will vary).	For healing and improved immune function.
Vitamin D or cod liver oil	400 IU or more daily. As directed on label.	Needed for healing and absorption of minerals, especially calcium.
Vitamin E emulsion or capsules	200 IU daily.	Increases tissue oxygenation and reduces fever. Emulsion form is recommended for easier assimilation.

Herbs

❑ Bayberry bark, burdock root, milk thistle, nettle, pau d'arco, sage, and yellow dock purify the blood, fight infection, and aid in recuperation after the trauma of illness.

Caution: Do not use sage if you suffer from any type of seizure disorder, or are pregnant or nursing.

❑ Birch leaves and lobelia both help to reduce pain.

Caution: Lobelia is only to be taken under supervision of a health care professional as it is potentially toxic. People with high blood pressure, heart disease, liver disease, kidney disease, seizure disorders, or shortness of breath should not take lobelia. Pregnant and lactating women should avoid lobelia as well.

❑ Catnip tea is a nerve tonic. It can also be used as an enema to reduce fever. (*See* ENEMAS in Part Three.)

❑ Cordyceps, a Chinese herb, is beneficial for the heart. It can slow the heart rate, increase blood supply to the arteries and heart, and lower blood pressure.

❑ Dandelion has a long history in the treatment of fever.

❑ Ginkgo biloba can benefit the cardiovascular system by preventing the formation of free radicals. Use a ginkgo extract containing 24 percent ginkgo flavone glycosides.

Caution: Do not take ginkgo biloba if you have a bleeding disorder, or are scheduled for surgery or a dental procedure.

❑ Goldenseal is a natural antibiotic.

Caution: Do not take goldenseal internally on a daily basis for more than one week at a time. Do not use it during pregnancy or if you are breast-feeding, and use with caution if you are allergic to ragweed. If you have a history of cardiovascular disease, diabetes, or glaucoma, use it only under a doctor's supervision.

❑ Hawthorn leaf, myrrh gum, and red clover detoxify and deacidify the blood.

❑ Wintergreen oil can be applied to the chest in compress form to relieve pain.

Recommendations

❑ Drink plenty of fresh juices and distilled water.

❑ Eat no solid food until the fever subsides and joint pain begins to ease. Then keep to a light diet, including fresh fruits and vegetables, yogurt, cottage cheese, and fruit juices.

❑ Do not consume any caffeine, carbonated soft drinks, fried foods, processed or refined foods, salt, or sugar in any form during the recovery period. These foods slow healing.

❑ Get plenty of bed rest. This is vital for recovery.

❑ If antibiotics are prescribed, take acidophilus following antibiotic treatment to replace the needed "friendly" bacteria. Antibiotics are usually necessary to combat the underlying *Streptococcus* infection and help prevent permanent heart damage. Do not take the acidophilus at the same time as the antibiotics, however, or the antibiotics will kill the friendly bacteria.

❑ Do not give aspirin to a child with a fever. Use acetaminophen or ibuprofen instead.

❑ If you (or your child) are experiencing symptoms of strep throat, see a physician to be tested and, if appropriate, treated. Symptoms of strep throat include a severe sore throat accompanied by a fever of over 101°F without any other cold symptoms, or a mild sore throat that does not dissipate after several days.

❑ Use homeopathic treatments to ease symptoms. Homeopathic remedies that have been used to treat rheumatic fever include *Aconite, Bryonia, Pulsatilla,* and *Rhus toxicodendron.*

Considerations

❑ Massage therapy and mild exercise such as yoga can be helpful for preventing muscle atrophy during bed rest. (*See* MASSAGE THERAPY in Part Three.)

❑ If you develop rheumatic heart disease, you may need surgery to repair the damage to the heart.

❑ *See also* ARTHRITIS; FEVER; and/or SORE THROAT, all in Part Two.

RHEUMATOID ARTHRITIS

See under ARTHRITIS.

RICKETS/OSTEOMALACIA

Rickets and osteomalacia are two terms for the disorder caused by vitamin D deficiency. In children, this disease is called rickets, and results either from inadequate intake of vitamin D or from too little exposure to sunlight (sunlight causes vitamin D to be synthesized in the skin). The lack of vitamin D in turn affects the body's ability to absorb calcium and phosphorus. Early signs include nervousness, painful muscle spasms, leg cramps, and numbness in the extremities. Ultimately, bone malformations may develop due to softening of the bones—bowed legs, knock-knees, scoliosis (abnormal curvature of the spine), a narrow rib cage, a protruding breastbone, and/or beading at the ends of the ribs—as well as decaying teeth, delayed walking, irritability, restlessness, and profuse sweating. Rickets is now virtually eliminated in the United States. It was most often seen in children aged six to twenty-four months old.

In adults, vitamin D deficiency disease is referred to as osteomalacia and is usually related to the body's inability to absorb phosphorus and calcium properly. It is most likely to occur in pregnant women and nursing mothers, whose nutritional requirements are higher than normal, or in people with malabsorption problems. It may also affect individuals who do not get enough exposure to sunshine or those whose diets are so low in fat that adequate bile cannot be manufactured and vitamin D cannot be absorbed. This condition can be caused by chronic renal failure. Osteomalacia is difficult to diagnose and is often misdiagnosed as osteoporosis.

Unless otherwise specified, the dosages recommended in this section are for adults. For children between the ages of twelve and seventeen, reduce the dose to three-quarters the recommended amount. For children between six and twelve, use one-half the recommended dose, and for children under the age of six, use one-quarter the recommended amount.

NUTRIENTS

SUPPLEMENT	SUGGESTED DOSAGE	COMMENTS
Essential		
Boron	3 mg daily. Do not exceed this amount.	Enhances calcium absorption.
Calcium	1,500 mg daily.	Necessary to remineralize bone. Do not use bone meal or dolomite as a source of calcium, as these may contain lead.
Phosphorus	As directed on label.	Needed for bone and tooth formation.
Silica	500 mg daily.	Supplies silicon, which strengthens bones and connective tissue. Aids calcium absorption.
Vitamin D	400–600 IU daily. Do not exceed this amount.	Necessary for utilization of calcium and phosphorus.
Important		
Betaine hydrochloride (HCl)	As directed on label.	May be needed for proper digestion.
Fish oil	As directed on label.	A good source of vitamins A and D.
Multivitamin and mineral complex plus extra vitamin B$_{12}$	As directed on label. 1,000–2,000 mcg daily.	If malabsorption is a problem, take higher amounts of all vitamins and minerals.
Proteolytic enzymes	As directed on label. Take between meals.	Important in digestion.
Vitamin A with mixed carotenoids	10,000 IU daily.	Necessary for growth.
Zinc	30 mg daily.	Needed for calcium absorption. Use zinc gluconate lozenges or OptiZinc for best absorption.

Herbs

❑ Dandelion root, nettle, and oat straw promote bone building and are all good sources of calcium and magnesium.

Recommendations

❑ Change your diet. To get rickets your diet would have to be very deficient in calcium and vitamin D. The best sources are milk and some other dairy products. All dairy products have calcium, but not all have vitamin D. Eat more raw fruits and vegetables, raw nuts and seeds, yogurt and cottage cheese, and sardines. A diet high in calcium is essential.

❑ Sunlight exposure is important as well, if a guaranteed source of vitamin D is not available from foods.

❑ Do not consume sugar, junk foods, or carbonated beverages.

❑ Have a hair analysis done to check for mineral deficiencies. (*See* HAIR ANALYSIS in Part Three.)

❑ Be watchful if a child has severe allergies, celiac disease, asthma, bronchitis, or colon disturbances. These conditions can result in absorption problems. This may be difficult to detect at first because growth and weight are usually normal with these conditions.

Considerations

❑ Food allergy testing may be beneficial.

❑ There are a number of combination supplement products available that contain many of the nutrients recommended in the table above. Bone Builder from Ethical Nutrients, Bone Defense from KAL, and Cal Apatite from Metagenics are good products for promoting proper bone growth.

❑ *See also* OSTEOPOROSIS in Part Two.

RINGWORM

See under FUNGAL INFECTION.

ROSACEA

Rosacea is a chronic skin disorder that most often affects the forehead, nose, cheekbones, and chin. Groups of capillaries close to the surface of the skin become dilated, resulting in blotchy red areas with small bumps and, sometimes, pimples. The redness can come and go, but eventually may become permanent if blood vessels under the skin become dilated, a phenomenon known as telangiectasia. The skin tissue can swell and thicken, and may be tender and sensitive to the touch.

The inflammation of rosacea can look a great deal like acne, but it tends to be more chronic, and blackheads and whiteheads are almost never present. It is a fairly common disorder—about 14 million Americans have it to some degree—but many never realize they have it. Rosacea usually begins with frequent flushing of the face, particularly the nose and cheeks. The flushing is caused by the swelling of the blood vessels under the skin. This "red mask" can serve as a flag for attention. Inflammation can then spread across the face, and small bumps may appear. Later, swelling of the nose may occur. However, it can take years from the beginnings of this condition before the later stages develop. Rosacea can also cause a persistent burning and feeling of grittiness in the eyes or inflamed and swollen eyelids. In severe cases, vision can be impaired.

The underlying cause or causes of rosacea are not understood, but certain factors are known to aggravate the condition, including the consumption of alcohol, hot liquids, and/or spicy foods; exposure to sunlight; humidity; extremes of temperature; and the use of makeup and skin care products containing alcohol. Stress, vitamin deficiencies, and infection can be contributing factors. The things that aggravate one person's rosacea may have no effect on another person.

Rosacea is most common in white women between the ages of thirty and fifty. One survey showed that 44 percent developed the disease between thirty and fifty years of age; 39 percent developed it after fifty years; and 17 percent before thirty years of age. When it does occur in men, rosacea tends to be more severe, and is usually accompanied by rhinophyma (a nose that becomes chronically red and enlarged). Fair-skinned individuals seem to be more susceptible to this condition than darker-skinned people. People who flush easily seem to be more prone than others to develop rosacea.

In rare cases, rosacea may affect the skin in other parts of the body as well as the face. It is not a dangerous condition, but it is chronic and can be distressing for cosmetic reasons. Without proper care, it can develop into a disfiguring condition.

The dosages recommended below are for adults.

NUTRIENTS

SUPPLEMENT	SUGGESTED DOSAGE	COMMENTS
Very Important		
Primrose oil	500 mg 3 times daily.	A good healer for many skin disorders. Contains linoleic acid, which is needed by the skin.
Pycnogenol	As directed on label.	Powerful antioxidant that moderates allergic and inflammatory responses by reducing histamine production.
Vitamin A with mixed carotenoids	25,000 IU daily for 3 months, then reduce to 15,000 IU daily. If you are pregnant, do not exceed 10,000 IU daily.	Necessary for healing and construction of new skin tissue.
Vitamin B complex	100 mg of each major B vitamin 3 times daily (amounts of individual vitamins in a complex will vary).	Antistress vitamins that are necessary in all cellular functions and help to maintain healthy skin.
plus extra vitamin B₂ (riboflavin) and	50 mg daily.	B vitamins that have been shown to be particularly useful
vitamin B₁₂	1,000–2,000 mcg daily.	in the treatment of rosacea.

Important		
Kelp	1,000–1,500 mg daily.	Supplies balanced minerals needed for good skin tone.
Multivitamin and mineral complex	As directed on label.	To ensure optimum nutrition and guard against deficiencies.
Vitamin E	200 IU daily.	Protects against free radicals. Use d-alpha-tocopherol form.
Zinc	50 mg daily. Do not exceed a total of 100 mg daily from all supplements.	For tissue repair. Enhances immune system response. Use zinc gluconate lozenges or OptiZinc for best absorption.
Helpful		
Ageless Beauty from Biotec Foods	As directed on label.	Protects the skin from free radical damage.
Chlorophyll or alfalfa	As directed on label.	Aids in cleansing the blood, preventing infections. Also supplies needed balanced minerals. *See under* Herbs, below.
Flaxseed oil capsules or liquid	1,000 mg daily. 1 tsp daily.	To supply needed essential fatty acids.
Herpanacine from Diamond-Herpanacine Associates	As directed on label.	Contains antioxidants, amino acids, and herbs that promote skin health.
L-cysteine	500 mg daily, on an empty stomach. Take with water or juice. Do not take with milk. Take with 50 mg vitamin B₆ and 100 mg vitamin C for better absorption.	Contains sulfur, needed for healthy skin. (*See* AMINO ACIDS in Part One.)
Lecithin granules or capsules	1 tbsp 3 times daily, before meals. 1,200 mg 3 times daily, before meals.	Aids absorption of the essential fatty acids.
Proteolytic enzymes	As directed on label. Take between meals.	Helps to reduce inflammation.
Selenium	200 mcg daily. Do not exceed this amount. If you are pregnant, do not exceed 40 mcg daily.	Encourages tissue elasticity and is a powerful antioxidant.
Superoxide dismutase (SOD)	As directed on label.	A free radical destroyer.
Vitamin C with bioflavonoids	3,000–5,000 mg daily, in divided doses.	Promotes immune function, strengthens capillaries, and acts as a mild anti-inflammatory.

Herbs

❑ Alfalfa is a good source of chlorophyll, which has detoxifying properties. It also supplies many needed vitamins and minerals.

❑ Aloe vera has excellent healing properties. Apply pure aloe vera gel topically to dry skin as directed on the product label or as needed.

Note: Some people with rosacea may experience irritation as a result of using aloe vera. If this occurs, discontinue use.

❑ Borage seed, dandelion root, dong quai, parsley, sarsaparilla, and yellow dock root improve skin tone.

❑ Bromelain and turmeric (curcumin) help to control inflammation.

❑ Burdock root and red clover are powerful blood cleansers. Burdock also helps to improve skin tone.

❑ Calendula, cayenne (capsicum), fennel seed, ginger, marshmallow root, sage, and slippery elm bark nourish the skin and promote healing.

Caution: Do not use sage if you suffer from any type of seizure disorder, or are pregnant or nursing.

❑ Milk thistle aids the liver in cleansing the blood.

❑ Nettle and rosemary improve skin tone, nourish the skin, and promote healing.

Recommendations

❑ Eat a diet that emphasizes raw vegetables and grains, organically grown if possible.

❑ Avoid fats, especially saturated fats, and all animal products. Saturated fats promote inflammation. Also avoid alcohol, caffeine, cheese, chocolate, cocoa, dairy products, eggs, fish, salt, sugar, and spicy foods.

❑ Do not drink hot beverages such as coffee or tea. Allow your food to cool to room temperature before eating it.

❑ Investigate the possibility of food allergies. Keep a food diary for one month to see which foods may be aggravating the condition. Then avoid those foods. (*See* ALLERGIES in Part Two for further information.)

❑ Once a month, follow a fasting program. (*See* FASTING in Part Three.)

❑ Keep the skin scrupulously clean, but treat it gently. Use a mild natural soap and lukewarm to cool (never cold or hot) water for cleansing. Pat the skin dry after washing—do not rub it. Avoid touching the skin except when cleansing it.

❑ Avoid extremes of temperature, especially heat. Keep baths and showers short, and use water that is as cool as you can tolerate comfortably. Avoid saunas (including the type used for facials and steam inhalations), steam baths, and hot tubs. If you need to increase the humidity in your home, use only a cool mist humidifier.

❑ As much as possible, avoid wearing makeup. If you do use cosmetics, choose all-natural, water-based products.

❑ *Do not* use topical steroid creams. These only make the condition worse.

❑ Friction is extremely irritating, so avoid wearing tight clothing such as turtlenecks that can rub against the skin. Be careful about anything that comes close to or into contact with your face. Even holding the telephone receiver against your face for a while can raise the local temperature and irritate sensitive skin.

❑ In severe cases, a laser or electrical device can be used to remove the excess tissue. Dermabrasion also has helped some people with rosacea.

Considerations

❑ There is no known cure for rosacea. Topical and/or oral antibiotics, usually tetracycline, are often prescribed to keep the inflammation under control. As with any drug, these can have side effects, especially with long-term use. Moreover, if you stop taking the antibiotics, the condition may rebound. More information is available from the National Rosacea Society. (*See* Health and Medical Organizations in the Appendix.)

❑ An underlying vascular disorder may be involved in the development of rosacea. Several findings support this theory. First, there are structural abnormalities in the small blood vessels in the facial skin of people with rosacea. Second, the condition is exacerbated by the use of drugs that dilate blood vessels, such as theophylline and nitroglycerin. Finally, people with rosacea are more likely than most to suffer from migraines, a type of headache also linked to vascular malfunction.

❑ *Demodex folliculorum,* a type of microscopic mite that lives on cast-off skin cells and is normally present on human skin, has been found in significantly higher than normal numbers in skin samples taken from people with rosacea. Researchers speculate that this organism, or some type of reaction to it, may be involved in rosacea.

SCABIES

Scabies is a parasitic infection that causes a persistent, itchy rash. It is caused by a tiny mite that burrows into the top layer of the skin to lay its eggs. This results in groups of small red lumps. The scabies skin mite, so small it can hardly be seen without a microscope, infects over 300 million people worldwide every year. When the rash first appears, you may see fine, wavy lines emanating from some of the lumps if you look closely. The skin may then become dry and scaly, and the itching can be intense, especially at night. Scratching can set the stage for a bacterial infection as well.

Scabies can be a particular problem in institutional settings such as nursing homes and day care centers. It is spread primarily by skin-to-skin contact, and it is highly contagious. The areas most commonly affected are the buttocks, genitals (in men), nipples (in women), wrists, and armpits, as well as the skin between the toes and fingers.

To diagnose the condition, a physician usually takes a scraping of skin from the affected area and examines it under a microscope. Children under the age of fifteen have the highest incidence of scabies, and are usually the first in the family to contract it. It is also considered to be a sexually transmitted disease.

Unless otherwise stated, the dosages recommended here are for adults. For children between the ages of twelve and seventeen, reduce the dose to three-quarters of the recommended amount. For children between the ages of six and twelve, use one-half the recommended dose, and for children under six, use one-quarter of the recommended amount.

NUTRIENTS

SUPPLEMENT	SUGGESTED DOSAGE	COMMENTS
Very Important		
Garlic (Kyolic from Wakunaga)	2 capsules 3 times daily, with meals.	Has antiparasitic and antibiotic properties.
Primrose oil	1,000 mg 3 times daily.	A good healer for most skin disorders.
Vitamin A with mixed carotenoids	25,000 IU daily for 3 months, then reduce to 15,000 IU daily. If you are pregnant, do not exceed 10,000 IU daily.	Necessary for healing and for construction of new skin tissue.
Important		
Kelp	1,000–1,500 mg daily.	Supplies balanced minerals.
Zinc	50 mg daily. Do not exceed a total of 100 mg daily from all supplements.	For tissue repair. Enhances immune system response. Use zinc gluconate lozenges or zinc methionate (OptiZinc) for best absorption.
Helpful		
Colloidal silver	Apply topically as directed on label.	To prevent secondary infection.
Vitamin E	200 IU daily.	Promotes healing. Use d-alpha-tocopherol form.

Herbs

❏ Aloe vera has excellent healing properties. Apply gel topically to the affected area as directed on the product label.

❏ Balsam of Peru, goldenseal, and/or tea tree oil can be applied topically to fight the infection.

❏ Goldenseal can also be taken internally to bolster the immune system.

Caution: Do not take goldenseal internally on a daily basis for more than one week at a time. Do not use it during pregnancy or if you are breast-feeding, and use with caution if you are allergic to ragweed. If you have a history of cardiovascular disease, diabetes, or glaucoma, use it only under a doctor's supervision.

❏ Black walnut, garlic, and wormwood are useful for parasitic infections.

Caution: Do not use wormwood in high doses or for extended periods because it contains the chemical compound thujone that can be poisonous. Do not use wormwood if you suffer from any type of seizure disorder or are pregnant.

❏ Comfrey and/or calendula salve helps to soothe itching and irritation.

Caution: Comfrey is recommended for external use only.

❏ Rhubarb helps the body to rid itself of parasitic infections.

Recommendations

❏ Diet alone cannot cure scabies. To get rid of the mites, apply permethrin cream 5 percent (Elemite) topically to the entire body from the neck down, as directed on the label or as prescribed by your physician Other medications include sulfur ointment and crotamiton (Eurax). All are fine for children as young as two years of age.

❏ Because scabies is easily spread from one person to another by close contact, if one household member develops it, thoroughly wash all clothing, towels, and bed linens in the house.

❏ Practice scrupulous personal hygiene. Avoid contact with infested persons or their clothing.

❏ To promote healing, eat plenty of foods high in zinc, such as soybeans, sunflower seeds, wheat bran, whole-grain products, yeast, and blackstrap molasses.

❏ Do not drink soft drinks or alcoholic beverages. Consume no sugar, chocolate, or junk foods.

❏ Drink at least ten 8-ounce glasses of clean water a day.

❏ Avoid fried foods and all animal products. Use cold-pressed vegetable oils only.

Considerations

❏ A topical scabicide called lindane (gamma benzene hexachloride, found in the product Kwell) was once considered a standard treatment for scabies. In recent years, however, it has largely been replaced by permethrin, which is believed to be safer and cause fewer side effects. Do not use lindane unless the permethrin is not working.

❏ Scabicides are not recommended for children under the age of six or for pregnant women. In such cases, a milder sulfur solution is usually recommended.

❏ It may take one to two weeks for the itching to subside, even after treatment. An antihistamine or a cortisone cream may be recommended to provide relief. Calendula salve, cool compresses, and cool oatmeal baths are natural alternatives to those medications.

❏ Crowded, unsanitary, or institutional living conditions are conducive to the spread of scabies.

SCHIZOPHRENIA

Schizophrenia is a disorder that makes it impossible to differentiate between what is imagined and what is real. The characteristic symptoms include disordered thinking, speech, and perception; a lack of curiosity; diminishing emotional contact with others; lethargy; emotional changes such as tension and/or depression; and more dramatic behavioral disturbances, ranging from catatonia to violent outbursts and delusions. People with schizophrenia lose, to some degree, their hold on reality, and many seem to withdraw into their own worlds. Hallucinations are not uncommon.

There are five basic types of schizophrenia:

1. *Catatonic schizophrenia* is characterized by unusual rigid postures, lack of movement, or frenzied movement.

2. *Disorganized schizophrenia*, which used to be called hebephrenic schizophrenia, is characterized by a lack of the normal range of emotions along with speech that displays a disorganized way of thinking.

3. *Paranoid schizophrenia* is characterized by hallucinatory and delusional symptoms.

4. *Undifferentiated schizophrenia* involves a mixture of different symptoms from the types above.

5. *Residual schizophrenia* is a type of schizophrenia in which the severity of schizophrenia symptoms has decreased. Hallucinations, delusions, or other symptoms may still be present but are considerably less than when the schizophrenia was originally diagnosed.

While the onset of the disorder is often related to a stressful life event, the underlying cause or causes of schizophrenia are not known. Some researchers believe that schizophrenia is hereditary, and there is evidence that some cases of schizophrenia are the result of an inherited defect in body chemistry in which brain chemicals called neurotransmitters function abnormally. Others theorize that schizophrenia results from external factors, such as complications during birth; head injury; a reaction to a virus, including the influenza virus; or environmental poisons that reach and damage the brain. There is a high incidence of childhood head injuries and birth complications among people with schizophrenia. A wide range of drugs also can cause schizophrenic-type symptoms.

Yet another theory focuses on nutritional factors. There is some indication that schizophrenia might be associated with high copper levels in body tissues. When copper levels are too high, the levels of vitamin C and zinc in the body drop. A zinc deficiency may result in damage to the pineal area of the brain, which normally contains high levels of zinc, which in turn may make an individual vulnerable to schizophrenia or other psychoses. Other clues come from the seasonality of the disorder. The incidence of schizophrenic episodes tends to peak in cold-weather months, when zinc intake tends to be lower. Magnesium deficiency could also be a factor. Some research has shown that magnesium levels in the blood of people with active schizophrenia are lower than normal and that the levels are higher in persons whose schizophrenia is in remission. It has been hypothesized that a type of vicious cycle may be at work here; the high level of stress experienced by those with severe psychiatric disorders may lead to magnesium deficiency, which in turn would exacerbate symptoms such as anxiety, fear, hallucinations, weakness, and physical complaints.

Levels of, and the balance between, the neurotransmitters dopamine, serotonin, epinephrine, and norepinephrine, and the way in which the brain responds to these substances, are thought to play a profound role in the development of schizophrenia.

Approximately 2.4 million American adults, or about 1.1 percent of the population age eighteen and older, have schizophrenia. It affects men and women evenly; it first appears in men in their late teens or early twenties, in contrast to women, who generally are affected in their twenties or early thirties. One interesting thing that was found is that there seems to be more schizophrenia in the developed countries than in developing nations. Researchers advise extreme caution in drawing any conclusions from this, however, as there could be numerous social and economic factors skewing the results.

Unless otherwise specified, the dosages recommended here are for adults. For children between the ages of twelve and seventeen, reduce the dose to three-quarters the recommended amount.

NUTRIENTS

SUPPLEMENT	SUGGESTED DOSAGE	COMMENTS
Essential		
5-hydroxy L-tryptophan (5-HTP)	As directed on label.	Increases the body's production of serotonin, a vital brain chemical.
Flaxseed oil	As directed on label.	To supply essential fatty acids, needed for proper brain and nerve function.
Folic acid	2,000 mcg daily.	Deficiency has been found in approximately 25 percent of those hospitalized for psychiatric disorders.
and vitamin B$_{12}$	1,000 mcg twice daily.	Folic acid works best when taken with vitamin B$_{12}$ and vitamin C.
and vitamin C with bioflavonoids	5,000 mg daily.	
Gamma-aminobutyric acid (GABA)	As directed on label, on an empty stomach. Take with water or juice. Do not take with milk. Take with 50 mg vitamin B$_6$ and 100 mg vitamin C for better absorption.	Essential for brain metabolism. Aids in proper brain function. (*See* AMINO ACIDS in Part One.)
Garlic (Kyolic from Wakunaga)	As directed on label.	Enhances brain function.
Glutathione or	As directed on label.	Deficiency can affect the nervous system.

cysteine plus	As directed on label.	
glutamic acid and	As directed on label.	Nutrients used to synthesize glutathione.
glycine	As directed on label.	
L-asparagine	As directed on label.	Maintains balance in the central nervous system.
L-glutamic acid	As directed on label.	Important in brain metabolism. Acts as a neurotransmitter.
L-methionine	As directed on label.	Helps to counteract histamine, which is found in high levels in people with schizophrenia.
L-phenylalanine	As directed on label.	An amino acid that is converted into tyrosine, which is important for synthesis of both dopamine and norepinephrine.
Pycnogenol or	As directed on label.	Antioxidants useful for dementia and other
grape seed extract	As directed on label.	syndromes of the brain.
Zinc	Up to 80 mg daily. Do not exceed 100 mg daily from all supplements.	Balances copper, often found in high concentrations in people with this disorder.
plus manganese	As directed on label. Take separately from calcium.	Enhances action of B vitamins necessary for brain function.

Very Important		
Free form amino acid	As directed on label. Take on an empty stomach.	Needed for normal brain function. Use a formula containing all the essential amino acids.
Raw liver extract injections or vitamin B complex injections plus extra vitamin B$_6$ (pyridoxine) and vitamin B$_{12}$ or vitamin B complex	1 cc 3 times weekly for 3 weeks, then twice weekly for 3 months. Then reduce to 1 cc once weekly. 1 cc 3 times weekly for 3 weeks, then twice weekly for 3 months. Then reduce to 1 cc once weekly. ½ cc 3 times weekly for 3 weeks, then twice weekly for 3 months. Then reduce to ½ cc once weekly. 1 cc 3 times weekly or as prescribed by physician. 100 mg of each major B vitamin 3 times daily (amounts of individual vitamins in a complex will vary).	To supply B vitamins and other valuable nutrients. B vitamin deficiencies are related to brain malfunction. Many people with brain disorders have found this program helpful. All injectables can be combined in a single shot. If injections are not available, use a sublingual form.
plus extra vitamin B$_6$ (pyridoxine) plus vitamin B$_3$ (niacin) or niacinamide	100 mg twice daily. 100 mg 3 times daily. Do not exceed this amount. 1,000 mg daily.	Required by the nervous system; necessary for normal brain function. Deficiency has been linked to schizophrenia. Injections (under a doctor's supervision) are best. *Caution:* Do not take niacin if you have a liver disorder, gout, or high blood pressure.
Vitamin E emulsion or capsules	200 IU daily.	An antioxidant that improves brain circulation. Emulsion form is recommended for easier assimilation and greater safety at high doses.

Important		
Dimethylglycine (DMG) (Aangamik DMG from FoodScience of Vermont)	As directed on label.	Enhances cerebral oxygen utilization.
Essential fatty acids (black currant seed oil or primrose oil)	As directed on label 3 times daily.	Helps cerebral circulation.
Lecithin granules or capsules	1 tbsp 3 times daily, before meals. 1,200 mg 3 times daily, before meals.	Improves brain function. Contains choline and inositol. Works well with vitamin E.
L-glutamine	1,000–4,000 mg daily, on an empty stomach. Take with water or juice. Do not take with milk. Take with 50 mg vitamin B$_6$ and 100 mg vitamin C for better absorption.	Needed for normal brain function. (*See* AMINO ACIDS in Part One.)

Helpful		
Kelp	1,000–1,500 mg daily.	Contains balanced essential minerals.
Multivitamin and mineral complex with calcium and magnesium	As directed on label.	All nutrients are needed for normal brain function.
Raw thyroid glandular	As directed on label.	Reduced thyroid function results in poor cerebral function. (*See* HYPOTHYROIDISM in Part Two and GLANDULAR THERAPY in Part Three.)

Herbs

❏ Ginkgo biloba improves brain function and cerebral circulation, and enhances memory.

Caution: Do not take ginkgo biloba if you have a bleeding disorder, or are scheduled for surgery or a dental procedure.

❏ Kava kava and passionflower are good for relief of stress and depression.

Caution: Kava kava can cause drowsiness. It is not recommended for pregnant women or nursing mothers, and it should not be taken together with other substances that act on the central nervous system, such as alcohol, barbiturates, antidepressants, and antipsychotic drugs.

Recommendations

❏ Eat a high-fiber diet that includes plenty of fresh raw vegetables and quality protein, and try eating more frequent small meals rather than three larger ones each day. This helps to keep blood sugar levels stable, which in turn has a stabilizing influence on mood and behavior. *See* HYPOGLYCEMIA in Part Two for additional suggestions.

❑ Include the following in your diet: breast of chicken or turkey, brewer's yeast, halibut, peas, sunflower seeds, and tuna. Also eat foods rich in niacin, such as broccoli, carrots, corn, eggs, fish, potatoes, tomatoes, and whole wheat.

Caution: Brewer's yeast can cause an allergic reaction in some individuals. Start with a small amount at first, and discontinue use if any allergic symptoms occur.

❑ Do not consume caffeine. It promotes the release of unwanted norepinephrine, a stimulating neurotransmitter.

❑ Avoid alcohol. Alcohol consumption depletes the body of zinc. Many psychological disorders are known to be adversely affected by zinc deficiencies.

❑ Keep environmental pressures under control. Overstimulation from very strong emotions or an excessive workload can exacerbate symptoms. Also avoid understimulation.

Considerations

❑ Sometimes extremely high doses of certain vitamins are needed to keep the mind functioning well.

❑ Hair analysis reveals mineral imbalances that may contribute to mental difficulties. (*See* HAIR ANALYSIS in Part Three.)

❑ Some experts believe that many suicides among the young may be related to undiagnosed schizophrenia.

❑ Psychiatrists found a link between schizophrenia and pellagra, a vitamin B$_3$ (niacin) deficiency disease. Taking several grams of niacinamide daily (under a doctor's supervision) has been tried with good results.

❑ Undiagnosed celiac disease, caused by an intolerance to gluten, can cause symptoms similar to those of schizophrenia. Gluten intolerance can also cause severe depression. (*See* CELIAC DISEASE in Part Two.)

❑ Drug therapy is usually the medical treatment of choice for schizophrenia. However, there is no single medication that is effective in all cases. It may be necessary to try several different drugs in order to find the one that works best to keep symptoms under control.

❑ With newer drugs there is a tendency to gain weight and develop a condition called metabolic syndrome. This causes increases in blood sugar, cholesterol, and blood pressure. Be sure that your doctor is monitoring your weight and these medical tests, so that if treatment is needed, it can be provided early.

❑ Olanzapine (Zyprexa) has been used since the mid-1990s to treat schizophrenia. When using this drug, tell your doctor if you eat grapefruit or drink grapefruit juice because of potential interactions, and be sure to drink plenty of water. This drug was supposed to reduce tremors associated with older drugs such as haloperidol (Haldol). It is highly effective, but does promote weight gain. Monitor your weight if you are taking this drug.

❑ Some people are prescribed ziprasidone (Geodon). It is best absorbed with a meal that contains at least 500 calories and any amount of fat. If you are gaining weight with this drug, opt for low-fat meals (less than 30 percent of calories).

❑ The essential fatty acids in the red blood cells and spinal fluid of patients with schizophrenia differ from those without the condition. In one study, the omega-3 fat DHA was lower in the brain and higher in the spinal fluid of those with schizophrenia. This finding will likely provoke new research into the area of fatty acids and brain function.

❑ If you are taking prescription drugs for schizophrenia, do not stop taking your medication without first consulting a physician. Do not take any of the supplements listed above that might affect dopamine, serotonin, or norepinephrine synthesis without consulting a physician.

❑ Some cases of schizophrenia have been linked to food allergies. Many people find their symptoms improve after they fast. (*See also* ALLERGIES in Part Two and FASTING in Part Three.)

❑ For more information concerning schizophrenia, you can consult www.schizophrenia.com. (*See* Health and Medical Organizations in the Appendix).

SCIATICA

See under BACKACHE.

SCOTOMA

See under EYE PROBLEMS.

SEASONAL AFFECTIVE DISORDER (SAD)

See under DEPRESSION.

SEBACEOUS CYST

Sebaceous cysts are skin growths that contain a mixture of sebum (oil) and skin proteins. They generally appear as small, slowly growing swellings on the face, scalp, or back. A whitehead is actually a tiny sebaceous cyst.

These nodules feel firm but movable and rarely hurt unless they become infected. If infection sets in, there may be redness and swelling, and the area may become sensitive to the touch. Sebaceous cysts are benign, but they can become a site of chronic, usually bacterial, infection. With chronic infection, an abscess may form.

Unless otherwise stated, the dosages recommended here are for adults. For children between the ages of twelve and seventeen, reduce the dose to three-quarters of the recommended amount. For children between the ages of six and twelve, use one-half the recommended dose, and for children under six, use one-quarter of the recommended amount.

NUTRIENTS

SUPPLEMENT	SUGGESTED DOSAGE	COMMENTS
Very Important		
Primrose oil	1,000 mg 3 times daily.	A good healer for most skin disorders.
Vitamin A	25,000 IU daily for 3 months, then reduce to 15,000 IU daily. If you are pregnant, do not exceed 10,000 IU daily.	Necessary for healing and construction of new skin tissue.
plus carotenoid complex with beta-carotene	As directed on label.	Used by the body to make vitamin A as needed.
Vitamin B complex plus extra	As directed on label.	Antistress and antiaging vitamins.
vitamin B₁₂	1,000–2,000 mcg daily.	Needed for healthy skin.
Important		
Garlic (Kyolic from Wakunaga)	2 capsules 3 times daily, with meals.	Has anti-infective properties.
Kelp	1,000–1,500 mg daily.	Supplies balanced minerals needed for good skin tone.
Zinc	50 mg daily. Do not exceed a total of 100 mg daily from all supplements.	For tissue repair. Enhances immune system response. Use zinc gluconate lozenges or OptiZinc for best absorption.
Helpful		
Superoxide dismutase (SOD)	As directed on label.	A free radical destroyer.

Herbs

❑ Aloe vera is soothing and healing. Apply pure aloe vera gel to the affected area as directed on the product label.

❑ Burdock root and red clover are both powerful blood cleansers.

❑ Goldenseal extract or tea tree oil can be applied topically to fight infection.

❑ Milk thistle aids the liver in cleansing the blood.

❑ Witch hazel, applied to the skin, is excellent for absorbing oil.

Recommendations

❑ Avoid fats, especially saturated fats, and all fried foods. Also avoid alcohol, caffeine, chocolate, cocoa, dairy products, eggs, fat, fish, meat, salt, and sugar.

❑ Follow a fasting program. (*See* FASTING in Part Three.)

❑ Apply warm compresses several times daily.

❑ Use hot water when washing your skin. This helps to dissolve skin oil.

Considerations

❑ If the cyst is inflamed, your doctor may inject it with a steroid medicine to reduce swelling.

❑ If an antibiotic is prescribed, be sure to take an acidophilus supplement to replace necessary "friendly" bacteria. Do not take acidophilus at the same time of day as the antibiotic.

❑ If you develop an inflamed or infected sebaceous cyst, you physician may suggest surgical drainage, a procedure that is performed in the doctor's office.

❑ *See also* OILY SKIN in Part Two.

SEBORRHEA

Seborrhea, or seborrheic dermatitis, is characterized by scaly patches of skin that result from a disorder of the sebaceous (oil-secreting) glands. Seborrhea most often occurs on the scalp, face, and chest, but can appear on other parts of the body as well. It may or may not be itchy.

Seborrheic skin may be yellowish and/or greasy or dry and flaky. The scaly bumps may coalesce to form large plaques or patches. Seborrheic dermatitis can occur at any age, but is most common in infancy ("cradle cap") and middle age. The exact cause is not known, but it may be linked to nutritional deficiencies (especially a lack of biotin and vitamin A) or the effects of a yeast organism, *Pityrosporum ovale,* which normally lives in the hair follicles. Heredity and climate probably also play a role. Adult seborrheic dermatitis, which usually affects the scalp and face, is often associated with stress and anxiety. Other factors associated with an increased chance of developing seborrhea include infrequent shampooing, oily skin, obesity, Parkinson's disease, AIDS, and other skin disorders, such as acne, rosacea, and psoriasis.

Unless otherwise specified, the dosages recommended here are for adults. For children between the ages of twelve and seventeen, reduce the dose to three-quarters the recommended amount. For children between six and twelve, use one-half the recommended dose, and for children under the age of six, use one-quarter the recommended amount.

NUTRIENTS

SUPPLEMENT	SUGGESTED DOSAGE	COMMENTS
Essential		
Essential fatty acids (primrose oil or Ultimate Oil from Nature's Secret)	As directed on label.	Important for many skin disorders; contains needed linoleic acid.
Vitamin B complex plus extra	As directed on label.	The B vitamins, especially vitamin B₆, are needed for protein metabolism, which is essential for healing and repair. Use a super-high-potency formula. A sublingual form is recommended for best absorption. Consider injections (under a doctor's supervision).
vitamin B₆ (pyridoxine)	50 mg 3 times daily.	
and biotin	300–400 mcg 3 times daily.	Deficiency has been linked to seborrhea.

Zinc	50 mg daily. Do not exceed a total of 100 mg daily from all supplements.	Important for healing. Enhances immunity. Use zinc gluconate lozenges or OptiZinc for best absorption.
Important		
ConcenTrace from Trace Minerals Research	As directed on label.	Contains essential trace minerals to nourish the skin.
Herpanacine from Diamond-Herpanacine Associates	As directed on label.	Contains amino acids, vitamins, and herbs that promote skin health and remove toxins.
Methylsulfonyl-methane (MSM)	As directed on label.	Possesses healing and nutritional properties for the skin.
Panoderm I from American Biologics	As directed on label.	Contains squalene, a substance found in healthy skin. Acts as a natural antioxidant and prevents damage to the skin due to cosmetics, wind, sun, and pollutants.
Pycnogenol or grape seed extract	As directed on label. As directed on label.	Powerful antioxidants that strengthen the skin to resist disease.
Vitamin A plus carotenoid complex with beta-carotene plus vitamin E	Up to 50,000 IU daily. If you are pregnant, do not exceed 10,000 IU daily. As directed on label. 200 IU daily.	Deficiency may cause or contribute to seborrhea. Speeds healing. Increases oxygen intake.
Helpful		
Acidophilus (Kyo-Dophilus from Wakunaga)	As directed on label. Take on an empty stomach.	To replenish "friendly" bacteria. Especially important if antibiotics are prescribed. Use a nondairy formula.
Coenzyme Q10 plus Coenzyme A from Coenzyme-A Technologies	60 mg daily. As directed on label.	An important free radical scavenger that supplies oxygen to the cells. Works effectively with coenzyme Q10 to support the immune system's detoxification of many dangerous substances.
Dimethylglycine (DMG) (Aangamik DMG from FoodScience of Vermont)	As directed on label.	Increases oxygenation of tissues.
Free form amino acid	As directed on label.	For healing and repair of tissues.
Kelp	1,000–1,500 mg daily.	Contains balanced minerals. A good source of iodine.
Lecithin granules or capsules	1 tbsp 3 times daily, with meals. 1,200 mg 3 times daily, with meals.	For cellular protection.
Multivitamin and mineral complex	As directed on label.	All nutrients are necessary in balance.

Herbs

❑ Dandelion, goldenseal, and red clover, taken internally, are good for most skin disorders.

Caution: Do not take goldenseal internally on a daily basis for more than one week at a time. Do not use it during pregnancy or if you are breast-feeding, and use with caution if you are allergic to ragweed. If you have a history of cardiovascular disease, diabetes, or glaucoma, use it only under a doctor's supervision.

❑ Emu oil, applied topically, has an anti-inflammatory effect on skin tissues.

❑ Oat straw may be used in a bath to reduce symptoms, especially inflammation and itching.

❑ Olive leaf extract has healing properties for the skin.

❑ Tea tree oil is a natural antiseptic and antifungal that can be applied directly to the affected area. If it is too strong, it can be diluted with an equal amount of jojoba oil (available in health food stores) or distilled water.

❑ Wild pansy (*Viola tricolor*) grows wild in parts of Europe, the Near East, and Africa, as well as in parts of North America. The aerial parts can be dried and used topically to treat various skin ailments, including seborrhea, cradle cap, and eczema. To make a compress or rinse, pour ½ cup of boiling water over 2 teaspoons of wild pansy, steep for ten minutes, and strain. Use the resulting liquid to make a hot compress, to be removed from the affected area when dry or cold. Use this treatment several times a day.

Recommendations

❑ Eat a diet composed of 50 to 75 percent raw foods and soured products such as low-fat yogurt.

❑ Avoid chocolate, dairy products, white flour, fried foods, seafood, nuts, and anything containing sugar.

❑ Do not eat any foods containing raw eggs. Egg whites contain high levels of avidin, a protein that binds biotin and prevents it from being absorbed. Biotin is needed for healthy hair and skin. Eating uncooked eggs also poses a risk of *Salmonella* poisoning (*see* FOODBORNE/WATERBORNE ILLNESS in Part Two).

❑ If antibiotics are prescribed, take extra B-complex vitamins and an acidophilus supplement to replace the "friendly" bacteria destroyed by the antibiotics.

❑ Try changing your hair products. Choose products without chemicals.

❑ To minimize the frequency and severity of flare-ups, dry your skin thoroughly after bathing, and wear loose-fitting clothing made of natural fibers that "breathe."

❑ *Echinacea purpurea*, a homeopathic preparation, can be used to reduce symptoms.

❑ Avoid using over-the-counter ointments to treat seborrhea. Use can cause an overload on the skin.

❏ Do not pick at or squeeze the affected skin.

❏ Avoid using irritating soaps, but make sure you keep the affected areas clean. Avoid greasy ointments and creams.

❏ Keep your hair clean and make sure you use a non-oily shampoo.

❏ If dietary changes and nutritional supplementation do not produce an improvement, seek the advice of a qualified health care professional.

❏ Follow a fasting program once a month. (*See* FASTING in Part Three.)

Considerations

❏ Dermatologists usually prescribe topical steroids to reduce inflammation and control itching. Anti-fungal shampoos are available without a prescription such as Selsun Blue (with selenium sulfide) and Head and Shoulders (with pyrithione zinc).

❏ An absence of intestinal flora may be responsible for biotin deficiency in infants. Studies have shown that treating both the nursing mother and her infant with biotin can be successful in resolving cradle cap. For adults, treatment with biotin alone does not appear to be effective, but supplementation with biotin combined with the whole vitamin B complex and essential fatty acids produces improvement in many cases. Do not give your infant anything without speaking to a pediatrician first.

❏ Consuming raw egg whites has produced seborrheic dermatitis in laboratory tests.

❏ Colloidal silver is a natural topical antibiotic that has been known to fight skin conditions such as seborrhea.

❏ Some findings suggest that many skin disorders, including eczema and psoriasis, may be related to gluten allergy. A gluten-free diet may be helpful. *See* CELIAC DISEASE in Part Two for dietary suggestions.

❏ Taking supplemental vitamin B complex has been shown to be the most effective treatment in many cases.

❏ *See also* DANDRUFF and DERMATITIS in Part Two.

SEIZURE

See under EPILEPSY.

SENILITY (DEMENTIA)

Senility was once considered an inevitable consequence of aging. However, we now know that it is a physically based disease resulting from a loss of brain cells. Brain function, or certain aspects of brain function, decline to the point that mental disability results. Forgetfulness, fearfulness, depression, agitation, difficulty absorbing new information, loss of normal emotional responses, and an ability to remember things that happened years ago, but not things

that took place a few minutes ago, are typical. Other signs include mood swings, jealousy, paranoia, frustration, anger, insensitivity to the feelings of others, fear of being alone, repeating conversations, inability to make decisions or complete a task, lack of a sense of time, hoarding, failure to recognize people, and self-neglect. The disorder usually gets progressively worse. Complications that may occur include injuries (primarily due to falls), inadequate nutrition, constipation, and a variety of infections.

Dementia can be caused by several diseases affecting brain function, among them alcoholism, Alzheimer's disease, kidney or liver failure, hypothyroidism, multiple strokes, atherosclerosis, multiple sclerosis, or diabetes, to name a few. It can also result from nutritional deficiencies, especially deficiencies of vitamins B_1 (thiamine), B_3 (niacin), B_6 (pyridoxine), and B_{12}. Older adults who develop gait abnormalities seem to be more prone to getting vascular or other non–Alzheimer's type dementia according to one study. This is a valid early warning signal because such individuals are more than three and a half times more likely to develop dementia as compared with those who have the same basic risk factors but who do not have the gait problem. Blood pressure medication, dietary changes, and nutritional therapy aimed at lessening the risk of stroke might help.

Many people diagnosed as senile actually suffer from *pseudodementia*—symptoms that mimic dementia but that are actually caused by depression, deafness, brain tumors, thyroid problems, liver or kidney problems, the use of certain drugs, or other disorders. A thorough medical and psychological examination by a qualified professional, preferably a specialist in the field, is necessary for an accurate diagnosis.

Dementia is considered incurable. However, because generally declining health contributes to the problem, proper diet and nutritional supplements can help. The following supplements are helpful for improving brain function. When choosing supplements, avoid heavily coated or sustained-release products. These are difficult to break down. Instead, choose liquids, powders, or sublingual forms.

NUTRIENTS

SUPPLEMENT	SUGGESTED DOSAGE	COMMENTS
Essential		
Dimethylglycine (DMG) (Aangamik DMG from FoodScience of Vermont)	As directed on label.	Helps to maintain mental acuity and enhances immune function.
Essential fatty acids (flaxseed oil or primrose oil)	As directed on label.	Promotes brain and nerve function as well as a healthy immune system.
Free form amino acid	As directed on label.	To supply protein, needed for normal brain function. Protein deficiency is common among older adults.

Gamma-amino-butyric acid (GABA)	As directed on label, on an empty stomach. Take with water or juice. Do not take with milk. Take with 50 mg vitamin B_6 and 100 mg vitamin C for better absorption.	Essential for brain function and metabolism. Has a calming effect. (*See* AMINO ACIDS in Part One.)
Garlic (Kyolic from Wakunaga)	As directed on label.	Enhances brain function; helps to reduce stress and anxiety.
L-asparagine	As directed on label, on an empty stomach.	To maintain balance in the brain and central nervous system.
L-phenylalanine	As directed on label, on an empty stomach.	Promotes alertness, aids memory, and helps overcome depression. *Caution:* Do not take this supplement if you are taking an MAO inhibitor drug, or if you suffer from panic attacks, diabetes, high blood pressure, or PKU.
L-tyrosine	As directed on label, on an empty stomach.	Promotes brain function and helps fight depression. *Caution:* Do not take tyrosine if you are taking an MAO inhibitor drug, commonly prescribed for depression.
Melatonin	2–3 mg daily, taken 2 hours or less before bedtime.	Aids sleep, helps maintain equilibrium, and strengthens the immune system.
Nicotinamide adenine dinucleotide (NADH)	As directed on label.	A coenzyme form of niacin that is essential for production of energy and various neurotransmitters.
Phosphatidyl choline	As directed on label.	Aids in treating neurological disorders, memory loss, and depression. Is safe and effective. However, if you have bipolar mood disorder, you should not take large amounts.
Phosphatidyl serine	As directed on label.	Has been known to reverse depression and symptoms of Alzheimer's disease, and to enhance memory and learning abilities. The brain normally produces it, but production dwindles with age.
Pregnenolone	As directed on label.	May treat symptoms of aging, increase brain function, and enhance mood, memory, and thinking.
Vitamin B complex injections	1 cc once weekly or as prescribed by physician.	All B vitamins are necessary for brain and nerve health. Older adults often have deficiencies because the ability to absorb the B vitamins declines with age. Injections (under a doctor's supervision) are best.
plus extra vitamin B_6 (pyridoxine) and	½ cc once weekly or as prescribed by physician.	Vital for mental health and for maintaining proper electrolyte balance in the body.
vitamin B_{12} injections plus	As prescribed by physician.	
liver extract injections or vitamin B complex	1 cc once weekly or as prescribed by physician. 100 mg of each major B vitamin 3 times daily (amounts of individual vitamins in a complex will vary).	A good source of B vitamins and other valuable nutrients. If injections are not available, use a sublingual form.
plus extra		

vitamin B_3 (niacin) and	100 mg daily. Do not exceed this amount. Take with 100 mg niacinamide to reduce flushing.	Improves cerebral circulation and lowers cholesterol levels. *Caution:* Do not take niacin if you have a liver disorder, gout, or high blood pressure.
vitamin B_6 (pyridoxine) and	50 mg daily.	
vitamin B_{12}	2,000 mcg daily.	Needed to prevent anemia. Also prevents nerve damage and may assist memory and learning. Use a lozenge or sublingual form.

Very Important

S-Adenosylmethionine (SAMe)	400 mg 2 times daily.	Aids in relieving stress and depression, eases pain, and produces antioxidant effects. *Caution:* Do not use if you have bipolar mood disorder or take prescription antidepressants.
Trimethylglycine (TMG)	500–1,000 mg in the morning.	Assists the body in utilizing vitamin B_6, vitamin B_{12}, and folic acid. Also helps to rid the body of toxic elements (such as homocysteine) and increases levels of the natural mood elevator S-adenosylmethionine.
Vitamin C with bioflavonoids	3,000–10,000 mg daily, in divided doses.	Reduces blood clotting tendency, improving cerebral circulation.
Vitamin E	200 IU daily.	Improves cerebral circulation and boosts immunity, which declines with age. Use d-alpha-tocopherol form.

Important

GH3 from Gero Vita	As directed on label.	Helps to promote brain function. Consider injections (under a doctor's supervision). *Caution:* Do not use GH3 if you are allergic to sulfites.

Helpful

Coenzyme Q_{10} plus	100–200 mg daily.	Free radical scavenger and immunostimulant. Increases cellular oxygen levels.
Coenzyme A from Coenzyme-A Technologies	As directed on label.	Works effectively with coenzyme Q_{10} to support the immune system's detoxification of many dangerous substances.
Kelp	As directed on label.	Reported to be very beneficial to brain tissue, the membranes surrounding the brain, the sensory nerves, and the spinal cord.
Lecithin granules or capsules	1 tbsp 3 times daily, before meals. 1,200 mg 3 times daily, before meals.	For brain cell protection and function.
L-glutamine	As directed on label, on an empty stomach. Take with water or juice. Do not take with milk. Take with 50 mg vitamin B_6 and 100 mg vitamin C for better absorption.	Needed for normal brain function. (*See* AMINO ACIDS in Part One.)
Multivitamin complex	As directed on label.	For necessary vitamins. Use a high-potency formula.

Zinc	50–80 mg daily. Do not exceed a total of 100 mg daily from all supplements.	Aids in heavy metal detoxification and enhancing immunity. Use zinc gluconate lozenges or OptiZinc for best absorption.

Herbs

❏ Anise, blessed thistle, and blue cohosh appear to sharpen brain power.

❏ Ginkgo biloba improves cerebral circulation, enhances brain function and memory, and destroys free radicals to protect brain cells. Three times a day, place ½ dropperful of alcohol-free liquid extract under your tongue and hold it there for a few minutes before swallowing. Or take 400 milligrams in capsule form three times daily.

Caution: Do not take ginkgo biloba if you have a bleeding disorder, or are scheduled for surgery or a dental procedure.

❏ Gotu kola, ginseng, and mullein oil all aid with memory function.

Caution: Do not use ginseng if you have high blood pressure or are pregnant or nursing.

❏ Kava kava and St. John's wort help to calm people who anger easily.

Cautions: Kava kava can cause drowsiness. It is not recommended for pregnant women or nursing mothers, and it should not be taken together with other substances that act on the central nervous system, such as alcohol, barbiturates, antidepressants, and antipsychotic drugs. St. John's wort may cause increased sensitivity to sunlight. It may also produce anxiety, gastrointestinal symptoms, and headaches. It can interact with some drugs including antidepressants, birth control pills, and anticoagulants.

❏ The Chinese herb qian ceng ta (*Huperzia serrata*) increases memory retention. It is the source of the compound huperzine A. Pure standardized extracts of this compound have been shown to increase mental sharpness, language ability, and memory in a significant percentage of people with Alzheimer's disease. It is a potent blocker of acetylcholinesterase, an enzyme that regulates the activity of acetylcholine, which is an important brain chemical involved in maintaining healthy learning and memory functions.

❏ Valerian root promotes better sleep patterns when taken at bedtime.

Recommendations

❏ Eat a diet consisting of 50 to 75 percent raw foods, along with seeds, whole-grain cereals and breads, raw nuts, and low-fat yogurt and other soured products. Eat Swiss cheese, brown rice, and plenty of fiber daily.

❏ Drink plenty of liquids, even if you are not thirsty—as we grow older, our "thirst system" does not work as well.

❏ Move the bowels daily. Oat bran, rice bran, and a high-fiber diet are important. ABC Aerobic Bulk Cleanse from Aerobic Life Industries, a colon cleanser, is very helpful. Enemas may be needed. (*See* ENEMAS in Part Three.)

❏ Keep active. Exercising, walking, engaging in mental activity, and doing things you enjoy, like pursuing a hobby, are important. Seek out companionship and new experiences. Some people withdraw and keep to themselves as they get older because it seems easier and/or safer, but this can lead to loneliness and depression. If getting out and about is a problem, consider investing in and learning to use a computer. There are a number of online services geared to seniors that can serve as a source of companionship as well as information.

❏ Be sure to maintain a safe environment at home.

❏ Protect against head injury by wearing your seat belt and by wearing protective headgear when participating in activities such as bicycle riding.

❏ Have a complete physical examination to rule out the possibility of underlying illness as a cause of symptoms.

Considerations

❏ To make an accurate diagnosis of senile dementia, a physician needs to be thoroughly informed about symptoms—exactly what they are, how often they occur and under what circumstances, and any factors that have been noted to improve or worsen them. He or she will also need to know about any medical conditions you may have and what types of medications (prescription and over-the-counter) and supplements you are taking, as these can have an effect on memory. To rule out other conditions, the doctor may perform a number of tests, including blood tests, memory testing, an electrocardiogram (EKG) to measure heart activity, an electroencephalogram (EEG) to measure brain waves, brain scans, and/or a spinal tap.

❏ There is no cure for most types of dementia. Often, treatment is aimed at controlling anger, depression, delusions, and other symptoms that are present as a result of the condition. Antidepressants and tranquilizers are some of the types of medications that may be recommended.

❏ Evidence suggests that many cases of dementia may be prevented by "stroke reduction" measures—not smoking, controlling high blood pressure, pursuing chelation therapy to remove toxic metals from the body, adhering to a proper diet, and taking appropriate nutritional supplements.

❏ Ultimately, a person with long-term dementia is unable to live independently, and often requires full-time nursing care.

❏ Feelings of isolation, loneliness, frustration, anger, fatigue, and loss of a social life often accompany this condition—and this can be overwhelming. Frequent time spent with family members and friends, along with psychological care, can help to alleviate these feelings.

❏ Smoking may increase your chance of getting dementia.

❑ People who have atherosclerosis and high blood pressure have a higher risk of developing senility. (*See* ARTERIO-SCLEROSIS/ATHEROSCLEROSIS and HIGH BLOOD PRESSURE in Part Two.)

❑ Food allergies can cause mental as well as physical symptoms. (*See* ALLERGIES in Part Two.)

❑ Toxic metals in the body can produce symptoms similar to those of senility. A hair analysis can reveal whether the body is incurring damage due to the presence of toxic levels of metals like aluminum and lead. (*See* HAIR ANALYSIS in Part Three.)

❑ *See* ALUMINUM TOXICITY; ALZHEIMER'S DISEASE; and PARKINSON'S DISEASE, all in Part Two.

❑ *See also* BINSWANGER'S DISEASE and PICK'S DISEASE *under* RARE DISORDERS in Part Two.

SEXUAL DYSFUNCTION IN WOMEN

Sexual dysfunction is the inability to experience pleasure from sexual intercourse, characterized by a general lack of sexual desire and responsiveness. The term frigidity was once commonly used to describe sexual dysfunction in women. However, the term sexual dysfunction is preferred. It is usually of psychological origin, stemming from fear, anxiety, guilt, depression, conflict with one's mate, and/or feelings of inferiority. Early traumatic sexual experience or other unpleasant childhood and adolescent episodes are often factors.

Sexual dysfunction may also be a result of physiological factors. Some women find intercourse painful due to insufficient lubrication, inadequate stimulation, underlying illness or infection, or some other physical cause. The pain causes them to fear and shrink from sexual contact. Vitamin deficiency can cause a deficiency in estrogen levels and result in improper lubrication. A chronic illness, some medications, low testosterone levels, and certain medical conditions can also greatly diminish sexual desire. The supplement program outlined below should help.

NUTRIENTS

SUPPLEMENT	SUGGESTED DOSAGE	COMMENTS
Very Important		
Kelp	2,000–2,500 mg daily.	A good source of iodine and other important minerals.
Vitamin B complex	100 mg of each major B vitamin twice daily (amounts of individual vitamins in a complex will vary).	Calms the nervous system and aids in reducing anxiety.
Vitamin E	200 IU daily.	Necessary for the functioning of the reproductive system and glands. Use d-alpha-tocopherol form.
Helpful		
Fish liver oil	As directed on label. Take with meals.	Supplies vitamins A and D.
Lecithin granules or capsules	1 tbsp 3 times daily, with meals. 2,400 mg 3 times daily, with meals.	Contains essential fatty acids and aids in proper nerve function.
L-phenylalanine and L-tyrosine	500 mg each daily, on an empty stomach. Take with water or juice. Do not take with milk. Take with 50 mg vitamin B6 and 100 mg vitamin C for better absorption. Do not exceed the recommended dosage.	Amino acids needed for synthesis of crucial neurotransmitters involved in mood and nervous system function. Cautions: Do not take phenylalanine if you are pregnant or nursing a baby, or if you suffer from panic attacks, diabetes, high blood pressure, or PKU. Do not take tyrosine if you are taking an MAO inhibitor drug.
Para-aminobenzoic acid (PABA)	100 mg daily.	A B vitamin that stimulates vital life functions.
Vitamin C with bioflavonoids	3,000–6,000 mg daily, in divided doses.	Important in glandular function and stress response.
Zinc plus copper	50–80 mg daily. Do not exceed a total of 100 mg daily from all supplements. 3 mg daily.	Zinc deficiency can result in impaired sexual function. Use zinc gluconate lozenges or OptiZinc for best absorption. Needed to balance with zinc.

Herbs

❑ Chives (*Allium schoenoprasum*) contain minerals required for the manufacture of sex hormones.

❑ Damiana (*Turnera aphrodisiaca*) is the "woman's sexuality herb"—one of the most popular of plant aphrodisiacs. It contains alkaloids that directly stimulate the nerves and organs and have a testosterone-like effect. Damiana is excellent for supporting the sexual organs and enhancing sexual pleasure. For best results, place a dropperful of damiana extract under your tongue an hour or two before sexual activity. It may take several days for the difference to become apparent.

❑ Kava kava, traditionally valued for its mellowing effects, may help with issues of anxiety and nervousness.

Caution: Kava kava can cause drowsiness. It is not recommended for pregnant women or nursing mothers, and it should not be taken together with other substances that act on the central nervous system, such as alcohol, barbiturates, antidepressants, and antipsychotic drugs.

❑ Wild yam contains a natural steroid called dehydroepiandrosterone (DHEA) that rejuvenates and gives vigor to lovemaking. Take it for two weeks, then stop for two weeks, and so on.

❑ Other herbs that are good for promoting energy and sexuality include fo-ti, gotu kola, sarsaparilla, saw palmetto, and Siberian ginseng.

Caution: Do not use Siberian ginseng if you have hypoglycemia, high blood pressure, or a heart disorder.

Recommendations

❑ Make sure to include the following in your diet: alfalfa sprouts; avocados; eggs that come fresh from hens (not those stored cold in the supermarket); olive oil; pumpkin seeds and other seeds and nuts; soy and sesame oil; and wheat.

❑ Try taking supplemental bee pollen to increase energy.

Caution: Bee pollen may cause an allergic reaction in some people. Start with a small amount at first, and discontinue use if a rash, wheezing, discomfort, or other symptom occurs.

❑ Avoid poultry, red meat, and sugar products. Get your protein from vegetable-based foods like soy and legumes.

❑ Avoid smoggy conditions. Smog is highly toxic and dangerous; it adversely affects immune function and hormonal activity, as well as a host of other body functions.

Considerations

❑ There are medical alternatives that can help some women by alleviating painful intercourse. Painful intercourse may also be a sign of certain gynecological diseases.

❑ If sexual dysfunction is due to interpersonal conflict or psychological causes, help from a couples counselor or other mental health professional is advised.

❑ Sexual dysfunction in men can be caused by psychological issues. Psychological erectile dysfunction in men can be based on early sexual trauma, anxiety, fear, guilt, and other psychological conflicts. (*See* ERECTILE DYSFUNCTION in Part Two.)

❑ Depression or hypothyroidism may be the underlying problem. (*See* DEPRESSION and HYPOTHYROIDISM in Part Two.)

SEXUALLY TRANSMITTED DISEASE (STD)

There are numerous diseases that are passed on either exclusively or primarily through intimate sexual contact. These include acquired immunodeficiency syndrome (AIDS), chancroid, chlamydia, genital herpes, gonorrhea, lympho-granuloma venereum (LGV), granuloma inguinale, some types of hepatitis, syphilis, and trichomoniasis. Genital candidiasis also can be transmitted through sexual contact.

Crabs (pubic lice) and scabies also are sexually transmitted, but are considered parasitic infestations rather than infectious diseases. This section deals primarily with two of the more common sexually transmitted diseases, gonorrhea and syphilis.

Gonorrhea is caused by a microorganism called *Neisseria gonorrhoeae.* These bacteria are commonly referred to as gonococci. The U.S. Centers for Disease Control and Prevention (CDC) estimates that there are some 700,000 new cases of gonorrhea in the United States each year, but that only half are reported. Most, about 75 percent of the cases, are found in people aged fifteen to twenty-nine years. The rate of gonorrheal infection is 121 people per 100,000. In women, gonorrhea often causes no symptoms. When it does, they include frequent and painful urination, vaginal discharge, abnormal menstrual bleeding, acute inflammation in the pelvic area, and rectal itching. Men with gonorrhea usually do experience symptoms, including a yellow discharge of pus and mucus from the penis and slow, difficult, and painful urination. Symptoms usually appear between two and twenty-one days after sexual contact.

If not treated, the infection can travel through the bloodstream and go into the bones, joints, tendons, and other tissues, causing a systemic illness with mild fever, achy feeling, inflamed joints, and, occasionally, skin lesions. At this stage, the organism is difficult to detect, and the condition is often misdiagnosed as simple arthritis. In men, complications of gonorrhea can include sterility and urethral stricture. In women, the infection can spread into the uterus and fallopian tubes, resulting in pelvic inflammatory disease (PID). This can cause ectopic pregnancy and infertility in as many as 10 percent of affected women.

Syphilis is fairly rare in the United States, but it seems to be making a comeback. Between 2005 and 2006, the number of reported cases increased 12 percent. Health officials have had over 36,000 cases reported to them. Most cases occurred in persons aged twenty to thirty years.

Syphilis is caused by a type of bacteria called *Treponema pallidum.* This disease is occasionally contracted through close physical contact such as kissing, as well as through sexual intercourse. If not treated, the illness progresses, usually over the course of many years, through three basic stages. In the first stage, ten to ninety days after contact, a chancre (pronounced SHAN-ker)—a red, painless ulcer—appears at the spot where the bacteria entered the body. In the second stage, perhaps four to ten weeks after contact, a rash and patches of flaking tissue appear in the mouth, palms of the hands, soles of the feet, or genital area. There may be systemic symptoms, usually mild, as well—headache, nausea, and general discomfort. If the disease progresses to its third stage (which is quite rare in the United States), a year or more after the initial infection, brain damage, hearing loss, heart disease, and/or blindness can occur. This disease can remain dormant for up to twenty years.

Unless otherwise stated, the dosages recommended here are for adults. For children between the ages of twelve and seventeen, reduce the dose to three-quarters of the recommended amount.

NUTRIENTS

SUPPLEMENT	SUGGESTED DOSAGE	COMMENTS
Very Important		
Acidophilus (Kyo-Dophilus from Wakunaga)	As directed on label 3 times daily, on an empty stomach.	To restore "friendly" bacteria. Important when taking antibiotics, which are usually prescribed for STDs. Use a nondairy formula.

Free form amino acid	As directed on label.	Needed for tissue repair. Use free form amino acids for quicker absorption and assimilation.
Garlic (Kyolic from Wakunaga)	2 capsules 3 times daily.	A natural antibiotic and immune system stimulant.
Vitamin C with bioflavonoids	750–2,500 mg 4 times daily.	Boosts immune system function and is an antiviral agent.
Zinc	100 mg daily. Do not exceed this amount from all supplements.	Important for the health of the reproductive organs. Promotes wound healing and boosts immune function to fight a broad range of microbes. Use zinc gluconate lozenges or OptiZinc for best absorption.
Important		
Colloidal silver	Use topically as directed on label.	An antiseptic that rapidly reduces inflammation and promotes healing of lesions.
Kelp	1,000–1,500 mg daily.	Supplies balanced vitamins and minerals.
Vitamin B complex	50 mg of each major B vitamin 3 times daily (amounts of individual vitamins in a complex will vary).	Necessary in all cellular enzyme system functions.
Helpful		
Coenzyme Q$_{10}$	30–60 mg daily.	A powerful free radical scavenger.
Multivitamin and mineral complex	As directed on label.	All nutrients are necessary in balance. Use a high-potency formula.
Raw glandular complex plus	As directed on label.	Promote immune function.
raw thymus glandular	As directed on label.	
Vitamin K or alfalfa	100 mcg daily.	Antibiotics destroy the intestinal bacteria that produce vitamin K, which is necessary for blood clotting. *See under* Herbs, below.

Herbs

❑ Alfalfa is a good source of vitamin K, which is needed for blood clotting and healing. This vitamin is depleted by antibiotics.

❑ Astragalus helps to protect the immune system.

Caution: Do not use astragalus in the presence of a fever.

❑ Echinacea, goldenseal, pau d'arco, and suma may alleviate symptoms. Alternate among two or more of these herbs. Consume three cups of herbal tea daily or take herbs in capsule or extract form as directed on the product label.

Cautions: Do not take echinacea for longer than three months. It should not be used by people who are allergic to ragweed. Do not take goldenseal internally on a daily basis for more than one week at a time. Do not use it during pregnancy or if you are breast-feeding, and use with cau-

tion if you are allergic to ragweed. If you have a history of cardiovascular disease, diabetes, or glaucoma, use it only under a doctor's supervision.

❑ Hops helps to relieve pain and stress.

❑ Red clover acts as an antibiotic and anti-inflammatory agent, and aids relaxation.

❑ Suma enhances the immune system and helps prevent stress. This herb is sometimes referred to as Brazilian ginseng.

Recommendations

❑ Use a latex (not sheepskin) condom for any sexual activity until the infection has cleared completely. These diseases are highly contagious. Be aware, however, that even the use of a condom does not guarantee protection against STDs. Abstinence is the only way to avoid any chance of transmitting the infection.

❑ If you are taking penicillin or another antibiotic for a sexually transmitted disease, be sure to add some form of acidophilus to your diet to replace lost "friendly" bacteria.

Considerations

❑ Antibiotics are the usual treatment for both syphilis and gonorrhea. It is important to take any prescribed antibiotic for the full course, even if symptoms abate. Do not stop taking the medication early.

❑ In a child of any age, the presence of a sexually transmitted disease is automatically considered to be a sign of sexual abuse, which should be pursued accordingly.

❑ *See also* AIDS (ACQUIRED IMMUNODEFICIENCY SYNDROME); CANDIDIASIS; CHLAMYDIA; HERPES INFECTION; WARTS; and/or YEAST INFECTION, all in Part Two.

SHINGLES (HERPES ZOSTER)

Shingles, also known as herpes zoster, is a disease caused by the varicella-zoster virus, the same virus that causes chickenpox. It affects the nerve endings in the skin. Shingles can appear anywhere on the body; however, it is most commonly found on the skin of the abdomen underneath the ribs, leading toward the navel. Other commonly affected areas are the vaginal tissues and the inside of the mouth.

Most adults have already contracted chickenpox. This common childhood disease causes a fever and a rash that itches maddeningly but rarely does any permanent damage. However, once the varicella-zoster virus enters the body and has caused chickenpox, it doesn't go away. It may lie dormant in the spinal cord and nerve ganglia for years until activated, usually by a weakening (temporary or permanent) of the immune system. Then the varicella-zoster infection spreads to the very ends of the nerves, causing them to send impulses to the brain that are interpreted as severe

Early Symptoms of Sexually Transmitted Diseases

It is important to detect sexually transmitted diseases in their early stages so that prompt treatment can begin and, in the case of some diseases, irreparable damage to the body can be prevented. Use the table below to familiarize yourself with the beginning stages of various STDs.

Disease	First Symptoms
AIDS (acquired immunodeficiency syndrome)	Headache, night sweats, unexplained weight loss, fatigue, swollen lymph glands, persistent fever, oral thrush (a heavy, whitish coating on the tongue and the insides of the mouth), recurrent vaginal yeast infections, persistent diarrhea, lung infections.
Candidiasis	Itching in the genital area, pain when urinating, a thick odorless vaginal discharge.
Chlamydia	For women: a white vaginal discharge that resembles cottage cheese, a burning sensation when urinating, itching, painful intercourse. For men: a clear, watery urethral discharge. Often, however, there are no symptoms at all.
Genital herpes	Itching, burning in the genital area, discomfort while urinating, a watery vaginal or urethral discharge, weeping, fluid-filled eruptions in the vagina or on the penis.
Genital warts	Soft, cauliflower-like growths appearing either singly or in clusters in and around the vagina, anus, penis, groin, and/or scrotal area.
Gonorrhea	For women: frequent and painful urination, a cloudy vaginal discharge, vaginal itching, inflammation of the pelvic area, rectal discharge, abnormal uterine bleeding. For men: a yellowish, pus-filled urethral discharge.
Pelvic inflammatory disease (PID)	A pus-filled vaginal discharge with fever and lower abdominal pain.
Syphilis	A sore on the genitalia, rash, patches of flaking tissue, fever, sore throat, sores in the mouth or anus.
Trichomoniasis	For women: vaginal itching and pain, with a foamy, greenish or yellow foul-smelling discharge. For men: a clear urethral discharge.

pain, itching, or burning, and rendering the overlying skin much more sensitive than usual. One out of every five people who has had chickenpox is likely to get shingles. Those who have never had chickenpox have very little chance of developing shingles because it is not very contagious.

An attack of shingles is often preceded by three or four days of chills, fever, and achy feelings. There may also be pain in the affected area. Then crops of tiny fluid-filled blisters surrounded by a red rim appear. The affected area becomes excruciatingly painful and sensitive to the touch. Other symptoms can include numbness, fatigue, depression, tingling, shooting pains, swollen and painful lymph nodes, fever, and headache. This phase of shingles lasts seven to fourteen days. The blisters eventually form crusty scabs and drop off. Scarring can occur in severe cases.

The chance of an attack of shingles can be increased by many factors, including stress; cancer; the use of anticancer drugs; spinal cord injuries; and conditions that suppress the immune system, such as the human immunodeficiency virus (HIV); or the use of medications such as corticosteroids or cyclosporine. However, serious illness is not required to activate the virus. Any type of physical or emotional stress can make one susceptible. Often, something as innocuous as a minor injury or a mild cold can lead to an attack in an otherwise healthy person. In most cases, it is never determined just what the trigger is.

Ten to 20 out of every 100 persons will get shingles in their lifetime. Most get it only once; about 4 in every 100 persons will have it more than once. It can appear at any age, but is most common in people over the age of fifty, when immune function naturally begins to decline as a result of aging. Most cases of shingles run their course within a few weeks. More severe cases may last longer and require aggressive treatment.

In some cases, the pain continues for months, even years, after the blisters have disappeared. This syndrome, called postherpetic neuralgia (PHN), is more likely to occur in older people. If shingles develop near the eyes, the cornea may be affected and blindness may result. The acute pain of shingles and the chronic pain of PHN are called neuropathic pain. Both originate in the nerve cells, but their duration and the reaction to treatment is different. Pain that occurs with the initial outbreak responds to treatment and is limited in duration. In contrast, PHN lasts longer, is often difficult to treat, and can be incapacitating. The skin of many people with PHN becomes so sensitive that they cannot tolerate wearing clothing or even feeling a light breeze on the affected area. Described as agonizing, excruciating, and burning, the pain can have a severe impact on daily living, leading to a loss of independence and, ultimately, to depression and isolation.

For people with immune deficiencies, shingles and its aftermath can be devastating. The disease is capable of affecting the internal organs, attacking even the lungs, kidneys, and liver. Disseminated shingles can cause permanent injury—including blindness, deafness, or paralysis, depending upon the area of the body that is served by the infected nerves—if it goes unchecked. Death can occur as the result of a secondary bacterial infection or viral pneumonia brought on by shingles.

Unless otherwise specified, the dosages recommended here are for adults. For children between the ages of twelve and seventeen, reduce the dose to three-quarters the recommended amount. For children between six and twelve, use one-half the recommended dose, and for children under the age of six, use one-quarter the recommended amount.

NUTRIENTS

SUPPLEMENT	SUGGESTED DOSAGE	COMMENTS
Essential		
L-lysine	500 mg twice daily, on an empty stomach. Take with water or juice. Do not take with milk. Take with 50 mg vitamin B$_6$ and 100 mg vitamin C for better absorption.	Important for healing and for fighting the virus that causes shingles. (*See* AMINO ACIDS in Part One.) *Caution:* Do not take this supplement for longer than 6 months at a time.
Vitamin C with bioflavonoids	2,000 mg 4 times daily.	Aids in fighting the virus and boosting the immune system.
Very Important		
Beta-1,3-D-glucan	As directed on label.	Useful for treating bacterial, viral, and fungal infections.
Vitamin B complex plus extra vitamin B$_{12}$	100 mg of each major B vitamin 3 times daily (amounts of individual vitamins in a complex will vary). 1,000 mcg twice daily.	Needed for nerve health and to counteract deficiencies. Injections (under a doctor's supervision) may be necessary. Use a lozenge or sublingual form.
Zinc	80 mg daily for 1 week, then reduce to 50 mg daily. Do not exceed a total of 100 mg daily from all supplements.	Enhances immunity and protects against infection. Use zinc chelate lozenges or zinc picolinate in sublingual form for faster absorption.
Important		
Calcium plus magnesium	1,500 mg daily. 750 mg daily.	For nerve function and healing, and to combat stress. Use chelate forms.
Garlic (Kyolic from Wakunaga)	2 capsules 3 times daily, with meals.	Excellent for building the immune system.
S-Adenosylmethionine (SAMe) (SAMe Rx-Mood from Nature's Plus)	As directed on label.	Aids in reducing pain and inflammation. A natural antidepressant. *Caution:* Do not use if you have bipolar mood disorder or take prescription antidepressants. Do not give this supplement to a child under twelve.
Vitamin A emulsion or capsules plus carotenoid complex with beta-carotene	50,000 IU daily for 2 weeks, then reduce to 25,000 IU daily. If you are pregnant, do not exceed 10,000 IU daily. 10,000 IU daily. As directed on label.	Boosts the immune system and protects against infection. Emulsion form is recommended for easier assimilation and greater safety at higher doses. To protect immune function and enhance healing.
Vitamin D	1,000 IU twice daily for 1 week, then reduce to 400 IU daily.	Aids in tissue healing and is needed for calcium absorption.
Vitamin E	200 IU daily. You can also open a capsule and apply the oil directly to the affected areas of skin.	Helps prevent formation of scar tissue. Also helps to alleviate pain from long-term cases of shingles. Use d-alpha-tocopherol form.
Helpful		
Acidophilus (Kyo-Dophilus from Wakunaga)	As directed on label.	Provides "friendly" bacteria to the intestines and stimulates immune function. Use a nondairy formula.
Coenzyme Q$_{10}$ plus Coenzyme A from Coenzyme-A Technologies	60 mg daily. As directed on label.	A free radical scavenger that boosts immune function. Works effectively with coenzyme Q$_{10}$ to support the immune system's detoxification of many dangerous substances.
Colloidal silver	As directed on label.	A natural antibiotic that has shown effectiveness in treating shingles. Use topically only.
Essential fatty acids (flaxseed oil or primrose oil)	As directed on label.	Promotes healing of skin and nerve tissue.
Grape seed extract	As directed on label.	A powerful antioxidant that protects skin cells and decreases the number of outbreaks of blisters.
Herpanacine from Diamond-Herpanacine Associates	As directed on label.	Builds the immune system and fights infection.
Inf-zyme Forte from American Biologics	4 tablets 3 times daily, with meals.	Has antioxidant properties and aids in proper breakdown of proteins, fats, and carbohydrates.
Maitake extract or reishi extract or shiitake extract	As directed on label. As directed on label. As directed on label.	Has immune-boosting and antiviral properties.
Multivitamin and mineral complex	As directed on label.	All nutrients are necessary in balance.

Herbs

❑ Alfalfa, chamomile, and dandelion promote healing by helping to restore the body's normal acid/alkaline balance. Dandelion also helps to detoxify and support the liver. A cool chamomile compress can aid in soothing the blisters.

Caution: Do not use chamomile if you are allergic to ragweed. Do not use during pregnancy or nursing. It may interact with warfarin or cyclosporine, so patients using these drugs should avoid it.

❏ Astragalus root and echinacea boost immune function.

Cautions: Do not use astragalus in the presence of a fever. Do not take echinacea for longer than three months. It should not be used by people who are allergic to ragweed.

❏ Bi phaya yaw (*Clinacanthus nutans*), an herb used in traditional Thai medicine, has been shown in clinical studies to shorten the time it takes to recover from shingles in some cases. It is applied in cream form.

❏ Burdock and red clover cleanse both the lymph nodes and the bloodstream.

❏ Cayenne (capsicum) contains a substance called capsaicin, which relieves pain and aids in healing. It also acts as a detoxifier. Cayenne is available in tablet and capsule form.

❏ Goldenseal has powerful antibiotic properties and reduces infection.

Caution: Do not take goldenseal internally on a daily basis for more than one week at a time. Do not use it during pregnancy or if you are breast-feeding, and use with caution if you are allergic to ragweed. If you have a history of cardiovascular disease, diabetes, or glaucoma, use it only under a doctor's supervision.

❏ Green tea has antiviral, anti-inflammatory, and antioxidant properties. The polyphenols it contains have been found to fight herpesviruses.

Caution: Green tea contains vitamin K, which can make anticoagulant medications less effective. Consult your health care professional if you are using them. The caffeine in green tea could cause insomnia, anxiety, upset stomach, nausea, or diarrhea.

❏ Licorice extract can be used topically to treat shingles and postherpetic neuralgia. It appears to interfere with the growth of the virus.

Caution: Licorice root should not be used during pregnancy or nursing. It should not be used by persons with diabetes, glaucoma, heart disease, high blood pressure, or a history of stroke.

❏ Milk thistle protects the liver and promotes healthy liver function.

❏ A combination of oat straw, St. John's wort, and skullcap helps to reduce stress and itching. Mix equal amounts of oat straw, St. John's wort, and skullcap tinctures together, and take 1 teaspoon of this mixture four times daily.

Caution: St. John's wort may cause increased sensitivity to sunlight. It may also produce anxiety, gastrointestinal symptoms, and headaches. It can interact with some drugs including antidepressants, birth control pills, and anticoagulants.

❏ Olive leaf extract aids in fighting the virus.

❏ Rose hips are high in vitamin C and are good for preventing infections on the skin.

❏ Valerian root calms the nervous system. Taken at bedtime, it acts as a sleep aid.

Recommendations

❏ Eating fruits and vegetables is particularly important to prevent developing shingles. In one study, those who ate no fruits had three times the risk of developing shingles as those who ate three servings a day. In those over sixty years of age, eating both fruits and vegetables reduced the risk.

❏ Include in the diet brewer's yeast, brown rice, garlic, raw fruits and vegetables, and whole grains.

Caution: Brewer's yeast can cause an allergic reaction in some individuals. Start with a small amount at first, and discontinue use if any allergic symptoms occur.

❏ Eat plenty of foods that contain vitamin B_6, including bananas, nuts, potatoes, and sweet potatoes.

❏ Go on a cleansing fast. (*See* FASTING in Part Three.)

❏ Use bee pollen or propolis, chlorophyll, and/or kelp to fight the virus and promote healing.

Caution: Bee pollen may cause an allergic reaction in some individuals. Start with a small amount, and discontinue use if a rash, wheezing, discomfort, or other symptoms occur.

❏ Keep stress to a minimum. Stress reduces the immune system's effectiveness in fighting off infection. Studies have found that people with shingles report having recently been through stressful periods more often than other people.

❏ Avoid drafts. Allow the affected area to be exposed to sunlight for fifteen minutes each day. Wash the blisters gently when bathing, and otherwise avoid touching or scratching them.

❏ If you are suffering from a rash or blisters of an unknown origin, see a dermatologist—he or she can administer a test for shingles that only takes a few minutes.

❏ See an ophthalmologist if the shingles appear on the forehead, near the eyes, or on the tip of the nose. Untreated ophthalmic herpes zoster can lead to vision loss.

❏ Try using essential oils. Bergamot oil, calophyllum oil (related to St. John's wort), eucalyptus oil, geranium oil, goldenseal oil, and lemon oil can be used singly or in combination. These highly concentrated plant essences have strong antiviral properties. The best way to use them is to add a few drops of essential oil to a tablespoon of a carrier oil such as almond, peanut, or olive oil, and apply the mixture directly to the lesions at the first sign of an outbreak. In most instances, the lesions dry up and disappear completely within three to five days after this treatment.

❏ Consider using homeopathic remedies to alleviate symptoms. *Apis mellifica, Arsenicum album, Clematis erecta, Iris versicolor,* and *Rhus toxicodendron* are homeopathic remedies that may be helpful.

Considerations

❏ The severity and duration of a shingles attack can be reduced by immediate treatment with antiviral drugs such as acyclovir (Zovirax), valcyclovir (Valtrex), or famcyclovir (Famvir). Steroids, antidepressants, anticonvulsants, and topical creams are sometimes prescribed for the aftermath.

❑ In 2006, the FDA approved a vaccine (Zostavax) for people over sixty years of age who have had chickenpox. Its use cut the number of people developing shingles in half, and there was a decrease in the severity of the virus in those who developed it. The vaccine seems to be less effective with advancing age. If you are over sixty and are concerned about the possibility of developing shingles, ask your doctor for more information.

❑ Adenosine monophosphate (AMP), a compound that occurs naturally in the body, has been found to be effective against shingles.

❑ In treating postherpetic neuralgia, doctors often must resort to treating only the residual pain, whether with medication or other approaches.

❑ Pain medication such as acetaminophen (Tylenol, Datril, and others) or nonsteroidal anti-inflammatory drugs (NSAIDs) may be used to control inflammation and mild or moderate pain. Narcotics may be needed for severe pain.

❑ Capsaicin has been attracting attention for its ability to relieve pain in persons suffering from postherpetic neuralgia. Capsaicin is not a product of chemical engineering, but a component found in plants of the same family as red peppers. Researchers in Toronto found that 56 percent of people with postherpetic neuralgia who were treated with capsaicin cream (Zostrix) for four weeks experienced significant relief of pain, and that 78 percent had at least some improvement in pain. Clinical studies suggest that capsaicin directly reduces the amount of substance P, a neurotransmitter responsible for the transmission of pain impulses. If there is a deficiency of substance P, the nerves are unable to transmit sensations of pain. Capsaicin is easy to use—you simply apply it topically to the affected area three or four times a day. In addition, capsaicin does not interact with any other drugs or medications, which makes it an especially attractive option for elderly people, who are often taking one or more drugs on a regular basis. Capsaicin cream is sold over the counter in most drugstores and health food stores. It should not be applied until the blisters caused by shingles have healed completely, however, or extreme burning pain may result.

❑ Topical lidocaine (Lidoderm) may be prescribed for pain that has been going on for longer than one month. The medication in the patch penetrates the skin, reaching the damaged nerves just under the skin without being absorbed significantly into the bloodstream. This means that the patch can be used for long periods of time without serious side effects. Possible side effects of this drug include redness and swelling. However, this is usually mild and does not last long.

❑ People with compromised immune systems may be given serum or other biological products obtained from the pooled blood of people who have recently recovered from shingles to assist their own immune systems in resisting the virus. Physicians are now more likely to administer huge doses of antiviral drugs to try to destroy or cripple the virus.

❑ Dimethylsulfoxide (DMSO) has been used with success to relieve the pain of shingles and promote healing of the lesions. This liquid, a by-product of wood processing, is applied topically to the affected area as needed. Only DMSO from a health food store can be used for therapeutic purposes.

Caution: Only pure DMSO from a health food store should be used. Commercial-grade DMSO such as that found in hardware stores is not suitable for healing purposes. Any contaminants on the skin or in the product can be taken into the tissues by action of the DMSO.

Note: The use of DMSO may result in a garlicky body odor. This is temporary, and is not a cause for concern.

❑ Transcutaneous electrical nerve stimulation (TENS) therapy uses a device that generates low-level pulses of electrical current. The TENS unit is applied to the skin's surface, causing tingling sensations and offering some people pain relief. One theory as to how TENS works is that the electrical current stimulates production of endorphins, the body's natural painkillers. (*See* TENS UNIT THERAPY *under* PAIN CONTROL in Part Three.)

❑ As a last resort, nerve blocks may be used to provide temporary relief. These procedures usually entail the injection of a local anesthetic into the area of the affected nerves. Postherpetic neuralgia (PHN) most commonly affects older adults; because they are often unable to tolerate medication, the nerve block becomes a viable option.

❑ An injection directly into the spine is another option for relief of pain. A Japanese clinical study reported in *The New England Journal of Medicine* (November 2000) found that an injection of the steroid methylprednisone combined with the anesthetic lidocaine reduced pain by more than 70 percent in one patient group compared with groups that received lidocaine alone or an inactive substance.

❑ While shingles itself is not very contagious, a person with shingles may infect previously uninfected persons, particularly children, with chickenpox.

❑ If conservative measures are not effective, an antidepressant such as amitriptyline (Elavil, Endep) may be prescribed. These drugs not only ease the emotional impact of unrelenting pain, but they seem to alleviate the pain itself. They appear to do this by causing an increase in the production of endorphins, the body's own natural painkillers.

❑ Experiments are being conducted in which live chickenpox vaccine is given intravenously in an attempt to prevent shingles. Since you cannot develop shingles if you never contract chickenpox, researchers theorize that a vaccine that prevents chickenpox would therefore also prevent shingles. Detractors argue that while this approach may produce immunity in those who have never had chickenpox, the virus in the vaccine may also take refuge in the central nervous system and cause shingles years or decades later.

❏ One of the biggest obstacles to researchers in learning more about the varicella-zoster virus is the fact that there are no animals in which it can be studied; chickenpox and shingles occur only in humans, and the virus grows poorly in laboratory cultures. Nonetheless, research continues into the biology of varicella-zoster, with the hope of developing a better understanding of how the immune system controls it and perhaps finding ways to ease the suffering caused by shingles and postherpetic neuralgia.

❏ See also PAIN CONTROL in Part Three.

❏ For names and addresses of organizations that can offer further information about shingles, and on pain control, see Health and Medical Organizations in the Appendix.

SINUSITIS

Sinusitis is an inflammation of the nasal sinuses. There are sinuses located above the eyes (frontal sinuses); to either side of the nose, inside the cheekbones (maxillary sinuses); behind the bridge of the nose (sphenoid sinuses); and in the upper nose (ethmoid sinuses). Sinuses are air-filled pockets in the skull that are connected to the nose and throat by passages designed to drain away mucus. The sinuses are the first line of defense in protecting the lungs against infection. Most cases of sinusitis affect the frontal and/or maxillary sinuses, but any or all of the sinuses may be involved, and each individual tends to have problems with a particular set of sinuses. If the sinuses are too small or poorly positioned to handle the volume of mucus produced, they can become clogged. Pressure in the sinuses increases, causing pain. Sinuses that are clogged for a long time seem to invite infection.

Sinusitis can be either acute or chronic. Acute sinusitis is frequently caused by bacterial or viral infections of the nose, throat, and upper respiratory tract, such as the common cold. Air travel also can lead to acute inflammation of the sinuses, because of changes in air pressure. Chronic sinusitis problems may be caused by small growths in the nose, injury of the nasal bones, air pollution, dental complications, emotional stress, smoking, and exposure to irritant fumes and smells. Allergic sinusitis may be caused by hay fever or food allergies, especially allergies to milk and dairy products. People with compromised immune systems (such as those with HIV) or with abnormal mucus production (such as in cystic fibrosis) are susceptible to fungal sinusitis, a potentially dangerous condition that requires aggressive treatment.

Symptoms of sinusitis include fever (usually low-grade, but higher in some cases), cough, headache, earache, toothache, facial pain, cranial pressure, difficulty breathing through the nose, loss of the sense of smell, and tenderness over the forehead and cheekbones. If tapping the forehead just over the eyes, the cheekbones, or the area around the bridge of the nose causes pain, the sinuses may be infected. Sometimes sinusitis produces facial swelling followed by a stuffy nose and thick discharge of mucus. The symptoms suffered by those with sinusitis can have other unpleasant effects such as pain. Postnasal drip can cause a sore throat, nausea, and bad breath; difficulty breathing can cause snoring and loss of sleep.

Unless otherwise stated, the dosages recommended here are for adults. For children between the ages of twelve and seventeen, reduce the dose to three-quarters of the recommended amount. For children between the ages of six and twelve, use one-half the recommended dose, and for children under six, use one-quarter of the recommended amount.

NUTRIENTS

SUPPLEMENT	SUGGESTED DOSAGE	COMMENTS
Very Important		
Acidophilus (Kyo-Dophilus from Wakunaga)	As directed on label.	Replaces good bacteria in the colon. Important if antibiotics are prescribed. Use a nondairy formula.
Bee pollen	Start with ½ tsp daily and increase slowly to 1 tbsp daily, taken in juice.	Increases immunity and speeds healing. *Caution:* Bee pollen may cause an allergic reaction in some individuals. Discontinue use if at any time a rash, wheezing, discomfort, or other symptoms occur.
Flaxseed oil	As directed on label.	Reduces pain and inflammation. Enhances all body functions.
Multivitamin and mineral complex	As directed on label.	To improve overall health and assure proper nutrition.
Quercetin plus	As directed on label.	Protects against allergens and increases immunity.
bromelain or	As directed on label.	Enhances the effectiveness of quercetin.
Anti-Allergy formula from Freeda Vitamins	As directed on label.	Contains quercetin, calcium pantothenate, and calcium ascorbate to provide nutritional support and reduce allergic response.
Raw thymus glandular	500 mg twice daily.	Protects immune function and health of the mucous membrane cells.
SinuCheck from Enzymatic Therapy	2 capsules 4 times daily.	A natural decongestant to help clear blocked nasal passages due to colds and sinusitis.
Vitamin A with mixed carotenoids	10,000 IU daily.	Enhances the immune system; protects against colds, flu, and other infections. Helps maintain the health of the mucous membranes.
including natural beta-carotene	15,000 IU daily.	Precursor of vitamin A.
Vitamin B complex plus extra	75–100 mg of each major B vitamin 3 times daily, with meals (amounts of individual vitamins in a complex will vary).	Helps to maintain healthy nerves and reduce stress. A sublingual form is best.

vitamin B₅ (pantothenic acid) and	100 mg 3 times daily, with meals.	Aids in the formation of antibodies.
vitamin B₆ (pyridoxine) and	50 mg 3 times daily, with meals.	Aids immune system function.
vitamin B₁₂	1,000 mcg 3 times daily.	
Vitamin C with bioflavonoids	3,000–10,000 mg daily, in divided doses.	Boosts immune function and aids in preventing infection and decreasing mucus.
Vitamin E	200 IU daily.	Improves circulation and speeds healing. Use d-alpha-tocopherol form.
Helpful		
Coenzyme Q₁₀	60 mg daily.	Valuable immune system stimulant. Increases cellular oxygenation.
Colloidal silver	As directed on label.	A natural antibiotic.
Dimethylsulfoxide (DMSO)	As directed on label.	Relieves pain and strengthens the immune system. Use only DMSO from a health food store.
Garlic (Kyolic from Wakunaga)	2 capsules 3 times daily.	An immune system stimulant that helps to keep infection in check.
Methylsulfonyl-methane (MSM)	As directed on label.	Use for pain relief and to reduce inflammation.
Proteolytic enzymes (Novenzyme from International Health Products)	As directed on label. Take with meals and between meals.	Destroys free radicals. Also aids in digestion of foods.
Pycnogenol or grape seed extract	As directed on label. As directed on label.	Powerful antioxidants that reduce inflammation and the frequency of colds and flu, and neutralize allergic reactions.
Sea mussel	As directed on label.	Provides needed amino acids and aids in the functioning of the mucous membranes. Reduces inflammation.
Zinc lozenges	1 15-mg lozenge every 2 to 4 waking hours for 1 week. Do not exceed this amount.	Antiviral agent and immunity booster.

Herbs

❑ Anise, fenugreek, marshmallow, and red clover help to loosen phlegm and clear congestion.

❑ Bayberry is a decongestant and astringent.

❑ Bitter orange oil can be used to swab nasal passages for local relief.

❑ Cat's Claw Defense Complex from Source Naturals contains a combination of herbs designed to strengthen the body and help the body deal with outside elements.

Caution: Do not use cat's claw during pregnancy.

❑ ClearLungs from RidgeCrest Herbals contains Chinese herbal ingredients to restore free breathing, ease mucus accumulation, and enhance tissue repair. Echinacea boosts the immune system and fights viral infection.

Caution: Do not take echinacea for longer than three months. It should not be used by people who are allergic to ragweed.

❑ P.S.I. from Terra Maxa relieves nasal and sinus congestion.

❑ Ginger root can be crushed and applied as a poultice to the forehead and nose to stimulate circulation and drainage.

❑ Goldenseal is effective in combating sinusitis. Its benefits can be enhanced by combining it with 250 to 500 milligrams of bromelain, an enzyme present in fresh pineapple. Goldenseal can be taken as a tea, or the tea can be used as an intranasal douche. Or put a dropperful of alcohol-free goldenseal extract in your mouth, swish it around for a few minutes, then swallow. Do this three times daily.

Caution: Do not take goldenseal internally on a daily basis for more than one week at a time. Do not use it during pregnancy or if you are breast-feeding, and use with caution if you are allergic to ragweed. If you have a history of cardiovascular disease, diabetes, or glaucoma, use it only under a doctor's supervision.

❑ Horehound helps to relieve symptoms.

❑ Mullein reduces inflammation and soothes irritation.

❑ Nettle is good for all types of allergies and respiratory problems.

❑ Olive leaf extract has antibacterial and anti-inflammatory properties.

❑ Rose hips are a good source of vitamin C.

Recommendations

❑ Eat a diet consisting of 75 percent raw foods.

❑ Drink plenty of distilled water and fresh vegetable and fruit juices. Also consume plenty of hot liquids such as soups and herbal teas. These help the mucus to flow, relieving congestion and sinus pressure. Adding cayenne pepper, garlic, ginger, horseradish, and raw onion to soups or teas may bring even faster relief.

❑ Eliminate sugar from your diet. Reduce your salt intake.

❑ Do not eat dairy foods, except for low-fat soured products like yogurt and cottage cheese. Dairy products increase mucus formation.

❑ Go on a cleansing fast. (*See* FASTING in Part Three.)

❑ Mix a solution of 1 cup warm water, ½ teaspoon of sea salt, and a pinch of bicarbonate of soda. Use a squeeze spray bottle (available over the counter in drugstores) or an eyedropper to instill the solution in the nostrils, one side at a time. Repeat this procedure three or four times a day as necessary for relief from stuffiness.

❑ Try using a menthol or eucalyptus pack applied over the sinuses to relieve pain and swelling. Stop if the packs cause irritation.

❑ Use a vaporizer to ease breathing and clear secretions.

❑ Use steam inhalations to promote drainage and ease pressure. Boil a pot of water and add a few drops of eucalyptus oil or rosemary oil. Remove the pot from the heat and lean your face over it at a distance of about six inches to inhale the steam. (Be careful not to get so close that irritation or scalding results.) Place a towel over your head to capture the steam and breathe in deeply. Do this several times daily for five to ten minutes at a time. Or simply take a hot shower to help relieve the pain and pressure of sinusitis.

❑ You can also use a Neti pot, a small teapot-like device especially designed for nasal irrigation. They are available in many health food stores. Fill the pot with sea salt and water (2 teaspoons salt to one pint water) and rinse out your nose with this solution. This should reduce inflammation and congestion.

❑ Use warm compresses or ice packs to help relieve pain (experiment to see which works best for you).

❑ Try homeopathic remedies to alleviate symptoms. *Belladonna* is good for infections accompanied by fever and pain in the face and forehead. *Kali bichromicum* is useful if there is an overabundance of mucus in the throat.

❑ If you are taking antibiotics for a sinus infection, be sure to add an acidophilus supplement to your program. Do not take the acidophilus and the antibiotic at the same time.

❑ If you use decongestants, use them only as directed and for the prescribed amount of time. If possible, avoid using nose drops and sprays. These can become addictive and interfere with normal sinus function. In addition, drops and sprays, as well as inhalers, can shrink blood vessels in the nose, eventually causing the vessels to weaken. Moreover, withdrawal from decongestants can cause a rebound effect, in which the swelling becomes worse after use is discontinued than it was to begin with. They can also cause dangerous elevations in blood pressure. Do not use these medications if you have high blood pressure or heart problems.

❑ If sinusitis causes your eyes to become swollen, red, or itchy, or to begin tearing, try a product called OcuDyne. Made by NutriCology, this is a complex containing vitamins, minerals, antioxidants, key amino acids, active bioflavonoids, and the herbs bilberry and ginkgo biloba to protect the eyes and boost immune function.

Caution: Do not take ginkgo biloba if you have a bleeding disorder, or are scheduled for surgery or a dental procedure.

❑ Do not use force when blowing your nose, as this forces mucus back into the sinus cavities. Instead, draw secretions to the back of the throat by sniffing, then expel them.

❑ Do not smoke, and avoid secondhand smoke. If you live in a smoggy area, consider getting an air purifier or moving to a less polluted area. Air Supply from Wein Products is a personal air purifier. Worn around the neck, it sets up a defensive shield against microorganisms and microparticles in the air wherever you go.

❑ If you notice swelling around the eyes, consult your physician. This is a serious sign.

❑ Have regular dental examinations. Infections in the mouth can easily spread to the sinuses.

Considerations

❑ If nasal secretions turn clear after a week, you probably do not have an infection; if the mucus is greenish or yellowish, you probably do. If secretions are clear and you have no other symptoms of a cold, you probably have allergies.

❑ Antibiotics may be necessary to clear a bacterial infection. Always take antibiotics for the full course prescribed, even if symptoms seem to improve earlier. Stopping prematurely can lead to antibiotic-resistant bacteria and a worse infection.

❑ Sometimes physicians prescribe antibiotics even if they cannot confirm a bacterial infection. The reasoning for this is that it is very difficult to ascertain whether bacteria are causing the sinusitis, and that it may be worth it to prevent a bacterial infection from appearing later. As with any medication, it is important to know the benefits, risks, and costs of using and of not using an antibiotic.

❑ If sinus trouble is chronic and severe, and medication fails to relieve it, surgery may be needed to drain the sinuses, not only to relieve discomfort but to guard against serious consequences.

❑ Endoscopic surgery, a treatment sometimes recommended for chronic, severe sinusitis, clears nasal passages without external incisions or scars. The procedure can be performed using local anesthesia and results in minimal pain and swelling.

❑ While they are uncommon, polyps and benign cysts that retain mucus can develop in the sinuses, especially in the large maxillary or frontal sinuses. Intrusive or malignant growths require surgical removal.

❑ Anyone suffering from unremitting sinusitis should consult a health care provider to rule out an underlying immune dysfunction. In a University of Miami study, 50 percent of chronic sinusitis patients were found to be suffering from immunologic disorders.

SKIN CANCER

Skin cancer affects more people in the United States than any other form of cancer. It is estimated that there are 1 million cases of non-melanoma skin cancer diagnosed yearly in the United States. Melanoma, the most serious type of skin cancer, accounted for about 68,720 cases of skin cancer in 2009 and most (about 8,650) of the 11,590 deaths due to skin cancer each year. This is more than twice the number diagnosed twenty years ago. Because of the dramatic increases over the past two decades, mostly because of overexposure to ultraviolet radiation from the sun, the National Cancer Institute has warned that 40 to 50 percent of all Americans who live to the age of sixty-five will eventually develop at least one skin cancer. There are several different types of skin cancer. The two most common skin cancers are basal cell carcinoma and squamous cell carcinoma; most people who are diagnosed with skin cancer have one or the other of these types of the disease. Both are highly curable if treated early. The third major type of skin cancer is malignant melanoma, which is a more serious disease. There are approximately 15,000 new cases of malignant melanoma diagnosed each year, and half of the patients survive six to seven years.

Basal cell carcinoma is the most common of the three major types of skin cancer. It is most prevalent in blond, fair-skinned people. Unlike many other malignant growths, it does not spread until it has been present for a long period of time. The cell damage results in an ulcerlike growth that spreads slowly as it destroys tissue. A large, pearly-looking lump, most often on the face by the nose, neck, or ears, is usually the first sign. About six weeks after it appears, the lump becomes ulcerated, with a raw, moist center and a hard border that may bleed. Scabs continually form over the ulcer and then come off, but the ulcer never really heals. Sometimes basal cell carcinomas show up on the back or chest as flat sores that grow slowly. Basal cell carcinomas do not usually spread throughout the body and generally are curable. However, recurrences are common. If they are not treated, they can do substantial damage to the lower layers of skin and bone.

In squamous cell carcinoma, the underlying skin cells are damaged, and this leads to the development of a tumor or lump under the skin, most often on the ears, hands, face, or lower lip. The lump may resemble a wart or a small ulcerated spot that never heals. This type of skin cancer occurs most frequently in fair-skinned people over fifty years old. The risk is higher for those who have had long-term outdoor employment and for those who reside in sunny climates. This is a very treatable type of skin cancer if it is detected and dealt with in the early stages.

Malignant melanoma is rarer than either squamous cell or basal cell carcinoma, but is much more serious. With this type of skin cancer, a tumor arises from the pigment-producing cells of the deeper layers of the skin. It is estimated that as many as half of all cases of melanoma originate in moles. People in some families seem to have a genetically based higher risk of developing melanoma. They often have odd moles, called *dysplastic nevi,* that are irregular in shape and color and can be as large as half an inch in diameter. Dysplastic nevi may be precursors to skin cancer. This cancer can also appear in the form of a new mole. In men, melanomas tend to occur anywhere from the neck to the waist; in women, the arms and legs seem to be affected most.

If not treated at an early stage, melanoma can be life-threatening, spreading through the bloodstream and lymphatic vessels to the internal organs. However, if the disease is treated early, the chances of recovery are quite good. There are four types of melanoma, each with slightly different characteristics:

1. *Superficial spreading melanoma* (SSM), the most common type; 70 percent of the cases fall into this category. It occurs primarily in younger people. An SSM lesion typically begins as a flat mole, most often on the lower legs or upper back, that develops a raised, irregular surface. As it grows, its borders usually become asymmetrical and notched.

2. *Acral lentiginous melanoma,* most common among people of African and Asian descent. The lesions have flat, dark-brown areas with bumpy portions that are brown-black or blue-black in color. They are most likely to appear on the palms of the hands, the soles of the feet, the nail beds of fingers and toes, and the mucous membranes.

3. *Lentigo maligna melanoma,* a type of cancer in which lesions usually occur on the face, neck, ears, or other areas that have been heavily sun-exposed for a long period of time. This type of melanoma rarely occurs before the age of fifty, and it is usually preceded by a precancerous stage called *lentigo maligna* that appears years in advance of the melanoma.

4. *Nodular melanoma,* a type of the disease that attacks the underlying tissue without first spreading across the surface of the skin. It is more common in men than in women, and the elderly get it more than the young. The lesions may resemble blood blisters, and they may range in coloration from pearly white to blue-black. Nodular melanoma tends to metastasize (spread to other sites in the body) sooner than the other types of melanoma.

Melanoma tends to progress through four different stages. The so-called *TNM system* is often used to determine the stages. In the TNM system, *T* stands for the existence of a *t*umor, *N* represents the fact that the tumor has spread to the lymph *n*odes, and *M* stands for *m*etastasis, or spread of the cancer to other places in the body.

The four stages of melanoma are the following:

1. *Stage one.* The cancer is found in the top of the inner layer of skin but has not spread.

2. *Stage two.* The cancer has spread into the inner layer of skin but not yet into the lymph nodes.

3. *Stage three.* The tumor has spread to body tissue beneath the skin's outer and inner layers. There may be additional tumors near the site of the original tumor. The cancer may have spread to the lymph nodes near the tumor.

4. *Stage four.* The cancer has spread to other parts of the body, away from the original site of the melanoma.

Overexposure to the sun's ultraviolet (UV) rays is the major factor in basal cell carcinoma, squamous cell carcinoma, and melanoma. These rays disrupt the genetic material in the skin cells, causing tissue damage. They also harm the skin's normal repair mechanism. Normally, after UV exposure, this mechanism causes damaged cells to immediately cease reproducing, die, and be sloughed off to be replaced by new, healthy skin cells—this is why skin peels after a sunburn. If this repair system is impaired, damaged cells may continue to reproduce, and the skin becomes increasingly vulnerable to injury from subsequent exposure to UV rays. There are two types of UV radiation, designated ultraviolet-A (UVA) and ultraviolet-B (UVB). UVA is ultraviolet radiation with a wavelength of 320 to 400 nanometers. It passes right through the Earth's ozone layer. UVB is ultraviolet radiation with a wavelength of 280 to 320 nanometers. The ozone layer absorbs most of this radiation, but a small amount gets through to the earth's surface, where it poses the same risks as UVA radiation.

UV exposure is not only the major cause of wrinkles; it is the major risk factor of most forms of skin cancer. People who have had severe or blistering sunburns, especially in childhood, are twice as likely to develop the disease later in life. People with blond or red hair, blue or green eyes, and fair skin, who sunburn or freckle easily, are at the greatest risk for skin cancer because they have less protective pigment in their skin. One sign that cumulative sun damage may have reached dangerous levels is the development of spots called *actinic* or *solar keratoses*. Considered precancerous lesions, these appear most often in and around the face, neck, and head, and take the form of rough bumps or flat patches that may be itchy or tingly. Later, these spots may become hard to the touch and grayish or brown in color. Although these abnormalities may not be dangerous in themselves, they should be evaluated and, if need be, treated, as they can develop into more serious skin cancers.

In addition to the three major types of skin cancer, there are a number of other, less common types of cancer that affect the skin. *Mycosis fungoides* is technically a type of lymphoma (lymphatic cancer), but its main effects are on the skin. Initially, it appears as an itchy rash that may last for several years. Over time, the lesions spread, become firmer, and ulcerate. Eventually, if untreated, the disease may spread to the lymph nodes and other internal organs. Mycosis fungoides is a rare, slow-growing cancer that can be difficult to diagnose, especially early in the disease. A skin biopsy should make correct diagnosis possible.

A type of skin cancer that has become increasingly common in recent years is Kaposi's sarcoma. This type of cancer causes raised lesions that may be pink, red, brown, or purplish in color. They may appear anywhere on the body, but the most common sites are the legs, toes, upper torso, and mucous membranes. Kaposi's sarcoma was once a rare, very slowly progressing disease seen primarily in older men of Mediterranean descent. Since the AIDS epidemic began, however, it is no longer uncommon, and is primarily associated with a poorly functioning immune system. People with AIDS tend to get a more aggressive variety of this cancer that eventually affects the lymph nodes and other internal organs. However, a new treatment called HAART (highly active antiretroviral therapy) has decreased the incidence of Kaposi's sarcoma and can keep it from advancing.

In recent years, the incidence of skin cancer has been rising steadily, and the average age of people with skin cancer has been getting lower. Women under forty are developing the disease twice as fast as men in the same age group. Fortunately, skin cancer is quite curable when treated early.

Unless otherwise stated, the dosages recommended here are for adults. For children between the ages of twelve and seventeen, reduce the dose to three-quarters of the recommended amount. For children between the ages of six and twelve, use one-half the recommended dose, and for children under six, use one-quarter of the recommended amount.

NUTRIENTS

SUPPLEMENT	SUGGESTED DOSAGE	COMMENTS
Essential		
Beta-1,3-D-glucan	As directed on label.	Can stimulate immune cells to digest cellular debris.
Coenzyme Q10 plus	100 mg daily.	Improves cellular oxygenation.
Coenzyme A from Coenzyme-A Technologies	As directed on label.	Works with coenzyme Q10.
Dimethylglycine (DMG) (Aangamik DMG from FoodScience of Vermont)	As directed on label.	Improves cellular oxygenation.
Essential fatty acids (primrose oil)	As directed on label 3 times daily, before meals.	For cellular protection.
Garlic (Kyolic from Wakunaga)	2 capsules 3 times daily.	Enhances immune function.
Histidine	As directed on label.	May help to increase the skin's immunity to damage from the sun's rays.
Proteolytic enzymes	As directed on label. Take with meals.	Powerful free radical scavengers that also reduce inflammation and aid in proper breakdown of foods.
Quercetin	As directed on label.	A flavonoid that has antioxidant properties.
Selenium	200 mcg daily. If you are pregnant, do not exceed 40 mcg daily.	Powerful free radical scavenger. Protects against UV damage.
Superoxide dismutase (SOD)	As directed on label.	Destroys free radicals. Consider injections (under a doctor's supervision).
Vitamin A	10,000–50,000 IU daily for 10 days or for as long as you are on the program. If you are pregnant, do not exceed 10,000 IU daily.	Powerful antioxidants that destroy free radicals. Use emulsion form for easier assimilation and greater safety at high doses.
plus natural beta-carotene and	15,000 IU daily.	Precursor of vitamin A.
carotenoid complex (Betatene)	As directed on label.	
Vitamin B complex	100 mg of each major B vitamin daily (amounts of individual vitamins in a complex will vary).	Necessary for normal cell division and function.
and/or brewer's yeast	2 20-grain tablets 3 times daily.	A good source of B vitamins.
Vitamin C with	5,000–20,000 mg daily, in divided doses.	Powerful anticancer agent. Boosts immunity.

bioflavonoids	(*See* ASCORBIC ACID FLUSH in Part Three.)	
Vitamin E	200 IU daily.	Promotes healing and tissue repair. Use d-alpha-tocopherol form.

Important

Maitake extract or reishi extract or shiitake extract	4,000–8,000 mg daily. As directed on label. As directed on label.	These mushrooms contain substances that inhibit the growth and spread of cancerous tumors and also boost immune response.
Phytocharged nutritional supplements from Schiff	As directed on label.	Dietary supplements that protect against damage from sunlight and promote health.
Pycnogenol or grape seed extract	As directed on label. As directed on label.	Antioxidants that protect against UV-induced oxidative changes in skin.
Zinc	As directed on label. Do not exceed 100 mg daily from all supplements.	Important in activity of enzymes; cell division, growth, and repair; and proper immune function. Use zinc gluconate lozenges or zinc methionate (OptiZinc) for best absorption.

Helpful

Acidophilus	As directed on label. Take on an empty stomach.	Has an antibacterial effect on the body. Use a nondairy formula.
Aerobic 07 from Aerobic Life Industries	As directed on label.	Antimicrobial agents.
ConcenTrace from Trace Minerals Research	As directed on label.	To nourish skin and hair.
Dimethylsulfoxide (DMSO)	Apply topically as directed on label.	Promotes healing. Use only DMSO from a health food store.
Herpanacine from Diamond-Herpanacine Associates	As directed on label.	Contains antioxidants, amino acids, and herbs that promote skin health.
Kelp	1,000–1,500 mg daily.	For mineral balance. Use kelp in tablet form and/or eat sea vegetables.
L-cysteine and L-methionine	As directed on label, on an empty stomach. Take with water or juice. Do not take with milk. Take with 50 mg vitamin B_6 and 100 mg vitamin C for better absorption.	To detoxify harmful substances. (*See* AMINO ACIDS in Part One.)
Multienzyme complex	As directed on label. Take with meals.	To aid digestion.
Multivitamin and mineral complex	As directed on label, with meals.	All nutrients are necessary in balance. Do not use a sustained-release formula.

N-Acetylglucosamine (N-A-G from Source Naturals)	As directed on label.	Supplies glucosamine, which helps in the formation of mucous membrane and connective tissues.
Para-aminobenzoic acid (PABA)	25 mg daily.	Helps to protect against skin cancer.
Raw glandular complex plus raw thymus glandular	As directed on label. As directed on label.	Stimulates glandular function, especially that of the thymus, an important component of the immune system.
Taurine	As directed on label.	Functions as foundation for tissue and organ repair.
Vitamin B_3 (niacin) plus choline and folic acid	100 mg daily. Do not exceed this amount. 500–1,000 mg daily. 400 mcg daily.	B vitamins that improve circulation, build red blood cells, and aid liver function. *Caution:* Do not take niacin if you have a liver disorder, gout, or high blood pressure.
Vitamin B_{12} injections or vitamin B_{12}	As prescribed by physician. 1,000 mcg 3 times daily.	To prevent anemia. Injections (under a doctor's supervision) are best. If injections are not available, use a lozenge or sublingual form.

Herbs

❏ Alfalfa, burdock, dandelion root, Irish moss, marshmallow root, oat straw, rose hips, and yellow dock are all beneficial for tissue repair. Rose hips are also a good source of vitamin C.

❏ Astragalus generates anticancer cells in the body and boosts the immune system.

Caution: Do not use astragalus in the presence of a fever.

❏ Bilberry, cayenne (capsicum), ginger, goldenseal, nettle, sarsaparilla, and turmeric stimulate the liver and help to stabilize blood composition, and may retard the proliferation of cancer cells.

Caution: Do not take goldenseal internally on a daily basis for more than one week at a time. Do not use it during pregnancy or if you are breast-feeding, and use with caution if you are allergic to ragweed. If you have a history of cardiovascular disease, diabetes, or glaucoma, use it only under a doctor's supervision.

❏ Burdock root and red clover aid in cleansing the blood and lymph nodes.

❏ The seeds and peel of the Chinese cucumber inhibit cancer cells.

❏ Skin cancers may respond to treatment with poultices combining comfrey, pau d'arco, ragwort, and wood sage. (*See* USING A POULTICE in Part Three.)

Cautions: Comfrey is recommended for external use only. Do not use sage if you suffer from any type of seizure disorder, or are pregnant or nursing.

❏ Ginkgo biloba, pau d'arco, and curcumin (a naturally occurring pigment isolated from turmeric) are powerful antioxidants with immune-enhancing capabilities.

Caution: Do not take ginkgo biloba if you have a bleeding disorder, or are scheduled for surgery or a dental procedure.

❏ Studies have shown that green tea has anticancer properties. Drink 4 cups daily.

Caution: Green tea contains vitamin K, which can make anticoagulant medications less effective. Consult your health care professional if you are using them. The caffeine in green tea could cause insomnia, anxiety, upset stomach, nausea, or diarrhea.

❏ Tea tree oil cream, applied topically, is a natural antiseptic and antifungal that enhances healing.

Recommendations

❏ Eat a diet that is low in fat and high in antioxidants, such as beta-carotene–rich carrots, sweet potatoes, squash, and spinach; cruciferous vegetables such as broccoli, Brussels sprouts, cabbage, kale, and turnips; and citrus fruits.

❏ Be aware of the warning signs of skin cancer:

- An open sore that bleeds, crusts over, and does not heal properly.

- A reddish, irritated spot, usually on the chest, shoulder, arm, or leg. It may itch or hurt, or cause no discomfort.

- A smooth growth with an elevated border and an indented center. As it becomes bigger, tiny blood vessels develop on the surface.

- A shiny scarlike area that is white, yellow, or waxy, with a shiny, taut appearance.

- An enlarging, irregular, "angry-looking" lesion on the face, lips, or ears.

❏ Examine your skin regularly. The Skin Cancer Foundation recommends performing a full-body self-examination every three months. To do this, you need a full-length mirror, a handheld mirror, and ample lighting. Look for any changes in any moles or marks on your body, using the following A-B-C-D checklist:

- *Asymmetry.* Both sides of the mole should be shaped similarly. If not, the mole is suspect.

- *Border.* The edges of mole should be smooth, not blurred or ragged.

- *Color.* Tan, brown, and dark brown are normal. Red, white, blue, and black are not.

- *Diameter.* Any mole that is larger than ¼ inch in diameter, or whose diameter seems to be increasing, is suspicious.

In addition to keeping track of moles, look carefully for other unusual spots or growths. Any irregularities you find should be evaluated by a dermatologist. Many people over fifty years of age see a dermatologist yearly.

❏ Stay away from tanning salons. Their equipment is sometimes said to be safer than the sun because tanning beds emit ultraviolet-A (UVA) rays, the so-called cool rays, rather than the ultraviolet-B (UVB) rays, which are most often implicated in sunburn. It has been established, however, that UVA rays can cause skin cancer just as UVB rays can. Do not be misled by claims to the contrary. The essential differences between UVA and UVB rays are that UVA rays are more likely to penetrate deeper into the skin, and are more likely to lead to skin damage such as wrinkling and collagen damage and, perhaps, melanoma. UVB rays are more likely to burn the top layer of skin and cause skin cancers such as basal and squamous cell cancers, are at their strongest at low and high altitudes, and have a shorter wavelength than UVA rays. A study reported in the *Journal of the National Cancer Institute* indicated that women who frequented tanning salons more than once a month had a 55 percent higher chance of developing malignant melanoma. The study also revealed that natural blondes were twice as likely, and redheads four times as likely, to develop melanoma than were brown- or black-haired women.

❏ Beware of new moles that appear after age forty. Be suspicious of any mole that appears unusual; is irregularly shaped or changes in size or color; or one that is pearly white, translucent, black, or multicolored; and that has a ridge around the edge. A mole that spreads, bleeds, or itches, or that is constantly irritated by clothing, is also suspect.

❏ Check for discharge from moles. Have any suspicious mole evaluated by a professional.

❏ See your health care provider if you find a growth that fits any of the descriptions in this section. Early detection is the key to successful treatment of skin cancer.

❏ Include in the diet plenty of foods that are high in vitamin E. A diet rich in vitamin E may protect your skin against damage from UV rays. Good food sources of vitamin E include asparagus, green leafy vegetables, raw nuts, wheat germ, and organic, cold-pressed vegetable oils.

❏ Get plenty of vitamin A in your diet and apply creams containing vitamin A on your skin as supplements. Vitamin A and related compounds stimulate skin cell renewal by increasing the rate of cell division. Natural vitamin A also may inhibit the growth of skin tumors, according to animal studies. Topical application of vitamin A can easily saturate the upper layers of the skin.

❏ To protect against skin cancer, take protective measures. The sun's ultraviolet rays are strongest between 10:00 A.M. and 3:00 P.M. Stay out of the sun as much as possible between these hours. When spending time outdoors, wear light-colored clothing made of tightly woven material (you can buy clothing made of materials that act as a sunblock). Wear a hat and sunglasses that block ultraviolet rays. Always use sunscreen. By themselves, sunscreens might not be effective in protecting you from the most dangerous forms of skin cancer. However, sunscreen use is an important part of your sun protection program. Used properly, certain sunscreens help protect human skin from some of the sun's damaging UV radiation. Choose a product with a sun protection factor (SPF) of 15 or higher and one that specifies *broad-spectrum* protection. When choosing a sunscreen, it's important to know that an SPF of 30 is not twice as protective as an SPF of 15; rather, when properly used, an SPF of 15 protects the skin from 93 percent of UVB radiation, and an SPF 30 sunscreen provides 97 percent protection. Even if a sunscreen is water-resistant, you should reapply it every three or four hours for as long as you are outside—more often if you go swimming or if you are perspiring heavily. (Sunscreens can claim only to be water-*resistant*, not water*proof*.) Wear sunscreen on cloudy days. Nearly 85 percent of the sun's UV rays penetrate through clouds. Be sure to protect your lips with a lip balm that has an SPF of 15, too. To increase awareness of the damaging potential of UV radiation, the U.S. Environmental Protection Agency and the National Weather Service have developed a UV index for use in weather reports to help individuals evaluate the level of danger from sun exposure on any given day. Following are the risk levels associated with exposure to UV rays as given in the index numbers:

Scale	Exposure level
• 0–2	Low
• 3–5	Moderate
• 6–8	High
• 9–10	Very high
• 11 or higher	Extreme

❏ If you have a family history of melanoma, avoid the sun as much as possible and use a sunblock every day.

❏ Avoid exposure to halogen lighting at close range. Halogen lights also emit UV radiation. The National Foundation for Cancer Research advises maintaining a distance of at least twenty inches from a 20-watt halogen bulb and three to six feet from 50 watt bulbs. However, the information was based on animal studies, and the FDA did not think the health risks were great enough at this time to warrant immediate action.

Considerations

❏ Skin cancer often originates in moles, but moles are not necessarily a cancer risk. They are extremely common (most people have them), and the overwhelming majority of them do *not* become cancerous.

❏ Medical treatment for skin cancer often involves surgery. Excisional biopsy (removal of the growth for analysis) cures skin cancer in its early stages in about 95 percent of cases. More radical surgery may be necessary if excision is delayed, and if the growth is large, a skin graft may be necessary.

❏ Other treatments sometimes used for skin cancer include:

- *Cryosurgery,* a method that uses liquid nitrogen to freeze and kill the diseased tissue, which later flakes away. This type of treatment is used frequently for people with bleeding disorders and for those who cannot tolerate anesthesia.

- *Electrosurgery,* in which the cancer is scooped out with a curette (a circular blade) and an electric current burns a border around the site to kill remaining cancer cells.

- *Laser surgery,* in which a laser is used to cut away the damaged tissue and seal off surrounding blood vessels as it goes.

- *Moh's microsurgery,* in which a surgeon shaves off cancerous tissue one thin layer at a time until healthy tissue is reached. Each layer is then examined under a microscope so that the doctor can be assured that he or she has gotten all the cancer while taking a minimum of healthy skin. This surgery is most effective for recurrent cancers and for cases in which the tumor is large or the extent of the cancer is unknown.

- *Radiation therapy,* which involves training an X-ray or an electron beam on the diseased area to kill cancerous tissue. This alternative is good for cases in which surgery poses particular risks.

❏ A treatment called *photodynamic therapy* has been approved in the United States. A photosensitizing agent is injected into the bloodstream, which remains in cancer cells but not healthy ones. A concentrated light beam is then applied, which kills the cancer cells. The cosmetic results appear to be much better than with surgical treatments; however, there is concern that the cancer could recur.

❏ Actinic keratoses may be treated by curettage/electrodesiccation, in which the lesion is scraped and a biopsy is taken, or shave removal or dermabrasion to remove the upper layers of skin.

❏ Seborrheic keratoses are slightly raised, brownish spots on the skin that may appear waxy, scaly, or wartlike. They seem to be stuck on the skin and are most often found on the chest and back. They are harmless—neither cancerous nor precancerous—and appear normally as people age. They result from irregular clumping together, rather than even distribution, of skin pigment. The tendency to develop seborrheic keratoses is inherited. People often mistake these growths for melanomas. If there is any doubt as to the nature of a spot on the skin, a dermatologist should take a scraping of the area and examine the sample for cancer cells. Treatment, if any is necessary, can include curettage, cryosurgery, chemosurgery, or electrosurgery. Actinic keratoses are flatter and redder than seborrheic keratoses, and are considered a precursor of cancer. They tend to appear on areas of skin that are normally exposed to the sun.

❏ With early detection and treatment, most people recover from skin cancer, but regular checkups are advised for at least the next five years.

The average person incurs between 25 and 80 percent of all sun exposure prior to the age of eighteen. Thus, even though skin cancer is rare in children, the childhood years have a major influence on a person's tendency to develop skin cancer later in life. An infant under the age of six months should never be exposed to direct sunlight or have sunscreen applied to his or her skin. Infants should always be dressed in protective clothing when they are outside. Sunscreen can be used on a baby over six months old (choose a PABA-free formula, preferably one meant for young children), but sun exposure should still be limited, and the child should still be dressed in protective clothing. For toddlers and young children, limit time in the sun and apply sunscreen regularly whenever they are outdoors. Older children should be taught the importance of applying sunscreen regularly—an important lifelong habit.

Certain medications may make the skin more susceptible to sun damage. These include antibiotics, antidepressants, diuretics, antihistamines, sedatives, estrogen, and acne medications such as retinoic acid. Ask your health care provider or pharmacist if any medication that you take might have such an effect.

A study reported in the *Journal of the American Academy of Dermatology* found that well-educated white-collar men have the highest risk of developing melanoma. Researchers surmise that a pattern of many months of little sun exposure (a result of working indoors) with occasional overexposure and sunburn (such as that acquired at sunny resort vacations) may be responsible.

The prescription medication tretinoin (Retin-A) may be able to reverse precancerous sun damage in skin. Skin care products containing alpha-hydroxy acids, which are available over the counter, may have a similar effect, although they are less potent.

The U.S. Food and Drug Administration has approved for marketing as a sun protectant a line of clothing produced by Sun Precautions, Inc., of Everett, WA. The clothing, which carries an SPF rating of 30, is sold under the brand name Solumbra. (*See* Manufacturer and Distributor Information in the Appendix.)

Preliminary research into the potential of beta-carotene, folic acid, retinoic acid, vitamin C, vitamin E, and minerals as inhibitors of skin cancer is encouraging.

Garlic may be effective in fighting basal cell carcinoma by boosting the body's immune response.

A worldwide rise in the incidence of skin cancer has been linked to the destruction of the earth's ozone layer. The ozone layer acts as a protective atmospheric sunscreen. As it becomes thinner and holes develop in it, more of the sun's harmful rays reach the earth.

More information about skin cancer is available from the American Cancer Society. (*See* Health and Medical Organizations in the Appendix.)

SKIN PROBLEMS

See ACNE; AGE SPOTS; ATHLETE'S FOOT; BEDSORES; BOIL; BRUISING; BURNS; CANKER SORES; COLD SORES (FEVER BLISTERS); CORNS AND CALLUSES; DANDRUFF; DERMATITIS; DRY SKIN; HIVES; INSECT BITE; LEG ULCERS; OILY SKIN; PSORIASIS; ROSACEA; SCABIES; SEBACEOUS CYST; SEBORRHEA; SKIN CANCER; SKIN RASH; SUNBURN; VITILIGO; WRINKLES. *See also under* FUNGAL INFECTION; PREGNANCY-RELATED PROBLEMS.

SKIN RASH

The skin is the body's largest organ. It consists of three layers—the epidermis (outer layer), the dermis (middle layer), and the subcutaneous layer (inner layer). The skin acts as a shield between the body and the millions of foreign substances that exist in our environment. It also functions as a means of excreting toxins and other substances from the body, as do the kidneys and bowels. As a result, the skin is subject to the development of various bumps and blisters, as well as to changes in color, cracking, dryness, flaking, itching, redness, roughness, scaling, thickening, and a host of other problems.

There are many reasons for skin reactions. Some of the most common include allergies to molds, foods, chemicals, cosmetics, and other substances. Insect bites, exposure to certain plants (such as poison ivy), fungi, diaper rash, sun and wind exposure, drugs, and alcohol can pose problems as well. Reactions to detergents, jewelry, and fragrances; nervous tension; and friction, either from two parts of the body rubbing against each other or from contact with ill-fitting clothing or shoes, also contribute. (*See* Common Types of Rashes on page 722.)

A rash should not be taken lightly, as it can sometimes be an indication of an underlying illness—sometimes a potentially serious illness. Certain types of rashes can be valuable as early warning signals.

Unless otherwise stated, the dosages recommended here are for adults. For children between the ages of twelve and seventeen, reduce the dose to three-quarters of the recommended amount. For children between the ages of six and twelve, use one-half the recommended dose, and for children under six, use one-quarter of the recommended amount.

NUTRIENTS

SUPPLEMENT	SUGGESTED DOSAGE	COMMENTS
Bee pollen	As directed on label.	Has antioxidant properties that can aid in healing. *Caution:* Do not use if you are allergic to bee stings.
Beta-1,3-D-glucan	As directed on label.	Can attack organisms that do not belong on the body, including bacteria, viruses, and fungi.
Colloidal silver	As directed on label.	A powerful antibiotic that has been shown to be effective in fighting many skin rashes. *Caution:* Only use topically.

Common Types of Rashes

The best way to approach treatment for a rash is to eliminate the underlying cause. Following are descriptions of some of the conditions most often responsible for skin rashes. This list is not exhaustive, and it is not meant as a substitute for diag- nosis by a qualified health care practitioner. Any rash that persists for longer than one week, that seems to be getting worse, or that is accompanied by other symptoms, such as fever, should be evaluated by a professional.

Cause of Rash	Characteristic Features
Athlete's foot	Inflammation, scaling, cracking, and blisters on the feet, especially between the toes. Burning and/ or itching may be severe.
Chickenpox	Crops of small round blisterlike pimples that crust over as they heal. Usually appears first on the torso, following a day or so of fever and headache, and then spreads to the face and extremities. Extremely itchy. Most common in children.
Dermatitis (eczema)	There are several types of dermatitis, including atopic dermatitis, nummular dermatitis, seborrheic dermatitis, and hand dermatitis. General features include patches of scaling, flaking, and thickening skin that may appear anywhere on the body. Skin color in the affected area may change. Itching is common. One type of dermatitis causes round lesions on the limbs.
Food or drug allergy	A flat pink or red rash, with possible swelling and/or itching.
Fungal infection (Candida)	Moist, possibly itchy, red patches that may appear anywhere on the body, but are most common in areas where skin surfaces rub together. In babies, an inflamed, shiny diaper rash.
Herpes infection	Painful fluid-filled blisters that erupt periodically around the mouth and/or genitals.
Hives	A rash that usually appears suddenly and can take the form of patches of tiny, goose bump-like spots or red, itchy welts that cover significant areas of the body—or anything in between.
Lyme disease	A red, circular lesion that gradually expands as the center appears to clear up. This may be followed by a rash composed of small raised bumps on the torso. The rash may or may not be accompanied by flulike symptoms of fever, chills, and nausea.
Measles	A raised red rash that usually begins on the forehead and ears and spreads to the rest of the body. The rash usually follows several days of viral symptoms including fever, cough, sneezing, runny nose, and possibly conjunctivitis. There may be tiny red spots with white centers in the mouth as well.
Mononucleosis	A lumpy red rash accompanied by headache, achiness, low-grade fever, sore throat, and persistent fatigue.
Poison ivy/poison oak/poison sumac	A red, intensely itchy rash with swelling and oozing blisters. If scratched, the rash can spread.
Psoriasis	Silvery, scaly patches that may appear anywhere on the body, but are most common on the scalp, ears, arms, legs, knees, elbows, and back. The rash follows a pattern of periodic flare-ups followed by healing. It may or may not be itchy.
Ringworm	Small, itchy round red spots that grow to be approximately ¼ inch in diameter, with scaly, slightly raised borders. They tend to clear in the center as they expand.
Rosacea	Reddening, small bumps, and pimples, usually affecting the nose and the center of the face. It resembles acne, but is chronic and is more common in middle-aged and older individuals.
Scabies	A persistent itchy rash with small red lumps that may become dry and scaly. Fine, wavy dark lines may emanate from some lumps. Most often occurs between the fingers, on the wrists and/or forearms, and on the breasts and/or genitals.
Seborrhea	Greasy yellowish, flaky patches of skin that form scales and crusts. It can appear anywhere on the body, but most often affects the scalp, face, and/or chest. It may or may not be itchy.
Shingles	Crops of tiny blisters that are extremely painful and sensitive to the touch and that eventually crust, scab, and are shed. Most common on the abdomen below the ribs, but it can occur anywhere on the body. May be preceded and/or accompanied by flulike symptoms of chills, fever, and achiness.

Grape seed extract	As directed on label.	Has antioxidant properties that can aid in healing.
Vitamin A and	As directed on label.	Vitamins that are thought to improve the health of the skin.
vitamin C and	As directed on label.	
vitamin E plus	As directed on label.	
niacinamide and	As directed on label.	
panthenol	As directed on label.	

Herbs

❑ Aloe vera gel, ginkgo biloba extract, and green tea extract have antioxidant properties that can aid in healing.

❑ Calendula, chamomile, elderflower, and tea tree oil can be used externally as a soothing wash on rashes.

❑ A poultice made with dandelion, and yellow dock root benefits many types of skin rashes. (*See* USING A POULTICE in Part Three.)

❑ Itch Relief Lotion from Derma-E Skin Care contains chamomile, tea tree oil, and vitamin E. It offers quick relief of skin irritation.

❑ Soak a washcloth in malva tea and apply it as a warm compress to the infected area to reduce inflammation.

❑ Oat straw may be used topically in a bath to reduce symptoms, especially inflammation and itching.

❑ Olive leaf extract has healing properties for the skin.

Recommendations

❑ For quick relief of itching and inflammation, soak a clean cloth in cool water (or, for even greater soothing effect, in comfrey tea that has cooled), wring it out, and apply it to the affected area for ten minutes. Repeat this procedure as often as necessary for relief.

Caution: Comfrey is recommended for external use only.

❑ Take lukewarm showers instead of baths, and try not to shower every day during the duration of the rash. Also avoid using the same washcloth, sponge, or shower pouf each time you shower, as bacteria and fungi can grow in these moist areas.

❑ Whenever possible, use hypoallergenic skin care products, deodorants, shaving creams, soaps, hair products, cosmetics, household products, and laundry detergents. Keep in mind, however, that *hypoallergenic* means only that a product *is not likely to* cause allergies; not that it *will not*. Also, when choosing products, look for "fragrance-free" formulas rather than "unscented" ones.

❑ Wear cool, loose clothing. Next to the skin, cotton is best.

❑ Avoid prolonged contact with known skin irritants including chemicals, dust, direct sunlight, and water.

❑ Radiation and chemotherapy treatments can cause skin to become more sensitive to allergens and irritants. Occasion-ally, radiation can also cause the skin to thin, lose elasticity, and become lighter or darker in color. Emollients and high-SPF sunscreens should be used generously on affected areas.

❑ Many medications cause skin rashes in people when they are exposed to sunlight. If your medication causes photosensitivity, ask your doctor if there are any alternatives.

❑ *See* Common Types of Rashes on page 722 to help you identify possible causes of a rash, and refer to the appropriate sections in Part Two for advice on treatment.

Considerations

❑ Four of the most serious diseases in which skin rash is an early warning signal are Rocky Mountain spotted fever, meningococcal disease, staphylococcal toxic shock syndrome, and streptococcal toxic shock syndrome.

❑ Skin rashes in children are often caused by food allergies, especially to chocolate, dairy products, eggs, peanuts, milk, wheat, fish, chicken, pork, or beef. Some experts estimate that allergies to eggs, peanuts, and milk account for as many as 75 percent of all skin rashes in children.

❑ Many doctors recommend hydrocortisone cream for minor irritations, poison ivy, itchy insect bites, and diaper rash. Antihistamines and antibiotics are also common treatments prescribed by doctors for various types of rashes. In severe cases, a doctor may prescribe an oral steroid (such as prednisone, prednisolone, or hydrocortisone) or the use of phototherapy (procedures involving the use of ultraviolet radiation).

❑ Allergy testing is advised, particularly for persistent rashes. (*See* ALLERGIES in Part Two.)

❑ *See also* ACNE; ALLERGIES; ATHLETE'S FOOT; CANDIDIASIS; CHEMICAL ALLERGIES; CHICKENPOX; DERMATITIS; ENVIRONMENTAL TOXICITY; FUNGAL INFECTION; GANGRENE; HERPES INFECTION; HIVES; INSECT BITE; LUPUS; LYME DISEASE; MEASLES; MONONUCLEOSIS; POISON IVY/POISON OAK/POISON SUMAC; PSORIASIS; RHEUMATIC FEVER; ROSACEA; SCABIES; SEBORRHEA; SHINGLES (HERPES ZOSTER); VITILIGO; and/or WARTS, all in Part Two.

SLEEP PROBLEMS

See under INSOMNIA; NARCOLEPSY.

SMOKING DEPENDENCY

Every time a person smokes, he or she inhales more than 4,800 different chemicals (69 are carcinogens), including nicotine. Nicotine, which is extremely addictive, increases levels of the pleasure-inducing brain chemicals serotonin, dopamine, and norepinephrine. Tobacco has been used as a mood-altering substance for centuries. It has been ingested by various means, including chewing, sniffing, and smoking. Today it is most commonly consumed by smoking cigarettes.

Nicotine acts as a stimulant on the central nervous system. When nicotine is ingested, adrenaline production increases, raising the blood pressure and heart rate. Nicotine also affects the overall metabolic rate, the regulation of body temperature, the degree of tension in the muscles, and the levels of certain hormones. These and other metabolic changes create a pleasurable sensation in the user that often—and paradoxically—is experienced as a feeling of relaxation. This pleasurable sensation is one of the factors that makes tobacco so addictive. Another is the fact that tolerance to the effects of nicotine develops quite rapidly. That is, the dose needed to achieve the desired effect begins to rise almost immediately, encouraging you to increase the amount you smoke—which in turn increases the likelihood of addiction. Once you become addicted, your body depends on the presence of nicotine. If you then refrain from smoking, withdrawal symptoms occur. These include irritability, frustration, anger, anxiety, difficulty concentrating, restlessness, increased appetite, headache, stomach cramps, a slowed heart rate, a rise in blood pressure, and, most of all, an intense craving for nicotine.

Once the smoking habit has been acquired, it is difficult to break. Some authorities have stated that addiction to tobacco may be harder to overcome than addiction to heroin or cocaine. This is because smoking creates both physical *and* psychological dependency. It may be easier to overcome the physical addiction than the psychological dependency. Acute physical withdrawal, while unpleasant, lasts for a limited period of time, usually no more than several weeks. Long-term cravings are more likely a matter of psychological dependency, and require an ongoing effort to master. By the time an individual has become addicted to nicotine, the act of smoking itself has become a source of pleasure, and it may be so intertwined in your mind with other activities—having your morning coffee, reading the newspaper, working, socializing, whatever—that you find yourself unable to imagine engaging in these activities without a cigarette in hand. In addition, smoking provides a convenient excuse for taking a momentary break, especially during times of stress, and may help to smooth over awkward moments. Many smokers also are afraid of what might happen if they stopped; they fear withdrawal symptoms, weight gain, or a decreased ability to concentrate. All of these factors combine to make quitting difficult.

Even though it can be difficult to stop smoking, many people do it every day. There is certainly no shortage of reasons to quit. There are 440,000 deaths due to cigarettes in the United States every year. This is more than the number of deaths from alcohol, illegal drugs, traffic accidents, suicide, and homicide combined. Tobacco smoking causes an estimated 30 percent of all cancer deaths, 20 percent of fatal heart attacks, and 73 percent of deaths from chronic obstructive pulmonary disease. It also accounts for at least 90 percent of lung cancer cases. Many other health problems have been linked to smoking as well, including angina, arteriosclerosis, cataracts, chronic bronchitis, circulatory ailments, colorectal cancer, diarrhea, emphysema, heartburn,

high blood pressure, impotence, peptic ulcers, respiratory ailments, urinary incontinence, and cancers of the mouth and throat, especially among cigarette smokers who also consume alcohol and/or use mouthwash containing alcohol. Smoking increases the risk of catching colds and lengthens recovery time. Tobacco smoke paralyzes the cilia (hairlike protrusions lining the nose and throat), reducing their capacity to clear the passages by moving mucus—and the cold viruses trapped within it—to the outside.

Nicotine has long been known to be a deadly toxin. A single pinhead-sized drop of liquid nicotine, introduced directly into the bloodstream, would be fatal. At the doses normally ingested by smokers, nicotine makes the heart pump faster and work harder, increasing the likelihood of heart disease. It also constricts the peripheral blood vessels, contributing to circulatory disorders such as Raynaud's phenomenon and hardening of the arteries.

And nicotine is not the only ingredient in cigarettes that poses a danger to health. In addition to nicotine, cigarette smoke contains carbon monoxide, benzene, cyanide, ammonia, nitrosamines, vinyl chloride, radioactive particles, and other known irritants and carcinogens. Carbon monoxide binds to hemoglobin, interfering with the transport of oxygen throughout the body. Carbon monoxide also promotes the development of cholesterol deposits on artery walls. These two factors increase the risk of heart attack and stroke. Hydrogen cyanide causes bronchitis by inflaming the lining of the bronchi. Over the long term, smoking dramatically reduces the flow of blood to the brain.

Men who have smoked for years are more likely to have abnormally low penile blood pressure, which contributes to impotence. This is probably because smoking damages the blood vessels, including the tiny blood vessels that supply the penis. It also contributes to sterility; the sperm of men who smoke have less ability than that of nonsmokers to penetrate, and thus to fertilize, an egg.

Female cigarette smokers tend to experience menopause earlier, face a greater risk of osteoporosis after menopause, and have a much higher risk of developing cervical or uterine cancer. They also appear less fertile and have more difficulties during pregnancy. Smokers tend to have more miscarriages, stillbirths, and premature deliveries. Their babies often are smaller and have more health problems than babies of nonsmokers. Infants whose mothers smoke both during pregnancy and after childbirth appear to be three times as likely to die of sudden infant death syndrome (SIDS) as infants of nonsmokers. Children whose fathers smoke also face an increase in health problems.

Smoking has a detrimental effect on nutrition. Smokers break down vitamin C about twice as fast as nonsmokers. This can deprive the body of adequate amounts of one of the most powerful and versatile antioxidants at our disposal. Other antioxidant vitamins are depleted as well. Cigarette smoke contains high concentrations of nitrogen dioxide ozone, a compound that oxidizes the antioxidant vitamins and is also known to do damage to DNA. The accelerated antioxidant usage, in combination with the DNA damage, speeds the aging process.

Finally, smoking is increasingly a social problem. More and more nonsmokers are becoming concerned about the effects of "secondhand" smoke on their own health, and justifiably so. There is a growing body of evidence that secondhand smoke may be even more dangerous than the smoke the smoker breathes. Smoking is now prohibited in many workplaces and public buildings.

The dangers of smoking are well known today, yet people continue to smoke. Why? Some people started smoking before the hazards were widely known; others start in adolescence, when people generally feel invulnerable and are more likely to engage in risk-taking behavior—especially if it seems "adult," helps them fit in with a particular social group, and/or provokes their parents. However, surveys consistently show that no matter when or why they started, most current smokers do not smoke because they want to (well over 50 percent say they wish they had never started), but because they are addicted.

The good news is that this addiction can be overcome, and that health benefits begin almost immediately. In just twenty-four hours after your last cigarette, your blood pressure and pulse rate should return to normal, as should the levels of oxygen and carbon monoxide in your blood. Within a week, your risk of heart attack begins to decrease, your senses of smell and taste improve, and breathing becomes easier.

The nutrients and dietary suggestions below are recommended to correct probable smoking-related deficiencies and damage while you work to kick the habit. They are recommended also if you cannot avoid being a passive smoker.

Unless otherwise stated, the dosages recommended here are for adults. For children between the ages of twelve and seventeen, reduce the dose to three-quarters of the recommended amount.

NUTRIENTS

SUPPLEMENT	SUGGESTED DOSAGE	COMMENTS
Essential		
Coenzyme Q10	200 mg twice daily.	Aids oxygen flow to the brain; protects heart tissue. Also acts as an antioxidant to protect cells and lung tissue.
plus Coenzyme A from Coenzyme-A Technologies	As directed on label.	Works well with coenzyme Q10 to rid the body of toxic substances.
Oxy-5000 Forte from American Biologics	2 tablets 3 times daily.	A powerful antioxidant. Destroys free radicals produced in the smoke.
Pycnogenol or grape seed extract	As directed on label. As directed on label.	Helps to protect and repair the lungs.
Vitamin B complex plus extra	100 mg of each major B vitamin daily (amounts of individual vitamins in a complex will vary).	Necessary in cellular enzyme systems often damaged in smokers. Use sublingual form.
vitamin B12 and folic acid	1,000 mcg twice daily. 400 mcg daily.	Increases energy; needed for liver function. Use a lozenge or sublingual form. Needed for the formation of red blood cells; important for healthy cell division and replication.
Vitamin C with bioflavonoids	5,000–20,000 mg daily. (See ASCORBIC ACID FLUSH in Part Three.)	Important antioxidant that protects against cell damage. Smoking drastically depletes the body of vitamin C.
Vitamin E	200 IU daily.	One of the most important antioxidants, needed to protect cells and organs from damage by the smoke. Use d-alpha-tocopherol form.
Very Important		
Vitamin A	25,000 IU daily. If you are pregnant, do not exceed 10,000 IU daily.	Antioxidants that aid in the healing of mucous membranes. Important for lung protection. *Caution:* Vitamin A supplements should include only vitamin A and not beta-carotene, which has been shown to increase the risk of dying in smokers.
Zinc	50–80 mg daily. Do not exceed a total of 100 mg daily from all supplements.	Important in immune function. Use zinc gluconate lozenges or OptiZinc for best absorption.
Helpful		
Cell Guard from Biotec Foods	As directed on label.	Provides high levels of antioxidant enzymes for cellular health.
Dimethylglycine (DMG) (Aangamik DMG from FoodScience of Vermont)	As directed on label.	Detoxifies the body and helps the body maintain high energy levels.
Herpanacine from Diamond-Herpanacine Associates	As directed on label.	Detoxifies the body, balances the nervous system, and boosts immunity.
L-cysteine and L-methionine plus glutathione	As directed on label, on an empty stomach. Take with water or juice. Do not take with milk. Take with 50 mg vitamin B6 and 100 mg vitamin C for better absorption. As directed on label.	Potent detoxifiers that protect the lungs, liver, brain, and tissues from cigarette smoke. Protects the liver.
Maitake extract	1,000–4,000 mg daily.	Inhibits carcinogenesis and protects against metastasis through the lungs.
Multivitamin and mineral complex with selenium	As directed on label. 200 mcg daily. If you are pregnant, do not exceed 40 mcg daily.	Necessary for immune system function. Helps to prevent cell damage. Make sure the supplement contains folic acid, as it has been shown to reduce strokes related to smoking.
Raw thymus glandular	As directed on label.	A glandular that improves immune function.

Herbs

❏ Burdock root and red clover help to cleanse the bloodstream of toxins.

❏ Cayenne (capsicum) desensitizes respiratory tract cells to irritants from cigarette smoke.

❏ Catnip, hops, lobelia, skullcap, and/or valerian root can be used to help reduce the nervousness and anxiety that may accompany nicotine withdrawal.

Caution: Lobelia is only to be taken under supervision of a health care professional as it is potentially toxic. People with high blood pressure, heart disease, liver disease, kidney disease, seizure disorders, or shortness of breath should not take lobelia. Pregnant and lactating women should avoid lobelia as well.

❏ Dandelion root and milk thistle protect the liver against harmful toxins from cigarette smoke.

❏ Ginger causes perspiration, which helps the body to shed some of the poisons ingested through smoking. It also soothes the stomach irritation occasionally experienced with the use of cayenne or lobelia.

Recommendations

❏ Consume more asparagus, broccoli, Brussels sprouts, cabbage, cauliflower, spinach, sweet potatoes, and turnips.

❏ Eat plenty of grains, nuts, seeds, and unpolished brown rice. Millet cereal is a good source of protein. Eat wheat, oat, and bran. Also consume yellow and deep-orange vegetables such as carrots, pumpkin, squash, and yams. Apples, berries, Brazil nuts, cantaloupe, cherries, grapes, legumes (including chickpeas, lentils, and red beans), and plums are also helpful.

❏ Eat onions and garlic, or take garlic in supplement form.

❏ Drink fresh carrot juice daily as a preventive measure against lung cancer. Also drink fresh beet juice (made from both the roots and the greens) and asparagus juice. All dark-colored juices are good, as are black currants. Also beneficial is apple juice, if it is fresh. Drink fruit juices in the morning and vegetable juices in the afternoon.

❏ Cook all sprouts slightly except for alfalfa sprouts, which should be eaten raw.

❏ *Do not* consume junk foods, processed refined foods, saturated fats, salt, sugar, or white flour.

❏ Instead of salt, use a kelp or potassium substitute. If you must, use a *small* amount of blackstrap molasses or pure maple syrup as a natural sweetener in place of sugar. Use whole wheat or rye instead of white flour. Eliminate alcohol, coffee, and all teas except for herbal teas.

❏ Do not eat any animal protein except for broiled fish (up to three servings per week). *Never* eat luncheon meat, hot dogs, or smoked or cured meats. Limit your consumption of dairy products to a little low-fat yogurt, kefir, or raw cheese on an occasional basis.

❏ Do not eat any peanuts. Limit, but do not eliminate altogether, your intake of soybean products; they contain enzyme inhibitors.

❏ Keep in mind that the acute craving for a cigarette usually lasts only three to five minutes. Focusing on this fact may make it easier to wait it out. Also remember that it gets easier and easier as time goes by. When cravings strike, try taking a walk, doing some sit-ups, or engaging in any activity that can momentarily take your mind off cigarettes.

❏ To accelerate toxin elimination, *see* FASTING in Part Three, and follow the program.

❏ Take coffee enemas daily. Use cleansing enemas with lemon and water or garlic and water two or three times weekly. Enemas are not for children. (*See* ENEMAS in Part Three.)

❏ Drink spring or steam-distilled water only.

❏ As much as possible, avoid stress.

❏ If you take any medications, consult with your physician about the possible need for an adjustment in dosage after you quit smoking. Tobacco alters the absorption and utilization of many medications, including insulin, asthma drugs, and certain antidepressants, blood pressure medications, and painkillers.

Considerations

❏ The difficulty of quitting appears to be related less to how many packs a day you smoke than to how early in life you started smoking.

❏ Many people have been successful in the quest to stop smoking by going on a fast using only live juices and quality steam-distilled water. A live juice fast can quickly remove nicotine and other damaging chemicals from the body. Adhering to a five-day live juice fast can have amazing results.

❏ There are several natural products on the market that may help you deal with withdrawal symptoms, such as Smoking Withdrawal from Natra-Bio.

❏ A lack of beta-carotene and the B-complex vitamins has been linked to lung and throat cancer. However, the beta-carotene data is controversial. One major study (called ATBC study) published in the *Journal of the National Cancer Institute* found that smokers who take a high dose of beta-carotene (20 milligrams per day) had an increased risk of developing lung cancer, especially for heavy smokers who drink alcohol. The authors stated that smokers should avoid high-dose beta-carotene supplementation.

❏ Taking vitamin C and E supplements is controversial in smokers. One study showed a 19 percent increase in mortality in users of these supplements who were aged fifty to sixty-two years. However, in the same study, mortality was *decreased* by 41 percent among those aged sixty-six to sixty-nine years. Further study is needed to determine why there was this apparent age-related discrepancy.

☐ In one study, broccoli (about 1 cup a day) was shown to protect cells against damage in smokers. Other investigators have shown that eating a wide variety of fruits and vegetables containing lycopene, lutein/zeaxanthin, total carotenoids, and other natural compounds reduced the risk of developing lung cancer in smokers by 15 to 28 percent.

☐ A study cosponsored by the British and Norwegian governments found that DNA taken from the lungs of female smokers showed significantly more damage than that taken from men. DNA damage is a marker of increased cancer risk.

☐ Research at the University of Indiana found that people who drank six cups of tea a day were protected from the toxic effects cigarette smoke has on the lungs by up to 50 percent. Still, quitting is preferable since you still can get lung cancer if you smoke and drink tea.

☐ Smoking a pack of cigarettes a day or more triples the risk of needing surgery for a herniated disk, but quitting smoking reduces that risk, according to researchers at the Medical College of Wisconsin.

☐ According to a study reported in the *Archives of Internal Medicine*, smoking increases the risk of developing leukemia by 30 percent.

☐ There are alternative sources of nicotine for those who wish to quit smoking. They are available either in transdermal patch form, as chewing gum, and as nasal sprays and inhalers. Some of these are available over the counter, while others require a prescription.

☐ In July 2009, the U.S. Food and Drug Administration (FDA) announced that it is requiring manufacturers to put a Boxed Warning on the prescribing information for the smoking-cessation drugs Chantix (varenicline) and Zyban (buproprion). The warning highlights the risk of serious mental health events, including changes in behavior, depressed mood, hostility, and suicidal thoughts when taking these drugs.

☐ A diagnostic procedure called a sputum cytology test can sometimes detect the presence of cancer before there are symptoms and before other tests show the disease. In this test, sputum coughed up from the lungs and the bronchial tubes is examined for signs of tumor cells.

SNAKEBITE

There are four types of poisonous snakes in the United States: copperheads, coral snakes, cottonmouths (or water moccasins), and a variety of rattlesnakes. Approximately 4,000 to 7,000 Americans are bitten by poisonous snakes each year, most commonly in the summer months, in grassy or rocky environments. However, only about 25 percent of these bites involve venom—that is, the snake saves its venom for its prey, not necessarily for defense. If you encounter a snake that is large enough to consider *you* prey, your problems far outweigh a simple bite!

The toxicity of snake venom, which varies from species to species, can kill local tissue and release toxins into the body that can cause serious problems with blood pressure, heart rate, and pain. A person who has been bitten by a poisonous snake may exhibit mild to severe symptoms, which can include swelling or discoloration of the skin in the area of the bite, a racing pulse, weakness, shortness of breath, nausea, and vomiting. In extreme cases, pain and swelling can be severe, the pupils may dilate, and shock and convulsion may occur. The person may twitch and his or her speech may become slurred. In the most severe cases, paralysis, unconsciousness, and death can result. There are only about four deaths in the United States each year due to snakebite, yet this is a situation feared universally by hikers, paddlers, climbers, fishermen, hunters, and campers. Most deaths occur in children because of their smaller body mass and lack of sufficient immune system development. Improper treatment causes many injuries, and there is a lot of misinformation concerning first aid. (*See* What to Do in Case of Snakebite on page 728.)

It is worth emphasizing that the majority of snakes are *not* poisonous. Nevertheless, anyone who has been bitten by a snake should be seen by a professional immediately, because the severity of initial symptoms does not always reflect the seriousness of the bite. If you have a pet snake that bites, make sure that it cannot get out to harm anyone, especially small children.

The nutrients and other measures outlined here are intended to alleviate pain and hasten healing *after appropriate medical care has been administered*. They are *not* meant to substitute for it. Unless otherwise stated, the dosages recommended here are for adults. For children between the ages of twelve and seventeen, reduce the dose to three-quarters of the recommended amount. For children between the ages of six and twelve, use one-half the recommended dose, and for children under six, use one-quarter of the recommended amount.

NUTRIENTS

SUPPLEMENT	SUGGESTED DOSAGE	COMMENTS
Helpful		
Calcium	500 mg every 4 to 6 hours until pain begins to ease.	To relieve pain. Acts as a sedative. Use calcium gluconate form.
and magnesium	1,000 mg with the first 500 mg of calcium.	Works with calcium.
Charcoal tablets	8 tablets every 3 hours until the swelling subsides. Take with a large glass of water. If possible, start immediately after being bitten.	A powerful detoxifying agent.
Colloidal silver	Apply topically as directed on label.	An antiseptic that reduces inflammation and promotes healing of skin sores.
L-serine	As directed on label, on an empty stomach. Take with water or juice. Do not take with milk. Take with 50 mg vitamin B6 and 100 mg vitamin C for better absorption.	Helps maintain a healthy immune system and aids in the production of antibodies.

What to Do in Case of Snakebite

If you or someone with you is bitten by a snake, it is vital to seek appropriate medical treatment. It is equally vital to avoid making inappropriate attempts at treatment; such mistakes can cause more problems than they solve.

What to do in any particular case depends on the circumstances surrounding the bite.

What to Do

While not all snakebites are life-threatening, it is important to follow these simple steps:

- Remain calm (or, if the victim is someone other than yourself, calm him or her).

- If possible, call for emergency assistance.

- Gently wash the area with soap and water.

- Apply a cold, wet cloth over the bite.

- Get yourself or the victim to the nearest hospital emergency room for further treatment.

What *Not* to Do

The list of measures that should be *avoided* in response to snakebite include:

- *Do not* apply a tourniquet. This has been the cause of numerous amputations. It is possible that the application of a tourniquet is more dangerous than the snakebite itself.

- *Do not* pack the entire bitten area in ice. This can block circulation and cause injury to tissue, or even gangrene. An ice pack or some cubes wrapped in cloth, applied periodically to the skin, is the maximum you want to use.

- *Do not* cut the wound with a knife or razor. Older first-aid kits often contain cutters, but excessive bleeding can cause more damage. If you happen to cut an artery, the victim can bleed to death. Unless you happen to be a vascular surgeon, leave the razor blades in your pack.

- *Do not* use your mouth to try to "suck out" the venom. The average human mouth has so many bacteria in it that infection of the wound would be almost certain, complicating treatment in the long run.

- *Do not* drink alcohol (or give it to the victim).

- *Do not* use an electric shock, Taser, stun gun, cattle prod, or any such device applied to the snakebite. All you will do is make the victim more miserable, and the venom will not be broken down by the electricity.

Other Measures

If you can *safely* kill the snake, do so and decapitate it. Bury the head and bring the body with you to the emergency room for identification. The correct *antivenin* can then be selected at the hospital. *Do not bring the head, however,* as even a decapitated snake head can bite up to an hour after its death.

There is one type of snakebite kit that is worthwhile. It is called Sawyer Extractor Pump Kit, and is available from Sawyer Products. (*See* Manufacturer and Distributor Information in the Appendix.) It contains a syringe-like device that does work to suck out venom without requiring you to open up the fang wounds with a tool. This prevents excessive bleeding and contamination of the wound. This kit will probably get out about half the venom if it is used quickly (within five minutes is recommended). These are available from many sporting goods stores and on the Internet for less than twenty dollars. If you are going to be someplace in snake country that is *really* far from civilization, having one of these kits in your backpack is a necessity. After you use it, transport to the nearest hospital is still required so that proper care can be administered.

Multivitamin and mineral complex	As directed on label.	All nutrients work together to promote health.
Ultimate Cleanse from Nature's Secret	As directed on label.	A two-part body-cleansing program that detoxifies the organs, blood, and the channels of elimination.
Vitamin A with mixed carotenoids including beta-carotene	10,000 IU daily.	Enhances immunity and promotes tissue healing.
Vitamin B$_5$ (pantothenic acid)	500 mg every 4 hours for 2 days.	The antistress vitamin.
Vitamin C with bioflavonoids	2,000 mg every hour for 5 to 6 hours, up to a total of 15,000 mg daily.	A powerful detoxifier. Relieves pain and discomfort and fights infection.
Vitamin E	200 IU daily.	Promotes healing and reduces blood pressure. Use d-alpha-tocopherol form.
Zinc	30 mg daily.	Boosts immune function. Use zinc gluconate lozenges or OptiZinc for best absorption.

Herbs

❏ Black cohosh syrup helps to relieve pain. Take ½ to 1 tablespoon of the syrup three times daily.

Caution: Do not use black cohosh if you are pregnant or have any type of chronic disease. Black cohosh should not be used by those with liver problems.

❏ Poultices of comfrey, slippery elm, or white oak leaves and bark can be used. (*See* USING A POULTICE in Part Three.) Comfrey salve, plantain poultice, or plantain salve can also be used.

Caution: Comfrey is recommended for external use only.

❏ Echinacea, taken in tea and/or capsule form, boosts the immune system.

Caution: Do not take echinacea for longer than three months. It should not be used by people who are allergic to ragweed.

❏ Olive leaf extract has antibacterial properties.

❏ Yellow dock can be used to alleviate symptoms. Drink a cup of yellow dock tea or take 2 capsules of yellow dock every hour until the symptoms are gone.

Recommendations

❏ Prevention is the best cure! To reduce the possibility of snakebite, always remain on paths and hiking trails when in wooded areas.

❏ Wear leather boots and long pants if walking in tall grass.

❏ Carry a walking stick, especially in rattlesnake country. A snake often will strike at the stick first.

❏ Be alert. If you see a snake, do not approach it. Stay at least six feet away.

❏ If you come across a log, step onto the log and then over it. Never step directly over it.

❏ If you are walking in a tall grassy area, use a long walking stick or other object to tap the ground in front of you before you step.

❏ Take special caution when walking near or through a wet marshy area, as water moccasins can occupy these areas.

Considerations

❏ A poisonous snakebite is a medical emergency. In the United States, treatment is a complex process that may include the administration of antivenin plus fluid and electrolyte replacement, the administration of oxygen, and other supportive measures. If possible, it is wise to call ahead to the emergency room and alert them of the situation before your arrival so that the proper antivenin can be ready for treatment as soon as possible.

❏ Snakebite is more likely to be life-threatening for children and for elderly people.

❏ In a life-threatening situation, massive doses of vitamin C may save the victim's life. (*See* ASCORBIC ACID FLUSH in Part Three.)

❏ Most cases of snakebite occur between sunrise and sunset. Snakes are cold-blooded and are more likely to be out then, basking in the warmth of the day.

❏ Nonpoisonous snakebites are usually treated with antibiotics in order to prevent infection.

SORE THROAT

Sore throats are one of the most common health complaints. They are characterized by a raw, burning, and/or scratchy feeling at the back of the throat. Most sore throats are caused by viral infections such as the common cold. Bacterial infection, especially *Streptococcus* infection, can also be responsible. In addition, a sore throat can be caused by anything that irritates the sensitive mucous membranes at the back of the throat and mouth. Some irritants include medications, surgery, radiation therapy, dust, smoke, fumes, extremely hot foods or drinks, tooth or gum infections, dental work, and abrasions. Chronic coughing and excessive loud talking also irritate the throat.

An acute sore throat usually runs its course within a few days to a few weeks. Sore throats are seldom serious, but quite often are the first symptom of another disorder. Sore throats can signal a cold, flu, strep, mononucleosis, Epstein-Barr virus, herpes simplex, as well as many childhood illnesses such as measles and chickenpox. More rarely, a sore throat may indicate chronic fatigue syndrome, diphtheria, epiglottitis, gingivitis, laryngeal cancer, or an abscess around the tonsils.

Unless otherwise stated, the dosages recommended here are for adults. For children between the ages of twelve and seventeen, reduce the dose to three-quarters of the recommended amount. For children between the ages of six and twelve, use one-half the recommended dose, and for children under six, use one-quarter of the recommended amount.

NUTRIENTS

SUPPLEMENT	SUGGESTED DOSAGE	COMMENTS
Helpful		
Acidophilus (Kyo-Dophilus from Wakunaga)	As directed on label. Take on an empty stomach.	To replenish "friendly" bacteria. Especially important if antibiotics are prescribed. Use a nondairy formula.
Bee propolis	As directed on label.	Protects mucous membranes of the mouth and throat. *Caution:* Do not use if you are allergic to bee stings.
Garlic (Kyolic from Wakunaga) or	2 capsules 3 times daily, with meals.	For improved immune function.
Kyo-Green from Wakunaga	As directed on label.	Contains live enzymes, amino acids, vitamins, minerals, and chlorophyll for healing.
Maitake extract or	As directed on label.	To boost immunity and fight viral infection.

reishi extract or	As directed on label.	
shiitake extract	As directed on label.	
Multivitamin and mineral complex	As directed on label.	To maintain a balance of all necessary nutrients.
Vitamin A emulsion or capsules plus	100,000 IU daily for 1 week, then 50,000 IU daily for 1 week, then reduce to 25,000 IU daily. If you are pregnant, do not exceed 10,000 IU daily. 25,000 IU daily for 1 week; then reduce to 10,000 IU daily. If you are pregnant, do not exceed 10,000 IU daily.	Aids healing and potentiates immune function. Emulsion form is recommended for easier assimilation and greater safety at high doses.
carotenoid complex with beta-carotene	As directed on label.	Provides important antioxidant protection. Enhances immunity.
Vitamin C with bioflavonoids	5,000–20,000 mg daily, in divided doses. (See ASCORBIC ACID FLUSH in Part Three.)	Has antiviral properties.
Vitamin E	200 IU daily.	Promotes healing and tissue repair. Use d-alpha-tocopherol form.
Zinc lozenges	As directed on label.	For pain relief, healing, and improved immune function.

Herbs

❑ Bee pollen, blackberry, calendula, and cayenne all have been known to soothe or heal a sore throat.

Caution: Bee pollen may cause an allergic reaction in some people. Start with a small amount; discontinue if rash, wheezing, discomfort, or other symptom occurs.

❑ Catnip tea enemas help to reduce fever. (*See* ENEMAS in Part Three.)

❑ Echinacea and goldenseal fight bacterial and viral infection.

Cautions: Do not take echinacea for longer than three months. It should not be used by people who are allergic to ragweed. Do not take goldenseal internally on a daily basis for more than one week at a time. Do not use it during pregnancy or if you are breast-feeding, and use with caution if you are allergic to ragweed. If you have a history of cardiovascular disease, diabetes, or glaucoma, use it only under a doctor's supervision.

❑ Fenugreek used as a gargle can relieve a sore throat and reduce the pain of swollen glands. Add 20 drops of extract to 1 cup water and gargle with the mixture three times daily.

❑ Licorice soothes a sore, hoarse throat. Lungwort soothes throat irritation. Licorice can be found in lozenge form.

Caution: Licorice root should not be used during pregnancy or nursing, or by persons with diabetes, glaucoma, heart disease, high blood pressure, or a history of stroke.

❑ Marshmallow root tea soothes a scratchy, itchy throat.

❑ Raspberry leaf tea is good for easing the pain of a sore throat as well as fever blisters.

❑ Hot mullein poultices are soothing to sore throats. (*See* USING A POULTICE in Part Three.)

❑ Olive leaf extract has been found to be a good remedy for a sore throat.

❑ Singer's Saving Grace from Herbs, Etc. is a soothing throat spray that contains a combination of several herbs, including echinacea, licorice, and ginger.

Recommendations

❑ Be sure to cook all your food until it is tender. Poaching and steaming are good methods of cooking to retain moisture.

❑ Cut your food into very small pieces—or, if necessary, grind or purée it. This will cause less irritation to the throat. Be sure to chew your food well before swallowing.

❑ Use frozen popsicles, ice cream, yogurt, and sherbet to soothe a sore throat.

❑ Avoid eating foods that are spicy, hot, salty, or acidic. These can be irritating to the throat.

❑ If you are having an especially difficult time swallowing and are not able to get the proper intake of nutrients, try drinking an instant breakfast drink.

❑ If your physician prescribes antibiotics for a bacterial throat infection, eat yogurt and take an acidophilus supplement to replace the "friendly" bacteria. Do not take the acidophilus at the same time as the antibiotic, however.

❑ Liquid vitamin C, made by dissolving vitamin C powder in water or juice, is good to sip. Allow it to drip down the throat slowly.

❑ Gargle alternately with chlorophyll liquid and sea salt (½ teaspoon in a glass of warm water) every few hours.

❑ Drink plenty of liquids. Fresh juices are best.

❑ Sip tea made from chamomile or sage, or some chicken or vegetable broth to keep your throat lubricated.

Cautions: Do not use chamomile if you are allergic to ragweed. Do not use during pregnancy or nursing. It may interact with warfarin or cyclosporine, so patients using these drugs should avoid it. Do not use sage if you suffer from any type of seizure disorder, or are pregnant or nursing.

❑ Use a mixture of raw honey and lemon juice to coat and soothe the throat.

Caution: Do not give raw honey to infants or to people with poor immune systems.

❑ Try using homeopathic remedies to relieve symptoms. *Aconite, Belladonna, Ferrum phosphoricum,* and *Gelsemium* are some of the homeopathic remedies that have been used to treat sore throat.

❑ *See* FASTING in Part Three, and follow the program.

❑ If you smoke, stop. Smoking is a major cause of sore throats. (*See* SMOKING DEPENDENCY in Part Two.)

Snoring can make a sore throat much more painful. If you snore, try sleeping on your side or using adhesive strips that hold the nostrils open. These can be found in drugstores and many supermarkets.

Seek a physician's care if your sore throat is accompanied by any of the following:

- *High or persistent fever.* A fever that is higher than 101°F should be evaluated by a physician.

- *Rash.* This can be a sign of strep throat or other potentially serious conditions.

- *Severe headache and stiff neck.* This can be a symptom of meningitis.

- *Prolonged hoarseness.* This may indicate an underlying medical problem such as throat cancer or oral cancer.

Considerations

A constant tickle or chronic irritating cough can be an indication of food allergies. (*See* ALLERGIES in Part Two.)

If sore throat recurs or lasts for longer than two weeks, you may have an underlying illness such as mononucleosis.

Many sore throats and infections are contracted from bacteria on toothbrushes. Toothbrushes should be replaced once monthly and after any type of infectious illness. Between uses, store your toothbrush in hydrogen peroxide or grapefruit seed extract to kill germs (if you use hydrogen peroxide, rinse the toothbrush well before brushing).

Breathing in dry air can sometimes worsen the soreness. A humidifier or vaporizer can help by adding more moisture to the air.

See also COMMON COLD; MONONUCLEOSIS; SINUSITIS; and TONSILLITIS, all in Part Two.

SPIDER BITES AND SCORPION STINGS

The bites of all spiders can be poisonous and painful. However, most spiders are not big enough to cause serious harm. Infants, older adults, and people of any age who have allergies are at greatest risk of having more serious reactions.

A bite from a poisonous spider may produce a wide variety of symptoms, including intense pain, numbness, redness, and swelling in the affected area, as well as generalized convulsions, difficulty breathing, dizziness, fever or chills, headache, impaired speech, itching, joint pain, muscle spasms, muscular cramping, nausea, stiffness, sweating, vomiting, and weakness.

Two types of spider—the black widow and the brown recluse—are more poisonous than most and can cause serious reactions. The black widow spider has a black body with a distinctive red hourglass shape on the main body segment. It injects a neurotoxin (nerve poison) that can cause a variety of symptoms, including immediate pain, burning, swelling, and redness at the site of the bite (dou-

ble fang marks may be visible); cramping pain and muscle rigidity in the stomach, chest, shoulders, and back; abdominal pain similar to that of appendicitis; spastic muscle contractions; headache; dizziness; rash and itching; restlessness and anxiety; sweating; swelling of the eyelids; nausea and/or vomiting; salivation and/or tearing of the eyes; weakness, tremors, or paralysis, especially in the legs; and localized tissue death. In about 1 percent of cases, black widow bites lead to anaphylactic shock and death. It is important to note, however, that symptoms similar to those of a black widow spider bite can resemble those of other conditions or medical problems. If you suspect a black widow bite, always consult your physician for a diagnosis and, if appropriate, emergency treatment.

The brown recluse spider is about an inch across, including the legs. Its body is only about 3/8-inch long and has a violin-like marking (the neck of the violin is pointed toward the rear of the spider). The venom of the brown recluse spider is necrotic (causes local tissue damage or death), and it usually creates a blister encircled by red and white rings—it looks like a deep-blue or purple area located around the bite, surrounded by a whitish ring and large red outer ring). This "bull's-eye" appearance is used to distinguish it from other spider bites. Other common symptoms include burning, pain, itching, or redness at the site that may develop as soon as several hours or as long as several days after the bite; an ulcer or blister that turns black; headache and/or body aches; rash; fever; and nausea and/or vomiting. Death from this type of bite is even rarer than from black widow bites, but if you think you may have been bitten by a poisonous spider, you should seek medical help immediately. As with black widow bites, the symptoms of a brown recluse spider bite may resemble those of other conditions or medical problems, and a physician should be consulted for diagnosis and treatment.

Scorpions can be identified by their elongated bodies and curled tails, the ends of which are equipped with a curved "fang" or stinger. There are more than 1,500 species of scorpions, which are related to spiders. In the United States, dangerous scorpions are usually limited in range to the southwestern states, and while their stings are not necessarily deadly, they are extremely painful. Some people describe a scorpion bite as feeling like a hornet sting followed by having a nail driven through the sting site. Other symptoms may follow a scorpion sting as well, among them malaise, sweating, heart palpitations, rise in blood pressure, salivation, nausea, vomiting, and diarrhea. Compared with their U.S. counterparts, Mexican scorpions are another matter altogether; some 1,000 people a year die from their stings. Any type of scorpion sting requires emergency medical attention and should be approached in the same way as snakebite. (*See* What to Do in Case of Snakebite on page 728.) It is possible for hyperacute (typically allergic) reactions to occur in susceptible individuals, taking the form of blurring of consciousness, unconsciousness, convulsions, a rapid drop in blood pressure, shock, and, in extreme cases, death.

The recommendations for nutritional supplements and herbs outlined here are intended to alleviate pain and hasten healing *after appropriate medical care has been administered*. They are *not* meant to substitute for it. Unless otherwise stated, the dosages recommended here are for adults. For children between the ages of twelve and seventeen, reduce the dose to three-quarters of the recommended amount. For children between the ages of six and twelve, use one-half the recommended dose, and for children under six, use one-quarter of the recommended amount.

NUTRIENTS

SUPPLEMENT	SUGGESTED DOSAGE	COMMENTS
Helpful		
Calcium and magnesium	1,000–2,000 mg daily until the wound heals. 500–1,000 mg daily until the wound heals.	Helps relieve pain. Use calcium gluconate form. Needed to balance with calcium.
Charcoal tablets	6–10 capsules as soon as possible after the bite or sting, taken with a large glass of water.	A powerful detoxifying agent. Take immediately after being bitten/stung if possible.
Colloidal silver	Apply topically as directed on label.	An antibiotic that reduces inflammation, promotes healing, and inhibits infection.
Dimethylglycine (DMG) (Aangamik DMG from FoodScience of Vermont)	As directed on label.	Enhances immunity and detoxifies the body.
Flaxseed oil	As directed on label.	Reduces pain and inflammation and aids recovery.
Herpanacine from Diamond-Herpanacine Associates	As directed on label.	Promotes good skin health and detoxifies the body.
Multivitamin and mineral complex	As directed on label.	To maintain a balance of all essential nutrients.
Pycnogenol or grape seed extract	As directed on label. As directed on label.	Protects the skin, reduces inflammation, and enhances immunity.
Ultimate Cleanse from Nature's Secret	As directed on label.	Stimulates and detoxifies the organs and blood.
Vitamin A plus carotenoid complex with beta-carotene	10,000 IU daily. As directed on label.	Enhances immunity and protects protects the body from bacteria. Powerful antioxidants that boost the immune system.
Vitamin B complex plus extra Vitamin B₅ (pantothenic acid)	As directed on label. 500 mg daily.	Maintains healthy nerves and skin. A sublingual form is recommended. Has antiallergenic and antistress properties.
Vitamin C with bioflavonoids	1,000 mg every hour until pain and swelling subside.	Aids in detoxifying the venom and eliminating it from the body. Very important in crisis allergy situations.
Vitamin E oil	Apply topically to the affected area 3 to 4 times daily.	Aids healing and relieves discomfort. Purchase in oil form or cut open a capsule to release the oil.
Zinc	60–90 mg daily. Do not exceed a total of 100 mg daily from all supplements.	Boosts immune response. Also acts as a natural insect repellent. Use zinc gluconate lozenges or OptiZinc for best absorption.

Herbs

❑ Any of the following poultices may be beneficial (*see* USING A POULTICE in Part Three):

- A combination of dandelion and yellow dock relieves itchy skin.

- Fenugreek and flaxseed mixed with slippery elm bark is useful for treating inflammation.

- Goldenseal is good for inflammations of all kinds.

  Caution: Do not take goldenseal internally on a daily basis for more than one week at a time. Do not use it during pregnancy or if you are breast-feeding, and use with caution if you are allergic to ragweed. If you have a history of cardiovascular disease, diabetes, or glaucoma, use it only under a doctor's supervision.

- A mixture of lobelia and crushed charcoal tablets is beneficial for insect bites and most wounds.

  Caution: Lobelia is only to be taken under supervision of a health care professional as it is potentially toxic. People with high blood pressure, heart disease, liver disease, kidney disease, seizure disorders, or shortness of breath should not take lobelia. Pregnant and lactating women should avoid lobelia as well.

❑ A tincture made from calendula buds and alcohol should be on hand for stings and other "surface" injuries. A poultice made from the fresh flower heads is also good. (*See* USING A POULTICE in Part Three.)

❑ A cream containing 5 percent tea tree oil helps to heal insect bites, sunburn, cuts, rashes, and other skin irritations.

❑ Echinacea, taken in tea or capsule form, boosts the immune system.

Caution: Do not take echinacea for longer than three months. It should not be used by people who are allergic to ragweed.

❑ Ginkgo biloba helps to relieve muscle pains.

Caution: Do not take ginkgo biloba if you have a bleeding disorder, or are scheduled for surgery or a dental procedure.

❑ Yellow dock purifies the blood and is beneficial for many problems affecting the skin. Drink as much yellow dock tea as you can, or take 2 capsules of yellow dock every hour until symptoms are relieved.

Recommendations

❑ Use essential oils of basil, cinnamon, lavender, lemon, sage, savory, or thyme for their antitoxic and antivenin properties. Apply a drop of essential oil on the sting.

Caution: Do not use sage if you suffer from any type of seizure disorder, or are pregnant or nursing.

Considerations

❑ Specific treatment for a brown recluse spider bite will be determined by your physician. Treatment may include washing the area well with soap and water; applying a cold or ice pack wrapped in a cloth, or a cold, wet washcloth to the site; applying an antibiotic lotion or cream to protect against infection (especially for children); taking acetaminophen (Tylenol or the equivalent) for pain; elevating the site of the bite if possible to help prevent swelling; and, depending on the severity of the bite, administration of corticosteroids and other medications and/or surgery on the ulcerated area. Hospitalization may be needed.

❑ Specific treatment for a black widow spider bite will be determined by your physician. Treatment may include washing the area well with soap and water; applying a cold or ice pack wrapped in a cloth, or a cold, wet washcloth to the site (ice should *not* be applied directly to the skin); application of an antibiotic lotion or cream to protect against infection (especially for children); taking acetaminophen (Tylenol or the equivalent); treatment with muscle relaxants, pain relievers, and/or other medications; plus supportive care. Antivenin may be needed, although it is usually not required. In some cases, hospitalization may be required.

❑ Treatment of a scorpion sting may include applying an ice pack wrapped in cloth to ease pain at the site of the sting; injections of a morphine-based painkiller; and, in the case of more serious symptoms, treatment similar to those used for snakebite. The individual must receive treatment, including supportive medical treatment, as quickly as possible. There is antivenin available for scorpion venom. Its use must be overseen by a doctor.

❑ In life-threatening cases of spider bite, massive injections of vitamin C and vitamin B$_5$ (pantothenic acid), administered by a medical professional, may be invaluable. This is something only a medical professional can decide.

❑ For bites that do not appear to be life-threatening, a doctor may administer calcium gluconate to relieve muscle soreness and an antianxiety medication for muscle spasms.

❑ Hydrocortisone ointment, calamine lotion, or a paste made from baking soda may be used to soothe the wound.

❑ Rattlesnake and black widow venom are similar in many respects. Treatment for a black widow bite is therefore similar to that for snakebite.

❑ If you have been bitten by any type of spider, it is important to be sure that your tetanus immunization is current.

❑ *See also* BEE STING; INSECT ALLERGY; and/or SNAKEBITE in Part Two.

SPRAINS, STRAINS, AND OTHER INJURIES OF THE MUSCLES AND JOINTS

A sprain is not the same thing as a strain. If a muscle is stressed beyond its capability, it becomes *strained*. Putting undue weight on the muscles and using the muscles for prolonged periods without rest can create muscle strain. A strained muscle may go into spasms or knot up instead of relaxing normally. Localized pain (during movement), swelling, and loss of mobility occur.

If one of the ligaments, the tissues that connect bones to muscles, is wrenched or stretched excessively, the ligament may tear, causing a *sprain*. There is likely to be a brief sharp pain followed by rapid swelling. Soft tissue surrounding the joint may be sore and bruised. Sprains can result from unexpected movement or twisting of the affected area, or from a hard fall. The joints most often sprained are the ankle, back, finger, knee, and wrist.

These types of injuries are common in athletes. In most cases, they heal on their own. The following supplement program can help these injuries heal. Unless otherwise stated, the dosages recommended here are for adults. For children between the ages of twelve and seventeen, reduce the dose to three-quarters of the recommended amount. For children between the ages of six and twelve, use one-half the recommended dose, and for children under six, use one-quarter of the recommended amount.

NUTRIENTS

SUPPLEMENT	SUGGESTED DOSAGE	COMMENTS
Very Important		
Chondroitin sulfate	500–1,000 mg daily.	Nutritional support for strengthening joints, ligaments, and tendons.
Glucosamine sulfate (GS-500 from Enzymatic Therapy) or N-Acetylglucosamine (N-A-G from Source Naturals)	As directed on label.	Very important for the formation of bones, tendons, ligaments, cartilage, and synovial (joint) fluid.
Inf-zyme Forte from American Biologics	As directed on label. Take between meals.	To destroy free radicals released during injury.
Methylsulfonyl-methane (MSM)	500–1,000 mg 3 times daily.	A sulfur compound needed for reducing pain and inflammation; also for joint and tissue repair.
Helpful		
Bromelain	400 mg 3 times daily, between meals.	An enzyme that helps to stimulate production of prostaglandins and reduces inflammation.

Calcium	1,500–2,000 mg daily.	Needed for repair of connective tissue. Use both calcium chelate and calcium gluconate forms to assure assimilation. Very important for the skeletal system. Calcium supplementation may increase the risk of prostate cancer.
and magnesium	750–1,000 mg daily.	
Curcumin	600 mg 3 times daily.	Reduces inflammation and aids in healing.
Desiccated liver	As directed on label.	Aids in building healthy blood cells.
Dimethylglycine (DMG) (Aangamik DMG from FoodScience Labs)	As directed on label.	Increases tissue oxygenation.
Essential fatty acids (flaxseed oil or Ultimate Oil from Nature's Secret)	As directed on label.	Promotes cellular and cardiovascular health; improves stamina and speeds recovery.
Free form amino acid	As directed on label, on an empty stomach.	To help repair and strengthen connective tissue, reduce body fat, and increase energy.
Grape seed extract	As directed on label.	A powerful anti-inflammatory.
L-leucine plus L-isoleucine and L-valine	As directed on label, on an empty stomach. Take with water or juice. Do not take with milk. Take with 50 mg vitamin B$_6$ and 100 mg vitamin C for better absorption.	Branched-chain amino acids that promote the healing of bones, skin, and muscle tissue. (See AMINO ACIDS in Part One.)
Manganese	15 mg daily.	Strengthens wounded ligaments and/or tendons.
Multivitamin and mineral complex	As directed on label.	To promote good health, nutritional balance, and tissue repair.
Neonatal Multi-Gland from Biotics Research	As directed on label.	To stimulate healing of connective tissue.
Potassium	99 mg daily.	Vital for tissue repair.
S-Adenosyl-methionine (SAMe) (SAMe Rx-Mood from Nature's Plus)	400 mg 2 times daily.	Deficiency results in the inability to maintain cartilage properly. Aids in reducing pain and inflammation. Caution: Do not use if you have bipolar mood disorder or take prescription antidepressants. Do not give to a child under twelve.
Silica	500 mg daily.	Supplies silicon, needed for connective tissue repair and calcium absorption.
Vitamin A plus carotenoid complex with beta-carotene	10,000 IU daily. As directed on label.	Enhances immunity and aids in protein utilization. Powerful antioxidants that boost the immune system.
Vitamin B complex plus extra vitamin B$_5$ (pantothenic acid)	100 mg of each major B vitamin daily (amounts of individual vitamins in a complex will vary). 500 mg daily.	All the B vitamins are important during stressful situations. Use a high-potency formula. The most important antistress vitamin.
Vitamin C with	5,000–20,000 mg daily, in divided doses.	An antioxidant required for tissue growth and repair.
bioflavonoids	(See ASCORBIC ACID FLUSH in Part Three.)	Calcium ascorbate is the best source of vitamin C to use for these injuries.
Vitamin E	200 IU daily.	A free radical scavenger. Use d-alpha-tocopherol form.
Zinc	50 mg daily. Do not exceed a total of 100 mg daily from all supplements.	Important in tissue repair. Use zinc gluconate lozenges or OptiZinc for best absorption.

Herbs

❏ Boswellia, an Ayurvedic herb, is good for reducing inflammation. Choose a product standardized to contain 150 milligrams of boswellic acids per dose. Boswellia cream can be good for relieving pain as well. Boswellin Cream from Nature's Herbs is a good product.

❏ Fenugreek and flaxseed powder can be combined with slippery elm bark to make a poultice for swelling. (See USING A POULTICE in Part Three.)

❏ Feverfew and ginger are good for pain and soreness.

Caution: Do not use feverfew when pregnant or nursing. People who take prescription blood-thinning medications should consult a health care provider before using feverfew, as the combination can result in internal bleeding.

❏ Ginger is also a powerful antioxidant that has anti-inflammatory effects.

❏ Green tea and nettle leaf have anti-inflammatory properties.

Caution: Green tea contains vitamin K, which can make anticoagulant medications less effective. Consult your health care professional if you are using them. The caffeine in green tea could cause insomnia, anxiety, upset stomach, nausea, or diarrhea.

❏ Goldenseal poultices are good for reducing inflammation.

Caution: Do not take goldenseal internally on a daily basis for more than one week at a time. Do not use it during pregnancy or if you are breast-feeding, and use with caution if you are allergic to ragweed. If you have a history of cardiovascular disease, diabetes, or glaucoma, use it only under a doctor's supervision.

❏ Horse chestnut extract gel, applied topically to the injured area, can reduce swelling and inflammation.

❏ Mustard poultices are good for swelling and can relax tense muscles.

❏ After the initial treatment of applying ice to the injury, combine turmeric and a little hot water to make a paste. Apply this mixture to the injured area with a gauze dressing. This treatment helps to reduce swelling. It is also good for bruising.

Sports Nutrition for the Serious Bodybuilder

Nutrition and dietary supplements have become a focus of serious attention from athletes of all types, especially bodybuilders. Many of them have found that the combination of proper diet, appropriate supplements, and a good comprehensive workout plan work together to help them achieve their personal goals. There are three basic approaches to the use of supplements to build muscle: providing the body with protein that it can use to make the muscle; promoting the body's production of androgenic hormones such as testosterone so that it is inclined to build itself up in response to exercise; and providing nutrients that increase endurance, so that more—and more strenuous—exercise is possible.

Note: This regimen is an advanced supplementation program intended for the serious bodybuilder who has some knowledge of sports nutrition, not for the person who has just begun to exercise or tone his or her muscles.

SUPPLEMENT	SUGGESTED DOSAGE	COMMENTS
Beta-hydroxy-beta-methylbutyrate (HMB)	As directed on label. Take sublingually, as directed on label.	Potent cortisol inhibitor. Cortisol is an anti-anabolic agent released as a result of strenuous physical exertion. *Caution:* Do not use if you are suffering from joint problems.
Calcium D-gluconate	200–400 mg. daily.	Blocks conversion of testosterone to estrogen.
Calcium pyruvate	2,000–6,000 mg daily, with meals.	Enhances endurance by as much as 20 to 50 percent. Increases metabolism, resulting in fat loss of up to 48 percent. Increases protein uptake.
Chrysin	500–2,000 mg daily, with meals.	Prevents excess testosterone precursors from being converted to estrogen in the body. This increases lean muscle mass development.
Colostrum	2,000–3,000 mg daily.	Helps stimulate growth, regeneration, and repair of muscle, skin, bone, and cartilage. Stimulates body to catabolize adipose (fat) tissue rather than lean muscle tissue.
Conjugated linoleic acid (CLA)	750–1,500 mg daily, with meals.	Decreases body fat, improves muscle tone, and increases lean muscle mass gain and exercise tolerance.
Creatine	Loading phase: 30 g daily. Maintenance: 5 g daily.	Use micronized effervescent or micronized creatine monohydrate form. These are more easily digested than ordinary creatine. Avoid products from Asia due to quality issues.
Cross-flow microfiltered whey protein isolates (IsoPure from Nature's Best or Pro Complex from Optimum Nutrition)	1 g for every 2.2 lbs of body weight.	To promote protein synthesis. Provides glycomacropeptides, low molecular weight oligopeptides, and branched-chain amino acids.
D-ribose	2,200 mg daily. Can be taken with creatine to boost its effectiveness.	Increases effectiveness of creatine monohydrate. A precursor to ATP (the cellular energy source). Complements creatine monohydrate in its ability to generate lean muscle mass, endurance, and muscular energy.
GH Stak from Muscle-Link	As directed on label.	Increases lean muscle mass, reduces adipose (fat tissue), supports cardiac output, increases libido, increases energy. Improves blood lipid levels, slows down overall body deterioration associated with aging. Use effervescent or sublingual forms only.
Glucosamine sulfate	1,500–4,000 mg daily.	To improve joint integrity, function, and range of motion.
Human growth hormone (HGH) (Humagro or Testatropinol from Advanced Sports Nutrition)	As directed on label.	Homeopathic growth hormone 4c impacts testosterone, growth hormone, adrenaline, adrenocorticotropic hormone, luteinizing hormone, FSH, and TSH.
Methylsulfonyl-methane (MSM)	1,000–4,000 mg daily.	To improve tissue integrity in the joints.
Ornithine alpha-ketoglutarate (OKG)	1,300–2,600 mg daily, before exercise or at bedtime.	Helps prevent muscle tissue breakdown. Aids in muscle growth and stimulates growth hormone release.
7 Keto-DHEA	50–150 mg daily.	The best form of DHEA—it is not converted into estrogens in the body. Slows overall body deterioration. Enhances fat loss and lean muscle mass development.
Sodium phosphate and potassium bicarbonate	As directed on label.	Delay onset of muscular fatigue by buffering lactic acid, improving muscular power and endurance.

HERBS

❑ *Tribulus terrestris* (an herb whose common name is puncture vine) increases production of luteinizing hormone and testosterone in men, thereby increasing strength and lean muscle mass.

❑ Yohimbe is a central nervous system stimulant that increases testosterone levels. It is used to increase strength and lean muscle mass, as well as to enhance libido.

Caution: Yohimbe should not be used by women who are pregnant or nursing. Do not use yohimbe if you have high blood pressure, heart disease, stomach ulcers, depression, or other psychiatric conditions. There have been cases of people dying from taking too much yohimbe.

RECOMMENDATIONS

❑ For bruises, muscle strain, and other workout-related injuries, use homeopathic *Arnica montana.*

CONSIDERATIONS

❑ Research performed at the University of Toronto in Canada demonstrated that by mixing a specified amount of water with a creatine monohydrate mixture containing creatine and carbohydrates, you can vastly increase the speed at which the creatine and carbohydrates enter the bloodstream, thus enhancing your training. This is known as the osmotic acceleration principle. The following schedule applies:

Body Weight	Creatine mix	Water
0–170 lbs	9 g creatine 65 g carbohydrate	10 oz, followed by 10 oz 10 minutes later.
170 220 lbs	10 g creatine 75 g carbohydrate	20 oz, followed by 10 oz 10 minutes later.
220–300 lbs	12 g creatine 85 g carbohydrate	20 oz, followed by 12 oz 10 minutes later.

Cell-Tech from MuscleTech is a premade creatine product that can be used for this purpose.

Recommendations

❑ Immediately after the injury, raise the affected area—above heart level if possible—and apply ice for no longer than twenty minutes. *Do not* use heat immediately following an injury. On the first day, apply ice for twenty minutes and then remove ice for twenty minutes. Continue this throughout the day. On day two, apply ice intermittently every four hours. Then, after the inflammation has subsided, apply heat for twenty-minute periods two or three times a day. If possible, use a splint or sling to immobilize and protect the injured area.

❑ If there is significant swelling, call your physician right away or go to a hospital emergency room to have the injury evaluated. Especially with injuries to the wrists and ankles, it is wise to have X-rays taken to make sure no bones have been broken.

❑ Consume plenty of juices made from fresh raw vegetables, including beets, garlic, and radishes. Raw vegetables are high in valuable vitamins and enzymes.

❑ Use homeopathic remedies to ease the discomfort. Homeopathic remedies used to treat symptoms of sprains, strains, and other types of injuries include *Aconitum napellus, Arnica montana, Hypericum, Rhus toxicodendron, Ruta graveolens,* and *Symphytum officinalis.*

❑ To prevent sprains and strains, do stretching exercises both before and after exercise and other physical activity.

Considerations

❑ Minor sprains can usually be treated at home. However, anytime an injury becomes painful and swollen, you should see a medical professional—especially if you hear a popping sound and find that you cannot use the injured joint normally.

❑ Aromatherapy can be helpful. Cold compresses made with essential oils of camphor, chamomile, eucalyptus, lavender, and/or rosemary are good. Add 10 drops or so of essential oil to 1 quart of cool water and use the mixture to make the compresses.

❑ Clay poultices can be used to treat sprains and fractures. (*See* USING A POULTICE in Part Three.)

❑ The risk of injury to the muscles and joints is higher in contact sports than in other types of activity.

❑ *See* Sports Nutrition for the Serious Bodybuilder, the preceding table.

❑ *See* BRUISING and FRACTURE, both in Part Two.

❑ *See also* PAIN CONTROL in Part Three.

STRESS

The term "stress" refers to any reaction to a physical, mental, social, or emotional stimulus that requires a response or alteration to the way we perform, think, or feel. Change is stressful—whether the change is good or bad. Worry produces stress. Indeed, stress is an unavoidable part of life. It can result from many things, both physical and psychological. Pressures and deadlines at work, problems with loved ones, the need to pay the bills, and getting ready for the holidays are obvious sources of stress for many people. Less obvious sources include everyday encounters with crowds, noise, traffic, pain, extremes of temperature, and even welcome events such as starting a new job or the birth or adoption of a child. Overwork, lack of sleep, and physical illness put stress on the body. Excessive alcohol consumption and smoking are usually increased as a reaction to stress and yet create more stress for the body. Some people create their own stress; whether there is anything objectively wrong in their lives or not, they find things to worry about. For such people, stress becomes almost an addiction.

Some people handle stress well, and it has little impact on their emotional or physical health. Others are very negatively influenced by it. Stress can cause fatigue, chronic headaches, irritability, changes in appetite, memory loss, low self-esteem, withdrawal, teeth grinding, cold hands, high blood pressure, shallow breathing, nervous twitches, lowered sexual drive, insomnia or other changes in sleep patterns, and/or gastrointestinal disorders. Stress creates an excellent breeding ground for illness. Researchers estimate that stress contributes to many major illnesses, including cardiovascular disease, cancer, endocrine and metabolic disease, skin disorders, and infectious ailments of all kinds. Many psychiatrists believe that the majority of back problems—one of the most common adult ailments in the United States—are related to stress. Stress is also a common precursor of psychological difficulties such as anxiety and depression.

Stress is often viewed as a psychological problem, but it has very real physical effects. The body responds to stress with a series of physiological changes that include increased secretion of adrenaline, elevation of blood pressure, acceleration of the heartbeat, and greater tension in the muscles. Digestion slows or stops, fats and sugars are released from stores in the body, cholesterol levels rise, and the composition of the blood changes slightly, making it more prone to clotting. This in turn increases the risk of stroke or heart attack.

Almost all body functions and organs react to stress. The pituitary gland increases its production of adrenocorticotropic hormone (ACTH), which in turn stimulates the release of the hormones cortisone and cortisol. These have the effect of inhibiting the functioning of disease-fighting white blood cells and suppressing the immune response. This complex of physical changes is called the "fight or flight" response and is apparently designed to prepare one to face an immediate danger. Today, most of our stresses are not the result of physical threats, but the body still responds as if they were.

The increased production of adrenal hormones is responsible for most of the symptoms associated with stress. It is also the reason that stress can lead to nutritional deficiencies. Increased adrenaline production causes the body to step up its metabolism of proteins, fats, and carbohydrates to quickly produce energy for the body to use. This response causes the body to excrete amino acids, potassium, and phosphorus; to deplete magnesium stored in muscle tissue; and to store less calcium. Stress also triggers the release of cortisol, an adrenal hormone that regulates carbohydrate metabolism and blood pressure. It also ages brain cells and builds fat around the body's midsection. Further, stress increases the level of an immune system protein called interleukin-6 (IL-6), which has direct effects on most of the cells in the body and is associated with many disorders, including diabetes, arthritis, cancer, osteoporosis, Alzheimer's disease, periodontal disease, and cardiovascular disease. IL-6 has also been linked to frailty and functional decline in older adults. IL-6 has been shown to be affected by several controllable factors. For example, being obese compared to lean causes a greater release of IL-6 after meals. In addition, high-glycemic-load carbohydrates like potatoes evoke a greater release of IL-6 than high-fiber foods like bran. In one study, both waist circumference and cortisol release were associated with high IL-6 levels. Achieving a normal body weight and eating a low-glycemic-load diet, rich in fruits, vegetables, and whole grains, can reduce the release of IL-6 and the risk of developing the diseases associated with it.

As a result of a complex of physical reactions, the body does not absorb nutrients well when it is under stress. The result is that, especially with prolonged or recurrent stress, the body becomes at once deficient in many nutrients and unable to replace them adequately. Many of the disorders that arise from stress are the result of nutritional deficiencies, especially deficiencies of the B-complex vitamins, which are very important for proper functioning of the nervous system, and of certain electrolytes, which are depleted by the body's stress response. Stress also promotes the formation of free radicals that can become oxidized and damage body tissues, especially cell membranes.

Anxiety, panic attacks, obsessive-compulsive disorder, post-traumatic stress disorder (PTSD), dissociative disorders, and phobic disorders are among the more serious emotional manifestations of stress. They are often a result of an event that the individual was unable to deal with at the time. Post-traumatic stress disorder in particular seems to be becoming increasingly common in our stress-filled world. The key sign of PTSD involves mentally reliving past traumatic events in a manner and to an extent that this interferes with normal life. (*See* Is It Stress or Is It PTSD? on page 739.)

Many people attribute their stress-related symptoms to "nerves," and in fact stress usually does affect the parts of the body that are related to the nervous system first, especially through the digestive organs. Symptoms of stress-related digestive disorders may be a flare-up of an ulcer or irritable bowel syndrome. If stress that produces such symptoms is not handled properly, more serious illnesses may result.

Stress can be either acute or long-term. Long-term stress is particularly dangerous. A state of continual stress eventually wears out the body. Because of its effect on the immune response, stress increases susceptibility to illness and slows healing.

Unless otherwise stated, the dosages recommended here are for adults. For children between the ages of twelve and seventeen, reduce the dose to three-quarters of the recommended amount. For children between the ages of six and twelve, use one-half the recommended dose, and for children under six, use one-quarter of the recommended amount.

NUTRIENTS

SUPPLEMENT	SUGGESTED DOSAGE	COMMENTS
Essential		
ACES + Zn from Carlson Labs	2 capsules daily.	Contains beta-carotene, selenium, and vitamins C and E, which work together as antioxidants to disarm damaging free radicals caused by stress.
Gamma-amino-butyric acid (GABA)	750 mg twice daily. Take with 50 mg inositol and 500 mg niacinamide to enhance effectiveness.	Acts as a tranquilizer and is important for proper brain function. (*See* AMINO ACIDS in Part One.)
Glutathione	As directed on label.	An antioxidant that protects the cells against damage.
Inositol	250 mg twice daily.	A nutrient related to the B-vitamins. It can help with panic attacks, obsessive-compulsive disorder, and depression.
Nicotinamide adenine dinucleotide (NADH)	10 mg daily first thing in the morning.	Important in the creation and transfer of chemical energy, especially during breathing.
S-Adenosyl-methionine (SAMe)	As directed on label.	Can ease depression. *Caution:* Do not use if you have bipolar mood disorder or take prescription antidepressants. Do not give to a child under twelve.
Taurine (Taurine Plus from American Biologics)	As directed on label.	Essential amino acid for brain and heart protection. Use a sublingual form.
Trimethylglycine (TMG)	As directed on label.	Reduces homocysteine levels in the blood and acts like SAMe to ease depression.
Vitamin B complex injections plus extra vitamin B₆ (pyridoxine) injections and vitamin B₁₂ injections and/or vitamin B complex plus extra vitamin B₅ (pantothenic acid)	1 cc weekly or as prescribed by physician. ½ cc weekly or as prescribed by physician. 1 cc weekly or as prescribed by physician. 100 mg of each major B vitamin daily (amounts of individual vitamins in a complex will vary). 500 mg daily.	All B vitamins are necessary for health and proper functioning of the nervous system. Intramuscular injections (under a doctor's supervision) give fast results. Take oral supplements either in addition to injections or alone, if injections are unavailable. Use a sublingual form. An antistress vitamin needed by the thymus gland.
Vitamin C with bioflavonoids	3,000–10,000 mg daily.	Essential to adrenal gland function. Stress depletes the gland hormones, the antistress hormones.
Very Important		
Anti-Stress Enzymes from Biotec Foods	As directed on label.	Enzymes that remove toxic wastes and restore balance and equilibrium to the system.
Calcium and magnesium	2,000 mg daily. 1,000 mg daily.	Lost when stress is present. Use calcium chelate form. Deficiency is common in highly stressed individuals, and can result in anxiety, fear, and even hallucinations.
Coenzyme Q₁₀ plus Coenzyme A from Coenzyme-A Technologies	As directed on label. As directed on label.	Both of these coenzymes work to increase energy and protect the heart and immune system.
L-tyrosine	500 mg twice daily, during the day and at bedtime. Take with water or juice on an empty stomach. Do not take with milk. Take with 50 mg vitamin B₆ and 100 mg vitamin C for better absorption.	Helps to reduce stress on the body. An effective and safe sleeping aid. Also good for depression. (*See* AMINO ACIDS in Part One.) *Caution:* Do not take this supplement if you are taking an MAO inhibitor drug.
Melatonin	Start with 1.5 mg daily, taken 2 hours or less before bedtime. If this is not effective, gradually increase the dosage until an effective level is reached (up to 5 mg at night).	A natural hormone that promotes sound sleep; helpful if stress leads to occasional sleeplessness.
Helpful		
Fiber (oat bran or psyllium husks)	As directed on label. Take separately from other supplements and medications.	For bowel cleansing and improved bowel function. Stress often causes diarrhea and/or constipation.
Free form amino acid (Amino Balance from Anabol Naturals)	As directed on label.	To supply protein, which is used rapidly by the body at stressful times. Use a formula containing both essential and nonessential amino acids.
Lecithin granules or capsules	1 tbsp 3 times daily, with meals. 2,400 mg 3 times daily, with meals.	For cellular protection and brain function.
L-lysine	As directed on label. Take with 50 mg vitamin C and 1 15-mg zinc gluconate lozenge.	For cold sores, often an early indicator of stress. Reduces stress so it is better handled. *Caution:* Do not take for longer than six months at a time.
Maitake extract or reishi extract or shiitake extract	As directed on label. As directed on label. As directed on label.	Adaptogens that help the body adapt to stress and normalize body functions.
Multivitamin and mineral complex with natural beta-carotene and potassium and selenium	As directed on label. 25,000 IU daily. 99 mg daily. 200 mcg daily.	Especially necessary during stress. An important antioxidant. To replace potassium lost due to excretion during stress. A potent antioxidant that decreases anxiety attacks.
Raw adrenal glandular and raw thymus glandular	As directed on label. As directed on label.	To stimulate the adrenal and thymus glands, important in the body's stress reaction.
Vitamin E	200 IU daily. Take with meals.	Needed for immune function. A powerful antioxidant. Use d-alpha-tocopherol form.
Zinc	50 mg daily. Do not exceed a total of 100 mg daily from all supplements.	Needed for immune function and to protect the cells from free radical damage. Use zinc gluconate lozenges or OptiZinc for best absorption.

Is It Stress or Is It PTSD?

Post-traumatic stress disorder, or PTSD, is a serious illness that needs professional intervention and treatment. To help decide whether you (or a loved one) might have this disorder, the following five questions are important:

1. Have you ever experienced or witnessed a life-threatening event that caused you to feel intense fear, helplessness, or horror?

2. Do you reexperience this event in at least one of the following ways?

- Repeated distressing memories or dreams.

- Flashbacks or a sense of reliving the event.

- Intense physical and/or emotional distress when exposed to things that remind you of the event.

3. Do you avoid reminders of the event and feel numb, compared with the way you felt before, in three or more of the following ways?

- Avoiding thoughts, feelings, or conversation concerning it.

- Avoiding activities, places, and people who remind you of it.

- Being unable to remember important parts of it.

- Losing interest in significant activities in your life.

- Feeling detached from other people.

- Feeling that your range of emotions is restricted.

- Feeling as if you have no future, and that you cannot expect to have a career, long life, successful marriage, or achieve other important goals.

4. Are you troubled by two or more of the following?

- Problems sleeping.

- Irritability or outbursts of anger.

- Problems with concentration.

- Feeling "on guard" all the time.

- Exaggerated startle response (jumpiness).

5. Do your symptoms interfere with your daily life?

Herbs

❑ Ashwagandha is an Ayurvedic herb that acts as a sedative and nerve tonic.

❑ Bilberry prevents destruction, mutation, and premature death of cells throughout the body.

❑ Ginkgo biloba aids in proper brain function and good circulation.

Caution: Do not take ginkgo biloba if you have a bleeding disorder, or are scheduled for surgery or a dental procedure.

❑ Milk thistle cleanses and protects the liver, and has antioxidant properties.

❑ Many plants produce their own antioxidants, which they use as protection against environmental stresses. Specific herbs tend to protect specific parts of the body. However, because of their strong antioxidant properties, most have important influences on other parts of the body as well. For a robust antistress tonic, mix ½ teaspoon of any three of the herbs listed below and steep in 2 cups of almost-boiling distilled water, or use alcohol-free extracts mixed in water.

❑ Catnip is an effective antistress herb that also causes drowsiness.

❑ Chamomile is a gentle relaxant. It is a good nerve tonic, soothing to the digestive tract, and a pleasant sleep aid.

Caution: Do not use chamomile if you are allergic to ragweed. Do not use during pregnancy or nursing. It may interact with warfarin or cyclosporine, so patients using these drugs should avoid it.

❑ Dong quai, rehmannia, and schizandra support the kidneys, adrenal glands, and central nervous system. These organs are among the most susceptible to the effects of stress.

❑ Holy basil (*Ocimum sanctum*), an Indian herb known locally as *tulsi*, is related to but not the same as culinary basil. It appears to lower stress and cortisol levels. A Thai derivative is known as bai gkaprow.

❑ Hops helps to ease nervousness, restlessness, and stress. It also decreases the desire for alcohol.

❑ For some people, kava kava may relax the mind as well as the entire body.

Caution: Kava kava can cause drowsiness. It is not recommended for pregnant women or nursing mothers, and it should not be taken together with other substances that act on the central nervous system, such as alcohol, barbiturates, antidepressants, and antipsychotic drugs.

❑ Essential oil of mandarin, used in conjunction with bergamot oil in an aromatherapy lamp, is a proven stress reducer. Mix 5 drops of mandarin oil with 3 drops of bergamot oil.

❑ Passionflower is calming and is a potent addition to any antistress formula.

❑ Polygala root and sour jujube seed are powerful Chinese herbs known to soothe and calm the spirit.

❑ For some individuals, St. John's wort is good for depression and nerve pain.

Caution: St. John's wort may cause increased sensitivity to sunlight. It may also produce anxiety, gastrointestinal symptoms, and headaches. It can interact with some drugs including antidepressants, birth control pills, and anticoagulants.

❑ Siberian ginseng helps the body cope with stress.

Caution: Do not use Siberian ginseng if you have hypoglycemia, high blood pressure, or a heart disorder.

❑ Skullcap is good for nervous disorders. It also relieves headaches and aids sleep.

❑ Valerian keeps the nervous system from being overwhelmed. It also is a powerful sleep aid when taken at bedtime and helps to ease stress-related headaches.

❑ Wild oat is said to restore balance to the nervous system.

Recommendations

❑ Eat a diet composed of 50 to 75 percent raw foods. Fresh fruits and vegetables not only supply valuable vitamins and minerals, but are rich in compounds called flavonoids, many of which scavenge and neutralize dangerous free radicals.

❑ Avoid processed foods and all foods that create stress on the system, such as artificial sweeteners, carbonated soft drinks, chocolate, eggs, fried foods, junk foods, pork, red meat, sugar, white flour products, foods containing preservatives or heavy spices, and chips and similar snack foods.

❑ Eliminate dairy products from your diet for three weeks. Then reintroduce them slowly—and watch for returning symptoms of your "nervous" condition. During this time, make a point to get adequate calcium, magnesium, and vitamin D from other foods or supplements, as they are found primarily in dairy products.

❑ Limit your intake of caffeine. Caffeine contributes to nervousness and can disrupt sleep patterns.

❑ Avoid alcohol, tobacco, and mood-altering drugs. While these substances may offer temporary relief from stress, they do nothing to really address the problem, and they are harmful to your health. The stress will still be there the next day.

❑ Follow a monthly fasting program. (*See* FASTING in Part Three.)

❑ Get regular exercise. Physical activity can clear your mind and keep stress under control. Some people like to run or walk by themselves, while others prefer team sports or group workouts. Any type of exercise will do the trick, as long as it is *regular*. Exercising only once a month will not do much to relieve stress.

Caution: If you are thirty-five or older and/or have been sedentary for some time, consult with your health care provider before beginning an exercise program.

❑ Learn to relax. Relaxation is often difficult for people suffering from the effects of stress, but it is necessary. A technique called *progressive relaxation* can be helpful. This involves tightening and relaxing the major muscle groups one at a time, being aware of each sensation. Start at your feet and work up to your head. Tense the muscles for a count of ten, concentrating on the tension, then let the muscles go lax and breathe deeply, enjoying the sensation of release.

❑ Get sufficient sleep each night. This may be difficult, because stress can keep you up at night (unless you are one of those people who welcomes sleep as an escape), but it is very important. The less sleep you get, the more stress will affect you, the more your immune system will weaken, and the greater your chance of becoming ill will be.

❑ Try meditation. Many people find that regular meditation helps them to relax and handle stress. Meditation does not have to have spiritual or religious connotations. For example, you can meditate on a word such as "peace," "calm," "relax," or "warm." Or you may find it helpful to meditate on a pleasant person, place, or event. It is good to have a store of pleasant thoughts to draw on during stressful times. While meditation can have some short-term benefits, it is more effective when practiced on a daily basis. Try meditating twice a day for ten to twenty minutes each time.

❑ Practice deep breathing. This can be done when facing a stressful situation—at home, at work, in your car, or elsewhere. Holding your breath is also good for relieving stress. Inhale deeply with your mouth closed, hold your breath for a few seconds (do not wait until you are uncomfortable), then exhale slowly through your mouth, with your tongue placed at the top of your teeth, next to the gum line. Do this four or five times, or until the tension passes. (*See* Breathing Exercises *under* PAIN CONTROL in Part Three.)

❑ Monitor your internal conversations. The way we talk to ourselves has a lot to do with how we feel about ourselves and our environments. Telling yourself things like "I should be able to handle this better," or "I shouldn't have let that idiot cut me off in traffic," or "I'll never get the hang of this computer" only adds to the stressfulness of situations and does nothing to resolve them. Learn to listen for—and then make yourself stop—these futile inner conversations. Some therapists recommend shouting "Get out!" (or any other phrase you choose) immediately when any intrusive and unpleasant worries enter your thoughts.

❑ Identify the sources of stress in your life. This can be an important first step in managing stress. Take a stress inventory periodically to help you understand what is causing your problems. You can use the following list of major stressors as a starting point:

- Death of a spouse or other close family member.
- Divorce.
- Death of a close friend.
- Financial problems.
- Legal separation from spouse.
- Job loss.
- Major injury.

- New marriage.
- Scheduled surgery.
- Change in family member's health.
- Serious trouble at work.
- Increased responsibility at work or at home.
- Sexual problems.
- Change of jobs.
- Child leaving home.
- Change in residence.
- Major change in diet.
- Vacation.
- Allergies.

Remember that this list is not exhaustive and that different people react to the same events differently. Also remember that children and young adults have different lists of stressful situations, which are just as serious for them as those above are for adults.

❑ Take a day off—that's what weekends are for. Take a drive, listen to music, go to the beach or lake, read—whatever you find rewarding and relaxing. Try to keep your thoughts in the present during this time so that you do not think about whatever it is that is causing the stress.

❑ Pursue a hobby. Hobbies are great for relieving stress. Take the time to do what you enjoy. Don't feel guilty about spending time doing something for yourself. Your health is worth it.

❑ Avoid hassles. Identify the things that are making you feel stressed out and either eliminate them from your life or prepare yourself to cope with them. If rush hour traffic causes you stress, see if you can change your work hours slightly to avoid it. If that isn't possible, join a carpool or listen to a book on tape or a favorite piece of music while driving.

❑ Do not repress or deny your emotions. This only compounds stress. Admit your feelings and accept them. Keeping strong feelings bottled up only causes them to resurface later as illness. Don't be afraid to cry. Learning to cry can help you to manage stress. Crying can relieve anxiety and let loose bottled-up emotions.

❑ Work on creating a stress-free home environment. Keep the noise level down—noise contributes to stress. Turn down the radio, stereo, and television. Throw rugs and wall hangings absorb noise and are good additions to decor. Color is another important element of your environment to consider. Certain colors are much more calming and soothing than others. (See COLOR THERAPY in Part Three.) Also, use as much natural lighting in your home as possible. Unnatural fluorescent lighting can be especially aggravating.

❑ Investigate aromatherapy. This is the art of using highly concentrated distilled plant essences, called essential oils, for healing purposes. Essential oils affect both the mind and the body by means of olfactory stimulation of the brain. Essential oils that are particularly good for relieving stress include chamomile, bergamot, sandalwood, lavender, and sweet marjoram. Add 10 to 20 drops of one or more of these oils to a warm bath and relax in the tub, or simply dab a couple of drops of oil on a tissue or handkerchief and inhale the aroma periodically during the day. (See AROMATHERAPY AND ESSENTIAL OILS in Part Three.)

❑ Try not to take life too seriously. Learn to laugh.

❑ If stress-related symptoms become chronic or recurrent, consult your doctor to rule out an underlying illness.

❑ If you feel you simply cannot handle the stresses in your life, consider seeking outside help. It may be worth it to consult a qualified counselor or other practitioner who can help you to handle your problems and learn effective stress-reduction techniques. It is often enlightening and beneficial to talk with someone who can offer an objective response, whether a trusted friend or a professional counselor.

Considerations

❑ A study done at the University of Washington Medical School rated stressful situations according to their negative effects on physical and mental health. Rated highest was the death of a spouse. Divorce is next, followed by such circumstances as getting married, personal illness, and so on. The study found that the more stressful situations a person is experiencing, the greater the chance of illness.

❑ Stress in young people should never be underestimated. Problems at school, changing schools, peer pressures, personal image problems, sexual identity issues, the addition of a family member, or problems with boyfriends or girlfriends all can lead to anxiety in young children and adolescents. Moreover, young people generally have fewer mechanisms or resources to cope with these situations than adults do. Often, adolescents or young children act out their feelings of stress in ways that are difficult for adults to understand.

❑ Evidence shows that stress can trigger reactions to allergens and make allergic symptoms more severe.

❑ Stress can aggravate certain skin disorders, such as psoriasis and skin cancer, by damaging immune cells in the skin. The damage is done by a chemical released when nerve cells respond to stress.

❑ Dr. Hans Selye, stress expert and author of *Stress Without Distress* (Signet Books, 1991) said that it is not stress that is harmful—it is *distress*. Distress occurs when unresolved emotional stress is prolonged and not dealt with in a positive way.

❑ A group of Dutch researchers studied a group of eighty people for a period of six months. They found that individuals with high levels of stress had fewer than half the antibodies in their systems than subjects under less stress did.

❑ In a study done at the University of Pennsylvania, people who considered themselves chronic worriers found that they could reduce their anxiety levels by setting aside a specific time to worry each day. They reserved thirty minutes each day to worry and did not permit themselves to worry at other times.

❏ Stress-related digestive problems often defy conventional treatment, but there are many mind-body techniques that can help you relax and provide a safe alternative to never-ending medication. A book entitled *Character Strengths and Virtues: A Handbook and Classification* by Christopher Peterson and Martin E. P. Seligman (Oxford University Press, 2004) categorizes and analyzes twenty-four key traits associated with mental health and happiness. A rather scholarly work that is much too large to summarize here, this book is nevertheless recommended reading. The authors argue that stress reduction is key to regaining good mental health, and that one vital element of this is simple meditation or contemplation the first thing in the morning or just before bedtime, which helps relax the body and gain control over stress. Of equal importance is good nutrition.

❏ Heavy metal intoxication and food allergies can both cause symptoms that mimic those of stress. A hair analysis can reveal heavy metal poisoning. (*See* HAIR ANALYSIS in Part Three; *see also* ALLERGIES in Part Two.)

❏ The symptoms of hypoglycemia may mimic those of stress. (*See* HYPOGLYCEMIA in Part Two.)

❏ *See also* ANXIETY DISORDER and DEPRESSION in Part Two.

STRETCH MARKS

See under PREGNANCY-RELATED PROBLEMS.

STROKE

See under ARTERIOSCLEROSIS/ATHEROSCLEROSIS; and CARDIO-VASCULAR DISEASE.

STYE

See under EYE PROBLEMS.

SUBSTANCE ABUSE

See ALCOHOLISM; DRUG ADDICTION (SUBSTANCE ABUSE); and SMOKING DEPENDENCY.

SUNBURN

Sunburn is caused by excessive exposure to the sun's ultraviolet (UV) rays. The amount of exposure required to cause a burn depends on the individual, the geographical location, the time, and the atmospheric conditions. There are two types of ultraviolet rays, designated ultraviolet-A (UVA) and ultraviolet-B (UVB). Both are dangerous. UVB rays attack the skin's outer layers, while UVA rays attack the underlying layers.

Most sunburns are first-degree burns that cause the skin to become red, warm, and tender to the touch. Depending on the severity of the burn and the individual's skin type, the burn may subsequently "cool" into a suntan or thin layers of skin may peel off. A more serious sunburn can be a second-degree burn, causing extreme reddening, swelling, pain, and even blisters. This is a sign that the burn has gone deeper than just the surface layer of the skin and has caused damage and the release of fluids from cells in the lower layers of the skin. This results in eruptions and breaks in the skin where bacteria and other infectious organisms can enter. In the most severe cases, the burn may be accompanied by chills, fever, nausea, and/or delirium. Sunburn such as this is extremely painful and, for children, extremely dangerous. Dehydration often accompanies sunburn.

Fair-skinned people are more prone to sunburn than darker-skinned individuals, but no matter what your skin color, you will burn if you get enough exposure. Symptoms do not necessarily appear while you are in the sun; they may begin from one hour to twenty-four hours after sun exposure, and usually reach their peak in two to three days.

Today, the effects of sun exposure are becoming an increasing concern because of the decline in the earth's ozone layer. The ozone layer screens out the most harmful ultraviolet rays, but it is becoming steadily thinner all over the world, and holes that fluctuate in size have developed in various places. The incidence of skin cancer is growing at an alarming rate. Having a few bad episodes of sunburn as a child makes you much more likely to develop skin cancer as an adult. (*See* SKIN CANCER in Part Two.)

Unless otherwise stated, the dosages recommended here are for adults. For children between the ages of twelve and seventeen, reduce the dose to three-quarters of the recommended amount. For children between the ages of six and twelve, use one-half the recommended dose, and for children under six, use one-quarter of the recommended amount.

NUTRIENTS

SUPPLEMENT	SUGGESTED DOSAGE	COMMENTS
Important		
Cell Guard from Biotec Foods	As directed on label.	Provides high levels of antioxidants to protect and nourish the cells.
Coenzyme Q$_{10}$	60 mg daily.	Free radical scavenger that also increases the supply of oxygen to the cells.
Colloidal silver	Apply topically as directed on label.	Antiseptic to prevent infection. Subdues inflammation and promotes healing.
ConcenTrace from Trace Minerals Research	As directed on label.	Nourishes the skin by providing needed trace minerals.
Dimethylglycine (DMG) (Aangamik DMG from FoodScience of Vermont)	As directed on label.	Increases tissue oxygenation.

Free form amino acid (Amino Balance from Anabol Naturals)	As directed on label.	To supply protein, needed for tissue repair.
Herpanacine from Diamond-Herpanacine Associates	As directed on label.	Promotes skin health, detoxifies the body, and enhances immunity.
L-cysteine	500 mg daily, on an empty stomach. Take with water or juice. Do not take with milk. Take with 50 mg vitamin B$_6$ and 1,500 mg vitamin C.	Promotes healing of burns.
Multivitamin and mineral complex	As directed on label.	All nutrients are necessary in balance.
Potassium	99 mg daily.	Potassium lost through sunburn must be replaced.
Pycnogenol	As directed on label.	An antioxidant that has circulatory benefits and may reduce skin damage risks.
Vitamin A with mixed carotenoids including beta-carotene plus	25,000 IU daily for 2 weeks, then reduce to 10,000 IU daily until healed. If you are pregnant, do not exceed 10,000 IU daily.	To destroy free radicals released by sun exposure and aid in tissue repair and healing.
vitamin E	Start with 100 IU daily and increase to 200 IU daily until healed.	Use d-alpha-tocopherol form.
Vitamin C with bioflavonoids	10,000 mg and up daily, in three fairly equal doses.	Needed for tissue repair and healing. Also reduces scarring. Use calcium ascorbate form.
Helpful		
Calcium and	2,000 mg daily.	Necessary for proper pH balance and potassium utilization. Also reduce stress on tissues.
magnesium	1,000 mg daily.	
Essential fatty acids (primrose oil or Ultimate Oil from Nature's Secret)	As directed on label.	Needed for tissue healing.
Silica	As directed on label.	Supplies silicon, needed for repair of skin tissue.
Vitamin B complex	100 mg of each major B vitamin daily, with meals (amounts of individual vitamins in a complex will vary).	Important for tissue healing, especially for serious burns. A sublingual form is best.
plus extra vitamin B$_6$ (pyridoxine) and	50 mg 3 times daily, with meals.	Needed for protein metabolism.
para-aminobenzoic acid (PABA)	25 mg daily, with meals.	Good for protecting the skin.
Vitamin E oil or ointment	Once the burn has cooled and healing has begun, apply topically to the affected area 3 to 4 times daily.	Promotes healing and helps prevent scarring. Purchase in oil or ointment form, or open a capsule to release the oil.
Zinc	100 mg daily for 1 month; then reduce to 50 mg daily. Do not exceed 100 mg daily from all supplements.	Boosts the immune system and aids in tissue healing. Use zinc gluconate lozenges or OptiZinc for best absorption.

Herbs

❑ Aloe vera gel is a remarkably effective treatment for any kind of burn. It is even used in the burn units of some hospitals. Aloe relieves discomfort, speeds healing, and also helps to moisturize the skin and relieve dryness. Gently apply a thin layer of aloe vera gel to the sunburned area. Reapply it every hour until the pain is gone. Pulp taken directly from inside the fresh plant is best. If you use a commercial aloe product, make sure to choose one that contains no mineral oil, paraffin waxes, alcohol, or coloring.

❑ Apply a salve of calendula flowers and St. John's wort to badly burned areas. These two herbs have antiseptic properties, act as painkillers for burns, and promote healing of skin wounds.

Caution: St. John's wort may cause increased sensitivity to sunlight. It may also produce anxiety, gastrointestinal symptoms, and headaches. It can interact with some drugs including antidepressants, birth control pills, and anticoagulants.

❑ An herbal bath can help minimize the stinging and pain of sunburn. Add 6 cups of chamomile tea or 6 drops of chamomile oil to a lukewarm tubful of water. Soak in the bath for thirty minutes or more. Lavender oil is also good and can be used in place of chamomile oil if you wish.

❑ Make a large pot of strong comfrey or gotu kola tea and let it cool. Soak sterile cotton gauze in the tea to make a compress and apply it to the affected area. Leave the compress in place for up to thirty minutes.

Caution: Comfrey is recommended for external use only.

❑ A cream containing at least 5 percent tea tree oil helps to heal sunburn and other skin irritations.

❑ Make a wash of apple cider vinegar diluted with an equal amount of water. Wash the area with this mixture, then rub an herbal infusion of St. John's wort oil onto the affected sunburned area.

Caution: St. John's wort may cause increased sensitivity to sunlight. It may also produce anxiety, gastrointestinal symptoms, and headaches. It can interact with some drugs including antidepressants, birth control pills, and anticoagulants.

Recommendations

❑ Eat high-protein foods for tissue repair, and raw fruits and vegetables to supply needed vitamins and minerals.

❑ For immediate relief of sunburn pain, use cool-water compresses or cold clay poultices. (*See* USING A POULTICE in Part Three.) Or dissolve 1 pound of baking soda in a tubful of cool water, and soak in the bath for about thirty minutes. The herbal treatments described above are also excellent for relieving pain and stinging.

❑ Strictly avoid any further sun exposure until the burn is completely healed.

❏ When it comes to sunburn, prevention is better than cure. While most sunburns are minor burns that heal on their own, a history of sunburn is strongly linked to the development of skin cancer. Take precautions to prevent yourself from getting sunburned:

- Avoid spending time outdoors between the hours of 10:00 A.M. and 3:00 P.M.

- When you do spend time outdoors, wear a sun hat, protective clothing, and sunglasses that specify UV protection. The best type of clothing is made of light-colored, lightweight, tightly woven material.

- Always use a sunscreen with a sun protection factor (SPF) of 15 or higher. Apply the sunscreen to all exposed areas of skin. Reapply it frequently, at least every three to four hours, more often if you are swimming or perspiring. Make sure the sunscreen protects against both UVA and UVB rays. Keep in mind that the SPF number refers only to the level of protection against UVB rays. Avobenezone appears to provide the best protection against UVA damage.

- Add to your sunscreen the contents of 1 capsule each of vitamin A, vitamin C, vitamin E, and selenium to help prevent free radical damage to the skin. After sunning, add these antioxidants to whatever skin cream you use for added protection and to aid in preventing wrinkles.

- Don't neglect your lips. The lips also are susceptible to sunburn. Use a sun protection product designed for the lips as well as a sunscreen for your face and body. Choose a formula containing natural ingredients such as aloe vera and vitamin E. Your health food store should carry such products in handy stick form.

- Do not rely on the weather to judge how strong the sun is. Cloudy or hazy days do not afford protection against sunburn; approximately 80 percent of the sun's ultraviolet rays pass through clouds. Reflections from water, metal, sand, or snow may increase—even double—the amount of ultraviolet rays you absorb. Take the same precautions on cloudy or hazy days that you do on bright, sunny days. Almost 90 percent of sunburn is caused by incidental sun exposure, not sunbathing. If you work outdoors, always wear sunscreen and protect yourself by wearing a hat.

❏ To prevent dehydration, drink plenty of water while spending time in the sun.

❏ If you desire a tan, start with only fifteen-minute periods of sun exposure, and increase your exposure slowly, adding no more than fifteen more minutes every few days. This helps to prevent burning and results in a longer-lasting tan. Self-tanning lotions may be the safest way to get a tan.

❏ Always wear sunglasses to protect your eyes. Make sure your glasses protect your eyes from both UVA and UVB rays.

❏ For ordinary sunburn apply cool—not cold—compresses to the affected area(s) as often as needed. If the burn is se-

vere, see a physician. If a child is sunburned, take special care. Do not apply any creams or anything to the burned area other than cool water or, *sparingly*, a bit of aloe vera gel twice a day. The burn will heal more readily if left exposed to the air.

❏ If you take any medications, ask your physician or pharmacist if they may increase your sensitivity to the sun.

Considerations

❏ Tretinoin (vitamin A acid), the active ingredient in the prescription medication Retin-A, is sometimes prescribed to help repair skin that has been damaged by sun exposure. However, the use of tretinoin renders the skin significantly more vulnerable to additional sun damage. If you use this medication, you should *always* use a high-SPF sunblock and avoid sun exposure as much as possible. This product should not be used during pregnancy, as it may cause birth defects.

❏ For a severe burn, a physician may prescribe silver sulfadiazine (Silvadene) cream and/or antibiotics to prevent infection, debridement to remove dead tissue, and/or hydrotherapy to loosen dead skin. Depending on the location and extent of the burn, physical therapy may be prescribed to keep muscles flexible. Muscle contractures can result from overlying skin damage and contraction.

❏ Your doctor may recommend taking an anti-inflammatory agent such as acetaminophen (Tylenol, Datril, and others) or ibuprofen (Advil, Nuprin, and others) to help relieve pain and inflammation. You should not give an aspirin-based product to a child with a sunburn.

❏ Berlock dermatitis is a heightened reaction to the sun caused by oil of bergamot, a common ingredient in perfumes, pomades, and colognes.

SWEATING

See under PREGNANCY-RELATED PROBLEMS.

SWIMMER'S EAR

See under EAR INFECTION.

TEMPOROMANDIBULAR JOINT SYNDROME

See TMJ SYNDROME.

TENDINITIS

See under BURSITIS.

THROMBOPHLEBITIS

Phlebitis means inflammation of a vein. This problem usually occurs in the extremities, particularly the legs. If the inflammation is associated with the formation of a thrombus (a blood clot) in the vein, the condition is called *thrombophlebitis.*

Thrombophlebitis can be either superficial or deep. It is considered superficial if it affects a subcutaneous vein, one of the veins near the skin's surface. In superficial thrombophlebitis, the affected vein can be felt (it feels harder than normal), and may be seen as a reddish line under the skin, with localized swelling, pain, and tenderness to the touch. If there is widespread vein involvement, the lymphatic vessels (thin-walled vessels carrying fluid from the tissues to the bloodstream) may become inflamed. Superficial thrombophlebitis is a relatively common disorder. A superficial clot may be brought about by trauma, infection, standing for long periods of time, lack of exercise, and intravenous drug use. Pregnancy, varicose veins, obesity, and smoking increase the risk of superficial thrombophlebitis. Thrombophlebitis may also be associated with environmental sensitivities or allergies. Diagnosis of the condition is usually based on physical findings and/or a medical history indicating an increased risk.

Deep thrombophlebitis (known also as deep venous thrombosis, or DVT) affects the intermuscular or intramuscular veins farther below the skin's surface. DVT is a much more serious condition than superficial thrombophlebitis because the veins affected are larger and located deep within the musculature of the leg. These are the veins responsible for the transport of 90 percent of the blood that flows back to the heart from the legs. Symptoms of DVT may include pain, warmth, swelling, and/or bluish discoloration of the skin of the affected limb. These symptoms are sometimes, but not often, accompanied by fever and chills. The pain is typically felt as a deep soreness that is worse when standing or walking and that gets better with rest, especially with the leg elevated. The veins directly under the skin may become dilated and more visible. Inflammation situated in a vein in the pelvis is called pelvic vein thrombophlebitis.

Any long period of immobility—whether from being bedridden or sitting during extended periods of travel—is a risk factor for DVT. DVT has been dubbed the "economy class syndrome" due to its association with long-distance air travel, but it can just as often affect people who frequently take trips on buses or trains or in cars. Unusual and tragic cases, such as the death of thirty-nine-year-old NBC reporter David Bloom, caused by his riding for days in a cramped military vehicle while covering the Iraq war, occasionally bring DVT to the attention of the public. In fact, any situation that creates restricted blood flow—certain types of cancer, obesity, inherited clotting disorders, pregnancy, damage to the veins due to injury or orthopedic surgery, or anything else—can lead to DVT.

The primary risk associated with DVT is a sharp restriction in blood flow through the veins that can result in chronic venous insufficiency, a condition characterized by swelling, increased pigmentation, dermatitis, and ulcer-

ation of the affected leg. DVT can become life-threatening if a blood clot breaks off from the venous lining and travels through the bloodstream to the heart, lungs, or brain, where it may lodge in a blood vessel and cut off circulation to those vital organs. If the clot blocks blood flow to the heart, the result is a heart attack; if it blocks the supply of blood to the brain, a stroke may occur. If blood flow to a lung is blocked, the result is a pulmonary embolism, a less well known but equally serious scenario. Chest pain can be a symptom of both heart attack and pulmonary embolism. Other common symptoms of pulmonary embolism are unexplained shortness of breath and the coughing up of blood. If you have any symptoms of pulmonary embolism, you need emergency medical help at once. However, despite its potential seriousness, DVT can be completely without symptoms. Indeed, nearly half of all people who have it have no symptoms at all. Nine out of ten cases of pulmonary embolism are caused by blood clots that form in the legs and travel to the lungs. More than 300,000 people in the United States have a pulmonary embolism each year; 2 percent die within the first day and 10 percent have recurrent pulmonary embolism, of which 45 percent die. Pulmonary embolism occurs equally in men and women, but the risk of having pulmonary embolism increases after age sixty.

The reason or reasons for the formation of clots in the veins are often unknown. In most cases, clots are probably the result of a minor injury to the inside lining of a blood vessel. If the vessel lining receives a microscopic tear, for instance, this initiates clotting—a normal part of the body's repair processes. Platelets clump together to protect the injured area, and a series of biochemical events is initiated that results in the transformation of fibrinogen, a circulating blood protein, into strands of insoluble fibrin, which are deposited to form a net that traps blood cells, plasma, and yet more platelets. The result is a blood clot. Other possible causes of deep thrombus formation include abnormal clotting tendencies; poor circulation; certain types of cancer; and Behçet's syndrome, a condition affecting the small blood vessels that predisposes an individual to the formation of clots. Factors that increase the risk of DVT include recent childbirth, surgery, trauma, the use of birth control pills, and prolonged bed rest. For some patients, a hospital stay with a decrease in activity level also can increase their DVT risk.

A potential complication of DVT is postphlebitic syndrome, a permanent condition caused by valves in the leg veins that no longer work properly. For people with this syndrome, clotting takes a long time to clear up, and the result is sometimes an inflammatory reaction that can scar the veins, particularly the valves. These valves act as check valves, allowing the blood to flow only one way (back to the heart). If the valves are defective or become damaged, blood can flow backward, which allows it to pool in the legs to cause pain, swelling, and, sometimes, skin ulceration and varicose veins.

Unless otherwise stated, the dosages recommended here are for adults. For children between the ages of twelve and seventeen, reduce the dose to three-quarters of the recommended amount. For children between the ages of six and twelve, use one-half the recommended dose, and for children under six, use one-quarter of the recommended amount.

NUTRIENTS

SUPPLEMENT	SUGGESTED DOSAGE	COMMENTS
Important		
Acetyl L-carnitine	500 mg daily.	Protects the brain and blood vessels from fat accumulation.
Coenzyme Q$_{10}$	100–200 mg daily.	Improves circulation and protects the heart.
Flaxseed oil or Ultimate Oil from Nature's Secret	2 tsp daily. As directed on label.	To supply essential fatty acids that minimize blood clot formation and keep veins and arteries soft and pliable, promoting cellular and cardiovascular health.
Garlic (Kyolic from Wakunaga)	2 capsules 3 times daily, with meals.	Improves circulation and thins the blood.
Heart Science from Source Naturals	As directed on label.	Contains powerful antioxidants and artery lining protectors.
L-cysteine and L-methionine	500 mg each daily, on an empty stomach. Take with water or juice, not milk. Take with 50 mg vitamin B$_6$ and 100 mg vitamin C for better absorption.	Protects and preserves cells; and prevents accumulation of fat in the blood vessels. (*See* AMINO ACIDS in Part One.)
Lecithin granules or capsules	1 tbsp 3 times daily, before meals. 1,200 mg 3 times daily, before meals.	Fat emulsifier; to increase circulation.
L-histidine	500 mg daily.	Important blood vessel dilator.
Magnesium and calcium	1,000 mg daily. 1,500 mg daily.	A natural blood-thinner that reduces abnormal clotting. Works with magnesium.
Methylsulfonyl-methane (MSM)	As directed on label.	Relieves pain and inflammation.
Pycnogenol or grape seed extract	50 mg 3 times daily. As directed on label.	Antioxidants that restore flexibility to arterial walls and reduce the risk of blood vessel disease and thrombophlebitis.
Vitamin C with bioflavonoids	4,000–6,000 mg daily.	Aids circulation and reduces clotting tendencies. Prevent bruising and promote healing.
Vitamin E	200 IU daily.	Thins the blood and reduces platelet "stickiness." Use d-alpha-tocopherol form. Emulsion form is recommended for easier assimilation and greater safety at high doses.
Zinc	50 mg daily. Do not exceed a total of 100 mg daily from all supplements.	Aids in healing of ulcers and boosts immune function. Needed to maintain proper concentration of vitamin E in the body. Use zinc gluconate lozenges or OptiZinc for best absorption.

Helpful		
Advanced Carotenoid Complex from Solgar	As directed on label.	Contains antioxidants, immune system enhancers, free radical scavengers, potential cancer fighters, and heart disease protectors.
Body Essential Silica Gel from Natureworks	As directed on label.	Good for healing of veins and skin tissues.
Vitamin B complex	As directed on label.	Speeds healing time and aids all bodily functions.

Herbs

❑ Alfalfa, pau d'arco, red raspberry, rosemary, and yarrow are antioxidant herbs that improve blood oxygenation.

❑ Butcher's broom improves circulation.

❑ Cayenne (capsicum) thins the blood, eases blood pressure, and improves circulation. It can also be combined with ginger, plantain, and witch hazel in a poultice and applied directly on the affected area.

❑ Ginger, skullcap, and valerian root dilate the blood vessels and aid circulation.

❑ Ginkgo biloba improves circulation and brain function, and is a powerful antioxidant.

Caution: Do not take ginkgo biloba if you have a bleeding disorder, or are scheduled for surgery or a dental procedure.

❑ Leg ulcers can be treated with alcohol-free goldenseal extract. Moisten a sterile piece of gauze with a dropperful of extract and place it over the affected area.

Caution: Do not take goldenseal internally on a daily basis for more than one week at a time. Do not use it during pregnancy or if you are breast-feeding, and use with caution if you are allergic to ragweed. If you have a history of cardiovascular disease, diabetes, or glaucoma, use it only under a doctor's supervision.

❑ Hawthorn dilates the blood vessels, lowers cholesterol levels, and protects the heart.

❑ Olive leaf extract aids in preventing infection.

Recommendations

❑ Eat plenty of fresh fruits and vegetables; raw nuts and seeds; soybean products; and whole grains.

❑ Reduce your consumption of red meat. Better yet, eliminate it from your diet.

❑ Do not consume any dairy products, fried or salty foods, or processed or partially hydrogenated vegetable oils.

❑ Get regular moderate exercise. Walking, swimming, and other exercise improve circulation and prevent sluggishness in the veins, lessening the tendency to form clots.

Caution: If you are thirty-five or older and/or have been sedentary for some time, consult with your health care provider before beginning an exercise program.

❏ Take alternating hot and cold sitz baths, or apply alternating hot and cold compresses using the herbs recommended above. (*See* SITZ BATH in Part Three.)

❏ Lie on a padded slant board with your feet higher than your head for fifteen minutes a day. This is particularly helpful if you stand on your feet a lot.

❏ Ask your pharmacist about special elastic support stockings (anti-embolism stockings) to improve circulation.

❏ If you smoke, *stop.* Smoking constricts the blood vessels, resulting in poor circulation and weakened blood flow. This is especially important if you are taking birth control pills. (*See* SMOKING DEPENDENCY in Part Two.)

❏ Avoid wearing tight-fitting clothing that cuts off circulation, such as girdles and knee socks with tight bands.

❏ If you experience a swollen, painful vein that does not get better within two weeks, talk to a health care professional.

❏ If symptoms of pulmonary embolism develop, sit down at once and call for emergency help (if someone is with you, have that person make the call). Getting to an emergency room quickly is your best bet.

❏ If you are confined to bed, move your legs as much as possible to counteract pooling of the blood in the veins.

❏ Clean your legs daily to remove germs that can cause infection.

❏ Avoid using products that can dry your skin. Contact your health care provider if you notice any redness or swelling in the legs—these may be signs of infection.

❏ If you develop leg ulcers, keep the ulcers clean and germ-free to prevent infection. Follow your physician's recommendations concerning proper care for your ulcers, and be forewarned that leg ulcers may take three months to a year to heal. (*See* LEG ULCERS in Part Two.)

❏ Avoid wearing socks with tight elastic at the top, which constricts the veins.

❏ When traveling, take the following preventive measures:

• Do not sit inactive for an entire trip or flight. Get up, move around, stretch. Some airplanes are large enough to allow walking up one aisle and down another. Some airlines offer leaflets suggesting leg exercises that passengers can do in their seats. If you are traveling by car, stop, get out, walk around, and stretch every couple of hours.

• Drink plenty of fluids to prevent dehydration. Dehydration causes the blood vessels to narrow and blood to thicken, increasing the risk of DVT.

• Avoid consuming alcohol and coffee, particularly on a long trip. Both contribute to dehydration.

• Avoid sitting with your legs crossed for long periods.

Considerations

❏ To make a definitive diagnosis of DVT, a doctor must rule out a number of other disorders, including cellulitis and occlusive arterial disease. One test commonly used to diagnose DVT is duplex ultrasound. In this procedure, a handheld ultrasonic device is passed over the affected area, and a picture of the blood flow is displayed on a computer screen. A less common test is venography, in which dye is injected into a vein to make blood flow visible on an X-ray. Duplex ultrasound, chest X-ray, and other tests can be used to diagnose pulmonary embolism, as required.

❏ Treatment of thrombophlebitis primarily consists of using anticoagulant (blood-thinning) medications. Blood-thinners such as heparin and warfarin (Coumadin) do not dissolve clots that have already formed, but can prevent the formation of new clots. More invasive treatments, such as the use of filters that can be inserted into the veins, and the use of potent "clot buster" drugs, which can dissolve large clots quickly, are available for difficult or life-threatening situations.

❏ Superficial thrombophlebitis is usually treated by elevating the affected limb; applying warm moist compresses; and bed rest. A doctor may also prescribe anti-inflammatory drugs.

❏ DVT is a potentially serious health problem, and hospitalization may be recommended. An anticoagulant such as heparin or warfarin (Coumadin) is usually given, both intravenously and orally. Surgery may be needed to tie off the affected vein to prevent the clot from traveling to the lungs, a condition known as a pulmonary embolism. Recovery time varies, depending on the severity of the disease.

Note: Do not combine vitamin E and prescription blood-thinning drugs.

❏ Being overweight, having low good cholesterol (HDL), or having a diagnosis of metabolic syndrome increases your risk of a venous thrombosis by about 50 percent. If you are overweight, lose weight; if your blood cholesterol and other tests are abnormal, seek medical advice on how to correct them.

❏ In one study, gamma tocopherol (the major form of vitamin E in the American diet) was shown to decrease the risk of thrombic events by reducing platelet activity.

❏ Behçet's syndrome is a chronic multisystem disease distinguished by thrombophlebitis, plus arthritis, iritis, uveitis, and ulceration of the mouth and genitalia. This disease is found worldwide, but is most common in young men of eastern Mediterranean and eastern Asian descent.

❏ Persons with Behçet's syndrome should avoid needle punctures because these can induce inflammatory skin lesions.

❏ *See also* CIRCULATORY PROBLEMS and LEG ULCERS, both in Part Two.

THRUSH

See under FUNGAL INFECTION.

THYROID PROBLEMS

See HYPERTHYROIDISM; HYPOTHYROIDISM.

TIC DOULOUREUX

See under HEADACHE.

TINNITUS

See under HEARING LOSS.

TMJ SYNDROME

About 75 percent of Americans will at some time suffer from symptoms associated with temporomandibular joint (TMJ) syndrome, a condition in which the temporomandibular joint does not function properly. Of this group, 5 to 10 percent actually meet the medical criteria for the condition. Women outnumber men 4 to 1, and Caucasians are more likely to develop it than African Americans. The temporomandibular joint is the joint that connects the temporal bone (the bone that forms the sides of the skull) with the mandible (the jawbone). This painful affliction produces pain in the muscles and joints of the jaw that sometimes radiates to the face, neck, and shoulder. There may also be difficulty opening the mouth all the way, and clicking, grinding, and popping noises may occur during chewing and movement of the joint. Headaches, muscle spasms, toothaches, dizziness, feelings of pain and pressure behind the eyes, pain and ringing in the ears, and difficulty opening and closing the jaw normally are other possible symptoms.

The jaw joint is embedded in an intricate web of nerves and muscle. The force of chewing and of clenching or gritting the teeth creates enormous tension and pressure in that region of the face. The cartilage disk that cushions the joint may become displaced or wear out. This causes the bones of the temporomandibular joint to rub against one another, rather than gliding smoothly past each other. In some instances, a misalignment of the jaw and teeth prevents smooth operation of the joint.

The most common underlying causes of TMJ syndrome are stress and a poor bite, together with clenching and grinding of the teeth (bruxism), especially at night. TMJ syndrome can also be caused by bad posture, habits such as cradling the telephone between the shoulder and jaw, repeated or hard blows to the jaw or chin, or whiplash. Poor dental work and orthodontia may aggravate the problem, as can habits such as gum chewing, thumb sucking, and chewing exclusively on one side of the mouth. A common contributing factor is hypoglycemia; people tend to clench and grind their teeth more when their blood sugar is low.

To diagnose TMJ syndrome, a physician may use X-rays and a technique called arthrography, in which an opaque dye is injected into the joint and then viewed with fluoroscopy.

A correct diet and the proper supplements, possibly in conjunction with other treatments, are valuable for TMJ syndrome and often solve the problem. They are also helpful for bruxism (teeth grinding).

Unless otherwise stated, the dosages recommended here are for adults. For children between the ages of twelve and seventeen, reduce the dose to three-quarters of the recommended amount. For children between the ages of six and twelve, use one-half the recommended dose, and for children under six, use one-quarter of the recommended amount.

TMJ Self-Test

Place your little fingers in your ears so that hearing is obstructed. Then slowly and steadily open and close your jaw. If at any point you hear a clicking, popping, and/or grinding noise, the jaw joints may be out of alignment, and examination by a professional experienced in diagnosing and treating TMJ syndrome is advisable.

NUTRIENTS

SUPPLEMENT	SUGGESTED DOSAGE	COMMENTS
Essential		
Calcium and magnesium	2,000 mg daily. 1,500 mg daily, in divided doses, after meals and at bedtime.	For proper muscular function and calming effect. Prevents bone softening and relieves stress. Use chelate forms.
Chondroitin sulfate plus glucosamine sulfate	500–1,000 mg daily. As directed on label.	Nutritional support for strengthening joints, ligaments, and tendons.
Kyolic-EPA from Wakunaga	As directed on label.	Increases activity of anti-inflammatory prostaglandins.
Methylsulfonyl-methane (MSM)	500–1,000 mg 3 times daily.	A sulfur compound that can reduce inflammation and aid in joint and tissue repair.
S-Adenosylmethionine (SAMe) (SAMe Rx-Mood from Nature's Plus)	400 mg 2 times daily.	Deficiency results in an inability to maintain cartilage properly. Aids in reducing pain and inflammation. *Caution:* Do not use if you have bipolar mood disorder or take prescription antidepressants. Do not give to a child under twelve.
Vitamin B complex plus extra vitamin B₅ (pantothenic acid)	100 mg of each major B vitamin 3 times daily (amounts of individual vitamins in a complex will vary). 100 mg twice daily.	Antistress vitamins. Sublingual forms are recommended for best absorption.

Helpful		
Coenzyme Q₁₀ plus	60 mg daily.	Improves oxygenation of affected tissues.
Coenzyme A from Coenzyme-A Technologies	As directed on label.	Works effectively with coenzyme Q₁₀ to support the immune system's detoxification of many dangerous substances.
L-tyrosine	500 mg daily. Take at bedtime on an empty stomach with water or juice. Do not take with milk. Take with 50 mg vitamin B₆ and 500 mg vitamin C for better absorption.	Improves the quality of sleep and relieves anxiety and depression. (*See* AMINO ACIDS in Part One.) *Caution:* Do not take tyrosine if you are taking an MAO inhibitor drug.
Multivitamin and mineral complex	As directed on label.	For balanced nutrients. A hypoallergenic product is best.
Vitamin C with bioflavonoids	4,000–8,000 mg daily.	Combats stress and is necessary in adrenal gland function. Also necessary for healing and repair of connective tissue.

Herbs

❑ Blue violet, catnip, chamomile, hops, kava kava, lobelia, St. John's wort, skullcap, thyme, passionflower, red raspberry, valerian root, and wild lettuce have calming and antistress properties.

Cautions: Do not use chamomile if you are allergic to ragweed. Do not use during pregnancy or nursing. It may interact with warfarin or cyclosporine, so patients using these drugs should avoid it. Kava kava can cause drowsiness. It is not recommended for pregnant women or nursing mothers, and it should not be taken together with other substances that act on the central nervous system, such as alcohol, barbiturates, antidepressants, and antipsychotic drugs. Lobelia is only to be taken under supervision of a health care professional as it is potentially toxic. People with high blood pressure, heart disease, liver disease, kidney disease, seizure disorders, or shortness of breath should not take lobelia. Pregnant and lactating women should avoid lobelia as well. St. John's wort may cause increased sensitivity to sunlight. It may also produce anxiety, gastrointestinal symptoms, and headaches. It can interact with some drugs including antidepressants, birth control pills, and anticoagulants.

❑ Boswellia, an Ayurvedic herb, helps to restore blood vessels around inflamed connective tissue. It also reduces inflammation.

❑ Feverfew and ginger are good for pain and soreness. Ginger is also a powerful antioxidant that has anti-inflammatory effects.

Caution: Do not use feverfew when pregnant or nursing. People who take prescription blood-thinning medications should consult a health care provider before using feverfew, as the combination can result in internal bleeding.

❑ Nettle leaf has anti-inflammatory properties.

❑ Nerve Blend SP-14 from Solaray Products combats stress and is also beneficial.

❑ Turmeric and willow bark are good for pain and inflammation.

Recommendations

❑ Eat a diet including lightly steamed vegetables, fresh fruits, whole-grain products, whitefish, skinless chicken and turkey, brown rice, and homemade soups and breads.

❑ Also eat more sulfur-containing foods, such as asparagus, eggs, garlic, and onions. Sulfur is needed for the repair and rebuilding of bone, cartilage, and connective tissue. It also aids in the absorption of calcium.

❑ Eat fresh pineapple frequently. Bromelain, an enzyme found in pineapple, is excellent for reducing inflammation. To be effective, the pineapple must be fresh. Freezing and canning destroy enzymes.

❑ Avoid high-stress foods: all forms of sugar, all white flour products, all junk foods, candy, colas, potato chips, pies, and fast foods.

❑ Do not consume any foods or beverages containing caffeine. As a stimulant, caffeine can increase tension, which often aggravates the problem. Also avoid taking over-the-counter medications containing decongestants, which can have a similar effect.

❑ Do not consume alcoholic beverages. These are a common contributing factor in bruxism (teeth grinding), which can cause or aggravate TMJ syndrome.

❑ If you work at a desk, check your posture periodically throughout the day. Do not lean over the desk; keep your back comfortably straight, with your ears not too far in front of your shoulders. Try to keep your head aligned so that your cheekbones are over your collarbone.

❑ Sleep on your back to give your back, shoulder, and neck muscles plenty of rest. Do not sleep on your side or lie on your stomach with your head turned to the side. Avoid propping your head at a sharp angle to read or watch television in bed.

❑ Fast at least once a month to give the body and jaws a rest. (*See* FASTING in Part Three.)

❑ Do not chew gum. Avoid overly chewy foods such as red meat and bagels.

❑ Experiment with heat and cold therapy, and use hot or cold packs—whichever works best—for relief of pain, especially pain in the neck and shoulders.

❑ Be wary of any practitioner who rigidly adheres to one single approach in treating TMJ syndrome. A multidisciplinary approach is a better choice. This could include: self-care practices, physical therapy, psychotherapy, relaxation techniques, biofeedback, hypnotherapy, and acupuncture.

❏ If possible, seek help from practitioners associated with a university dental or medical school.

Considerations

❏ TMJ syndrome is often treated with a special bite plate that is worn over the teeth to stabilize the bite and prevent tooth-clenching. To permanently correct the bite, you may have to have teeth reshaped, undergo orthodontia, or get crowns or a permanent oral appliance. Rarely, surgery is required to repair a damaged joint.

❏ Stress management, combined with heat and muscle relaxants, often relieves the symptoms of TMJ syndrome.

❏ Physical therapy is becoming a widely recognized, viable treatment for TMJ syndrome. This may involve jaw and tongue exercises to retrain stressed muscles and/or the use of a transcutaneous nerve stimulation (TENS) unit; ultrasound, which promotes tissue healing; and electrogalvanic stimulation, which helps relax muscles. These types of therapy should be prescribed in conjunction with an exercise and stress-reduction program.

❏ Some TMJ syndrome sufferers have been helped by biofeedback readings taken from the masseter muscle (the muscle that opens and closes the jaw). This treatment, combined with relaxation techniques such as controlled breathing, has proved effective.

❏ Orthodontists, dentists, physical therapists, and many other "specialists" now offer various treatments for TMJ syndrome. However, it is estimated that 70 to 90 percent of all cases of TMJ syndrome respond to simple, inexpensive treatments, such as those recommended in this section. It therefore makes sense to try such measures *before* investing in expensive medical or dental treatment.

❏ TMJ syndrome is not the only disorder that can cause jaw pain. Another possible cause is rheumatoid arthritis. In this disorder, the symptoms are more severe in the morning and tend to ease somewhat as the day goes on. (*See* ARTHRITIS in Part Two.) This is not usually the case with TMJ syndrome.

❏ A displaced disk can also cause jaw pain. Treatment for this disorder involves realigning the ligaments with a plastic splint.

❏ *See also* BRUXISM and STRESS, both in Part Two.

TONSILLITIS

Tonsillitis is an inflammation of the palatine tonsils, which are the accumulations of lymphatic tissue on the right and left sides of the upper throat. It can be caused by either viral or bacterial infection. Generally, younger children tend to get viral tonsillitis, while older children and adults tend to get bacterial tonsillitis—usually caused by *Streptococcus* bacteria. Symptoms include sore throat, difficulty swallowing, hoarseness, coughing, and redness, pain, and swelling of the tonsils. Other possible symptoms include headache, earache, fever and chills, nausea and vomiting, nasal obstruction and discharge, and enlarged lymph nodes throughout the body.

This disorder is most common in children, but it can occur at any age. In adults, it may be a sign that the body's resistance to disease is lower than it should be. An improper diet that is high in refined carbohydrates and low in protein and other nutrients may also predispose one to developing tonsillitis. Some people have repeated bouts of tonsillitis, and it can become a chronic condition. If untreated, tonsillitis can lead to a very severe condition called a *peritonsillar abscess*, in which the airways become obstructed, making breathing difficult. The infection can also spread into the neck and chest area. In general, the more repeated bouts of tonsillitis a person has, the more difficult it is to cure. Each time the tonsils become inflamed, scar tissue accumulates on the tonsils. If you are concerned, see a doctor, especially with the care of children.

Unless otherwise specified, the dosages recommended here are for adults. For children between the ages of twelve and seventeen, reduce the dose to three-quarters the recommended amount. For children between six and twelve, use one-half the recommended dose, and for children under the age of six, use one-quarter the recommended amount.

NUTRIENTS

SUPPLEMENT	SUGGESTED DOSAGE	COMMENTS
Important		
Vitamin C with bioflavonoids	5,000–20,000 mg daily. (*See* ASCORBIC ACID FLUSH in Part Three.)	To fight infection and boost the immune response.
Zinc lozenges	1 15-mg lozenge every 2 to 3 waking hours for 3 days, then reduce to 1 lozenge 4 times daily until healed.	An immunostimulant that aids healing.
Helpful		
Acidophilus (Kyo-Dophilus from Wakunaga)	As directed on label. Take on an empty stomach.	Necessary if antibiotics are prescribed. Use a nondairy formula.
Chlorophyll	Use as a gargle, as directed on label.	Has an antibiotic effect and can heal irritations in the mouth and throat. Use a liquid form.
Cod liver oil	As directed on label.	Aids immune response and healing of tissue.
Maitake extract or shiitake extract or reishi extract	As directed on label. As directed on label. As directed on label.	Mushroom extracts with immune-boosting and antiviral properties.
Proteolytic enzymes	As directed on label. Take between meals.	Aids in reducing inflammation.
Pycnogenol or grape seed extract	As directed on label. As directed on label.	Antioxidants that protect the skin, reduce inflammation, and enhance immunity.

Vitamin A with mixed carotenoids including beta-carotene	10,000 IU daily for 3 days, then reduce to 5,000 IU daily.	Needed for repair of tissue. Aids healing. Emulsion form is recommended for easier assimilation.
Vitamin B complex	50 mg of each major B vitamin 3 times daily, with meals (amounts of individual vitamins in a complex will vary).	To help maintain a healthy mouth and throat.
plus extra vitamin B$_5$ (pantothenic acid) and	100 mg daily.	Plays a role in the production of the formation of antibodies and aids in the utilization of other vitamins.
vitamin B$_6$ (pyridoxine)	50 mg daily.	Helps reduce swelling.
Vitamin E	200 IU daily.	Destroys free radicals and enhances the immune system. Use d-alpha-tocopherol form.

Herbs

❑ Catnip tea enemas are good for reducing fever. (*See* ENEMAS in Part Three.)

❑ Chamomile relieves fever, headaches, and pain.

Caution: Do not use chamomile if you are allergic to ragweed. Do not use during pregnancy or nursing. It may interact with warfarin or cyclosporine, so patients using these drugs should avoid it.

❑ ClearLungs from RidgeCrest Herbals is an herbal combination that helps to strengthen the immune system, enhances tissue repair, and controls inflammation.

❑ Echinacea fights infection and boosts the immune system. Make echinacea tea and drink as much of it as you can. Or take it in tincture form, ½ teaspoon every three to four hours until your symptoms improve.

Caution: Do not take echinacea for longer than three months. It should not be used by people who are allergic to ragweed.

❑ A hot infusion made from equal parts of dried elderflower, peppermint, and yarrow eases the pain of tonsillitis. Drink this throughout the day.

❑ Flaxseed oil reduces pain and inflammation, and aids recovery.

❑ Marshmallow tea coats inflamed mucous membranes. Steep 3 heaping teaspoons of marshmallow blossoms in 3 cups of cold water for twelve hours, then heat and strain. Drink 2 to 3 cups daily.

❑ Hot mullein poultices are soothing. (*See* USING A POULTICE in Part Three.)

❑ Pau d'arco is a natural antibiotic and potentiates immune function. It is also a powerful antioxidant.

❑ Sage tea, made with a bit of alum, can be used as a gargle. It can also be prepared with hot malt vinegar and taken orally in 2- to 3-ounce doses.

Caution: Do not use sage if you suffer from any type of seizure disorder, or are pregnant or nursing.

❑ For sore throat, take alcohol-free extract of goldenseal or St. John's wort. Place 6 drops or ½ dropperful of extract under your tongue and leave it there for a few minutes before swallowing. Do this four times daily for three days.

Cautions: Do not take goldenseal internally on a daily basis for more than one week at a time. Do not use it during pregnancy or if you are breast-feeding, and use with caution if you are allergic to ragweed. If you have a history of cardiovascular disease, diabetes, or glaucoma, use it only under a doctor's supervision. St. John's wort may cause increased sensitivity to sunlight. It may also produce anxiety, gastrointestinal symptoms, and headaches. It can interact with some drugs including antidepressants, birth control pills, and anticoagulants.

❑ Thyme reduces fever, headaches, and mucus. It is good for chronic respiratory problems and sore throat.

Recommendations

❑ Use a warm saltwater gargle. Dissolve ½ teaspoon of salt in 1 cup of warm water and gargle with the mixture three times a day to help reduce swelling, relieve pain, and remove mucus.

❑ Apply hot or cold compresses, whichever one provides more relief, to the throat area.

❑ Do not smoke, and avoid secondhand smoke. Tobacco smoke irritates the throat.

❑ Add humidity to the air at home with a humidifier, a pan of water placed on a radiator, or boiling a pot of water on the stove. Moistening steam stimulates the blood flow to the mucous membranes, promoting healing.

❑ For relief of tonsillitis pain, inhale essential oils of bergamot, lavender, tea tree, thyme, benzoin, and lemon.

❑ If you have a sore throat that does not improve within two weeks, consult your health care provider to determine what type of sore throat you have.

❑ If your physician prescribes antibiotics for bacterial tonsillitis, eat yogurt and take an acidophilus supplement to replace the "friendly" bacteria. Do not take the acidophilus at the same time as the antibiotic, however.

❑ Rest and drink plenty of fluids.

Considerations

❑ A cleansing juice fast for three days with vegetable broth can be helpful. (*See* FASTING in Part Three.)

❑ Bee propolis is good for treating tonsillitis.

Caution: Do not take bee propolis if you are allergic to bee stings. Do not give this supplement to a young child.

❑ If an abscess develops, surgical drainage may be required.

☐ If tonsillitis becomes recurrent or chronic, tonsillectomy (removal of the tonsils) may be recommended. In the past, doctors removed tonsils on a very frequent basis. Today we know that the tonsils are important for the proper functioning of the immune system. Tonsils should not be removed unless absolutely necessary.

TOOTH DECAY

Tooth decay rivals the common cold as the most prevalent human disorder. It is not a natural process, as many people believe, but a bacterial disease. This bacteria can enter the bloodstream and cause other problems in the body. Bacteria in the mouth combine with mucus and food debris to create a sticky mass called plaque that sticks to the surfaces of the teeth. The bacteria in the plaque feed on ingested sugars and produce an acid that leaches calcium and phosphate from the teeth. Gradually, if the sticky deposits are not removed, the teeth erode—first the enamel (the outer layer) and then the dentin (the body of the tooth). If unchecked, decay can progress even further, into the pulp that contains the nerve in the center of the tooth, resulting in a toothache. Infection may result, leaving the tooth vulnerable to abscess.

Tooth decay depends on three factors: the presence of bacteria, the availability of sugars for the bacteria to feed on, and the vulnerability of tooth enamel. Poor nutrition and poor oral hygiene are probably the main factors behind most cavities. In particular, people who consume large quantities of refined carbohydrates—especially sticky-textured foods that cling to tooth surfaces—or who snack frequently without cleaning their teeth afterward are much more likely to have a problem with tooth decay. There are also some people who, for reasons not yet understood, seem to have unusually acidic saliva and/or higher than normal levels of bacteria present in their mouths, and they too are more prone to tooth decay.

Tooth decay normally causes no symptoms until it is rather far advanced. Then the tooth may become sensitive to heat, cold, and the consumption of sugar. In later stages, a toothache may occur.

Unless otherwise specified, the dosages recommended here are for adults. For children between the ages of twelve and seventeen, reduce the dose to three-quarters of the recommended amount. For children between six and twelve, use one-half of the recommended dose, and for children under the age of six, use one-quarter of the recommended amount.

NUTRIENTS

SUPPLEMENT	SUGGESTED DOSAGE	COMMENTS
Important		
Acidophilus (Kyo-Dophilus from Wakunaga)	As directed on label.	Important if taking antibiotics; protects "friendly" bacteria in the colon. Use a nondairy formula.
Calcium and magnesium	1,500 mg daily. 750 mg daily.	Necessary for strong, healthy teeth. Needed to balance with calcium.
Grape seed extract	As directed on label.	A powerful antioxidant and anti-inflammatory.
L-tyrosine	As directed on label, on an empty stomach. Take with water or juice. Do not take with milk. Take with 50 mg vitamin B_6 and 500 mg vitamin C for better absorption.	Use for relief of pain and anxiety. (*See* AMINO ACIDS in Part One.) *Caution:* Do not take this supplement if you are taking an MAO inhibitor drug.
Vitamin A with mixed carotenoids including beta-carotene	10,000 IU daily.	Important for healing and for tooth formation.
Vitamin B complex	As directed on label.	Helps maintain healthy nerves and gums. A sublingual type is best.
Vitamin C with bioflavonoids	3,000 mg daily, in divided doses.	Protects against infection and inflammation. Do not use a chewable form, as this may erode tooth enamel.
Vitamin D	400 mg daily.	Needed for absorption of calcium and healing of gum tissue.
Vitamin E	200 IU daily.	Promotes healing.
Vitamin K	As directed on label.	May aid in preventing tooth decay.
Helpful		
Coenzyme Q_{10} plus Coenzyme A from Coenzyme-A Technologies	As directed on label. As directed on label.	Provides energy needed for gum cell growth and healing of gum tissue. Works effectively with coenzyme Q_{10} to support the immune system's detoxification of many dangerous substances.
Multivitamin and mineral complex	As directed on label.	All nutrients are needed in balance.
S-Adenosylmethionine (SAMe) (SAMe Rx-Mood from Nature's Plus)	400 mg twice daily.	Deficiency results in an inability to maintain cartilage properly. Aids in reducing pain and inflammation. *Caution:* Do not use if you have bipolar mood disorder or take prescription antidepressants. Do not give to a child under twelve.
Shark cartilage	Start with 1 gram per 15 lbs of body weight daily, divided into 3 doses. When relief is achieved, reduce the dosage to 1 gm per 40 lbs of body weight daily.	Treats pain and inflammation. Aids in repairing joints and bones.
Zinc	30 mg daily. Do not exceed a total of 100 mg daily from all supplements.	Boosts immune function. Use zinc gluconate or OptiZinc for best absorption.

Herbs

❑ Calendula, chamomile, peppermint, and yarrow are naturally anti-inflammatory.

Caution: Do not use chamomile if you are allergic to ragweed. Do not use during pregnancy or nursing. It may interact with warfarin or cyclosporine, so patients using these drugs should avoid it.

❑ Essential oil of clove, available in most drugstores, is helpful for toothache pain. Apply 1 or 2 drops to the affected tooth with a cotton swab as needed. If you find the clove oil too strong, dilute it with olive oil.

❑ Alcohol-free goldenseal extract can be used as an antibacterial mouthwash. If inflammation is present, put a few drops of goldenseal extract on a piece of sterile cotton and press it against the gum by the affected tooth, pushing it in place tightly, at bedtime. Leave the cotton in place overnight. Do this for three consecutive nights to destroy bacteria and reduce inflammation.

Caution: Do not take goldenseal internally on a daily basis for more than one week at a time. Do not use it during pregnancy or if you are breast-feeding, and use with caution if you are allergic to ragweed. If you have a history of cardiovascular disease, diabetes, or glaucoma, use it only under a doctor's supervision.

❑ Kava kava, St. John's wort, white willow bark, and wintergreen have analgesic properties. White willow bark is also an anti-inflammatory.

Cautions: Kava kava can cause drowsiness. It is not recommended for pregnant women or nursing mothers, and it should not be taken together with other substances that act on the central nervous system, such as alcohol, barbiturates, antidepressants, and antipsychotic drugs. St. John's wort may cause increased sensitivity to sunlight. It may also produce anxiety, gastrointestinal symptoms, and headaches. It can interact with some drugs including antidepressants, birth control pills, and anticoagulants.

❑ Sage is good for its anti-inflammatory properties. Bring to a boil 2 tablespoons of dried, crushed sage leaves in 1 cup of water. Steep for twenty minutes and strain. Cool to a comfortable temperature and use the mixture to rinse your mouth several times daily.

Caution: Do not use sage if you suffer from any type of seizure disorder, or are pregnant or nursing.

❑ Thyme is a natural antiseptic that reduces the level of bacteria in the mouth.

Recommendations

❑ Eat plenty of raw fruits and vegetables. These contain minerals that help to keep the saliva from becoming too acidic.

❑ Avoid carbonated soft drinks. These are high in phosphates, which promote the loss of calcium from the tooth enamel.

❑ Avoid all refined sugars.

❑ Do not smoke.

❑ Practice good oral hygiene. Brush your teeth after each meal and snack, if possible, and floss between the teeth daily. This is the only way to remove cavity-causing plaque. There are also mouth rinses available to enhance the plaque-removing power of brushing and flossing. Do not brush too hard. Brushing either too hard or too much can cause the gums to recede, exposing the root areas of the teeth, which are more prone to decay than the rest of the tooth. Use a soft-bristle toothbrush and replace it with a new one every month.

❑ Do not use chewable vitamin C supplements, which can erode tooth enamel. Tablets or powders designed for swallowing do not pose this danger.

❑ To ease the pain of toothache or abscess until you can see your dentist, rinse the affected area with warm salt water (add ½ teaspoon of salt to 8 ounces of warm water).

Considerations

❑ Stim-U-Dent, found in most drugstores, is beneficial for keeping the gums massaged and clean. It also aids in removing plaque. Before using one, to avoid damaging your gums, soak it in water or hold it in your mouth until it softens. Massage between all your teeth.

❑ Regularly scheduled dental checkups are recommended at least every six months for cleaning.

❑ Researchers are looking into adding cranberry extract to toothpaste and/or mouthwash. Evidence developed at Tel Aviv University in Israel suggests that a compound present in cranberries may reduce plaque formation.

❑ Researchers in Britain believe that they have developed a vaccine that prevents tooth decay by eliminating bacteria from the mouth. The American Dental Association's (ADA) Division of Science may be optimistic about the findings, but it has not been approved yet.

❑ At present, the only known way to stop tooth decay once it has started is to remove the decayed area and cover it with some type of filling. Fillings are made of various materials, such as tooth-colored composite resins, porcelain, or combinations of several materials. Silver amalgam fillings contain a variety of materials, including small amounts of mercury. Some people don't like using mercury fillings because they fear possible adverse health effects. While some medical studies have shown these fillings to be safe, they remain controversial. You may wish to discuss concerns about filling materials with your dentist before treatment.

❑ It was once believed that having dental work done posed a risk of endocarditis, a heart infection, for some people. The American Heart Association still believes there is a risk involved in tooth-cleaning and other dental work, even though there is not yet enough evidence to conclusively prove a link. Endocarditis rarely occurs in people with normal hearts. However, if you have certain preexisting heart conditions, you can be at increased risk if bacteria enter the bloodstream. Some of these preexisting conditions include the presence of an artificial (prosthetic) heart valve, a history of previous endocarditis, heart valves that are damaged (scarred) by conditions such as rheumatic fever, congenital heart or heart valve defects, and hypertrophic cardiomyopathy (an enlarged heart). Some congenital heart defects, including ventricular septal defect, atrial septal defect, and patent ductus arteriosus, can be successfully repaired surgically. If this is done, the individual is no longer at increased risk of developing endocarditis due to dental work.

❑ Fluoride increases resistance to tooth decay. It is added to many toothpastes and community drinking water supplies, as discussed in WATER in Part One. Many dentists recommend routine fluoride treatments to prevent cavities, especially for children. Fluoride is a chemical compound containing the element fluorine. Fluorine is a deadly and highly reactive chemical, but the fluoride compounds used in toothpaste and in water supplies are not believed to be dangerous in small amounts. However, there is still some debate as to whether or not fluoride is a risk factor for cancer, and if you are sensitized to the issue you will probably consider fluoride in all its forms a pollutant. Before removing fluoride from your child's water, discuss the pros and cons with your child's pediatrician and pediatric dentist. Avoiding decay is the best way to avoid having to have a tooth filled.

❑ Many Americans get medical or dental X-rays every year. These peeks inside the body can be valuable, even lifesaving, tools for diagnosing health problems. But X-rays are sometimes ordered when they are not needed. Other times, failure to follow precautions may expose people to more radiation than necessary. Our general advice is to keep X-rays to a minimum, especially ones taken for less than critical reasons. But, on the grand scale of things to worry about, dental X-rays aren't it. Below is a comparison of exposures from different sources of radiation:

Source	Estimated Exposure (millisievert [mSv])
Dental X-rays	
• Bitewings	0.038
• Full-mouth series (19 films)	0.150
Medical x-rays	
• Lower GI series	4.06
• Upper GI series	2.44
• Chest	0.08
Average in U.S. (natural sources)	3.00 (per year)

❑ Air abrasive technology uses a targeted spray of powder to remove tooth decay with no drilling sound or vibrations.

❑ Laser technology may be used as an alternative to the conventional dental drill.

TOXICITY

See ALUMINUM TOXICITY; ARSENIC POISONING; CADMIUM TOXICITY; CHEMICAL POISONING; COPPER TOXICITY; ENVIRONMENTAL TOXICITY; FOODBORNE/WATERBORNE ILLNESS; LEAD POISONING; MERCURY TOXICITY; NICKEL TOXICITY.

TUBERCULOSIS

Tuberculosis (TB) is a very old and highly contagious disease caused by the bacteria *Mycobacterium tuberculosis*. It is primarily a disease of the lungs, but it can affect any body organ, including the bones, kidneys, intestines, spleen, and liver. One of the most lethal among infectious diseases, TB is found throughout the world. It kills about 2 million people a year worldwide, and one-third of the world is infected. It is especially devastating in places such as Asia and Africa, where HIV and AIDS are widespread and have compromised the immune systems of so many people that the tuberculosis bacteria often meet with little or no resistance. It is the leading killer of people around the world who are infected with HIV. It is estimated that by the year 2020, there will be 1 billion new cases of this disease, 150 million will get sick, and 36 million people worldwide will die from it.

TB is usually spread by infected airborne droplets that are coughed up by individuals with the active disease and then inhaled by susceptible persons. Once inhaled, the bacteria normally lodge in the lungs. The body may successfully battle the infection at this point. If the immune system is not functioning optimally, however, or if another onslaught of the bacteria reaches the lungs, chances are the bacteria will multiply and proceed to liquefy and destroy lung tissue. Overcrowded, poorly ventilated housing and overpopulated prisons are fertile breeding grounds for the spread of TB. Studies in India have confirmed that smoking contributes to half the deaths from TB in that country, perhaps by weakening the immune system. Tuberculosis may also be contracted from contaminated food or from milk that has not been pasteurized. In such cases, the primary focus of the infection usually is in the digestive tract. This type of tuberculosis is more common in developing countries. It is rare in the Western world.

Not everyone infected with TB bacteria becomes sick. Some people have what is called latent TB infection. People with latent TB infection have TB germs in their bodies, but the germs are not active. A person with latent TB does not have symptoms, does not feel sick, cannot spread the TB bacteria to others, usually has had a skin test or blood test result indicating TB infection, and has had a normal chest X-ray and a negative sputum smear. These people must be treated for latent TB infection to prevent active TB disease. Usually, only one drug—isoniazid (INH)—is needed to treat latent TB infection. INH is typically taken for nine months in order to kill the TB bacteria in the body. Without treatment, however, TB bacteria may become active and multiply, and the person will get sick with TB disease.

Symptoms of TB may be slow in developing and initially resemble those of influenza—general malaise, coughing, loss of appetite, night sweats, chest pain, and low-grade fever. At first, the cough may be nonproductive, but as the disease progresses, increasing amounts of sputum are produced. As the condition worsens, fever, night sweats, chronic fatigue, weight loss, chest pain, and shortness of breath may occur, and the sputum may become bloody. In advanced cases, TB of the larynx can occur, making it impossible to speak above a whisper.

Antibiotic regimens that could successfully combat the disease have been developed, and living standards have risen so that the poor nutrition and inadequate hygienic standards that had once helped TB to spread and flourish are less prevalent in the United States. In spite of the fact that multidrug-resistant strains of TB exist (if a strain of TB is resistant to both of the drugs most often widely prescribed for TB, it is considered multidrug-resistant), rates of TB have declined. For example, between 2001 and 2002, the number of reported cases of TB declined 5.7 percent (a 43 percent decline from 1992 when it was at its peak). In 2006, the reported cases of TB were 13,299 (a rate of 4.4 per 100,000), which represented a 3.3 percent decline from the previous year. But the global epidemic of tuberculosis, together with the migration of people from one country to another, probably means that unless aggressive action is taken to eradicate TB everywhere in the world, the United States will again see an upsurge of this disease in coming decades. The best defense against tuberculosis is a strong immune system and a healthy diet.

Unless otherwise specified, the dosages recommended here are for adults. For children between the ages of twelve and seventeen, reduce the dose to three-quarters of the recommended amount. For children between six and twelve, use one-half of the recommended dose, and for children under the age of six, use one-quarter of the recommended amount.

NUTRIENTS

SUPPLEMENT	SUGGESTED DOSAGE	COMMENTS
Very Important		
Coenzyme Q$_{10}$	75 mg daily.	Helps carry oxygen to tissues for healing.
Free form amino acid	As directed on label.	Needed for tissue repair. Free form amino acids are rapidly absorbed and assimilated by the body.
Garlic (Kyolic from Wakunaga)	2 capsules 3 times daily, with meals.	Acts as a natural antibiotic; keeps infection in check and stimulates immune function.
Grape seed extract	As directed on label.	A powerful antioxidant that enhances immunity.
L-cysteine and L-methionine	500 mg each twice daily, on an empty stomach. Take with water or juice. Do not take with milk.	To protect the lungs and liver by detoxifying harmful toxins. (*See* AMINO ACIDS in Part One.)
	Take with 50 mg vitamin B$_6$ and 1,500 mg vitamin C for better absorption and prevention of cysteine kidney stones.	
Selenium	200 mcg daily. If you are pregnant, do not exceed 40 mcg daily.	Protects against free radicals and promotes a healthy immune system.
Vitamin A plus natural carotenoid complex (Betatene) plus vitamin E	25,000 IU daily. If you are pregnant, do not exceed 10,000 IU daily. 25,000 IU daily. 200 IU daily.	Use d-alpha-tocopherol form.
Vitamin B complex plus extra vitamin B$_5$ (pantothenic acid) and vitamin B$_6$ (pyridoxine)	100 mg of each major B vitamin 3 times daily (amounts of individual vitamins in a complex will vary). 100 mg 3 times daily. 50 mg 3 times daily.	Needed for production of red blood cells and antibodies. Aids in utilization of oxygen. Use a high-stress formula. Injections (under a doctor's supervision) may be necessary. If injections are not available, use a sublingual form. The antistress vitamin. Some drugs used to fight TB can cause a deficiency of this vitamin.
Vitamin D	Start with 1,000 IU daily and decrease slowly to 400 IU daily over the course of 1 month.	Essential for utilization of calcium and phosphorus. People with TB need sunlight daily and/or vitamin D for healing.
Important		
ACES + Zn from Carlson Labs	As directed on label. Do not exceed 100 mg of zinc daily from all sources.	A formula that fights free radicals with enzymes and antioxidants.
CTR Support from PhysioLogics	As directed on label.	To diminish damage caused by inflammation.
Essential fatty acids (Ultimate Oil from Nature's Secret)	As directed on label.	Important in formation of all cells, including lung tissue.
Glutathione	500 mg daily, on an empty stomach.	Protects the lungs and cells from free radical damage.
Kelp	2,000–3,000 mg daily.	For a natural supply of minerals. Rich in iodine.
L-serine	500 mg daily, on an empty stomach. Take with water or juice. Do not take with milk. Take with 50 mg vitamin B$_6$ and 100 mg vitamin C for better absorption.	Helps the body maintain immune function. (*See* AMINO ACIDS in Part One.)
Multienzyme complex plus proteolytic enzymes	As directed on label. Take with meals. As directed on label. Take between meals.	Needed to keep inflammation down, to digest essential nutrients, and to improve absorption.
Multimineral complex with boron and calcium and magnesium and silica	3 mg daily. Do not exceed this amount. 1,000 mg daily. 750 mg daily. 25–100 mg daily.	All nutrients are needed for strength and healing. Take with meals. Use a high-potency formula. Do not use a sustained-release formula.

Multivitamin complex	As directed on label.	To provide a balance of needed nutrients.
Oxy-5000 Forte from American Biologics	As directed on label.	An antioxidant formula with superoxide dismutase (SOD).
Zinc	50–80 mg daily. Do not exceed a total of 100 mg daily from all supplements.	Promotes immune function and healing. Use zinc gluconate lozenges or OptiZinc for best absorption.

Herbs

❑ Butcher's broom, calendula, cayenne (capsicum), chamomile, peppermint, and yarrow have anti-inflammatory properties.

Caution: Do not use chamomile if you are allergic to ragweed. Do not use during pregnancy or nursing. It may interact with warfarin or cyclosporine, so patients using these drugs should avoid it.

❑ Elecampane (*Inula helenium*), taken as a tea, goldenseal root, horehound, licorice, lobelia, marshmallow root, mullein, myrrh gum, and thyme have decongestant and expectorant properties.

Cautions: You should not take elecampane if you have had a known allergic reaction to inulin or if you are pregnant or breast-feeding. Do not take goldenseal internally on a daily basis for more than one week at a time. Do not use it during pregnancy or if you are breast-feeding, and use with caution if you are allergic to ragweed. If you have a history of cardiovascular disease, diabetes, or glaucoma, use it only under a doctor's supervision. Licorice root should not be used during pregnancy or nursing. It should not be used by persons with diabetes, glaucoma, heart disease, high blood pressure, or a history of stroke. Lobelia is only to be taken under supervision of a health care professional as it is potentially toxic. People with high blood pressure, heart disease, liver disease, kidney disease, seizure disorders, or shortness of breath should not take lobelia. Pregnant and lactating women should avoid lobelia as well.

❑ A combination echinacea and pau d'arco tea is beneficial. Echinacea is a powerful antioxidant and bolsters the immune system; pau d'arco benefits the body by cleansing the blood and acting as an antibacterial agent, as well as possessing antitumor agents. Drink 3 cups of this tea daily. Or combine echinacea tincture with equal parts of tinctures of elecampane and mullein, and take 1 teaspoon of this mixture three times daily.

Caution: Do not take echinacea for longer than three months. It should not be used by people who are allergic to ragweed.

❑ ClearLungs from RidgeCrest Herbals is a Chinese herbal formula that relieves bronchial and lung congestion.

❑ Lung Tonic from Herbs, Etc. supports lung function.

Recommendations

❑ If you suspect that you may have tuberculosis, or that you may have been exposed to it, see your health care provider. Prompt proper treatment is essential.

❑ Follow the prescribed treatment regimen exactly. If any medications cause side effects, contact your physician. *Do not* discontinue taking the medications on your own.

❑ To promote healing, eat a diet consisting of at least 50 percent raw vegetables and fruits. Also eat alfalfa sprouts, fish, fowl, pomegranates, raw cheeses, raw seeds and nuts, whole grains, and garlic.

❑ Drink fresh pineapple and carrot juice and a "green drink" daily. Drink fresh raw potato juice; potato juice contains compounds called protease inhibitors, which block carcinogens and prevent cell mutation. (*See* JUICING in Part Three.)

❑ Make a purée of steamed asparagus in a blender. Refrigerate and take 4 tablespoons twice a day with meals. Asparagus stimulates immune function and is anticarcinogenic.

❑ Make kefir, buttermilk, and fresh sugar-free yogurt a part of your daily diet. Also take an acidophilus supplement for as long as you are taking antibiotics, to relieve stress on the gastrointestinal tract and enhance nutrient absorption. Do not take the acidophilus at the same time as the antibiotic, but do make sure you take it.

❑ Do not smoke, consume alcohol, or use recreational drugs. All of these affect the ability of the immune system to fight infection. Smoking is even more dangerous than usual in the presence of a lung infection.

❑ Avoid stress. Rest, sunshine, and fresh air are most important. A dry climate is recommended.

Considerations

❑ There are two kinds of tests that can be used to help detect TB infection—the TB skin test (TST) and special TB blood tests. A positive TB skin test or TB blood test only tells that a person has been infected with TB bacteria. It does not tell whether or not the person has progressed to TB disease. Other tests, such as a chest X-ray and a sample of sputum, are needed to see whether the person has TB disease.

❑ Modern treatment regimens include long-term treatment with the antibiotics isoniazid (INH), rifampin (Rifadin), pyrazinamide, streptomycin, and/or ethambutol (Myambutol). Whatever antibiotic treatment is prescribed, it is important to take it for the full course recommended, even if you start to feel better.

❑ If you are taking one of the drugs for TB and have lost weight before treatment as a result of the disease, be sure to consume adequate protein so that you restore muscle mass. In one study, weight gain was mostly as fat during the first six months. Muscle takes a lot longer to rebuild.

❑ People infected with TB should not use cortisone preparations. Cortisone suppresses immune function and makes the infection more difficult to treat.

❑ Vaccines and drugs cannot control TB if poor lifestyle practices are followed. Cleanliness and proper nutrition are vital in combating this disease.

❑ One large-scale study of 30,000 people found that taking 50 milligrams of vitamin E with more than 90 milligrams of vitamin C increased the risk of developing TB after exposure by 60 percent. It seems prudent to avoid taking vitamin E and C in supplement form if you live in a high-risk TB area. It is fine to obtain these vitamins from foods.

❑ Experts estimate that up to 90 percent of the population may have encountered the tubercle bacillus sometime in their lives, but in the majority of cases, the immune system successfully keeps a full-blown infection from developing. People who do not defeat it outright often carry the germ in a dormant state, sometimes for decades, before immunity weakens and the bacteria begin replicating and infect the host.

❑ The Air Supply personal air purifier from Wein Products is a small unit worn around the neck. It sets up an invisible pure air shield against microorganisms (such as viruses, bacteria, and mold) and microparticles (including dust, pollen, and pollutants) in the air. It also eliminates vapors, smells, and harmful volatile compounds in the air.

❑ The tubercle bacillus has an incredible capacity for reproduction. A single organism is capable of producing billions of descendants within one month.

❑ People with AIDS are more likely than most to have tuberculosis at some point during their illness.

❑ The Bacillus Calmette-Guérin vaccine (BCG), which consists of a weakened form of tubercle bacilli, can be used for vaccination against tuberculosis. This vaccine is not widely used in the United States, but it is often given to infants and small children in other countries where TB is common. The vaccine provides immunity against TB, and may be given to persons at high risk of developing TB such as those with HIV. A TB skin test may indicate if you are carrying TB bacteria even before you have symptoms of the disease. However, if you were vaccinated with BCG, you may have a positive reaction to a TB skin test.

❑ In 2006, the World Health Organization set new guidelines for reducing the number of new TB cases and deaths by 2015 in 196 countries and territories. The goal is a 50 percent reduction.

TUMOR

A tumor, or neoplasm, is an abnormal new growth of tissue. It may be localized to one area or present in many sites in the body. Tumors can appear nearly anywhere in or on the body, and can be cancerous (malignant) or noncancerous (benign). Polyps and papillomas are examples of benign tumors. Squamous cell and basal cell carcinomas are examples of malignant tumors.

Unlike benign tumors, malignant tumors are usually serious and are likely to grow, take over other organs, and metastasize (spread). They can be a life-threatening problem if they are not detected and treated at an early stage. The prognosis for a person who develops a malignant tumor depends on the location of that tumor. If it is difficult to detect and there are few discernable symptoms, then treatment may not begin soon enough to prevent the tumor from metastasizing.

Environmental factors and diet seem to play an important role in the development of tumors of all types. Tumors have been known to decrease in size and even disappear in response to dietary changes and supplementation with high-quality vitamins and minerals. If you have a tumor, discuss your options with your doctor. Most cancer treatments like chemotherapy, radiation therapy, and surgery work better when the patient is well nourished. Thus, supplementation is important regardless of how you wish to be treated. The suggestions here are designed to enhance immune function and suppress the growth of tumors—both benign and malignant.

Unless otherwise specified, the dosages recommended here are for adults. For children between the ages of twelve and seventeen, reduce the dose to three-quarters of the recommended amount. For children between six and twelve, use one-half of the recommended dose, and for children under the age of six, use one-quarter of the recommended amount.

NUTRIENTS

SUPPLEMENT	SUGGESTED DOSAGE	COMMENTS
Important		
Coenzyme Q10 plus	100 mg daily.	Promotes immune function; carries oxygen to the cells.
Coenzyme A from Coenzyme-A Technologies	As directed on label.	Works with coenzyme Q10.
Garlic (Kyolic from Wakunaga)	2 capsules 3 times daily, with meals.	May help to reduce the size of tumors.
Maitake extract or reishi extract or shiitake extract	As directed on label. As directed on label. As directed on label.	Mushroom extracts that strengthen the body and improve overall health; have immunostimulant properties, have antitumor action, and reverse T cell suppression caused by tumors.
Melatonin	5–10 mg daily, at bedtime.	People with brain tumors may have an increased survival rate if they take melatonin along with their radiation therapy.
Proteolytic enzymes or Inf-zyme Forte from American Biologics	As directed on label. As directed on label.	To help the immune system and aid in the breakdown of undigested foods.

Shark liver oil	100 mg 3 times daily for 20 days, then 10 to 15 days off. Maintain this schedule.	Immune system booster that can help protect the body from radiation damage.
Vitamin C with bioflavonoids	3,000–10,000 mg daily, in divided doses.	Promotes immune function.
Zinc	30–80 mg daily. Do not exceed a total of 100 mg daily from all supplements.	Promotes a healthy immune system and wound healing, and helps maintain the proper concentration of vitamin E in the blood. Use zinc gluconate lozenges or OptiZinc for best absorption.
Helpful		
Kelp	1,000–1,500 mg daily.	Promotes immune function. Supplies balanced minerals.
L-arginine and	500 mg daily, on an empty stomach. Take with water or juice. Do not take with milk. Take with 50 mg vitamin B6 and 100 mg vitamin C for better absorption.	Retards tumor growth by enhancing immune function. (See AMINO ACIDS in Part One.)
L-cysteine plus	500 mg daily, on an empty stomach. Take with 1,500 mg vitamin C to prevent cysteine kidney stones.	Detoxifies harmful toxins, protects the body against radiation, and acts against carcinogens.
glutathione plus	500 mg daily, on an empty stomach.	Helps to reduce side effects of chemotherapy and protect the liver.
taurine	500 mg daily, on an empty stomach.	Used in some clinics for treatment of breast cancer.
Lecithin granules or capsules	1 tbsp 3 times daily, with meals. 1,200 mg 3 times daily, with meals.	An important component of healthy cell membranes.
Multivitamin and mineral complex	As directed on label, with meals.	For necessary vitamins and minerals. Use a high-potency formula.
Primrose oil or flaxseed oil or salmon oil	1,000 mg 3 times daily, before meals. As directed on label. As directed on label.	To supply essential fatty acids, specifically useful for breast tumors. Both eicosapentaenoic acid (EPA) and docosahexaenoic acid (DHA) are helpful in protecting the body against toxic effects of some cancer treatments.
Raw thymus glandular	As directed on label.	Stimulates the thymus gland, which is important for immune function. (See GLANDULAR THERAPY in Part Three.)
Vitamin A plus natural carotenoid complex (Betatene) plus vitamin E or ACES from Carlson Labs	25,000 IU daily. If you are pregnant, do not exceed 10,000 IU daily. 25,000 IU daily. 200 IU daily. As directed on label.	Powerful immunostimulants and antioxidants. Emulsion forms are recommended for easier assimilation and greater safety at higher doses. Use d-alpha-tocopherol form. Supplies vitamin C in addition to vitamins A and E and selenium.
Vitamin B complex plus extra vitamin B6 (pyridoxine)	As directed on label. 50 mg 3 times daily.	Vital in intracellular metabolism and normal cell multiplication. A sublingual type is best. Required for normal cell growth and brain and nervous system function. Enhances immunity.
plus vitamin B5 (pantothenic acid)	100 mg daily.	Consider injections (under a doctor's supervision). An antistress vitamin that plays a role in hormone and antibody production, energy production, vitamin production, and in treating depression and anxiety.

Herbs

❑ Cat's claw boosts the immune system and has anti-tumor properties. Cat's Claw Defense Complex from Source Naturals is a combination of cat's claw and other herbs, plus antioxidant nutrients such as beta-carotene, N-acetylcysteine, vitamin C, and zinc.

Caution: Do not use cat's claw during pregnancy.

❑ Many people with external tumors have responded well to poultices made from comfrey, pau d'arco, ragwort, and wood sage. (See USING A POULTICE in Part Three.)

Caution: Comfrey is recommended for external use only.

❑ For breast lumps, try using poultices made of poke root, which is effective in combating glandular swelling. (See USING A POULTICE in Part Three.)

Note: Poke root is recommended for external use only.

❑ Other beneficial herbs include barberry, burdock root, dandelion, milk thistle, pau d'arco, and red clover. These herbs purify the blood, stimulate liver activity, act as natural antibiotics, and generally help healing.

Caution: Do not use barberry during pregnancy.

Recommendations

❑ Eat a diet consisting of 50 percent raw fruits and vegetables. If possible, purchase produce from an organic source. Nuts, seeds, whole grains, and low-fat yogurt and yogurt products also should be included in the diet. Do not consume animal protein (eat soy protein instead), dairy products (except for yogurt), processed and packaged foods, salt (if you do use salt, use sea salt, which still retains its mineral content), sugar, white flour, or white flour products. If you are eliminating dairy, be sure to get calcium, magnesium, and vitamin D from other foods or supplements.

❑ See CANCER in Part Two and follow the recommended diet.

❑ See FASTING in Part Three and follow the program.

Considerations

❑ Although benign tumors are generally limited in growth, they usually should be removed; a small percentage may later become malignant.

❑ Malignant tumors must be treated as early as possible. Depending on the site and size of the tumor, there are many different methods of treatment. (See CANCER in Part Two.)

❑ Dietary intake from foods may impact cancer outcomes. A study where all existing data on the subject were reviewed found that a low-glycemic-load diet reduced the risk of both colorectal and endometrial cancer. A low-glycemic-load diet consists of eating an abundance of fruits and vegetables and whole grains, and limiting the intake of simple sugars, fats, and nutrient-poor foods. High-glycemic-load diets are purported to promote tumor growth because they cause a high surge in insulin response following ingestion. Insulin stimulates insulin-like growth factor-1, which is a known tumor inducer. An earlier study found that following a low-glycemic-load diet seemed to have no effect on prostate, ovarian, lung, and colorectal cancer risk.

❑ Which vitamins and minerals promote and arrest tumor growth is an area of intense interest for nutritional scientists. Iron deficiency has been linked to the development of tumors. However, iron supplements should be taken only if tests show a deficiency. People with cancer should *not* take supplemental iron. Similarly, vitamin E has been shown to increase the risk of lung cancer. However, for bladder cancer, taking selenium (about 100 micrograms per day) reduced its risk.

❑ In one study, a reduction in the risk of two types of esophageal cancer was seen as a result of eating fruits and vegetables. Those foods that seemed to provide the most protection were: apples, peaches, nectarines, plums, pears, strawberries, citrus fruits, and spinach.

❑ Plants contain lignans, which may protect against cancer. Good sources include legumes, seeds, cereals/grains, berries, dried fruit, and vegetables. In one study, the risk of colorectal cancer was reduced by 30 percent with a lignan-rich diet. High intakes of vegetables, fruit, and total dietary fiber each were associated with a lower risk for rectal cancer.

❑ In one study of long-term survivors of colorectal, breast, and prostate cancer, those who participated in a regular exercise program and followed a healthy diet had a better quality of life and slower decline compared to a matched group who did not adopt a healthy lifestyle and diet.

❑ Scientists studying a genetic disorder have found that a rare, noncancerous heart tumor, called a *myxoma,* also has a genetic cause. This is the same genetic defect that causes Usher syndrome, a leading cause of deafness and blindness in young children.

❑ VEGF Trap, a type of drug known as a vascular endothelial growth factor (VEGF) blocker, is used to prevent angiogenesis—the formation of blood vessels that feed tumors. It is a class of drugs called monoclonal antibodies. It has shown promise in treating tumors. Drugs in this category also include bevacizumab (Avastin), which has been approved for treating colorectal cancer and lung cancer. VEGF Trap is currently undergoing clinical trials.

❑ Curcuminoids, the yellow pigments found in the spice turmeric (*Curcuma longa*), appear to have properties that block the gene expression leading to tumor formation. A member of the ginger family, turmeric is widely used in southeast Asia as a culinary spice, especially in curries. Brand-name products that contain curcuminoids include Turmeric Special Formula from Solaray.

❑ Scientists at the University of California–Los Angeles School of Medicine have found that sodium linoleate, a compound that contains the amino acid linoleic acid, has the ability to fight cancer cells in the laboratory.

❑ Studies done in Japan suggest that taking garlic supplements may help reduce the size of tumors.

❑ Regular physical checkups and tests for various cancers, such as breast, colon, cervical, prostate, and skin cancer, should be part of your routine, especially after the age of forty. All of these cancers are more easily treated and better outcomes occur with early detection.

❑ *See also* BREAST CANCER; CANCER; FIBROCYSTIC BREASTS; FIBROIDS, UTERINE; POLYPS; PROSTATE CANCER; SKIN CANCER; and/or WARTS, all in Part Two.

ULCER

See BEDSORES; CANKER SORES (APHTHOUS ULCERS); LEG ULCERS; PEPTIC ULCER. *See also under* EYE PROBLEMS.

ULCERATIVE COLITIS

Ulcerative colitis is a chronic disorder in which the mucous membranes lining the colon become inflamed and develop ulcers, causing bloody diarrhea, pain, gas, bloating, and, at times, hard stools. The colon muscles then have to work harder to move these hardened stools through the colon. This can cause the mucous membrane lining of the colon wall to bulge out into small pouchlike projections called *diverticula.* This usually occurs in the lower left section of the large intestine, called the *sigmoid* (S-shaped) *colon,* although it can occur in any part of the colon. Enteritis and ileitis are types of inflammation of the small intestine often associated with colitis.

Ulcerative colitis can occur in people of any age, but it usually starts between the ages of fifteen and thirty, and less frequently between fifty and seventy years of age. It affects men and women equally and appears to run in families, with up to 20 percent of people with ulcerative colitis having a family member or relative with ulcerative colitis or Crohn's disease. A higher incidence of ulcerative colitis is seen in Caucasians and people of Jewish descent. Ulcerative colitis can range from relatively mild to severe. Common complications are diarrhea and bleeding, often causing the loss of vital nutrients and fluids. A rarer complication is toxic megacolon, in which the intestinal wall weakens and balloons out, threatening to rupture.

The cause or causes of most cases of colitis are unknown, but possible contributing factors include poor eating habits, stress, and food allergies. Colitis can also be caused by infectious agents such as bacteria. This type of colitis is often associated with the use of antibiotics, which alter the normal bowel flora and permit microorganisms that are normally held in check to proliferate. The symptoms can range from simple diarrhea to the more severe type of symptoms associated with ulcerative colitis.

Unless otherwise specified, the dosages recommended here are for adults. For children between the ages of twelve and seventeen, reduce the dose to three-quarters of the recommended amount. For children between six and twelve, use one-half of the recommended dose, and for children under the age of six, use one-quarter of the recommended amount. With ulcerative colitis, the colon is highly inflamed, so it is best to only add one or two new supplements at a time so as to not further irritate the colon.

NUTRIENTS

SUPPLEMENT	SUGGESTED DOSAGE	COMMENTS
Essential		
Iron	As directed by physician.	Usually depleted in people with chronic inflammatory bowel disease. *Note:* Do not take supplemental iron unless anemia has been diagnosed.
Proteolytic enzymes plus	As directed on label. Take between meals.	Vital for proper digestion of proteins and helps to control inflammation.
multienzyme complex with pancreatin	As directed on label. Take after meals.	Anti-inflammatory enzymes. Use a formula that is high in pancreatin and low in hydrochloric acid (HCl).
Vitamin B complex plus extra	As directed on label.	Essential for the breakdown of fats, protein, and carbohydrates and for proper digestion. Use a hypoallergenic formula.
vitamin B$_6$ (pyridoxine) and	50 mg 2 times daily.	
vitamin B$_{12}$ and	1,000 mcg twice daily.	A sublingual form is best.
folic acid	400 mcg twice daily.	Often depleted in people with this disorder. May protect against colon cancer.
Very Important		
Acidophilus (Kyo-Dophilus from Wakunaga) or bifidus (Bio-Bifidus from American Biologics)	As directed on label twice daily, on an empty stomach	To normalize the intestinal bacteria. Very important if you are taking antibiotics. Use a nondairy formula.
ABC Aerobic Bulk Cleanse from Aerobic Life Industries or psyllium husks	1 tbsp in water or juice on an empty stomach in the morning. Drink it quickly, before it thickens. Take separately from other supplements and medications. As directed on label.	To keep the colon walls clean of toxic wastes.
Free form amino acid	As directed on label twice daily, on an empty stomach.	To supply needed protein for tissue healing.
L-glutamine	500 mg twice daily, on an empty stomach. Take with water or juice. Do not take with milk. Take with 50 mg vitamin B$_6$ and 100 mg vitamin C for better absorption.	A major metabolic fuel for the intestinal cells; maintains the villi, the absorption surfaces of the intestines. (*See* AMINO ACIDS in Part One.)
Vitamin A with mixed carotenoids including natural beta-carotene plus	25,000 IU daily. If you are pregnant, do not exceed 10,000 IU daily.	An antioxidant that protects the mucous membranes and aids in healing. An antioxidant that promotes healing.
vitamin E	200 IU daily.	Deficiency has been associated with bowel cancer. Use d-alpha-tocopherol form.
Helpful		
Aerobic 07 from Aerobic Life Industries	As directed on label twice daily.	Provides stabilized oxygen to the colon and destroys unwanted bacteria.
Colloidal silver	As directed on label.	A natural broad-spectrum antiseptic that fights infection, subdues inflammation, and promotes healing. Apply topically.
Essential fatty acids (flaxseed oil or primrose oil)	As directed on label.	Important in cell formation. Protects the lining of the colon.
Garlic (Kyolic from Wakunaga)	2 capsules 3 times daily, with meals.	A natural antibiotic that has a healing effect on the colon.
Glucosamine sulfate or N-Acetylglucosamine (N-A-G from Source Naturals)	As directed on label. As directed on label.	An important component in the protective mucous secretions of the digestive tract.
Multimineral complex with calcium and chromium and magnesium and zinc	As directed on label.	Malabsorption of these essential minerals is a problem with colitis. Calcium also is needed for the prevention of cancer, which may occur due to constant irritation. Use a high-potency formula.
Raw thymus glandular	500 mg twice daily.	Important in immune function. (*See* GLANDULAR THERAPY in Part Three.)
Shark cartilage	As directed on label.	
Vitamin C with bioflavonoids	3,000–5,000 mg daily, in divided doses.	Needed for immune function and healing of mucous membranes. Use a buffered form.

Herbs

❑ ABC Aerobic Bulk Cleanse from Aerobic Life Industries contains healing herbs that cleanse the colon. Take it mixed with half fruit or vegetable juice and half aloe vera juice, before meals.

Note: Always take this product separately from other supplements and medications.

❑ Alfalfa, taken in capsule or liquid form, supplies vita-

Diet for Colitis

Ulcerative colitis can be an extremely painful and even temporarily disabling condition. Diet is probably the most significant factor in achieving and maintaining remission. Shari Lieberman, nutritionist and author, recommends the following dietary guidelines for people with colitis:

- The most important thing to do is keep a daily record of what you eat and what symptoms you experience. This way you can see which foods have aggravated or improved your condition. Some people are sensitive only to certain foods, such as yeast products, wheat products, or dairy products.

- Eat a high protein diet, containing proteins mainly from vegetable sources. Non-vegetable sources that are also acceptable include baked or broiled fish and chicken and turkey (without the skin).

- Eat lots of vegetables. If you cannot tolerate raw vegetables, steam them.

- Eat a high-fiber diet. Oat bran, brown rice, barley and other whole grains, lentils, and related products such as rice cakes are good. Be sure grains are well cooked.

- Keep excess fats and oils out of your diet, and stay away from high-fat milk and cheeses. Fats and oils exacerbate the diarrhea that comes with colitis.

- Include garlic in the diet for its healing and antibiotic properties.

- Eat cooked foods that are broiled or baked, not fried or sautéed. Avoid sauces made with butter.

- Avoid carbonated soft drinks, spicy foods, and anything containing caffeine. These substances can irritate the colon. Also avoid red meat, sugar, and processed foods.

- Try soy-based cheese instead of dairy cheese; try soymilk instead of cow's milk. If you do eat dairy foods, use nonfat types. If you are a lactose intolerant, try lactose-free milk. Many lactose-intolerant people can tolerate low-fat yogurt. Yogurts with active probiotic cultures like *Lactobacillus rhamnosus GR-1* have been shown to reduce inflammation.

- Drink plenty of liquids—at least ten 8-ounce glasses of water daily to make up for the fluid lost with diarrhea. Carrot and cabbage juices and "green drinks" are also good. Or add chlorophyll liquid to juices.

- Do not eat fruit on an empty stomach. Eat it between meals instead. Avoid acidic fruits such as oranges and grapefruit. Fruit juices should be diluted with water and taken during or after meals.

---

min K and chlorophyll, needed for healing. Take it as directed on the product label three times daily.

❏ Aloe vera aids in healing the colon, thereby easing pain. Drink ½ cup of aloe vera juice in the morning and again at bedtime.

❏ Boswellia, bromelain, buchu leaves, and turmeric (curcumin) reduce inflammation.

❏ Burdock root, milk thistle, and red clover aid in cleansing the blood. Milk thistle also improves liver function.

❏ Chamomile, dandelion, feverfew, papaya, red clover, and yarrow extract or tea are beneficial for colitis, as is pau d'arco tea.

Cautions: Do not use chamomile if you are allergic to ragweed. Do not use during pregnancy or nursing. It may interact with warfarin or cyclosporine, so patients using these drugs should avoid it. Do not use feverfew when pregnant or nursing. People who take prescription blood-thinning medications should consult a health care provider before using feverfew, as the combination can result in internal bleeding.

❏ Lobelia tea is good to drink. Also use it as an enema for inflammation of the colon; it gives quick relief. (*See* ENEMAS in Part Three.)

Caution: Lobelia is only to be taken under supervision of a health care professional as it is potentially toxic. People with high blood pressure, heart disease, liver disease, kidney disease, seizure disorders, or shortness of breath should not take lobelia. Pregnant and lactating women should avoid lobelia as well.

❏ Nettle and quercetin aid in inhibiting allergic reactions.

Recommendations

❏ Do not wear clothing that is tight around the waist.

❏ For acute pain, try drinking a large glass of water. This aids in flushing out particles caught in the crevices of the colon, relieving pain.

❏ During a flare-up, consume only soft foods until the pain has subsided. Put oat bran or steamed vegetables through a blender. Add 1 tablespoon of oat or rice bran daily to cereals and juice to add the bulk needed for cleansing the colon. Or add 1 tablespoon of Aerobic Bulk Cleanse to juice and drink it on an empty stomach upon arising.

❏ Eat plenty of dark green leafy vegetables. These are rich sources of vitamin K. Vitamin K deficiency has been linked to ulcerative colitis.

❏ Try eating junior baby foods for two weeks. Baby foods are easy to digest. Earth's Best baby foods are organic and are available in many health food stores and supermarkets. (*See* Manufacturer and Distributor Information in the Appendix.) While on the baby-food diet, take extra fiber such as glucomannan.

❏ Glucomannan should be taken one-half to one hour before meals with a large glass of water.

Note: Always take supplemental fiber separately from other supplements and medications.

❏ Do stretching exercises and take proteolytic enzymes to improve digestion.

❏ Use cleansing enemas made with 2 quarts of lukewarm water. This helps to rid the colon of undigested foods and relieve pain. Use wheatgrass juice as a retention enema. For severe gas and bloating, use a *B. bifidus* enema. (*See* ENEMAS in Part Three.)

❏ For long-term management of ulcerative colitis and to prevent flare-ups, *see* Diet for Colitis on the previous page and follow the suggestions there.

❏ *See* FASTING in Part Three, and follow the program once a month.

Considerations

❏ A food sensitivity test is advised for anyone who suffers from colitis. We have seen many people with colitis do well once they make changes in their diet and lifestyle.

❏ Some patients with irritable bowel syndrome responded to an elimination diet and probiotics. It is possible that this sort of therapy would be effective in ulcerative colitis as well.

❏ When magnesium is given intravenously with vitamin B_6, it relaxes the muscles in the walls of the bowels and can control an attack of spastic colon.

❏ If serious complications arise and all other treatments have failed, surgery may be required.

❏ Vitamin K deficiency has been linked to ulcerative colitis. Sulfa drugs and mineral oil deplete vitamin K.

❏ Ulcerative colitis and Crohn's disease are both classified as inflammatory bowel diseases. Irritable bowel syndrome (IBS), although capable of causing some similar symptoms, is a condition that involves no inflammation. (*See* IRRITABLE BOWEL SYNDROME in Part Two.) Some investigators have shown a link between breast-feeding and a lower risk of inflammatory bowel disease. Babies who were breast-fed had a 23 percent reduced rate of developing Crohn's disease and a 13 percent lower risk of ulcerative colitis.

❏ The earliest signs of ulcerative colitis sometimes mimic the symptoms of arthritis—an achy feeling and joint pain. These symptoms may or may not be accompanied by the abdominal discomfort typical of colitis. If you start experiencing arthritis-like symptoms, it may be beneficial to change your diet and see if improvement results. (*See* Diet for Colitis, previous page.)

❏ Anyone who has had ulcerative colitis for at least five years—even if it is mild or inactive for a long time—should undergo regular colonoscopy, since people with this disease run a much greater than usual risk of developing colon cancer. A colonoscopy is an examination performed with a long, flexible instrument that allows a physician to see inside the length of the colon.

❏ Several nutrients have been identified to lower the risk of developing colon cancer, so those with ulcerative colitis may wish to include these in their diet. In one study, both riboflavin (5 milligrams) and folic acid (400 micrograms) normalized nutrient levels in the body. Vitamin B_6 has been shown to improve the effectiveness of folic acid. Because other studies have found that folic acid alone does not reduce the risk of colon cancer, there appears to be some benefit to taking folic acid with riboflavin and vitamin B_6. Vitamin D at intakes of 1,000 to 2,000 IU per day have been shown to reduce the risk of colon cancer by 50 percent. In another study, calcium also was protective at 1,200 milligrams per day in both men and women. In fact, the benefits lasted five years after the study concluded. However, men should consult with their physicians before using calcium supplements, as they have been shown to increase the risk of prostate cancer. Lycopene (30 milligrams per day) may lower colon cancer risk by blocking insulin-like growth factor-1, which is thought to be responsible for colon cancer.

❏ Omega-3 fats from fish appear to be protective against colon cancer by decreasing the formation of inflammatory eicosanoids. Eating just two servings of fish a week was shown to reduce the risk by about 25 percent. It is also helpful in controlling inflammation associated with ulcerative colitis.

❏ *See also* DIVERTICULITIS and MALABSORPTION SYNDROME, both in Part Two.

UNDERWEIGHT/WEIGHT LOSS

Some people are thinner than average all their lives and are perfectly healthy that way. For others, however, underweight may be associated with health problems. This is particularly true if the condition results from unintended, perhaps sudden, weight loss. Unintended weight loss can result from a malabsorption problem; intestinal parasites; certain types of cancer, a colon disorder such as Crohn's disease, ulcerative colitis, or diverticulitis; or a chronic illness such as diabetes, chronic diarrhea, or hyperthyroidism. Surgery, stress, or trauma, such as the loss of a loved one, can also contribute to loss of appetite and weight loss.

Underweight can also be caused by treatments such as cancer chemotherapy and radiation therapy, whose side effects include nausea, vomiting, and loss of appetite. An individual who is underweight but believes he or she weighs too much may be suffering from an eating disorder. Some patients with AIDS who are not getting the newer HAART therapy may suffer from what is known as "wasting syndrome," in which they become more and more emaciated as the disease progresses.

Weight loss may in turn cause nutritional deficiencies that further impair health and complicate recovery. Two age groups for whom poor nutrition is a special problem are the very young and the very old. Malnutrition in childhood, especially in infancy, can have permanent effects because it interferes with normal growth and development. Children also have less in the way of nutritional reserves in their bodies to draw upon if intake or absorption of nutrients is inadequate. At the other end of the life span, many elderly people find themselves less and less interested in eating as time goes by, and reduced financial resources may add to the incentive to skip meals. As a result, older people have an increased risk of becoming malnourished.

The suggestions in this section are intended for older people who require nutritional rehabilitation. The dosages are intended for adults. They may also be useful for people who have higher than normal nutritional requirements, such as people who have hepatitis or are undergoing cancer treatment, and those who are recovering from burns or trauma. A child who is undernourished or stops gaining weight should be seen by a physician.

NUTRIENTS

SUPPLEMENT	SUGGESTED DOSAGE	COMMENTS
Essential		
Raw liver extract	As directed on label.	Excellent source of B vitamins and minerals. Use liver extract from organically raised beef. Use a liquid form for easy assimilation.
Vitamin A plus carotenoid complex with natural beta-carotene	10,000 IU daily. As directed on label.	Antioxidants that enhance immunity and aid in fat storage. Essential for protein utilization.
Vitamin B complex	100 mg of each major B vitamin daily, with meals. (amounts of individual vitamins in a complex will vary).	Increases the appetite and aids in digestion of fats, carbohydrates, and protein. Use a sublingual form for best absorption. Injections (under a doctor's supervision) may be necessary.
Vitamin C with bioflavonoids	3,000 mg daily, in divided doses.	Helps to prevent cancer, protects against infection, and enhances immunity.
Vitamin D	400 IU daily.	Necessary for healthy bone formation.
Vitamin E	200 IU daily.	A powerful antioxidant that helps helps prevent cancer and inhibits the formation of free radicals. Use d-alpha-tocopherol form.
Zinc	80 mg daily. Do not exceed 100 mg daily from all supplements.	Improves the senses of taste and smell. Use zinc gluconate lozenges or OptiZinc for best absorption.`
Important		
Essential fatty acids (Ultimate Oil from Nature's Secret)	As directed on label.	A most important element of the diet.
Free form amino acid	As directed on label.	To supply needed protein in a form that is readily available and easily metabolized. Use a formula containing all the essential amino acids.
Garlic (Kyolic from Wakunaga)	2 capsules 3 times daily, with meals.	Provides protection against free radicals. Contains many essential nutrients.
Inf-zyme Forte from American Biologics	4 tablets 3 times daily, with meals.	Aids in the proper breakdown of proteins, fats, and carbohydrates for better absorption of foods.
Quercetin plus bromelain	As directed on label. As directed on label.	Aids in preventing reactions to certain foods, pollens, and other allergens. Increases immunity. Enhances the effectiveness of quercetin.
Helpful		
Brewer's yeast	As directed on label.	Stimulates the appetite and supplies B vitamins.
Floradix Iron + Herbs from Salus Haus	As directed on label. But only if your physician says you need iron.	Increases appetite and helps digestion.
Multienzyme complex	As directed on label.	Aids digestion.
Multivitamin and mineral supplement	As directed on label.	To supply a balance of all needed vitamins and minerals. Use a high-potency formula.
Spiru-tein from Nature's Plus	As directed on label. Take between meals.	A safe protein supplement.

Herbs

❑ Alfalfa, blessed thistle, caraway, cayenne (capsicum), celery, dill, fennel, hyssop, and lady's mantle all work to stimulate the appetite.

❑ Astragalus protects the immune system, helps with digestion, and combats fatigue.

Caution: Do not use astragalus in the presence of a fever.

❑ Fenugreek and ginseng have long been used as appetite stimulants and digestive aids, especially for older adults.

Caution: Do not use ginseng if you have high blood pressure, or are pregnant or nursing.

Recommendations

❑ If you think you may be underweight, and particularly if you are experiencing unintended weight loss, have a complete medical examination to check for an underlying physical disorder. You may have a health problem that requires treatment. An unintentional weight loss of five pounds in an adult should be a trigger to seek help. Be concerned about an infant or young child who suddenly seems to stop gaining weight normally.

❑ Eat a diet consisting of at least 300 grams of complex carbohydrates, 100 grams of protein, and 2,500 to 3,000 calories a day. Include starchy vegetables, such as potatoes and beans, as well as grains, turkey, chicken, fish, eggs, avocados, olive oil, safflower oil, raw cheeses, nuts, and seeds. Eat only whole-grain breads, pasta, crackers, and hot and cold cereals.

❑ Eat nondairy soy-based cream soups. Soymilk can be used in the same ways as cow's milk. Cream soups are usually higher in protein and calories than broth soups.

❑ Drink herbal teas, fruit and vegetable juices, and mineral water. When drinking non-caloric beverages such as water and tea, add some honey to increase calorie intake.

❑ Eat frequent but small meals and snacks, and eat them slowly. If you are undernourished, you may lose your appetite if confronted with large amounts of food at one sitting. You can always have additional servings if you are still hungry after the first.

❑ Do not eat fried or junk foods for extra calories. Instead, eat high-calorie snacks such as the following between meals or before bedtime: raw cheese; banana soy pudding; turkey, chicken, or tuna sandwiches with cheese; raw nuts; rice crackers with nut butter; yogurt; yogurt fruit shakes; carob soymilk; almond milk; buttermilk; custard; nuts; and avocados.

❑ Eliminate from the diet coffee, tea, and anything else (such as soft drinks) that contains caffeine.

❑ If possible, get regular moderate exercise. Walking and similar activities are good. Moderate exercise helps in the assimilation of nutrients and in increasing the appetite. Avoid strenuous exercise.

❑ Eat in relaxed surroundings. Do not try to eat when you are upset or nervous.

❑ If you smoke, stop.

❑ Investigate the possibility of food allergies. (*See* ALLERGIES in Part Two.) Avoid any foods you think you may be allergic to.

❑ Consult your physician about any medications you may be taking. Some medications can cause a decrease in appetite that can result in weight loss.

❑ If other people comment on your thinness but you feel you actually could stand to lose weight, consider professional evaluation for an eating disorder. (*See* ANOREXIA NERVOSA and/or BULIMIA in Part Two.)

Considerations

❑ Unexplained (and perhaps unwanted) weight loss among older adults can have a variety of causes, many of them physiological. These can include the following:

• As people grow older, food can lose its appeal as the senses of taste and smell diminish.

• Dental problems may hinder eating habits.

• Older people who live alone may suffer depression,

loneliness, and paranoia, and thus neglect their personal diets.

• Medications can reduce appetite or change how people taste food.

• Older people on fixed incomes may not be able to afford their favorite foods.

• Health problems associated with aging, such as cancer, often retard the appetite.

❑ Consideration of the appearance and smell of the food, as well as the eating environment, is important when trying to stimulate a poor appetite.

❑ The color red helps to stimulate taste buds. (*See* COLOR THERAPY in Part Three.)

❑ *See also* APPETITE, POOR.

URINARY TRACT INFECTION

See BLADDER INFECTION (CYSTITIS); KIDNEY DISEASE (RENAL FAILURE); and VAGINITIS.

UTERINE PROLAPSE

See PROLAPSE OF THE UTERUS.

UVEITIS

See under EYE PROBLEMS.

VAGINITIS

The symptoms of vaginitis, or inflammation of the mucous membranes lining the vagina, include a burning and/or itching sensation and abnormal vaginal discharge. Vaginitis may be caused by bacterial or fungal infection, vitamin B deficiency, or irritation from excessive douching or the use of such products as deodorant sprays. Infectious vaginitis is often caused by trichomonas, gonococci, or other sexually transmitted organisms. Other factors, such as poor hygiene and tight, nonporous clothing, may contribute to the problem. Pregnancy, diabetes, and the use of antibiotics disturb the body's natural balance, creating an environment in which infectious organisms can thrive. Oral contraceptives also can produce vaginal inflammation.

Atrophic vaginitis is a condition primarily found in postmenopausal women and those whose ovaries have been surgically removed. This disorder can result in the formation of adhesions and a high susceptibility to infection. Common symptoms include itching or burning, painful intercourse, and a thin, watery discharge, occasionally tinged with blood.

Unless otherwise specified, the dosages recommended here are for adults. For a girl between the ages of twelve and seventeen, reduce the dose to three-quarters of the recommended amount.

NUTRIENTS

SUPPLEMENT	SUGGESTED DOSAGE	COMMENTS
Very Important		
Acidophilus (Kyo-Dophilus from Wakunaga)	As directed on label 3 times daily, with meals. Also open 3 capsules and dissolve in 1 qt warm water with 6 drops tea tree oil added to use as a douche.	To replenish normal "friendly" bacteria. Use a nondairy formula.
Biotin	300 mcg 3 times daily.	Inhibits yeast.
Essential fatty acids	As directed on label.	Aids healing.
Garlic (Kyolic from Wakunaga)	1 capsule 3 times daily, with meals.	Has antifungal properties.
Vitamin B complex	50–100 mg of each major B vitamin, 3 times daily, with meals (amounts of individual vitamins in a complex will vary).	Regulates metabolism and promotes good health. Often deficient in people with vaginitis. Use a high-potency formula.
plus extra vitamin B$_6$ (pyridoxine)	50 mg 3 times daily.	Especially important if using estrogen cream for treatment of atrophic vaginitis.
Yeast-Gard from Lake Consumer Products	As directed on label.	Excellent antifungal agent. Reduces pain.
Helpful		
N-Acetylglucosamine (N-A-G from Source Naturals)	As directed on label.	Amino acid compound. Forms the basis of complex molecular structures that are key parts of mucous membrane tissue.
Vitamin A with mixed carotenoids including beta-carotene	25,000 IU daily. If you are pregnant, do not exceed 10,000 IU daily.	Powerful antioxidants that aid healing.
plus vitamin E	200 IU daily.	Use d-alpha-tocopherol form.
Vitamin C with bioflavonoids	2,000–5,000 mg daily, in divided doses.	Important immune system stimulant. Necessary for tissue healing.
Vitamin D with extra calcium and magnesium	1,000 mg daily. 1,500 mg daily. 1,000 mg daily.	To relieve stress. Women need supplements of these nutrients at this time.
Zinc	30 mg daily. Do not exceed a total of 100 mg daily from all supplements.	To increase immunity and promote proper utilization of vitamin A. Also reduces severity of herpes outbreaks. Use zinc gluconate lozenges or OptiZinc for best absorption.

Herbs

❑ Aloe vera is helpful for infections and is known for its healing effects. Aloe vera gel can be applied topically to relieve itching. It can also be taken internally or used in a douche.

❑ Barberry has remarkable infection-fighting properties.

❑ Douche with infusions made from antiseptic herbs such as calendula, garlic, goldenseal, fresh plantain, St. John's wort, or tea tree oil, along with herbs such as comfrey leaves, to soothe irritation. Echinacea and goldenseal can also be taken orally.

Cautions: Comfrey is recommended for external use only. Do not take echinacea for longer than three months. It should not be used by people who are allergic to ragweed. Do not take goldenseal internally on a daily basis for more than one week at a time. Do not use it during pregnancy or if you are breast-feeding, and use with caution if you are allergic to ragweed. If you have a history of cardiovascular disease, diabetes, or glaucoma, use it only under a doctor's supervision. St. John's wort may cause increased sensitivity to sunlight. It may also produce anxiety, gastrointestinal symptoms, and headaches. It can interact with some drugs, including antidepressants, birth control pills, and anticoagulants.

❑ Calendula and vitamin A vaginal suppositories are soothing and healing to irritated tissues. Goldenseal suppositories are useful for all types of infection.

Caution: Do not take goldenseal internally on a daily basis for more than one week at a time. Do not use it during pregnancy or if you are breast-feeding, and use with caution if you are allergic to ragweed. If you have a history of cardiovascular disease, diabetes, or glaucoma, use it only under a doctor's supervision.

❑ Chamomile has antifungal properties.

Caution: Do not use chamomile if you are allergic to ragweed. Do not use during pregnancy or nursing. It may interact with warfarin or cyclosporine, so patients using these drugs should avoid it.

❑ Cinnamon and dandelion inhibit the growth of *Candida albicans.* They can be used as a douche or taken internally.

Caution: Do not use cinnamon in large quantities during pregnancy.

❑ Echinacea has antifungal properties and enhances the immune system. It can be taken internally or used as a douche.

Caution: Do not take echinacea for longer than three months. It should not be used by people who are allergic to ragweed.

❑ Pau d'arco contains natural antibiotic agents and has a healing effect. It can be taken in capsule form, made into a tea, or used as a douche.

❑ Tea tree oil is good for vaginitis. Topical tea tree oil cream is effective against fungal infection, herpes blisters, warts, and other types of infection. Tea tree oil suppositories have been used successfully for vaginal yeast infections.

Recommendations

❑ Eat plain yogurt that contains live yogurt cultures, or apply plain yogurt directly to the vagina. This can help fight infection and soothe inflammation. Also consume brown rice, millet, and acidophilus.

❑ Consume fiber daily. Oat bran is a good source.

❑ Eat a diet that is fruit-free, sugar-free, and yeast-free.

❑ Avoid aged cheeses, alcohol, chocolate, dried fruits, fermented foods, all grains containing gluten (wheat, oats, rye, and barley), ham, honey, nut butters, pickles, raw mushrooms, soy sauce, sprouts, sugar in any form, vinegar, and all yeast products. Also eliminate citrus and acidic fruits (grapefruits, lemons, limes, oranges, pineapple, and tomatoes) from your diet until the inflammation subsides.

❑ Keep clean and dry. Wear cotton underwear, which absorbs moisture and allows air to circulate. Avoid tight clothing and synthetic fabrics. Change into dry clothing as soon as possible after swimming. Do not spend prolonged periods of time in a wet bathing suit.

❑ To relieve itching, open a vitamin E capsule and apply the oil to the inflamed area.

❑ Add 3 cups of pure apple cider vinegar to bathwater to treat vaginitis. Soak in the tub for twenty minutes, allowing the water to flow into the vagina.

❑ Do not use corticosteroids or oral contraceptives until your condition improves. Oral contraceptives can upset the balance of microorganisms in the body.

❑ Do not use sweet-smelling douches. Try douching with 2 capsules of garlic or with 1 cup of fresh garlic juice added to a quart of warm water. Alternate this treatment with acidophilus douches: Open 2 acidophilus capsules and add them to either 1 quart of warm water or to 1 cup of plain yogurt. The garlic fights infection while the acidophilus helps to restore normal flora and acid balance.

❑ Avoid taking iron supplements until the inflammation subsides. Infectious bacteria require iron for growth. If a bacterial infection is present, the body naturally "hides" iron by storing it in the liver, spleen, and bone marrow to inhibit the growth of the bacteria.

Caution: Check with your physician before taking iron supplements.

❑ Drink steam-distilled water only.

Considerations

❑ You may need antibiotics to clear the infection, if it is bacterial. Check with your physician if your pain and/or itching lasts more than a week. Refrain from intercourse until your infection has cleared.

❑ Atrophic vaginitis is often treated with prescription estrogen ointments. The use of these products increases the body's need for vitamin B_6. Vaginal absorption of synthetic estrogen may be dangerous.

❑ Natural progesterone cream applied to the vagina is beneficial for atrophic vaginitis.

❑ *See also* BLADDER INFECTION (CYSTITIS); CANDIDIASIS; KIDNEY DISEASE (RENAL FAILURE); and SEXUALLY TRANSMITTED DISEASE (STD), all in Part Two.

VARICOSE VEINS

Varicose veins are abnormally enlarged, bulging, bluish, and lumpy-looking veins, often associated with dull, nagging aches and pains. This is the result of malfunctioning valves inside the veins. When blood pulses through the arteries, powered by the beating of the heart, to provide nutrients and oxygen to the body tissues, it returns to the heart by means of the veins. Like the arteries, the veins are tube-shaped vessels in graduated sizes, but unlike the arteries, the veins have tiny valves on their inner walls to prevent the blood from flowing backward, toward the arteries. If the valves do not work properly, circulation is impaired and blood accumulates in the veins, stretching them. Swelling, restlessness, leg sores, itching, leg cramps, and a feeling of heaviness in the legs are characteristic of varicose veins.

Because poor circulation contributes to the formation of varicose veins, they are more common in people who sit or stand in one position for prolonged periods of time, people who habitually sit with their legs crossed, and those who lack proper regular exercise. Excess weight, heavy lifting, and pregnancy put increased pressure on the legs, increasing the likelihood of developing varicose veins. Constipation, heart failure, liver disease, and abdominal tumors can also play a role in the formation of varicose veins. A deficiency of vitamin C and bioflavonoids (mainly rutin) can weaken the collagen structure in the vein walls, which can lead to varicose veins. A tendency toward varicose veins may also run in families. Some experts believe that hormone replacement therapy (HRT) and birth control pills can contribute to the formation of varicose veins. It is estimated that approximately 50 to 55 percent of all middle-aged American women and 40 to 45 percent of men have at least some varicosities. More women than men are affected.

Most cases of varicose veins do not pose a serious problem and can be managed with simple home measures. In some cases, however, if varicose veins are not treated properly, complications such as bleeding under the skin, deep vein blood clots, an eczema-like condition near the affected veins, or ulcerated spots near the ankles may occur. Other possible, and more serious, complications that can arise include phlebitis (inflammation of a vein), thrombophlebitis (formation of a clot in an inflamed vein), post-thrombotic syndrome (indicated by a number of symptoms including leg ulcers), hemorrhage from a ruptured vein, or pulmonary embolism (a blood clot that travels to the lung and lodges there).

Unless otherwise specified, the dosages recommended here are for adults. For children between the ages of twelve and seventeen, reduce the dose to three-quarters of the recommended amount.

NUTRIENTS

SUPPLEMENT	SUGGESTED DOSAGE	COMMENTS
Very Important		
Coenzyme Q10	100 mg daily.	Improves tissue oxygenation, increases circulation, and enhances immunity
plus Coenzyme A from Coenzyme-A Technologies	As directed on label.	Works with coenzyme Q10 to support the immune system's detoxification of many dangerous substances.
Dimethylglycine (DMG) (Aangamik DMG from FoodScience of Vermont)	50 mg 3 times daily.	Improves oxygen utilization in the tissues.
Essential fatty acids (Ultimate Oil from Nature's Secret)	As directed on label.	Reduces pain and helps to keep blood vessels soft and pliable.
Glutathione	As directed on label.	Protects the heart, veins, and arteries from oxidant damage.
Pycnogenol or grape seed extract	As directed on label. As directed on label.	Stimulates blood circulation, boosts immunity, neutralizes free radicals, and strengthens connective tissue, including that of the cardiovascular system.
Vitamin C plus	3,000–6,000 mg daily.	Aids circulation by reducing blood clotting tendencies.
bioflavonoid complex plus extra	100 mg daily.	To promote healing and prevent bruising.
rutin	50 mg 3 times daily.	A potent noncitrus bioflavonoid that helps maintain the strength of blood vessels.
Important		
Vitamin E	200 IU daily.	Improves circulation and aids in preventing heavy feeling in the legs. Use d-alpha-tocopherol form.
Helpful		
Aerobic Bulk Cleanse from Aerobic Life Industries	As directed on label. Take separately from other supplements and medications.	Keeping the colon clean is important.
Brewer's yeast	As directed on label.	Contains needed protein and B vitamins.
Lecithin granules or capsules	1 tbsp 3 times daily, with meals. 1,200 mg 3 times daily, with meals.	Fat emulsifier that aids circulation.
Multivitamin and mineral complex	As directed on label.	To maintain a balance of all necessary nutrients.
Vitamin A plus natural carotenoid complex (Betatene)	10,000 IU daily. As directed on label.	To enhance immunity, protect the cells, and slow the aging process.
Vitamin B complex plus extra vitamin B6 (pyridoxine) and vitamin B12	50–100 mg of each major B vitamin 3 times daily, with meals (amounts of individual vitamins in a complex will vary). 50 mg daily. 300–1,000 mcg daily.	B vitamins are needed to help in digestion of foods. Sublingual forms are best for all the B vitamins.
Vitamin D plus calcium and magnesium	1,000 mg daily, at bedtime. 1,500 mg daily, at bedtime. 750 mg daily, at bedtime.	This combination helps to relieve leg cramps. Use calcium chelate form.
Zinc plus copper	80 mg daily. 3 mg daily.	Aids healing. Needed to balance with zinc.

Herbs

☐ Aloe vera gel is a cooling and soothing topical treatment for varicose veins.

☐ Bilberry supports the health of connective tissue, including that of the veins.

☐ Bromelain can reduce the risk of clot formation in the blood vessels.

☐ Butcher's broom, ginkgo biloba, gotu kola, and hawthorn berries improve circulation in the legs.

☐ Cayenne helps to relieve pain and inflammation, and also expands blood vessels, reducing stress on the capillaries. It is available in capsule and cream forms.

☐ Dandelion alleviates tissue swelling by reducing water retention.

☐ Horse chestnut makes a good treatment for the discomfort of varicose veins. Mix ½ teaspoon of horse chestnut powder with 2 cups of water, and moisten a sterile cotton gauze cloth with the mixture. Rub the cloth gently over the affected area. This is soothing to inflamed veins. Witch hazel can be used in the same way to reduce discomfort.

☐ Horse Chestnut Cream from Planetary Formulas is a topical formula containing horse chestnut, butcher's broom, witch hazel, white oak, and myrrh. It can be used to reduce the appearance of varicose veins.

☐ Herbs used in traditional Chinese medicine that are helpful in alleviating symptoms include magnolia flower (*Magnolia liliflora,* also known as xho yi hua), scutellaria (*Scutellaria baicalensis,* or huang qin; also known as Baikal skullcap), trichosanth (*Trichosanthes kirilowii*), and wild angelica (*Angelica dahurica,* or bai zhi).

☐ Bathing your legs or other affected area in white oak bark tea three times a day helps to stimulate blood flow. Simmer (but do not boil) a strong tea and use the tea to make compresses. Apply the compresses to affected areas.

Recommendations

☐ Eat a diet that is low in fat and refined carbohydrates and includes plenty of fish and fresh fruits and vegetables.

☐ Eat as many blackberries and cherries as you can. These may help prevent varicose veins, or ease the symptoms if you already have them.

❑ Include garlic, ginger, onions, and pineapple in your diet.

❑ Make sure that your diet contains plenty of fiber to prevent constipation and keep the bowels clean.

❑ Avoid animal protein, processed and refined foods, sugar, ice cream, fried foods, cheeses, peanuts, junk foods, tobacco, alcohol, and salt.

❑ Maintain a healthy weight and get regular moderate exercise. Walking, swimming, and bicycling all promote good circulation. Change your daily routine to allow more time for exercise and movement for your legs.

❑ Wear loose clothing that does not restrict blood flow. It is a good idea to wear supportive elastic stockings; these help to support the varicose veins and prevent swelling.

❑ Elevate your legs above heart level for twenty minutes at least once a day to alleviate symptoms.

❑ Avoid long periods of standing or sitting. Avoid crossing your legs, doing heavy lifting, and putting any unnecessary pressure on your legs.

❑ If you sit at a desk all day at work, make sure to get up and walk around periodically. You can also flex your leg muscles and wiggle your toes to increase blood flow. If possible, try to rest your feet on an object that is elevated from the floor when seated.

❑ If you have to stand for long periods of time, shift your weight between your feet, stand on your toes, or take short walks to alleviate pressure.

❑ Elevate your feet in front of you while sitting down to read or watch television.

❑ After bathing, apply castor oil directly over the problem veins and massage the oil into your legs from the feet up.

❑ To help improve circulation and ease pain, fill a tub with cold water. Stand in the water and simulate walking.

❑ Try using homeopathic remedies to ease symptoms. Homeopathic remedies that have been used to treat varicose veins include *Ferrum metallicum*, *Hamamelis virginiana*, and *Pulsatilla*.

❑ Avoid scratching the itchy skin above varicose veins. This can cause ulceration and bleeding.

Considerations

❑ Cellulose is an indigestible carbohydrate found on the outer layer of vegetables and fruits. Good for alleviating symptoms, it can be found in apples, beets, Brazil nuts, broccoli, carrots, celery, green beans, lima beans, pears, peas, and whole grains.

❑ Some physicians treat varicose veins by injecting a sodium tetradecyl sulfate (saline) solution into the affected vein and applying compression bandages for a period of time. The solution fuses the vein walls together permanently, closing the defective vein. The body compensates for lost vessels by finding an alternate route for blood flow.

Tell your doctor if you are pregnant or want to become pregnant. Also tell your doctor what medications you are taking; some medicines may interact with this treatment.

❑ Spider veins are chronically dilated capillaries near the surface of the skin. They are harmless and rarely cause any problems, although they can be distressing for cosmetic reasons.

❑ Hemorrhoids are actually varicose veins of the anus or rectum. Symptoms of hemorrhoids include rectal itching, pain, and blood in the stool. (*See* HEMORRHOIDS in Part Two.)

❑ Massage therapy can aid in stimulating the legs. You should not massage the veins directly, but instead massage the area around them and upward toward the heart.

❑ Compression therapy, in which a compression garment of some type is used to exert pressure on the legs in an effort to help the venous valves close properly, may be helpful in alleviating symptoms.

❑ Dimethylsulfoxide (DMSO) has been used to relieve the swelling and pain of severe varicose veins. This liquid, a by-product of wood processing, is applied topically to the affected area as needed.

Cautions: Do *not* apply DMSO to hemorrhoids. Only pure DMSO from a health food store should be used. Commercial-grade DMSO such as that found in hardware stores is not suitable for healing purposes. Any contaminants on the skin or in the product can be taken into the tissues by action of the DMSO.

Note: The use of DMSO may result in a garlicky body odor. This is temporary, and is not a cause for concern.

❑ The symptoms of varicose veins are similar to those of thrombophlebitis. In addition, the chances of developing varicose veins increase greatly if you suffer from thrombophlebitis. (*See* THROMBOPHLEBITIS in Part Two.)

❑ Sclerotherapy is a treatment sometimes recommended for varicose veins. In this procedure, an irritant is injected into the vein, causing it to become nonfunctional, and subsequently shrink and fade. There are potential mild complications with this procedure.

❑ Surgical removal of varicose veins is a treatment option that may be recommended if the veins are causing a considerable amount of discomfort. The operation results in scarring.

❑ Vein stripping is a medical treatment in which a main superficial vein is removed and the veins connected to it tied off, forcing the blood to return to the heart through the deeper leg veins.

❑ A more recent technique involves inserting a catheter into the vein, then heating it with radio-frequency or laser-generated heat. As the catheter is slowly withdrawn, it collapses the damaged vein. These veins then are gradually absorbed into the body. Large veins must still be removed surgically later, but the additional procedure adds little to the pain and inconvenience overall. However, this procedure is performed by only a handful of surgeons and is still considered experimental.

❑ Valve repair is another treatment option for varicose veins. In this procedure, a synthetic material is used to restore the valve.

❑ *See* CIRCULATORY PROBLEMS in Part Two.

❑ *See also under* PREGNANCY-RELATED PROBLEMS in Part Two.

VENEREAL DISEASE

See SEXUALLY TRANSMITTED DISEASE (STD).

VERTIGO

Vertigo is a sensation of dizziness, faintness, or lightheadedness that results from an impaired sense of balance and equilibrium. The term comes from *vertere,* the Latin verb meaning "to turn." A person suffering from vertigo may feel that he or she is sinking or falling and/or that the room and objects in it are spinning around. In some cases, the individual may feel that he or she is spinning, too. Vertigo is sometimes accompanied by nausea and hearing loss. Vertigo is not an illness in itself—it is a symptom of another condition.

Vertigo occurs when the central nervous system receives conflicting messages from the inner ears, eyes, muscles, and skin pressure receptors. This may result from any of a variety of causes including:

• Benign paroxysmal positional vertigo (BPPV). It is the most common form of vertigo and is characterized by the sensation of motion initiated by sudden head movements.

• Inflammation within the inner ear. This is known as labyrinthitis. This condition is characterized by the sudden onset of vertigo and may be associated with hearing loss.

• Ménière's disease. It is composed of a triad of symptoms: episodes of vertigo, ringing in the ears, and hearing loss. People have the abrupt onset of severe vertigo and fluctuating hearing loss, as well as periods in which they are symptom-free.

• Acoustic neuroma. A type of tumor. Symptoms include vertigo with one-sided ringing in the ear and hearing loss.

• Decreased blood flow to the brain and base of the brain. Bleeding into the back of the brain is known as cerebellar hemorrhage and is characterized by vertigo, headache, difficulty walking, and inability to look toward the side of the bleed. The result is that the person's eyes gaze away from the side with the problem. Walking is also extremely impaired.

• Multiple sclerosis. Vertigo is often the presenting symptom in MS. The onset is usually abrupt, and examina-

tion of the eyes may reveal the inability of the eyes to move past the midline toward the nose.

• Head trauma and neck injury. This vertigo usually goes away on its own.

• Migraine, a severe form of headache. The vertigo is usually followed by a headache. There is often a prior history of similar episodes but no lasting problems.

Because of the effects of aging on the body, older people are more prone than others to vertigo. The body maintains a sense of balance through a complex mechanism involving both the inner ears and visual input. Within the canals of the inner ears, there are structures called *otoliths,* which are minute calcium carbonate crystals that press upon the hairlike cells that line the inner membranes. Gravity acts on the otoliths so that they shift in response to head movements. This bends the hairlike cells, which, in turn, transmit signals to the brain. The brain then uses these signals to calculate the positioning of the head. As people age, tiny bits of debris may accumulate in the inner ears and press against the hairlike cells, resulting in false signals being sent to the brain. This can interfere with the sense of balance and result in vertigo. In addition, with increasing age, nerve impulses require more time to travel from the eyes to the brain and spinal cord. This can cause dizziness and loss of balance upon sudden movement.

Dizziness is not synonymous with vertigo. Anyone may occasionally experience a feeling of lightheadedness, dizziness, unsteadiness, or the sensation of feeling faint. Those with low blood pressure may have this feeling upon rising quickly from a sitting or lying position. In some cases, dizziness can be a warning sign of a heart attack, stroke, concussion, or brain damage.

Unless otherwise specified, the dosages recommended here are for adults. For children between the ages of twelve and seventeen, reduce the dose to three-quarters of the recommended amount. For children between six and twelve, use one-half of the recommended dose, and for children under the age of six, use one-quarter of the recommended amount.

NUTRIENTS

SUPPLEMENT	SUGGESTED DOSAGE	COMMENTS
Very Important		
Dimethylglycine (DMG) (Aangamik DMG from FoodScience of Vermont)	As directed on label.	Increases oxygen supply to the brain.
Vitamin B complex	100 mg of each major B vitamin 3 times daily, with meals (amounts of individual vitamins in a complex will vary).	B vitamins are necessary for normal brain and central nervous system function. Consider injections (under a doctor's supervision) for better absorption. If injections are not available, use sublingual forms.
plus extra vitamin B₃ (niacin)	100 mg 3 times daily. Do not exceed this amount.	Improves cerebral circulation and lowers cholesterol.

and vitamin B₆ (pyridoxine)	50 mg daily.	*Caution:* Do not take niacin if you have a liver disorder, gout, or high blood pressure.
and vitamin B₁₂	1,000–2,000 mcg daily.	A sublingual form is recommended.
Vitamin C with bioflavonoids	3,000–10,000 mg daily, in divided doses.	Antioxidants that also improve circulation.
Vitamin E	200 IU daily.	Improves circulation. Use d-alpha-tocopherol form.

Important		
Choline and inositol and/or lecithin	As directed on label, 3 times daily. / As directed on label.	Necessary in nerve function. Help to prevent hardening of the arteries and improve brain function.
Coenzyme Q₁₀ plus Coenzyme A from Coenzyme-A Technologies	100–200 mg daily. / As directed on label.	Improves circulation to the brain. Works well with coenzyme Q₁₀ to support the immune system's detoxification of many dangerous substances.
Vitamin A with mixed carotenoids including natural beta-carotene	10,000 IU daily.	Enhances immunity and acts as an antioxidant.
Zinc	30 mg daily. Do not exceed a total of 100 mg daily from all supplements.	Promotes a healthy immune system and helps maintain vitamin E levels. Use zinc gluconate lozenges or OptiZinc for best absorption.

Helpful		
Brewer's yeast	½ tsp daily for 3 days, then increase to 1 tbsp daily.	Contains balanced B vitamins.
Calcium and magnesium	1,500 mg daily. / 750 mg daily.	Important in maintaining regular nerve impulses. To help prevent dizziness.
Kelp	1,000–1,500 mg daily.	For necessary balanced minerals and vitamins.
Melatonin	1.5–5 mg daily, taken 2 hours or less before bedtime.	Helps to maintain equilibrium.
Multivitamin and mineral complex	As directed on label.	For necessary balance of vitamins and minerals.

Herbs

❑ Black cohosh lowers blood pressure.

Caution: Do not use black cohosh if you are pregnant or have any type of chronic disease. Black cohosh should not be used by those with liver problems.

❑ Butcher's broom and cayenne (capsicum) help improve circulation.

❑ Dandelion tea or extract is very good for high blood pressure.

❑ Ginger relieves dizziness and nausea.

❑ Ginkgo biloba improves circulation and improves brain function by increasing the supply of oxygen to the brain. Take 120 milligrams of ginkgo biloba extract daily.

Caution: Do not take ginkgo biloba if you have a bleeding disorder, or are scheduled for surgery or a dental procedure.

Recommendations

❑ Avoid making rapid or extreme movements and rapid changes in body position.

❑ Limit your total sodium intake to about 2,000 milligrams per day. Too much sodium can disrupt the workings of the inner ear.

❑ Avoid alcohol, caffeine, nicotine, and all fried foods.

❑ To subdue dizziness, sit in a chair with your feet flat on the floor and stare at a fixed object for a few minutes.

❑ If you begin to experience dizziness soon after taking new medication, the problem may be drug related. Discuss the problem with your physician or pharmacist.

❑ If vertigo is a recurring problem, consult your health care provider. It may be a sign of an underlying problem that requires treatment.

Considerations

❑ People who have vertigo sometimes experience a phenomenon called nystagmus, involuntary rapid or jerky eye movements. It may occur spontaneously or as a result of changing positions. Nystagmus, or any other unusual eye movement, always requires the attention of a physician.

❑ Dizziness can be caused by many different things, some of them serious. If you feel dizzy and find it difficult to speak, swallow, or think clearly, seek medical attention. These may be the symptoms of a stroke. Numbness and tingling or loss of vision accompanied by dizziness also can be signs of a stroke.

❑ If dizziness is accompanied by nausea, sweating, and paleness of complexion with a racing heartbeat, seek medical attention. This can be a sign of a number of different health problems, including a heart attack, or, if you have diabetes, a hypoglycemic (low blood sugar) episode. Hypotension, or a sudden drop in blood pressure, also can cause sudden dizziness, especially after meals.

❑ Air contains less oxygen at altitudes high above sea level. Lower oxygen levels can cause mild, temporary dizziness or light-headedness.

❑ Certain activities, such as taking amusement park rides, watching action movies, sailing, or playing video games, may bring on vertigo or dizziness. In such cases, symptoms diminish soon after the activity ceases.

❑ Treatment for benign paroxysmal positional vertigo usually entails special exercises and, sometimes, surgery.

☐ *See also* ARTERIOSCLEROSIS/ATHEROSCLEROSIS; CARDIOVAS-CULAR DISEASE; and MENIÉRÈ'S DISEASE in Part Two.

VITILIGO

Vitiligo, also called leukoderma, is a skin condition characterized by chalky white patches of skin surrounded by a dark border. The spots can be few or many; they may be tiny or cover the body. They usually appear on both sides of the body in approximately the same place (for example, you may have exactly the same white patches on the top of your left and right feet), and they do not hurt or itch. These spots occur because, for some reason, the cells that normally produce the skin pigment melanin are absent. If the affected area is on the scalp, the hair that grows from it is likely to be white as well.

Vitiligo itself is not a threat to health. However, it has been linked with other diseases in some cases, including Addison's disease, pernicious anemia, and alopecia areata (patches of hair loss). The exact cause of vitiligo is not known, but it can run in families and may be related to an autoimmune problem. A thyroid gland malfunction may be involved as well. Vitiligo can also occur after physical trauma to the skin. Chemical agents such as catechol (used for tanning and dyeing) and phenol (often found in disinfectants) may be involved in the development of this condition. Physical and emotional stress may aggravate the condition. The unpigmented spots are a concern primarily for cosmetic reasons and are highly vulnerable to sunburn.

Unless otherwise specified, the dosages recommended here are for adults. For children between the ages of twelve and seventeen, reduce the dose to three-quarters of the recommended amount. For children between six and twelve, use one-half of the recommended dose, and for children under the age of six, use one-quarter of the recommended amount.

NUTRIENTS

SUPPLEMENT	SUGGESTED DOSAGE	COMMENTS
Very Important		
Vitamin B complex	50 mg and up of each major B vitamin, 3 times daily (amounts of individual vitamins in a complex will vary).	Needed for proper skin tone and texture. Helps to combat stress. A sublingual form is recommended.
plus extra vitamin B₅ (pantothenic acid) and	300 mg daily, in divided doses.	The antistress vitamin. Important in skin pigmentation. A sublingual form is best.
para-aminobenzoic acid (PABA)	100 mg and up, 3 times daily.	Aids in stopping discoloration of the hair. Consider injections (under a doctor's supervision).
Important		
Essential fatty acids (primrose oil or Ultimate Oil from Nature's Secret)	As directed on label.	Stimulates hormone function and contains all the needed essential fatty acids.
Helpful		
Ageless Beauty from Biotec Foods	As directed on label.	Protects the skin from free radical damage.
Calcium and magnesium	1,000 mg daily. 500 mg daily.	Deficiency contributes to fragility of the skin. Needed to balance with calcium.
Methylsulfonyl-methane (MSM)	As directed on label.	Possesses remarkable therapeutic properties for the skin. Helps to detoxify the body on a cellular level.
Multivitamin and mineral complex	As directed on label.	To maintain a balance of all essential nutrients.
S-Adenosyl-methionine (SAMe)	As directed on label.	Aids in relief of stress and depression, eases pain, and has antioxidant effects. *Caution:* Do not use if you have bipolar mood disorder or take prescription antidepressants. Do not give to a child under twelve.
Silica	As directed on label.	Important for developing skin's strength and elasticity; stimulates collagen formation.
Vitamin A plus carotenoid complex with beta-carotene	10,000 IU daily. As directed on label.	To promote healing and construction of new skin tissue.
Vitamin C with bioflavonoids	3,000–5,000 mg daily, in divided doses.	Necessary for the formation of collagen, a protein that gives skin its flexibility. Also fights free radicals and strengthens the capillaries that feed the skin.
Vitamin E	200 IU daily.	Protects against free radicals that can damage the skin. Use d-alpha-tocopherol form.
Zinc plus copper	50 mg daily. Do not exceed a total of 100 mg daily from all supplements. 3 mg daily.	For tissue strength and repair. Use zinc gluconate lozenges or OptiZinc for best absorption. Needed for collagen production and healthy skin. Also needed to balance with zinc.

Herbs

☐ The use of picrorrhiza (an Indian herb used in Ayurvedic medicine) has been shown to reduce the number and size of unpigmented skin patches.

☐ St. John's wort can help reduce stress and anxiety.

Caution: St. John's wort may cause increased sensitivity to sunlight. It may also produce anxiety, gastrointestinal symptoms, and headaches. It can interact with some drugs, including antidepressants, birth control pills, and anticoagulants.

☐ Ginkgo biloba (40 milligrams, three times a day) was shown to arrest the progression of the condition. Ginkgo is a potent antioxidant and immune booster.

Caution: Do not take ginkgo biloba if you have a bleeding disorder, or are scheduled for surgery or a dental procedure.

Recommendations

❑ Consult a nutritionally oriented physician for vitamin B complex plus PABA injections (*see under* Nutrients, above).

❑ Treat the affected area gently—cleanse gently, apply moisturizers liberally, and protect exposed areas from cleansing agents or other chemicals by wearing protective gloves or clothing.

❑ Expose patches of affected skin to the sun—this may promote repigmentation—but don't overdo it. Use adequate sun protection on the affected area, and always apply a sunscreen with a sun protection factor (SPF) of 15 or higher to any unpigmented areas. They have no natural protection against the sun's ultraviolet rays.

Considerations

❑ Vitiligo sometimes responds to the use of PABA and magnesium. Small spots of pigment appear gradually, like freckles. The spots gradually merge until normal color is restored. Some people with vitiligo have prematurely gray or white hair. A small percentage of such people treated with PABA and magnesium have experienced a return of both skin and hair to the original color.

❑ Vitiligo lesions may be de-emphasized by the use of commercial cosmetics that cover the affected area with an opaque, waterproof layer. DermaBlend is one widely available product. (*See* Manufacturer and Distributor Information in the Appendix.)

❑ Creams and lotions that contain antioxidants such as ginkgo biloba, green tea, vitamin C, and carotenes may be helpful.

❑ Creams containing fluorinated steroids may be prescribed to stimulate repigmentation of the skin.

❑ For persons with widespread vitiligo, bleaching of the unaffected skin with hydroquinone (a weak but safe depigmenting agent) may be recommended. (A commonly used form is 20 percent monobenzyl ether.) This is done to minimize the difference in color between pigmented and depigmented areas. The process is irreversible, and it can take from several months to years to complete.

❑ Psoralen plus ultraviolet light A (PUVA) therapy is often used to treat vitiligo. This therapy combines ultraviolet light with an oral drug, and has proven to be effective, even for those with advanced symptoms. However, this treatment has many potential side effects for some individuals, including eye problems, liver damage, nausea, and skin blistering. Often hundreds of procedures are necessary. PUVA seems to work better when combined with a prescription vitamin D_3 cream. One study showed that light therapy was enhanced with L-phenylalanine and alpha-lipoic acid.

❑ B_{12} and folic acid were shown to be ineffective at improving the treatment outcome of vitiligo with narrowband UVB phototherapy.

❑ For mild forms of vitiligo, topical corticosteroids may be used to restore small patches of nonpigmented skin.

❑ Autologous melanocyte transplant is a procedure in which a sample of your normal pigmented skin is placed in a laboratory dish containing a special cell-culture solution to grow melanocytes. When the melanocytes in the culture solution have multiplied, the doctor transplants them to your depigmented skin patches. This procedure is currently experimental and is impractical for the routine care of people with vitiligo. It is also very expensive, and its side effects are not known.

❑ GH3 cream from Gero Vita International has given good results for many skin problems. This face cream is for adult use only.

❑ Hypnosis by a trained clinician may help with treatment in some patients. This alternative therapy was used in ancient times to treat all sorts of skin disorders.

WARTS

Warts are small growths that are caused by human papillomaviruses (HPVs). There are at least forty known types of HPV. Warts may appear singly or in clusters. This section addresses three types of warts: common warts, plantar warts, and genital warts.

Common warts can be found anywhere on the body, but are most common on the hands, fingers, elbows, forearms, knees, face, and the skin around the nails. Most often, they occur on skin that is continually exposed to friction, trauma, or abrasion. They can also occur on the larynx (the voice box) and cause hoarseness. Common warts may be flat or raised, dry or moist, and have a rough and pitted surface that is either the same color as or slightly darker than the surrounding skin. They can be as small as a pinhead or as large as a small bean. Highly contagious, the virus that causes common warts is acquired through breaks in the skin. Common warts can spread if they are picked, trimmed, bitten, or touched. Warts on the face can spread as a result of shaving. Common warts typically do not cause pain or itching.

Plantar warts occur on the soles of the feet and the undersides of the toes. They are bumpy white growths that may resemble calluses, except that they can be tender to the touch and often bleed if the surface is trimmed. They also often have an identifiable hard center. Plantar warts do not tend to spread to other parts of the body.

Genital warts are soft, moist growths found in and around the vagina, anus, penis, groin, thigh, and/or scrotum. They are usually pink or red in color and resemble tiny heads of cauliflower. Genital warts most often occur in clusters, but they can appear singly as well; these are referred to as low-risk human papillomavirus (HPV) warts. They are transmitted through vaginal, oral, or anal sex, and are highly contagious. Because the warts do not usually appear until three months or more after an individual becomes infected with the HPV that causes them, the virus can be spread before the carrier is even aware that he or she has it. Genital warts are not cancerous. If left untreated, they may go away or increase in size and number. An infant born to a mother with genital warts may contract the virus, although this is rare.

High-risk warts caused by HPV are cancerous, but no symptoms appear until the cancer is quite advanced. If the high-risk HPV infections are not cleared by the body's own immune system, the wart cells turn into cancer cells. About 10 percent of women with high-risk HPV infections are at risk for cervical cancer. High-risk HPV can also linger and infect the cells of the penis, anus, vulva, or vagina, where it can cause cancer. HPV affects 20 million Americans, and 6.2 million become infected each year. About 4,000 women die each year from cervical cancer caused by HPV. At least 50 percent of sexually active men and women contract HPV at some time in their lives. Cervical cancer affects 11,070 women each year.

Besides developing cervical cancer, women also need to worry about head and neck cancer later in life from HPV. Men with HPV do as well. Each year, more than 1,700 women and 5,700 men are diagnosed with head and neck cancer (in the oral cavity and oropharynx). This means that the virus may appear to lie dormant, but in fact is actively promoting cancer growth specifically in the mouth and neck area. No other parts of the body seem to develop cancer from HPV. Thus, it is important to get checked and treated for HPV as early as possible, and often, if engaged in repeated unprotected sex. Other cancers caused by HPV affect smaller numbers of patients per category but about the same total number.

A new vaccine called Gardasil can prevent women from getting HPV. It is the only vaccine that helps protect against four types of HPV: two that cause 70 percent of cervical cancers and two more that cause 90 percent of genital warts. The vaccine is for females aged nine to twenty-six years. The vaccine is less effective in preventing HPV-related diseases in young women who already have been exposed to one or more HPV types. It does not treat existing HPV; it can only prevent HPV before a person gets it. Thus, young girls need to get this vaccine before they become sexually active. The vaccine comes in three doses spread out over six months, and all need to be taken to assure maximal effect. Studies on thousands of girls around the world have found no serious side effects. Some girls reported fainting after the shots, so doctors were recommended to keep the patients in their offices for fifteen minutes afterward. Women still need to be screened for cervical cancer by regular PAP tests even if they have been vaccinated. The vaccine is not approved for males. Men who are concerned that they may have genital warts should be evaluated by their health care providers at routine physical exams. Genital warts affect about 1 percent of sexually active adults in the United States. Warts in both men and women can be removed by patient-applied medications or treated by a doctor.

Unless otherwise specified, the dosages recommended here are for adults. For children between the ages of twelve and seventeen, reduce the dose to three-quarters of the recommended amount. For children between six and twelve, use one-half of the recommended dose, and for children under the age of six, use one-quarter of the recommended amount.

NUTRIENTS

SUPPLEMENT	SUGGESTED DOSAGE	COMMENTS
Very Important		
Vitamin B complex	50 mg of each major B vitamin 3 times daily (amounts of individual vitamins in a complex will vary).	Important in normal cell multiplication.
Vitamin C with bioflavonoids	4,000–10,000 mg daily, in divided doses.	Has powerful antiviral capacity.
Important		
L-cysteine	500 mg twice daily, on an empty stomach. Take with water or juice. Do not take with milk. Take with 50 mg vitamin B_6 and 100 mg vitamin C for better absorption.	Supplies sulfur, needed for prevention and treatment of warts. (*See* AMINO ACIDS in Part One.)
Methylsulfonyl-methane (MSM)	As directed on label.	MSM and vitamin C are used by the body to build healthy new cells.
Vitamin A with mixed carotenoids including natural beta-carotene	100,000 IU daily for 1 month, then 50,000 IU daily for 1 month, then reduce to 25,000 IU daily for 1 month or until warts disappear. If you are pregnant, do not exceed 10,000 IU daily.	Needed for normalizing skin and epithelial membranes. Use emulsion form for easier assimilation and greater safety at higher doses.
Vitamin E	200 IU daily. Can be applied topically; cut open capsule to release oil. Apply to warts daily.	Improves circulation and promotes tissue repair and healing. Use d-alpha-tocopherol form.
Zinc	50–80 mg daily. Do not exceed a total of 100 mg daily from all supplements.	Increases immunity against viruses. Use zinc gluconate lozenges or OptiZinc for best absorption.
Helpful		
Multivitamin and mineral complex	As directed on label.	Needed for normal cell division.
Reishi extract or shiitake extract	As directed on label. As directed on label.	Has antiviral properties.

Herbs

❑ Aloe vera gel; myrrh; essential oils of clove, lemongrass, peppermint, tea tree, or wintergreen; and tinctures of black walnut, chickweed, goldenseal, and pau d'arco have all been used externally to treat warts. Aloe vera gel has both antibacterial and antiviral properties. Place a small dab of oil or extract on the wart two or three times daily until the wart is gone. If irritation occurs, dilute the oil or extract with distilled water or cold-pressed vegetable oil.

❏ Astragalus protects the immune system, which is important in warding off warts.

Caution: Do not use astragalus in the presence of a fever.

❏ Black walnut has healing properties. It is particularly useful for warts in the mouth and throat.

Recommendations

❏ To remove common warts, try one or more of the following remedies:

* Crush a garlic clove and apply the garlic directly on the wart, avoiding the surrounding skin. Cover it with a bandage and leave it in place for twenty-four hours. Blisters should then form, and the wart should fall off in about a week.

* Apply a paste made from castor oil and baking soda to the wart. Put the mixture on each night and cover it with a bandage. This may remove the wart in three to six weeks.

* The best treatment for plantar warts is to apply an appropriately sized strip of duct tape or adhesive tape over the wart for a maximum of two months (changing the tape periodically). This treatment has been proven as effective as using liquid nitrogen treatment, which is done in a doctor's office for up to six sessions two or three weeks apart. The treatment is called tape occlusion. Allergic reactions to the adhesive on the tape may make it unsuitable for use by certain sensitive individuals, however.

❏ Increase the amount of sulfur-containing amino acids in your diet by eating more asparagus, citrus fruits, eggs, garlic, and onions. Desiccated liver tablets are also good.

❏ If you suspect you may have genital warts, see your health care provider promptly. This is especially important for women, because genital warts have been linked to cervical cancer. An immediate Pap test is advised.

❏ Keep genital warts dry. After bathing, use a hair dryer on a low setting to dry the area. Do not rub or irritate it. Wear only cotton underwear. Do not have sexual intercourse until the warts are completely healed.

❏ Do not cut or burn a wart off yourself. These are procedures that must be done by a qualified health care provider.

Considerations

❏ Plantar warts may not require treatment. However, if a wart is painful and interferes with walking, treatment is warranted. Several treatment sessions may be necessary to eliminate them, but doctors can usually eradicate even the most stubborn plantar warts.

❏ Adequate daily vitamin C intake is most important in maintaining effective immunity against the viruses that cause warts. In one study, women who had diets rich in mixed tocopherols, vitamin E, and cryptoxanthin had a 30 percent decreased risk for cervical cancer. Oils and seeds contain mixed forms of vitamin E, and foods with cryptoxanthin include red bell peppers, papaya, cilantro, corn, oranges, avocados, and grapefruit.

❏ People who take medications to suppress the immune system, such as those who have received organ transplants or who have certain autoimmune disorders, are more prone to develop warts.

❏ Most common warts disappear within a year or two, even without treatment. Unless a common wart becomes bothersome, there is no need to do anything about it. Commonly used medical treatments for common and plantar warts include fulguration (using electric current to destroy wart tissue), freezing with liquid nitrogen, and topical applications of some chemicals, such as salicylic acid.

❏ Cantharidin is another chemical your physician may apply to get rid of warts.

❏ For larger genital warts, carbon dioxide (CO_2) laser surgery may be recommended. Interferon injections may be used for genital warts that do not go away with other treatment.

❏ Common warts can be treated with a mild acid solution such as salicylic acid or acetic acid (vinegar). It is thought that the acid weakens the walls of the wart enough to allow some of the virus to enter the bloodstream, causing the production of antibodies that eventually attack and destroy the warts. Removal does not allow the body to build up immunity to the virus.

❏ There are a variety of treatments for genital warts, but none is a perfect cure and all have side effects. Treatment falls into three categories: prescription topical preparations that destroy wart tissue; surgical methods to remove wart tissue; and biological approaches that target the virus.

❏ Women who have been diagnosed with genital warts should have a vaginal and uterine Pap smear every six months, as these warts are associated with an increased risk of cervical cancer.

WEAKENED IMMUNE SYSTEM

Modern conventional medicine battles disease directly by means of drugs, surgery, radiation, and other therapies, but true health can be attained only by maintaining a healthy, properly functioning immune system. It is the immune system that fights off disease-causing microorganisms and that engineers the healing process. The immune system is the key to fighting every kind of insult to the body, from that little shaving nick to the myriad of mutated viruses that seem to abound these days. Even the aging process may be more closely related to the functioning of the immune system than to the passage of time.

Weakening of the immune system results in increased susceptibility to virtually every type of illness. Some common signs of impaired immune function include fatigue, listlessness, repeated infections, inflammation, allergic reactions, slow wound healing, chronic diarrhea, and infections that represent an overgrowth of some normally present organism, such as oral thrush, or vaginal yeast infections. It is estimated that even healthy Americans collectively get one billion colds per year. People who have significantly more colds and infectious illnesses are likely to have some problem with immune function. By understanding some of the basic elements of the immune system and how they work, plus the overall role the immune system plays in your health, you can take responsibility for your own health.

In its simplest terms, the task of the immune system is to identify those things that naturally belong in the body and those that are foreign or otherwise harmful material, and then to neutralize or destroy the foreign material. The immune system is unlike other bodily systems in that it is not a group of physical structures but a system of complex interactions involving many different organs, structures, and substances, among them white blood cells, bone marrow, the lymphatic vessels and organs, specialized cells found in various body tissues, and specialized substances, called serum factors, that are present in the blood. Ideally, all of these components work together to protect the body against infection and disease.

The human immune system is functional at birth, but it does not yet function well. This is termed *innate immunity*—the immunity you are born with. Immune function develops and becomes more sophisticated as the system matures and the body learns to defend itself against different foreign invaders called antigens. This is termed *adaptive immunity.*

The immune system has the ability to learn to identify, and then to remember, specific antigens that have been encountered. It does this through two basic means, known as *cell-mediated immunity* and *humoral immunity.* In cell-mediated immunity, white blood cells called T lymphocytes identify and then destroy cancerous cells, viruses, and microorganisms like bacteria and fungi. The T lymphocytes, or T cells, mature in the thymus gland (hence the "T" designation). The thymus, a small gland located behind the top of the breastbone, is a major gland of the immune system. In the thymus, each T cell is programmed to identify one particular type of invading enemy. Not all prospective T cells make a successful passage through the thymus. Those whose programming is imperfect are eliminated. The ones that do make it are released into the bloodstream to search out and destroy antigens that correspond to their programming. They attack the antigens in part

through the secretion of proteins called cytokines. Interferon is one of the better-known cytokines.

Humoral immunity involves the production of antibodies. These are not cells, but special proteins whose chemical structures are formed to match the surfaces of specific antigens. When they encounter their specific antigens, antibodies either damage the invasive cells or alert the white blood cells to attack. The antibodies are produced by another group of white blood cells, the B lymphocytes, which are manufactured by and mature in the bone marrow. When a B lymphocyte is presented with a particular antigen, it engineers an antibody to match it and stores a blueprint of the invader so that it can initiate the production of antibodies in case of subsequent exposure, even if a long period of time elapses in between. For this system to work, each B cell must come into existence prepared to produce an almost infinite variety of different antibodies, so that it can match whatever antigen it is presented with. This is made possible by a mechanism known as "jumping genes." Inside the B cells, the genes that determine the chemical structure of the protein to be produced can be shuffled around and linked up in an astronomical number of different combinations. As a result, any B cell is capable of producing an antibody molecule to match virtually any foreign invader. It is the phenomenon of humoral immunity that makes immunization possible.

Because of their crucial role in all aspects of immunity—both cell-mediated and humoral—white blood cells are considered the body's first line of defense. White blood cells are larger than red blood cells. In addition, they can move independently in the bloodstream and are able to pass through the cell walls. This enables them to travel quickly to the site of an injury or infection. There are different categories of white blood cells, each of which performs a specific function. These include the following:

- *Granulocytes.* There are three types of granulocytes:

  1. *Neutrophils,* the most abundant type of white blood cell, whose function is to ingest and destroy microorganisms such as bacteria.

  2. *Eosinophils,* which ingest and destroy antigen-antibody combinations (formed when antibodies intercept antigens) and also moderate hypersensitive (allergic) reactions by secreting an enzyme that breaks down histamine. High levels of eosinophils in the blood are often present in individuals with allergic disorders, presumably because the body is attempting to tame the allergic reaction.

  3. *Basophils,* which secrete compounds such as heparin or histamine in response to contact with antigens.

- *Lymphocytes.* The lymphocytes are responsible for the development of specific immunities. Three important types of lymphocytes are T cells, B cells, and NK cells.

  1. *T cells* undergo maturation in the thymus gland and play a major role in cell-mediated immunity.

2. *B cells* mature in the bone marrow and are responsible for the production of antibodies.

3. *NK (natural killer) cells* destroy body cells that have become infected or cancerous.

- *Monocytes.* The largest cells in the blood, monocytes act as the "garbage collectors" of the body. They engulf and digest foreign particles as well as damaged or aging cells, including tumor cells. After spending about twenty-four hours circulating in the bloodstream, most monocytes enter the tissues and perform similar functions there. At this point, they are known as macrophages.

Another important component of immunity is the lymphatic system. This is a system of organs (including the spleen, the thymus, the tonsils, and the lymph nodes) and fluid, called lymph, that circulates through the lymphatic vessels in the body and also bathes the body's cells. The lymphatic system provides a kind of continuous cleansing that operates at the cellular level. It is through the lymphatic system that fluid from the spaces between cells is drained, taking with it waste products, toxins, and other debris from the tissues. The lymph flows through the lymph nodes, where the macrophages filter out the undesirables, and from there it returns to the venous circulation.

Other elements of the immune system include the spleen, the thymus, and the bone marrow. The spleen filters the blood and removes old red blood cells that need replacing. The spleen is populated by macrophages, dendritic cells (white blood cells that collect bits of antigens so that T cells can learn to recognize them), red blood cells, natural killer cells, and B and T cells. In the spleen, antigens are brought to the B cells, which use them to learn to manufacture the appropriate antigen response. People whose spleens have been removed tend to be more prone to illness because these important functions are no longer performed.

The T cells play a role in immunity by secreting interleukin-1, interleukin-2, and interferon, as well as activating B cells so that they produce antibodies. These secretions are known as cytokines. We need cytokines to survive, but sometimes too many are secreted and they create a highly immune-charged system. For example, obesity causes the excess release of cytokines and puts the body in an inflammatory state, which makes it more prone to heart disease and diabetes.

The bone marrow produces new white blood cells, platelets, B cells, natural killer cells, granulocytes, and thymocytes. All white blood cells are made from stem cells. Stem cells are embryonic cells that have the capacity to mature into virtually any type of cell. Some of the white blood cells made in the bone marrow leave the bone marrow and mature elsewhere in the body, while others mature where they are and support the immune system. All the cells of the immune system come originally from the bone marrow. Both the appendix and the tonsils also support the immune system.

Marvelous as it is, the immune system can work as it should only if it is cared for properly. This means getting all the right nutrients and providing the right environment, plus avoiding those things that tend to depress immunity.

Many elements of the environment we live in today compromise our immune systems' defensive abilities. The chemicals in the household cleaners we use; the overuse of antibiotics and other drugs; the antibiotics, pesticides, and myriad additives present in the foods we eat; and exposure to environmental pollutants all place a strain on the immune system. Another factor that adversely affects the immune system is stress. Stress results in a sequence of biochemical events that ultimately suppresses the normal activity of white blood cells and places undue demands on the endocrine system, as well as depleting the body of needed nutrients. The result is impaired healing ability and lowered defense against infection.

Proper immune function is an intricate balancing act. While inadequate immunity predisposes one to infectious illness of every type, it is also possible to become ill as a result of an immune response that is too strong or directed at an inappropriate target. Many different disorders, including allergies, lupus, pernicious anemia, rheumatic heart disease, rheumatoid arthritis, and type 1 diabetes have been linked to inappropriate immune system activity. Consequently, they are known as autoimmune, or "self-attacking-self," disorders.

While much is known about the functioning of the immune system, much more remains to be learned. Only in the past ten to fifteen years have many facets of immune function begun to be studied and understood by physicians and researchers. The field of immunology (the study of the immune system) is one of the fastest-growing fields in medicine today.

The program of supplements outlined here is designed to strengthen the immune system, whether it is damaged as a result of disease, stress, inadequate nutrition, poor living habits, chemotherapy, or a combination of one or more of these factors. The dosages recommended are for adults. For children between the ages of twelve and seventeen, reduce the dose to three-quarters of the recommended amount. For children between six and twelve, use one-half of the recommended dose, and for children under the age of six, use one-quarter of the recommended amount.

NUTRIENTS

SUPPLEMENT	SUGGESTED DOSAGE	COMMENTS
Acetyl-L-carnitine	As directed on label.	An energy carrier, metabolic facilitator, and cell membrane protectant. Protects the heart.
Acidophilus (Kyo-Dophilus from Wakunaga)	As directed on label. Take on an empty stomach.	Restores important bacteria to the intestinal tract. Use a nondairy formula.
Aerobic 07 from Aerobic Life Industries	9 drops twice daily, taken in water.	For tissue oxygenation.
Béres Drops Plus from Nupharma Nutraceuticals	As directed on label.	Contains minerals and trace elements that boost and nourish the immune system.

Supplement	Dosage	Comments
Beta-1,3-D-glucan	As directed on label.	Stimulates macrophages to remove cellular debris and, possibly, to recognize and kill tumor cells.
Bovine colostrum	As directed on label.	Contains immunoglobulins and antibody-stimulating factors. Enhances immunity.
Coenzyme Q$_{10}$	100 mg daily.	Supports the immune system. An oxygen enhancer to protect the cells and heart function.
plus Coenzyme A from Coenzyme-A Technologies	As directed on label.	Works well with coenzyme Q$_{10}$ to support the immune system and increase energy.
Essential fatty acids (Ultimate Oil from Nature's Secret)	As directed on label.	A most important element in the diet. Necessary for a healthy immune system.
Free form amino acid (Amino Balance from Anabol Naturals)	As directed on label, on an empty stomach.	Protein that is broken down into a form the body can use. Use a formula containing all the essential amino acids.
Garlic (Kyolic from Wakunaga)	2 capsules 3 times daily.	Stimulates the immune system.
Glutathione	As directed on label.	Inhibits the formation of free radicals; aids in red blood cell integrity; reduces quantities of hydrogen peroxide; protects immune cells.
Kelp	2,000–3,000 mg daily.	Supplies a balance of minerals needed for immune system integrity.
Kyo-Green from Wakunaga	As directed on label.	Supplies nutrients and chlorophyll needed for tissue repair, and cleanses the blood. Important in immune response.
L-arginine and L-ornithine	As directed on label, on an empty stomach. Take with water or juice. Do not take with milk. Take with 50 mg vitamin B$_6$ and 100 mg vitamin C for better absorption.	To enhance the immune system and retard the growth of tumors and cancer. Necessary for the immune system. (See AMINO ACIDS in Part One.)
L-cysteine and L-methionine plus L-lysine	500 mg each twice daily, on an empty stomach.	To destroy free radicals and viruses and protect the glands, especially the liver. (See AMINO ACIDS in Part One.)
Lecithin granules or capsules	1 tbsp 3 times daily, with meals. 1,200 mg 3 times daily, with meals.	Aids in cellular protection.
Maitake extract or reishi extract or shiitake extract	As directed on label. As directed on label. As directed on label.	Mushrooms that build immunity and fight viral infections and cancer.
Manganese	2 mg daily.	Necessary for proper immune function. Works with the B vitamins to provide a general feeling of well-being.
Multivitamin and mineral complex	As directed on label.	All vitamins and minerals are necessary in balance. Use a high-potency formula.
Proteolytic enzymes or Inf-zyme Forte from American Biologics	As directed on label. 4 tablets 3 times daily, with meals.	To aid in proper breakdown of proteins, fats, and carbohydrates for better absorption of nutrients.
Pycnogenol and/or grape seed extract	As directed on label 3 times daily, with meals. As directed on label.	A unique bioflavonoid that is a potent antioxidant and immune system enhancer. One of the most potent antioxidants; protects the cells.
Quercetin plus bromelain	As directed on label. As directed on label.	Helps to prevent reactions to certain foods, pollens, and other allergens. Increases immunity. Enhances the effectiveness of quercetin.
Raw thymus glandular plus multiglandular complex with raw spleen glandular	As directed on label. As directed on label.	To enhance T cell production. Glandulars from lamb source are best.
Selenium	200 mcg daily. If you are pregnant, do not exceed 40 mcg daily.	Important free radical destroyer.
Squalene (shark liver oil)	As directed on label.	Aids in rebuilding and functioning of cells; has anticancer properties.
Superoxide dismutase (SOD) plus dimethylglycine (DMG) (Aangamik DMG from Food-Science of Vermont)	As directed on label. As directed on label.	To improve oxygenation of tissues.
Taurine Plus from American Biologics	As directed on label.	An antioxidant and immune regulator necessary for white blood cell activation and neurological function.
Vitamin A plus natural carotenoid complex with beta-carotene	10,000 IU daily. As directed on label.	Needed for proper immune function. Powerful antioxidants, free radical scavengers, and immune system enhancers. May protect against cancer and heart disease.
Vitamin B complex plus extra vitamin B$_6$ (pyridoxine) and vitamin B$_{12}$ plus raw liver extract	100 mg of each major B vitamin 3 times daily, with meals (amounts of individual vitamins in a complex will vary). 50 mg 3 times daily. 1,000–2,000 mcg daily. As directed on label.	Antistress vitamins, especially important for normal brain function. Consider injections (under a doctor's supervision). If injections are not available, use a sublingual form. Vitamins B$_6$ and B$_{12}$ potentiate amino acids and are necessary for best absorption of amino acids and for proper functioning of enzymes in the body. A good source of B vitamins and iron. Consider injections (under a doctor's supervision).
Vitamin C with bioflavonoids	5,000–20,000 mg daily, in divided doses. (See ASCORBIC ACID FLUSH in Part Three.)	An important antioxidant that decreases susceptibility to infection.
Vitamin E	200 IU daily.	An antioxidant that is an integral part of the body's defense system. Use d-alpha-tocopherol form. Use an emulsion form for easier assimilation.
Zinc plus copper	50–80 mg daily. Do not exceed this amount. 3 mg daily.	Very important for the immune system. Use zinc chelate form. Needed to balance with zinc.

Herbs

❑ Astragalus boosts the immune system and generates anticancer cells in the body. It is also a powerful antioxidant and protects the liver from toxins.

Caution: Do not use astragalus in the presence of a fever.

❑ Bayberry, fenugreek, hawthorn, horehound, licorice root, and red clover all enhance the immune response.

Caution: Licorice root should not be used during pregnancy or nursing. It should not be used by persons with diabetes, glaucoma, heart disease, high blood pressure, or a history of stroke.

❑ BioStrath, an herbal tonic produced by Nature's Answer, contains vitamins, minerals, and essential amino acids, plus adenosine triphosphate (ATP), a key cellular energy source. This supplement is good for fighting illness and for long-term vitality.

❑ Black radish, dandelion, and milk thistle help to cleanse the liver and the bloodstream. The liver is *the* organ of detoxification and must function optimally.

❑ Boxthorn seed, ginseng, suma, and wisteria contain germanium, a trace element that aids immune function and has anticancer properties.

Caution: Do not use ginseng if you have high blood pressure or are pregnant or nursing.

❑ Echinacea boosts the immune system and enhances lymphatic function. The echinacea supplement Echinaforce from Bioforce USA has been studied regarding reduction of common cold symptoms. It was found to be 60 percent more effective than a placebo.

Caution: Do not take echinacea for longer than three months. It should not be used by people who are allergic to ragweed.

❑ Esberitox from Enzymatic Therapy is a combination of different herbs designed to promote a healthy immune system. It is also effective against the common cold.

❑ Ginkgo biloba is good for the brain cells, aids circulation, and is a powerful antioxidant.

Caution: Do not take ginkgo biloba if you have a bleeding disorder, or are scheduled for surgery or a dental procedure.

❑ Goldenseal strengthens the immune system, cleanses the body, and has antibacterial properties.

Caution: Do not take goldenseal internally on a daily basis for more than one week at a time. Do not use it during pregnancy or if you are breast-feeding, and use with caution if you are allergic to ragweed. If you have a history of cardiovascular disease, diabetes, or glaucoma, use it only under a doctor's supervision.

❑ ImmunoCare from Himalaya Herbal Healthcare is a combination formula containing Ayurvedic herbs that may protect white blood cells.

❑ Ligustrum (known in Chinese herbology as *nu zhen zi*) inhibits tumor growth in a cancer cell line in a Petri dish, but not in humans.

❑ Moducare from Essential Sterolin Products has proven effective in balancing T cell activity, which has the potential to increase immune system function. This supplement also improves symptoms of various autoimmune disorders. Moducare is a 100 to 1 mixture of sitosterol and sitosterolin derived from an original South African herbal traditional remedy. The usual dosage is three 20-milligram capsules daily.

❑ Rather than taking shiitake, reishi, and other mushroom extracts separately, you can take them in combination formulas such as Mushroom Optimizer from Jarrow Formulas. This product combines reishi, turkeytail, maitake, cordyceps, blazei, shiitake, and white woodear extracts to work on immune system problems.

❑ Picrorrhiza, an Indian herb used in Ayurvedic medicine, is a powerful immunostimulant that boosts all aspects of immune function.

❑ St. John's wort is a natural blood purifier and may fight viruses.

Caution: St. John's wort may cause increased sensitivity to sunlight. It may also produce anxiety, gastrointestinal symptoms, and headaches. It can interact with some drugs including antidepressants, birth control pills, and anticoagulants.

Recommendations

❑ Take an inventory of the factors that may be compromising your immune system and take steps to correct them. Two of the most common immune suppressors include stress and an incorrect diet, especially a diet high in fat and refined processed foods. Obesity also dampens immune function.

❑ Supply your immune system with adequate amounts of nutrients that promote proper immune function. Some of the most valuable include:

- Vitamin A is the anti-infection vitamin. If used properly and in moderate doses, vitamin A is rarely toxic and is very important in the body's defense system.

- Vitamin C may be the single most important vitamin for the immune system. It is essential for the formation of adrenal hormones and the production of lymphocytes. It also has a direct effect on bacteria and viruses. Vitamin C should be taken with bioflavonoids, natural plant substances that enhance absorption and reinforce the action of this vitamin.

- Vitamin E interacts with vitamins A and C and the mineral selenium, acting as a primary antioxidant and scavenger of toxic free radicals. Vitamin E activity is an integral part of the body's defense system.

- Zinc boosts the immune response and promotes the healing of wounds when used in appropriate doses (100 milligrams or less daily). It also helps to protect the liver. Doses over 100 milligrams per day may actually depress immune function, however.

❑ Begin a diet of fresh fruits and vegetables (preferably raw) plus nuts, seeds, grains, and other foods that are high in fiber.

❑ Include in your diet chlorella, garlic, and pearl barley. These foods contain germanium, a trace element beneficial for the immune system. Also add kelp to the diet, in the form of giant red kelp or brown kelp. Kelp contains iodine, calcium, iron, carotene, protein, riboflavin, and vitamin C, which are necessary for the immune system's functional integrity.

❑ Consume "green drinks" daily. The best contain a wide variety of plants and are organic.

❑ Avoid animal products, processed foods, sugar, and soda.

❑ Follow a fasting program once a month to rid your body of toxins that can weaken the immune system. Children should not fast. (See FASTING in Part Three.)

❑ Use spirulina, especially while fasting. Spirulina is a naturally digestible food that aids in protecting the immune system. It supplies many nutrients needed for cleansing and healing.

❑ Be sure to get sufficient sleep. As much as possible, avoid stress.

❑ Get regular moderate exercise (but don't overdo it). Exercise reduces stress and elevates mood, which has a positive effect on immune response. In addition, T lymphocyte production is stimulated by exercise.

Caution: If you are thirty-five or older and/or have been sedentary for some time, consult with your health care provider before beginning an exercise program.

❑ Avoid overeating.

❑ Do not smoke or consume beverages containing alcohol or caffeine.

❑ Do not take any recreational drugs.

Considerations

❑ White blood cells are an indicator of health. Since the beginning of the AIDS epidemic, we have all become aware of the importance of a good immune system. White blood cell counts—and the implications of low numbers of white blood cells—are very important. The normal range of white blood cells in a person with a strong immune system is anywhere from 4,000 to 12,000 cells per microliter (μL, the equivalent of one-millionth liter) of blood.

❑ Marijuana use weakens the immune system. Delta-9 tetrahydrocannabinol (THC), the most active compound in marijuana, alters the normal immune response, making the white blood cells less effective than normal.

❑ A person's mental state can suppress his or her immune system. A positive frame of mind is important in building up the immune system. (See ANXIETY DISORDER; DEPRESSION; and/or STRESS in Part Two.)

❑ An underactive thyroid results in immune deficiency. (See HYPOTHYROIDISM in Part Two.)

❑ Food allergies and adverse food reactions can place stress on the immune system. (See ALLERGIES in Part Two.)

❑ Research has shown that dehydroepiandrosterone (DHEA), a hormone, may enhance the functioning of the immune system. (See DHEA THERAPY in Part Three.)

❑ Human growth hormone (HGH) is another naturally occurring hormone that strengthens the immune system. Treatment with HGH requires the supervision of a physician, but it is not typically used to treat immune problems. (See GROWTH HORMONE THERAPY in Part Three.)

❑ *See also* AIDS (ACQUIRED IMMUNODEFICIENCY SYNDROME) in Part Two.

WEIGHT PROBLEMS

See ANOREXIA NERVOSA; APPETITE, POOR; BULIMIA; OBESITY; and UNDERWEIGHT/WEIGHT LOSS.

WILSON'S DISEASE

Wilson's disease, also called *hepatolenticular degeneration* or *inherited copper toxicosis,* is an uncommon inherited disorder that affects approximately 1 in 40,000 persons worldwide. In people with Wilson's disease, the body is unable to metabolize the trace element copper as it should, with the result that excess copper accumulates in the brain, kidneys, liver, and the corneas of the eyes. This causes organ damage and other complications, including neurological problems and psychotic behavior. Untreated, Wilson's disease leads to brain damage, cirrhosis of the liver, hepatitis, and, ultimately, death. Fortunately, early detection and treatment of the disease can minimize the symptoms and complications and possibly even prevent them altogether.

Symptoms of Wilson's disease may include bloody vomit; difficulty speaking, swallowing, and/or walking; drooling; an enlarged spleen; jaundice; loss of appetite; loss of coordination; progressive fatigue and/or weakness; progressive intellectual impairment; psychological deterioration manifested as personality changes and/or bizarre behavior; rigidity, spasms, or tremors of the muscles; swelling and/or fluid accumulation in the abdomen; and unexplained weight loss. Sometimes the first sign is the development of a pigmented ring, known as a Kayser-Fleischer ring, at the outer margin of the cornea, which may be detected during a routine eye examination. In the advanced stages of the disease, symptoms due to chronic active hepatitis or cirrhosis may appear, menstrual cycles may cease, and an individual may experience chest pains, heart palpitations, light-headedness, pallor, and shortness of breath as a result of exertion.

Although people who have Wilson's disease are born with the disorder, symptoms are rarely seen before the age of six and most often do not appear until adolescence or even later. However, to prevent complications, treatment is required whether symptoms have appeared or not. Diagnosis is usually based on a study of individual and family medical history plus blood tests to determine levels of ceruloplasmin (a copper-carrying protein in the blood) and to check for anemia, plus a urine test to reveal elevated levels of copper in the urine. A liver biopsy to evaluate the amount of copper in liver tissue may be done to confirm the diagnosis.

The dosages recommended here are for adults. For children between the ages of twelve and seventeen, reduce the dose to three-quarters of the recommended amount. For children between six and twelve, use one-half of the recommended dose, and for children under the age of six, use one-quarter of the recommended amount.

NUTRIENTS

SUPPLEMENT	SUGGESTED DOSAGE	COMMENTS
Very Important		
Garlic (Kyolic from Wakunaga)	As directed on label.	A powerful antioxidant that protects liver and heart function. Promotes normal healing and prevents cell damage.
Iron	As directed by physician. Take with 100 mg vitamin C for better absorption.	To correct and protect against anemia. *Caution:* Do not take iron unless anemia is diagnosed.
Multivitamin and mineral complex with	As directed on label.	A balance of all nutrients is essential for healing.
potassium and	99 mg daily.	Necessary for proper muscle contraction.
selenium	200 mcg daily. If you are pregnant, do not exceed 40 mcg daily.	Needed for proper adrenal gland function.
Vitamin A with mixed carotenoids including beta-carotene	10,000 IU daily.	Powerful antioxidants that also enhance immunity.
Vitamin B complex	75 mg of each major B vitamin 3 times daily (amounts of individual vitamins in a complex will vary).	Protects the liver and is needed for proper brain function.
plus extra vitamin B$_6$ (pyridoxine)	50 mg 3 times daily.	Helps to prevent damage to the nervous system and guard against anemia. Also combats fluid retention.
Vitamin C with bioflavonoids	3,000–5,000 mg daily, in divided doses.	Protects against inflammation, anemia, and hepatitis, and reduces copper levels in the body. Use an esterified form.
Vitamin E	100 IU daily. Take separately from iron.	Promotes normal healing and prevents cell damage. Use d-alpha-tocopherol form.

Zinc	75 mg daily. Do not exceed this amount.	Decreases copper levels and enhances immunity. Zinc balances copper in the body.
Important		
Acetyl-L-carnitine	As directed on label.	Protects liver and heart function.
Advanced Carotenoid Complex from Solgar	As directed on label.	Contains powerful free radical scavengers and immune system enhancers.
Calcium and magnesium	1,500–2,000 mg daily. 750–1,000 mg daily.	Minerals that work together to prevent muscle spasms.
Coenzyme Q$_{10}$ plus Coenzyme A from Coenzyme-A Technologies	As directed on label. As directed on label.	A powerful antioxidant that also increases circulation and energy. Works with coenzyme Q$_{10}$.
Flaxseed oil	As directed on label.	To supply essential fatty acids, which are vital for brain and nerve function and enhance immunity.
Free form amino acid	As directed on label, on an empty stomach.	Necessary for protein synthesis. Use a formula containing all the essential amino acids.
Gamma-amino-butyric acid (GABA)	As directed on label, on an empty stomach.	Essential for proper brain function. Also has a tranquilizing effect. (*See* AMINO ACIDS in Part One.)
L-arginine and L-ornithine plus L-cysteine	As directed on label, on an empty stomach. Take at bedtime with water or juice. Do not take with milk. Take with 50 mg vitamin B$_6$ and 100 mg vitamin C for better absorption. As directed on label, on an empty stomach.	To aid in liver and kidney detoxification. (*See* AMINO ACIDS in Part One.) Reduces the body's absorption of copper.
Methylsulfonyl-methane (MSM)	As directed on label.	Contains sulfur, which aids in removing copper from the body.
Pycnogenol and/or grape seed extract	As directed on label. As directed on label.	Powerful antioxidants that lessen mental deterioration.

Herbs

❑ Alfalfa, ginkgo biloba, gotu kola, kava kava, lobelia, parsley, oat straw, periwinkle, and skullcap are good for overall good health and the functioning of the brain and nervous system.

Caution: Do not take ginkgo biloba if you have a bleeding disorder, or are scheduled for surgery or a dental procedure. Kava kava can cause drowsiness. It is not recommended for pregnant women or nursing mothers, and it should not be taken together with other substances that act on the central nervous system, such as alchohol, barbiturates, antidepressants, and antipsychotic drugs. Lobelia is only to be taken under supervision of a health care professional as it is potentially toxic. People with high blood pressure, heart disease, liver disease, kidney disease, seizure disorders, or shortness of breath should not take lobelia. Pregnant and lactating women should avoid lobelia as well.

❑ Astragalus, echinacea, and pau d'arco are helpful for fatigue.

Cautions: Do not use astragalus in the presence of a fever. Do not take echinacea for longer than three months. It should not be used by people who are allergic to ragweed.

❑ Black radish and red clover strengthen the liver.

❑ Burdock, dandelion, milk thistle, and suma cleanse and support the liver and help to fight fatigue.

❑ Cat's claw is an anti-inflammatory, antioxidant, immune system enhancer, and internal cleanser. Cat's Claw Defense Complex from Source Naturals is a good source of this herb and also contains other beneficial ingredients.

Caution: Do not use cat's claw during pregnancy.

❑ Cayenne (capsicum) eases blood pressure, fights fatigue, and helps support the nervous system.

❑ Goldenseal is helpful if symptoms include difficulty swallowing, and it can ease fatigue as well. Licorice is also beneficial for swallowing difficulties, as is gargling with thyme tea.

Cautions: Do not take goldenseal internally on a daily basis for more than one week at a time. Do not use it during pregnancy or if you are breast-feeding, and use with caution if you are allergic to ragweed. If you have a history of cardiovascular disease, diabetes, or glaucoma, use it only under a doctor's supervision. Licorice root should not be used during pregnancy or nursing. It should not be used by persons with diabetes, glaucoma, heart disease, high blood pressure, or a history of stroke.

❑ St. John's wort is beneficial for the nervous system and also helps to overcome fatigue and difficulty swallowing.

Caution: St. John's wort may cause increased sensitivity to sunlight. It may also produce anxiety, gastrointestinal symptoms, and headaches. It can interact with some drugs including antidepressants, birth control pills, and anticoagulants.

❑ Siberian ginseng is a tonic herb that helps reduce fatigue and supports brain and nervous system function.

Caution: Do not use this herb if you have hypoglycemia, high blood pressure, or a heart disorder.

❑ Valerian root is calming and is good for the brain and nervous system. It can also be beneficial for swallowing difficulties.

Recommendations

❑ Increase your consumption of onions. They contain sulfur, which helps to rid the body of copper.

❑ Eat fresh (not canned) pineapple frequently. It contains bromelain, an enzyme that helps to keep down swelling and inflammation.

❑ Have the copper level of your drinking water tested. Look in the yellow pages of your local telephone directory or consult your state's environmental agency for laboratories that can do this type of testing. If your tap water contains more than 1 part per million of copper, drink quality bottled water instead (steam-distilled is best) or check the pipes in your home; if you can determine that all or most of the copper in your water is coming from the pipes, it may be worthwhile to replace them with copper-free ones.

❑ If you take a multivitamin and/or mineral supplement, be sure to choose a formula that does *not* contain copper.

❑ Eliminate from the diet foods high in copper. These include barley, beets, blackstrap molasses, broccoli, chocolate, enriched cereals, garlic, lentils, liver, mushrooms, nuts, organ meats, salmon, and shellfish, as well as avocados, beans and other legumes, egg yolks, oats, oranges, pecans, raisins, soybeans, whole grains, and green leafy vegetables.

❑ If you suffer from tremors, avoid caffeine.

❑ Avoid alcohol consumption. Wilson's disease increases the risk of cirrhosis of the liver.

❑ Do not use copper cookware or utensils.

Considerations

❑ Wilson's disease can be neither prevented nor cured. With appropriate management, however, the prognosis is excellent. Anyone with a family history of Wilson's disease should undergo diagnostic testing—the sooner the better, and whether or not symptoms are present—so that treatment, if necessary, may begin as soon as possible.

❑ Treatment of Wilson's disease is a lifelong proposition. Most often, it involves taking penicillamine (Cuprimine, Depen), a drug that removes copper from the body by increasing its excretion in the urine. Possible side effects of this drug include deficiencies of vitamin B_6 (pyridoxine) and iron, and many people experience an allergic reaction to the drug within ten days of taking it. The most serious potential side effects of this medication include kidney disease, blood cell problems, and Goodpasture's syndrome (a potentially life-threatening syndrome characterized by bleeding of the lungs and kidney failure). Penicillamine has also been suspected of being linked to leukemia development in at least two cases. A person with a sensitivity to penicillamine may also be given a steroid such as prednisone (Deltasone and others) to decrease the reaction to the penicillamine, or the drug trientine (Syprine) may be prescribed instead. This medication also chelates copper so that it can be eliminated from the body.

❑ Some doctors prescribe high doses of zinc in place of, or in conjunction with, conventional drugs to keep copper levels under control. Zinc naturally balances with copper in the body. Zinc acetate (Galzin) is another medication that may be prescribed. It should be taken exactly as the doctor has prescribed.

❑ Regardless of the treatment regimen, regular checkups are required to monitor possible side effects from medication and to check the level of copper in the urine.

❑ If you develop any personality changes or problems linked to Wilson's disease, consulting a psychologist or other mental health professional may be helpful.

❑ Elevated copper levels in the body result in the depletion of vitamin C and zinc. Persons with Wilson's disease therefore always require a higher than normal intake of these nutrients.

❑ Wilson's disease is not the only cause of elevated levels of copper in the body. Toxic levels of copper can also accumulate in the body as a result of excessive exposure to the metal. If a person with elevated copper levels has normal liver function and no corneal abnormalities, it is likely that the toxicity is due to something other than Wilson's disease. In addition, copper toxicity as a result of excessive copper ingestion can be demonstrated by hair analysis, whereas persons with Wilson's disease do not exhibit elevated levels of copper in the hair.

❑ Tetrathiomolybdate is an experimental drug that shows promise in treating Wilson's disease.

❑ Without proper treatment Wilson's disease is usually fatal by age thirty. However, if treatment is begun early enough, symptomatic recovery is usually complete, and a life of normal length and quality can be expected.

❑ *See also* COPPER TOXICITY in Part Two. The Wilson's Disease Association offers aid and support to people with Wilson's and related diseases. (*See* Health and Medical Organizations in the Appendix.)

WILSON'S SYNDROME

See under HYPOTHYROIDISM.

WORMS (PARASITES)

Worms are parasites that live in the gastrointestinal tract. The most common types of worms are roundworms (including ascarids, hookworms, pinworms, and threadworms) and tapeworms. Roundworms are contagious intestinal parasites that are shaped like earthworms but are smaller in size. They can easily be seen with the naked eye. Pinworms are white, threadlike worms about one-third inch long. In the United States, pinworm infestation in young children is by far the most prevalent parasitic worm problem. Tapeworms vary in length from an inch up to thirty feet and can survive for up to twenty-five years in the body.

Depending on the type of worm involved and the severity of the infestation, there may be a variety of symptoms.

In some cases, there may be no perceptible symptoms at all. In other cases, worms may be seen in the stool.

Pinworms can cause severe anal itching (especially at night, as the worms tend to migrate outside the anus to lay their eggs), insomnia, and restlessness. Hookworms can cause itching on the soles of the feet, and in some cases, bloody sputum, fever, rash, and loss of appetite. Threadworms can cause coughing or bronchitis, abdominal pain, diarrhea, and gas, preceded by tiny red abrasions that sometimes itch. Small tapeworms can cause weight and appetite loss, abdominal pain, vomiting, and diarrhea. Large tapeworms can cause similar symptoms, but usually without weight loss. Ascariasis, caused by ascarids, is characterized by bloating, stomach pain, vomiting, and difficulty breathing. Trichinosis is a disease caused by a microscopic roundworm that, if left untreated, can lead to muscle damage and cardiac or neurological complications.

Worm infestations can range from mild to severe, even life-threatening, particularly in children. They result in poor absorption of essential nutrients, and in some cases, loss of blood from the gastrointestinal tract. They can therefore lead to such deficiency-related disorders as anemia and growth problems. Malabsorption resulting from parasitic infection makes one susceptible to many diseases because it results in diminished immune function.

Worms can be contracted through a variety of mechanisms, including improper disposal of human or animal waste, walking barefoot on contaminated soil, and ingestion of eggs or larvae from uncooked or partially cooked meat. In some cases, eggs may become airborne and be inhaled.

Parasites are more common than most people suppose, and they can be behind many illnesses, including colon disorders. They are more common in children than in adults. They are also common in people with AIDS, chronic fatigue syndrome, candidiasis, and many other disorders. Unfortunately, physicians often do not check for worm infestation.

The dosages recommended here are for adults. For children between the ages of twelve and seventeen, reduce the dose to three-quarters of the recommended amount. For children between six and twelve, use one-half of the recommended dose, and for children under the age of six, use one-quarter of the recommended amount.

NUTRIENTS

SUPPLEMENT	SUGGESTED DOSAGE	COMMENTS
Important		
Acidophilus (Kyo-Dophilus from Wakunaga)	As directed on label.	Restores normal intestinal flora. Use a nondairy formula.
Beta-carotene	50,000 IU daily until you are healed.	Acts as an anti-infective.
Essential fatty acids (Ultimate Oil from Nature's Secret)	As directed on label.	Helps to protect the gastrointestinal tract.

Garlic (Kyolic from Wakunaga)	2 capsules 3 times daily, with meals.	Has antiparasitic properties. A fresh clove of garlic can also be put in the shoes to be absorbed through the skin.
Kyolic-EPA from Wakunaga	As directed on label.	Restores proper fatty acid balance. Repairs tissues and aids in healing.
Liquid Kyolic with B_1 and B_{12}	As directed on label.	An excellent blood builder.
Multivitamin and mineral complex	As directed on label.	To promote overall health and proper nutrition. All nutrients are needed by persons with these disorders.
Parasitin from Växa International	As directed on label.	To cleanse and detoxify the body of parasites and worms.
Vitamin B complex plus extra vitamin B_{12}	50 mg of each major B vitamin 3 times daily, with meals (amounts of individual vitamins in a complex will vary). 1,000–2,000 mcg twice daily.	To prevent anemia associated with parasitic infestation. Use sublingual forms to assure absorption.
Vitamin C with bioflavonoids	3,000 mg daily.	Protects against infection and enhances immune function.
Zinc	50 mg daily. Do not exceed a total of 100 mg daily from all supplements.	Promotes a healthy immune system and proper wound healing.

Herbs

❏ Aloe vera juice, taken twice daily as directed on the product label, has an alkalinizing and anti-inflammatory effect.

❏ Black walnut extract destroys many types of worms. Take black walnut extract on an empty stomach three times per day.

❏ Butternut bark, fennel seed, flaxseed, licorice root, and senna leaf are good for bowel and colon cleansing.

Caution: Licorice root should not be used during pregnancy or nursing. It should not be used by persons with diabetes, glaucoma, heart disease, high blood pressure, or a history of stroke.

❏ Calendula ointment or witch hazel can be used to help relieve anal itching and irritation.

❏ Cascara sagrada, chamomile, ficus, gentian root, mugwort, mullein oil, parsley, pau d'arco, rhubarb root, slippery elm, thyme, valerian, and wormwood are effective against many types of worms.

Cautions: Do not use chamomile if you are allergic to ragweed. Do not use during pregnancy or nursing. It may interact with warfarin or cyclosporine, so patients using these drugs should avoid it. Do not use wormwood in high doses or for extended periods because it contains the chemical compound thujone that can be poisonous. Do not use wormwood if you suffer from any type of seizure disorder or are pregnant.

❏ Cayenne (capsicum), garlic, and turmeric help to strengthen the immune system and destroy many types of worms.

❏ Grapefruit seed extract is very effective for destroying parasites. It can be taken internally and is also good for washing vegetables before eating (mix 10 drops of extract in 2 quarts of water) to remove any bacteria or parasites.

❏ Pinkroot works well against roundworms.

❏ Pumpkin extract contains zinc and aids in expelling worms.

Recommendations

❏ Eat a high-fiber diet consisting primarily of raw vegetables and whole grains.

❏ Eat pumpkin seeds, sesame seeds, and figs (or drink fig juice) on an empty stomach three times per day. This can be combined with the black walnut extract mentioned under Herbs, above.

❏ Drink only filtered or bottled steam-distilled water.

❏ Monitor your intake and output of fluids, and replace fluids as needed.

❏ Eliminate *all* sugar, refined carbohydrates, fruits (except figs and pineapples), and pork and pork products from the diet until the worms have been completely eradicated. Worms thrive on sugar.

❏ For tapeworms, fast for three days on raw pineapple. (*See* FASTING in Part Three.) The bromelain in pineapple destroys tapeworms.

❏ Drink plenty of papaya juice.

❏ For pinworms, eat bitter melon, a cucumber-shaped vegetable found in Asian markets. This is effective against pinworms and is a good immune system strengthener. Eat one or two melons a day for seven to ten days. Do this again after two months to ensure that the infestation has not returned.

❏ *Never* eat meat, fish, or poultry that is not fully cooked or that has been left out at room temperature for too long. Sushi is usually safe, but not always. (*See* FOODBORNE/ WATERBORNE ILLNESS in Part Two.)

❏ Take a warm bath using ½ cup of Epsom salts per gallon of water. Before getting into the water, apply zinc oxide to the opening of the anus. Repeat for three days in a row.

❏ Have pet cats and dogs checked and, if appropriate, treated for parasites when you first get them, and in the spring and fall of each year thereafter.

❏ Always wear shoes in soiled areas.

❏ Maintain meticulous personal hygiene. Avoid scratching the anal area, and wash your hands frequently, preferably with antibacterial soap, scrubbing well under the

THE DISORDERS | Part Two

fingernails. If children are affected, teach them proper hygiene as well.

❑ Wash all utensils and surfaces that come in contact with raw meat, pork, or fish with antibacterial soap.

❑ Wash underwear, bed linens, and towels after each use in very hot water with chlorine bleach added, if possible. Change linens and towels daily.

❑ For a severe infestation, use high colonics (also known as colonic irrigation). This procedure is usually performed in a professional office. If this treatment is not available, follow the procedure for colon cleansing described in this book. Speak to your child's pediatrician before using colonics. (*See* COLON CLEANSING and ENEMAS, both in Part Three.) A product called 10-Day Colon Cleanse from Aerobic Life Industries is also recommended.

Considerations

❑ Worm infestations can be persistent and stubborn. It may be necessary to treat all members of the household to finally eradicate the parasites. All family members should be examined for possible infection. In addition, it is a good idea to compile a list of people who have been in close contact with the affected individual and advise them to seek the evaluation and advice of a health care provider.

❑ The following are the different types of worms and the routes through which they can enter the body:

- *Ascarids:* Through the soil, or in contaminated raw or undercooked food.

- *Hookworms and threadworms:* Through the feet or drinking water.

- *Pinworms:* Eggs can be transferred by touch from an infected individual who has eggs on the fingers from scratching the affected area.

- *Tapeworms:* In raw or undercooked beef, fish, or pork, or through inadvertently swallowing infested fleas or lice that live on pets.

❑ Doctors treat most types of worms with prescription medications such as mebendazole (Vermox) or thiabendazole (Mintezol), or with pyrantel pamoate (Antiminth), which is available over the counter. Creams or ointments may be prescribed to relieve anal itching and irritation.

❑ Some sushi has been found to be contaminated with a wormlike parasite called anisakis, which can cause illness similar to Crohn's disease if ingested. This parasite is a tightly coiled, clear worm, about one-half to three-quarters inch in length. It commonly embeds itself in herring and other fish. Fortunately, an experienced sushi chef can spot this parasite easily, so its presence in sushi is relatively rare.

❑ The risk of parasitic infection is increased by travel to places with inadequate public sanitation, personal hygiene levels, and/or food-handling practices.

❑ Because of the generalized nutritional deficiency associated with this disorder, good nutrition is vital. Foods high in protein and iron are particularly important.

WRINKLES

Wrinkles form when the skin thins and loses its elasticity. As long as the skin is supple, any creasing of the skin disappears as soon as you stop making the expression that caused it. But skin that has lost its suppleness retains the lines formed by smiling or frowning, for instance, even after you have assumed a more neutral expression. Over time, these lines deepen into wrinkles.

Some amount of wrinkling is a result of aging and is probably inevitable; no matter what you do, you will develop some lines if you simply live long enough. With aging, all skin cells begin to produce excess amounts of free radicals—unstable atoms and molecules that are normally removed by naturally occurring antioxidants within the skin cells. In aging skin cells, antioxidants are in short supply. The free radicals generated are left unchecked to cause damage to cell membranes, proteins, and DNA. These free radicals eventually break down collagen, a protein substance in connective tissue, and release chemicals that cause skin inflammation. It is a combination of these cellular and molecular events that leads to skin aging and the formation of wrinkles.

The first signs of wrinkles usually appear in the delicate tissue around the eyes—smile lines or "crow's feet." The cheeks and lips show damage next. As we age, our skin becomes thinner and dryer, both of which contribute to the formation of wrinkles. But other factors help to determine the rate and the extent of wrinkling, including diet and nutrition, muscle tone, habitual facial expressions, stress, proper skin care (or lack thereof), exposure to environmental pollutants, and lifestyle habits such as smoking. Heredity probably also plays a role.

The most important factor of all is sun exposure, which not only dries out the skin but also leads to the generation of free radicals that can damage skin cells. The sun is your skin's worst enemy. It is estimated that much of what we think of as signs of age are actually signs of overexposure to sunlight. Furthermore, overexposure does not necessarily mean sunbathing or sunburn; approximately 70 percent of sun damage is incurred during such everyday activities as driving and walking to and from your car. The ultraviolet-A (UVA) rays that do this damage are present all day long and in all seasons. These rays erode the elastic tissues in the skin, causing wrinkling. Worse, the effects of the sun are cumulative, although they may not be obvious for many years.

Unless otherwise specified, the dosages recommended here are for adults.

NUTRIENTS

SUPPLEMENT	SUGGESTED DOSAGE	COMMENTS
Very Important		
Methylsulfonyl-methane (MSM)	As directed on label.	Has been shown to help prevent wrinkling of the skin.
Primrose oil or black currant seed oil	1,000 mg 3 times daily. As directed on label.	Good healers for dermatitis, acne, and most other skin disorders. These oils contain linoleic acid, which is needed by the skin.
Vitamin A	25,000 IU daily for 3 months, then reduce to 15,000 IU daily. If you are pregnant, do not exceed 10,000 IU daily.	Necessary for healing and construction of new skin tissue.
plus natural carotenoid complex (Betatene)	As directed on label.	Antioxidants and vitamin A precursors.
Vitamin B complex plus extra vitamin B$_{12}$	As directed on label. 1,000–2,000 mcg daily.	Antistress and antiaging vitamins. Sublingual forms are best.
Important		
Kelp	1,000–1,500 mg daily.	Supplies balanced minerals needed for good skin tone.
Selenium	200 mcg daily. If you are pregnant, do not exceed 40 mcg daily.	An antioxidant that works with vitamin E.
Silica	As directed on label.	Important for skin strength and elasticity. Stimulates collagen formation.
Topical vitamin C (Hyper-C Serum from Jason Natural Cosmetics)	As directed on label. Apply topically to the face after washing and before applying moisturizer for best absorption.	Studies have shown that applying vitamin C topically promotes collagen production, improves skin tone, and can slightly reduce the appearance of fine wrinkles.
Vitamin C with bioflavonoids	3,000–5,000 mg daily, in divided doses.	Necessary for the formation of collagen, a protein that gives the skin its flexibility. Also fights free radicals and strengthens the capillaries that feed the skin.
Vitamin E	200 IU daily.	Protects against free radicals that can damage the skin and contribute to aging. Use d-alpha-tocopherol form.
Zinc	50 mg daily. Do not exceed a total of 100 mg daily from all supplements.	For tissue strength and repair. Use zinc gluconate lozenges or OptiZinc for best absorption.
plus copper	3 mg daily.	Needed for collagen production and healthy skin. Also needed to balance with zinc.
Helpful		
Ageless Beauty from Biotec Foods	As directed on label.	Protects the skin from free radical damage.
Calcium and magnesium	1,500 mg daily. 750 mg daily.	Deficiency contributes to fragility of the skin. Needed to balance with calcium.
Collagen cream	Apply topically as directed on label.	Good for very dry skin. A nourishing cream.
Elastin cream	Apply topically as directed on label.	Helps smooth existing wrinkles and prevent formation of new ones.
Flaxseed oil capsules or liquid or Ultimate Oil from Nature's Secret	1,000 mg daily. 1 tsp daily. As directed on label.	To supply needed essential fatty acids.
Glucosamine sulfate or N-Acetylglucosamine (N-A-G from Source Naturals)	As directed on label. As directed on label.	Important for the formation of healthy skin and connective tissue.
Grape seed extract	As directed on label.	An antioxidant that protects the skin from damage.
Herpanacine from Diamond-Herpanacine Associates	As directed on label.	Contains antioxidants, amino acids, and herbs that promote skin health.
Pycnogenol	As directed on label.	A free radical scavenger that also strengthens collagen.
Superoxide dismutase (SOD)	As directed on label.	A free radical destroyer. Also good for brown age spots.
Tretinoin (Retin-A)	As prescribed by physician.	Removes fine lines and smooths out wrinkles; also excellent for age spots, precancerous lesions, and sun-damaged skin. Available by prescription only. Takes around six months to show results.
Vitamin D	400 IU daily.	Deficiency can contribute to aging of the skin.

Herbs

❏ Acerola hydrates the skin.

❏ Alfalfa, borage, burdock root, chamomile, oat straw, red raspberry, and thyme are all good for general nourishment of the hair, skin, and nails.

Caution: Do not use chamomile if you are allergic to ragweed. Do not use during pregnancy or nursing. It may interact with warfarin or cyclosporine, so patients using these drugs should avoid it.

❏ Aloe vera has soothing, healing, and moisturizing properties. Apply pure aloe vera gel to dry skin as directed on the product label.

❏ Comfrey is good for alleviating dry skin.

Caution: Comfrey is recommended for external use only.

❏ Witch hazel is very useful in skin care.

❏ Other herbs that are beneficial for skin tone include borage seed, cranberry, flaxseed, ginger root, lavender, lemongrass, parsley, and pumpkin seed.

Recommendations

❏ Eat a well-balanced diet that includes many and varied fruits and vegetables, preferably raw, to provide your skin with the nutrients it needs. Also eat whole grains, seeds, nuts, and legumes.

❑ Drink at least 2 quarts of water every day, even if you do not feel thirsty. This helps to keep the skin hydrated and to flush away toxins, discouraging the formation of wrinkles.

❑ Obtain fatty acids from cold-pressed vegetable oils. Avoid saturated and animal fats.

❑ Do not smoke, and avoid alcohol and caffeine. All of these substances dry out the skin, making it more vulnerable to wrinkling. In addition, the smoking habit means pursing one's lips hundreds of times each day. The creases that form when you inhale from a cigarette often develop into wrinkles at a comparatively early age.

❑ No matter what your age or skin type, protect yourself from the sun. Always apply a sunscreen with a sun protection factor (SPF) of at least 15 to all exposed areas of skin, especially your face, regardless of the season or the weather. Sun exposure is the single greatest source of skin damage.

❑ Get regular exercise. Like other organs of the body, skin gets its nourishment from the bloodstream. Exercise increases the circulation of blood to the skin.

❑ Exercise your face. Sit in a chair and extend your jaw in an exaggerated chewing motion. Stretch the muscles under your chin and the front of your neck. Lying on a slant board for fifteen minutes a day is also good.

❑ Avoid alcohol-based toning products. Use witch hazel or an herbal/floral water instead.

❑ Pay attention to your facial expressions. If you find yourself squinting, raising your eyebrows, or making some other potentially wrinkle-inducing expression over and over again, you can make a conscious effort to stop.

❑ Practice good skin care and keep your skin well lubricated, especially if it is dry. (*See* DRY SKIN in Part Two.)

❑ Avoid using harsh soaps or solid cleansing creams such as cold cream on your face. Use natural oils such as avocado oil instead to remove dirt and old makeup. Apply it gently to your face and rinse it off with warm water. E-Gem Skin Care Soap from Carlson Laboratories is also good. Use a facial sponge or loofah (also spelled loofa or luffa) several times a week to remove dead, dry skin cells and stimulate circulation.

❑ Open a capsule of ACES + Zn from Carlson Labs and add the contents to your moisturizing cream before applying. This will help protect the skin from free radical damage. Do the same with your sunscreen.

❑ Do not apply heavy oils around the eye area before going to bed. This may cause eyes to be puffy in the morning.

❑ Limit your use of cosmetics, and choose the ones you do use carefully. Do not share your cosmetics, and replace them every three months.

Considerations

❑ Selecting good skin care products can be confusing. We recommend that you seek out products containing natural ingredients, and avoid those that contain petrolatum, mineral oil, or any hydrogenated oils. Some good ingredients to look for in skin care products include the following:

- *Allantoin,* a soothing agent derived from comfrey.

- *Aloe vera,* which is rich in nutrients and softens the skin.

- *Alpha-hydroxy acids,* natural fruit acids that encourage the shedding of dead surface skin cells and the formation of fresh, new skin cells.

- *Arnica,* an herb with both astringent and skin-soothing properties.

- *Burdock,* an herb that helps the body eliminate poisons from the skin.

- *Calendula,* an herb that promotes skin cell formation and stimulates tissue growth, and also soothes and softens sensitive skin.

- *Chamomile,* an anti-inflammatory, antibacterial herb that is good for sensitive skin.

- *Collagen,* a protein found in healthy young skin tissue.

- *Comfrey,* an herb that aids healing and soothes chapped, irritated, or blemished skin.

  Caution: Comfrey is recommended for external use only.

- *Cucumber,* which contains amino and organic acids that cool and refresh the skin and tighten the pores.

- *Essential fatty acids* (including linoleic, linolenic, and arachidonic acids), which smooth rough skin, protect against moisture loss, and prevent invasion by free radicals.

- *Ginkgo biloba,* an antioxidant that helps skin stay younger looking.

- *Glycerine,* a soap by-product that attracts and holds moisture in the skin.

- *Ivy,* an herb that stimulates circulation and aids other ingredients in penetrating the skin.

- *Liposomes,* microscopic bubbles that deliver active ingredients deep into the skin.

- *Panthenol (provitamin B_5),* a nutrient that builds moisture and soothes irritation.

- *Retinoic acid,* a form of vitamin A that smooths skin, promotes cell renewal, and improves circulation to the skin.

- *Sage,* an herb with astringent properties that can help relieve dry, itchy skin.

  Caution: Do not use sage if you suffer from any type of seizure disorder, or are pregnant or nursing.

- *Witch hazel,* a natural astringent that tones the skin.

- *Yarrow,* an astringent herb that acts as an anti-inflammatory and tightens and firms saggy skin.

❑ There are many excellent home facial treatments that can help with specific skin problems. Some of the best include:

- *To add color to sallow skin,* mash ½ cup or so of strawberries in a blender and apply them to your face. Leave them on for ten minutes, then rinse with tepid water.

- *To alleviate puffiness in the eye area,* place cool cucumber slices over your eyes for ten minutes or more, as needed.

- *To cleanse the pores,* rub mashed tomato over your face.

- *To moisturize your skin,* mash together grapes (a natural source of collagen and alpha-hydroxy acids) with enough honey to make a paste, and apply the mixture to your face as a mask. Leave it in place for twenty to thirty minutes while you relax, then rinse it off.

- *To remove dead surface skin cells and improve skin texture,* gently rub a small handful of dry short-grain rice against your face for a few minutes. This technique has been used by Japanese women for centuries.

- *To soften and nourish the skin,* mash half of an avocado and apply it to your face. Leave it on until it dries, then rinse off with warm water. Avocado contains essential fatty acids and other nutrients that help prevent premature wrinkling.

- *To tighten and refine pores,* whip up the white of an egg with a pinch of alum and apply it to your face as a mask. After fifteen to twenty minutes, rinse it off with lukewarm water.

❑ Wrinkle lines from the lips toward the nose may be due to a deficiency of vitamin B_2 (riboflavin).

❑ Researchers studying premature aging have found that vitamin E, carotenoids, and selenium may help prevent wrinkling.

❑ Antioxidant supplements improve skin integrity, making it appear younger looking longer.

❑ Chemical peels, used by many dermatologists and skin care professionals, trigger collagen production deep underneath the skin by destroying the upper layer of skin cells. The new collagen produced helps to improve elasticity and give the skin a more youthful look. Chemical peels can irritate the skin, and they can also cause sun sensitivity.

❑ Alpha-hydroxy acids (AHAs) are acids derived from various fruits that act in much the same way, but they are natural, less irritating to the skin, and do not produce sun sensitivity. Glycolic acid (the best for exfoliation), citric acid, and malic acid are all AHAs. While these are gentler than chemical peels, they still can irritate sensitive or fair skin.

❑ Ester-C Gel with E Skin Recovery Complex from Derma-E Skin Care is a good product that combines esterified vitamin C, vitamin E, borage oil, green tea extract, and herbs that help repair dull, aging, sun-damaged skin.

❑ Dermatologists are constantly searching for ways to prevent or treat wrinkles. Doctors perform a wide range of treatments for wrinkles, including facial peels; cosmetic skin surgery; laser resurfacing; local injections with purified botulinum toxin (Botox), collagen injections, or new soft-tissue fillers such as hyaluronic acid (Restylane); and fat transfers, to name a few. Many, if not all, of these treatments can cause unpleasant side effects. If you are considering medical treatment for this condition, do plenty of research and discuss your options with a qualified dermatologist.

❑ Surgical treatment is an expensive but effective option as well. If you are bothered by your wrinkles, speak to a board-certified plastic surgeon. Get a second opinion or ask around before committing to a procedure.

XEROPHTHALMIA

See under EYE PROBLEMS.

YEAST INFECTION (YEAST VAGINITIS)

See under CANDIDIASIS; FUNGAL INFECTION; and VAGINITIS.

PART THREE

Remedies
and
Therapies

Introduction

In Part Two, various treatment programs were recommended for each of the health problems discussed. Part Three explains how to implement some of the remedies and therapies discussed earlier, as well as providing information about some cutting-edge technologies that are showing promise in the treatment of various disorders. It covers when each treatment can be beneficial, and, when appropriate, offers instructions for effective use. You can learn about the more traditional treatments offered by homeopathic medicine and chiropractic; ancient techniques offered by Ayurvedic medicine, fasting, juicing, and poultices; less well-known treatment approaches such as aromatherapy, hyperbaric oxygen therapy, and magnetic field therapy; and a potpourri of more innovative treatments that may be helpful depending on the condition you are trying to treat. These remedies should all be used in conjunction with a healthy diet and supplementation program.

After learning about what is available out there, you will be able to choose the options that are most suitable for you and your situation.

ACUPRESSURE

See under PAIN CONTROL.

ACUPUNCTURE

See under PAIN CONTROL.

AROMATHERAPY AND ESSENTIAL OILS

Aromatherapy is the use of pure essential oils to enhance physical and mental well-being. Essential oils are aromatic, highly concentrated distilled essences of plants. These oils can have many different applications in our lives. They can sometimes be used as a natural adjunct to, or substitute for, prescription or over-the-counter drugs. We can also use them simply to make ourselves feel better.

Aromatherapy uses the sense of smell to enrich our experience of the world. Smell plays a significant role in our daily perceptions and how we react physically, emotionally, and mentally to what is going on around us. Various scents help us orient ourselves to the season of the year, our location, and situations of danger. Essential oils not only affect the physical but also the mental and emotional aspects of our lives. The inhalation of certain essential oils has been associated with the release of brain chemicals that stimulate various emotions. For example, lavender oil has the ability to evoke and increase the release of serotonin, thus producing a calming effect on the body. Some essential oils also have healing properties when applied topically to the skin.

When purchasing essential oils, make sure they are 100 percent pure botanical extracts, not chemical reproductions of different fragrances. Chemical reproductions are not effective in aromatherapy because they do not evoke the same biochemical response as natural, pure essential oils.

Pure essential oils are extracted directly from various parts of different plants. The oils can be obtained by a variety of methods, including distillation, solvent extraction, carbon dioxide extraction, expression (pressing), and enfleurage (a process in which some type of odorless oil is used to extract essential oil from flower petals). The type and part of the plant being used determines which type of extraction process is appropriate.

The following are some helpful hints to keep in mind when shopping for essential oils:

- Buy in small quantities (the oxygen in partially filled bottles deteriorates the oil).
- Read the label carefully and make sure it says "pure essential oil."
- Be aware that the availability of different plants and the extraction methods used affect prices, so there can be great variations in the costs of different oils. This is normal.

- Certain plant oils, such as apple blossom and peach blossom, cannot be extracted. If you find oils with such scents, they are not true essential oils.

Using essential oils is really very simple. Basically, you dilute a small amount of essential oil in a base of some kind (either water or another oil, termed a carrier oil, depending on the intended use), and apply or inhale it. For inhalation therapy, there are special devices available, including diffusers, simmer pots, aromatherapy lamps, and lightbulb rings. When using one of these devices, follow the manufacturer's instructions. Or you can inhale an essential oil directly from the bottle. For topical applications, you can use any of the following to dilute essential oils:

- Almond oil.
- Apricot oil.
- Grape seed oil.
- Jojoba oil.
- Olive oil.
- Water.

The following are some suggested dilution ratios for topical applications:

- Baths. Add 8 drops essential oil to 1 cup water and add to the bath.
- Body lotion. Add 25 drops essential oil to 8 ounces of unscented lotion.
- Carpet freshener. Add 25 drops essential oil to 16 ounces of water.
- Cleaning. Add 25 drops essential oil to 2 gallons of water.
- Facial oil. Add 6 drops essential oil to 1 ounce of jojoba oil.
- Hair conditioner. Add 1 drop essential oil to 4 to 6 ounces of unscented conditioner.
- Hair rinse. Add 10 drops essential oil to 16 ounces water.
- Massage oil. Add 25 drops essential oil to 2 ounces almond, apricot, grape seed, jojoba, or olive oil.
- Perfume. Add 12 drops essential oil to ½ ounce water or jojoba oil.
- Room deodorizer. Add 25 drops essential oil to 16 ounces water.
- Shampoo. Add 12 drops essential oil to 16 ounces unscented shampoo.

When using essential oils, be aware that they are highly concentrated and very potent. Keep the following commonsense precautions in mind:

- Do not use oils full strength. Always dilute them first. Some essential oils can be toxic if used at full strength.
- Do not use oils near the eyes.

Common Essential Oils

There are many different essential oils available, each with its own special properties. The table below lists some of the more commonly used oils and their qualities. Use it to determine which essential oil or oils you might like to try.

Essential Oil	Uses
Bergamot	Contains statin-like compounds and may help with blood disorders.
Cedarwood	Has antibacterial properties.
Chamomile	An analgesic, anti-inflammatory, and anticonvulsive. Excellent for headaches (apply as a compress to head). Good in baths, hair rinse, and massage oil. *Caution:* Do not use chamomile if you are allergic to ragweed. Do not use during pregnancy or nursing. It may interact with warfarin or cyclosporine, so patients using these drugs should avoid it.
Cinnamon bark	Useful for scent enhancement in the home or office. Makes a good air freshener and is also antifungal.
Clary sage	A very aromatic oil that is enjoyed by both men and women. An antioxidant, anti-inflammatory, and anti-microbial. Good when used in skin and hair care products. *Caution:* Should not be used in the first months of pregnancy.
Cypress	An antifungal and may promote hair growth.
Eucalyptus	Antifungal, antibacterial, and anti-inflammatory. May promote good dental health and reduce decay and cavities. Improves lung function. Used as an ointment for muscular aches and pains. Good for repelling insects, and for use on insect bites or stings. Has a normalizing, balancing effect.
Frankincense	An anti-inflammatory. Helpful for asthma and breathing. Reduces pain and improves physical function in arthritis. Controls diarrheal disease in patients with colitis.
Geranium	Immune system booster, blood-pressure-lowering agent, hormone balancer, and insect repellent. A normalizing and balancing, mildly sedating oil good for PMS, as a bath additive.
Grapefruit	Acts as an antioxidant and antiproliferation agent, which may reduce cancer risk. Useful in baths, skin care products, and colognes.
Hyssop	Helps reduce anxiety and stress; promotes alertness, calmness, and a feeling of contentedness. May reduce risk of dental decay and cavities. Helps induce sleep and prevent insomnia. Improves circulation. *Caution:* Do not use if you have epilepsy or other seizure disorders.
Jasmine	An antibacterial agent and antioxidant. Has been used for apathy, hysteria, uterine disorders, coughs, and as a muscle relaxant for childbirth because it is an antispasmodic.
Juniper	An antioxidant and antibacterial, and increases blood flow. *Caution:* Do not use during pregnancy. Do not use if you have kidney problems.
Lavender	Reduces pain related to postsurgical procedures, and neck and back pain. Can act as a sedative to aid in falling asleep and promoting deep sleep. May reduce situational stress.
Lemon	An antioxidant that reduces oxidative stress to the bad cholesterol (LDL). Retards tumor growth in a cancer cell line. Emulsifies and disperses grease and oil. Helpful in cleaning products and hair rinses and for wound cleansing.
Linden	A calming, sedating, and soothing tonic.
Mandarin	A sweet, light, and tangy fragrance. Helps decrease platelet clumping. Acts as an antioxidant and inhibits human cancer cell line growth. Is also used as a digestive aid and is commonly found in soaps, cosmetics, perfumes, and colognes.
Orange	Has antifungal properties. Useful in relieving short-term knee pain. *Caution:* This oil increases sensitivity to the sun. Do not use it if you will be spending considerable time outdoors.
Patchouli	An earthy scent used in personal fragrances, baths, and hair care products. Good for dry skin. Is effective against mosquito bites.
Peppermint	Helps digestion, which could help people who experience nausea. Reduces symptoms of irritable bowel syndrome such as diarrhea. Reduces fatigue and improves mood. Promotes better sleep. Good for use in baths and oral care products.

Pine	May reduce appetite by modulating satiety hormones.
Rosemary	An antioxidant and anti-inflammatory, and inhibits *H. pylori* in a Petri dish. Helps keep bones strong, and was shown to have anticancer effects on human cell lines. Used in hair care products as a conditioner and shine enhancer. *Caution:* If irritation occurs, discontinue use. Do not use directly on the skin without diluting. Use caution inhaling it if you have asthma or bronchitis. Do not use if you have epilepsy.
Sandalwood	Acts as an anticancer agent in cells and helps support the liver by increasing glutathione, which is a potent antioxidant. Good in skin care blends.
Tea tree	A potent antibacterial, antimicrobial, anti-inflammatory, antiviral, and fungicide. Good for athlete's foot, dandruff, and yeast infections. May reduce gingivitis and support healthy gums.
Thyme	An antibacterial, antioxidant, and antifungal. Helps support bone health.
Ylang ylang	Lifts mood, eases anxiety, relaxes, reduces stress, normalizes the heartbeat, and lowers blood pressure. Has a harmonizing effect. May be used on the skin or for aromatherapy.

- Do not touch your face, mucous membranes, or genitals if your hands have been in direct contact with the oils.

- Keep essential oils out of the reach of children.

- Be cautious about using essential oils for children, especially young children. If you do use essential oils on a child, reduce the concentration of the essential oil by half or more.

- Be cautious using essential oils during pregnancy.

- Avoid sun exposure when using bergamot and other citrus oils.

To help you determine which essential oil or oils may be suited to your particular needs, *see* Common Essential Oils on the previous page.

ASCORBIC ACID FLUSH

Because vitamin C (ascorbic acid) promotes the healing of wounds and protects the body from bacterial infection, allergens, and other pollutants, it is often beneficial to flush the body with ascorbic acid. This therapy may help treat chemical allergies, influenza, and sprains, and it can help prevent other illnesses. Your intake will likely exceed the upper limit of safety, which is 2,000 milligrams for adults over age nineteen, 1,200 to 1,800 milligrams for children age nine to eighteen, and 400 to 650 milligrams for children age one to eight.

Procedure for Adults

Place 1,000 milligrams of ascorbic acid in a cup of water or juice. To make this drink, use ascorbic acid in the form of either esterified vitamin C, such as Ester-C, or a buffered product, such as calcium ascorbate. Take every half hour, keeping track of how much has been taken, until diarrhea results. Count the number of teaspoons needed to produce diarrhea. Subtract 1 teaspoon from this amount, and take

the resulting ascorbic acid drink every four hours for one to two days. During therapy, make sure the stool retains a tapioca-like consistency. If it again becomes watery, decrease dosage as necessary. Repeat therapy once a month.

AYURVEDIC REMEDIES

Ayurvedic medicine is one of the oldest forms of medicine in the world. It incorporates tools such as diet, exercise, breathing exercises, meditation (yoga), mental visualization, therapeutic massage, and herbs to treat illness and maintain health. This ancient healing method also uses color therapy, sound therapy, and aromatherapy to help create balance within the body.

In Ayurveda, the fundamental healing philosophy is the concept of the three *doshas,* or basic types of energy or functional principles. These are vata (from ether and air), pitta (from fire and water), and kapha (from water and earth), and according to the principles of Ayurveda, they are present in everyone and everything. Vata is the energy of movement. Pitta is the energy of digestion or metabolism. Kapha is the energy of lubrication and structure. All three doshas are present in everyone, but one is usually predominant in any given individual. Ayurvedic medicine sees disease as a result of excess or deficiency in vata, pitta, or kapha, and also the presence of toxins. Good health indicates a balance of these three energies in a body that is relatively toxin-free. Herbs are used to treat illness by restoring this balance. Herbs that deal with energy or movement are used to increase vata. Herbs that treat digestion, assimilation, absorption, and metabolism are pitta, and those involved with structure and the musculoskeletal system—the "glue" that holds the body together—are kapha.

Ayurvedic medicine regards the human body as a manifestation of cosmic energy that is transferred to all levels, both mental and physical. This can be difficult for people from Western cultures to grasp, but practitioners believe the two systems of energy are closer than we can conceive.

At Ayurveda's core is the belief that we are a totality of body and soul within the universe, and if we can live in harmony with nature and our inner beings, we will stay healthy.

BIOFEEDBACK

See under PAIN CONTROL.

BLOOD PURIFICATION

Blood is composed of four components: plasma; red blood cells; white blood cells; and platelets. Through these components, the blood performs several life-sustaining functions. The plasma is the watery, colorless liquid in which the other components float. The red blood cells transport oxygen to the cells. The white blood cells destroy bacteria and other disease-producing organisms. The platelets are needed for the blood-clotting process.

In addition, blood transports nutrients to the cells and carries away wastes; transports hormones from the endocrine glands to other parts of the body; helps regulate the amounts of acids, bases, salts, and water in the cells; and helps regulate body temperature. If any of these functions is impaired, the consequences can have a direct bearing on your health.

There are several ways in which the functions carried out by the blood may be hampered. First, hundreds of chemicals ranging from gases such as carbon monoxide to toxic metals such as lead to natural substances such as fat—can find their way into the blood and impair its function. These foreign substances enter the body through the air we breathe, the water we drink, the food we eat, and the surfaces with which we come in contact through the skin. Because these substances act on the blood in different ways, the adverse effects they produce may vary widely.

Second, the performance of the blood may be hampered by a lack of specific nutrients. A classic example is an iron deficiency that results in anemia. However, there are many nutrients that the blood requires on a daily basis if it is to perform normally. Finally, genetics can play a role in creating blood disorders. Sickle-cell anemia and hemophilia are two common examples of such disorders.

Blood purification techniques can act in two ways. Some help draw foreign substances out of the body, while others provide important nutrients to help restore the blood's normal structure and maximize its performance.

Procedure

Blood purification is achieved through the use of a special fast. (This is for healthy adults only. If you have a chronic condition, please check with your health care provider first. Pregnant and lactating women should only do this with a physician's consent.) Once you have decided to follow a blood purification program, it is vital to choose an appropriate time for the fast. Consider that fasting requires the conservation of energy. Therefore, avoid fasting on a week when, for instance, you are moving your office or participating in a sports event. Also keep in mind that the cold-weather months are not an ideal time for a fast, as some of the heat you need to withstand the cold is created during the digestive process. Most important is the need to be mentally prepared. If you are "psyched up" for the fast, it is the right time to fast.

Once you have chosen the time for the fast and have prepared yourself mentally, you can begin to prepare yourself physically. For one week prior to the fast, follow a raw vegetable diet, including lots of "green drinks." Chlorophyll, obtained from tablets or fresh juice, "pre-cleanses" the body, making the fast less of a shock to your system.

While on the fast, consume only steam-distilled water; juices; and dandelion, milk thistle, licorice root, yellow dock root, burdock root, or red clover tea or extract. Drink at least 8 to 10 cups of distilled water daily to aid in cleansing and to help carry toxins out of the body. The best juices for blood purification are lemon juice, beet juice and its tops, carrot juice, and the juices of all leafy greens. Leafy green juices are particularly important because they supply chlorophyll, an essential part of any blood purification therapy. Chlorophyll not only cleanses the blood of impurities, but also builds up the blood with important nutrients, promotes regularity, and inhibits cellular damage from radiation. This makes chlorophyll helpful in the treatment of many disorders. Wheatgrass, barley, and alfalfa juices are all rich in chlorophyll. This fast provides very little salt. Most diets provide too much salt, but too little can make you lightheaded and dizzy. If you feel either of these, take some clear broth.

Stay on the fast for three days, or as directed by your health care provider. Once you have completed the fast, avoid white flour and all sugars—substances that are highly refined and hard to digest. The stress placed on your body by such foods can "undo" all of the good accomplished by the fast. Ideally, these foods should be avoided all of the time. At the very least, eliminate them—as well as heated fats and oils—for at least one month after your fast.

NUTRIENTS

SUPPLEMENT	SUGGESTED DOSAGE	COMMENTS
Very Important		
Chlorophyll tablets or	As directed on label.	Cleanses and refurbishes red blood cells.
liquid chlorophyll or	As directed on label. Take with juice.	Aids immune system function.
fresh wheatgrass juice	As directed on label.	
Important		
Cell Guard from Biotec Foods	As directed on label.	A good antioxidant formula.

Helpful		
Kyo-Green from Wakunaga	As directed on label.	Good for the liver and the colon. Contains wheatgrass and barley grass.
Ultimate Cleanse from Nature's Secret	As directed on label.	A two-part system that helps to stimulate and detoxify the organs, blood, and channels of elimination.

Herbs

❑ Barberry, black radish, eyebright, lobelia, milk thistle, Oregon grape, pau d'arco, wild yam, and yellow dock cleanse and detoxify the liver and the endocrine system. You can use these herbs independently or in any combination.

Cautions: Lobelia is only to be taken under supervision of a health care professional as it is potentially toxic. People with high blood pressure, heart disease, liver disease, kidney disease, seizure disorders, or shortness of breath should not take lobelia. Pregnant and lactating women should avoid lobelia as well. Do not use Oregon grape during pregnancy.

❑ Borage seed, chamomile, dandelion, ginkgo biloba, and sarsaparilla help to restore the acid/alkaline balance to the bloodstream. Ginkgo biloba is also a powerful antioxidant and improves circulation.

Cautions: Do not use chamomile if you are allergic to ragweed. Do not use during pregnancy or nursing. It may interact with warfarin or cyclosporine, so patients using these drugs should avoid it. Do not take ginkgo biloba if you have a bleeding disorder, or are scheduled for surgery or a dental procedure.

❑ Burdock, dandelion, hawthorn, licorice, pau d'arco, red clover, rhubarb, sage, shiitake mushroom, and Siberian and other ginsengs detoxify and cleanse the blood. These herbs can be used independently or in any combination.

Cautions: Licorice root should not be used during pregnancy or nursing. It should not be used by persons with diabetes, glaucoma, heart disease, high blood pressure, or a history of stroke. Do not use sage if you suffer from any type of seizure disorder, or are pregnant or nursing. Do not use Siberian ginseng if you have hypoglycemia or a heart disorder. Do not use ginseng if you have high blood pressure or are pregnant or nursing.

❑ Echinacea cleanses the lymphatic glands.

Caution: Do not take echinacea for longer than three months. It should not be used by people who are allergic to ragweed.

❑ Goldenseal cleanses the mucous membranes.

Caution: Do not take goldenseal internally on a daily basis for more than one week at a time. Do not use it during pregnancy or if you are breast-feeding, and use with caution if you are allergic to ragweed. If you have a history of

cardiovascular disease, diabetes, or glaucoma, use it only under a doctor's supervision.

❑ Green tea is a powerful antioxidant. Drink two or three cups daily.

Caution: Green tea contains vitamin K, which can make anticoagulant medications less effective. Consult your health care professional if you are using them. The caffeine in green tea could cause insomnia, anxiety, upset stomach, nausea, or diarrhea.

Considerations

❑ *See also* ENEMAS and FASTING in Part Three.

CHELATION THERAPY

Chelation (pronounced *key-LAY-shun*) therapy is a safe, nonsurgical treatment used to rid the body of excess toxins, particularly metals. Chelating agents used in this therapy are available in over-the-counter formulas that can be taken orally at home, and in intravenous solutions that must be administered under the supervision of a physician. These chelators draw out toxic metals and other harmful substances that impair body function, and help the body eliminate these toxins via the kidneys. Oral chelating agents can often prevent problems from occurring by restoring circulation to the body's tissues. If serious health problems already exist, intravenous therapy is usually necessary.

Chelation therapy is used to treat a variety of health problems. First, chelating agents are used to bind with heavy toxic metals such as cadmium, lead, and mercury— substances that enter the body through food, water, and other means—and excrete these metals from the body. As certain minerals accumulate in the body, they interact with other minerals, promoting the actions of some and inhibiting the actions of others. Lead, for instance, has been shown to inhibit the actions of calcium, iron, and potassium, all of which are important nutrients. When chelating agents are used to eliminate toxic metals such as lead from the body, essential nutrients are better able to do their job.

Chelation therapy is also used in the treatment of atherosclerosis and other circulatory disorders, as well as in the treatment of gangrene, which often is the result of poor circulation. In atherosclerosis, deposits of cholesterol, fats, and other substances collect on the walls of large and medium-sized arteries in the form of hard plaque. It has been found that calcium acts as the "glue" that holds the atherosclerotic plaque together. Chelating agents bind with this calcium and carry it out of the body, potentially breaking up the plaque deposits, unclogging the arteries, and permitting more normal blood flow.

ORAL CHELATION THERAPY

Oral chelating agents offer a safe, convenient alternative for persons who are at risk for circulatory problems or problems caused by toxic metal accumulation. Among the many disorders that may be helped by chelation therapy are multiple sclerosis, Parkinson's disease, Alzheimer's disease, and arthritis. This should be only an adjunct to the conventional treatment prescribed by your doctor. Some people have reported dramatic improvement in arterial circulation after chelation treatment. However, the medical literature cannot support its use. A review of all published medical research on the subject concluded that it is not effective for treating cardiovascular disease. The American Heart Association does not endorse it and the FDA has not approved this method for treating cardiovascular disease. It is always wise to consult a health care professional first if you have one of these chronic conditions.

Procedure

The following chelating agents can be used to prevent many degenerative illnesses and can often alleviate the symptoms of existing conditions. These agents can be purchased in the combinations shown below in health food stores and drugstores. Follow package directions regarding dosage.

- Alfalfa, fiber, rutin, and selenium.

- Calcium and magnesium chelate with potassium.

- Chromium, garlic, pectin, and potassium.

- Coenzyme A.

- Coenzyme Q_{10}.

- Copper chelate, iron, sea kelp, and zinc chelate.

In addition, the following supplements can act as oral chelating agents to rid the body of excess toxic metals and minerals. Mineral supplements can be used with intravenous chelation to replace lost minerals and to control free radical damage, which has been linked to heart disease.

NUTRIENTS

SUPPLEMENT	SUGGESTED DOSAGE	COMMENTS
Aangamik DMG from FoodScience of Vermont	200 mg daily.	Increases available oxygen and prevents cellular and tissue oxidation.
Alfalfa liquid or tablets	Double the amount directed on the label.	Detoxifies the liver and alkalizes the body. Chelates toxic substances from the body.
Apple pectin and rutin	As directed on label. As directed on label.	To bind with unwanted toxic metals and remove them from the body through the intestinal tract.
Calcium plus magnesium	1,500 mg daily. 700–1,000 mg daily.	Replaces calcium lost by using chelating substances. Use calcium citrate form. Displaces calcium within the cells of the artery walls.
Coenzyme Q_{10}	60–90 mg daily.	Improves circulation, lowers blood pressure, and acts as a chelating agent.
Garlic (Kyolic from Wakunaga)	2 capsules twice daily, with meals.	A good chelating agent and detoxifier.
L-cysteine and L-methionine	500 mg each twice daily, on an empty stomach. Take with water or juice. Do not take with milk. Take with 50 mg vitamin B_6 and 100 mg vitamin C for better absorption.	Two of the most important natural dietary chelators. Cysteine is effective for nickel toxicity.
L-lysine plus glutathione	500 mg each daily.	Aids in detoxifying harmful toxins and metals. Powerful free radical scavengers and antioxidants that remove unwanted substances from the body. *Caution:* Do not take lysine longer than six months at a time.
Selenium	200 mcg daily. If you are pregnant, do not exceed 40 mcg daily.	A powerful free radical scavenger.
Vitamin A with mixed carotenoids including natural beta-carotene or carotenoid complex	25,000 IU daily. If you are pregnant, do not exceed 10,000 IU daily. As directed on label.	To aid in excreting toxic substances. Use emulsion forms for easier assimilation.
Vitamin B complex plus extra vitamin B_3 (niacin) and vitamin B_5 (pantothenic acid) and vitamin B_{12} and folic acid	100 mg of each major B vitamin 3 times daily (amounts of individual vitamins in a complex will vary). 50 mg 3 times daily. 50 mg 3 times daily. 1,000 mcg 3 times daily. As directed on label.	B vitamins aid in protecting the body from harmful substances and are needed for all cellular functions. *Caution:* Do not take niacin if you have a liver disorder, gout, or high blood pressure.
Vitamin C with bioflavonoids	5,000–15,000 mg daily, in divided doses.	Powerful chelating agents and immunostimulants.
Vitamin E	200 IU daily.	Removes toxic substances and destroys free radicals. Use d-alpha-tocopherol form. Emulsion form is recommended for easier assimilation and greater safety at higher doses.

Recommendations

❑ Follow a diet designed to treat heart disease and/or high cholesterol. Avoid fried foods; dairy products; mayonnaise; red meat; processed and fast foods; salt; and gravies. Limit vegetable oils. Drink only steam-distilled water.

❑ Eat as many fiber-rich foods as possible. Oats, brown rice, and wheat bran are all good sources of fiber. *See* CARDIOVASCULAR DISEASE and HIGH CHOLESTEROL in Part Two for more information.

❏ Add a high-protein drink to your diet, or take the essential amino acids in supplement form. A deficiency of any one essential amino acid will reduce the effectiveness of all the others.

❏ Increase your intake of manganese by eating Brazil nuts, pecans, barley, buckwheat, whole wheat, and dried split peas. Manganese is an important chelating agent when consumed in manganese-rich foods. It is a major factor in blocking calcium from entering the cells of the arterial lining.

Caution: Brazil nuts contain very high amounts of selenium, over 500 micrograms per ounce of nuts. If you are pregnant, do not consume Brazil nuts.

❏ Incorporate onions into your daily meals. Onions produce a natural chelating effect in the body and tend to decrease the "clotting power" of blood.

❏ When using chelation therapy, make sure to replace any essential minerals that might be displaced by chelating agents. Alfalfa, iron (with your doctor's approval), kelp, and zinc supplements are recommended. Use a natural source of iron, such as blackstrap molasses or Floradix Iron + Herbs from Salus Haus.

❏ If you take zinc supplements, eat sulfur-rich foods, like garlic, onions, and legumes. Zinc inhibits the action of sulfur.

INTRAVENOUS CHELATION THERAPY

Intravenous chelation therapy is often used to remove calcified, hardened plaque from the arterial walls, improving circulation. When done under the care of a physician, this procedure can be a safe alternative to vascular surgery. This therapy is also used to remove heavy metals, such as lead, from the body. Most serious illnesses require repeated injections of the chelating agents.

The most common chelating agent now used in intravenous therapy is ethylenediaminetetraacetic acid (EDTA). A strong substance, EDTA attracts lead, strontium, and many other metals, as well as calcium. Although there is controversy surrounding the use of this agent, it has not been found to be toxic when used correctly.

Prior to beginning a course of EDTA chelation therapy, you must undergo a thorough physical examination. This includes a series of laboratory tests, including evaluations of cholesterol, blood, kidney function, liver function, glucose, and electrolytes. In addition, electrocardiogram and chest X-rays are routinely performed. Other studies often assess vitamin B_{12} and mineral status. Typically, kidney function studies are repeated several times during the course of chelation therapy. Blood studies may have to be repeated, too, depending on the initial laboratory results.

The course of chelation therapy varies from person to person, but a typical course includes two treatments per week, each of three hours' duration. In addition to EDTA, physicians frequently administer supplements—including vitamin C, magnesium, and trace minerals—with the intravenous infusion, depending on the individual's particular illness and the results of the laboratory studies.

Recommendations

❏ While undergoing EDTA chelation therapy, be sure to take supplemental vitamins and minerals, particularly zinc, chromium, and the B-complex vitamins. This is important, as chelation agents are known to bind with and remove certain vitamins and minerals from the body. Make sure that your physician knows you are doing this. During therapy, take these supplements as directed in NUTRITION, DIET, AND WELLNESS in Part One.

Considerations

❏ When supervised by a qualified physician, EDTA intravenous chelation therapy is safe and causes few side effects.

❏ Hair analysis is an excellent means of determining the concentration of minerals in the body. (*See* HAIR ANALYSIS in Part Three.)

❏ There are hundreds of doctors in the United States who are certified by the American Board of Clinical Metal Toxicology as approved chelation therapists. For information on the approved physicians in your area, you can contact them directly. (*See* Health and Medical Organizations in the Appendix.)

CHINESE MEDICINE

Traditional Chinese medicine (TCM) is an ancient form of medicine. It is based mainly on the prevention of illness, although it has helped many people to find a cure for a wide variety of health problems.

Chinese medicine uses herbs, acupuncture, acupressure, massage, and diet to promote health. It especially emphasizes changing lifestyle habits. The key to understanding Chinese medicine is to understand the idea of *balance.* The goal in using any of the tools of Chinese medicine, including herbs, is to supply the body with what it requires to regulate the flow of *chi,* or vital energy, and to promote a state of equilibrium, or balance, and harmony. Once balance is attained, the person regains health.

For centuries, the Chinese have taught how to achieve balance in life using the concept of yin and yang, which are present in human beings and in all of nature. Yang is characterized as heat and light; yin as shadow and cold. Dryness and summer are yang; wetness and winter are yin. Chinese philosophy also classifies energy as yang and blood as yin. A person with an excess of yang might be overweight, have an angry temperament, and high blood pressure. Such an individual would benefit from such foods as asparagus, bananas, cucumbers, soy products (tofu), and watermelon.

A person with a quiet personality, who is listless or tires easily, may have an excess of cooling yin. Foods recommended for this type of person include beef, garlic, ginger, lamb, and pepper. Yin foods are cooling and have a cooling effect, whereas yang foods are warming. Neutral foods include black beans, cabbage, carrots, lemons, and rice and other whole-grain foods. These foods provide balance. To maintain health, one must consume the proper balance of yin, yang, and neutral foods.

Like foods, medicinal herbs are seen in terms of yin and yang. Chinese herbs are very powerful and should be used under the advice of a healer trained in traditional Chinese medicine. There are more than 5,000 herbs in the Chinese pharmacopoeia, many of them unknown to Western practitioners. Along with commonly known herbals, such as astragalus (which enhances immune function) and reishi (the mushroom of immortality), traditional Chinese remedies that have been becoming more widely available in the United States include cordyceps and velvet antler (also sometimes called antler velvet). Cordyceps (also called caterpillar fungus) is a plant that is found only in certain isolated places in southwest China and Tibet, at elevations of more than 12,000 feet above sea level. Chinese researchers have found more than two hundred species of wild cordyceps. Studies on this herb suggest that it can reduce the ill effects of radiation treatment, lower blood pressure, reduce symptoms of asthma and other respiratory problems, increase energy levels, improve memory, and improve male sexual ability. Velvet antler has been reported to increase energy, mental alertness, and sex drive; decrease blood pressure and cholesterol levels; and reduce PMS symptoms. Velvet antler also may be effective as an anti-inflammatory.

If you are interested in exploring traditional Chinese medicine, we suggest that you work with a qualified practitioner of Oriental medicine, certified by the National Certification Commission for Acupuncture and Oriental Medicine (NCCAOM) rather than simply buying Chinese remedies on your own. The NCCAOM can help you to locate a qualified practitioner in your area. (See Health and Medical Organizations in the Appendix.) Many of the over-the-counter remedies that are available are not actually traditional and/or may be adulterated.

CHIROPRACTIC

See under PAIN CONTROL.

COLON CLEANSING

Retained debris in the colon leads to the absorption of toxins, resulting in systemic intoxication (poisoning). Symptoms of this condition can include mental confusion, depression, irritability, fatigue, gastrointestinal irregularities, and even allergic reactions such as hives, sneezing, and coughing. Many nutritionists and researchers believe that this toxicity can eventually lead to more serious disorders.

Colon cleansing can rid the colon of debris, and help prevent and treat a variety of health problems. This is for adults, and it is wise to check with your health care professional first.

Procedure

The best means of removing toxins and wastes from the body is a fast. This should be the first step in any colon-cleansing program. (*See* BLOOD PURIFICATION and FASTING in Part Three.) In addition to following a fast, use a wheatgrass, fresh lemon juice, garlic, or coffee enema. (*See* ENEMAS in Part Three.) If bowel problems or related symptoms are chronic, repeat this program once monthly.

The following supplements aid in cleansing the colon.

NUTRIENTS

SUPPLEMENT	SUGGESTED DOSAGE	COMMENTS
Very Important		
Fiber (ground flaxseeds, oat bran, or psyllium seed husks)	1 capsule or 1 teaspoon 4 times daily. Take separately from other supplements and medications.	Essential for a clean colon. Not habit forming.
Important		
Acidophilus or Kyo-Dophilus from Wakunaga	As directed on label. Take on an empty stomach. As directed on label. Take on an empty stomach.	Restores the normal "friendly" bacteria in the colon. If you are allergic to dairy products, use a nondairy formula.
Aloe vera juice	½ cup 3 times daily. Use a pure form.	Heals colon inflammation.
Bio-Bifidus from American Biologics	As directed on label. For fast results, also use as an enema. (do this only once).	Replaces the bowel flora.
Helpful		
Apple pectin	As directed on label.	A source of quality fiber. Helps to detoxify heavy metals.
Kyo-Green from Wakunaga or ProGreens from Nutricology or wheatgrass juice or capsules	As directed on label. As directed on label. As directed on label. As directed on label.	To assist in keeping the colon clear of toxic debris and aid in healing of an inflamed colon.
Sonne's #7 Detoxificant from Sonne Organic Foods	As directed on label.	An intestinal cleanser. Contains liquid bentonite, which absorbs and eliminates toxins.
Ultimate Cleanse from Nature's Secret	As directed on label.	An excellent detoxification program.
Vitamin C with bioflavonoids	6,000–10,000 mg daily, in divided doses. (*See* ASCORBIC ACID FLUSH in Part Three.)	Protects the body from pollutants. Use a buffered or esterified form.

Herbs

❑ Aloe vera, calendula, and peppermint help to restore the acid/alkaline balance of the colon and promote healing.

❑ Burdock, echinacea, and licorice have detoxifying properties. Licorice also supports the organs.

Cautions: Do not take echinacea for longer than three months. It should not be used by people who are allergic to ragweed. Licorice root should not be used during pregnancy or nursing. It should not be used by persons with diabetes, glaucoma, heart disease, high blood pressure, or a history of stroke.

❑ Barberry, butternut bark, cascara sagrada (a natural laxative made from the bark of *Rhamnus purshiana*), flaxseed, red raspberry, rhubarb, and senna can be used to flush the colon and release waste.

Caution: Do not use barberry during pregnancy.

❑ Boneset, elecampane, fenugreek, lobelia, and yarrow loosen and flush mucus from the intestines.

Caution: Do not use boneset on a daily basis for more than one week, as long-term use can lead to toxicity. Lobelia is only to be taken under supervision of a health care professional as it is potentially toxic. People with high blood pressure, heart disease, liver disease, kidney disease, seizure disorders, or shortness of breath should not take lobelia. Pregnant and lactating women should avoid lobelia as well.

❑ Burdock root, milk thistle, and red clover cleanse the blood and support the liver.

❑ Fennel restores the acid/alkaline balance of the colon, promotes healing, flushes the colon, and releases waste.

❑ Garlic eliminates certain parasites.

❑ Marshmallow restores the acid/alkaline balance of the colon, promotes healing, and loosens and flushes mucus from the intestines.

❑ Pau d'arco restores the acid/alkaline balance of the colon, promotes healing, and has detoxifying properties.

❑ Slippery elm bark soothes inflammation and cleanses excess waste from the colon. For quick relief, use slippery elm tea as an enema.

Recommendations

❑ Eat only raw foods for two weeks, and then maintain a diet of 50 percent raw foods, including plenty of raw vegetables and non-citrus fruits such as apples, bananas, berries, grapes, and pears.

❑ Drink at least ten 8-ounce glasses of water each day, even if you are not thirsty. Insufficient liquid intake promotes hard stools, which can stay in the colon for weeks or even months, causing symptoms such as headache, fatigue, and depression, and resulting in a toxic bloodstream.

❑ Avoid saturated fats, sugar, and highly processed foods. Avoid oils and fried foods until the colon returns to normal

and the stools are normal. Use olive oil, canola oil, or essential fatty acids sparingly during this cleansing period. Dairy products should be avoided because they create excess mucus in the colon. The nutrients in dairy—calcium, magnesium, and vitamin D—should be obtained from other foods or supplements. This diet helps to maintain a clean colon.

❑ If you have a blood sugar problem, avoid sweet fruits.

❑ Upon arising and at bedtime, drink the juice of a fresh lemon squeezed into a cup of warm water to cleanse the bloodstream and detoxify and neutralize the system.

❑ Each morning, take a brisk walk and drink fresh carrot and apple juice, "green drinks," or fresh pineapple and papaya juice.

❑ Make a colon-cleansing drink by mixing 1 tablespoon of bentonite with 1 teaspoon of psyllium seed, ½ cup of apple juice, ½ cup of aloe vera juice, and ½ cup of steam-distilled water. Drink this mixture once daily until the colon is clean and not foul smelling.

❑ Use a fiber supplement such as psyllium seed on a daily basis. Mix the supplement with water or juice, and drink it immediately, as the mixture thickens quickly. Avoid fiber supplements in capsule and pill form.

COLOR THERAPY (CHROMATHERAPY)

Scientists have studied the effects of color on our moods, health, and way of thinking for years. Even an individual's preference for one color over another may be related to the way that color makes the individual feel.

Color can be described as light—visible radiant energy—of certain wavelengths. Photoreceptors in the retina, called cones, translate this energy into colors. The retina contains three kinds of cones: one for blue, one for green, and one for red. We perceive other colors by combining these colors in the brain.

The colors you choose for your clothes and for your home, office, car, and other surroundings can have a profound effect on you. Colors have been known to ease stress, to fill you with energy, and even to alleviate pain and other physical problems. This idea, it should be noted, is far from new. In fact, the "color your world" concept is part of the ancient Chinese design technique *feng shui.*

When selecting a color to effect a change in mood or to relieve discomfort, it is vital to choose the color suited to your particular objective. For instance, blue has a relaxing, peaceful, and calming effect. Blue may slightly lower blood pressure, the heart rate, and respiration. In one study, children prone to aggressive behavior became calmer when placed in a blue classroom. Blue has also been found to make people feel cooler in hot and humid environments. To help relieve the pain of ulcers, back problems, insomnia, rheumatism, and inflammatory disorders, surround yourself with blue, and focus your mind on the body part you want to heal while looking at the color. One good place to do this is in the countryside, where the blue of the sky and the water can impart a feeling of calming "oneness" with the universe.

As another of nature's most abundant colors, green, like blue, has a soothing and relaxing effect on the body as well as on the mind. People who are depressed or anxious can benefit from green surroundings. Green also helps nervous disorders, exhaustion, heart problems, and cancer. When you are ill, try sitting on a hillside or by a green pasture, and focus on the body part you want to heal. Green may also be a good environmental color for the dieter.

Like blue and green, violet creates a peaceful environment. Violet also suppresses the appetite and is good for scalp and kidney problems and for migraine headaches.

The color red stimulates, excites, and warms the body. Red increases the heart rate, brain wave activity, and respiration. The color of passion and energy, red is also good for sexual dysfunction, as well as for anemia, bladder infections, and skin problems. Those who have poor coordination should avoid wearing the color red. In addition, people suffering from hypertension (high blood pressure) should avoid rooms with a red decor, as this can cause their blood pressure to rise. Conversely, red has a good effect on those with hypotension (low blood pressure).

Pink has a soothing effect on the body, relaxing the muscles. Because it has been found to have a tranquilizing effect on aggressive and violent people, pink is often used in prisons, hospitals, and juvenile and drug centers. Those suffering from anxiety or withdrawal symptoms can benefit from pink surroundings. Pink is also a good color for the bedroom, where it can help evoke feelings of romance.

Orange is the color of choice for stimulating the appetite and reducing fatigue. Use this color in place mats and tablecloths, for instance—to encourage a finicky eater or to pique the appetite of a person who is ill. This color should be avoided by those who are trying to lose weight. If you are feeling tired or run down, try wearing an orange garment to lift your energy level. General weakness, allergies, and constipation may also improve.

Yellow is the most memorable of all the colors. Whenever you want to remember something, jot it down on yellow paper. This color also raises the blood pressure and increases the pulse rate, but to a lesser degree than red does. As the color of sunshine, yellow has an energizing effect; it can help relieve depression. A chromotherapist may use this color to treat muscle cramps, hypoglycemia, overactive thyroid, and gallstones.

Black is a "power" color. Try wearing black clothes for a feeling of strength and self-confidence. Black also suppresses the appetite. If you want to lose weight, cover your dining table with a black tablecloth.

CRYSTAL AND GEMSTONE THERAPY

Some people believe colorful crystals hold incredible powers. For example, Thomas Edison is said to have believed that his success was due in part to a pocketful of quartz crystals he always carried with him. He felt that the stones allowed him the opportunity to take notice of his inner self and his creativity. Gemstone therapists believe that gems possess a specific healing energy that can be transferred to the body.

Certain gemstones are used for healing specific organs by contact with the body's related energy centers, called *chakras*. Certain stones also direct energies toward emotional states. Quartz crystals are probably the most popular. Quartz can be a beautiful white, such as milk quartz, or colorless and shiny like rock crystal. The rock crystal's therapeutic properties are aimed at soothing resentment and envy. It is also used to calm weak kidneys, cardiac pain, and upset stomachs.

In some cases, the healing properties of gems are used to stimulate energy flow to certain areas of the body. Amber (yellow to brown) is believed to aid in kidney and bladder function. Agate (gray, blue, and beige) promotes self-confidence and energy. Amethyst (purple) is used to unlock blocked energy, bring calm in times of grief, and promote positive thinking. Diamonds (many colors) protect energy fields and cleanse the blood. Emerald (green) improves memory and intellect. Jade (green or white) attracts loyal friends, brings good fortune, composure, peacefulness, and wisdom. Onyx (black) improves devotion and concentration. Ruby (red) increases energy, improves circulation, and promotes intuitive thinking. Sapphire (blue) gives the wearer self-esteem, purity of mind, and contentment. Turquoise is used to protect against harmful energy. Black onyx aids in changing bad habits. These are only a few examples of the powers ascribed to gemstones.

All crystals and gemstones should be "cleansed" periodically in running water to wash away the negative energies they may have picked up, particularly if they have been used for healing.

DHEA THERAPY

The most abundant hormone found in the bloodstream, dehydroepiandrosterone (DHEA) is produced by the adrenal glands, which sit atop the kidneys. Much like human growth hormone (HGH) and melatonin—two other hormones now known to have antiaging properties—DHEA is produced abundantly during youth, with production peaking around age twenty-five. After this, though, production wanes. By the age of eighty, people are thought to have only 10 to 20 percent of the DHEA they had at twenty.

Research has shown that DHEA has many functions in the body pertaining to health and longevity. Among other things, it may help to generate the sex hormones estrogen and testosterone. If testosterone increases, then so does the percentage of muscle mass, and the percentage of body fat decreases. If estrogen is increased, new bone deposition can occur, thereby helping to prevent osteoporosis. As the production of DHEA declines with age, the structures and systems of the body appear to decline with it. This leaves the body vulnerable to various cancers, including cancer of the breast, prostate, and bladder, as well as to atherosclerosis, high blood pressure, Parkinson's disease, diabetes, nerve degeneration, and other age-related conditions.

Some research suggests that DHEA replacement therapy can have a number of highly beneficial effects. In a 1986 study based on twelve years of research involving 242 middle-aged and elderly men, small doses of DHEA appeared to be linked with a 48 percent reduction in death from heart disease, and a 36 percent reduction in death from other causes. In one twenty-eight-day study, DHEA therapy enabled men to lose 31 percent of mean body fat without changing body weight. However, a 2006 randomized controlled study at the Mayo Clinic in Rochester, Minnesota, showed that elderly women taking DHEA had no changes in body composition, muscle strength, or how well they could handle glucose, and showed no improvement in quality of life. The authors concluded that DHEA has no physiological relevant benefit in aging.

DHEA comes both in nonprescription-strength pills and capsules, and in higher-dosage prescription-strength pills and capsules. Most of the DHEA that you can buy is made in laboratories from substances extracted from wild yams, the most common substance being *diosgenin*. Also available are extracts of the wild yams that have *not* been processed into DHEA, but that the body may convert into DHEA.

DHEA therapy should be undertaken with caution. Some physicians believe that high doses of DHEA suppress the body's natural ability to synthesize the hormone. Women should take no more than 10 milligrams daily. Sometimes changing estrogen levels and making them higher will stimulate the growth of breast and prostate cancers. Before using this therapy, check with your doctor, who knows your health risk and your family history. Animal studies have indicated that high doses can also lead to liver damage. For this reason, while undergoing DHEA replacement therapy, it is important to take supplements of the antioxidants vitamin C, vitamin E, and selenium to prevent oxidative damage to the liver. A better source of DHEA might be 7-Keto DHEA. This substance plays the same role as DHEA in the body, such as strengthening the immune system and enhancing memory, but, unlike ordinary DHEA, it is not converted into estrogens or testosterone.

ENEMAS

Over time, toxic wastes can accumulate in the colon and liver, and then circulate throughout the body via the bloodstream. A clean and healthy colon and liver, then, are essential for the health of all the organs and tissues of the body.

There are two types of enemas—the retention enema and the cleansing enema. Retention enemas, also known as suppositories or implants, are held in the body for about fifteen minutes. Their primary action is to help rid the liver and colon of impurities. Cleansing enemas, which are retained for only a few minutes, are used to flush and cleanse the colon.

When using any enema, keep in mind that enemas should never be used if there is rectal bleeding. In such a case, contact a physician immediately.

If you experience tension or spasms in the bowel while using an enema, proceed slowly and try using warmer water—99°F is a good temperature—to help relax the bowel. If the bowel is weak or flaccid, try using colder water—75°F to 80°F—to help strengthen it.

After using any enema, be sure to wash and sterilize the tip of the enema bag. Enemas are for adults, and it is always wise to check with a health care professional first.

THE CATNIP TEA ENEMA

Catnip tea enemas are a good way to bring a high fever down quickly and keep it down. These also relieve constipation and congestion, which keep fever up. Repeat the procedure every four to six hours, and continue taking the enemas twice daily as long as fever persists. If the fever does not correct itself after twenty-four hours, seek medical attention. Catnip tea enemas should *not* be given to children.

Procedure

To make the solution for the catnip tea enema, place about 8 tablespoons of fresh or dried catnip leaves in a glass or enameled pot. (If you are using bagged catnip tea, use the amount recommended on the package to make 1 quart of tea.) In a separate pot, bring 1 quart of steam-distilled water to a boil. Remove the water from the heat and pour it over the herbs. Cover the pot and let the tea steep for five to ten minutes. Then strain out the catnip and allow the tea to cool to a comfortable, slightly warm temperature.

Place all of the solution in an enema bag. Do not use petroleum jelly to lubricate the tip of the enema bag. Instead, use vitamin E oil (buy it in oil form or pierce the end of a vitamin E capsule and squeeze the liquid onto the tip). The liquid will both ease insertion and have a healing effect on the anus and the lining of the colon, if these areas are inflamed. Aloe vera may also be used for this purpose.

The best position to assume when receiving the enema is "head down and rear up." If you experience any pain during insertion, stop the flow of the enema bag and, remaining in the same position, take deep breaths until the pain subsides. Then resume the enema flow. If you expel the liquid before all of it has been inserted, simply begin the process over again. If pain persists, discontinue the enema procedure.

After the liquid has been inserted, roll onto your back, and finally roll over and lie on your right side. As you are doing this, massage your colon to help loosen any fecal matter. Start on your right side and gradually move your fingers up toward the bottom of your rib cage, then across your abdomen and down the left side. Hold the solution in your body for three or four minutes before expelling it.

THE COFFEE OR WHEATGRASS RETENTION ENEMA

This type of enema is not hard to retain, since it is only a pint of liquid. When used as a retention enema—an enema that is held in the body for a specified period of time—coffee does not go through the digestive system and does not affect the body as a coffee beverage does.

A coffee retention enema is quite helpful during a serious illness, after hospitalization, and after exposure to toxic chemicals. This enema can also be used while fasting to relieve the headaches sometimes caused by the quick release of toxins. Ask your doctor before doing this if you are recovering from a major illness or have a chronic condition.

Some alternative clinics use fresh wheatgrass retention enemas for the treatment of cancer and other chronic illnesses, using 1 ounce of fresh wheatgrass juice in 1 cup of warm water. Wheatgrass contains nearly all the nutrients and enzymes the body needs for healing. If you cannot obtain fresh wheatgrass, Sweet Wheat from Sweet Wheat, Inc., a freeze-dried product, is a good alternative. Try using coffee and wheatgrass enemas on alternating days.

Procedure

To make the coffee enema solution, place 2 quarts of steam-distilled water in a pan, and add 6 heaping tablespoons of ground coffee (do not use instant or decaffeinated). Boil the mixture for fifteen minutes, cool to a comfortable temperature, and strain. Use only 1 pint of the strained coffee at a time, and refrigerate the remainder in a closed jar.

Place 1 pint of the enema solution in an enema bag. Do not use petroleum jelly to lubricate the tip of the enema bag. Instead, use vitamin E oil (buy it in oil form or pierce the end of a vitamin E capsule and squeeze the liquid onto the tip). The liquid will both ease insertion and have a healing effect on the anus and the lining of the colon, if these areas are inflamed. Aloe vera gel may also be used for this purpose.

The best position to assume when receiving the enema is "head down and rear up." After the liquid has been inserted, roll onto your right side and hold the solution in your body for fifteen minutes before allowing the fluid to be expelled. Do not roll from side to side.

Do not be concerned if the liquid is not expelled after fifteen minutes. Simply stand up and move around as usual until you feel the urge to expel the liquid.

Recommendations

❑ Use steam-distilled water, not tap water. This is especially important for retention enemas—you do not want to absorb any chemicals from the tap water.

❑ To maximize the benefits of this or any other retention enema, use a cleansing enema first.

❑ Do not abuse coffee enemas by using them too often. Use them only once daily while following a program for a specific disorder, unless you are being treated for cancer. People with cancer may need up to three enemas a day. You may also use coffee and wheatgrass enemas occasionally as needed.

❑ Remember that excessive use of coffee enemas over six months or more may deplete the body's stores of iron, as well as other minerals and vitamins, causing anemia. Do not use coffee enemas for longer than four to six weeks at a time. If you develop anemia during treatment—or whenever you use this enema daily for a long period of time—be sure to take desiccated liver tablets as directed on the label.

Caution: Only a doctor can diagnose anemia by a blood test, so seek medical attention if you are feeling sluggish. Do not take iron or products with iron until anemia is diagnosed.

❑ If you have cancer, AIDS, or another serious illness, or if you have a malabsorption problem, add 1 cc of B-complex vitamins or 2 cc of injectable liver extract, plus an eyedropperful of liquid kelp or sea water concentrate (found in health food stores) to the enema solution. If you are unable to locate injectable forms of these supplements, open 2 capsules of a B-complex supplement and add the contents to the enema solution, making sure it dissolves before use. You can open up a capsule of probiotics and add the contents to the solution. Used daily, these supplements replace any lost B vitamins, help rebuild the liver, and provide an extra boost of energy. You can also add burdock root and milk thistle extract to the enema. Use only alcohol-free liquid extract and 5 drops of each to the enema solution. This will help to cleanse the blood and the liver. Consult your doctor before doing this.

❑ To kill unwanted bacteria in the colon—or for any type of colon disorder, including diarrhea and constipation—add 5 drops of Aerobic 07 from Aerobic Life Industries to the enema solution.

THE LEMON JUICE CLEANSING ENEMA

The lemon juice enema is an excellent means of cleansing the colon of fecal matter and other impurities and of detoxifying the system. This enema also balances the pH of the colon and is useful whenever cleansing of the colon is desired, as well as for colon disorders, such as constipation.

Procedure

To make the solution for the lemon enema, add the juice of 3 lemons to 2 quarts of lukewarm steam-distilled water. (Be sure to avoid using either very cold or very warm water.) If desired, add 2 eyedroppers of liquid kelp to boost the mineral content of the solution.

Place all of the solution in an enema bag. Do not use petroleum jelly to lubricate the tip of the enema bag. Instead, use vitamin E oil (buy it in oil form or pierce the end of a vitamin E capsule and squeeze the liquid onto the tip). The liquid will both ease insertion and have a healing effect on the anus and the lining of the colon, if these areas are inflamed. Aloe vera gel may also be used for this purpose.

The best position to assume when receiving the enema is "head down and rear up." After the liquid has been inserted, roll onto your back, and finally roll over and lie on your left side. As you are doing this, massage your colon to help loosen any fecal matter. Start on your right side and gradually move your fingers up toward the bottom of your rib cage, then across your abdomen and down the left side.

Note that 2 quarts is a lot of liquid. If you experience any pain during insertion, stop the flow of the enema bag and, remaining in the same position, take deep breaths until the pain subsides. Then resume the enema flow. If you expel the liquid before all of it has been inserted, simply begin the process over again. If pain persists, discontinue the enema procedure.

Hold the solution in your body for three or four minutes before allowing it to be expelled. After two or three such sessions, you will find it easier to insert and hold the liquid.

Recommendations

❏ If you have trouble with constipation, use the lemon juice enema once a week, and the coffee retention enema once a week. The bowels will soon move, the colon will be clean, and the stool will not be foul-smelling. Constipation is also treated with fiber-rich foods like fruits, vegetables, and whole grains, and plenty of water.

❏ If you suffer from colitis, use the lemon juice enema once a week. Any time pain from colitis is experienced, this enema will quickly relieve the discomfort. But check with your health care professional first, if you have been diagnosed with colitis.

❏ If you are allergic to lemons, prepare the enema solution with 1 to 2 ounces of wheatgrass juice or 1 ounce of liquid aged garlic extract (Kyolic) in 2 quarts of steam-distilled water. Or fill the enema bag with plain steam-distilled water.

THE PROFLORA WHEY ENEMA

This remedy may be beneficial if you have used high colonics or taken antibiotics over a long period of time—practices that can kill the body's "friendly" bacteria. The whey enema may help the body fight yeast infections and improves digestion and the assimilation of nutrients.

Procedure

To make the enema solution, mix 2 quarts of lukewarm steam-distilled water and 5 tablespoons of ProFlora whey.

Pour the mixture into the enema bag. Release any air from the enema tube before insertion, and lubricate the tip with vitamin E oil (buy it in oil form or pierce the end of a vitamin E capsule and squeeze the liquid onto the tip). Do not use petroleum jelly to lubricate the tip of the bag.

For best results, use a plain water enema before using the ProFlora whey enema, as this makes it easier to retain the solution for the necessary period of time. Do not use this type of enema on a daily basis. Limit it to three times a year.

To replace the friendly bacteria in the colon, do a probiotic retention enema after the ProFlora whey enema. Open up 8 capsules of Kyo-Dophilus from Wakunaga and add the contents to 1 cup of lukewarm (body-temperature) water. The best position to assume when receiving the enema is "head down and rear up." This enema will normalize the pH of the colon and restore healthy bacteria so that constipation will be eliminated. After the liquid has been inserted, roll onto your right side and hold the solution in your body for fifteen minutes before allowing the fluid to be expelled. Do not roll from side to side.

Do not be concerned if the liquid is not expelled after fifteen minutes. Simply stand up and move around as usual until you feel the urge to expel the liquid. Do not use this type of enema on a daily basis. Limit it to three times a year.

EXERCISE

The closest thing to a "magic bullet" for maintaining youth and optimal health is a well-balanced combination of exercise and proper nutrition. The entire body benefits from this formula, both physically and psychologically.

Regular exercise improves digestion and elimination, increases endurance and energy levels, promotes lean body mass while burning fat, and lowers overall blood cholesterol while increasing the proportion of "good" cholesterol (HDL) to "bad" cholesterol (LDL). Exercise also reduces stress and anxiety, which are contributing factors to many illnesses and conditions. In addition to the physical benefits, studies have shown that regular exercise elevates mood, increases feelings of well-being, and reduces anxiety and depression.

The power of exercise in maintaining health was underscored by the continuing Aerobics Center Longitudinal Study, which was designed to examine the effects of different fitness levels. According to a report on the study published in the *Journal of the American Medical Association*, low fitness may pose as great a risk to health as smoking, and a greater risk than high cholesterol, high blood pressure, or obesity. It was reported that smokers who are moderately physically fit, but have high blood pressure and high cholesterol, live longer than nonsmokers who are healthy but sedentary. Moderate fitness, it was stated, can be achieved in ten weeks through many different forms of exercise, including daily sessions of walking, bicycling, or even gardening.

Exercise includes a variety of movements and different activities. *Recreational* exercise is meant for enjoyment and relaxation, while *therapeutic* exercise is intended to alleviate or prevent a particular problem. Sometimes an exercise can be both recreational and therapeutic. Take swimming, for example. With careful attention to arm and shoulder movements, swimming can meet both the recreational and therapeutic needs of someone who has arthritis of the shoulder.

There are a number of exercise types, each of which has a specific purpose:

- *Aerobic or endurance exercise* improves the body's capacity to use fuel and oxygen. Swimming, bicycle riding, jogging, and power walking are examples of this type of exercise. The body's cardiovascular system benefits through increased blood supply to the muscles and enhanced oxygen delivery throughout the body. Just thirty minutes a day of sustained aerobic activity can lower blood pressure and strengthen heart function.

- *Range-of-motion exercise* helps maintain a joint's complete movement by putting a body part through its maximum available range of motion. Extending and moving one's arms in wide circular motions is an example of this. Some degree of flexibility is required to perform range-of-motion exercises, so stretching beforehand is recommended.

- *Strengthening exercise* helps a muscle's ability to contract and do work. Doing sit-ups, for example, is a way of strengthening abdominal muscles.

One exercise rarely achieves two goals. For instance, a strengthening exercise will not significantly affect endurance, and range-of-motion exercises will not necessarily improve strength. A total exercise program must consider the individual's goals and include activities designed to achieve those goals. (*See* PAIN CONTROL in Part Three for other types of exercises that can be used for relaxation, meditation, and healing.)

Exercise should not be looked at as a chore. Try to select activities that you enjoy and look forward to doing. Whatever you choose, start out slowly, listen to your body, and gradually increase the intensity and duration of your workout.

A word of caution: If you are over thirty-five and/or have been sedentary for some time, consult with your health care provider before beginning any new exercise program.

FASTING

Over time, toxins build up in the body as the result of the pollutants in the air we breathe, the chemicals in the food and water we consume, and other means. Periodically, the body seeks to rid itself of these toxins and releases them from the tissues. The toxins then enter the bloodstream, causing the body to experience a "low" or "down" cycle.

During such a cycle, you may suffer from headaches, diarrhea, or depression. Fasting is an effective and safe method of helping the body detoxify itself and move through this low cycle with greater speed and fewer symptoms. In fact, fasting is recommended for any illness, as it gives the body the rest it needs to recover. Acute illnesses, colon disorders, allergies, and respiratory diseases are most responsive to fasting, while chronic degenerative diseases are the least responsive. By relieving the body of the work of digesting foods, fasting permits the system to rid itself of toxins while facilitating healing.

But fasting is helpful not just in times of poor health or during the body's low cycles. By fasting regularly, you give all of your organs a rest, and thus help reverse the aging process and live a longer and healthier life. During a fast, the following happens:

- The natural process of toxin excretion continues, while the influx of new toxins is reduced. This results in a reduction of total body toxicity.

- The immune system's workload is greatly reduced, and the digestive tract is spared any inflammation due to allergic reactions to food.

- Due to a lowering of serum fats that thins the blood, tissue oxygenation is increased and white blood cells are moved more efficiently.

- Fat-stored chemicals, such as pesticides and drugs, are released.

- Physical awareness and sensitivity to diet and surroundings are increased.

Due to these effects of fasting, a fast can help you heal with greater speed; cleanse your liver, kidneys, and colon; purify your blood; help you lose excess weight and water; flush out toxins; clear the eyes and tongue; and cleanse the breath. It is recommended that you fast at least three days a month, and follow a ten-day fast at least twice a year. Fasting is for healthy adults; those with chronic conditions should ask their physician first. Children cannot afford this much time without nourishment and should not be put on a fast.

Depending on the length of the fast, it accomplishes different things. A three-day fast helps the body rid itself of toxins and cleanses the blood. A five-day fast begins the process of healing and rebuilding the immune system. A ten-day fast can take care of many problems before they arise, and may help to fight off illness, including the degenerative diseases that have become so common in our chemically polluted environment.

Certain precautions should be taken during fasts. First, *do not* fast on water alone. An all-water fast releases toxins too quickly, causing headaches and worse. Instead, follow the live-juice diet detailed below, as this both removes toxins and promotes healing by supplying the body with vitamins, minerals, and enzymes. Such a fast is also more likely to lead to a continued healthy diet once the fast is over, as it will accustom you to the taste of raw vegetables and the vitality that this diet promotes. Second, whenever you fast for more than three days, do so only under the supervision of a qualified health care professional. If you have diabetes, hypoglycemia, or another chronic health problem, even short fasts should be supervised by a doctor. Pregnant and lactating women should *never* fast.

A final word of advice: It took years to wear your body down, and it will take time to build it back up to its peak condition. But believe that it can be done. Then, whenever you start to feel unwell, fast and feel better. Although a typical diet usually provides too much salt, when you fast your body gets very little salt (sodium)—a necessary nutrient. If you feel lightheaded or dizzy, include some broth in your diet.

Procedure

To prepare for the fast, eat only raw vegetables and fruits for two days. This will make the fast less of a shock to the system.

While on the fast, consume at least ten 8-ounce glasses of steam-distilled water a day, plus pure juices and up to 2 cups of herbal tea a day. Dilute all juices with the water, adding about 1 part water to 3 parts juice. Do not drink orange or tomato juice, and avoid all juices made with sweeteners or other additives.

The best juice to use during your fast is fresh lemon juice made by adding the juice of one lemon to a cup of warm water. Fresh apple, beet, cabbage, carrot, celery, and grape juices are also good, as are "green drinks," which are made from green leafy vegetables. These green drinks are excellent detoxifiers. Raw cabbage juice is particularly good for ulcers, cancer, and all colon problems. Just be sure to drink the cabbage juice as soon as it is prepared. As this juice sits, it loses its vitamin content.

As a general rule, you should not combine fruit and vegetable juices. Apples are the only fruit that should be added to vegetable juices.

Follow the juice-water-and-tea fast with a two-day diet of raw fruits and vegetables. The desired effects of the fast can be ruined by eating cooked foods immediately afterward. Because both the size of the stomach and the amount of secreted digestive juices may decrease during fasting, the first meals after a fast should be frequent and small.

Herbs

❏ Herbal teas may be consumed throughout the fast, once or twice per day or more if you wish. Try the following teas:

- Use alfalfa, burdock, chamomile, dandelion, milk thistle, red clover, and rose hips tea to rejuvenate the liver and cleanse the bloodstream.

Caution: Do not use chamomile if you are allergic to ragweed. Do not use during pregnancy or nursing. It may interact with warfarin or cyclosporine, so patients using these drugs should avoid it.

- Drink 2 parts echinacea and pau d'arco tea mixed with 1 part unsweetened cranberry juice. Used four times a day, this will rebuild the immune system, aid in bladder function, and rid the colon of unwanted bacteria.

Caution: Do not take echinacea for longer than three months. It should not be used by people who are allergic to ragweed.

- Use peppermint tea for its calming and strengthening effect on the nerves, and for indigestion, nausea, and flatulence.

- Use slippery elm tea for inflammation of the colon. This tea also is beneficial when used as an enema solution.

❏ Take 2 capsules of garlic twice a day. If you prefer a liquid supplement, add 1 tablespoon of liquid aged garlic extract (Kyolic) to a cup of water. Garlic supplements may be taken on a daily basis before, during, and after a fast to promote overall health, aid in the healing process, and rid the colon of many types of parasites.

Recommendations

❏ When fasting, you may not be getting enough salt. If you feel lightheaded or dizzy, take some broth with sodium and/or add salt to your food.

❏ If you must have something to eat during the fast, eat a piece of watermelon. Always eat watermelon by itself, with no additional foods. You can also try applesauce—fresh, not canned—made in a blender or food processor. Leave the skin on the apples, and do not cook them.

❏ Take a fiber supplement on a daily basis before and after your fast, but not during the fast. To promote cleansing of the colon before and after your fast, be sure to make extra fiber a part of your daily diet. Bran, especially oat bran, is an excellent source of fiber. Try to avoid supplements containing wheat bran, as they may be irritating to the colon wall. Another good fiber source is ABC Aerobic Bulk Cleanse from Aerobic Life Industries. To use this colon cleanser, mix it with half aloe vera juice and half natural cranberry juice. This mixture adds fiber and has a healing and cleansing effect also. Psyllium seed husks and ground flaxseed are other good-quality fiber products. Be certain to accompany any fiber capsule with a large glass of water, because the capsules expand and soak up a good deal of water.

❏ Do not chew gum while on the fast. The digestive process starts when chewing prompts the body to secrete enzymes into the gastrointestinal tract. If there is no food in the stomach for the enzymes to digest, trouble occurs.

❏ If desired, take spirulina during the fast. Spirulina is high in protein and contains a wide range of vitamins and minerals, plus chlorophyll for cleansing. If you are using tablets, take 5 tablets three times daily. If you are using powder, take 1 teaspoon three times daily, mixing the powder with a cup of unsweetened juice.

❑ If you have hypoglycemia, consult a qualified health care professional before starting any fast.

❑ If you are over sixty-five, or if you need daily supplements for another reason, continue taking your vitamin and mineral supplements during the fast. Older people need certain vitamins and minerals daily. When you are drinking fresh juices, reduce the dosage of supplements that you take.

❑ If desired, before, during, and after your fast, use Kyo-Green from Wakunaga of America and ProGreens from Nutricology. These products contain all the nutrients needed to aid in the healing process. If used during the fast, these products should replace a cup of "green drink."

❑ During a fast, as toxins are released from your body, you may experience fatigue; body odor; dry, scaly skin; skin eruptions; headaches; dizziness; irritability; anxiety; confusion; nausea; coughing; diarrhea; dark urine; dark, foul-smelling stools; body aches; insomnia; sinus and bronchial mucus discharge; and/or visual or hearing problems. These symptoms are not serious and should pass quickly. To alleviate any of these symptoms, use a daily lemon juice enema to cleanse the colon, and a daily coffee enema to rid the liver of impurities. Also, you may be lacking in salt; use salted broth. (*See* ENEMAS in Part Three.)

❑ During your fast, be sure to get adequate rest. If necessary, try napping during the day to recharge your batteries.

❑ If desired, before, during, and after your fast, use Desert Delight from Aerobic Life Industries. This product, which contains crabapple, papaya, and aloe vera juice, helps keep the colon clean, and also supports kidney and bladder function, aids digestion, and has a healing effect on ulcers. If used during the fast, substitute this product for a cup of juice.

❑ To make an excellent juice for healing many illnesses, juice together 3 carrots, 3 kale leaves, 2 stalks celery, 2 beets, 1 turnip, ¼ pound spinach, ½ head of cabbage, ¼ bunch of parsley, ¼ of an onion, and ½ clove of garlic. If you don't have a juicer, place the vegetables in pure water and gently boil them, adding no seasonings. A cup of this juice may be substituted for any other juice while fasting. Save the vegetables from the broth to eat after your fast. Remember that no solid food is allowed during the fast.

❑ During a fast, as toxins are released from your body, you will probably experience a coated tongue and an unpleasant taste in your mouth. To relieve this problem, try rinsing your mouth with fresh lemon juice.

❑ If you are a denture wearer, keep your dentures in your mouth throughout the fast to prevent shrinkage of the gums.

❑ While fasting, continue your normal daily routine, including moderate exercise. Avoid any strenuous exercise.

❑ Be aware that when you fast during a low phase, you help your body experience the "up" phase of the cycle—a period during which you feel great. This occurs because the body has been cleansed of impurities. However, when you start to pollute your body again, the toxins once again begin to build up, and, in time, you will again have a low phase. When this occurs, the fast should be repeated.

❑ Before, during, and after your fast, use dry-brush massages to help rid the skin of toxins and dead cells. Perform the massage with a *natural* bristle brush that has a long handle, so that you can reach your back. Always brush toward the heart—from wrist to elbow, elbow to shoulder, ankles to knees, knees to hips, and so on. This massage will flake away large amounts of dead skin, freeing the pores of impediments, and, in turn, helping the skin to excrete poisons. It will also greatly improve circulation. *Do not* use this technique on areas of the body affected by acne, eczema, or psoriasis. Also avoid brushing areas that are broken or recently scarred, or that have protruding varicose veins.

GLANDULAR THERAPY

The glandular system is both important and complex. Virtually all body functions—from digestion to reproduction to growth—depend on a healthy glandular system.

To a large degree, the health of the glands, like the health of any organ of the body, can be greatly improved by adequate vitamin and mineral supplementation. Glandular therapy, the use of concentrated forms of various raw animal glands, can also improve the health of specific glands. If you have a chronic condition that affects one of your glands, ask your doctor before using any glandular supplements. Most have not been tested in children, so ask your child's pediatrician before using them.

Early endocrinologists hypothesized that glandulars worked by providing nutrients the body lacked. Once supplied with the missing nutrients, the malfunctioning organ was able to repair itself and function properly.

Some of the most important glandulars are the following:

• Raw adrenal glandular.

• Raw brain glandular.

• Raw heart glandular.

• Raw kidney glandular.

• Raw liver glandular.

• Raw lung glandular.

• Raw mammary glandular.

• Raw ovary glandular.

• Raw pancreas glandular.

• Raw pituitary glandular.

- Raw spleen glandular.
- Raw thymus glandular.
- Raw thyroid glandular.

Care should be taken in the purchase of glandulars. Many glandular products are by-products of the meat-processing industry and are taken from adult animals that show the effects of aging and exposure to toxins. This impairs the quality of the glandular. For best results, make sure that the glandulars you buy come from young, organically raised free-range animals that have not received hormones.

MAINTAINING A HEALTHY GLANDULAR SYSTEM

A gland is an organ that manufactures and releases fluids and other substances into the body for the body's use. The function of these fluids is so wide-ranging that virtually all body processes depend on a healthy glandular system. An imbalance or malfunction of any one glandular substance or gland can create tremendous problems throughout the body.

Glands fall into two categories: the exocrine glands and the endocrine glands. The exocrine glands, each of which secretes a specialized substance, open onto a surface of an organ or other structure through a duct. Examples of such glands are the salivary glands of the mouth, and the sweat and oil glands of the skin. Other exocrine glands can be found in the kidneys, the mammary glands, and the digestive tract. These glands perform a variety of functions. The salivary glands, for instance, secrete saliva, which aids in the digestion of food, while the sweat glands help rid the body of waste products.

Unlike the exocrine glands, the endocrine glands are ductless, and thus secrete the substances they produce—specifically, hormones—directly into the bloodstream. Examples of these glands include the adrenal glands, found atop the kidneys; the gonads, found in the reproductive organs; the pancreas, found behind the stomach; the pituitary gland, found at the base of the brain; the thyroid and parathyroid glands, found in the neck; and the thymus gland, found below the thyroid. The pineal gland, which is attached to the brain, is also thought to be an endocrine gland.

By secreting hormones—chemicals that start or control the activity of an organ or group of cells—the endocrine glands help regulate practically all body functions. For instance, the pancreas secretes insulin, an important regulator of sugar metabolism. The female gonads, called the ovaries, produce hormones like estrogen, which aids the development of secondary sex characteristics, prepares the walls of the uterus to receive a fertilized egg, and performs many other important functions. The thymus secretes thymosin, a hormone that is critical to proper immune system function. The pituitary gland, which is often called the "master gland," regulates the functions of the other glands, and also produces a hormone that stimu-lates body growth. It should be noted that the pituitary gland, like many of the other endocrine glands, produces more than one hormone. Similarly, some hormones, such as estrogen, are secreted by more than one gland.

Like all organs, the glands need nutritional support, especially when stress depletes the body's stores of nutrients. Glandulars—concentrated forms of various organic animal glands—are one means of improving the health of the glands. In addition, nutritional supplements can help maintain the health of these glands, and thereby ensure proper functioning of the glandular system.

NUTRIENTS

SUPPLEMENT	SUGGESTED DOSAGE	COMMENTS
Very Important		
Kelp	Up to 200 mg daily.	Rich in minerals and the element iodine, which are necessary for thyroid function.
L-arginine plus	500 mg daily.	Increases the size and activity of the thymus gland.
L-lysine	500 mg daily.	Add this supplement if you are prone to herpes outbreaks.
L-glycine	500 mg daily.	Essential for the health of the thymus gland, spleen, and bone marrow.
L-tyrosine	500 mg daily.	Important to the health and function of the adrenal, thyroid, and pituitary glands.
Manganese	As directed on label. Take separately from calcium.	Crucial to the production of thyroxine, the hormone that regulates the metabolic process. This nutrient is stored in and used by the liver, kidneys, pancreas, lungs, prostate gland, and brain.
Vitamin A plus natural beta-carotene and other carotenoids	As directed on label. As directed on label.	Nutrients that nourish the thymus gland and increase antibody production. All organs with duct systems require these nutrients.
Vitamin B complex plus extra vitamin B₂ (riboflavin) and vitamin B₅ (pantothenic acid)	100 mg of each major B vitamin twice daily (amounts of individual vitamins in a complex will vary). 50 mg 3 times daily 50 mg 3 times daily.	B vitamins work best when all are taken together. Especially important if you are under stress. Vital to the health of the entire glandular system, especially the adrenal glands. The antistress vitamin.
Vitamin C with bioflavonoids	1,500 mg daily.	Important for adrenal function, and should be taken when using L-cysteine to prevent formation of cystine kidney stones.
Zinc plus copper	50 mg daily. Do not exceed 100 mg daily from all supplements. 3 mg daily.	Needed by the immune system, and for thymus and pancreas health. Especially important for the gonads (sex glands). Needed to balance with zinc.

Important		
Lecithin granules or capsules	1 tsp 3 times daily, before meals. 1,200 mg 3 times daily, before meals.	All cells and organs have lecithin surrounding them for protection. Also helps cleanse the liver.
Raw thymus glandular plus multiglandular complex	As directed on label. As directed on label.	To stimulate immune function and aid glandular function. Sublingual forms are best.
Helpful		
Essential fatty acids (flaxseed oil, primrose oil, or salmon oil)	As directed on label.	Needed to nourish the glands.
L-cysteine and L-methionine plus glutathione	500 mg each daily, on an empty stomach. Take with water or juice. Do not take with milk. Take with 50 mg vitamin B_6 and 100 mg vitamin C for better absorption.	Aid in detoxifying glands of harmful pollutants. Also necessary for insulin production, and act as powerful antioxidants.
Selenium	As directed on label. If you are pregnant, do not exceed 40 mcg daily.	Nourishes the liver and pancreas.
Silica or oat straw	500 mg twice daily.	To supply silicon, a trace mineral that aids in healing the glands and tissues. *See* under Herbs, below.
Superoxide dismutase (SOD) or Cell Guard from Biotec Foods	As directed on label, on an empty stomach. Take with a large glass of water. As directed on label.	A potent detoxifier that also transports oxygen for healing in the glandular system. An antioxidant complex that contains SOD.
Vitamin E	200 IU daily.	Rids the body of toxic substances when combined with vitamin C and selenium. Use d-alpha-tocopherol form.

Herbs

❏ Black cohosh, black radish extract, goldenseal, licorice, lobelia, mullein, and red clover, taken in tea form, help strengthen and rebuild the liver, and restore glandular balance.

Cautions: Do not use black cohosh if you are pregnant or have any type of chronic disease. Black cohosh should not be used by those with liver problems. Do not take goldenseal internally on a daily basis for more than one week at a time. Do not use it during pregnancy or if you are breastfeeding, and use with caution if you are allergic to ragweed. If you have a history of cardiovascular disease, diabetes, or glaucoma, use it only under a doctor's supervision. Licorice root should not be used during pregnancy or nursing. It should not be used by persons with diabetes, glaucoma, heart disease, high blood pressure, or a history of stroke. Lobelia is only to be taken under supervision of a health care professional as it is potentially toxic. People with high blood pressure, heart disease, liver disease, kidney disease, seizure disorders, or shortness of breath should not take lobelia. Pregnant and lactating women should avoid lobelia as well.

❏ Burdock root and red clover aid in cleansing the lymphatic glands and ridding the body of toxins.

❏ Cedar stimulates pancreatic function.

❏ Celery seed and hydrangea are diuretics that can be used to stimulate the kidneys.

❏ Chicory, milk thistle, and stillingia root stimulate and cleanse the liver.

❏ Cordyceps exerts its primary effects on the kidneys and increases lung capacity.

❏ Dandelion stimulates and cleanses the liver. It also stimulates bile production, thereby benefiting the spleen and improving the health of the pancreas.

❏ Echinacea cleanses and strengthens the kidneys, liver, pancreas, and spleen.

❏ *Caution:* Do not take echinacea for longer than three months. It should not be used by people who are allergic to ragweed.

❏ Gentian contains elements that are known to normalize the functions of the thyroid gland.

❏ Oat straw is a good source of silicon, which aids in healing, and is also high in calcium. It can be taken in tea or capsule form.

❏ Parsley is a diuretic that stimulates kidney function. It also helps strengthen and rebuild the liver, and maintain glandular balance.

❏ Uva ursi is a diuretic that stimulates kidney function. It also has a germicidal effect, and thereby destroys any bacteria that may be present. It is a tonic for a weakened liver, kidneys, and other glands.

Recommendations

❏ *See* BLOOD PURIFICATION in Part Three and follow the instructions.

❏ Use alfalfa, beet, black radish, and dandelion juice for cleansing the liver. (*See* JUICING in Part Three.)

❏ Use olive oil and lemon juice (3 tablespoons of olive oil mixed with the juice of a fresh lemon), plus plenty of pure apple juice, to stimulate the gallbladder and help excrete bile and even small gallstones. (*See* GALLBLADDER DISORDERS in Part Two.)

❏ *See* FASTING in Part Three and follow the program once monthly to allow glands time to heal and rest.

❏ *See* HYPOTHYROIDISM in Part Two and follow the temperature self-test to determine how well your thyroid gland is functioning.

Considerations

❑ When toxic substances circulate through the bloodstream due to poor eating habits, the use of drugs, or other factors, the presence of these substances is reflected in the lymphatic system. The lymph glands act as a filter, removing poisons from the body.

GROWTH HORMONE THERAPY

Human growth hormone (HGH) is secreted by the pituitary gland in the brain. Like all hormones, HGH works to regulate the activities of vital organs, and thus helps maintain health throughout the body. HGH was originally called a growth hormone because it is produced in greatest amounts during adolescence, when growth is most rapid. HGH does indeed help to regulate growth. Because of the link between this hormone and the growth process, HGH therapy was first used to treat children who were failing to grow normally because of a deficiency of this hormone. Without HGH therapy, these children would have become dwarfs; with it, their growth was normal.

However, it has been found that HGH controls more than just growth. It is probably the most complex hormone the body uses. Tissue repair, healing, cell replacement, organ health, bone strength, brain function, enzyme production, and the health of nails, hair, and skin all require adequate amounts of HGH. In addition, this hormone strengthens the immune system and helps the body resist oxidative damage.

After adolescence, levels of HGH begin to decline at a rate of about 14 percent per decade. As production of the hormone decreases, so does the function of all vital organs. Because of this correlation between declining HGH production and aging, another application of HGH therapy has developed—the use of the hormone to reverse or retard age-related symptoms of physical and mental decline, and to treat some non-age-related disorders as well.

According to reports in scientific literature, benefits from HGH replacement therapy include a reversal of declining pulmonary function, decreased body fat, increased capacity to exercise, increased bone mass in people with osteoporosis, and the improvement or reversal of many other age related symptoms and disorders. HGH has also been shown to strengthen the immune system and to improve the quality of life for people with AIDS by treating "wasting syndrome"—severe weight and muscle loss. People receiving HGH have reported a general enhancement of health and well-being, including a more positive outlook.

Although HGH injections may be self-administered, therapy must be prescribed and supervised by a physician. This is particularly important in light of the fact that as the therapy promotes tissue repair and other processes, the need for many nutrients increases. Therefore, treatment should include the supplementation of various vitamins, minerals, and, in some cases, other hormones.

As long as the dosage remains low—4 to 8 international units of the hormone per week—HGH therapy appears to be free of significant side effects. Those side effects that do occur usually pass as the body adjusts to the therapy.

HGH is extremely expensive, and a program of HGH therapy can cost upwards of $20,000 a year. Many people turn to the Internet in an attempt to buy HGH at savings. Unfortunately, supplements sold online that purport to contain pure HGH are probably not worth the money. Any amount of HGH they contain is quite small—too small to have much of an effect. We recommend proper injections, or failing that, use of supplements that might stimulate the body to produce more HGH. Do not give HGH to children without consulting a pediatrician.

Recommendations

❑ Avoid the consumption of excessively sweet foods, as it results in a blood sugar level that is counterproductive to the release and utilization of HGH. High-sugar foods should especially be avoided before going to bed, as the primary supply of HGH is released during sleep.

❑ Avoid eating immediately before exercising. Although vigorous exercise usually stimulates the production of HGH, blood sugar levels must be stable during exercise for HGH release to take place. Drinking a protein-rich shake an hour before a workout is fine.

❑ To stimulate the body's production of HGH, take the amino acid arginine, which has been shown to encourage HGH production. This amino acid is best taken in supplement form (500 milligrams daily), as foods that are high in arginine also contain amino acids that inhibit its ability to reach the pituitary gland, the site of HGH release.

Considerations

❑ Doctor's Growth Hormone Triple Strength from Fountain of Youth Technologies is an Ayurvedic herbal formula whose ingredients include naturally occurring levodopa (L-dopa) and Ayurvedic herbs to stimulate the pituitary gland to release human growth hormone (HGH).

❑ The use of some brands of HGH has resulted in the production of antibodies to growth hormone.

❑ For information about other antiaging hormones, *see* MELATONIN *under* NATURAL FOOD SUPPLEMENTS in Part One, and DHEA THERAPY in Part Three.

GUIDED IMAGERY

See under PAIN CONTROL.

HAIR ANALYSIS

Hair analysis offers an accurate assessment of the concentration of minerals in the body—those that are toxic in any amount, those that are essential, and those that are needed in small amounts, but toxic in larger amounts. By allowing early detection of toxic substances such as mercury, lead, cadmium, and aluminum, hair analysis makes it possible to identify and treat toxicity before overt symptoms appear. By showing levels of minerals such as calcium, it makes it possible to identify and treat a range of nutritional deficiencies well before health problems become serious.

Before the technique of hair analysis was developed, medical practitioners who were interested in the concentration of trace elements in the body had to rely on urine and serum sampling. Unfortunately, these tests do not reflect the concentration of minerals in the cells and organs, but instead show the level of *circulating minerals.* The correlation between mineral concentrations in the internal organs of the body and concentrations in hair has been found to be much more reliable. In fact, hair analysis has been found to be such an accurate measure of substance exposure that it is often used to detect drug use.

Hair analysis begins with the removal of a small amount of hair, usually from the nape of the neck. Because harsh chemical treatment of the hair through coloring, bleaching, and permanent-waving can result in inaccuracies, a pubic hair specimen may be used instead. The hair sample is chemically washed and stripped of all substances found on it. A specific amount (by weight) of the resulting sample is then dissolved in a known volume of acid. Finally, using a method of chemical analysis called atomic absorption photospectrometry, each mineral is isolated and measured on a parts-per-million (ppm) basis.

Hair analysis also provides a relatively permanent record of mineral concentrations, which can be analyzed by computer to determine the correlation between various elements in the hair. Treatment of any identified problems, using chelation therapy and/or other programs, can then be designed and implemented before the condition becomes irreversible. (*See* CHELATION THERAPY in Part Three.) Later, follow-up hair analyses can be compared with the initial results to learn the effectiveness of the treatment. Your health care provider should be able to help you obtain an analysis of your hair from a reputable laboratory.

HEAT AND COLD THERAPY

See under PAIN CONTROL.

HOMEOPATHY

The practice of homeopathic medicine was started two hundred years ago by Samuel Hahnemann, a German physician. The basic principles of homeopathy are that the natural state of the human body is one of health and that we possess the natural ability to heal ourselves. What we describe as symptoms are actually the body's efforts to protect itself against disease. Therefore, to effect a cure, we should not suppress the symptoms, but seek to stimulate the body's own natural healing processes.

Conventional Western medicine often seeks a cure by administering large doses of suppressant drugs. This can be a harmful approach for three reasons. First, suppressing symptoms can hamper the body's ability to cure itself. Second, the use of some drugs can have serious side effects. Third, this can rob the body of the opportunity to develop its own natural immunity.

It is possible to increase the healing power of a medicine and reduce its toxicity while at the same time proportionately and progressively diluting the medicine. In homeopathy, the more a remedy is diluted, the greater its potency. This allows homeopathic physicians to administer extremely powerful but minute therapeutic doses with no unpleasant side effects and no danger of toxic reactions. The reverse is often true in conventional medicine.

The individual and not the illness is the focal point in homeopathic medicine. Homeopathy considers the state of the whole individual—physical, mental, and emotional—whereas conventional physicians are often concerned only with the physical aspects of illness. Of course, no system of healing can cure all diseases. One can follow homeopathy as the general rule, backing it up with conventional medicine as required.

Homeopathic medicines are among the safest preparations known to medical science. Most of them (about 80 percent) are derived from plants. Some examples of plant-derived homeopathic remedies are *Bryonia* (wild hops), *Calendula* (marigold), and *Rhus toxicodendron* (poison ivy). Other remedies are derived from animals or animal products. These include *Apis mellifica* (honeybee) and *Sepia* (inky fluid from the cuttlefish). Still other remedies are prepared from minerals or mineral ores. Examples include *Natrum muriaticum* (sodium chloride), *Silicea* (flint), and *Sulfur.*

Homeopathic remedies are prepared by grinding the active ingredient and mixing it with alcohol and water, then allowing it to soften and steep. Finally, the liquid is filtered to produce a tincture. The medicines are then made more potent by progressive dilutions, which increase the healing power while decreasing the concentration. There are various potency ranges. The base, or mother tincture, has a potency of 1x. To make a 2x potency, one part of the base tincture is attenuated (mixed) with 9 parts of alcohol and shaken ten times. To make a 3x potency, one part of the 2x potency is mixed with 9 parts of alcohol and shaken again. This process is continued until the desired potency is attained.

Other mixing agents that can be used in addition to alcohol are glycerin, water, and lactose. In addition to x potencies, there are *c potencies*. These are prepared in the same way as the x potencies, except they are mixed at a ratio of 99 to 1, instead of 9 to 1. There are also *k potencies*. The 1,000k potency is labeled as 1m, a 10,000k potency as 10m, and so on.

Homeopathic remedies come in pellets, tablets, and dilutions (liquids). The strength of the medicine affects the way it works. Generally speaking, the lower potencies, such as 3x or 6x, have a greater effect on the organs and are suited to acute illness. Medium potencies, such as 12x and 30x, affect the senses and nervous system. High potencies, 60x and above, affect mental condition.

The following is a rough guide to the various potencies, their effects, and uses:

Potency	What It Affects	Frequency of Dosage
6x, 12x, 6c, 12c	Body organs. Used for symptoms of acute conditions.	One dose every ¼ hour to every 4 hours.
30x, 30c	Body organs plus the senses and nervous system. Used for symptoms of chronic conditions.	Once a day to 3 times a day.
200x, 1m, 10m, LM	Body organs, senses, nervous system, mind, and emotions.	Once a month to once a year.

A typical dose of a homeopathic remedy is 3 tablets or 10 pellets for adults, 2 tablets or 5 pellets for children. Remedies should be taken on an empty stomach. The tablets should be placed under the tongue and held there for as long as possible while they dissolve. If possible, you should not swallow the tablets. Most homeopathic remedies carry claims about what they are designed to treat, which have been reviewed by the FDA. This makes it easy to find what you are looking for.

HYDROTHERAPY

Hydrotherapy—the therapeutic use of water, steam, and ice—has been used for centuries to effectively treat injuries and a wide range of illnesses. Treatment techniques include baths (full body and specific body parts), compresses, showers, sitz baths, steam baths, and whirlpools. Hospitals, clinics, and spas worldwide use forms of hydrotherapy as safe and effective methods for managing such conditions as back pain, bronchitis and other respiratory problems, cancer, hypertension, muscle pain and inflammation, and rheumatoid arthritis. Hydrotherapy is also useful in treating the discomfort caused by spinal trauma.

There are three categories of external hydrotherapy: hot water, cold water, and alternating hot and cold water. *Hot water* stimulates the immune system and increases circulation, helping to relieve the body of toxins. By soothing nerves, hot water calms and relaxes the body. *Cold water*, which constricts blood vessels, is effective in reducing inflammation. Cold-water treatments are also used to reduce fever. *Alternating hot- and cold-water treatments* have been found to alleviate upper respiratory congestion and stimulate organ function through improved circulation.

Many hydrotherapy techniques for a range of conditions can be effectively performed at home. For instance, muscular pain and swelling caused by a sprain or strain respond favorably to an immediate application of cold. An ice pack, applied continually (up to twenty minutes on, followed by twenty minutes off) during the initial twenty-four hours following a trauma, can reduce swelling and provide relief.

Sitz baths, in which the pelvis is immersed in water, increase blood flow in the pelvic region and help to relieve problems in that area. Hot-water sitz baths are commonly used for the treatment of inflamed hemorrhoids, painful ovaries and testicles, muscular disorders, prostate disorders, and uterine cramps. They are often prescribed to a women who has just delivered a child vaginally. Cold-water sitz baths are used to treat constipation, sexual dysfunction, inflammation, sore muscles, and vaginal discharge. Alternating hot- and cold-water sitz baths are helpful in relieving abdominal disorders, blood poisoning, congestion, foot infection, headaches, muscle disorders, neuralgia, and swollen ankles. (*See* SITZ BATH in Part Three.)

Other effective hydrotherapy methods include simple, soothing baths and showers, body wraps, foot and hand baths, steam inhalation, and hot and/or cold compresses.

Although many hydrotherapy methods can be performed at home, certain treatments such as hyperthermia, neutral baths, and whirlpool baths are available only in clinics or hospitals. These treatments must be performed under the careful supervision of a licensed therapist or other health care provider:

- *Hyperthermia.* Fever stimulates the body's immune system to produce the antibodies necessary for fighting certain illnesses. Hyperthermia is a hot-immersion bath used to induce fever in those who cannot achieve one naturally.

- *Neutral bath.* This therapy, in which the body is submerged to the neck in warm water (92°F to 98°F), helps to soothe the body. Neutral baths are effective in calming nervousness and emotional upsets, reducing joint swelling, and helping the body rid itself of toxins.

- *Whirlpool bath.* Used effectively in treating muscle and joint injuries, whirlpool baths are also used to soothe burns and to stimulate circulation in patients with paralysis.

If you are interested in locating a hydrotherapy facility in your area, check with your local hospital. You can also look in the yellow pages of your local telephone directory under "Health Resorts" or "Physical Therapists."

A word of caution: If you have any health-related problems or conditions, be sure to consult with your health care provider before beginning *any* hydrotherapy treatment. All of the treatments presented in this section are recommended for those who are in generally good health.

HYPERBARIC OXYGEN THERAPY

All human tissues and organs need oxygen in order to function. Hyperbaric oxygen therapy (HBOT) is the administration of oxygen at high atmospheric pressure. This saturates the body with oxygen, increasing the total available amount. HBOT is useful in the treatment of a variety of conditions that are associated with an insufficient amount of oxygen in part or all of the body.

HBOT is administered by placing the individual being treated in a special chamber that delivers pure oxygen at three times the normal atmospheric pressure. In most cases, the entire chamber is pressurized for treatment, and then depressurized before the person is removed. In some cases, oxygen is delivered by mask, making pressurization and depressurization unnecessary.

In the United States, HBOT is most commonly used in cases of trauma, including burns, wounds, injuries from motor vehicle accidents, carbon monoxide poisoning, acute cyanide poisoning, smoke inhalation, and the death of tissues from radiation therapy. HBOT is also used to treat skin grafts that are failing to take, gangrene, decompression sickness, and certain cases of blood loss and anemia. HBOT is now being used by both conventional and alternative physicians, and continues to gain acceptance for new applications.

Although HBOT is strictly controlled for safety, it may not be appropriate for all individuals. People with a history of emphysema, middle ear infection, or spontaneous pneumothorax (accumulation of air in the chest cavity) may encounter problems with this therapy.

HYPNOTHERAPY

See under PAIN CONTROL.

JUICING

Fruits and vegetables are excellent sources of a wide range of vitamins, minerals, enzymes, and other nutrients, including phytochemicals—compounds that have been shown to combat cancer in a petri dish. Since more of the healthful substances found in fruits and vegetables are being discovered all the time, no supplement pill can contain all of these compounds. Also, because each plant appears to produce particular phytochemicals that work against cancer in particular ways, it is suggested that a rich assortment of fruits and vegetables be included in the diet. It is also recommended that you consume two glasses of live juices a day for health maintenance. Four glasses a day is recommended if you want to speed healing and recovery from illness.

Juicing is an excellent means of adding fruits and vegetables to your diet. Since juice contains the whole fruit or vegetable—except for the fiber, which is the indigestible part of the plant—it contains virtually all of the plants' health-promoting components. Because fresh juices are made from *raw* fruits and vegetables, all of the components remain intact. Vitamin C and other water-soluble vitamins can be damaged by overprocessing or overcooking. Fresh juice, however, provides all of the plants' healthful ingredients in a form that is easy to digest and absorb. In fact, it has been estimated that fruit and vegetable juices can be assimilated in twenty to thirty minutes.

Ideally, the juices recommended in this book should be made fresh in your kitchen and consumed immediately. Many commercial juices are heat-treated to lengthen shelf life. As just discussed, this process can destroy important nutrients. In addition, preservatives may have been added. Even pure, freshly made juices can lose some of their nutrients by being allowed to sit for long periods of time. By buying the best produce available, properly preparing it for juicing, and processing it in your own juicer, you will produce the most healthful, nutrient-rich drinks possible.

The individual entries in Parts Two and Three recommend the use of specific juices for the treatment of specific disorders. It is helpful, though, to be familiar with the three categories into which juices generally fall: green juices, vegetable juices, and fruit juices.

Green Juices or "Green Drinks"

Green juices cleanse the body of pollutants and have a rejuvenating effect. Made from a variety of green vegetables, green juices are rich in chlorophyll, which helps to purify the blood, build red blood cells, detoxify and heal the body, and provide the body with fast energy.

Green juices can be made with alfalfa sprouts, barley grass, cabbage, kale, dandelion greens, spinach, and other green vegetables, including wheatgrass. To sweeten and dilute your green juices, try adding fresh carrot and apple juice. (No other fruit juices should be added.) Steam-distilled water is another good addition.

Although green juices have great health benefits, they should be consumed in moderation. Try drinking about 8 to 10 ounces a day. The following is an excellent "green drink":

Ageless Cocktail

4–5 carrots
3 sprigs fresh parsley
1 large handful spinach
1 large handful kale
1 beet, including tops
1 clove garlic, peeled
¼ head cabbage

1. Thoroughly wash all vegetables, peeling the carrots and beet. Cut the vegetables into pieces small enough to fit into the juicer.

2. Process the vegetables in the juicer and drink immediately.

Safer Juice Processing

Juice products are enjoyed by many for their flavor and nutritional advantages. However, as evidenced by outbreaks, unpasteurized juice can also serve as a vehicle for foodborne illnesses. The California Department of Health Services, Food and Drug Branch developed a video in cooperation with the U.S. Food and Drug Administration (FDA), Centers for Disease Control and Prevention, university researchers, and industry representatives to assist the industry in producing a safer product.

Topics covered in the video:

Introduction to food safety, juice products as a special case.

Regulation, Requirements, and Guidance.

Personnel Practices.

Cleaning and Sanitizing.

Agricultural Practices and Raw Materials.

Processing, Design, and Packaging.

Performance Standards and Intervention.

To order the *Safer Processing of Juice* video, call the California Department of Health Services, Food and Drug Branch at 916-650-6500.

Vegetable Juices

Fresh vegetable juices are restorers. They boost the immune system, remove acid wastes, and alkalize the blood.

Among the most healthful and delicious of the vegetable juices are beet, cabbage, carrot, celery, cucumber, kale, parsley, turnip, spinach, watercress, and wheatgrass juice. Carrot juice is probably the most popular of the juices and is packed with carotenoids, including beta-carotene, the vitamin A precursor that helps fight cancer. Because carrots are the sweetest of the vegetables, their juice is not just delicious on its own, but is also great for mixing with other vegetables to increase their appeal. On the other hand, strong-flavored vegetables—broccoli, celery, onions, parsley, radishes, rutabaga, and turnips, for instance—should be used in small amounts only.

Garlic is a great addition to vegetable drinks. Before juicing, drop the garlic into vinegar for 1 minute to destroy any bacteria and mold on its surface. To avoid irritating the lining of the intestinal tract, use only 1 fresh garlic clove in 2 glasses of juice.

For the greatest health benefits, use many different vegetables when making your juices. That way, you will provide your body with a variety of important nutrients. The recipes that follow are just two of the many healthful vegetable juice drinks that you might want to try.

Potassium/Raw Potato Juice

1 pound potatoes (3 medium potatoes)
1 carrot or 1 stalk celery (optional)
6–8 ounces steam-distilled water

1. Scrub the potatoes well and cut out any eyes. Do not use potatoes that are part green.
2. Cut each potato in half. Cut the peel from the potato, making

sure to keep about ½ inch of potato on the peel. Set aside the potato center for another use.
3. Cut the potato skins into small enough pieces to fit into the juicer. Wash the carrot or celery, peeling the carrot if it was not grown organically. Cut into pieces.
4. Process the vegetables in the juicer. Add the water and drink immediately. Do not allow to stand.

Cabbage Juice for Ulcers

¼–½ head cabbage
1 apple or 2 carrots
¼ cup steam-distilled water

1. Thoroughly wash the vegetables and fruit, peeling the apple or carrots. Cut the produce into small enough pieces to fit into the juicer.
2. Process the vegetables and fruit in the juicer. Add the water and drink immediately. Do not allow it to stand, so as not to lose its benefits.

Fruit Juices

Fruit juices help cleanse the body and nourish it with important nutrients, including cancer-fighting antioxidants.

Although any fruit can be juiced, certain juices are particularly healthful and delicious. One favorite cleansing juice is watermelon. To make this refreshing drink, place a whole piece of watermelon—with the rind intact—in the juicer. Other delicious juices can be made with apples, apricots, bananas, berries, citrus fruits, kiwi, melons, pears—with just about any fruit that you want to use.

You can enjoy fruit juices at any time of the day. About 10 to 12 ounces per day is recommended. The following is just one of the delicious fruit juice drinks you can make at home.

Preparing Produce for Juicing

Juicing is an easy way to make delicious drinks that can boost your health and help you treat a number of disorders. By following these guidelines, you will ensure that your juices are as pure, nutrient-rich, and appetizing as possible:

- Whenever possible, buy and use organically grown produce—produce that is grown without the use of pesticides and other harmful chemicals. This prevents chemical residues from ending up in your juice.
- If you are unable to obtain organically grown fruits and vegetables, peel or thoroughly wash the produce, using a vegetable brush to remove chemical residues and waxes. Most health food stores carry vegetable washes that will help remove any residues.
- When purchasing potatoes for juicing, avoid those with a green tint, and be sure to remove any sprouts or eyes. The chemical solanine, which gives the potato its green cast, can cause diarrhea, vomiting, and abdominal pain.
- When using organically grown produce, feel free to leave the skin on in most cases. Do remove the skin, though, before juicing apricots, grapefruits, kiwis, oranges, papayas, peaches, and pineapples. The skins of oranges and grapefruits are quite bitter, and also con-

tain a toxic substance that should not be consumed in large amounts. Because kiwis and papayas are tropical fruits, their skins are likely to contain residues of the harmful sprays often used in foreign countries, where some chemicals outlawed in the United States may still be legal. (The FDA is doing its best to inspect foreign growers.) The skins of pineapples are too thick to be processed by most juicers.

- When juicing fruits, leave in small seeds, except when using apples. Apple seeds actually contain cyanide, a toxic substance. Because of their size and hardness, all pits *must* be removed.
- Juice most produce with stems and leaves intact. However, remove carrot and rhubarb greens, as they contain toxic substances.
- When using soft fruits that contain very little water—avocados, bananas, and papayas, for instance—purée the fruits in a blender rather than using a juicer. Then stir the purée into other juices.
- Remember to rotate vegetables and fruits so you get a variety of nutrients.

Kiwi Deluxe

1 firm kiwi, peeled
1 small bunch red grapes
1 green apple
½ cup berries (blueberries, blackberries,
and raspberries are good choices)

1. Wash all of the fruit thoroughly, peeling the apple. Cut the fruit into small enough pieces to fit into the juicer.

2. Process the fruit in the juicer. Pour over ice and drink.

   Variation: Frozen fruit mixes can take the place of ice. This will make the drink taste like a shake. Add a cup of frozen fruit mix to the recipe above. You can also add rice milk or soymilk and a banana if desired.

LIGHT THERAPY

The body's circadian rhythm—its inner clock—is regulated by the pineal gland. Affected by the absence or presence of light, the pineal gland is responsible for controlling such bodily functions as hormone production, body temperature, and the timing of sleep. Disturbances in the circadian rhythm can lead to depression as well as insomnia and other sleep disorders. The use of natural sunlight and various forms of light therapy has been effective in reestablishing the body's natural rhythm.

Natural sunlight contains the full wavelength spectrum needed for maintaining health. It triggers the impulses

that regulate most bodily functions. Artificial lighting—incandescent and fluorescent—lacks the complete balanced spectrum found in sunlight. Without certain wavelengths, the body cannot absorb some nutrients. Inadequate exposure to proper light can contribute to or worsen such illnesses and conditions as fatigue, depression, stroke, hair loss, suppressed immune function, cancer, hyperactivity, osteoporosis, and Alzheimer's disease.

A variety of light therapies have been used effectively in the treatment of a number of disorders. Some of the most common therapies are:

- *Bright light therapy.* This therapy involves the use of bright white light that ranges in intensity from 2,000 to 5,000 lux. (A lux is equal to the light of one candle; the average indoor light ranges from 50 to 500 lux.) Bright light therapy has proven helpful in treating cases of bulimia, sleep phase syndrome (a condition in which the person cannot fall asleep until the middle of the night), and irregular menstrual cycles.

- *Cold laser therapy.* Utilizing a low-intensity beam of laser light that stimulates the natural healing process at a cellular level, cold laser therapy is used in the treatment of pain, mild trauma, and orthopedic myofascial syndrome. It has also been used in dentistry, dermatology, and neurology.

- *Full-spectrum light therapy.* Exposure to natural sunlight and other forms of full-spectrum light is effective in relieving a number of disorders, including depression, hyperactivity, hypertension, insomnia, migraines, and premenstrual syndrome. Sunlight has long been used to treat babies with jaundice; however, do not put your baby in the sun for treatment—hospitals have special lamps. Full-spectrum light, as well as bright white light, is effective in the treatment of seasonal affective disorder (SAD). Common symptoms of SAD, which is also called the "winter blues," are depression, fatigue, overeating, and lowered libido.

- *Photodynamic light therapy (PDT).* This therapy uses drugs, called *photosensitizing agents*, along with light to kill cancer cells. Depending on the part of the body being treated, the photosensitizing agent is either injected into the bloodstream or put on the skin. Over a certain amount of time the drug is absorbed by the cancer cells. Then light is applied to the area to be treated. The light causes the drug to react with oxygen, which forms a chemical that kills the cancer cells. PDT may also work by destroying the blood vessels that feed the cancer cells and by alerting the immune system to attack the cancer.

- *Ultraviolet light therapy.* Ultraviolet light therapies are used to treat illnesses such as cancer, as well as conditions like high cholesterol and premenstrual syndrome.

- The sun's ultraviolet-A (UVA) rays, which have longer wavelengths than ultraviolet-B (UVB) and ultraviolet-C (UVC) rays, are considered the least harmful. There are a variety of ultraviolet light therapies.

- *UVA-1 therapy* isolates a portion of the UVA wavelength. It has been shown to be effective in the treatment of patients with atopic dermatitis. It is also used in the treatment of various connective tissues disorders including systemic lupus erythematosus (SLE) and systemic sclerosis (SS).

MAGNET THERAPY

See under PAIN CONTROL.

MASSAGE

See under PAIN CONTROL.

MEDITATION

See under PAIN CONTROL.

MUSIC AND SOUND THERAPY

Music therapy is the controlled use of music in the treatment of physical, mental, or emotional disorders. A variety of problems—including depression, high blood pressure, asthma, migraines, ulcers, and a range of physical disabilities—are currently managed using music.

In general, the nature of the problem dictates the precise form of the therapy. For some problems, specific musical pieces are played for the person being treated. In other instances, individuals actively participate in rhythm bands, group singing, individual or group music lessons, or music-accompanied physical activities.

Music has been shown to have various therapeutic capabilities. When played for individuals or groups with mental or emotional problems or with stress-related ailments, music can reduce anxiety and lessen irritability. In work with blind people, music has facilitated the development of better auditory perception. As a part of physical therapy, music has been used to stimulate or regulate movement. Also as a means of physical therapy, the playing of instruments has been employed both for its psychological benefits, such as greater self-confidence, and for its physical benefits, such as the strengthening of weak mouth and lip muscles.

Music is not the only type of sound that has been found to have therapeutic value. For many years, environmental sounds—the sound of a running stream, a waterfall, or bird songs—have been used by therapists and psychologists as a means of treatment. These sounds, it appears, can do much to relieve stress and lift depression.

Anyone can take advantage of the ability of music and other sounds to induce relaxation, with or without professional guidance. Soft music and soothing sounds, used alone or with relaxation techniques, can effectively alleviate stress, relax muscles, and evoke a positive mood. Researchers suggest that these sounds promote the production of endorphins, the body's own painkillers, and can thereby also help in the control of pain. In some cases—as when music is to be applied to physical therapy—an experienced practitioner should be consulted.

PAIN CONTROL

Pain is a message sent by the body to the brain, signaling that disease, injury, or strenuous activity has caused trouble in some area. Without pain, you would remain unaware of many problems—from torn ligaments to appendicitis—until the disorders became serious. At low levels, pain can motivate you to rest the injured area so that tissues can be repaired and additional damage can be prevented. When severe, pain can motivate you to seek treatment as well.

Not all pain appears to serve a useful function, though. While *acute pain,* the pain described above, can alert us to a problem that needs immediate attention, in some cases pain lasts long after an injured area has healed. In other instances, pain may be caused by recurring backache, migraines and other headaches, arthritis, and other disorders. Referred to as *chronic pain*—which may be defined as pain that occurs, continually or intermittently, for more than six months—this pain may signal an ongoing problem that cannot be eliminated through treatment. In such a case, pain management often becomes the treatment goal.

For some people, pain is cyclical. Pain produces anxiety,

and this anxiety intensifies the pain. Fear and anticipation of the physical problem can also heighten the pain, leading to feelings of depression and helplessness. When experiencing such pain, it is natural to limit one's activities. This can lead to a "chronic pain cycle," which can adversely affect one's confidence and self-esteem.

Being aware of the chronic pain cycle as well as understanding its psychological effects can help you avoid being drawn into it:

1. The cycle generally begins with prolonged periods of rest and inactivity, causing a loss in physical strength, endurance, and flexibility. As a result, you may begin to lose confidence in your ability to do things, causing a lowering of personal goals.

2. Inability to perform usual activities at home or work is likely to promote feelings of frustration, and you may begin perceiving yourself as unproductive. This sense of lowered self-esteem may further lead to depression.

3. During times when the pain subsides or is more tolerable than usual, you may overexert yourself in an effort to prove to yourself and others that you can still do the things you did before the chronic pain began.

4. As a result of the overexertion, the pain often returns and may be more severe than before. You may find yourself unable to finish tasks or accomplish goals. Discouraged and in pain, you begin limiting your activities, and the cycle begins again.

One way to keep from getting caught up in the chronic pain cycle is through pain management. Often, the reduction of physical pain can prevent the cycle from starting.

There are a variety of treatments that can help alleviate pain. Some do so on a purely physical level, perhaps by interrupting the pain process or desensitizing nerve endings. Others approach pain control on a psychological level, by affecting the mind's perception of the pain. When treating pain, the physical and psychological can be intertwined. Just as a physical reduction of pain may decrease anxiety and improve outlook, so can the mind be used to relax muscles and effect other physical changes that then reduce symptoms.

The discussions in this section are meant to introduce you to some of the many pain-control techniques now available. Depending on the cause of your pain, the level of your pain, and your own treatment preferences, you may want to try one or more of these techniques. While some of these approaches—like the use of hot and cold packs—can easily be used on your own, other techniques—such as biofeedback—require at least initial training by a qualified practitioner. Some, like chiropractic, must be performed by a professional. When possible, get referrals from your health care provider or from friends. If a reputable pain clinic is available to you, this can be a wonderful resource—one that offers a range of practitioners experienced in using a variety of pain-control techniques. Make sure that the pro-

fessional you consult has successfully treated a condition such as yours.

ACUPRESSURE

Based on the same beliefs that are the foundation of acupuncture (see the discussion below), acupressure—also known as "contact healing"—is actually the older of the two methods. Acupressure and the healing art of *shiatsu* (a massage technique) are commonly referred to as "acupuncture without needles." Like acupuncture, acupressure seeks to restore health by restoring the normal flow of *chi*, the life energy that flows through the body along pathways called meridians. While acupuncture uses the insertion of needles to promote energy flow, acupressure uses finger and hand pressure. During pressure stimulation, neurotransmitters, which help to inhibit the reception and transmission of pain, are released.

Acupressure is a safe, simple, and inexpensive treatment. Although it may be performed by a skilled practitioner, because of the treatment's noninvasive nature, acupressure may also be performed by the individual for the immediate relief of pain. In fact, a number of self-acupressure techniques, including Acu-Yoga, *Do-In*, and *Tui Na*, can help you control pain through finger pressure, massage, body positioning, and a variety of other means.

More information on acupressure is available from the Acupressure Institute. (*See* Health and Medical Organizations in the Appendix.)

ACUPUNCTURE

This ancient Chinese practice is based on the belief that health is determined by *chi*, the vital life energy that flows through every living thing. This energy is thought to move through the body along pathways called meridians, each of which is linked to a specific organ. If the flow of energy is balanced, the individual enjoys good health. If something interrupts this flow, however, various problems, including pain, can result. Acupuncture is used to restore proper energy flow, and, as a result, good health.

In acupuncture treatment, the acupuncturist inserts thin needles at specific points in the body. Although slight discomfort may occasionally be felt upon insertion of the needle, the treatment is virtually painless. The needles may be left in place for anywhere from a few minutes to a half hour. To support the acupuncture therapy, the practitioner may recommend taking herbs in the form of teas and capsules, and may also suggest specific lifestyle changes and exercises. Relief may be experienced after only one treatment or after a series of treatments.

Although used for a variety of health problems, including addictions and mental disorders, in the United States, acupuncture is perhaps most commonly used to relieve pain, including backache and migraine headaches. Studies have indicated that acupuncture may stimulate the production of endorphins, the body's own painkillers. Completely safe, acupuncture has no known side effects.

For more information on acupuncture and a list of practitioners in your area, you can contact the American Association of Acupuncture and Oriental Medicine. (*See* Health and Medical Organizations in the Appendix.)

AURICULAR THERAPY (AURICULOTHERAPY)

Auricular therapy (or auriculotherapy) involves stimulating the external surface of the ear, or auricle, to alleviate pathological conditions in other parts of the body. Various techniques are used, including electrical stimulation and the use of acupuncture needles.

The use of the auricle in diagnosis was first described in the early 1950s by the French neurologist Dr. Paul Nogier. Nogier first published his comprehensive systems of diagnosis and treatment in 1957, after years of observation demonstrated to him that points on the ears that had reduced electrical resistance corresponded to specific areas of the body. Since 1982, the World Health Organization (WHO) has been sponsoring working groups in an attempt to establish international consensus on the terminology and the auricular location points. WHO used research conducted by Terry Oleson, Ph.D., and Richard Kroening, M.D., at UCLA Pain Management Center, along with a Chinese ear acupuncture text by Helen Huang, as a guide to standardization.

There are two main schools of thought regarding the auricular points, one European and the other Oriental. While there is no complete agreement on auricular points between the two schools, forty-three points were adopted by the WHO in 1987. The use of auricular therapy for pain management and in the treatment of addiction is in widespread use in Europe and has been increasing steadily in the United States since the early 1970s. Its main use has been to enhance treatment of addiction, particularly nicotine addiction. Auriculotherapy seeks to restore a sense of well-being, reduce anxiety, and promote detoxification.

According to theory, there are meridians that run through the body. Along these meridians are pressure points—the same points used in acupressure. There are literally hundreds of these points located in the lobe of the ear. It has long been believed in Asia that when the meridians become unbalanced, illness results. Using a tiny battery-operated machine, a small charge of direct current can be applied, eliminating the need for acupuncture needles. Very brief stimulation—ten seconds at about 100 microamperes or less—on auricular points can often produce profound and immediate results. The key is to treat at the exact point on the front of the ear and the one directly behind it on the back associated with the regional area of pathology. These areas are called *corresponding points.* They are highly conductive and sensitive to pressure, sometimes long after the health problem is considered healed. This form of therapy has led to dramatic improvements in long-standing problems that were unresponsive to conventional medical therapy.

For more information, you can contact the Auriculotherapy Certification Institute. (*See* Health and Medical Organizations in the Appendix.)

BIOFEEDBACK

Biofeedback combines a variety of relaxation methods such as guided imagery and meditation with the use of instruments that monitor the individual's responses. Over time, this teaches you to consciously regulate a number of your own *autonomic functions*—heart rate, blood pressure, and other processes previously believed to be involuntary. By consciously regulating these functions, you can control a number of problems, including pain.

During a biofeedback session, electrodes connected to a monitoring unit are taped or otherwise painlessly attached to the skin. The machine may measure any one of a number of things, including skin temperature, pulse, blood pressure, muscle tension, and brain wave activity. As you use various techniques, such as relaxation, to create the desired response—lower blood pressure, for instance—the machine, through sound or images, provides moment-by-moment feedback on your progress. Eventually, with the practitioner's help, you should become able to create the desired response without the use of the machine.

Although biofeedback has been successfully used to help control a wide range of health problems, it is perhaps best known for its use in the treatment of headaches and migraines. In a large number of cases, biofeedback has been successfully used to avert the onset of migraines. It has also been used to treat injuries, as well as to relieve the pain of TMJ syndrome.

It should be noted that biofeedback only measures stress; it does not cure it. Sessions should be conducted in conjunction with other therapies under the watchful eye of a qualified health care practitioner.

If you are considering biofeedback training, you can consult the Association for Applied Psychophysiology and Biofeedback. (*See* Health and Medical Organizations in the Appendix.)

BREATHING EXERCISES

Shallow or poor breathing can contribute to many disorders. We need to learn to breathe deeply, and from the abdomen rather than from the chest, which produces short and shallow breathing. Learning this technique helps one to breathe in more oxygen, which then passes through the lungs and is absorbed into the bloodstream and into our bodies. Oxygen is needed for cellular respiration, cell metabolism, and proper brain function. If you breathe too shallowly, the body may not be able eliminate sufficient carbon dioxide for good health. Proper breathing technique increases lung capacity, increases energy levels, speeds the healing process of many disorders, and helps to relieve anxiety, asthma symptoms, insomnia, and stress.

To practice deep breathing, do the following:

1. Slowly breathe in through your nose and from your abdomen as deeply as you can and hold the breath for a count of ten.

2. Place your tongue between your front teeth and the roof of your mouth. Slowly breathe out through your mouth.

Do this for five minutes three times daily. Choose an environment with fresh air when doing this exercise, not a place with a lot of traffic or pollution.

If you want to relax quickly—say, if you are under tension or stress, or are having an anxiety attack—place your arms down along the sides of your body. As you are inhaling deeply, stretch your arms up and out as if to form a V-shape. Then exhale slowly through your mouth and bring your arms back down to your side. This is a stretching and breathing exercise at the same time. Repeat this as many times as is comfortable every hour until you find relief.

CHIROPRACTIC

Chiropractic is a form of treatment that seeks to eliminate pain—and, in some cases, other problems—through the manipulation of the spinal column. Chiropractors believe that if the spinal vertebrae are properly aligned, impulses from the brain are able to travel freely along the spinal cord to the various organs, maintaining healthy function throughout the body. If a misalignment of the spine occurs, however, the normal flow of impulses is disrupted, resulting in pain as well as other physical disorders. Chiropractors seek to return the spine's alignment to its normal, healthy state. This permits the nervous system to regain normal function, allowing the body to heal itself and eliminate the pain.

After the chiropractor locates any spinal misalignments, chiropractic adjustment is used to reestablish normal function. This adjustment may involve touch; active motion, in which the patient bends and stretches in specific ways; and passive movement, in which the doctor assists the patient's movements. A hand-held rubber-tipped instrument may be used to gently manipulate the vertebrae. Some chiropractors support adjustment therapy with applications of heat and cold, electrical stimulation, nutrition, and other natural therapies. Chiropractic does not use drugs or surgery.

After physicians and dentists, chiropractors are the third largest group of health care professionals in our nation. They are licensed in all fifty states, and most health insurance plans cover some part of the treatment they provide. Chiropractors are the most widely used practitioners in the alternative health care field. The U.S. Department of Health and Human Services lists spinal manipulation as a proven treatment for acute lower back pain. Chiropractic therapy is also used to treat arthritis, bursitis, and a variety of other disorders, including many nonpainful ailments. To locate a qualified chiropractor in your area, you can consult TheRightChiropractor.com. (*See* Health and Medical Organizations in the Appendix.)

GUIDED IMAGERY

Much research has indicated that bodily functions previously thought to be totally beyond conscious control can be modified using psychological techniques. Guided imagery, a technique that has grown in popularity in the last several years, uses this mind-body connection to help people cope with a variety of disorders, including pain.

Researchers have established a link between negative emotions and lowered immune function. Conversely, they have found a connection between positive emotions and a healthy immune response. Guided imagery—the mind thinking in pictures—is an effective tool for eliminating negative thoughts and replacing them with positive ones.

Through guided imagery, the mind conjures up mental pictures or scenes in order to better direct the body's energy. You can, for instance, close your eyes and visualize the pain as a sharp knife in the affected body area. Then you can imagine that the knife is being withdrawn, and that a cooling, soothing cream is being applied to the area. Through imagery, people with cancer commonly visualize the cancer cells in their bodies as weak and their white "fighter" cells as strong and destructive. In other instances, people have found that, rather than visualizing the pain, focusing on a pleasant scene, such as a beautiful day at the beach, promotes relaxation and substantially controls pain.

Used with some success in the treatment of rheumatoid arthritis and other illnesses, guided imagery has also been shown to reduce stress, slow the heart rate, and stimulate the immune system. Taught properly, guided imagery can be an effective form of self-care; however, it is not meant to replace your doctor's care or prescribed medication. Rather, it can be used to enhance your prescribed course of treatment.

HEAT AND COLD THERAPY

Hot and cold packs are simple-to-use pain-control tools that have been widely employed for many years. When applied singly or in combination, these techniques often provide relief not only from the pain itself, but, in some cases, from any accompanying swelling.

Heat

Pain from backaches, arthritis, and similar disorders often responds well to heat therapy. By increasing the temperature in selected areas of the body, this treatment enhances blood circulation and helps muscles to relax, reducing stiffness and increasing mobility.

Heat can be applied to the affected area through a number of means, including hot water bottles and electric heating pads. Often, moist heat works better than dry heat. Some electric heating pads are capable of producing moist heat, as are some gel packs. Hot showers and wet towels are other means of concentrating moist heat on a painful area. Poultices can also be effective and, for certain disorders, sitz baths are helpful. (*See* USING A POULTICE and SITZ BATH in Part Three.)

Use all forms of heat therapy with caution. Monitor the intensity of the heat and the duration and frequency of the treatment. Do not allow yourself to fall asleep while using an electric heating pad. Regardless of the heat source, a good rule of thumb is twenty minutes on, twenty minutes off. After removing the heat, firmly rub or massage the affected area. This will both dissipate the heat and help relieve tension. Do not massage the area if it is inflamed or has just sustained a serious injury. Never massage the area if you have phlebitis or other vascular problems.

Cold

Because of its ability to prevent swelling, cold packs are often the treatment of choice directly following a strain, sprain, or other injury. In such cases, cold packs alone should be used during the first twenty-four to thirty-six hours. Cold packs can also help relieve certain types of chronic pain.

Ice packs are probably the most common means of applying cold. These packs can simply be applied to the painful area, or they can be rubbed on the area using a circular motion for five to seven minutes. Lower back pain seems to be particularly responsive to ice rubs. Cold gel packs, which are kept in the freezer between uses, are also effective, and, because of their pliable consistency, are often more comfortable than ice packs. If none are available, a pack of frozen peas works just as well and can mold to the area. When you are done with it, mark the bag so it can be used over again for this purpose (do not eat them) and place it back in the freezer.

Like heat therapy, cold therapy should be used with caution. Wrap ice packs, gel packs, or frozen peas in a towel before applying them to the affected area. Then apply the packs for no more than twenty minutes at a time.

Heat and Cold

In some cases, alternating hot and cold treatments work best. For a painful and stiff neck, for instance, try using a warm shower to relieve tension. After the shower, use a five- to seven-minute ice massage to reduce swelling and further relieve pain.

Experimentation is the best way to discover whether heat, cold, or alternating heat and cold best relieves your discomfort. If several applications of one type of treatment—say, heat—do not provide any relief, try the opposite treatment. If your pain persists, and especially if you are not sure of its cause, consult your health care provider.

Counterirritants

A variety of over-the-counter topical products, such as capsaicin cream, Ben-Gay, and Icy Hot, can be used in lieu of a heat pack to treat localized pain. As counterirritants, these products stimulate blood flow to the affected area, acting much like heat. Glucosamine/Chondroitin MSM Ultra Rx-Joint Cream from Nature's Plus, Traumeel from Heel Inc., and many other natural products found in health food stores are good for arthritis, inflammation, bruising, and sprains. While such products may be relatively convenient and easy to use, they should be used with discretion. Do not apply anything but ordinary clothing to an area that has been treated with a counterirritant. Heating pads placed over treated areas can increase the medication's rate of absorption into the skin, thus causing serious damage.

HERBS

Many herbs have been used for centuries for their pain-relieving properties. Some of the best include:

- Angelica, black haw, cramp bark, kava kava, rosemary, and valerian root are good for pain related to cramps and muscle spasms.

    Caution: Kava kava can cause drowsiness. It is not recommended for pregnant women or nursing mothers, and it should not be taken together with other substances that act on the central nervous system, such as alcohol, barbiturates, antidepressants, and antipsychotic drugs.

- A tea made of blue violet, catnip, chamomile, gotu kola, licorice, rosemary, white willow, or wood betony is effective in relieving tension and nerve pain.

    Cautions: Do not use chamomile if you are allergic to ragweed. Do not use during pregnancy or nursing. It may interact with warfarin or cyclosporine, so patients using these drugs should avoid it. Licorice root should not be used during pregnancy or nursing. It should not be used by persons with diabetes, glaucoma, heart disease, high blood pressure, or a history of stroke.

- Capsaicin, an ingredient in cayenne (capsicum), can provide pain relief when regularly applied to the affected area. Now available in Zostrix, an over-the-counter topical cream, capsaicin is thought to relieve pain by limiting the production of a neural pain transmitter called substance P. Although the application of capsaicin may cause a burning sensation at first, repeated use keeps nerves from replenishing their supply of substance P, so that pain is not transmitted to the brain. In studies, capsaicin has been used to control the pain of neuralgia, diabetic neuropathy, rheumatoid arthritis, osteoarthritis, and cluster headaches. Cayenne may also help to alleviate pain if taken orally in capsule form.

- Hops, kava kava, passionflower, valerian root, wild lettuce, and wood betony have muscle-relaxing properties and may help to relieve lower back pain.

    Caution: Kava kava can cause drowsiness. It is not recommended for pregnant women or nursing mothers, and it should not be taken together with other substances that act on the central nervous system, such as alcohol, barbiturates, antidepressants, and antipsychotic drugs.

- Essential oils of jasmine, juniper, lavender, peppermint, rose, rosemary, and thyme have been effective in the treatment of a variety of types of pain.

- Migraine Relief from Natural Care is an herbal blend that has been effective in relieving migraines.

- Fresh papaya juice and/or fresh pineapple is highly recommended for the treatment of inflammation, heartburn, ulcers, back pain, and digestive disorders.

- Saffron has been found to be effective in treating abdominal pain after childbirth.

HYPNOTHERAPY

Like meditation and visualization, hypnotherapy is a method by which a qualified physician or therapist can induce a positive mental state in an individual. The therapist attempts to quiet the person's conscious mind to make the unconscious mind more accessible. Hypnosis is designed to generate a state of deep relaxation in which there is a heightened receptivity to suggestion through the calm repetition of words and statements. Once an individual is in this state, the practitioner provides simple verbal suggestions that help the mind block the awareness of pain and replace it with a more positive feeling, such as a feeling of warmth. If the pain is the result of an earlier injury, the practitioner may also help the individual more clearly remember the incident—a practice that often helps alleviate anxiety and thus reduce pain.

Hypnotherapy enhances positive imagery, helps to reduce anxiety, and induces a deep level of relaxation. During a hypnotic state, the mind is highly focused and fully aware of the situation, enabling the person to concentrate without being distracted. During hypnosis, breathing and pulse rate slow down, and blood pressure may drop.

No one can be forced into hypnosis. You must be a willing participant in the process. Good rapport between therapist and client is important.

Hypnosis has been used successfully to control back pain, joint pain, burn pain, and the pain of migraines and other headaches. This technique can be a valuable self-help tool, as you can learn to hypnotize yourself whenever you need it. However, self-hypnosis must first be learned from a licensed psychologist, a certified hypnotherapist, or another professional with experience in hypnotherapy.

MAGNET THERAPY

Magnet therapy has been used in the Far East and Europe for some time and is becoming popular in the United States. It is said that magnets can be used to provide relief from pain and to hasten healing. Double-blind studies on the effectiveness of magnet therapy have shown that there is no scientific basis to conclude that small magnets of the type sold for the purpose can relieve pain or influence the course of disease. Many of today's products actually produce no significant magnetic field at the skin's surface, and none beneath. The initial study that is cited by magnet marketers is the pilot study done at the Baylor College of Medicine in Houston, where researchers found that magnets could provide significant relief for the pain of post-polio syndrome. However, other subsequent studies, such as one done at the New York College of Podiatric Medicine, reported no effect on patients suffering from heel pain. Researchers at the Veterans Administration Medical Center in Prescott, Arizona, conducted an elaborate study on back pain and found no evidence to support the claims of the magnet manufacturers.

Magnets are believed to work by increasing circulation and blood flow to affected areas, which in turn reduces swelling and inflammation. Arthritis, asthma, carpal tunnel syndrome, fibromyalgia, infections, migraines, osteoporosis, ruptured disks, sports injuries, and tennis elbow are a few of the conditions that are said to be helped by magnet therapy. So far, studies have shown that blood circulation is not affected by magnets.

Despite the decidedly mixed results of scientific research, the decision to try magnet therapy is one that each individual must make for him- or herself. If you are using magnets for pain relief and they seem to be working, by all means do not discontinue their use. However, if you do choose to use magnets, understand that they should not be used during pregnancy or in the presence of pacemakers, insulin pumps, and automatic defibrillators. People who take anticoagulants or use drug patches also should not use magnets. And on a practical note, keep your magnets away from your computer's hard drive and storage disks.

MASSAGE

Massage involves the manipulation of muscles and other soft tissues. It is beneficial in treating a wide range of conditions, including muscle spasms and pain, soreness from injury, and headaches. Massage works to relieve pain in a number of ways: by promoting muscle relaxation; by increasing lymphatic circulation and thereby possibly reducing inflammation; by breaking up scar tissue and adhesions; by promoting blood flow through the muscles; and by promoting drainage of the sinus fluids.

Massage is not advisable for everyone. Those with a history of phlebitis, high blood pressure, or any other vascular disorder should not receive any type of deep muscle massage performed with strong pressure. Always check with a physician before receiving deep muscle massage. Massage should not be performed on inflamed areas or on individuals with malignant or infectious conditions.

A variety of massage therapies are currently in use. Each

is based on a different theory and utilizes specific techniques. The following bodywork systems represent some of those most widely used:

- *Deep tissue massage.* Used to release chronic muscular tension, deep tissue massage is applied with greater pressure and on deeper muscles than classic Swedish massage. It generally focuses on a specific problem area.

- *Esalen massage.* This massage technique attempts to bring about a sense of well-being through deep and beneficial states of consciousness. Esalen massage focuses on the mind and body as a whole. It is a hypnotic method that uses slow, rhythmic movements to bring about a general state of relaxation.

- *The Feldenkrais method.* The idea of "self-image" is central to the theory and technique of this method. Through exercise and "touch," the therapist helps eliminate negative muscle patterns and the feelings and thoughts associated with them. This method uses two approaches: *Awareness through Movement* and *Functional Integration.* Awareness through Movement employs a group approach in which the participants are guided through a slow, gentle sequence designed to replace old movement patterns with new ones. Functional Integration is an individualized approach that uses hands-on touch and movement. The Feldenkrais method differs from most other types of massage in that there is no attempt to alter the body's structure. Rather, it is through touch that the practitioner attempts to communicate a sense of improved self-image and movement.

- *Neuromuscular massage.* This form of deep tissue massage concentrates on a specific muscle. Through the use of concentrated finger pressure, sensitive "trigger points" are released and blood flow is increased.

- *Reflexology.* Reflexology originated thousands of years ago in China. It was taken up in the United States in the 1950s. Reflexologists apply pressure to different spots on the feet, hands, and ears that correlate with the body's organs. This opens a channel for energy to flow to the affected part of the body. There may be pain when pressure is applied to some spots, and in some cases it is necessary to use prolonged pressure. The reflexologist should inform you about which body part any pressure point represents so that if you feel pain, you can apply pressure and massage the spot yourself to reduce the pain.

- *Reiki.* In Japanese, *reiki* (ray-key) means "universal life energy." The practice of reiki promotes a return to health through "wholeness." The treatment consists of the health professional gently placing his or her hands on a relaxed body. You keep your clothes on for a reiki session. The practitioner's hands touch a variety of places, such as the head, chest, abdomen, and back, to promote energy to flow through the body. For some people, this treatment promotes deep relaxation, while to others it may be invigorating. Reiki originated many thousands of years ago and is easy to learn, but powerful. It is used to relieve stress, empower goals, overcome obstacles, and heal illness. It can also be a tool for spiritual growth.

- *Rolfing or structural integration.* This method is based on the belief that function is improved when body parts are properly aligned. Through manipulation of connective tissue linking muscles to bones, the therapist attempts to restore fuller movement, resulting in a more balanced body. The Rolfer applies deep tissue pressure to the muscles of the neck, head, back, pelvis, legs, and arms. This pressure stretches and guides the connective tissues, allowing for more flexible movement. Rolfing is also effective for muscle pain, neck tension, back pain, headaches, and increasing the range of motion. Before treating you, a Rolfer will evaluate your motion as you walk, bend, and turn.

- *Shiatsu.* Literally meaning "finger pressure" in Japanese, this Oriental massage technique focuses on acupressure points to restore and maintain health. Through firm, rhythmic pressure applied to specific points for three to ten seconds each, the shiatsu therapist attempts to unblock the energy that flows through the acupuncture meridians. The pressure used depends on the person's needs. Other techniques used include kneading, stroking, tapping, and stretching done by a shiatsu therapist.

- *Sports massage.* A combination of kneading, passive stretching, and range of deep-tissue motions, sports massage is designed to ease muscle strain and promote flexibility. It is most effective when applied before or after exercising.

- *Swedish massage.* The development of this technique is credited to Per Hendricks Ling, who in the early 1800s used kneading, stroking, tapping, and shaking to induce the body to relax. Swedish massage can also relieve soreness and swelling, as well as promote rehabilitation after an injury.

For organizations that can provide further information about massage therapy, *see* Health and Medical Organizations in the Appendix.

MEDICATION

Numerous over-the-counter medications are available to help control pain. Two of the simplest nonnarcotic pain relievers are acetylsalicylic acid (aspirin) and acetaminophen (found in Tylenol, Datril, and many other products). Both of these medications can help relieve mild to moderate pain. Aspirin can also reduce swelling and inflammation. If you take aspirin for pain relief, you should also take supplements of vitamin C, as this nutrient has been shown to make the effects of the analgesic last longer.

Nonsteroidal anti-inflammatory drugs (NSAIDs), another type of nonnarcotic analgesic, may also be helpful in the relief of aches and pains. These products include ibuprofen (Advil, Nuprin, and others), ketoprofen (Orudis), and naproxen (Aleve).

Although over-the-counter analgesics are generally regarded as safe, discretion should be exercised in their use. For instance, aspirin has been related to gastrointestinal bleeding. If you take acetaminophen, be sure to avoid consuming alcohol, as this can both decrease the effectiveness of the drug and cause damage to the liver. If you take aspirin, be aware that it may affect the stomach. More important, you should *never* give aspirin to a child, especially a child with a cold or flulike symptoms. If you do, you run the risk of having the child get a life-threatening condition called Reye's syndrome.

Regardless of the pain reliever being used, you should never take more than the dosage directed on the label without first consulting your health care provider. Virtually any medication can cause problems when used inappropriately.

MEDITATION

Meditation, which has been practiced for thousands of years, is an effective means of treating stress and managing pain. Broadly defined, meditation is an activity that calms the mind and keeps it focused on the present. In the meditative state, the mind is not cluttered with thoughts or memories of the past, nor is it concerned with future events.

There are hundreds of meditation techniques, most of which fall into one of two categories: *concentrative* and *mindfulness.* During concentrative meditation, attention is focused on a single sound, an object, or one's breath, to bring about a calm, tranquil mind. One simple, common technique involves sitting or lying comfortably in a quiet environment, closing your eyes, and focusing attention on your breath as you inhale through your nose for a count of three, then exhale through your mouth for a count of five. This focus on your breathing rhythm—slow, deep, regular breaths—allows your mind to become tranquil and aware.

During mindfulness meditation, the mind becomes aware of but does not react to the wide variety of sensations, feelings, and images tied in with a current activity. By sitting quietly and allowing the images of your surroundings to pass through your mind without reacting to or becoming involved with them, you can attain a calm state of mind.

Much research has been done on transcendental meditation (TM). TM brings about a state of deep relaxation in which the body is totally at rest, but the mind is highly alert. Studies show that meditation, especially TM, is effective in controlling anxiety, enhancing the immune system, and reducing conditions such as high blood pressure. Meditation has also been used successfully to treat chronic pain and to control substance abuse.

Meditation is an effective self-care technique that can be a useful part of your health care program. However, it is not an alternative to recommended medical treatment.

QI GONG

Qi gong (pronounced cheie-gong) is a slow-motion exercise that is older than tai chi. Both concentrate on movement and breath meditation. *Qi* means "life force, energy," and *gong* means "work, a skill of practice." Qi gong increases vital energy for emotional and physical health.

According to traditional Chinese medicine, this type of exercise wards off illness. It has been linked to reduced blood pressure and increased levels of endorphins, natural body chemicals that relieve pain and maintain mental health. Work with a trained professional to begin with, and in a half-hour you will be able to practice qi gong on your own. You will not find the exercises too strenuous. They are done as if in slow motion.

This particular discipline not only improves your mind, but also tones the muscles and joints, and improves your balance. Remember to move your body slowly, with concentration, and remove all other thoughts from your mind. Proper breathing also is a part of qi gong. You want to enable your physical and mental processes to operate in balance for healing, relaxation, and internal energy.

RELAXATION TECHNIQUES

Once pain occurs—whether from injury or another source—your psychological reaction to it can have a profound effect on the duration and intensity of the pain. In some people, pain is cyclical; pain produces anxiety and tension, and tension intensifies pain. In the case of disorders such as migraines, tension can be a significant cause of the initial pain. By releasing tension, relaxation techniques can greatly reduce certain types of pain and actually prevent some pain from occurring.

A variety of relaxation techniques are available, including biofeedback, deep breathing, guided imagery, meditation, progressive relaxation, and yoga. These techniques facilitate deep relaxation and reduce stress. The advantage of relaxation therapy is that you can easily master these methods, either on your own or with the help of a professional, and then use them whenever they are needed.

TAI CHI

Tai chi, known as "meditation in motion," is similar to qi gong. It is used for meditation and complete relaxation. Both techniques are characterized by slow, soft, flowing movements that emphasize energy forces. These arts are very unlike the "strong" martial arts, such as karate and kung fu (wushu). Tai chi releases the flow of energy throughout the body. When this energy becomes blocked, one becomes ill.

TENS UNIT THERAPY

Transcutaneous electrical nerve stimulation (TENS) units can be helpful in dealing with localized pain, and are widely used both in doctors' offices and physiotherapy clinics.

TENS therapy can also be performed at home. With this technique, electrodes are placed on the skin and joined to the TENS unit with wires. Electric signals are then sent to the nerve endings, blocking pain signals before they reach the brain. It is believed that these signals may also stimulate the production of endorphins, the body's natural painkillers. TENS therapy is not considered painful, although some people report feelings of mild discomfort.

Pain relief from TENS therapy can be long- or short-term in nature. Because the treatments are safe and have no known side effects, they can be repeated as necessary.

USING A POULTICE

A poultice is made of a soft, moist substance that is mixed to the consistency of a paste, and then spread on or between layers of cloth. The cloth is then placed on a body surface.

Poultices act by increasing blood flow, relaxing tense muscles, soothing inflamed tissues, or drawing toxins from an infected area. Thus, they can be used to relieve the pain and inflammation associated with abscesses; boils; bruises; carbuncles; fibrocystic disease; fractures; enlarged glands in the neck, breast, or prostate; leg ulcers; sprains; sunburn; tumors; and ulcerated eyelids. They are also used to break up congestion, draw out pus, and remove embedded particles from the skin. Check with your health care provider first if you have any of these conditions to determine their severity.

Procedure

An herbal poultice may be made with dried or fresh herbs. The two types of poultices are prepared in slightly different ways. For information on choosing the best herbal poultice for your condition, as well as cautions regarding the use of specific herbs, *see* Types of Poultices in this section.

Preparing a Dried Herb Poultice

If you are using dried herbs, use a mortar and pestle to grind the herbs to a powder. Place the herbs in a bowl, and add enough warm water to make a thick paste that can be easily applied. Make a quantity sufficient to cover the affected area. The ratio of ground herbs to water will vary according to the herb being used. Add the water in small increments, just until the mixture is thick but not stiff.

Arrange a clean piece of gauze, muslin, linen, or white cotton sheeting on a clean, flat surface. The material should be large enough to cover the affected area completely. Spread the herbal paste over the cloth. Cleanse the affected area with hydrogen peroxide, and place the poultice over the area. Wrap a towel or plastic wrap around the poultice to prevent the soiling of clothes or sheets. Use a pin or other fastener to secure the poultice in place.

Preparing a Fresh Herb Poultice

If using fresh herbs for your poultice, place 2 ounces of the whole herb—about ½ cup—and 1 cup of water in a small saucepan. Simmer for 2 minutes. Do not drain.

Arrange a clean piece of gauze, muslin, linen, or white cotton sheeting on a clean, flat surface. The material should be large enough to cover the affected area completely. Pour the herbal solution over the cloth. Cleanse the affected body part with hydrogen peroxide, and place the poultice over the area. Wrap a towel or plastic wrap around the poultice to prevent the soiling of clothes or sheets. Hydrogen peroxide changes hair color so be careful when using it on the head. Use a pin or other fastener to secure the poultice in place.

Treatment Duration

Herbal poultices should be kept in place for one to twenty-four hours, as needed. During this period, you may experience a throbbing pain. When the pain subsides, you will know that the poultice has accomplished its task and should be removed. Apply fresh poultices as needed until the desired level of healing has been reached. Wash the skin thoroughly after each poultice is removed.

Types of Poultices

By making your poultice with the appropriate herbs or other substances, you will help ensure that the treatment is effective. Note that when the mixture used to make the poultice contains an irritant, such as mustard, it should not come into direct contact with the skin, but should be placed between pieces of cloth.

Herbs commonly used in poultices are listed below, along with the conditions for which they are appropriate.

- Dandelion, and yellow dock can be used to treat skin disorders such as acne, eczema, itchy or dry skin, psoriasis, and rashes. You can use one herb or combine two or three. The greatest benefit will be obtained from using all three.

- Elderberry can relieve pain associated with hemorrhoids.

- Fenugreek, flaxseed, and slippery elm can be combined to treat inflammation. Slippery elm can also be used alone for the inflamed gangrenous sores often associated with diabetes, and for leg ulcers. The use of a slippery elm poultice upon the appearance of sores and ulcers can help prevent gangrene. Slippery elm can also be combined with lobelia to treat abscesses, blood poisoning, and rheumatism.

  Caution: Lobelia is only to be taken under supervision of a health care professional as it is potentially toxic. People with high blood pressure, heart disease, liver disease, kidney disease, seizure disorders, or shortness of breath should not take lobelia. Pregnant and lactating women should avoid lobelia as well.

- Goldenseal is good for inflammations of all kinds.

  Caution: Do not take goldenseal internally on a daily basis for more than one week at a time. Do not use it during pregnancy or if you are breast-feeding, and use with caution if you are allergic to ragweed. If you have a history of cardiovascular disease, diabetes, or glaucoma, use it only under a doctor's supervision.

- Lobelia and charcoal (available in health food stores) can be combined and used to treat insect bites, bee stings, and almost all wounds. Lobelia can be combined with slippery elm to treat abscesses, blood poisoning, and rheumatism.

  Caution: Lobelia is only to be taken under supervision of a health care professional as it is potentially toxic. People with high blood pressure, heart disease, liver disease, kidney disease, seizure disorders, or shortness of breath should not take lobelia. Pregnant and lactating women should avoid lobelia as well.

- Mullein is used for inflamed hemorrhoids, lung disorders, mumps, tonsillitis, and sore throat. To make the poultice, mix 4 parts mullein with 1 part hot vinegar and 1 part water.

- Mustard is beneficial for inflammation, lung congestion, and swelling, and can help relax tense muscles. Because mustard is an irritant, place the mixture between two pieces of cloth, rather than placing it in direct contact with the skin.

- Onion is good for ear infections and for boils and sores that have difficulty healing. To make this poultice, place finely chopped onion between two pieces of cloth, rather than placing it in direct contact with the skin.

- Pau d'arco, ragwort, and wood sage can be combined and used to treat tumors and external cancers.

- Poke root is good for an inflamed or sore breast.

- Sage, like poke root, can help relieve breast inflammation and soreness.

  Caution: Do not use sage if you suffer from any type of seizure disorder, or are pregnant or nursing.

SITZ BATH

As a form of hydrotherapy—the use of hot and cold water, steam, and ice to restore and maintain health—the sitz bath increases blood flow to the pelvic and abdominal areas, and thus can help reduce inflammation and otherwise alleviate a variety of problems. Sitz baths (from the German *sitzen*, meaning "to sit") can use hot or cold water only, or can alternate heat and cold. Hot sitz baths are particularly helpful for such disorders as hemorrhoids, muscular disorders, painful ovaries and testicles, prostate problems, and uterine cramps. Cold sitz baths may be helpful in the treatment of constipation, impotence, inflammation, muscle disorders, and vaginal discharge. Alternating hot and cold sitz baths can help relieve abdominal disorders, blood poisoning, congestion, foot infection, headaches, muscle disorders, neuralgia, and swollen ankles. If your condition is severe, seek medical attention.

Procedure

To prepare a sitz bath, fill a tub or basin so that the water covers the hips and reaches the middle of the abdomen. If possible, place the water in a basin that will allow you to immerse just the pelvic and abdominal regions. Special sitz bath basins are available on the Internet or at local home health care retailers, the same ones who supply wheelchairs and other medical appliances. You can fill another basin with water that is a few degrees warmer, and immerse your feet in it while sitting in the sitz bath. If no suitable basins are available, place the sitz bathwater in a bathtub. You may wish to cover your body with a sheet or blanket to increase your comfort.

As discussed above, the temperature of the water should vary according to the type of illness you are treating. When using a hot sitz bath, the bathtub or basin should be filled with water of about 104°F to 106°F. *Make sure that the temperature of the water does not exceed 110°F.* This is often given as the recommended temperature, but we think it is a bit too hot. You might want to make the water 90°F to 100°F at the beginning of the bath and then gradually increase the temperature to about 106°F. As already mentioned, your feet can be immersed in slightly hotter water. You might also wish to apply a cold compress to your forehead, as the compress will make it easier for you to withstand the heat of the bath. (Make sure that the sitz bath, foot bath, and cold compress are all prepared ahead of time.)

Stay in the bath for twenty to forty minutes. After the moist heat of the bath has soothed the area being treated, you can further stimulate the body by taking a quick cold shower or simply splashing your body with cool water. Then towel yourself dry.

When using a cold sitz bath, fill the bathtub or basin with ice water. Stay in the cold bath for thirty to sixty seconds only. By no means should you stay in the water for more than sixty seconds, as this added time will provide no additional benefits, and may even be harmful. Then towel yourself dry.

When using alternating hot and cold baths, fill one basin with water of about 106°F, and a second basin with ice water. Immerse yourself first in the hot sitz bath, and remain there for three to four minutes. Then move to the cold sitz bath, and remain there for thirty to sixty seconds. Repeat this two to four times, and towel yourself dry.

A final word of caution: If you have any health-related problems or conditions, be sure to consult with your health care provider before using any type of sitz bath. Sitz baths are not appropriate for children.

STEAM INHALATION

Steam inhalation therapy is helpful for relieving the congestion of bronchitis, the common cold, and a variety of other respiratory and sinus conditions. Steam inhalation opens up congested sinuses and lung passages, allowing you to discharge mucus, breathe more easily, and heal faster. To make the steam, you may use water only, or you may add dried or fresh herbs or herbal oils to enhance the effects of the treatment.

Procedure

To provide the steam for the inhalation treatment, you may place the hot water in either a sink or a pot. In most cases, you can choose whichever method you find most convenient and comfortable. But if you are using fresh or dried herbs, you should use a glass or enameled pot, rather than the sink, to hold the water.

Using a Sink

If using your bathroom sink to hold the water, fill the sink with very hot water. If desired, add 2 to 5 drops of herbal oil. Keep the water hot and steaming during the treatment by allowing a small, continuous trickle of hot water to flow into the basin. (The overflow outlet of your sink should prevent the water from spilling over.) As the water becomes diluted, add a few more drops of the herbal oil as needed.

Hold your head over the sink, and breathe in the steam. Usually, five to ten minutes of steam should be sufficient to clear your congestion. In some cases, you may choose to extend the session. Keep your face far enough from the water so that the steam does not irritate or burn your skin. This is particularly important when a child is being treated, as a child's skin is more sensitive to heat.

Using a Pot

If you choose to use a pot to hold the water, and you are using fresh or dried herbs, be sure to select glass or enameled cookware only. This is important, as a metal pot can cause herbs to lose some of their medicinal properties. If you are using water only, any type of pot is appropriate.

Fill a wide pot with water, and bring it to a boil. Then remove the pot from the heat source, and place it on a heat-proof pad or cutting board at a convenient height for the inhalation treatment.

Once the water stops bubbling, if desired, add fresh or dried herbs or several drops of essential oil to the water. Allow the water to cool slightly. Then hold your head over the pot, and breathe in the steam. Capture the steam by draping a towel over your head and the pot, creating a "tent." Usually, five to ten minutes of steam should be sufficient to clear your congestion. In some cases, you may choose to extend the session. Keep your face far enough from the water so that the steam does not irritate or burn your skin. This is particularly important when a child is being treated, as a child's skin is more sensitive to heat.

Whichever method you use, after each steam inhalation treatment, take several deep, full breaths to clear lung congestion.

Repeat the therapy as needed.

Herbs

❑ Coltsfoot, comfrey, elecampane, eucalyptus, fennel, fenugreek, horseradish, licorice, lobelia, lungwort, mullein, pleurisy root, thyme, vervain, and yerba santa are expectorants that facilitate the excretion of mucus from the throat, lungs, and sinuses. These herbs may be used singly, in combination with one another, or in combination with the demulcent herbs listed below.

Cautions: Comfrey is recommended for external use only. Licorice root should not be used during pregnancy or nursing. It should not be used by persons with diabetes, glaucoma, heart disease, high blood pressure, or a history of stroke. Lobelia is only to be taken under supervision of a health care professional as it is potentially toxic. People with high blood pressure, heart disease, liver disease, kidney disease, seizure disorders, or shortness of breath should not take lobelia. Pregnant and lactating women should avoid lobelia as well.

❑ Burdock, chickweed, coltsfoot, Irish moss, lungwort, marshmallow, mullein, peach bark, and slippery elm are demulcents—substances that soften and relieve irritation of the mucous membranes. These herbs may be used singly, in combination with one another, or in combination with the expectorant herbs listed above.

SURGERY: PREPARING FOR AND RECOVERING FROM

Although few people enjoy the prospect of surgery, sometimes surgery is the best available means of improving the quality of life or extending life. Thousands of Americans face surgery each year, often with fear and doubt. Not knowing what is involved can mean putting yourself through far more discomfort than is necessary. Whether you are undergoing surgery for the first time or the tenth, understanding why you need it and knowing about the risks involved, available alternative treatments, and the aftereffects will help you make the right decision. Being educated about your illness will enable you to deal more effectively with the outcome.

After you have been informed of all your options and have decided that surgery is the only viable alternative, use the nutritional guidelines provided in the table below to prepare for the surgery. (For more information on making the decision to have surgery, *see* Recommendations in this section.) By taking these nutrients both before and after surgery, you will support the healing process and lessen postsurgical discomfort and pain. Make sure that your diet is well balanced and healthy. Remember that your general health *after* surgery partly depends on your general health *before* surgery. Do not take any supplements or drugs, even aspirin, that thin the blood. Fish oil containing eicosapentaenoic acid (EPA) and docosahexaenoic acid (DHA), feverfew, garlic, ginger, ginkgo biloba, kava kava, and vitamin E are among the supplements that should not be used prior to surgery.

Cautions: Do not use feverfew when pregnant or nursing. People who take prescription blood-thinning medications should consult a health care provider before using feverfew, as the combination can result in internal bleeding. Do not take ginkgo biloba if you have a bleeding disorder, or are scheduled for surgery or a dental procedure. Kava kava can cause drowsiness. It is not recommended for pregnant women or nursing mothers, and it should not be taken together with other substances that act on the central nervous system, such as alcohol, barbiturates, antidepressants, and antipsychotic drugs.

Unless otherwise stated, the dosages recommended here are for adults. For a child between the ages of twelve and seventeen, reduce the dose to three-quarters of the recommended amount. For a child between the ages of six and twelve, use one-half the recommended dose, and for a child under six, use one-quarter of the recommended amount. Be sure to discuss any supplements you are taking with your surgeon prior to surgery.

NUTRIENTS

SUPPLEMENT	SUGGESTED DOSAGE	COMMENTS
Acidophilus (Kyo-Dophilus from Wakunaga)	As directed on label 3 times daily.	To stabilize the intestinal bacterial flora if antibiotics are used. Use a high-potency powdered form.
Coenzyme Q$_{10}$	60 mg daily.	A free radical destroyer that improves tissue oxygenation.
Essential fatty acids (salmon oil or Ultimate Oil from Nature's Secret)	As directed on label.	Important for proper cell growth and healing of all tissues. *Caution:* Do not take for three weeks prior to surgery. Take this supplement after the surgery.
Free form amino acid	As directed on label.	Aids in collagen synthesis and wound healing. Is a readily available form of protein, easily absorbed by the body.
Garlic (Kyolic from Wakunaga)	2 capsules 3 times daily.	A natural antibiotic that enhances immune function.
L-cystine	500 mg twice daily.	Speeds healing of wounds.
L-glutamine	500 mg 3 times daily and at bedtime.	Speeds healing of wounds.
L-lysine	500 mg daily.	Speeds healing of wounds and aids collagen formation. *Caution:* Do not take lysine for longer than six months at a time.
Methylsulfonyl-methane (MSM)	As directed on label.	Good for pain and healing of tissues.
Multivitamin complex with vitamin A and mixed carotenoids including natural beta-carotene	As directed on label.	Provides necessary vitamins and minerals. Vitamin A is needed for protein utilization in tissue repair and is a free radical scavenger.
Pycnogenol or grape seed extract	As directed on label. As directed on label.	Surgery depletes the body of antioxidants. These are powerful antioxidants.
Vitamin C with bioflavonoids	6,000–10,000 mg daily, in divided doses.	Aids in tissue repair and healing of wounds. Vital in immune function. Use a buffered form.
Vitamin E	Beginning the day after surgery, take 200 IU daily. Do not take any vitamin E during the 2 weeks before surgery, as it thins the blood.	Improves circulation and repairs tissues. Use d-alpha-tocopherol form.
Vitamin E oil	After the stitches are removed and healing has begun, apply topically to the area of the incision 3 times daily.	Promotes healing and reduces scar formation. Purchase in oil form or cut open a capsule to release the oil.
Zinc plus calcium and magnesium and silica and vitamin D	50 mg daily. 1,500 mg daily. As directed on label. As directed on label. 400 IU daily.	Important for tissue repair. Look for a supplement that contains all of these nutrients.

Herbs

❏ Herbal teas are highly recommended before and after surgery. Try the following teas:

- Alfalfa, dandelion, and nettle are high in vitamins and minerals, and can also increase the appetite. Alfalfa is also a good source of iron.

- Bromelain and turmeric (curcumin) have potent anti-inflammatory properties.

- Burdock root and red clover aid in cleansing the blood and the liver.

- Echinacea enhances immune system function.

    Caution: Do not take echinacea for longer than three months. It should not be used by people who are allergic to ragweed.

- Goldenseal is a natural antibiotic and helps to prevent infection.

Caution: Do not take goldenseal internally on a daily basis for more than one week at a time. Do not use it during pregnancy or if you are breast-feeding, and use with caution if you are allergic to ragweed. If you have a history of cardiovascular disease, diabetes, or glaucoma, use it only under a doctor's supervision.

- Green tea contains powerful antioxidants that aid in the healing process.

  Caution: Green tea contains vitamin K, which can make anticoagulant medications less effective. Consult your health care professional if you are using them. The caffeine in green tea could cause insomnia, anxiety, upset stomach, nausea, or diarrhea.

- Kelp, reishi, and St. John's wort may help protect against the adverse effects of X-ray radiation.

  Caution: St. John's wort may cause increased sensitivity to sunlight. It may also produce anxiety, gastrointestinal symptoms, and headaches. It can interact with some drugs including antidepressants, birth control pills, and anticoagulants.

- Milk thistle protects the liver from the toxic buildup of drugs and chemicals resulting from surgical procedures.

- Pau d'arco is a natural antibacterial herb. It enhances healing and cleanses the blood.

- Rose hips are a good source of vitamin C and enhance healing.

Recommendations

❑ Consult with your physician about minimally invasive surgery, also called laparoscopic, "keyhole," and "Band-Aid" surgery. This type of procedure—involving one or more small incisions rather than a large one—does less damage to the skin, muscles, and nerves than does conventional "open" surgery. It also involves a shorter hospital stay and less recovery time. Be aware that such procedures can be used for certain surgeries only. It is more difficult to perform these on overweight people, so if you are overweight, you may not have this option.

❑ If you are overweight and have sufficient time to diet before surgery, try to gradually lose the extra weight. Studies show that excess weight can increase both the difficulty of performing surgery and the length of the recovery time. It has also been linked to an increased likelihood of postoperative infection.

❑ If you smoke, stop. Smoking delays healing and interferes with the actions of certain drugs.

❑ Make sure your doctor and those who will care for you are aware of any allergies you have to drugs, chemicals, or foods.

❑ Ask your surgeon if there is anything that you can do to prepare for the surgery. In addition to the surgeon's recommendations, avoid taking vitamin E supplements, aspirin, all compounds containing aspirin, and fish oil for two weeks prior to surgery. These substances thin the blood.

❑ Make sure your doctor and those who will care for you are aware of any supplements and medications—including natural medicines—you take regularly.

❑ Because blood transfusions are sometimes required during surgery, explore the possibility of storing your own blood for use during the operation. By using your own blood, you will avoid the risk of contracting hepatitis or another bloodborne disease.

❑ Many operations require that you be shaved. The infection rate is lower for patients who are shaved the day of surgery when compared with those who are shaved the night before.

❑ Add fiber to your diet. It ensures better intestinal tract function.

❑ Keep a positive attitude about your surgery, and look forward to getting out of bed and back to normal as soon as possible. The sooner you get out of bed, the better your chances of avoiding postoperative infection.

The practice of ordering routine laboratory tests before admission for surgery is commonplace in most hospitals. Many doctors believe that urinalysis, chest X-rays, or complete blood counts, for example, can identify potential problems that might complicate the surgery if not detected and treated early. Discuss with your doctor the necessity of having certain tests performed prior to surgery.

❑ Before deciding to have surgery, ask your physician the following types of questions:

- Why do I need the operation?

- Are there alternatives to surgery?

- What are the benefits of having the operation?

- What are the risks of having the operation?

- What if I do not have this operation?

- What is your experience in performing this surgery?

- What has been your complication rate?

- What kind of anesthesia will I need?

- How will the surgery improve my quality of life and/or my chances for survival?

- Are there other forms of treatment that might be used instead of surgery?

- What percentage of the operations performed of this type are successful?

- What physical changes will result from this operation, and what improvements can I expect?

- How long is the recovery period?

- What is the cost of the operation?

❑ Ask about the potential risks and side effects of having anesthesia. Be sure to mention any medical problems you have, including allergies, and any medications you have been taking, since they may affect your response to the anesthesia. Be sure to tell your anesthesiologist if you smoke.

❑ After surgery, try to consume at least ten cups of liquids each day, including distilled water, herbal teas, juices, and protein drinks. The appetite is often poor after surgery, and large meals can be overwhelming. Try eating five to seven small, light, nutritious meals a day. Some people prefer liquids after surgery. You can make a healthy whey protein shake with milk or soymilk, or if you don't feel up to it, buy some prepared drinks at the drugstore.

❑ After surgery, exercise caution when engaging in strenuous activity such as lifting. Most doctors advise patients to avoid lifting anything in excess of ten pounds for two weeks after surgery. Ask your doctor when you can begin light exercise, which has been shown to aid circulation and speed physical recovery. Also ask if there are any specific exercises that can aid your recovery.

❑ After surgery, the homeopathic remedy *Arnica montana* is good for reducing swelling and promoting healing.

Considerations

❑ After major surgery, people generally experience a rapid breakdown of skeletal muscle, which increases any feelings of weakness. When you get home, the best way to restore the muscles and regain strength is eating adequate protein and, later, engaging in activities and exercise. In studies in which the amino acid glutamine was added to postsurgical intravenous solutions, muscle breakdown rates were greatly diminished.

❑ Some foods interfere with the actions of certain medications. Milk, dairy products, and iron supplements may interfere with some forms of antibiotics. Acidic fruits, such as oranges, pineapples, and grapefruits, could inhibit the action of penicillin and aspirin. *See* Substances That Rob the Body of Nutrients on page 391 for a list of the nutrients that are lost with the use of different drugs.

❑ Postsurgical depression is not uncommon. A healthy dietary program can help fight depression.

❑ It takes the body a few weeks to recover from the trauma of surgery. During this period, hormonal imbalances are corrected, and the rate of metabolism is adjusted. Many incisions close within two days and heal within a week to the point that the skin will hold together under normal stress and body movement. However, you should obtain your doctor's approval before engaging in any exercise or lifting anything over ten pounds in weight.

THERAPEUTIC LIQUIDS

The benefits of vegetables and grains are discussed throughout this book. This section offers two recipes that provide these benefits in broths that have healing properties.

The first of the broths derives its healthful properties—including its high potassium content—from potatoes and other vegetables. When purchasing potatoes, choose ones that do not have a green tint. The chemical solanine, which gives the potato its green cast, can interfere with nerve impulses and cause diarrhea, vomiting, and abdominal pain. Use Potato Peeling Broth as a nutritious drink when fasting. This broth is also good for heart disorders.

The second broth—barley water—has healing and fortifying properties, and is useful during convalescence from many different illnesses. You can also add powdered slippery elm bark to the water to make a drink that is not only nourishing, but also soothing to the throat and digestive tract.

Many other therapeutic liquids can also be made from vegetables and grains, as well as from fruits. (To learn about nutritious juices, *see* JUICING in Part Three.) These broths should not be your only source of nutrition, but a supplement to a healthy diet.

Potato Peeling Broth

---

3 potatoes
1 carrot, sliced
1 celery stalk, sliced
2 quarts steam-distilled water
1 onion, sliced, and/or 3 cloves garlic, peeled

1. Scrub the potatoes well and cut out any eyes.

2. Cut the potatoes in half. Cut the peel from the potatoes, making sure to keep about ½ inch of potato with the peel. Set aside the potato centers for another use.

3. Place the potato peelings, carrot, and celery in a large pot. Cover with the water. Add the onion and/or garlic to taste and boil for about 30 minutes.

4. Cool the broth. Strain out and discard the vegetables and serve the broth as desired.

Barley Water

---

1 cup barley
3 quarts steam-distilled water

1. Place the barley and the water in a large pot and boil for about 3 hours.

2. Cool the broth. Strain out and discard the barley and serve the broth as desired.

TRANSCUTANEOUS ELECTRICAL NERVE STIMULATION (TENS)

See under TENS UNIT THERAPY in PAIN CONTROL

YOGA

Yoga is not new; it was developed in India more than 5,000 years ago, and was used to unite the body, mind, and spirit. Often, people think of yoga as physical exercise. However, the progress of learning to still the mind and unify consciousness is also important in yoga exercises. It can be difficult to turn off the voices in your head, especially when your body is motionless.

Hatha is a Sanskrit word meaning "willful" and *yoga* is translated as "union" or "communion." This is understood as meditation in action. *Hatha yoga* is a term familiar to many who practice yoga, but it is not actually a particular style of yoga.

There are many different styles of yoga to choose from. Some are softer and easier to do, and some are strenuous and hard to do. If you are a beginner, it is probably best to try the easier forms, and it is necessary to work with a teacher. The following are a few approaches to choose from:

- *Ananda yoga* will appeal to the beginner who desires to cultivate spirituality and learn how to meditate. Ananda is a slower-paced style.

- *Ashtanga yoga* becomes more strenuous as the student progresses. The postures are linked together in a continuous flow, performed while practicing ujjayi breathing (a breath technique employed in a variety of Hindu and Taoist yoga practices). This builds stamina, strength, and flexibility. It is challenging, and not for the beginner.

- *Bikram yoga* is also not for the beginner. It requires a great deal of work. It is a sequential series of twenty-six postures done in a continuous flow. The room this practice is done in is heated to 100 degrees or more to promote sweating that helps cleanse the body of toxins.

- *Kundalini* and *tantra yoga* focus on activating the energy centers in the body called *chakras*. The chakras are seven cores of energy in the body. This type of yoga involves exploring the core of the body rather than the limbs—moving to the center and seeing the body as rivers of energy.

- *Raja yoga* concentrates more on meditation and less on strength and is good for the beginner.

- *Sivananda yoga* is a holistic approach. There are five basic principles that unite the body, mind (intellect), spirit, and heart. They include proper breathing (pranayama), a vegetarian diet, proper relaxation (savasana), study of the Vedic scriptures, and meditation.

- *Tivamukti yoga* focuses on spiritual teachings, postures, chanting, meditation, music, and readings, and are all incorporated into the class.

- There are many other types of yoga, including kripalu yoga, integral yoga, and phoenix rising yoga therapy. There are many unique techniques and teaching methods. The goals, however, are the same: to teach a greater understanding and awareness of the body; to free oneself from negative thoughts that drain one's energies; and to strengthen mental and spiritual balance. Yoga postures remove obstructions from the body to enhance energy and well-being and achieve inner peace.

Appendix

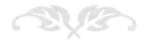

Introduction

As we know, many of our favorite foods contain incredible health benefits, and the scientific community continues to reinforce this fact. With a plethora of recent research, the specific healing properties of acai, pecans, almonds, grapes, cranberries, blueberries, kiwi, pomegranates, mushrooms, broccoli, cabbage, cinnamon, and a whole host of other popular foods have been revealed not just as anecdotal chatter but rather as documented medical facts.

According to a 2001 study published in the *Journal of Nutrition*, eating a handful of pecans daily reduces cholesterol and may be a viable alternative to using cholesterol-reducing drugs. In another study, doctors learned that niacin, or vitamin B_3, may boost levels of "good" cholesterol (HDL) when used in conjunction with a statin drug called simvastatin, which lowers levels of "bad" cholesterol (LDL). Some antioxidants also taken with vitamin B_3 in this study were found to have blunted niacin's effect, so discuss any supplementation you may be taking with your doctor before adding niacin to your medication regimen.

Among the more notable discoveries is the link between omega-3 fatty acids and cardiovascular health. Long thought to protect against heart disease, foods containing eiscosapentaenoic acid (EPA) and docosahexaenoic acid (DHA) were shown to reduce the risk of dying from a heart attack or dying from anything else. These nutrients are essential for life and are often lacking in the diet. The American Heart Association recommends eating fish at least twice a week. In addition, taking 1 gram of fish oil a day is a good idea. Fish and fish oil supplements help maintain proper blood flow and blood pressure, which is why it is particularly important for persons who are overweight or who have diabetes to include both in their diet because their blood tends to be too thick. However, don't overdo it—taking too many fish oil capsules could potentially lead to blood clotting problems.

Research has also led doctors to advise patients to drink cranberry juice to prevent and treat minor urinary tract infections. Of course, the antioxidants and other phytonutrients in cranberries may also help protect against heart disease, cancer, and other diseases. And the studies keep on coming. Blueberries have been shown to help improve memory, unclog arteries, enhance vision, strengthen blood vessels, stop urinary tract infections, promote weight control, and may reverse symptoms of aging.

Vegetables get in on the act as well. Broccoli contains high levels of vitamin C and beta-carotene—powerful antioxidants that fight age- and disease-causing free radicals. Broccoli is also high in fiber, which is important for bowel health and blood sugar control. This one vegetable contains as much calcium as dairy products and a high level of sulforaphane, which has been found (in laboratory studies) to reduce the number, size, and reproduction of malignant tumors, as well as delay their onset.

As science continues to confirm the health benefits of a fresh, natural diet, we've also learned that the way we eat these foods affects their benefits. The idea of food synergy is one that is not always talked about but is an important concept. For example, natural flavonoids found in certain foods can allow greater protection against cancer when ingested together than when taken individually. One specific instance occurs when you take the compound sulforaphane and the flavonoid polyphenol apigenin at the same time. When taken together, they are twelve times stronger than when ingested alone. Polyphenol apigenin can be found in fruits and vegetables such as apples, cherries, grapes, tomatoes, beans, broccoli sprouts, celery, leeks, onions, and parsley. Tea and wine also contain this antioxidant. You'll find sulforaphane in brassica vegetables such as broccoli, spinach, cabbage, cauliflower, Brussels sprouts, kale, collard greens, bok choy, and kohlrabi. Sulforaphane also positively interacts with selenium, a mineral that vegetables absorb through the soil. Because it can be hard to know how much selenium is present in store-bought vegetables, taking a supplement along with foods high in sulforaphane may be the best way to use this synergy to your advantage. Be sure not to exceed the upper limit of safety for selenium, which is 400 micrograms for those over fourteen years of age. Too much selenium can be harmful.

Many supplements are now available in liquid form. This delivery system has its advantages and disadvantages. Liquids are easy to swallow and offer quick absorption. However, they must be formulated properly so that they will remain stable in liquid form. Liquid concentrates require careful skill when manufactured, and may have preservatives added to keep them fresh. They should be refrigerated after opening. Liquid extracts are often very powerful, and small dosages are typically indicated.

You can learn more about liquid supplements, as well as about food synergy, nutritional practices, and so much more in the glossary, resources, and suggested reading that follow.

GLOSSARY

absorption. Nutritionally, the process by which nutrients are absorbed through the intestinal tract into the bloodstream to be used by the body. If nutrients are not properly absorbed, nutritional deficiencies can result.

acetic acid. A weak inorganic acid that is the active ingredient in vinegar; a 4 to 5 percent solution of acetic acid in water makes vinegar.

acid. Any of a class of compounds that share certain basic chemical characteristics. Acids have low pH (below 7), are usually sour to the taste, and, in their pure form, are often corrosive. They can be either organic or inorganic compounds. Some foods produce acids in the body (meat, dairy, grains) and some reduce acid (fruits, vegetables). Eating both assures a balance in the blood.

acidosis. A condition characterized by excessive acidity of bodily fluids.

acute illness. An illness that comes on quickly and may cause relatively severe symptoms, but is of limited duration.

adaptogen. A term for a substance, usually an herb, that produces suitable adjustments in the body. Adaptogens tend to normalize body functions, and when the job is completed, they are eliminated or incorporated into the body without side effects. Some beneficial adaptogens include garlic, ginseng, echinacea, ginkgo, goldenseal, and pau d'arco.

adrenal gland. One of a pair of glands situated atop the kidneys. The adrenal glands are the source of the stress hormones epinephrine (adrenaline) and cortisol, among others.

allergen. A substance that provokes an allergic response.

allergy. An inappropriate response by the immune system to a normally harmless substance. Allergies can affect any of the body's tissues. Hay fever is a common type of allergy.

allyl sulfides. Phytochemicals found in leeks, onions, garlic, and chives that act to detoxify the body.

alternative therapy. The treatment of disease by means other than conventional medical, pharmacological, and surgical techniques.

amino acid. Any of twenty-two nitrogen-containing organic acids from which proteins are made.

anabolic compound. A substance that allows the conversion of simple nutritive materials into complex materials that are part of living tissue during the constructive phase of metabolism.

analgesic. Tending to relieve pain, or a substance that relieves pain.

anemia. A deficiency in the blood's ability to carry oxygen to the body tissues.

anesthetic. Causing loss of sensation, or a substance that causes the loss of sensation, especially the ability to feel pain.

angina pectoris. A syndrome of chest pain from heart disease with sensations of suffocation, typically brought on by exertion, and may be relieved by rest. In some cases medical attention is needed.

antacid. A substance that neutralizes acid in the stomach, esophagus, or the first part of the duodenum.

antibiotic. Tending to destroy or inhibit the growth of microorganisms, especially bacteria.

antibody. A protein molecule made by the immune system that is designed to intercept and neutralize a specific invading organism or other foreign substance.

antigen. A substance that can elicit the formation of an antibody when introduced into the body.

antihistamine. A substance that interferes with the action of histamines by binding to histamine receptors in various body tissues (*see* histamine).

antioxidant. A substance that blocks or inhibits destructive oxidation reactions. Examples include vitamins C and E, the minerals selenium and germanium, the enzymes catalase and superoxide dismutase (SOD), coenzyme Q_{10}, and some amino acids.

antivenin. A serum that contains antitoxin specific for an animal or insect venom.

arrhythmia. *See* cardiac arrhythmia.

arteriosclerosis. A circulatory disorder characterized by a thickening and stiffening of the walls of large and medium-sized arteries, which impedes circulation.

artery. A blood vessel through which blood is pumped from the heart to all the organs, glands, and other tissues of the body.

ascorbate. A mineral salt of vitamin C. Taken as nutritional supplements, ascorbates are less acidic (and therefore less irritating) than pure ascorbic acid and also provide for better absorption of both the vitamin C and the mineral.

ascorbic acid. The organic acid more commonly known as vitamin C.

atherosclerosis. The most common type of arteriosclerosis, caused by the accumulation of fatty deposits in the inner linings of the arteries.

aura. A subjective sensation that precedes an attack of migraine or epilepsy. With epilepsy, it may precede the actual attack by hours or seconds, and may be of a psychic nature or sensory with olfactory, visual, auditory, or taste hallucinations. In a migraine attack, the aura immediately precedes the attack and primarily consists of visual sensory phenomena.

autoimmune disorder. Any condition in which the immune system reacts inappropriately to the body's own tissues and attacks them, causing damage and/or interfering with normal functioning. Examples include Bright's disease, type 1 diabetes, multiple sclerosis, rheumatoid arthritis, and systemic lupus erythematosus.

autologous transfusion. A transfusion of one's own blood that has been collected and kept for later use.

automatism. Automatic behavior or actions without conscious knowledge or control. Certain types of epileptic seizure may include automatisms. These may be complicated actions completed totally without the subject's control, and afterwards there will be no memory of having done them.

bacteria. Single-celled microorganisms. Some bacteria can cause disease; other ("friendly") bacteria are normally present in the body and perform such useful functions as aiding digestion and protecting the body from harmful invading organisms.

benign. Literally, "harmless." Used to refer to cells, especially cells growing in inappropriate locations that are not malignant (cancerous).

beta-carotene. A substance the body uses to make vitamin A.

bilary. Pertaining to bile or the bile duct.

bile. A bitter, yellowish substance that is released by the liver into the intestines for the digestion of fats.

biofeedback. A technique for helping an individual to become conscious of usually unconscious body processes, such as heartbeat or body temperature, so that he or she can gain some measure of control over them, and thereby learn to manage the effects of various disorders, including acute back pain, migraines, and Raynaud's disease.

bioflavonoid. Any of a group of biologically active flavonoids. They are essential for the stability and absorption of vitamin C. Although they are not technically vitamins, they are sometimes referred to as vitamin P.

bioidentical hormones. Custom-mixed female formulas containing various hormones that are chemically identical to those made naturally by the body.

biopsy. Excision of tissue from a living being for diagnosis.

biotin. A component of the B-vitamin complex formerly designated vitamin H. This is a water-soluble substance important in the metabolism of fats and carbohydrates. Present in many foods, it is particularly found in liver, kidney, milk, egg yolks, and yeast.

blood count. A basic diagnostic test in which a sample of blood is examined and the number of red blood cells, white blood cells, and platelets determined; or the results of such a test. It is sometimes referred to as CBC (complete blood count).

blood sugar. The glucose (a form of sugar) present in the blood.

blood-brain barrier. A mechanism involving the capillaries and certain other cells of the brain that keeps many substances, especially water-based substances, from passing out of the blood vessels to be absorbed by the brain tissue.

body mass index (BMI). A figure that represents the percentage of your body weight that is due to fat. It is determined from a calculation using body weight and height.

bowel tolerance. The amount of any substance the body can tolerate before it results in diarrhea.

BRCA1 and BRCA2 genes. Human genes that belong to a class of genes known as tumor suppressors. In normal cells they help ensure the stability of the cell's genetic material (DNA) and help prevent uncontrolled cell growth. Mutation of these genes has been linked to the development of hereditary breast and ovarian cancer.

bronchi. The two main branches of the trachea (windpipe) that lead to the lungs.

Candida albicans. A type of fungus normally present at some level in the body. If it is present in overabundance, it causes yeast infection. Known as candida.

capillaries. Tiny blood vessels (their walls are about one cell thick) that allow the exchange of nutrients and wastes between the bloodstream and the body's cells.

carbohydrate. Any one of many organic substances, almost all of them of plant origin, that are composed of carbon, hydrogen, and oxygen, and serve as one of the major sources of energy in the diet along with fats.

carcinogen. An agent that is capable of inducing cancerous changes in cells and/or tissues.

cardiac. Pertaining to the heart.

cardiac arrhythmia. An abnormal heart rate or rhythm.

carotene. A yellow to orange pigment that is converted into vitamin A in the body. There are several different forms, including alpha-, beta-, and gamma-carotene.

carotenoids. A group of phytochemicals that act as antioxidants and includes the carotenes as well as some other substances.

CAT scan. Computerized axial tomography scan. A computerized X-ray scanning procedure used to create a three-dimensional picture of the body, or part of the body, for the purpose of detecting abnormalities.

catatonia. A state in which an individual becomes unresponsive; a stupor.

cauterization. A technique used to stop bleeding that involves applying electrical current, a laser beam, or a chemical such as silver nitrate directly to a broken blood vessel.

cell. A very small but complex organic unit consisting of a nucleus, cytoplasm, and a cell membrane. All living tissues are composed of cells.

cellulose. An indigestible carbohydrate found in the outer layers of fruits and vegetables.

cerebral. Pertaining to the brain.

chancroid. A highly infectious sexually transmitted disease characterized by the presence of genital ulcers.

chelation. A chemical process by which a larger molecule or group of molecules surrounds or encloses a mineral atom.

chelation therapy. The introduction of certain substances into the body so that they will chelate, and then remove, foreign substances such as lead, cadmium, arsenic, and other heavy metals. Chelation therapy can also be used to reduce or remove calcium-based plaque from the linings of the blood vessels, easing the flow of blood to vital organs and tissues.

chemotherapy. Treatment of disease by the use of chemicals (such as drugs), especially the use of chemical treatments to combat cancer.

chiropractic. A system of healing based on the belief that many disorders result from misalignments (called subluxations) of the spinal vertebrae and other joints. Chiropractors primarily treat illness by using physical manipulation techniques to bring the body into proper alignment and thus restore normal health and functioning.

chlorophyll. The pigment responsible for the green color of plant tissues. It can be taken in supplement form as a limited source of magnesium and some trace elements.

cholesterol. A crystalline substance that is soluble in fats and that is produced by all vertebrates. It is a necessary constituent of cell membranes and facilitates the transport and absorption of fatty acids. Excess cholesterol, however, is a potential threat to health.

chromosome. Any of the threadlike strands of DNA in the nuclei of all living cells that carry genetic information. There are normally forty-six chromosomes (twenty-three pairs) in all human cells, with the exception of egg and sperm cells.

chronic illness. A disorder that persists or recurs over an extended period, often for life. Chronic illnesses can be as relatively benign as hay fever or as serious as multiple sclerosis.

citric acid. An organic acid found in citrus fruits. Often used to lower the pH of cosmetic products to bring them closer to the natural pH of the skin.

clotting factor. One of several substances, especially vitamin K, that are present in the bloodstream and are important in the process of blood clotting.

cocarcinogen. An agent that acts with another agent to cause cancer.

coenzyme. A molecule that works with an enzyme to enable the enzyme to perform its function in the body. Coenzymes are necessary in the utilization of vitamins and minerals.

cold-pressed. A term used to describe food oils that are extracted without the use of heat in order to preserve nutrients and flavor.

colic. Sharp abdominal pains that result from spasm or obstruction of certain organs or structures, especially the intestines, uterus, or bile ducts.

colonoscope. An instrument for examining the colon.

colonoscopy. A procedure in which a long flexible tube (a colonoscope) is threaded up through the rectum for the purpose of examining the entire colon and rectum and, if there is an abnormality, taking a biopsy or removing it. The procedure requires a thorough bowel cleansing. In some cases, surgery is required if the mass is too big.

complete protein. A source of dietary protein that contains a full complement of the eight essential amino acids and in the right ratios.

complex carbohydrate. A type of carbohydrate that, owing to its chemical structure, releases its sugar into the body relatively slowly and also provides fiber. The carbohydrates in starches and fiber are complex carbohydrates. Also called *polysaccharides.*

complication. A secondary infection, reaction, or other negative event that makes recovery from illness more difficult and/or longer.

congenital. Present from birth, but not necessarily inherited.

contraceptive. Tending to prevent conception, or a device, substance, or method used to prevent pregnancy.

contracture. Fibrosis of connective tissue in skin, fascia, muscle, or joint that prevents normal mobility.

contusion. A bruise; an injury in which the skin is not broken.

convulsion. A seizure characterized by intense, uncontrollable contraction of the voluntary muscles that results from abnormal cerebral stimulation.

coryza. The nasal symptoms of the common cold.

cradle cap. A type of seborrheic dermatitis found on infants, usually appearing on the scalp, face, and head, and consisting of thick, yellowish, crusted lesions. Scaling or fissuring often appears behind the ears and on the face.

cruciferous. Literally, "cross-shaped." A term used to refer to a group of vegetables—including broccoli, Brussels sprouts, cabbage, cauliflower, turnips, and rutabagas—that have characteristic cross-shaped blossoms and that contain substances that may help to prevent colon cancer.

cytokines. Protein substances that are made by cells of the immune system. Some cytokines can boost the immune response and others can suppress it.

cystoscope. Instrument used to examine the inside of the bladder.

daily value. DVs are made up of two sets of references: Daily Reference Values (DRVs) and Reference Daily Intakes (RDIs). Daily Value (DV) began to appear on FDA-regulated product labels in 1994. Today DVs appear on all packaged foods and dietary supplement labels for all essential nutrients. Non-essential compounds like herbs do not have corresponding DV percent.

dehydroepiandrosterone (DHEA). It is produced by the adrenal glands and is the most abundant hormone found in the bloodstream. DHEA serves as precursor to male and female sex hormones (androgens and estrogens).

dementia. A permanent acquired impairment of intellectual function that results in a marked decline in memory, language ability, personality, spatial skills, and/or cognition (orientation, perception, reasoning, abstract thinking, and calculation). Dementia may be transient, but is usually permanent, and can result from many different causes.

demulcent. Soothing, especially to mucous membranes.

dermis. The layer of skin that lies underneath the epidermis. Blood and lymphatic vessels and the glands that secrete perspiration and sebum are all found in the dermis.

detoxification. The process of reducing the buildup of various poisonous substances in the body. The liver is the major organ of the body involved with this process.

dietary reference intakes (DRIs). These can be used for planning and assessing diets for healthy people. The amounts of these nutrients defined by the DRI give us about twice the amount needed, so there is hardly any risk of frank vitamin deficiency such as beriberi, rickets, scurvy, and night blindness. What they do not account for are the amounts needed to maintain maximum health, rather than borderline health. Moreover, they are not good at providing an individual's need but rather population norms.

disorientation. The loss of a normal relationship to one's surroundings; the inability to comprehend time, people, and place.

dithiolthiones. Phytochemicals found in broccoli that increase levels of enzymes that help protect against certain types of cancer.

diuretic. Tending to increase urine flow, or a substance that promotes the excretion of fluids.

DNA. Deoxyribonucleic acid. Substance in the cell nucleus that genetically contains the cell's genetic blueprint and determines the type of life form into which a cell will develop.

docosahexaenoic acid (DHA). A fatty acid found in the meat of cold-water fish, including mackerel, herring, tuna, halibut, salmon, cod liver, whale blubber, and seal blubber. It has recently been shown to be effective at promoting brain health during infancy and is now found in many infant formulas.

dosha. Any of the three types of vital energy in Ayurvedic medicine. It is the balance between the doshas that determines health.

echocardiogram. A diagnostic test that uses ultrasound to detect structural and functional abnormalities of the heart.

edema. Retention of fluid and salt in the tissues that results in swelling.

EDTA. Ethylenediaminetetraacetic acid. An organic molecule used in chelation therapy.

EEG. Electroencephalogram. A test used to measure brain wave activity.

eicosapentaenoic acid (EPA). One of several omega-3 fatty acids used by the body. It is found in cold-water fatty fish and in fish oil supplements, along with docosahexaenoic acid (DHA). It serves as a precursor of bioactive compounds like prostaglandins.

EKC (or ECG). Electrocardiogram. A test that monitors heart function by tracing the conduction of electrical impulses associated with heart activity.

elastin. A protein that gives tissue its elasticity.

electrolyte. Soluble salts dissolved in the body's fluids. Electrolytes are the form in which most minerals circulate in the body. They are so named because they are capable of conducting electrical impulses.

ELISA. Enzyme-linked immunoadsorbent assay. A test that determines the presence of a particular protein, such as an antibody, by detecting the presence of an enzyme that is linked to that protein.

ellagic acid. A phytochemical found in strawberries and grapes that helps rid the body of free radicals.

embolus. A loose particle of tissue, a blood clot, or a tiny air bubble that travels through the bloodstream and, if it lodges in a narrowed portion of a blood vessel, can block blood flow.

emulsion. A combination of two liquids that do not mix with each other, such as oil and water; one substance is broken into tiny droplets and is suspended within the other. Emulsification is the first step in the digestion of fats.

endemic. Native to or prevalent in a particular geographic region. Often used to describe diseases.

endocrine system. The system of glands that secrete hormones into the bloodstream. Endocrine glands include the pituitary, thyroid, thymus, and adrenal glands, as well as the pancreas, ovaries, and testes.

endorphin. One of a number of natural hormonelike substances found primarily in the brain. One function of endorphins is to suppress the sensation of pain, which they do by binding to opiate receptors in the brain.

endoscope. Instrument for examining the interior of the intestine.

enteric. Pertaining to the small intestines.

enzyme. One of many specific protein catalysts that initiate or speed chemical reactions in the body without being consumed.

epidemic. An extensive outbreak of a disease, or a disease occurring with an unusually high incidence at certain times and places.

epidermis. The outer layer of the skin.

Epstein-Barr virus (EBV). A virus that causes infectious mononucleosis in 35 to 50 percent of patients and that may cause other health problems as well.

erythema. Reddening, especially of the skin.

essential. A term for nutrients needed for building and repair that cannot be manufactured by the body, and that therefore must be supplied in the diet. At present, there are some forty-two known essential nutrients.

essential fatty acids (EFAs). A term sometimes used to refer to three unsaturated fatty acids—arachidonic acid, linoleic acid, and linolenic acid—that are essential for health and cannot be manufactured by the body.

exacerbation. Aggravation of symptoms or an increase in the severity of a disease.

excision. Surgical cutting away and/or removal of tissue.

fat-soluble. Capable of dissolving in the same organic solvents as fats and oils.

fatty acid. Any one of many organic acids from which fats and oils are made.

FBS. Fasting blood sugar. The level of glucose present in a blood sample drawn at least eight hours after the last meal.

fiber. The indigestible portion of plant matter. Fiber is an important component of a healthy diet because it is capable of binding to toxins and escorting them out of the body. Fiber is often classified into two categories: those that don't dissolve in water (insoluble fiber) and those that do (soluble fiber).

flatulence. Excessive amounts of gas in the stomach or other parts of the digestive tract.

flavonoid. Any of a large group of crystalline compounds found in plants. Also called bioflavonoid.

free radical. An atom or group of atoms that is highly chemically reactive because it has at least one unpaired electron. Because they join so readily with other compounds, free radicals can attack cells and can cause a lot of damage in the body. Free radicals form in heated fats and oils, and as a result of exposure to atmospheric radiation and environmental pollutants, among other things.

free radical scavenger. A substance that removes or destroys free radicals.

fungus. One of a class of organisms that includes yeasts, mold, and mushrooms. A number of fungal species, such as *Candida albicans*, are capable of causing severe disease in immunocompromised hosts.

gastritis. Inflammation of the stomach lining.

gastroenteritis. Inflammation of the mucous lining of the stomach and the intestines.

gastrointestinal. Pertaining to the stomach, small and large intestines, colon, rectum, liver, pancreas, and gallbladder.

genetic. Inherited.

genistein. An isoflavone (a type of phytochemical) found in alfalfa sprouts, broccoli, cabbage, collard greens, kale, and soybeans. It aids with symptoms of perimenopause and may prevent some cancers.

GERD. Gastroesophageal reflux disease. Medical term for a syndrome characterized by frequent indigestion or heartburn.

gingivitis. Inflammation of the gums surrounding the teeth.

gland. An organ or tissue that secretes a substance(s) for use elsewhere in the body rather than for its own functioning.

globulin. A type of protein found in the blood. Certain globulins contain disease-fighting antibodies.

glucose. A simple sugar that is the principal source of energy for red blood cells and the brain.

gluten. A protein found in many grains, including wheat, rye, barley, and oats.

glycemic index. A numerical system of measuring how much of a rise in circulating blood sugar a carbohydrate triggers—the higher the number, the greater the blood sugar response. Only carbohydrate-containing foods have significant impact on blood sugar levels.

glycogen. A polysaccharide (complex carbohydrate) that is the main form in which glucose is stored in the body, primarily in the liver and muscles. It is converted back into glucose as needed to supply energy.

good manufacturing practices (GMP). FDA rules that ensure that all supplements are manufactured in a uniform way and that what appears on the label is what is in the product. This helps to assure safety.

hair analysis. A method of determining the levels of minerals, including both toxic metals and essential minerals, in the body by measuring the concentrations of those minerals in the hair. Unlike mineral levels in the blood, those in the hair reflect the person's status over several preceding months.

HDL cholesterol. A type of lipoprotein (a protein molecule that transports cholesterol in the bloodstream) that is commonly referred to as "good cholesterol" because high levels normally indicate a low risk for heart disease.

heavy metal. A metallic element whose specific gravity (a measurement of mass as compared with the mass of water or hydrogen) is greater than 5.0. Some heavy metals, such as arsenic, cadmium, lead, and mercury, are extremely toxic.

hematocrit. The percentage of blood (by volume) that is composed of red blood cells.

hematoma. A bulge or swelling that is filled with blood. Hematomas are usually the result of a blunt injury or other trauma that causes a blood vessel under the skin to break.

hemicellulose. An indigestible carbohydrate resembling cellulose, found in plant cell walls, that absorbs water.

hemoglobin. The iron-containing red pigment in the blood that is responsible for the transport of oxygen.

hemorrhage. Profuse or abnormal bleeding.

hepatic. Pertaining to the liver.

hepatitis. A general term for inflammation of the liver. It can result from infection or exposure to toxins.

herbal therapy. The use of herbal combinations for healing or cleansing purposes. Herbs can be used in tablet, capsule, tincture, or extract form, as well as in baths and poultices.

hernia. A condition in which part of an internal organ protrudes, inappropriately, through an opening in the tissues that are supposed to contain it.

highly active antiretroviral therapy (HAART). The new generation HIV/AIDS drug treatment. The aim of HAART is to reduce the amount of virus in the blood to very low or even nondetectable levels, although this doesn't mean the virus is gone. This is usually accomplished with a combination of three or more drugs. Treatment focuses on achieving the maximum suppression of symptoms for as long as possible.

histamine. A chemical released by the immune system that acts on various body tissues. It has the effect of constricting the smooth bronchial tube muscles, dilating small blood vessels, allowing fluid to leak from various tissues, and increasing the secretion of stomach acid.

HIV. Human immunodeficiency virus. The virus that causes AIDS.

Hodgkin's disease. A type of lymphoma (cancer of the lymphatic system).

homeopathy. A medical system based on the belief that "like cures like"—that is, that illness can be cured by taking a *minute* dose of a substance that, if taken by a healthy person, would produce symptoms like those being treated. Homeopathy employs a variety of plant, animal, and mineral substances in very small doses to stimulate the body's natural healing powers and to bring the body back into balance.

hormone. One of numerous essential substances produced by the endocrine glands that regulate many bodily functions.

hormone replacement therapy (HRT). Medications containing female hormones to replace the ones the body is no longer making.

host. An organism in or on which another organism lives and from which the invading organism obtains nourishment.

human growth hormone. Human growth hormone (HGH) is secreted by the pituitary gland in the brain. Like all hormones, HGH works to regulate the activities of vital organs, and thus helps maintain health throughout the body.

hyaluronic acid. An organic acid known as the most effective natural skin moisturizer. It is present in human skin and is able to hold five hundred times its own weight in water.

hydrochloric acid. A strong, corrosive inorganic acid that is produced in the stomach to aid in digestion.

hydrogenation. A chemical process used to turn liquid oils into more solid form by bombarding the oil molecules with hydrogen atoms. Hydrogenation destroys the nutritional value of the oil and also results in the formation of trans-fatty acids, strangely altered fatty acid molecules that do not occur in nature.

hypercalcemia. The presence of abnormally high amounts of calcium in the blood.

hyperglycemia. High blood sugar.

hypertension. High blood pressure. Generally, hypertension is defined as a regular resting pressure over 140/90.

hypoallergenic. Having a low capacity for inducing hypersensitive (allergic) reactions.

hypocalcemia. The presence of abnormally low amounts of calcium in the blood.

hypoglycemia. Low blood sugar.

hypotension. Low blood pressure.

hypothalamus. A portion of the brain that regulates many aspects of metabolism, including body temperature and the hunger response.

idiopathic. Term describing a disease of unknown cause.

immune globulin. A protein that functions as an antibody in the body's immune response. Immune globulins are manufactured by certain white blood cells and found in body fluids and on mucous membranes.

immune system. A complex system that depends on the interaction of many different organs, cells, and proteins. Its chief function is to identify and eliminate foreign substances such as harmful bacteria that have invaded the body. The gastrointestinal tract, liver, spleen, thymus, bone marrow, and lymphatic system all play vital roles in the proper functioning of the immune system.

immunity. The condition of being able to resist and overcome disease or infection.

immunodeficiency. A defect in the functioning of the immune system. It can be inherited or acquired, reversible or permanent. Immunodeficiency renders the body more susceptible to illness of every type, especially infectious illnesses.

immunology. The branch of medical science that deals with the functioning of the immune system.

immunotherapy. Treatment of disease by using techniques to stimulate or strengthen the immune system.

incubation period. The period of time between exposure to an infectious disease and the appearance of symptoms, during which the infection is developing.

infection. Invasion of body tissues by disease-causing organisms such as viruses, protozoa, fungi, or bacteria.

infestation. An invasion of the body by parasites such as insects, worms, or protozoa.

inflammation. A reaction to illness or injury characterized by swelling, warmth, pain, and redness.

inguinal. Pertaining to the groin.

insomnia. The inability to sleep.

insulin. A hormone produced by the pancreas that regulates the metabolism of glucose (sugar) in the body.

interaction. A phenomenon that occurs when two or more substances affect one another's activity or combine to create a different effect than any of them would have on its own. Any substance introduced into the body can potentially interact with another substance or substances already present. Drugs, foods, herbs, minerals, and vitamins can all interact with one another.

interferon. A protein produced by the cells in response to viral infection that prevents viral reproduction and is capable of protecting uninfected cells from viral infection. There are different types of interferon, designated alpha, beta, and gamma.

interleukin. Any of a number of immune system chemicals manufactured by the body to aid in fighting infection.

intestinal flora. Any bacteria present in the intestines that are essential for the digestion and metabolism of certain nutrients. They can be "friendly" or "pathogenic."

intolerance. Nutritionally, the inability to digest a particular food, usually due to a lack or deficiency of certain enzymes.

intravenous (IV) infusion. The use of a needle inserted in a vein to assist in fluid replacement, or to supply nutrition, electrolytes, or medication to the body.

ischemia. The condition of being starved for oxygenated blood. Ischemia affecting the heart or brain can cause a heart attack or stroke, respectively.

isoflavones. A class of phytochemical that have weak estrogen-like effects; their use should be discussed with a doctor in patients with estrogen-based cancers such as breast cancer.

IU. International unit. A measure of potency based on an accepted international standard. Dosages of vitamin A and E supplements, among others, are usually measured in international units. Because this is a measurement of potency, not weight or volume, the number of milligrams in an international unit varies, depending on the substance being measured.

ketogenic diet. A high-fat, low-carbohydrate diet that produces acetone or ketone bodies, or mild acidosis.

lactase. An enzyme that converts lactose into glucose and galactose. It is necessary for the digestion of milk and milk products.

lactic acid. An acid that results from anaerobic glucose metabolism. It is present in certain foods, including certain fruits and sour milk (when milk becomes sour, this means that some of the lactose, or milk sugar, it contained has been converted into lactic acid). Lactic acid is also produced in the muscles during anaerobic exercise. It is the buildup of lactic acid that causes muscle fatigue and cramping during strenuous activity. Synthetic lactic acid is used in food products as a flavoring and preservative.

lactobacilli. Any of a number of species of bacteria that are capable of transforming lactose (milk sugar) into lactic acid through fermentation. Lactobacilli are naturally present in the colon and are sometimes referred to as "friendly" bacteria because they aid in digestion and diminish the numbers of disease-causing microorganisms. The two species of lactobacilli most commonly available in supplement form are *L. acidophilus* and *L. bifidus*.

laser. Light amplification by stimulated emission of radiation. An instrument that focuses highly amplified light waves. Lasers are used in surgical procedures, especially eye surgery.

LDL cholesterol. A type of lipoprotein (a protein molecule that transports cholesterol in the bloodstream) that is commonly referred to as "bad cholesterol" because high levels normally indicate a high risk of heart disease. This is the form of cholesterol thought to clog arteries.

lecithin. A mixture of phospholipids that is composed of fatty acids, glycerol, phosphorus, and choline or inositol. All living cell membranes are largely composed of lecithin.

leukemia. Cancer of the blood-producing tissues, especially the bone marrow and lymph nodes, resulting in an overabundance of white blood cells. It can be either acute (most common in children) or chronic (most common in adults). It is similar in certain respects to Hodgkin's disease.

leukoderma. A deficiency of skin pigmentation, occurring usually in patches. Also known as vitiligo.

leukotrines. A group of hormones that are released in response to inflammation that can be caused by asthma or hay fever.

lignans. Phytoestrogens that are found in flaxseeds, whole wheat flour, tea, some fruits, and other cereal grains.

limbic system. A group of deep brain structures that, among other things, transmit the perception of pain to the brain and generate an emotional reaction to it.

limonoids. Phytochemicals found in citrus fruits that may inhibit the production of cancerous tumors.

lipid. Substances found in nature that are soluble in the same organic solvents as fats and oils are. Important nutritional lipids include choline, gamma-linolenic acid, inositol, lecithin, omega-6 fats (such as linoleic acid), and omega-3 fats (such as eicosapentaenoic acid [EPA]).

lipoprotein. A type of protein molecule that incorporates a lipid. Lipoproteins act as agents of lipid transport in the lymph and blood.

lipotropic. Any of a number of substances that help to prevent the accumulation of abnormal or excessive amounts of fat in the body and enhance fat metabolism. Commonly used lipotropics include choline, inositol, and methionine.

lutein. A phytochemical (one of the carotenoids) found in kale, spinach, and other dark green leafy vegetables that is beneficial for the eyes. It may help protect against macular degeneration.

lycopene. A phytochemical found in tomatoes that appears to afford protection against prostate cancer and to protect the skin against harm from ultraviolet rays.

lymph. A clear fluid derived from blood plasma that circulates throughout the body, is collected from the tissues, and flows through the lymphatic vessels, eventually returning to the bloodstream. Its function is to nourish tissue cells and return waste matter to the bloodstream.

lymph nodes. Organs located in the lymphatic vessels that act as filters, trapping and removing foreign material. They also form lymphocytes, immune cells that develop the capacity to seek out and destroy specific foreign agents.

lymphadenopathy. Enlargement of a lymph node or nodes as a result of the presence of a foreign substance or disease. This condition is often referred to as "swollen glands."

lymphocyte. A type of white blood cell found in lymph, blood, and other specialized tissues, such as the bone marrow and tonsils. There are several different categories of lymphocytes, designated B lymphocytes, T lymphocytes, and null (or non-B, non-T) lymphocytes. These cells are crucial components of the immune system. B lymphocytes are primarily responsible for antibody production, whereas the T lymphocytes are involved in the direct attack against invading organisms. It is the T-helper cell, a subtype of T lymphocyte, that is the primary cell infected and destroyed by human immunodeficiency virus (HIV), the virus that causes AIDS.

lymphokine. Any of a group of substances produced by the cells of the immune system when exposed to antigens. They are not antibodies, but rather perform such functions as stimulating the production of additional lymphocytes and activating other immune cells.

lymphoma. Cancer of the lymphatic tissues.

macrobiotics. A dietary approach adapted from Far Eastern philosophy whose basic principle consists of balancing the yin and yang energies of foods. Yin foods, such as water, are expansive; yang foods, such as salt or meat, are contractile. For the most part, the macrobiotic diet consists of whole grain cereals, millet, rice, soups, and vegetables, with beans and supplementary foods depending on the individual and the condition. Different conditions are considered either yin or yang, so the macrobiotic program must be adapted to each individual.

macrophage. A type of immune cell that surrounds and digests foreign materials and cellular debris in the body.

malabsorption. Nutritionally, a defect in the absorption of nutrients from the intestinal tract into the bloodstream.

malaise. An overall feeling of discomfort, unease, or indisposition that is often an indicator of infection.

malignant. Literally, "evil." Used to refer to cells or groups of cells that are cancerous and likely to spread.

mammography. An x-ray examination of the breast.

MAO. Monoamine oxidase, an enzyme that catalyzes the oxidation of monoamines. An abnormal amount of these enzymes can have adverse psychological effects. Some MAO inhibitors are drugs used as antidepressants.

melanoma. A malignant tumor originating from pigment cells in the deep layers of the skin.

menopause. The cessation of menstruation, caused by a sharp decrease in the production of the sex hormones estrogen and progesterone. Menopause usually occurs after the age of forty-five or following the removal of the female reproductive organs.

metabolic syndrome. A cluster of conditions—increased blood pressure, elevated insulin levels, excess body fat around the waist, and abnormal cholesterol levels—that occur together, increasing the risk of heart disease, stroke, and diabetes.

metabolism. The physical and chemical processes necessary to sustain life, including the production of cellular energy from foods, the synthesis of important biological substances, and degradation of various compounds.

metabolite. A substance produced as a result of a metabolic process.

metastasis. The spread of cancer to a site or sites away from the original tumor.

microgram. A measurement of weight equivalent to 1/1,000 milligram.

milligram. A measurement of weight equivalent to 1/1,000 gram (a gram is equal to approximately 1/28 ounce).

mineral. An inorganic substance required by the body in small quantities.

monoterpenes. Phytochemicals found in citrus fruits, eggplant, green vegetables, tomatoes, and yams that act as antioxidants and help protect the immune system.

motility. The power to move spontaneously.

MRI. Magnetic resonance imaging. A technique used in diagnosis that combines the use of radio waves and a strong magnetic field to produce detailed images of the internal structures of the body.

mucous membranes. Membranes that line the cavities and canals of the body that communicate with the air. Examples include the membranes lining the inside of the mouth, nose, anus, and vagina.

myelin sheath. A fatty covering that protects nerve cells. Myelin sheaths are noticeably damaged or missing in people with multiple sclerosis.

naturopathy. A form of health care that uses diet, herbs, and other natural methods and substances to cure illness. The goal is to produce a healthy body state without the use of drugs by stimulating innate defenses.

neuropathy. A complex of symptoms caused by abnormalities in motor or sensory nerves. Symptoms may include tingling or numbness, especially in the hands or feet, followed by gradual, progressive muscular weakness. It is common in people with diabetes.

neurotransmitter. A chemical that transmits nerve impulses from one nerve cell to another. Major neurotransmitters include acetylcholine, dopamine, gamma-aminobutyric acid, norepinephrine, and serotonin.

nonsteroidal anti-inflammatory drugs (NSAIDs). Drugs that block COX enzymes and reduce prostaglandins throughout the body, which reduces inflammation, pain, and fever.

nucleic acid. Any of a class of chemical compounds found in all viruses and plant and animal cells. Ribonucleic acid (RNA) and deoxyribonucleic acid (DNA), which contain the genetic instructions for every living cell, are two principal types.

nutraceutical. A food- or nutrient-based product or supplement designed and/or used for a specific clinical and/or therapeutic purpose.

nutrient. A substance that is needed by the body to maintain life and health.

occult blood test. A test that detects the presence of blood in bodily excretions such as stool, sputum, or urine. It can be one of the first tests used in screening for cancer.

oncologist. A cancer specialist.

oncology. The medical specialty dealing with cancer.

organic. A term used to describe foods that are grown without the use of synthetic chemicals, such as pesticides, herbicides, and hormones.

osteopathy. A system of medicine based on the belief that the body is a vital mechanical organism whose structural and functional integrity are coordinated and interdependent, and that disturbances in the musculoskeletal system can therefore cause disorders elsewhere in the body. Because of this philosophy, although osteopaths can prescribe drugs and perform surgery, they are more likely to recommend physical therapy or musculoskeletal manipulation as the treatment of first choice.

osteopenia. Low bone mass.

osteoporosis. A disorder in which minerals leach out of the bones, rendering them progressively more porous and fragile.

oxidation. A chemical reaction in which oxygen reacts with another substance, resulting in a chemical transformation. Many oxidation reactions result in some type of deterioration or spoilage.

Pap test. Microscopic examination of cells collected from the vagina and cervix to test for signs of cancer.

parasite. An organism that lives on or in another organism and obtains nourishment from it.

pathogen. A toxin or small organism that can cause disease.

peptide. A substance composed of two or more amino acids.

perimenopause. The period before menopause—possibly starting as much as ten years before—during which women may experience uncomfortable symptoms because of fluctuating hormones.

peristalsis. The rhythmic contractions of the muscles of the digestive tract that move matter into the stomach, through the intestines, and, ultimately, out of the body.

PET scan. Positron emission tomography scan. A method by which brain sections can be reconstructed using radioactive isotopes for diagnostic purposes. Using several types of isotope, cerebral blood flow, blood volume, oxygen uptake, glucose transport, glucose metabolism can be identified.

petrolatum. A semisolid mixture of hydrocarbons, such as Vaseline.

pH. Potential of hydrogen. A scale used to measure the relative acidity or alkalinity of substances. The scale runs from 0 to 14. A pH of 7 is considered neutral; numbers below 7 denote increasing acidity and numbers above 7 denote increasing alkalinity. Human blood is around 7.35 to 7.45.

pharyngitis. Sore throat.

phenylketonuria (PKU). An inherited disorder caused by a lack of an enzyme necessary to convert the amino acid phenylalanine into another amino acid, tyrosine, so that excesses can be eliminated from the body. A buildup of excess phenylalanine in the blood can lead to neurological disturbances and mental retardation.

phytochemical. Any one of many substances present in fruits and vegetables (*phyto* means "plant" in Greek). There are hundreds of phytochemicals, and more are being identified every day. Some appear to help protect the body against illness, including such serious diseases as cancer and heart disease.

pituitary. A gland located at the base of the brain that secretes a number of different hormones. Pituitary hormones regu-late growth and metabolism by coordinating the actions of other endocrine glands.

placebo. A pharmacologically inactive substance, primarily used in experiments to provide a basis for comparison with pharmacologically active substances.

plaque. An unwanted deposit of a certain substance on tissues, often with the potential to cause some type of health problem. The buildup of plaque in the arteries is a leading cause of cardiovascular disease; plaque deposits on the teeth can lead to gum disease; Alzheimer's disease is associated with the accumulation of characteristic plaques in brain tissue.

precancerous lesion. Abnormal tissue that is not malignant, but that may be in the process of becoming so.

probiotics. Elements that encourage the growth of beneficial bacteria in the intestine.

progesterone. A hormone whose functions include preparing a woman's body for pregnancy in the second half of the menstrual cycle. Progesterone cream is used in hormone replacement therapy to prevent vaginal atrophy.

prognosis. A forecast as to the likely course and/or outcome of a disorder or condition.

prostaglandin. Any of a number of hormonelike chemicals that are made in the body from essential fatty acids and that have important effects on target organs. They influence the secretion of hormones and enzymes, and are important in regulating the inflammatory response, blood pressure, and blood-clotting time.

protein. Any of many complex nitrogen-based organic compounds made up of different combinations of amino acids. Proteins are basic elements of all animal and vegetable tissues. Biological substances such as hormones and enzymes also are composed of protein. The body makes the specific proteins it needs for growth, repair, and other functions from amino acids that are either extracted from dietary protein or manufactured from other amino acids.

proteolytic enzymes. Enzymes that break down dietary proteins, yet do not attack the proteins that make up the normal cells of the body. Proteolytic enzymes may have value in fighting cancer and other diseases.

pruritus. Itching.

pterygia. A triangular thickening over the cornea of the eye, looking somewhat like a wing.

pulmonary. Pertaining to the lungs.

purulent. Containing or causing the production of pus.

radiation. Energy that is emitted or transmitted in the form of waves. The term is often used to refer to radioactivity; however, radioactivity is a specific type of radiation that comes from the decay of unstable atoms.

radiation therapy. A type of treatment, most often used for cancer, that involves the use of ionizing radiation, including Roentgen rays, radium, or other radioactive substances to destroy specific areas of tissue. Also called *radiotherapy*.

RAST. Radioallergosorbent test. A blood test that measures levels of specific antibodies produced by the body's immune system, used to test for allergic reactions.

RDA. Recommended dietary allowance. The amount of a vitamin or other nutrient that should be consumed daily in order to prevent nutritional deficiency. RDAs are determined by the U.S. Food and Drug Administration.

red blood cell. A blood cell that contains the red pigment hemoglobin and transports oxygen and carbon dioxide in the bloodstream.

remission. Lessening or reversal of the signs and symptoms of disease. This term is used particularly of serious and/or chronic illnesses such as cancer and multiple sclerosis.

renal. Pertaining to the kidneys.

retinoic acid. Vitamin A acid. A form of retinoic acid is the active ingredient in the medication Retin-A.

retrovirus. A type of virus that has RNA as its core nucleic acid and contains an enzyme called *reverse transcriptase* that permits the virus to copy its RNA into the DNA of infected cells, in effect taking over the cells' genetic machinery. Human immunodeficiency virus (HIV), the virus that causes AIDS, is a retrovirus. Retroviruses are also known to cause certain types of cancer in animals and are suspected of causing forms of cancers in animals.

RNA. Ribonucleic acid. A complex protein found in plant and animal cells. RNA carries coded genetic information from DNA, in the cell nucleus, to protein-producing cell structures called ribosomes, where these instructions are translated into the form of protein molecules—the basic component of all living tissue.

saturated fat. A fat that is solid at room temperature. Most saturated fats are of animal origin, although a few, such as coconut oil and palm oil, come from plants.

saturation. With regard to fats, the term "saturation" refers to the chemical structure of the fatty acid molecules, specifically the number of hydrogen atoms present. Fat molecules that cannot incorporate any additional hydrogen atoms are said to be *saturated*, and these have no double bonds holding the molecule together. Those that could incorporate one additional hydrogen atom and have one double bond are referred to as *monounsaturated*; and those that could incorporate two or more additional hydrogen atoms and have two or more double bonds are referred to as *polyunsaturated*.

scratch test. A procedure in which a small amount of a suspected allergen is applied to a lightly scratched area of skin to test for an allergic reaction.

sebum. The oily secretion produced by glands in the skin.

secondary infection. An infection that develops after and is made possible by the presence or effect of a previous infection, inflammation, or other condition, but that is not necessarily directly caused by it.

seizure. A sudden, brief episode characterized by changes in consciousness, perception, muscular motion, and/or behavior. A convulsion is a type of seizure.

selective serotonin reuptake inhibitors (SSRIs). A popular class of antidepressant medications.

serotonin. A neurotransmitter found principally in the brain that is considered essential for relaxation, sleep, and concentration.

serum. The fluid portion of the blood.

simple carbohydrate. A type of carbohydrate that, owing to its chemical structure, is rapidly digested and absorbed into the bloodstream. Glucose, lactose, and fructose are examples of simple carbohydrates.

sorbic acid. An organic acid used as a food preservative.

steroid. One of a group of fat-soluble organic compounds with a characteristic chemical composition. A number of different hormones, drugs, and other substances—including cholesterol—are classified as steroids.

sterols and stanols. Plant substances that occur naturally in small amounts in many grains, vegetables, fruits, legumes, nuts, and seeds. They have powerful cholesterol-lowering properties, and the FDA has granted a health claim to foods that contain an effective amount per serving. Manufacturers have started adding them to foods.

stroke. An attack in which the brain is suddenly deprived of oxygen as a result of interrupted blood flow. If it continues for more than a few minutes, brain damage and even death may result.

sublingual. Literally, "under the tongue." Sublingual medications and supplements often look like tablets or liquids meant for swallowing, but they are designed to be held in the mouth while the active ingredient is absorbed into the bloodstream through the mucous membranes.

sucralose. An artificial sweetener, six hundred times sweeter than sugar, used in diet foods. Sucralose is derived from sugar through a patented, multistep process that selectively substitutes three chlorine atoms for three hydrogen-oxygen groups on the sugar molecule. The tightly bound chlorine atoms create a molecular structure that is exceptionally stable and thus sucralose can be used in cooking.

symptom. An alteration in normal feeling or functioning experienced as a result of a bodily disorder.

syncope. Temporary loss of consciousness; fainting.

syndrome. A group of signs and symptoms that together are known or presumed to characterize a disorder.

synergy. An interaction between two or more substances in which their action is greater when they are together than the sum of their individual actions would be.

synthesize. To create a complex substance by combining simpler elements or compounds.

systemic. Pertaining to the entire body.

T cell. A type of lymphocyte that is a crucial part of the immune system. T cells can attack foreign cells, cancer cells, and cells infected with a virus.

telangiectasia. A vascular lesion formed by the dilation of a group of small blood vessels. A type of birthmark.

telomeres. The tips of chromosomes that keep them from shorting during cell division. Telomeres naturally shorten with age, and poor diet and poor health also can speed the process.

teratogen. An agent that causes malformation of a developing embryo or fetus.

thrombus. An obstruction in a blood vessel.

thrush. A fungal infection caused by *Candida albicans* that is characterized by small whitish spots on the tongue and the insides of the cheeks. It occurs most often in infants and in persons with compromised immune systems.

thymol. White crystals obtained from oil of thyme. This is an alternative treatment for hookworm.

topical. Pertaining to the surface of the body.

toxicity. The quality of being poisonous. Toxicity reactions in the body impair bodily functions and/or damage cells.

toxin. A poison that impairs the health and functioning of the body.

trace element. A mineral required by the body in extremely small quantities.

tremor. Involuntary trembling.

triglyceride. A compound consisting of three fatty acids plus glycerol. Triglycerides are the form in which fat is stored in the body and are the primary type of lipid in the diet. Too much of this type of fat can contribute to the hardening and narrowing of the arteries, and increase the risk of heart disease.

tumor. An abnormal mass of tissue that serves no function. Tumors are usually categorized as either benign or malignant (cancerous).

type A personality. A personality that tends to be impatient and aggressive. Persons with type A personalities tend to have stronger stress reactions and may be more susceptible to cardiovascular disease.

type B personality. A personality that tends to be relaxed and patient, and less reactive to stress. Those with type B personalities may be less prone to develop stress-related illnesses such as high blood pressure and heart disease.

ultrasound. Ultra-high-frequency sound waves. Ultrasound technology is used in a number of different medical diagnostic and treatment tools.

unsaturated fat. Any of a number of dietary fats that are liquid at room temperature. Unsaturated fats come from vegetable sources and are good sources of essential fatty acids. Examples include flaxseed oil, sunflower oil, safflower oil, and primrose oil.

urticaria. Hives.

vaccine. A preparation administered to achieve immunity against a specific agent by inducing the body to make antibodies to that agent. A vaccine may be a suspension of living or dead microorganisms, or a solution of an allergen or viral or bacterial antigens.

vascular. Pertaining to the circulatory system.

vein. One of the blood vessels that returns the blood from the body tissues to the heart.

venom. A poisonous substance produced by an animal, such as certain snakes and insects.

virus. Any of a vast group of minute, often disease-causing, structures composed of a protein coat and a core of DNA and/or RNA. Because they are incapable of reproducing on their own (they must reproduce inside the cells of an infected host), viruses are not technically considered living organisms. Unlike bacteria, viruses are not affected by antibiotics.

visualization. A technique that involves consciously using the mind to influence the health and functioning of the body. Also called creative visualization.

vital signs. Basic indicators of an individual's health status, including pulse, breathing, blood pressure, and body temperature.

vitamin. One of approximately fifteen organic substances that are essential in small quantities for life and health. Most vitamins cannot be manufactured by the body and so need to be supplied in the diet.

water-soluble. Capable of dissolving in water.

white blood cell. A blood cell that functions in fighting infection and in wound repair.

withdrawal. The process of adjustment that occurs when the use of a habit-forming substance to which the body has become accustomed is discontinued.

xenophthalmia. Inflammation of the eye caused by a foreign body.

yang. In Chinese medicine, one of the two vital principles that must be in balance to create harmony and balance in the body. Yang is heat, light, and dryness. Yang organs include the spleen, gallbladder, intestines, and the skin.

yeast. A type of single-celled fungus. Certain types of yeast can cause infection, most commonly in the mouth, vagina, or gastrointestinal tract. Common yeast infections include vaginitis and thrush.

yin. In Chinese medicine, one of the two vital principles that must be in balance to create harmony and balance in the body. Yin is cold, shadow, and moisture. Yin organs include the heart, liver, kidneys, lungs, and bones.

MANUFACTURER AND DISTRIBUTOR INFORMATION

Below are the manufacturers and distributors of some of the brand-name products mentioned in this book, plus their addresses, Web sites, and phone numbers. This list is not exhaustive. There are many other good products out there. We provide this contact information simply as a resource. None of the manufacturers or distributors mentioned have had any connection with the production of this book. Rather, we list these companies because we believe their products to be effective and of high quality.

Be aware that addresses and telephone numbers are subject to change. Often, your best bet is to use an Internet search engine, such as Yahoo or Google, to find the product using its name. You should find numerous hits that can steer you to a retailer or other supplier.

A. Vogel Homeopathic
See Bioforce USA.

Abbott Laboratories
100 Abbott Park Road
Abbott Park, IL 60064-3500
847-937-6100
www.abbott.com
Ensure; FreeStyle and Precision glucose monitors; Zone Bars.

AbDiagnostics
44 Darlington Avenue
Wilmington, NC 28403
910-815-0209
www.abdiagnostics.com
Allergy, cholesterol, diabetes, colon cancer, and other home testing products.

Abkit, Inc.
See Nature's Way Inc.

ABRA, Inc.
P.O. Box 795185
Dallas, TX 75379-5185
800-745-0761
www.abratherapeutics.com
VitaSerum and other organic skin care products.

Advanced Sports Nutrition (ASN), Inc.
1813 Cascade Avenue
Hood River, OR 97031
800-800-9119; 541-387-4500
www.a-s-n.com
Antioxidants, body-shaping products, Humagro; Testatropinol.

Aerobic Life Industries
2800 East Chambers, Suite 700
Phoenix, AZ 85040
800-798-0707
www.aerobiclife.com
ABC Aerobic Bulk Cleanse; ABC Max; Aerobic 07; China Gold; Colon Care Plus; Desert Delight; 45-Day MAX Colon Cleanse Kit; Mag 07; 10-Day Colon Cleanse.

AIM International
3923 East Flamingo Avenue
Nampa, ID 83687
800-456-2462; 208-465-5116
www.theaimcompanies.com
BarleyLife and other nutritional products.

AkPharma, Inc.
P.O. Box 111
Pleasantville, NJ 08232
609-645-5100
www.akpharma.com
Prelief (takes acids out of many foods). Inventors of Beano (now a GlaxoSmithKline product).

Alacer Corporation
80 Icon
Foothill Ranch, CA 92610
800-854-0249
www.emergenc.com
Emergen-C.

AllerGuard Corporation
40 Cindy Lane
Ocean, NJ 07712
800-234-0816
www.allerguard.com
X-MITE powder and other allergy relief products.

Allergy Control Products
22 Shelter Rock Lane
Danbury, CT 06810
800-255-3749
www.allergycontrol.com
Bedding, air filtration, other allergy products.

Allergy Research Group
NutriCology, Inc.
2300 North Loop Road
Alameda, CA 94502
800-545-9960; 510-263-2000
www.allergyresearchgroup.com

Allovedic Remedies
American Formulary, Inc.
140 Ethel Road West, Suite S-T
Piscataway, NJ 08854
732-985-9899
www.americanformulary.com
Herbal dietary supplements, including Antioxidant Formula; Blood Sugar Balance Formula; Cardiotonic Support Formula; Energy Formula; Joint Support Formula; Liver Support Formula; Memory Support Formula; Probiotic with B-Complex Formula; Rejuvenator Support Formula; Respiratory Support Formula.

American Biologics
1180 Walnut Avenue
Chula Vista, CA 91911
800-227-4473; 619-429-8200
www.americanbiologics.com
Bio-Bifidus Complex; Bio-Dophilus; Ultra Brain Power; GeOxy-132; Inf-zyme Forte; Micellized Vitamin A and E; Multi-Glandular; Oxy-5000 Forte; Panoderm I and II; Selenium Forte; Sub-Adrene; Taurine Plus; Ultra Connexin; Ultra Osteo Synergy.

America's Finest, Inc.
70 Ethel Road West, Suite 7
Piscataway, NJ 08854
800-350-3305
www.afisupplements.com
Bacopin & Ginkgo Complex, Herbal COX-2.

Amerifit Brands Inc.
55 Sebethe Drive, Suite 201
Cromwell, CT 06416
800-722-3476
www.amerifit.com
Culturelle; Estroven; FlexAble chewable wafers

Anabol Naturals
1550 Mansfield Street
Santa Cruz, CA 95062
800-426-2265; 831-479-1403
www.anabol.com
Amino Balance; crystalline free form amino acids; Muscle Octane.

Anurex Labs
8740 South West 21st Street
Ft. Lauderdale, FL 33324
305-757-7733
www.anurex.com
Anurex cryotherapy device for hemorrhoids.

Apollo Health, Inc.
A Division of Philips Home Healthcare Solutions
947 South 500, East Suite 210
American Fork, UT 84003
800-545-9667; 801-226-2370
www.lighttherapy.com
Brite Lite IV.

Ayurvedic Concepts
See Himalaya Herbal Healthcare.

Bayer Diabetes Care
555 White Plains Rd.
Tarrytown, NY 10591
914-366-1800
Bayer's Contour; Bayer's Breezez
www.simplewins.com

Bergstrom Nutrition
1000 West 8th Street
Vancouver, WA 98660
888-733-5676; 360-693-1883
www.bergstromnutrition.com
OptiMSM.

bioAllers
A division of Nutraceutical International Corporation
P.O. Box 5935
Bellingham, WA 98227-5935
800-243-0788
www.bioallers.com

BioChem Sports
See Country Life.

Bioforce USA
6 Grandinetti Drive
Ghent, NY 12075
800-641-7555; 518-828-9111
www.bioforceUSA.com
Distributor of Bioforce AG and A. Vogel herbal and homeopathic products, including Allergy Relief tablets; Calcium Absorption Formula; Cardiaforce; Echinaforce; Menopause tablets; Prostasan.

Biotec Foods
A Division of AgriGenic Food Corporation
5412 Bolsa Avenue, Suite C
Huntington Beach, CA 92649
800-788-1084
www.agrigenic.com
Ageless Beauty; Anti-Stress Enzymes; Bio-Gestin; Cell Guard.

Biotech Corporation
107 Oakwood Drive
Glastonbury, CT 06033
800-880-7188; 860-633-8111
www.biotechcorp.com
CelluRid; Dermasilk; Prostate Rx; Green Tea Rx.

Biotics Research
6801 Biotics Research Drive
Rosenberg, TX 77471
800-231-5777; 281-344-0909
www.bioticsresearch.com
Specialty nutritional products, vitamins, minerals, amino acids. Bio-Allay; A.D.P.; Betaine Plus HP; GlucoBalance; Bio-C Plus; Intenzyme Forte; Osteo-B Plus; and many other products.

Bluebonnet Nutrition Corporation
12915 Dairy Ashford
Sugar Land, TX 77478
800-580-8866; 281-240-3332
www.bluebonnetnutrition.com
Amino Acids, digestive enzymes, vitamins, minerals, herbs including Diet Chrome-Care.

Boiron
6 Campus Boulevard
Newtown Square, PA 19073
800-264-7661
www.boironusa.com
Homeopathic remedies, including Oscillococcinum.

Botanical Laboratories Inc.
1441 West Smith Road
Ferndale, WA 98248
800-232-4005; 360-384-5656
www.botlab.com
Wellesse and other brands.

CamoCare
See Abkit, Inc.

Carlson Laboratories, Inc.
15 College Drive
Arlington Heights, IL 60004-1985
888-234-5656; 847-255-1600
www.carlsonlabs.com
ACES; ACES + Zn; Amino Blend; Amino-VIL; D.A. #34; Co-Q-10; E-Gem Skin-Care Soap; E-Sel; fish oils; Glutathione Booster; Key-E suppositories; Super Daily Amino Blend.

Cayenne Company
2235 East 38th Street
Minneapolis, MN 55407-3083
800-229-3663; 612-724-5266
www.cayennecompany.com
Cayenne products, including Heart Food Caps; Power Caps; Power Plus.

CC Pollen Company
3627 East Indian School Road, Suite 209
Phoenix, AZ 85018
800-875-0096; 602-957-0096
www.ccpollen.com
Aller Bee-Gone; bee pollen, bee propolis; Royal Jelly products.

Century Systems, Inc.
P.O. Box 43725
120 Selig Drive
Atlanta, GA 30336
800-843-9662
www.1800thewoman.com
Miracle 2000.

CircAid Medical Products, Inc.
9323 Chesapeake Drive, Suite B-2
San Diego, CA 92123
800-247-2243; 858-576-3550
www.circaid.com
Compression garments and bandages for treating lymphedema, venous insufficiency, and venous ulcers.

Coenzyme-A Technologies
12512 Beverly Park Road, B1
Lynnwood, WA 98037
425-438-8586
www.coenzyme-a.com
Body Image; Clear Skin Image; Coenzyme A; Healthy Cholesterol Image; Healthy Joint Image.

cvc4health.com
4510 South Boyle Avenue
Vernon, CA 90058
800-421-6175
www.cvc4health.com
Superior Source sublingual nutritional supplements, including No Shot B-6/B-12/ Folic; Slumber Helper; Sweet-n-Natural Stevia Extract.

Country Life
180 Vanderbilt Motor Parkway
Hauppauge, NY 11788
800-645-5768
www.country-life.com
Biochem Sports & Fitness products; tea tree oil products; Herbal Mood Boost; Long Life Teas; Saw Palmetto & Pygeum Capsules; Soy-Licious, Iron-Tek, Country Life Vitamins.

Culligan International Company
9399 West Higgins Road
Rosemont, IL 60018
866-775-0260; 847-430-2800
www.culligan.com
WaterWatch Hot Line 800-285-5442
*Can put you in contact with a local
Culligan dealer to provide a free water-
testing service.*

Custom Probiotics
3000 Honolulu Avenue, Unit B
Glendale, CA 91214
800-219-8405; 818-248-3529
www.customprobiotics.com
*High-potency acidophilus (CP-1) and
bifidus dietary supplements.*

CWR Environmental Products Inc.
5155 Corporate Way, Suite G
Juniper, FL 33458
800-444-3563; 561-340-4000
www.cwrenviro.com
*Air purification and water-filtration
systems.*

DaVinci Laboratories
20 New England Drive, Suite 10
Essex Junction, VT 05452
800-325-1776
www.davincilabs.com
*Flora; Olivir, Spectra, CX-2 Solution,
Spectra-Reds. Products are available
through health professionals only.*

Derma-E Skin Care
4485 Runway Street
Simi Valley, CA 93063
800-521-3342; 805-582-2710
www.dermae.com
*Alpha Lipoderm; Clear Vein Crème Spider
Vein/Bruise Solution; Ester-C Gel; Itch
Relief Lotion; Peptides Plus Wrinkle
Reverse Crème; Pycnogenol Crème (or Gel);
Scar Gel; StopItch Instant Relief Crème;
Vitamin A with E Wrinkle Treatment;
Vitamin E 12,000 IU Deep Moisturizing
Crème.*

Diamond Herpanacine of PA, Inc.
1518 Grove Avenue, Suite #2B
Jenkintown, PA 19046
888-467-4200; 215-885-6880
*Herpanacine Skin Support; Diamond
MIND; Diamond Etern-L Anti-Aging;
Healthy Horizons—Award Winning
Formulas of Dr. Wayne Diamond.*

Doctor's Data, Inc.
3755 Illinois Avenue
St. Charles, IL 60174-2420
800-323-2784; 630-377-8139
www.doctorsdata.com
Hair analysis services.

Earth Essentials
P.O. Box 40339
Santa Barbara, CA 93140
800-347-5211; 805-684-4525
www.earthessentials.com
Natural skin and hair care products.

Earth's Best Baby Foods
The Hain Celestial Group, Inc.
4600 Sleepytime Drive
Boulder, CO 80301
800-434-4246
www.earthsbest.com
Organic baby foods.

Earth's Bounty
See Matrix Health Products, Inc.

Eclectic Institute
36350 Southeast Industrial Way
Sandy, OR 97055
800-332-4372
www.eclecticherb.com
*Freeze-dried botanicals, organic herbs,
herbal extracts, nutritional supplements.*

EcoNugenics, Inc.
2208 Northpoint Parkway
Santa Rosa, CA 95407
800-308-5518; 707-521-3370
www.econugenics.com
Padma Basic and other herbal supplements.

Eden Foods, Inc.
701 Tecumseh Road
Clinton, MI 49236
888-424-3336; 517-456-7424
www.edenfoods.com

Efamol, Ltd.
14, The Mole Business Park
Leatherhead, Surrey KT22 7BA
44 (0)1372 379828
www.efamol.com
Essential fatty acid supplements.

En Garde Health Products
7702 Balboa Boulevard, Building #10
Van Nuys, CA 91406
800-955-4633; 818-901-8505
www.engardehealth.com
DynamO2.

Enzymatic Therapy
825 Challenger Drive
Green Bay, WI 54311
800-783-2286
www.enzymatictherapy.com
*Acid-Ease; Asparagus Extract; Cell Forté
with IP-6; Cell Forté with IP-6 and Inositol;
Derma-Klear; Esberitox; GastroSoothe; GS-
500; Grape Seed Antioxidant; HyperiCalm;
Ivy Extract; Mega-Zyme; Remifemin;
SinuCheck; ThymuPlex; Vira-Plex.*

ESA Biosciences, Inc.
22 Alpha Road
Chelmsford, MA 01824
978-250-7000
www.esainc.com
LeadCare testing units.

Essential Phytosterolins Inc.
4 Commerce Crescent
Acton, Ontario Canada L7J 2X3
877-297-7332; 519-853-3511
www.moducare.com
*Moducare, a blend of plant sterols and
serolins.*

Esteem Products Ltd.
1800 136th Place NE, Suite 5
Bellevue, WA 98005
800-255-7631; 425-562-1281
www.esteemproducts.com
*CardioLife; Diet Esteem Plus; Senior Total
Woman; Senior Total Man.*

Ethical Nutrients
Metagenics Inc.
100 Avenida La Pata
San Clemente, CA 92673
800-692-9400; 949-366-0818
www.ethicalnutrients.com
*Antioxidants; phytonutrients; Bone
Builder; Bone Builder With Boron; Mycel
Baby Vites.*

Flora Inc.
805 East Badger Road
Lynden, WA 98264
800-446-2110
www.florahealth.com
*U.S. distributor of Salus Haus products,
including Floradix Iron + Herbs.*

FoodScience of Vermont
20 New England Drive
Essex Junction, VT 05453
800-874-9444; 802-878-5508
www.fslabs.com
*Aangamik DMG; Cardio-DMG; Coenzyme
Q10; Energy Now; Glucosamine Plus;
Immuno-DMG; Multi-Zyme; Neuro-
DMG; Olive Leaf Extract.*

Forest Herbs Research Ltd.
P.O. Box 912
Nelson, New Zealand
64 3 548 2741
www.forestherbs.co.nz
*Kolorex, containing both horopito and anise
seed.*

Forest Pharmaceuticals, Inc.
13600 Shoreline Drive
St. Louis, MO 63045
800-678-1605; 314-493-7000
www.forestpharm.com
*Aerobid; Armour Thyroid Tablets; Celexa;
Cervidil; Lexapro; Monurol; Namenda;
Tiazac.*

Fountain of Youth Technologies
P.O. Box 608
Millersport, OH 43046
800-939-4296; 740-467-3698
www.foytech.com
Doctor's Growth Hormone Triple Strength and other products.

Freeda Vitamins and Pharmacy
47-25 34th Street, 3rd Floor
Long Island City, NY 11101
718-433-4337
www.freedavitamins.com
Anti-Allergy Formula.

Futurebiotics, LLC
70 Commerce Drive
Hauppauge, NY 11788
800-645-1721; 631-273-6300
www.futurebiotics.com
AcneAdvance; Cholestatin; Colloidal mineral supplements; Vegetarian Enzyme Complex.

Gaia Herbs, Inc.
101 Gaia Herbs Drive
Brevard, NC 28712
800-831-7780
www.gaiaherbs.com
Liquid herbal extracts and gel caps; Saw Palmetto Supreme.

Garden of Life
5500 Village Boulevard, Suite 202
West Palm Beach, FL 33407
866-465-0051
www.gardenoflifeusa.com

Gero Vita International
1835 Newport Boulevard, Suite A 109 #439
Costa Mesa, CA 92627
800-535-9816
www.gvi.com
Arthro-7; GH3; Lung Support Formula; Prostata.

Global Marketing Associates, Inc.
3536 Arden Road
Hayward, CA 94545-3908
800-869-0763; 510-887-2462
www.gmaherbs.com
Garlitech.

Global Sweet
125 Tremont Street
Rehoboth, MA 02769
800-601-0688; 508-252-5294
www.globalsweet.com
Enamel-saver toothpaste plus other nutritional products.

Green Foods Corporation
220 Camino Del Sol
Oxnard, CA 93030
800-777-4430; 805-983-7470
www.greenfoods.com
Carrot Essence; Green Magma; Green Tea Barley Essence; MagmaSLIM, Veggie Magma.

Hain Celestial Group
4600 Sleepytime Drive
Boulder, CO 80301
800-434-4246
www.hain-celestial.com
Queen Helene products, including Footherapy and Batherapy; Spectrum Organics products.

Health From The Sun
200 Research Drive, Suite 4
Wilmington, MA 01887
800-447-2229
www.healthfromthesun.com
Borage oil; evening primrose oil; flaxseed oil; pumpkin seed oil; Total EFA Junior; Total EFA Womens; Omega-3-6-9.

Heel Inc.
10421 Research Road SE
Albuquerque, NM 87123-3423
800-621-7644; 505-293-3843
www.heelusa.com
Traumeel; Zeel.

HerbaSway Laboratories, LLC
101 North Plains Industrial Road
Wallingford, CT 06492
800-672-7322; 203-269-6991
www.herbasway.com
Cholestra; Diabetica Tea; HerbaGreen Tea; Kudja; Liver-Enhancer.

Herbs, Etc.
1345 Cerrillos Road
Santa Fe, NM 87505
888-694-3727; 505-982-1265
www.herbsetc.com
Alcohol-free herbal extracts, including Deep Health; Deep Sleep; Lung Tonic; Singer's Saving Grace.

Herbs for Kids
A Division of Nutraceutical International Corporation
P.O. Box 5935
Bellingham, WA 98227-5935
800-258-4463
www.herbsforkids.com
Alcohol-free organic herbal extracts.

Himalaya Herbal Healthcare
10440 West Office Drive
Houston, TX 77042
800-869-4640; 713-863-1622
www.himalayausa.com
GastriCare; GlucoCare; HeartCare; ImmunoCare; JointCare; LaxaCare; LeanCare; LiverCare; MindCare; ProstaCare; StressCare; UriCare; VeinCare; VigorCare.

Home Access Health Corporation
2401 West Hassell Road, Suite 1510
Hoffman Estates, IL 60195
800-448-8378; 847-781-2500
www.homeaccess.com
Home Access Express HIV-1 Test System; Home Access Hepatitis C; Check Up America Cholesterol Panel.

Hybrivet Systems
17 Erie Drive
Natick, MA 01760
800-262-5323; 508-651-7881
www.leadcheck.com
LeadCheck Aqua; LeadCheck Swabs.

Hyland's Inc.
210 West 131st Street
Los Angeles, CA 90061
800-624-9659; 310-768-0700
www.hylands.com
Homeopathic products, Calms Forte tablets, Nerve tonic.

Immune-Tree
1163 South 1680 West
Orem, UT 84058
888-484-8671; 801-434-8129
www.immunetree.com
Colostrum 6 Maximum Strength.

Integrated Health/Health Products Distributors, Inc.
P.O. Box 5600
Oracle, AZ 85623
800-228-4265; 520-896-9193
www.integratedhealth.com
Nutritional supplements, antioxidants, amino acids, minerals.

International Health Products
10050 Via de la Amistad #2468
San Diego, CA 92154
866-721-7405; 619-661-7400
www.internationalhealthgroup.com
Novenzyme; Trace Supreme; and other products.

InterNatural
P.O. Box 489
Twin Lakes, WI 53181
800-643-4221
www.internatural.com
Online supplier of health care and nutritional products.

Irwin Naturals
5310 Beethoven Street
Los Angeles, CA 90066
800-297-3273; 310-306-3636
www.irwinnaturals.com
Ginkgo Smart; Ginza-Plus; Green Tea Fat Metabolizer; Immuno-Shield; Maximum Strength Phase 2 Carb-Blocker; Prosta-Strong; System-Six; 3-in-1 Joint Formula; Triple-Boost.

Jarrow Formulas Inc.
1824 South Robertson Boulevard
Los Angeles, CA 90035
800-726-0886; 310-204-6936
www.jarrow.com
Bone-up; Colostrum Prime Life; IP6; Jarro-Dophilus; JarroSil; Q-Absorb; Mushroom Optimizer.

Jason Natural Cosmetics
Hain Celestial Group, Inc.
4600 Sleepytime Drive
Boulder, CO 80301
866-595-8917
www.jasoncosmetics.com
Hyper-C Serum; natural products for skin and hair.

Jo Mar Laboratories
583-B Division Street
Campbell, CA 95008
800-538-4545; 408-374-5920
www.jomarlabs.com
Crystalline free form amino acids.

Juvenon, Inc.
P.O. Box 432
Manateno, IL 60950
800-588-3666
www.juvenon.com
Juvenon Cellular Health Supplement.

KAL Dietary Supplements
See Nutraceutical Corporation.
Bone Defense; Kal Enhanced Energy Full Spectrum Multiple; Kal Lifestyle Formulas; Ultra Omega 3-6-9.

Kolorex
See Forest Herbs Research, Ltd.

LactAid, Inc.
McNeil Nutritionals, LLC
7050 Camp Hill Road
Fort Washington, PA 19034
800-522-8243
www.lactaid.com
LactAid.

Lake Consumer Products, Inc.
Subsidiary of Wisconsin
Pharmacal Co. LLC
1 Pharmacal Way
Jackson, WI 53037
800-635-3696; 262-677-7179
www.lakeconsumer.com
Women's products such as Yeast-Gard.

Lane Labs-USA, Inc.
3 North Street
Waldwick, NJ 07463
201-661-6000
www.lanelabs.com
Advacal; Noxylane.

Liddell Laboratories
1036 Country Club Road
Moraga, CA 94556
800-460-7733; 925-377-3000
www.liddell.net
Homeopathic remedies for a range of ailments.

Life Extension Foundation
P.O. Box 407198
Ft. Lauderdale, FL 33340-7198
800-678-8989; 954-766-8433
www.lef.org
Prolongevity supplements, including Gamma E Tocopherol; Pro Fem cream; Resveratrol with Pregnenolone; Super Carnosine.

Maharishi Ayurveda Products International
1680 Highway 1 North
Fairfield, IA 52556
800-345-8332; 719-260-5500
www.mapi.com
Amrit Ambrosia and Amrit Nectar Ayurvedic formulas.

Maitake Products, Inc.
1 Madison Street, Suite F6
East Rutherford, NJ 07073
800-747-7418; 973-470-0010
www.maitake.com
Grifron Maitake caplets; Grifron Maitake D-fraction; Mai Green Tea; Prost-Mate.

Matrix Health Products, Inc.
1101 Northeast 144th Street, Suite 109
Vancouver, WA 98685
800-736-5609; 360-816-1200
www.earthsbounty.com
Earth's Bounty supplements, including Longevatrol; Original and Organic Tahitian Noni; O2 Spray; Oxy-Caps; Oxy-Cleanse; Oxy-Max.

Medtronic
10 Medtronic Parkway
Minneapolis, MN 55432
800-328-2518; 763-514-4000
www.medtronic.com
Activa D Therapy System; Activa Parkinson's Control Therapy. Available through and implanted by qualified medical professionals only.

Medtronic Diabetes
18000 Devonshire Street
Northridge, CA 91325-1219
866-948-6633
www.minimed.com
Continuous glucose monitoring system.

MegaFood
8 Bowery Road
Derry, NH 03038
800-848-2542; 603-432-5022
www.megafood.com
Daily Foods; MegaFlora; MegaZymes.

Metabolic Maintenance Products
68994 North Pine Street
P.O. Box 940
Sisters, OR 97759
800-772-7873; 541-549-7800
www.metabolicmaintenance.com
Amino acids, antioxidants, herbals, vitamins, minerals. Products available through health-care professionals only.

Metagenics, Inc.
100 Avenue La Pata
San Clemente, CA 92673
800-692-9400; 949-366-0818
www.metagenics.com
Essentials, Ethical Nutrients, MetaBotanica, Metadocs, Metagenics, MetaPharma, and Unipro brand nutritional supplements, including: Cal Apatite; Collagenics; Endurabolic; Fibroplex; Metazyme; Omega EFA; Ultra Clear Sustain; Ultrabalance Protein. Available through health care professionals only.

Miller Pharmacal Group, Inc.
350 Randy Road, Suite 2
Carol Stream, IL 60188-1831
800-323-2935; 630-871-9557
www.millerpharmacal.com
A/G-Pro; Carozyme; Karbozyme; Milco-Zyme; MM-Zyme; Proteolytic Enzymes; Theramill Forte. Available through health-care professionals only.

MRM-USA
2665 Vista Pacific Drive
Oceanside, CA 92056
800-948-6296; 760-477-8177
www.mrm-usa.com
BioSorb Silymarin; Bone Maximizer; Colon Clear; LiverX; Neuro-Max II.

Muscle-Link
1701 Ives Avenue
Oxnard, CA 93033
800-667-4626; 805-385-3510
www.muscle-link.com
GH Stak.

MuscleTech
1785 South Park Avenue
Buffalo, NY 14220
800-443-4074
www.muscletech.com
Cell-Tech.

National Allergy Supply, Inc.
1620 Satellite Boulevard, Suite D
Duluth, GA 30097
800-522-1448; 770-623-3237
www.natlallergy.com
Drug-free allergy-relief products.

National Enzyme Company
15366 U.S. Highway 160
Forsyth, MO 65653
800-825-8545; 417-546-4796
www.nationalenzyme.com
Plant-derived digestive enzyme products.

NatraBio
A Division of Nutraceutical
International Corporation
P.O. Box 5935
Bellingham, WA 98227-5935
800-232-4005; 360-384-5656
www.natrabio.com
Homeopathic remedies: Adrenal Support; Acne Relief; Allergy Relief formulas.

Natren, Inc.
3105 Willow Lane
Westlake Village, CA 91361
866-462-8736
www.natren.com
Bifido Factor; Digesta-Lac; Gy-na-tren;
Healthy Trinity; LifeStart; Megadophilus.

Natrol Inc.
21411 Prairie Street
Chatsworth, CA 91311
800-262-8765; 818-739-6000
www.natrol.com
Cravex; DHEA; Digest Support; MSM;
Tonalin.

Natural Balance
1400 Kearns Boulevard
Park City, UT 84060
800-833-8737
www.naturalbalance.com
Brain Pep; Cobra; Colon Clenz; Diet Pep;
EROX, 5-HTP; HTP.Calm; MSM Cream;
Pyruvate; Turbo Charge.

Natural Organics
See Nature's Plus.

Naturally Vitamins
A Marlyn Nutraceuticals Inc. Company
4404 East Elwood
Phoenix, AZ 85040
888-766-4406; 480-991-0200
www.naturallyvitamins.com
Medizym.

NaturalMax
See Nutraceutical Corporation.

Nature's Answer
85 Commerce Drive
Hauppauge, NY 11788
800-439-2324; 631-231-7492
www.naturesanswer.com
Bio-Strath; For Kids herbal supplements,
including Bubble B-Gone; E-Kid-nacea;
E-Kid-nacea Plus; green tea; Kid B-Well
Tonic; Kid Catnip; Kid Chamomile; Tummie
Tonic.

Nature's Best Inc.
195 Engineers Road
Hauppauge, NY 11788
800-345-2378; 631-232-3355
www.naturesbest.com
IsoPure.

Nature's Life
900 Larkspur Landing Circle, Suite 105
Larkspur, CA 94939
800-247-6997; 435-655-6790
www.natureslife.com
Bromelain Joint Ease, Ginger & Curcumin
Joint Ease.

Nature's Path Foods
9100 Van Horne Way
Richmond, BC V6X 1W3 Canada
www.naturespath.com
Cereals, breads, organic products.

Nature's Path Supplements
P.O. Box 7862
North Port, FL 34287
800-326-5772; 941-426-3375
www.naturespathsupplements.com
Electrolyte products.

Nature's Plus
548 Broadhollow Road
Melville, NY 11747
800-645-9500; 631-293-0030
www.naturesplus.com
Rx Joint products; Spiru-tein; Source of
Life; Nature's Plus supplements, including
Bioperine 10; Bromelain; Candida Forte;
Coenzyme Q$_{10}$; Detoxygen; Glucosamine/
Chondroitin MSM Ultra Rx-Joint Cream;
Herbal Actives, including Artichoke;
ImmunActinZinc lozenges; Liv-R-Actin;
Ocu-Care; Prost-Actin; Quercetin Plus;
SAMe Rx-Mood; Spiru-tein; Ultra
Bromelain; Ultra Hair; Ultra Juice Green;
Ultra Nails.

Nature's Secret
5310 Beethoven Street
Los Angeles, CA 90066
800-297-3273; 310-306-3636 x3815
www.naturessecret.com
Ultimate Cleanse; Ultimate Fiber;
Ultimate Oil.

Nature's Sources, LLC
5665 W. Howard Street
Niles, IL 60714
800-827-7656
www.naturessources.com
AbsorbAid; Kolorex; Kolorex cream; Kolorex
Advanced Candida Care.

Nature's Way Inc.
1375 North Mountain Springs Parkway
Springville, UT 84663
800-962-8873; 801-489-1500
www.naturesway.com
Coenzyme Q$_{10}$; Kidney Bladder Formula;
Naturalax 2; Primadophilus; Silent Night
Formula.

NatureWorks
c/o Nature's Way Inc.
1375 North Mountain Springs Parkway
Springville, UT 84663
800-962-8873
www.naturework.com
Body Essential Silica gel; Calendula Cream.

New Chapter, Inc.
90 Technology Drive
Brattleboro, VT 05301
800-543-7279
www.newchapter.com
Everyman; Everywoman; Probiotic All-
Flora; Zyflamed.

Neways, Inc.
2089 Neways Drive
Springville, UT 84663
801-418-2000
www.neways.com
Nature's ScienCeuticals products, including
Cell Pill; Orbitol; Osteo Solutions.

Next Pharmaceuticals
360 Espinosa Road
Salinas, CA 93907
831-621-8712
www.nextpharmaceuticals.com
Flavoxine; Nexrutine.

Nordic Naturals
94 Hanger Way
Watsonville, CA 95076
800-662-2544; 831-724-6200
www.nordicnaturals.com
Essential fatty acids; Children's DHA;
EPA; Ultimate Omega.

North American Herb & Spice
P.O. Box 4885
Buffalo Grove, IL 60089
800-243-5242; 847-473-4700
www.oreganol.com
Oreganol P73; Oregamax; oil of rosemary.

NuMedica
9503 East 55th Place
Tulsa, OK 74145
866-787-5175; 918-665-1151
www.numedica.com

Nupharma Nutraceuticals, Inc.
4045 Sheridan Avenue, Suite 363
Miami Beach, FL 33140
305-861-3366; 866-888-8208
www.dldewey.com
Béres Drops Plus.

Nu Skin Enterprises
75 West Center
Provo, UT 84601
800-487-1000
www.nuskin.com

Nutraceutical Corporation
1400 Kearns Boulevard
Park City, UT 84060
800-669-8877
www.nutraceutical.com
Bioallers, Herbs for Kids; KAL, Natrabio;
Nature's Life, Natural Balance brands,
Solray, ZAND products, including L-5-HTP;
Kidney Blend SP-6; Heart Blend SP-8;
Nerve Blend SP-14.

Nutramax Laboratories, Inc.
2208 Lakeside Boulevard
Edgewood, MD 21040
800-925-5187; 410-776-4000
www.nutramaxlabs.com
Cosamin; Senior Moment.

Nutramedix
2885 Jupiter Park Drive, Suite 1600
Jupiter, FL 33458
800-730-3130; 561-745-2917
www.nutramedix.com
Maca; noni liquid extract; samento liquid extract.

Nutrapathic Products
See Parametric Associates, Inc.

Nutravitals
3005 Parkfield Loop South
Spring Hill, TN 38401
800-479-8994
www.nutravitals.com
Cinnulin PF.

NutriCology Inc.
2300 North Loop Road
Alameda, CA 94502
800-545-9960; 510-263-2000
www.nutricology.com
OcuDyne; Russian Choice Immune; Prima Uña de Gato; Progreens.

Nutri-Health USA, LLC
260 Justin Drive
Cottonwood, AZ 86326
800-914-6311
www.nutri-health.com
Flora Source.

Nutrition Now, Inc.
6350 Northeast Campus Drive
Vancouver, WA 98661
800-929-0418; 360-737-6800
www.nutritionnow.com
Quercetin Plus; PMS Support; PB 8; Pro-biotic Acidophilus; Rhino Gummy Bear vitamins.

Nutrition 21
4 Manhattanville Road
Purchase, NY 10577-2197
800-343-3082; 914-701-4500
www.nutrition21.com
Mineral supplements.

Olympian Labs
One Olympian Plaza
8445 East Hartford Drive
Scottsdale, AZ 85255
800-473-5883; 480-483-2302
www.olympian-labs.com
Asthma-X5, Biogra; Cold-X10, Fibro-X, Gastro-Calm; Glucosalage S04 (regular and extra strength); Herp-Eeze; Pedia-Calm.

Omega-Life, Inc.
P.O. Box 7
18752 Enterprise Drive
Muskego, WI 53005-0007
800-328-3529; 262-679-9850
www.fortifiedflax.com
Fortified Flax; Omega-Bars.

Omega Nutrition
1695 Franklin Street
Vancouver, BC V5L 1P5 Canada
800-661-3529; 604-253-4677
Mail orders in U.S.:
6515 Aldrich Road
Bellingham, WA 98226
www.omeganutrition.com
Flaxseed oil and other organic oil products.

Only Natural Inc.
31 Saratoga Boulevard
Island Park, NY 11558
800-866-2887; 516-897-7001
www.onlynaturalinc.com
Beauty aids; Glucosamine/Chondroitin Sulfate; horny goat weed; NONI, olive leaf extract; vitamins and other supplements.

Optimal Nutrients Inc.
1163 Chess Drive, Suite F
Foster City, CA 94404
800-966-8874; 650-525-0112
www.optimalnutrients.com
Earth Select and Enduroflex brands; Coenzyme Q_{10}; DHEA; 5-HTP; vanadyl sulfate.

Optimum Nutrition
700 North Commerce Street
Aurora, IL 60504
800-705-5226; 630-236-0097
www.optimumnutrition.com
Pro Complex.

Organogenesis, Inc.
150 Dan Road
Canton, MA 02021
781-575-0775
www.organogenesis.com
Apligraf wound dressings for diabetic foot ulcers.

Oxyfresh Worldwide, Inc.
1875 North Lakewood Drive
Coeur d'Alene, ID 83814
800-333-7374
www.oxyfresh.com
Oxyfresh Nutritionals.

Padma
See EcoNugenics, Inc.

Parametric Associates, Inc.
10934 Lin-Valle Drive
St. Louis, MO 63123
800-747-1601; 314-892-0988
www.nutrapathic.com
Nutrapathic products, including Brain Alert; Cardio-Power; Cold, Sinus & Allergy Season; Digest-All; Super Fat Metabolizer; Fatigue Free; Female Nutrients; G.O.U.T.; Male Formula; Mobility; Multiple "Plus"; Nutra-Mune; Para-Cleans; Pure & Regular; Stress Free; Super Antioxidant; Sweet Dreams.

Pharmanex, Inc.
75 West Center
Provo, UT 84601
800-487-1000; 801-345-1000
www.pharmanex.com
Cholestin.

PhysioLogics
2100 Smithtown Avenue
Ronkonkoma, NY 11779
800-765-6775
www.physiologics.com
Coloklysis; CTR Support, evening primrose oil. Products available through health care professionals and distributors.

P.L. Thomas & Co., Inc
1 Speedwell Avenue
Morristown, NJ 07960
973-984-0900
www.plthomas.com
5-LOXIN.

Planetary Herbals
P.O. Box 1760
Soquel, CA 95073
800-606-6226; 831-438-1700
www.planetaryherbals.com
Horse Chestnut Cream; Triphala.

Primary Source
c/o Sweetwater Natural Products
P.O. Box 278
Hancock, NH 03449
888-666-1188
www.psopc.com
OPC-branded products.

Progressive Research Labs, Inc.
9207 Heatherwood
Austin, TX 78748
800-877-0966
www.prlab.com
Diabetic Nutrition Rx; Hypoglycemic Nutrition Rx; Vision Nutrition Rx.

Prolongevity
See Life Extension Foundation.

Puritan's Pride
1233 Montauk Highway
Oakdale, NY 11769-9001
800-645-1030
www.puritanspride.com
Vitamin, mineral, and herbal supplements.

Q-Care International, LLC
680 Atlanta Country Club Drive
Marietta, GA 30067
800-992-4668; 770-953-2011
www.qcareintl.com
Q-103 needle management system.

Quantum, Inc.
P.O. Box 2791
Eugene, OR 97402
800-448-1448; 541-345-5556
www.quantumhealth.com
SuperLysine.

Queen Helene Products
See Hain Celestial Group.

Rainbow Light Nutritional Systems
125 McPherson Street
Santa Cruz, CA 95060
800-635-1233
www.rainbowlight.com

Rapid Nutrition
P.O. Box 66457
Los Angeles, CA 90066
800-297-3273
www.rapidnutritionproducts.com
Fast-release liquid soft-gels: Instant Energy; Rapid Joint Relief; Rapid Sleep; Multi-vitamin.

R-Garden Inc.
14 Enzyme Lane
Kettle Falls, WA 99141
800-800-1927; 509-738-2345
www.rgarden.com
Cordyceps.

Ridgecrest Herbals, Inc.
1151 South Redwood Road, Suite 106
Salt Lake City, UT 84104
800-242-4649; 801-978-9633
www.ridgecrestherbals.com
Asthmaclear; ClearLungs.

Right Foods (Bio-San Labs)
8 Bowers Road
Derry, NH 03038
800-634-6342; 603-432-5022
www.right-foods.com
JCTH.

RX Vitamins
150 Clearbrook Road, Suite 149
Elmsford, NY 10523
800-792-2222; 914-592-2323
www.rxvitamins.com
ARTH-9; DB-7; Menopause Formula; Ocular Formula. Marketed to health care professionals and selected pharmacies.

Sabinsa Corporation
70 Ethel Road West, #6
Piscataway, NJ 08854
732-777-1111
www.sabinsa.com
Ayurvedic extracts and nutraceuticals, including ashwagandha; Bacopin; Bioperine; Boswellin; Citrin; Coleus forskohlii; C3 Complex; Ginger Dry Extract; Ginger Soft Extract; Gymnema Sylvestre GS4.

Salus Haus
See Flora Inc.

Sawyer Products, Inc.
P.O. Box 188
Safety Harbor, FL 34695
800-356-7811
www.sawyerproducts.com
Extractor Pump kit.

Scandinavian Formulas, Inc.
140 East Church Street
Sellersville, PA 18960
800-688-2276; 215-453-2507
www.scandinavianformulas.com
Good Breath TMs; Saliva Sure; shark liver oil.

Schiff Products
P.O. Box 26708
Salt Lake City, UT 84126
800-526-6251
www.schiffvitamins.com
Phytocharged nutritional supplements.

Similasan Corporation
1745 Shea Center Drive, Suite 380
Highlands Ranch, CO 80129
800-426-1644
www.similasanusa.com
Similasan Eye Drops #1; Similasan Eye Drops #2.

Solaray Products
See Nutraceutical Corporation.

Solgar Vitamin and Herb Company, Inc.
301 Admiral Boulevard
Kansas City, MO 64106
800-544-8147; 816-221-3719
www.solgar.com
Advanced Carotenoid Complex; EarthSource Greens & More; MaxEPA; Whey to Go.

Sonne Organic Foods, Inc.
301 Admiral Blvd.
Kansas City, MO 64106
800-544-8147
816-221-3719
www.sonnes.com
Calphonite; Cod liver oil; Sonnes #7 Detoxificant; Wheat Germ Oil.

Source Naturals
23 Janis Way
Scotts Valley, CA 95066
888-815-2333; 831-438-1144
www.sourcenaturals.com
Activated Quercetin; Calcium Night; Cat's Claw Defense Complex; Coenzymate B Complex; Essential Enzymes; GlucosaMend; Heart Science; HotFlash; Lifeforce Multiple; N-A-G; Proanthodyn; Urban Air Defense; Visual Eyes; Wellness Formula.

Spectrum Organic Products, Inc.
The Hain Celestial Group, Inc.
4600 Sleepytime Drive
Boulder, CO 80301
800-434-4246
www.spectrumorganics.com
Organic and culinary oils, vinegars, and supplements.

Standard Homeopathic Company
See Hyland's, Inc.

Sun Chlorella USA
3305 Kashiwa Street
Torrance, CA 90505
800-829-2828
www.sunchlorellausa.com

Sun Precautions
2815 Wetmore Avenue
Everett, WA 98201
800-882-7860; 425-303-8585
www.sunprecautions.com
Solumbra sun-protective clothing.

The SunBox Company
19217 Orbit Drive
Gaithersburg, MD 20879
800-548-3968; 301-869-5980
www.sunbox.com
Dawn/Dusk Simulators.

Sundown Naturals
90 Orville Drive
Bohemia, NY 11716
888-848-2435; 561-241-9400
www.sundownnaturals.com

Superior Source
See cvc4health.com

Sweet Wheat, Inc.
P.O. Box 187
Clearwater, FL 33757
888-227-9338; 727-442-5454
www.sweetwheat.com
Sweet Wheat.

Symbiotics, Inc.
1 City Boulevard West, Suite 1440
Orange, CA 92868
888-784-4355; 714-860-7617
www.symbiotics.com
Colostrum Plus.

The Synergy Company
2279 South Resource Boulevard
Moab, UT 84532
800-723-0277; 435-259-5366
www.thesynergycompany.com
Pure Radiance C; Pure Synergy; Vita Synergy for Men; Vita Synergy for Women.

Terra Maxa, Inc.
3301 West Central Avenue
Toledo, OH 43606
800-783-7817
www.terramaxa.com
P.S.I.

Threshold Enterprises
23 Janis Way
Scotts Valley, CA 95066
800-777-5677; 831-438-6851
www.thresholdenterprises.com
Distributor of vitamin and mineral supplements.

Thunder Ridge Emu
9217 Center Street
Manassas, VA 20110
703-631-9074
www.thunderridgeemu.com
Emu oil.

Thursday Plantation (TP Health Ltd.)
Pacific Highway
Ballina, NSW 2478, Australia
61 (2)6620 5100
www.thursdayplantation.com
Tea tree oil.

Tom's of Maine
302 Lafayette Center
Kennebunk, ME 04043
800-367-8667; 207-985-2944
www.tomsofmaine.com
*Tom's of Maine Natural Toothpaste and
other natural body care products.*

Trace Minerals Research
1996 West 3300 South
Ogden, UT 84401
800-624-7145; 801-731-6051
www.traceminerals.com
*Arth-X; Complete Calcium & Magnesium;
ConcenTrace; Electrolyte Stamina Tablets.
Sells to retailers and other distributors, not
directly to consumers.*

TriMedica Inc.
1895 South Los Feliz Drive
Tempe, AZ 85281
800-800-8849; 480-998-1041
www.trimedica.com
*Alkamax Products; All Complete Enzymes;
Grobust; Oz Life; Pregnenolone 5 HTP;
Progesta; Pure MSM Liquid; Vitamin O2.*

Twinlab Corporation
600 East Quality Drive
American Fork, UT 84003
800-645-5626
www.twinlab.com
*Bone Support with Ostivone; Everslender;
OcuGuard; omega-3 fish oil softgels; Ripped
Fuel Extreme.*

Växa International, Inc.
600 North Westshore Boulevard,
Suite 800
Tampa, FL 33609
877-622-8292; 813 870 2904
www.vaxa.com
*Anti-Oxin; Attend; Buffer-pH; Clearin;
Medical pH-Test Strips; Parasitin;
Prostatin.*

Wakunaga of America Company, Ltd.
23501 Madero
Mission Viejo, CA 92691
800-421-2998; 949-855-2776
www.kyolic.com
*Arthritic Pain Relief Cream; Be Sure; Bifido
Factor; Cardio Logic; Ginkgo Biloba Plus;
Kyo-Chlorella; Kyo-Dophilus; Kyo-Green;
Kyolic aged garlic extract; Kyolic-EPA;
Kyolic Formula 102; Kyolic Formula 105;
Liquid Kyolic with B_1 and B_{12}; Kyolic
Neuro Logic; Kyo-Dophilus Vegetarian
Tablets.*

Warren Laboratories
1656 Interstate Highway 35 South
Abbott, TX 76621
254-580-9990
www.warrenlabsaloe.com
George's Aloe vera juice.

Waterwise
3608 Parkway Boulevard
Leesburg, FL 34748
800-874-9028; 352-787-5008
www.waterwise.com
*Showerwise filter with showerhead and
water distillation products.*

Wein Products Inc.
115 West 25th Street
Los Angeles, CA 90007
213-749-6049
www.weinproducts.com
Air Supply personal air purifier.

Windmill Health Products
6 Henderson Drive
West Caldwell, NJ 07006
800-822-4320
www.windmillvitamins.com
Menocom.

ZAND Herbal Formulas
A Division of Nutraceutical
Corporation
P.O. Box 5935
Bellingham, WA 98227-5935
800-241-0859
www.zand.com
*Allergy Season Formula; Cold and Flu
Formulas; Decongest Herbal; HerbalMist
throat spray; Herbs for Kids; Insure
Immune Support Liquids; Quick Cleanse
Program.*

HEALTH AND MEDICAL ORGANIZATIONS

The following is a list of organizations that can provide assistance for specific disorders and situations. The services offered by these organizations vary. Some provide information only; others offer various types of referrals, support groups, and even access to medical or social services. In most cases, the organizations' areas of interest are obvious from their names. Where this is not the case, a brief description of the organization's focus is offered. Be aware that contact information is subject to change.

RESOURCE ORGANIZATIONS

Academy of Chinese Healing Arts
3808 North Tamiami Trail
Sarasota, FL 34234
800-883-5528; 941-355-9080
http://universities.com/schools/A/
Academy_of_Chinese_Healing_Arts
.asp
Program includes acupuncture, Chinese herbology, and homeopathy.

Acupressure Institute
1533 Shattuck Avenue
Berkeley, CA 94709
800-442-2232; 510-845-1059
www.acupressureinstitute.com

Administration on Aging
One Massachusetts Avenue NW
Washington, DC 20001
800-677-1116; 202-619-0724
www.aoa.gov

Agency for Healthcare Research and Quality
540 Gaither Road
Rockville, MD 20850
301-427-1364
www.ahrq.gov
Federal agency charged with improving the quality, safety, efficiency, and effectiveness of health care for all Americans through health services research and information.

AIDS Action Committee of Massachusetts
294 Washington Street, 5th Floor
Boston, MA 02108
617-437-6200; 617-437-1394 (TTY)
Hotline: 800-235-2331
www.aac.org

Alcoholics Anonymous
P.O. Box 459
New York, NY 10163
212-870-3400
www.aa.org

Alexander Graham Bell Association for the Deaf
3417 Volta Place NW
Washington, DC 20007
202-337-5220 (voice); 202-337-5221 (TTY)
www.agbell.org

ALS Association
27001 Agoura Road, Suite 250
Calabasas Hills, CA 91301
818-880-9007
www.alsa.org

Alzheimer's Association
225 North Michigan Avenue, Floor 17
Chicago, IL 60601-7633
800-272-3900
www.alz.org

American Academy of Allergy, Asthma, and Immunology
555 East Wells Street, Suite 1100
Milwaukee, WI 53202-3823
800-822-2762; 414-272-6071
www.aaaai.org

American Academy of Anti-Aging Medicine
301 Yamato Rd, Suite 2199
Boca Raton, FL 33431
561 997-0112
www.worldhealth.net
Information on antiaging studies and assistance in finding a doctor specializing in this field.

American Academy of Child and Adolescent Psychiatry
3615 Wisconsin Avenue NW
Washington, DC 20016-3007
202-966-7300
www.aacap.org

American Academy of Dermatology
P.O. Box 4014
Schaumburg, IL 60618-4014
866 503-7546; 847-330-0230
www.aad.org

American Academy of Orthopaedic Surgeons
6300 North River Road
Rosemont, IL 60018-4262
800-346-AAOS; 847-823-7186
http://aaos.org

American Academy of Otolaryngology—Head and Neck Surgery
1650 Diagonal Street
Alexandria, VA 22314-2857
703-836-4444
www.entnet.org
Services include providing information about Ménière's disease.

American Academy of Pain Management
13947 Mono Way, #A
Sonora, CA 95370
209-533-9744
www.aapainmanage.org

American Academy of Sleep Medicine
One Westbrook Corporate Center, Suite 920
Westchester, IL 60154
708-492-0930
www.aasmnet.org

American Anorexia Bulimia Association of Philadelphia
P.O. Box 1287
Langhorne, PA 19047
215-221-1864
www.aabaphila.org

American Association of Acupuncture and Oriental Medicine (AAAOM)
P.O. Box 162340
Sacramento, CA 95816
866-455-7999; 916-443-4770
www.aaaomonline.org
Specializes in Oriental healing and exercise. Provides information on acupuncture and a list of practitioners in your area.

American Association of Clinical Endocrinologists
245 Riverside Avenue, Suite 200
Jacksonville, FL 32202
904-353-7878
www.aace.com
Provides information about thyroid and other glandular disorders.

American Association of Nutritional Consultants
401 Kings Highway
Winona Lake, IN 46590
888-828-2262
www.aanc.net
Offers certified nutritional counseling (CNC) certification.

American Association of Poison Control Centers
Poison Help Hotline
800-222-1222

American Board of Clinical Metal Toxicology
4889 Smith Road
West Chester, OH 45069
800-356-2228; 513-863-6277
www.abcmt.org
Can provide information on approved chelation therapists in your area.

American Botanical Council
6200 Manor Road
Austin, TX 78723
512-926-4900
http://abc.herbalgram.org
Provides information on the proper usage of herbs and medicinal plants.

American Brain Tumor Association
2720 River Road
Des Plaines, IL 60018
800-886-2282
www.abta.org

American Cancer Society
1599 Clifton Road
Atlanta, GA 30329
800-ACS-2345; 866-228-4327 (TTY)
www.cancer.org

American Chronic Pain Association, Inc. (ACPA)
P.O. Box 850
Rocklin, CA 95677-0850
800-533-3231; 916-632-0922
www.theacpa.org
Services include providing support and education for people with chronic pain.

American College for Advancement in Medicine (ACAM)
24411 Ridge Route, Suite 115
Laguna Hills, CA 92653
949-309-3520
www.acamnet.org
Provides a list of physicians who take an integral approach to medicine.

American College of Cardiology
Heart House
2400 N Street NW
Washington, DC 20037
800-253-4636; 202-375-6000
www.acc.org

American Council for Headache Education (ACHE)
819 Mantua Road
Mount Royal, NJ 08061
800-255-2243
www.achenet.org

American Council of the Blind
2200 Wilson Boulevard, Suite 650
Arlington, VA 22201
800-424-8666; 202-467-5081
www.acb.org

American Dental Association
211 East Chicago Avenue
Chicago, IL 60611-2678
312-440-2500
www.ada.org

American Diabetes Association
1701 North Beauregard Street
Alexandria, VA 22311
800-342-2383
www.diabetes.org

American Foundation for AIDS Research (AMFAR)
120 Wall Street, 13th Floor
New York, NY 10005-3908
212-806-1600
www.amfar.org

American Foundation for the Blind
11 Penn Plaza, Suite 300
New York, NY 10001
800-232-5463; 212-502-7600
www.afb.org

American Genetic Association
2030 SE Marine Science Drive
Newport, OR 97365
541-867-0334
www.theaga.org

American Heart Association
7272 Greenville Avenue
Dallas, TX 75231
800-242-8721; 214-373-6300
www.americanheart.org

American Hemochromatosis Society, Inc.
4044 West Lake Mary Boulevard, Unit #104, PMB 416
Lake Mary, FL 32746-2012
888-655-4766; 407-829-4488
www.americanhs.org

American Herbal Products Association
8630 Fenton Street, Suite 918
Silver Spring, MD 20910
301-588-1171
www.ahpa.org

American Industrial Hygiene Association
2700 Prosperity Avenue, Suite 250
Fairfax, VA 22031
703-849-8888
www.aiha.org
Provides information on occupational and environmental health and safety issues.

American Institute of Holistic Theology
2112 Eleventh Avenue South, Suite 520
Birmingham, AL 35205-2841
800-650-4325
www.aiht.edu
Provides instruction in a variety of natural approaches to health care and maintenance.

American Kidney Fund (AKF)
6110 Executive Boulevard, Suite 1010
Rockville, MD 20852
800-638-8299
www.akfinc.org

American Liver Foundation (ALF)
75 Maiden Lane, Suite 603
New York, NY 10038
800-465-4837; 212-668-1000
www.liverfoundation.org

American Lung Association
1301 Pennsylvania Avenue NW, Suite 800
Washington, DC 20004
800-548-8252; 212-315-8700
www.lungusa.org

American Medical Association (AMA)
515 North State Street
Chicago, IL 60654
800-621-8335
www.ama-assn.org

American Mental Health Foundation
1049 Fifth Avenue
New York, NY 10028
212-737-9027
www.americanmentalhealthfoundation.org

American Pain Foundation
201 North Charles Street, Suite 710
Baltimore, MD 21201-4111
888-615-7246
www.painfoundation.org

American Pain Society
4700 West Lake Avenue
Glenview, IL 60025
847-375-4715
www.ampainsoc.org

American Parkinson Disease Association
135 Parkinson Avenue
Staten Island, NY 10305
800-223-2732; 718-981-8001
www.apdaparkinson.org

American Reflexology Certification Board
P.O. Box 5147
Gulfport, FL 33737
303-933-6921
www.arcb.net
Can provide information on programs for learning this technique.

American Social Health Association
P.O. Box 13827
Research Triangle Park, NC 27709-9940
919-361-8400
www.ashastd.org
Provides information on sexually transmitted diseases.

American Society for Reproductive Medicine
1209 Montgomery Highway
Birmingham, AL 35216-2809
205-978-5000
www.asrm.org

American Society of Cataract and Refractive Surgery
4000 Legato Road, #700
Fairfax, VA 22033
703-591-2220
www.ascrs.org

American Speech-Language-Hearing Association
2200 Research Boulevard
Rockville, MD 20850-3289
800-638-8255; 301-296-5650 (TTY)
www.asha.org

American Tinnitus Association
P.O. Box 5
Portland, OR 97207-0005
800-634-8978; 503-248-9985
www.ata.org

American Thyroid Association
6066 Leesburg Pike, Suite 550
Falls Church, VA 22041
800-849-7643; 703-998-8890
www.thyroid.org

ANAD National Association of Anorexia Nervosa and Associated Eating Disorders
P.O. Box 7
Highland Park, IL 60035
847-831-3438
www.anad.org

Antiepileptic Drug Pregnancy Registry
149 CNY-MGH East, 10th Floor
Charlestown, MA 02129-2000
888-233-2334
www.aedpregnancyregistry.org

Anxiety Disorders Association of America
8730 Georgia Avenue, Suite 600
Silver Spring, MD 20910
240-485-1001
www.adaa.org

Arthritis Foundation
P.O. Box 7669
Atlanta, GA 30357-0669
800-283-7800; 404-872-7100
www.arthritis.org

Association for Applied Psychophysiology and Biofeedback
10200 West 44th Avenue, Suite 304
Wheat Ridge, CO 80033
800-477-8892; 303-422-8436
www.aapb.org

Association for the Education and Rehabilitation of the Blind and Visually Impaired
1703 North Beauregard Street, Suite 440
Alexandria, VA 22311
877-492-2708; 703-671-4500
www.aerbvi.org

Asthma and Allergy Foundation of America (AAFA)
1233 20th Street NW, Suite 402
Washington, DC 20036
800-727-8462; 202-466-7643
www.aafa.org

Attention Deficit Disorder Association (ADDA)
P.O. Box 7557
Wilmington, DE 19803-9997
800-939-1019
www.add.org

Auriculotherapy Certification Institute (ACI)
8033 Sunset Boulevard, PMB 265
Los Angeles, CA 90046-2427
323-656-2084
www.auriculotherapy.com

Autism Society of America
7910 Woodmont Avenue, Suite 300
Bethesda, MD 20814-3067
800-328-8476; 301-657-0881
www.autism-society.org

Brain Injury Association
1608 Spring Hill Road, Suite 110
Vienna, VA 22182
800-444-6443; 703-761-0750
www.biausa.org

Brain Research Foundation
111 W. Washington Street, Suite 1710
Chicago, IL 60602
312-759-5150
www.brainresearchfdn.org

Breast Cancer Network of Strength
212 West Van Buren Street, Suite 1000
Chicago, IL 60607-3903
800-221-2141; 312-986-8338
www.networkofstrength.org

Celiac Disease Foundation
13251 Ventura Boulevard, Suite 1
Studio City, CA 91604
818-990-2354
www.celiac.org

Center for the Study of Anorexia and Bulimia
1841 Broadway, 4th Floor
New York, NY 10023
212-333-3444
www.csabnyc.org

Centers for Disease Control
See U.S. Centers for Disease Control and Prevention (CDC).

Charlie Foundation to Help Cure Pediatric Epilepsy
1223 Wilshire Boulevard, Suite 815
Santa Monica, CA 90403
800-367-5386; 310-393-2347
www.charliefoundation.org

Children and Adults with Attention Deficit/Hyperactivity Disorder
8181 Professional Place, Suite 150
Landover, MD 20785
800-233-4050; 301-306-7070
www.chadd.org

Children of Aging Parents (CAPS)
P.O. Box 167
Richboro, PA 18954
800-227-7294
www.caps4caregivers.org

Children's PKU Network
3970 Via de la Valle
Del Mar, CA 92014
800-377-6677; 858-509-0767
www.pkunetwork.org

Children's Tumor Foundation
95 Pine Street, 16th Floor
New York, NY 10005
800-323-7938; 212-344-6633
www.ctf.org

CFIDS Association of America
P.O. Box 220398
Charlotte, NC 28222-0398
704-365-2343
www.cfids.org
Provides information and services related to chronic fatigue and immune dysfunction syndrome.

Citizens United for Research in Epilepsy (CURE)
730 North Franklin, Suite 404
Chicago, IL 60654
800-765-7118; 312-255-1801
www.CUREepilepsy.org

Clayton College of Natural Health
2140 11th Avenue South, Suite 305
Birmingham, AL 35205
800-659-8274
www.ccnh.edu
Provides degree programs in nutrition, naturopathy, and other holistic disciplines.

Crohn's and Colitis Foundation of America
386 Park Avenue South, 17th Floor
New York, NY 10016
800-932-2423
www.ccfa.org

Cystic Fibrosis Foundation (CFF)
6931 Arlington Road
Bethesda, MD 20814
800-344-4823; 301-951-4422
www.cff.org

Do It Now Foundation
www.doitnow.org
Publishes substance abuse and behavioral health information.

Dogs for the Deaf
10175 Wheeler Road
Central Point, OR 97502
541-826-9220 (voice and TDD)
www.dogsforthedeaf.org

Endometriosis Association
8585 North 76th Place
Milwaukee, WI 53223
414-355-2200
www.endometriosisassn.org

Environmental Protection Agency (EPA)
See U.S. Environmental Protection Agency.

Epilepsy Foundation of America
8301 Professional Place
Landover, MD 20785
800-332-1000
www.epilepsyfoundation.org

Epilepsy Foundation of Metropolitan New York
257 Park Avenue South, Suite 302
New York, NY 10010
212-677-8550
www.epilepsyinstitute.org

Esalen Institute
55000 Highway 1
Big Sur, CA 93920-9616
831-667-3000
www.esalen.org
Provides information on Esalen massage therapy.

Family Caregiver Alliance
180 Montgomery Street, Suite 1100
San Francisco, CA 94104
800-445-8106; 415-434-3388
www.caregiver.org

FDA Cancer Liaison Program
Office of Special Health Issues
U.S. Food and Drug Administration
5600 Fishers Lane, HF-12
Room 9-49
Rockville, MD 20857
888-463-6332; 301-827-4460
www.fda.gov/oashi/cancer/cancer
.html

Feingold Association of the United States
554 East Main Street, Suite 301
Riverhead, NY 11901
800-321-3287; 631-369-9340
www.feingold.org
Provides information on the effects of food and food additives on health, behavior, and learning.

Feldenkrais Guild of North America
5436 North Albina Avenue
Portland, OR 97217
800-775-2118; 503-221-6612
www.feldenkrais.com
Provides information on the Feldenkrais method of therapeutic touch.

Fibromyalgia Network
P.O. Box 31750
Tucson, AZ 85751
800-853-2929
www.fmnetnews.com

Food Allergy Network
11781 Lee Jackson Highway, Suite 160
Fairfax, VA 22033
800-929-4040
www.foodallergy.org

Food and Drug Administration (FDA)
See U.S. Food and Drug Administration

Foundation Fighting Blindness
11435 Cronhill Drive
Owings Mills, MD 21117-2220
800-683-5555; 410-568-0150
TDD: 800-683-5551; 410-363-7139
www.blindness.org
Provides information on retinal disorders, including macular degeneration, retinitis pigmentosa, and Usher syndrome.

The Genetic Alliance
4301 Connecticut Avenue NW, Suite 404
Washington, DC 20008-2369
202-966-5557
www.geneticalliance.org
Works to enhance the lives of people with genetic health conditions.

Gerontology Research Group
P.O. Box 905
Santa Clarita, CA 91380-9005
661-775-3995
www.grg.org
Physicians, scientists, and engineers dedicated to the quest to slow and ultimately reverse human aging.

Glaucoma Research Foundation
251 Post Street, Suite 600
San Francisco, CA 94108
800-826-6693; 415-986-3162
www.glaucoma.org

Guiding Eyes for the Blind
611 Granite Springs Road
Yorktown Heights, NY 10598
800-942-0149; 914-245-4024
www.guidingeyes.org

Harvard Medical School
Harvard University
25 Shattuck Street Boston, MA 02115
617-432-1000
www.hms.harvard.edu
Provides a variety of health-related publications and information.

Herpes Resource Center
See American Social Health Association.

Hudson Valley School of Classical Homeopathy
321 McKinstry Road
Gardiner, NY 12525
845-255-6141
www.classicalhomeopathy.com

Human Growth Foundation
997 Glen Cove Avenue, Suite 5
Glen Head, NY 11545
800-451-6434
www.hgfound.org

Immune Deficiency Foundation
40 West Chesapeake Avenue, Suite 308
Towson, MD 21204
800-296-4433
www.primaryimmune.org
Specializes in primary immunodeficiency diseases.

International Diabetes Center
3800 Park Nicollet Boulevard
St. Louis Park, MN 55416-2699
888-825-6315; 952-993-3393
www.idcdiabetes.org

International Essential Tremor Foundation
P.O. Box 14005
Lenexa, KS 66285-4005
888-387-3667; 913-341-3880
www.essentialtremor.org

International Foundation for Functional Gastrointestinal Disorders
P.O. Box 170864
Milwaukee, WI 53217-8076
888-964-2001; 414-964-1799
www.iffgd.org

International Radiosurgery Association
3002 North Second Street
Harrisburg, PA 17110
717-260-9808
www.irsa.org

Interstitial Cystitis Association
100 Park Avenue, Suite 108A
Rockville, MD 20850
800-435-7422; 301-610-5300
www.ichelp.org

Iron Disorders Institute, Inc.
P.O. Box 675
Taylors, SC 29687
888-565-4766; 864-292-1175
www.irondisorders.org

Juvenile Diabetes Research Foundation International
120 Wall Street
New York, NY 10005-4001
800-533-2873; 212-785-9500
http://jdrf.org

La Leche League International
957 North Plum Grove Road
Schaumberg, IL 60173
847-519-7730; 847-592-7570 (TTY)
www.llli.org

The Leukemia and Lymphoma Society
1311 Mamaroneck Avenue
White Plains, NY 10605
800-955-4572; 914-944-5213
www.leukemia-lymphoma.org

The Living Bank
P.O. Box 6725
Houston, TX 77265-6725
800-528-2971; 713-528-2971
www.livingbank.org
Provides information and maintains registry of donated organs, tissues, bones, and bodies for transplants or research.

Lung Line Information Service
National Jewish Health
1400 Jackson Street
Denver, CO 80206
800-222-5864; 303-388-4461
www.nationaljewish.org/about/
contact/lung-line.aspx
Provides information on asthma, allergies, and other disorders.

Lupus Foundation of America
2000 L Street NW, Suite 710
Washington, DC 20036
202-349-1155
www.lupus.org

March of Dimes National Foundation
1275 Mamaroneck Avenue
White Plains, NY 10605
888-663-4637; 914-997-4488
www.marchofdimes.com

Medic Alert Foundation
2323 Colorado Avenue
Turlock, CA 95382
888-633-4298; 209-668-3333
www.medicalert.org
Maintains files on individuals who wear a medical bracelet to provide information in case of an emergency.

Memorial Sloan-Kettering Cancer Center
1275 York Avenue
New York, NY 10065
212-639-2000
www.mskcc.org

Mental Health America
2001 North Beauregard Street, 6th Floor
Alexandria, VA 22311
800-969-6642; 703-684-7722;
800-433-5959 (TTY)
www.nmha.org

Mothers Against Drunk Driving (MADD)
511 East John Carpenter Freeway, Suite 700
Irving, TX 75062
800-438-6233; 214-744-6233
www.madd.org

Multiple Sclerosis Foundation
6350 North Andrews Avenue
Fort Lauderdale, FL 33309-2130
800-225-6495
www.msfacts.org

Muscular Dystrophy Association–USA
3300 East Sunrise Drive
Tucson, AZ 85718
800-572-1717
www.mdausa.org

Myasthenia Gravis Foundation of America
355 Lexington Avenue, 15th Floor
New York, NY 10017
800-541-5454; 212-297-2156
www.myasthenia.org

National Alopecia Areata Foundation
14 Mitchell Boulevard
San Rafael, CA 94903
415-472-3780
www.naaf.org

National Association for Continence
P.O. Box 1019
Charleston, SC 29402-1019
800-252-3337
www.nafc.org

National Association for Visually Handicapped
22 West 21st Street, 6th Floor
New York, NY 10010
212-889-3141
www.navh.org

National Association of People with AIDS (NAPWA)
8401 Coleville Road, Suite 505
Silver Spring, MD 20910
866-846-9366; 240-247-0880
www.napwa.org

National Association of the Deaf
8630 Fenton Street, Suite 820
Silver Spring, MD 20910
301-587-1788 (voice);
301-587-1789 (TTY)
www.nad.org

National Ayurvedic Medical Association
620 Cabrillo Avenue
Santa Cruz, CA 95065
800-669-8914
www.ayurveda-nama.org

National Cancer Institute
6116 Executive Boulevard, Room 3036A
Bethesda, MD 20892-8322
800-422-6237; 800-332-8615 (TTY)
www.cancer.gov

National Center for Chronic Disease Prevention and Health Promotion
U.S. Centers for Disease Control and Prevention (CDC)
Division of Diabetes Translation
4770 Buford Highway NE,
Mailstop K-10
Atlanta, GA 30341-3717
770-488-5000
www.cdc.gov/diabetes

National Center for Complementary and Alternative Medicine (NCCAM)
National Institutes of Health
9000 Rockville Pike
Bethesda, MD 20892
www.nccam.nih.gov
Provides information on complementary and alternative medicine and clinical trials for supplements.

National Center for Injury Prevention and Control (NCIPC)
U.S. Centers for Disease Control and Prevention (CDC)
4770 Buford Highway NE,
Mailstop F-63
Atlanta, GA 30341-3717
770-488-1506
www.cdc.gov/injury/
Services include providing information about fracture prevention and treatment and advice on making homes safer for elderly or frail individuals.

National Center on Sleep Disorders Research
P.O. Box 30105
Bethesda, MD 20824-0105
301-592-8573; 240-629-3255 (TTY)
www.nhlbi.nih.gov/about/ncsdr/

National Certification Commission for Acupuncture and Oriental Medicine (NCCAOM)
76 South Laura Street, Suite 1290
Jacksonville, FL 32202
904-598-1005
www.nccaom.org

National Clearinghouse for Alcohol and Drug Information
The Substance Abuse and Mental Health Services Administration (SAMHSA)
P.O. Box 2345
Rockville, MD 20847-2345
877-726-4727
www.ncadi.samhsa.gov

National Council on Aging
1901 L Street NW, 4th Floor
Washington, DC 20036
202-479-1200
http:www.ncoa.org

National Council on Alcoholism and Drug Dependence
244 East 58th Street, 4th Floor
New York, NY 10022
800-622-2255; 212-269-7797
www.ncadd.org

National Council on Patient Information and Education
4915 St. Elmo Avenue, Suite 505
Bethesda, MD 20814-6082
301-656-8565
www.talkaboutrx.org

National Diabetes Information Clearinghouse (NDIC)
1 Information Way
Bethesda, MD 20892-3560
800-860-8747
http://diabetes.niddk.nih.gov

National Down Syndrome Society (NDSS)
666 Broadway, 8th Floor
New York, NY 10012
800-221-4602; 212-460-9330
www.ndss.org

National Dysautonomia Research Foundation
P.O. Box 301
Red Wing, MN 55066-0301
651-267-0525
www.ndrf.org

National Eating Disorders Organization
603 Stewart Street, Suite 803
Seattle, WA 98101
206-382-3587
www.nationaleatingdisorders.org

National Eye Institute (NEI)
31 Center Drive MSC 2510
Bethesda, MD 20892-2510
301-496-5248
www.nei.nih.gov

National Foundation for the Treatment of Pain
P.O. Box 70045
Houston, TX 77270-0045
713-862-9332
www.paincare.org

National Headache Foundation
820 North Orleans, Suite 217
Chicago, IL 60610
888-643-5552
www.headaches.org

National Health Information Center
P.O. Box 1133
Washington, DC 20013-1133
800-336-4797; 301-565-4167
www.health.gov/nhic

National Heart, Lung, and Blood Institute
Information Center
P.O. Box 30105
Bethesda, MD 20824-0105
301-592-8573; 240-629-3255 (TTY)
www.nhlbi.nih.gov

National Hemophilia Foundation (NHF)
116 West 32nd Street, 11th Floor
New York, NY 10001
800-424-2634; 212-328-3700
www.hemophilia.org

National Hospice and Palliative Care Organization
1731 King Street, Suite 100
Alexandria, VA 22314
800-658-8898; 703-837-1500
www.nhpco.org

National Immunization Program
U.S. Centers for Disease Control and Prevention (CDC)
1600 Clifton Road NE
Atlanta, GA 30333
800-232-4636
www.cdc.gov/vaccines

National Institute for Occupational Safety and Health (NIOSH)
U.S. Centers for Disease Control and Prevention (CDC)
1600 Clifton Road
Atlanta, GA 30333
800-232-4636; 404-639-3311
www.cdc.gov/niosh

National Institute of Allergies and Infectious Diseases
National Institutes of Health
6610 Rockledge Drive
MSC 6612
Bethesda, MD 20892-6612
301-496-5717; 866-284-4107
www3.niaid.nih.gov

National Institute of Arthritis, Musculoskeletal, and Skin Diseases Information Clearinghouse
National Institutes of Health
1 Ams Circle
Bethseda, MD 20892
877-226-4267; 301-495-4848;
301-565-2966 (TTY)
http://niams.nih.gov
Services include providing information about fibromyalgia syndrome.

National Institute of Child Health and Human Development (NICHD)
National Institutes of Health
Building 31, Room 2A32, MSC 2425
31 Center Drive
Bethesda, MD 20892-2425
800-370-2943; 888-320-6942 (TTY)
www.nichd.nih.gov

National Institute of Diabetes and Digestive and Kidney Diseases (NIDDK)
National Institutes of Health
Building 31, Room 9A04, MSC 2560
31 Center Drive
Bethesda, MD 20892-2560
301-496-3583
www2.niddk.nih.gov

National Institute of Mental Health (NIMH)
National Institutes of Health
6001 Executive Boulevard, Room 8184
MSC 9663
Bethesda, MD 20892-9663
866-615-6464; 301-443-4513
www.nimh.nih.gov

National Institute on Aging
National Institutes of Health
Building 31, Room 5C27, MSC 2292
31 Center Drive
Bethesda, MD 20892
301-496-1752
www.nia.nih.gov

National Institute on Alcohol Abuse and Alcoholism
National Institutes of Health
5635 Fishers Lane
MSC 9304
Bethesda, MD 20892-9304
301-443-3860
www.niaaa.nih.gov

National Institute of Neurological Disorders and Stroke
National Institutes of Health
P.O. Box 5801
Bethesda, MD 20824
800-352-9424; 301-496-5751;
301-468-5981 (TTY)
www.ninds.nih.gov

National Institute on Drug Abuse
National Institutes of Health
6001 Executive Boulevard, Room 5213
Bethesda, MD 20892-9561
301-443-1124
www.nida.nih.gov

National Kidney Foundation
30 East 33rd Street
New York, NY 10016
800-622-9010; 212-889-2210
www.kidney.org

National Library Service for the Blind and Physically Handicapped
U.S. Library of Congress
1291 Taylor Street
Washington, DC 20011
888-657-7323; 202-707-5100;
202-707-0744 (TDD)
www.loc.gov/nls/

National Mental Health Information Center
P.O. Box 2345
Rockville, MD 20847
800-789-2647; 866-889-2647 (TDD)
http://mentalhealth.samhsa.gov/

National Multiple Sclerosis Society
733 Third Avenue
New York, NY 10017
800-344-4867
www.nationalmssociety.org

National Organic Program
U.S. Department of Agriculture
www.ams.usda.gov/nop

National Organization for Rare Disorders (NORD)
55 Kenosia Avenue
P.O. Box 1968
Danbury, CT 06813-1968
800-999-6673; 203-744-0100
www.rarediseases.org

National Osteoporosis Foundation
1232 22nd Street NW
Washington, DC 20037-1202
800-231-4222; 202-223-2226
www.nof.org

National Parkinson Foundation (NPF)
1501 Northwest Ninth Avenue
Miami, FL 33136-1494
800-327-4545; 305-243-6666
www.parkinson.org

National Pediculosis Association
P.O. Box 610189
Newton, MA 02461
866-323-5465
www.headlice.org

National Pesticide Information Center
Oregon State University
333 Weiniger
Corvallis, OR 97331-6502
800-858-7378
www.npic.orst.edu
Provides information on health hazards of and safety precautions against pesticides.

National Psoriasis Foundation
6600 Southwest 92nd Avenue, Suite 300
Portland, OR 97223-7195
800-723-9166; 503-244-7404
www.psoriasis.org

National Reye's Syndrome Foundation
P.O. Box 829
Bryan, OH 43506
800-233-7393; 419-636-2679
www.reyessyndrome.org

National Rosacea Society
800 South Northwest Highway, Suite 200
Barrington, IL 60010
888-662-5874
www.rosacea.org

National Safety Council
1121 Spring Lake Drive
Itasca, IL 60143-3201
630-285-1121
www.nsc.org

National Shingles Foundation
590 Madison Avenue, 21st Floor
New York, NY 10022
212-222-3390
www.vzvfoundation.org
Provides information about chicken pox, shingles, and postherpetic neuralgia.

National Stroke Association
9707 East Easter Lane, Building B
Centennial, CO 80112
800-787-6537; 303-649-9299
www.stroke.org

National Sudden and Unexpected Infant Death/Child Death and Pregnancy Loss Resource Center
2115 Wisconsin Avenue NW, Suite 601
Washington, DC 20007-2292
866-866-7437; 202-687-7466
www.sidscenter.org

National Testing Laboratories, Ltd.
6571 Wilson Mills Road
Cleveland, OH 44143
800-458-3330; 440-449-2525
www.ntllabs.com
Sells a kit to test for impurities, including lead, in your water.

National Vaccine Program Office
U.S. Department of Health and Human Services
200 Independence Avenue SW
Washington, DC 20201
877-696-6775; 202-619-0257
http://www.hhs.gov/nvpo

Natural Healing Institute
543 Encinitas Boulevard, Suites 105–108
Encinitas, CA 92024-2930
760-943-8485
www.naturalhealinginst.com
Offers license and certificate programs in naturopathic medicine, holistic health, nutrition, herbology, and massage.

Natural Resources Defense Council
40 West 20th Street
New York, NY 10011
212-727-2700
www.nrdc.org

NSF International, Inc.
P.O. Box 130140
789 North Dixboro Road
Ann Arbor, MI 48113-0140
800-673-6275; 734-769-8010
www.nsf.com
Standards development, product certification, education, and risk management for public health and safety.

Obsessive-Compulsive Anonymous
P.O. Box 215
New Hyde Park, NY 10040
516-739-0662
www.obsessivecompulsiveanonymous.org

Office of Women's Health
U.S. Food and Drug Administration
5600 Fishers Lane
Rockville, Maryland 20857
888-463-6332
www.fda.gov/womens

Osteoporosis and Related Bone Diseases—National Resource Center
National Institutes of Health
2 AMS Circle
Bethesda, MD 20892-3676
800-624-2663; 202-223-0344;
202-466-4315 (TTY)
www.niams.nih.gov/health_info/bone

Paget Foundation
120 Wall Street, Suite 1602
New York, NY 10005-4001
800-237-2438; 212-509-5335
www.paget.org

Parents Against Childhood Epilepsy (PACE)
7 East 85th Street, Suite A3
New York, NY 10028
212-665-7223
www.paceusa.org

Prevent Blindness America
211 West Wacker Drive, Suite 1700
Chicago, IL 60606
800-331-2020
www.preventblindness.org

Prevent Cancer Foundation
1600 Duke Street, Suite 500
Alexandria, VA 22314
800-227-2732; 703-836-4412
www.preventcancer.org

Project Inform
1375 Mission Street
San Francisco, CA 94103
800-822-7422; 415-558-8669
www.projectinform.org
Provides information to help educate people with HIV and their health care providers about treatment.

Rational Recovery
Box 800
Lotus, CA 95651
530-621-2667
www.rational.org
Abstinence-based recovery.

TheRightChiropractor
www.therightchiropractor.com
Can help you to contact a qualified chiropractor in your area.

Rolf Institute of Structural Integration
5055 Chaparral Court, Suite 103
Boulder, CO 80301
800-530-8875; 303-449-5903
www.rolf.org
Provides information on the Rolfing method of massage.

Schizophrenia.com
www.schizophrenia.com

Scleroderma Foundation
300 Rosewood Drive, Suite 105
Danvers, MA 01923
800-722-4673; 978-463-5843
www.scleroderma.org

Scoliosis Association
P.O. Box 811705
Boca Raton, FL 33481-1705
800-800-0669; 561-994-4435
www.scoliosis-assoc.org

Self Management and Recovery Training (SMART)
7537 Mentor Avenue, Suite 306
Mentor, OH 44060
866-951-5357; 440-951-5357
http://smartrecovery.org
Abstinence-based recovery using cognitive behavioral techniques.

Simon Foundation for Continence
P.O. Box 815
Wilmette, IL 60091
800-237-4666
www.simonfoundation.org
Provides information on dealing with incontinence.

Sjögren's Syndrome Foundation
6707 Democracy Boulevard, Suite 325
Bethesda, MD 20817
800-475-6473; 301-530-4420
www.sjogrens.org

Skin Cancer Foundation
149 Madison Avenue, Suite 901
New York, NY 10016
212-725-5176
www.skincancer.org

Spina Bifida Association of America (SBAA)
4590 MacArthur Boulevard NW, Suite 250
Washington, DC 20007-4226
800-621-3141; 202-944-3285
www.sbaa.org

Sudden Infant Death Syndrome Alliance
1314 Bedford Avenue, Suite 210
Baltimore, MD 21208
800-221-7437; 410-653-8226
www.sidsalliance.org

Unicorn Children's Foundation
3350 Northwest Boca Raton Boulevard, Suite A-28
Boca Raton, FL 33431
561-620-9377
www.unicornchildrensfoundation.org
Can provide a list of physicians who treat autistic disorders and learning disabilities.

United Cerebral Palsy Association
1660 L Street NW, Suite 700
Washington, DC 20036
800-872-5827; 202-776-0406
www.ucpa.org

United Ostomy Association
19772 MacArthur Boulevard, Suite 200
Irvine, CA 92612-2405
800-826-0826; 949-660-8624
www.uoa.org
A national network for bowel and urinary diversion support groups.

United Parkinson Foundation
833 West Washington Boulevard
Chicago, IL 60607
312-733-1893

University of Washington Virology Research Clinic
600 Broadway, Suite 400
Seattle, WA 98122
206-720-4340
www.depts.washington.edu/herpes

U.S. Centers for Disease Control and Prevention (CDC)
1600 Clifton Road
Atlanta, GA 30333
800-232-4636; 888-232-6348 (TTY)
http://www.cdc.gov

U.S. Environmental Protection Agency (EPA)
Ariel Rios Building
1200 Pennsylvania Avenue, N.W.
Washington, DC 20460
202-272-0167; 202-272-0165 (TTY)
www.epa.gov

U.S. Food and Drug Administration (FDA)
Food and Drug Administration
10903 New Hampshire Avenue
Silver Spring, MD 20993-0002
888-463-6332
www.fda.gov

U.S. National Library of Medicine MedlinePlus
8600 Rockville Pike
Bethesda, MD 20894
888-346-3656
http://medlineplus.gov

Vaccine Adverse Event Reporting System (FDA)
U.S. Department of Health and Human Services
P.O. Box 1100
Rockville, MD 20849-11008
800-822-7967
www.vaers.hhs.gov
Collects and analyzes information from reports of adverse events (possible side effects) that occur after the administration of U.S. licensed vaccines.

Water Quality Association
4151 Naperville Road
Lisle, IL 60532-3696
630-505-0160
www.wqa.org
Provides information on types of water and methods of water treatment.

Wilson Disease Association
1802 Brookside Drive
Wooster, OH 44691
888-264-1450
www.wilsonsdisease.org

Wilson's Temperature Syndrome
P.O. Box 1744
Lady Lake, FL 32158
800-621-7006
www.wilsonssyndrome.org

Women for Sobriety
P.O. Box 618
Quakerstown, PA 18951-0618
215-536-8026
www.womenforsobriety.org
Abstinence-based recovery for women only.

Women's Health America, Inc.
1289 Deming Way
Madison, WI 53717
800-558-7046
http://www.womenshealth.com
Provides information about PMS and hormone therapy.

Worldwide Education and Awareness for Movement Disorders (WE MOVE)
204 West 84th Street
New York, NY 10024
212-875-8312
http://wemove.org

HEALTH TREATMENT AND RETREAT CENTERS

The following are centers that can provide assistance in maintaining or improving upon your health. The services offered by these organizations vary.

Alegent Health
Bergan Mercy Medical Center
7500 Mercy Road
Omaha, NE 68124
402-398-6060

Immanuel Medical Center
6901 North 72nd Street
Omaha, NE 68122
402-572-2121
www.alegent.com
An integrated, not-for-profit community-based health care system with clinics, hospitals, and other facilities with a wide range of services and an emphasis on prevention, wellness, and health education.

Brigham and Women's Hospital
75 Francis Street
Boston, MA 02115
617-732-5500
www.brighamandwomens.org

BroMenn Healthcare
Department of Cardiology
P.O. Box 2850
Bloomington, IL 61702-2850
309-454-1400
www.bromenn.org

Broward General Medical Center
303 SE 17th Street, Suite 306
Fort Lauderdale, FL 33316
954-355-4400
www.browardhealth.org
Not-for-profit community health care system.

Dana-Farber Cancer Institute
44 Binney Street
Boston, MA 02115
866-408-3324; 617-632-3000
www.dana-farber.org

Dr. Dean Ornish
Preventative Medicine Research Institute
900 Bridgeway
Sausalito, CA 94965
415-332-2525
www.pmri.org
Offers health retreats for those interested in achieving a healthier lifestyle.

Fertility Research Foundation
877 Park Avenue
New York, NY 10021
888-439-2999; 212-744-5500
www.frfbaby.com
A treatment and research facility specializing in diagnosing and treating infertility problems.

The Hippocrates Health Institute
1443 Palmdale Court
West Palm Beach, FL 33411
800-842-2125; 561-471-8876
www.hippocratesinst.org
Practices a holistic approach to the treatment of cancer and other illnesses.

Johns Hopkins Breast Center
601 North Caroline Street
Baltimore, MD 21287
410-614-2853
www.hopkinsbreastcenter.org

Johns Hopkins Hospital
600 North Wolfe Street
Baltimore, MD 21287
410-955-9500
http://hopkinsmedicine.org

Massachusetts General Hospital Cancer Center
55 Fruit Street
Boston, MA 02108
800-320-0022
www.massgeneral.org/cancer/

Mayo Clinic
200 First Street SW
Rochester, MN 55905
507-284-2511; 507-284-9786 (TDD)
www.mayoclinic.org/rochester

Mayo Clinic Jacksonville
4500 San Pablo Road
Jacksonville, FL 32224
904-953-2000; 904-953-2300 (TDD)
http://mayoclinic.org/jacksonville

Mayo Clinic Scottsdale
13400 East Shea Boulevard
Scottsdale, AZ 85259
480-301-8000; 480-301-7683 (TDD)
www.mayoclinic.org/scottsdale

The McDougall Wellness Center
P.O. Box 14039
Santa Rosa, CA 95402
800-941-7111; 707-538-8609
www.drmcdougall.com
Offers a twelve-day health-improvement program focusing on diet and lifestyle modifications.

Memorial Sloan-Kettering Cancer Center
1275 York Avenue
New York, NY 10065
212-639-2000
www.mskcc.org

New York-Presbyterian Hospital
622 West 168th Street
New York, NY 10032
212-305-2500
www.nyp.org
Offers massage, hypnosis, acupressure, reflexology, and many other treatments.

Ornish Preventative Medicine Research Institute
See Dr. Dean Ornish.

Pritikin Longevity Center and Spa
19735 Turnberry Way
Aventura, FL 33180
800-327-4914; 305-935-7131
www.pritikin.com

St. John's Breast Center
St. John's Regional Health Center
1235 East Cherokee
Springfield, MO 65804
417-820-2000
www.stjohns.com

Scripps Center for Integrative Medicine
10820 North Torrey Pines Road
La Jolla, CA 92037
858-554-3000
www.scrippsintegrativemedicine.org

Swedish American Health System
1401 East State Street
Rockford, IL 61104
815-968-4400
www.swedishamerican.org

Swedish Medical Center
747 Broadway
Seattle, WA 98122-4307
206-386-6000
www.swedish.org

Walter Reed Army Medical Center
6900 Georgia Avenue NW
Washington, DC 20307
202-782-3501
www.wramc.amedd.army.mil
Services only for military health care beneficiaries on active duty or retired military beneficiaries and their spouses and children.

Weimar Center of Health and Education
P.O. Box 486
Weimar, CA 95736
800-525-9192
www.weimar.org
Offers an eighteen-day health-improvement program including hydrotherapy, massage, exercise, and lifestyle counseling.

Wildwood Lifestyle Center and Hospital
435 Lifestyle Lane
Wildwood, GA 30757
800-634-9355
www.wildwoodhealth.org

HEALTH SPAS

Cal-a-Vie Health Spa
29402 Spa Havens Way
Vista, CA 92084
866-772-4283
www.cal-a-vie.com

Canyon Ranch
165 Kemble Street
Lenox, MA 01240
800-742-9000
www.canyonranch.com

The Golden Door
P.O. Box 463077
Escondido, CA 92046-3077
800-424-0777; 760-744-5777
www.goldendoor.com/escondito

Green Valley Spa and Health Resort
871 West Canyon View Drive
Saint George, UT 84770
800-237-1068
www.greenvalleyspa.com

The Heartland Spa
1237 East 1600 North Road
Gilman, IL 60938
800-545-4853
www.heartlandspa.com

Lake Austin Resort
1705 South Quinlan Park Road
Austin, TX 78732
800-847-5637; 512-372-7300
www.lakeaustin.com

L'Auberge Del Mar Resort and Spa
1540 Camino Del Mar
Del Mar, CA 92014
800-245-9757; 858-259-1515;
800-901-9514 (TDD/TTY)
www.laubergedelmar.com

Mii Amo Spa
525 Boynton Canyon Road
Sedona, AZ 86336
888-749-2137; 928-203-8500
www.miiamo.com

The Raj
Maharishi Ayurveda Health Center
1734 Jasmine Avenue
Fairfield, IA 52556
800-248-9050; 641-472-9580
www.theraj.com

Spring Creek Ranch
1800 Spirit Dance Road
Jackson, WY 83001
800-443-6139; 307-733-8833
www.springcreekranch.com/spa

The Wiesbaden Hot Springs Spa and Lodgings
P.O. Box 349
Ouray, CO 81427
888-846-5191; 970-325-4347
www.wiesbadenhotsprings.com

SUGGESTED READING

The following list of books is provided for those who wish to explore a particular topic further. The books mentioned here are good sources of further information.

Airola, Paavo. *Cancer Causes, Prevention, and Treatment: The Total Approach.* Phoenix, AZ: Health Plus Publishers, 1972.

Airola, Paavo. *How to Get Well.* Phoenix, AZ: Health Plus Publishers, 1974.

Airola, Paavo. *How to Keep Slim, Healthy, and Young with Juice Fasting.* Phoenix, AZ: Health Plus Publishers, 1971.

Aladjem, Henrietta. *Understanding Lupus.* New York: Scribner, 1986.

Amen, Daniel G. *Magnificent Mind at Any Age.* New York: Harmony, 2009.

Antol, Marie Nadine. *Healing Teas.* Garden City Park, NY: Avery Publishing Group, 1996.

Appleton, Nancy. *Lick the Sugar Habit.* Garden City Park, NY: Avery Publishing Group, 1996.

Astor, Stephen. *Hidden Food Allergies.* Garden City Park, NY: Avery Publishing Group, 1989.

Balch, Phyllis A. *Prescription for Dietary Wellness.* Garden City Park, NY: Avery Publishing Group, 1995.

Balick, Michael J., Elaine Elisabetsky, and Sarah A. Laird. *Medicinal Resources of the Tropical Forest.* New York: Columbia University Press, 1996.

Barnes, Broda O., and Lawrence Galton. *Hypothyroidism: The Unsuspected Illness.* New York: Cromwell, 1976.

Becker, Robert O., and Gary Selden. *Body Electric: Electromagnetism and the Foundation of Life.* New York: William Morrow & Co., 1987.

Bell, Rachel, and Howard Peiper. *The A.D.D. and A.D.H.D. Diet!* Sheffield, MA: Safe Goods Publishing, 2004.

Bland, Jeffrey. *Medical Applications of Clinical Nutrition.* New Canaan, CT: Keats Publishing, 1983.

Bliznakov, Emile, and Gerry Hunt. *The Miracle Nutrient: Coenzyme Q10.* New York: Bantam Books, 1987.

Blumenthal, Mark, Josef Brinckmann, and Bernd Wollschlaeger (Editors). *The ABC Clinical Guide to Herbs.* Austin, TX: American Botanical Council, 2003.

Bradford, Robert W., and Michael Culbert. *Now That You Have Cancer.* Chula Vista, CA: The Bradford Foundation, 1992.

Brighthope, Ian. *The AIDS Fighters.* New Canaan, CT: Keats Publishing, 1988.

Brinkley, Ginny, Linda Goldberg, and Janice Kukar. *Your Child's First Journey.* Garden City Park, NY: Avery Publishing Group, 1989.

Buist, Robert. *Food Chemical Sensitivity.* Garden City Park, NY: Avery Publishing Group, 1988.

Cabot, Sandra. *Smart Medicine for Menopause.* Garden City Park, NY: Avery Publishing Group, 1995.

Calbom, Cherie. *Juicing, Fasting and Detoxing for Life.* New York: Wellness Central, 2008.

Campbell, Colin T., Howard Lyman (Preface), and John Robbins (Foreword). *The China Study.* Dallas, TX: Benbella Books, 2005.

Carter, Mildred, and Tammy Weber. *Body Reflexology: Healing at Your Fingertips.* West Nyack, NY: Parker Publishing Company, 1994.

Cass, Hyla, and Terrence McNally. *Kava: Nature's Answer to Stress, Anxiety, and Insomnia.* Rocklin, CA: Prima Publishing, 1998.

Cawood, Frank. *Super Life, Super Health.* Peachtree, GA: FC & A, 1999.

Check, William A., and Ann G. Fettner. *The Truth About AIDS: Evolution of an Epidemic.* New York: Holt, Rinehart & Winston, 1985.

Clare, Sally, and David Clare. *Creative Vegetarian Cookery.* Dorset, England: Prism Press, 1988.

Clark, Daniel, and Kaye Wyatt. *Colostrum: Life's First Food: The Ultimate Anti-Aging Weight Loss and Immune Supplement.* Salt Lake City, UT: CNR Publications, 1998.

Crook, William. *Help for the Hyperactive Child.* Jackson, TN: Professional Books, 1991.

Crook, William G. *The Yeast Connection Handbook.* Jackson, TN: Professional Books, 2001.

Cummings, Stephen, and Dana Ullman. *Everybody's Guide to Homeopathic Medicines.* New York: Tarcher, 2004.

D'Adamo, Peter J., and Catherine Whitney. *Eat Right 4 Your Type.* New York: Putnam, 1996.

Davidson, Paul. *Are You Sure It's Arthritis?* New York: Macmillan Publishing Co., 1985.

de Haas, Cherie. *Natural Skin Care.* Garden City Park, NY: Avery Publishing Group, 1989.

Editors of East West Journal. *Shopper's Guide to Natural Foods.* Garden City Park, NY: Avery Publishing Group, 1988.

Edwards, Linda. *Baking for Health.* Garden City Park, NY: Avery Publishing Group, 1988.

Erasmus, Udo. *Fats That Heal, Fats That Kill.* Burnaby, British Columbia, Canada: Alive Books, 1993.

Evans, Gary. *Chromium Picolinate: Everything You Need to Know.* Garden City Park, NY: Avery Publishing Group, 1996.

Evans, Richard A. *Making the Right Choice: Treatment Options in Cancer Surgery.* Garden City Park, NY: Avery Publishing Group, 1995.

Feingold, Ben F. *Why Your Child Is Hyperactive.* New York: Random House, 1985.

Feingold, Helene, and Ben Feingold. *The Feingold Cookbook for Hyperactive Children and Others with Problems Associated with Food Additives and Salicylates.* New York: Random House, 1979.

Fink, John. *Third Opinion: An International Directory to Alternative Therapy Centers for the Treatment and Prevention of Cancer.* Garden City Park, NY: Avery Publishing Group, 1997.

Foster, Cynthia. *Stop the Medicine.* Scottsdale, AZ: Break On Through Press, LLC., 1999.

Frankel, Paul. *The Methylation Miracle.* New York: St. Martin's Press, 1999.

Fujita, Takuo. *Calcium and Your Health.* Tokyo: Japan Publications, 1987.

Fulder, Stephen. *The Ginger Book.* Garden City Park, NY: Avery Publishing Group, 1996.

Fulder, Stephen. *The Ginseng Book.* Garden City Park, NY: Avery Publishing Group, 1996.

Germann, Donald R. *The Anti-Cancer Diet.* New York: Wyden Books, 1977.

Gittleman, Ann Louise. *The Gut Flush Plan.* New York: Avery, 2008.

Gittleman, Ann Louise. *The Fat Flush Plan.* New York: McGraw-Hill, 2002.

Gittleman, Ann Louise. *Guess What Came to Dinner: Parasites and Your Health.* Garden City Park, NY: Avery Publishing Group, 1993.

Gordon, Jay. *The ADD and ADHD Cure.* Hoboken, NJ: Wiley, 2008.

Graedon, Joe, and Teresa Graedon. *The People's Guide to Deadly Drug Interactions.* New York: St. Martin's Press, 1995.

Greene, Bob. *The Best Life Diet Revised and Updated.* New York: Simon & Schuster, 2008.

Gregory, Scott J., and Bianca Leonardo. *They Conquered AIDS!* True Life Publications, 1989.

Griffith, H. Winter. *Complete Guide to Symptoms, Illness and Surgery for People Over 50.* Los Angeles: The Body Press, 1992.

Grogan, Bryanna Clark. *Soyfoods: Cooking for a Positive Menopause.* Summertown, TN: Book Publishing Company, 1999.

Gutman, Jimmy, and Stephen Schettini. *The Ultimate GSH Handbook.* Montreal, Canada: Gutman & Schettini Enr, 1998.

Halpern, Georges. *Cordyceps: China's Healing Mushroom.* Garden City Park, NY: Avery Publishing Group, 1999.

Heidenry, Carolyn. *Making the Transition to a Macrobiotic Diet.* Garden City Park, NY: Avery Publishing Group, 1988.

Heinerman, John. *Aloe Vera, Jojoba & Yucca.* New Canaan, CT: Keats, 1982.

Heinerman, John. *Heinerman's Encyclopedia of Nature's Vitamins and Minerals.* Paramus, NJ: Prentice Hall, 1998.

Hobbs, Christopher. *The Ginsengs: A User's Guide.* Santa Barbara, CA: Botanica Press, 1996.

Howard, Mary Ann. *Blueprint for Health.* Grand Rapids, MI: Zondervan Publishing House, 1985.

Howell, Edward. *Enzyme Nutrition.* Garden City Park, NY: Avery Publishing Group, 1987.

Huggins, Hal A. *It's All in Your Head.* Garden City Park, NY: Avery Publishing Group, 1993.

Hyman, Mark, MD. *The UltraMind Solution.* New York: Scribner, 2008.

Jacobson, Michael. *Safe Food: Eating Wisely in a Risky World.* Washington, DC: Living Planet Press, 1991.

Jensen, Bernard. *Foods That Heal.* New York: Avery, 1988.

Kenney, Matthew. *Everyday Raw.* Layton, UT: Gibbs Smith, 2008.

Kingsolver, Barbara, Camille Kingsolver, and Steven L. Hopp. *Animal, Vegetable, Miracle: A Year of Food Life.* New York: Harper Perennial, 2008.

Krumholz, Harlan M., and Robert H. Phillips. *No If's, And's or Butts: The Smoker's Guide to Quitting.* Garden City Park, NY: Avery Publishing Group, 1993.

Kushi, Aveline, and Wendy Esko. *The Macrobiotic Cancer Prevention Cookbook.* Garden City Park, NY: Avery Publishing Group, 1987.

Kushi, Michio, with Edward Esko. *The Macrobiotic Approach to Cancer.* Garden City Park, NY: Avery Publishing Group, 1991.

Kushi, Michio. *The Macrobiotic Way.* Garden City Park, NY: Avery Publishing Group, 1993.

Lance, James W. *Migraine and Other Headaches.* New York: Scribner, 1986.

Lane, I. William, and Linda Comac. *Sharks Don't Get Cancer: How Shark Cartilage Could Save Your Life.* Garden City Park, NY: Avery Publishing Group, 1992.

Lane, I. William, and Linda Comac. *Sharks Still Don't Get Cancer.* Garden City Park, NY: Avery Publishing Group, 1996.

Lau, Benjamin. *Garlic for Health.* Wilmot, WI: Lotus Light Publications, 1988.

Lerman, Andrea. *The Macrobiotic Community Cookbook.* Garden City Park, NY: Avery Publishing Group, 1989.

Levenstein, Mary Kerney. *Everyday Cancer Risks and How to Avoid Them.* Garden City Park, NY: Avery Publishing Group, 1992.

Levitt, Paul, and Elissa Guralnick. *The Cancer Reference Book.* New York: Paddington Press, 1979.

Lundberg, Paul. *The Book of Shiatsu.* New York: Fireside, 1992.

Majeed, Muhammed, and Lakshmi Prakash. *Lactospore: The Effective Probiotic.* Piscataway, NJ: NutriScience Publishers, Inc., 1998.

Margolis, Simeon. *The Johns Hopkins Encyclopedia of Drugs.* New York: Medletter Associates, Inc., 1998.

Marks, Edith. *Coping with Glaucoma.* Garden City Park, NY: Avery Publishing Group, 1997.

McFarland, Judy Lindberg. *Aging Without Growing Old.* Palos Verdes, CA: Western Front, LTD, 2000.

Mcglothin, Paul, Meredith Averill, and Alison Hendrie. *The CR Way: Using the Secrets of Calorie Restriction for a Longer, Healthier Life.* New York: Collins Living, 2008.

Messina, Mark, and Virginia Messina, with Ken Setchell. *The Simple Soybean and Your Health.* Garden City Park, NY: Avery Publishing Group, 1994.

Meyerowitz, Steve. *Power Juices— Super Drinks.* New York: Kensington Publishing Corp., 2000.

Mindell, Earl. *Unsafe at Any Meal.* New York: Warner Books, 1986.

Minkin, Mary Jane. *What Every Woman Needs to Know About Menopause.* New Haven, CT: Yale University Press, 1986.

Moss, Ralph. *Cancer Therapy: The Independent Consumer's Guide to Non-Toxic Treatment & Prevention.* Brooklyn, NY: Equinox Press, 1995.

Murray, Michael. *Encyclopedia of Nutritional Supplements.* Rocklin, CA: Prima Publishing, 1996.

Murray, Michael. *How to Prevent and Treat Cancer with Natural Medicine.* New York: Riverhead, 2002.

Murray, Michael. *How to Prevent and Treat Diabetes with Natural Medicine.* New York: Riverhead, 2003.

Nestle, Marion. *Food Politics: How the Food Industry Influences Nutrition and Health.* Berkeley, CA: University of California Press, 2007 (2nd Edition).

Nestle, Marion. *What to Eat.* New York: North Point Press, 2006.

Northrup, Christiane. *The Wisdom of Menopause: Creating Physical and Emotional Health and Healing During the Change.* New York: Bantam, 2006.

Null, Gary Ph.D., and Shelly Null. *The Joy of Juicing.* New York: Avery, 2001.

Olkin, Sylvia Klein. *Positive Pregnancy Fitness.* Garden City Park, NY: Avery Publishing Group, 1987.

Ott, John N. *Light, Radiation, and You: How to Stay Healthy.* Old Greenwich, CT: Devin-Adair Publishers, 1982.

Oz, Mehmet, and Michael F. Roizen. *YOU: On A Diet: The Owner's Manual for Waist Management.* New York: Free Press, 2006.

Oz, Mehmet, and Michael Roizen. *YOU: The Owner's Manual.* New York: William Morrow; Updated and Expanded edition, 2008.

Packer, Lester, and Carol Colman. *The Antioxidant Miracle.* New York: Wiley, 1999.

Papon, R. Donald. *Homeopathy Made Simple.* Charlottesville, VA: Hampton Roads Publishing Company, Inc., 1999.

Passwater, Richard A., and Elmer Cranton. *Trace Elements, Hair Analysis and Nutrition.* New Canaan, CT: Keats Publishing, 1983.

Pearsall, Paul. *Superimmunity: Master Your Emotions and Improve Your Health.* New York: McGraw-Hill, 1987.

Peterson, Christopher, and Martin Seligman. *Character Strengths and Virtues: A Handbook and Classification.* New York: Oxford University Press, 2004.

Phillips, Robert H. *Coping with Osteoarthritis.* Garden City Park, NY: Avery Publishing Group, 1989.

Phillips, Robert H. *Coping with Prostate Cancer.* Garden City Park, NY: Avery Publishing Group, 1994.

Planck, Nina. *Real Food: What to Eat and Why.* New York: Bloomsbury USA, 2007.

Podell, Ronald M. *Contagious Emotions: Staying Well When Your Loved One Is Depressed.* New York: Pocket Books, 1993.

Pollan, Michael. *In Defense of Food.* New York: Penguin, 2008.

Pollan, Michael. *The Omnivore's Dilemma: A Natural History of Four Meals.* New York: Penguin, 2006.

Randolph, Theron G. *Human Ecology and Susceptibility to the Chemical Environment.* Springfield, IL: Charles C. Thomas, 1981.

Rapp, Doris J. *Allergies and the Hyperactive Child.* New York: Sovereign Books, 1979.

Robbins, John. *Diet for a New America.* Tiburon, CA: HJ Kramer, 1998.

Robbins, John. *The Food Revolution: How Your Diet Can Help Save Your Life and Our World.* Berkeley, CA: Conari Press, 2001.

Roizen, Michael F., and Mehmet Oz. *YOU: The Smart Patient: An Insider's Handbook for Getting the Best Treatment.* New York: Free Press, 2006.

Roizen, Michael F., and Mehmet Oz. *YOU: Staying Young: The Owner's Manual for Extending Your Warranty.* New York: Free Press, 2007.

Ross, Julia. *The Mood Cure.* New York: New York: Viking, 2002.

Sahelian, Ray. *DHEA: A Practical Guide.* Garden City Park, NY: Avery Publishing Group, 1996.

Sahelian, Ray. *5-HTP: Nature's Serotonin Solution.* Garden City Park, NY: Avery Publishing Group, 1998.

Schlosser, Eric. *Fast Food Nation.* New York: Harper Perennial, 2002 (1st Perennial Edition).

Sears, Barry. *Toxic Fat: When Good Fat Turns Bad.* Nashville, TN: Thomas Nelson, 2008.

Sears, Barry. *The Anti-Inflammation Zone.* New York: Regan Books, 2005.

Sears, Barry. *Omega Rx Zone.* New York: Regan Books, 2002.

Sears, Barry and Bill Lawren. *The Zone: A Dietary Road Map to Lose Weight Permanently.* New York: Regan Books, 1995.

Selye, Hans. *Stress Without Distress.* Philadelphia: J.B. Lippincott Co., 1974.

Shelton, Herbert M. *Fasting Can Save Your Life,* rev. ed. Natural Hygiene, 1981.

Shute, Wilfrid. *Dr. Wilfrid E. Shute's Complete Updated Vitamin E Book.* New Canaan, CT: Keats Publishing, 1975.

Smith, Lendon. *Feed Your Kids Right: Dr. Smith's Program for Your Child's Total Health.* New York: McGraw-Hill, 1979.

Steinman, David, and Samuel S. Epstein. *Diet for a Poisoned Planet.* New York: Running Press, 2006.

Svoboda, Robert. *Prakruti: Your Ayurvedic Constitution.* Albuquerque, NM: Geocom Limited, 1989.

Swanson, David. *Mayo Clinic on Chronic Pain.* New York: Kensington Publishing Corp., 1999.

Teitelbaum, Jacob. *From Fatigued to Fantastic.* Garden City Park, NY: Avery Publishing Group, 2007 (3rd. Edition).

Treben, Maria. *Health from God's Garden: Herbal Remedies for Glowing Health and Glorious Well-Being.* Rochester, VT: Thorsons Publishers, 1987.

Ulene, Art. *Complete Guide to Vitamins, Minerals, and Herbs.* New York: Avery Books (an imprint of Penguin Putnam), 2000.

University of California–Berkeley. *Wellness Letter: The Newsletter of Nutrition, Fitness, and Stress Management.* Berkeley, CA.

Wade, Carlson. *Carlson Wade's Amino Acids Book.* New Canaan, CT: Keats Publishing, 1985.

Walker, Lynne. *Nature's Pharmacy.* Paramus, NJ: Reward Books, 1998.

Walker, Morton. *The Chelation Way.* Garden City Park, NY: Avery Publishing Group, 1990.

Walters, Richard. *Options: The Alternative Cancer Therapy Book.* Garden City Park, NY: Avery Publishing Group, 1993.

Warren, Tom. *Beating Alzheimer's.* Garden City Park, NY: Avery Publishing Group, 1991.

Watson, Brenda. *The Fiber35 Diet: Nature's Weight Loss Secret.* New York: Free Press, 2007.

Weber, Marcea. *Macrobiotics and Beyond.* Garden City Park, NY: Avery Publishing Group, 1989.

Weber, Marcea. *Whole Meals.* Dorset, England: Prism Press, 1983.

Webster, David. *Acidophilus and Colon Health.* New York: Kensington Publishing Corp., 1999.

Weil, Andrew. *Eight Weeks to Optimum Health,* Revised Edition. New York: Knopf, 2006.

Weil, Andrew. *Healthy Aging.* New York: Knopf, 2005.

Weil, Andrew. *Natural Health, Natural Medicine.* Boston, MA: Houghton Mifflin, 2004 (Revised Edition).

Weiner, Michael A. *Maximum Immunity*. Boston: Houghton Mifflin Co., 1986.

Wigmore, Ann. *Recipes for Longer Life*. Garden City Park, NY: Avery Publishing Group, 1982.

Wigmore, Ann. *The Wheatgrass Book*. Garden City Park, NY: Avery Publishing Group, 1985.

Williams, Xandria. *What's in My Food?* Dorset, England: Prism Press, 1988.

Wilson, James L. *Adrenal Fatigue*. Petaluma, CA: Smart Publications, 2001.

Wilson, Roberta. *Aromatherapy for Vibrant Health and Beauty*. Garden City Park, NY: Avery Publishing Group, 1995.

Winter, Ruth. *A Consumer's Dictionary of Food Additives*: New York: Three Rivers Press, 2009 (7th Edition).

Wittenberg, Margaret M. *New Good Food Shopper's Pocket Guide*. Berkeley, CA: Ten Speed Press, 2008.

Wlodyga, Ronald R. *Health Secrets from the Bible*. Triumph Publishers, 1979.

Woessner, Candace, Judith Lauwers, and Barbara Bernard. *Breastfeeding Today*. Garden City Park, NY: Avery Publishing Group, 1988.

Wolfe, Sidney, and Rose-Ellen Hope. *Worst Pills, Best Pills II*. Washington, DC: Public Citizen's Health Research Group, 1993.

Zand, Janet, Robert Rountree, and Rachel Walton. *Smart Medicine for a Healthier Child*. New York: Avery, 2003 (2nd Edition).

Ziff, Sam. *Silver Dental Fillings: The Toxic Timebomb*. Santa Fe, NM: Aurora Press, 1984.

Index

Page numbers in italics refer to charts and tables.

wild cherry, 128
wild oregano, 128
wild pansy, 343, 702
wild yam, 129, 663, 706
Wilson's disease, 350, 779–82
Wilson's syndrome, 518–19
wines, 101
wintergreen, 129
witch hazel, 129
withdrawal, 175, 388
women
　　AIDS and, *167*
　　anemia and, 201
　　anorexia nervosa and, 203
　　chronic fatigue syndrome and, 330
　　fibromyalgia syndrome and, 435

heart disease and, 317
menopause and, 578
sexual dysfunction in, 706–7
smoking and, 398
See also pregnancy
Women's Health Initiative, 260–61, 316, 362, 580–82
wood betony, 129
workplace noise levels, 478
World Health Organization, 46, 99, 532, 620, 625, 757, 818
worms (parasites), 782–84
wormwood, 129
wrinkles, 784–87

X-ALD, 685–86

xerophthalmia, 429
X-rays, 242, 676, 754

Yale University, 359
yeast, 95
yellow dock, 130
yerba maté, 130
yoga, 830
yogurt, 8, 304
yohimbe, 130
yucca, 130

ZAND formulas, 95
zeaxanthin, 426
zinc, 42–43, 71, 345–46, 350, 779, 781–82
Zostavax vaccine, 712

ABOUT THE AUTHOR

Phyllis Balch was a certified nutritional consultant who received her certification from the American Association of Nutritional Consultants, and was a leading nutritional counselor for more than two decades. She came to the field as a result of experiencing directly the benefits of using diet and nutrition as remedies for sickness.

In the 1970s, Balch and her children suffered from a number of undiagnosed (or misdiagnosed) illnesses, and although they had expert medical knowledge very close at hand, their lives continued to be disrupted by these maladies. Balch felt there was something missing in the typical medical approach, which treated the symptoms rather than the cause of illness. Her introduction to the relationship between nutrition and well-being was through Paavo Airola, a well-known naturopath and writer. Balch then pursued her own intensive research into the science of nutrition, and by making radical changes in diet was able to transform her own health and the health of her children.

Convinced that nutrition was, in many cases, the answer to regaining and maintaining health, Balch opened a health food store called Good Things Naturally. In 1983, she published *Nutritional Outline for the Professional and the Wise Man*—now known as *Prescription for Nutritional Healing*—to share her knowledge with a broader audience. Through its first four editions, this book has had millions of readers in many countries, and it has been translated into seven foreign languages.

During her lifetime, Balch continually shared her knowledge with others and persuaded many traditionally schooled medical practitioners to incorporate nutritional healing methods of restoring health into their practice. She was highly sought after as a visiting lecturer and appeared on television and radio programs throughout North America. Balch, who lived in Fort Myers, Florida, and Greenfield, Indiana, died in December 2004 while working on the fourth edition of *Prescription for Nutritional Healing*.

About Stacey Bell, D.S.C.

In addition to revising the fifth edition of *Prescription for Nutritional Healing*, Stacey Bell has been a registered dietitian for thirty-five years, and has worked in that capacity and conducted clinical research studies for twenty years. She received a doctorate in nutrition from Boston University, with honors, in 1994. For her dissertation, she evaluated the effect of supplemental fish oil on immune function in patients with HIV infection and AIDS. Bell was on the faculty at Harvard Medical School in Boston, and has published more than seventy peer-reviewed scientific articles. Her research interests include obesity, diabetes, cancer, AIDS, burn patients, critical illness, and dietary supplements. A frequent lecturer around the world on many topics related to nutrition, she serves on the board of a nonprofit agency, Kids Can Cook, which offers basic cooking instruction and nutrition education to Boston middle-school-aged children.

BOOKS BY PHYLLIS A. BALCH, CNC

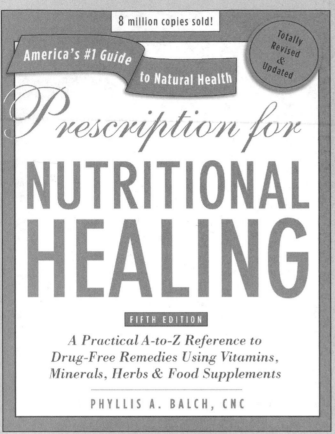
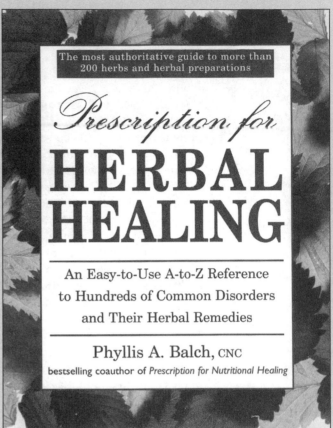
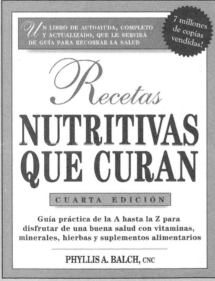
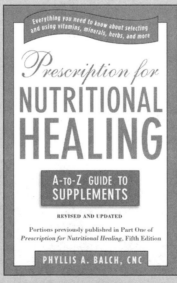
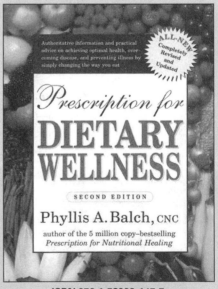
Natural remedies that work